Perfusion Imaging in Clinical Practice

A Multimodality Approach to Tissue Perfusion Analysis

Perfusion Imaging in Clinical Practice

A Multimodality Approach to Tissue Perfusion Analysis

Farhood Saremi, MD
Professor of Radiology and Medicine
Department of Radiology
University of Southern California
USC University Hospital
Los Angeles, California

Wolters Kluwer

Philadelphia • Baltimore • New York • London
Buenos Aires • Hong Kong • Sydney • Tokyo

Acquisitions Editor: Keith Donnellan
Product Development Editor: Nicole Dernoski
Editorial Coordinator: Kathryn Burress
Marketing Manager: Dan Dressler
Production Project Manager: Priscilla Crater
Design Coordinator: Joan Wendt
Manufacturing Coordinator: Beth Welsh
Prepress Vendor: SPi Global

9 8 7 6 5 4 3 2 1

Printed in China

Library of Congress Cataloging-in-Publication Data
Perfusion imaging in clinical practice : a multimodality approach to tissue perfusion analysis / editor, Farhood Saremi.
p. ; cm.
Includes bibliographical references and index.
ISBN 978-1-4511-9316-9 (alk. paper)
I. Saremi, Farhood, editor.
[DNLM: 1. Perfusion Imaging—methods. 2. Tissues—blood supply. 3. Tissues—radionuclide imaging. 4. Vascular Diseases—radionuclide imaging. WN 203]
QP110.V34
612.1'3—dc23

2014047934

LWW.com

RRS1504

CONTRIBUTORS

Mohammed Almekhlafi, MD
Calgary Stroke Program
Department of Clinical Neurosciences
Department of Radiology
University of Calgary
Calgary, Alberta, Canada
Department of Internal Medicine
King Abdulaziz University
Jeddah, Saudi Arabia

Constantinos D. Anagnostopoulos, MD, PhD, FRCP, FRCR, FESC
Research Director at the Center for Experimental Surgery, Clinical & Translational Research
Director of PET-CT Department & Small Animal Imaging Unit
Biomedical Research Foundation Academy of Athens
Athens, Greece

Erin Angel, PhD
Manager, Clinical Sciences, CT
Toshiba America Medical Systems
Tustin, California

Jun-ichi Asaumi, DDS
Professor of Oral and Maxillofacial Radiology
Department of Oral and Maxillofacial Radiology
Okayama University Graduate School of Medicine, Dentistry and Pharmaceutical Sciences
Okayama, Japan

Raymond Azab, MD
Abdominal Imaging Fellow
Keck Hospital of USC
University of Southern California
Los Angeles, California

Henryk Barthel, MD, PhD
Assistant Medical Director Neuro-PET and PET-MRI
Department of Nuclear Medicine
University Hospital Leipzig
Leipzig, Germany

Sotirios Bisdas, MD, PhD, MSc
Professor of Radiology
Consultant Neuroradiologist
Department of Neuroradiology
Eberhard Karls University Tübingen
Tübingen, Germany

Fernando Calamante, PhD
Associate Professor
Florey Institute of Neuroscience and Mental Health
Department of Medicine
Austin Health and Northern Health
University of Melbourne
Melbourne, Victoria, Australia

James D. Cameron, MBBS, MD
Professor of Medicine
Monash Cardiovascular Research Centre
Department of Medicine (Monash Medical Centre)
Monash University and Monash Heart
Clayton, Victoria, Australia

Hersh Chandarana, MD
Professor
Department of Radiology
NYU Langone Medical Center
New York, New York

Michael Chapell, PhD
Associate Professor
Institute of Biomedical Engineering
University of Oxford
Oxford, United Kingdom

Amedeo Chiribiri, MD, PhD
Senior Lecturer in Cardiovascular Imaging
King's College London
Division of Imaging Sciences and Medical Engineering
Rayne Institute, St. Thomas' Hospital
London, United Kingdom

Christopher D. d'Esterre, BMSc, PhD
Calgary Stroke Program
Department of Clinical Neurosciences
Postdoctoral Fellow
Department of Radiology
Foothills Medical Centre
Seaman Family MR Centre
University of Calgary
Calgary, Alberta, Canada

Jean-Luc Daire, PhD
INSERM U1149
Centre de Recherche Biomédicale Bichat-Beaujon
Paris, France

John A. Detre, MD
Professor
Departments of Neurology and Radiology
Director, Center for Functional Neuroimaging
University of Pennsylvania
Philadelphia, Pennsylvania

Mircea Cristian Dobre, MD, MS
Associate Physician, Radiology
Kaiser Permanente Santa Rosa Medical Center
Santa Rosa, California
Adjunct Clinical Faculty
Department of Radiology
Stanford School of Medicine
Stanford, California

Sharmila Dorbala, MD, MPH
Division of Nuclear Medicine and Molecular Imaging
Department of Radiology
Division of Cardiology
Department of Medicine
Noninvasive Cardiovascular Imaging Program
Departments of Medicine (Cardiology) and Radiology
Brigham and Women's Hospital
Boston, Massachusetts

Vinay Duddalwar, MD, FRCR
Associate Professor of Radiology
Section Chief, Abdominal Imaging, USC
Medical Director, Imaging, Norris Comprehensive Cancer Center
Keck Hospital of USC
USC Norris Cancer Center
University of Southern California
Los Angeles, California

Esmaeil Enjilela, PhD
Imaging Program
Lawson Health Research Institute
Imaging Research Lab
Robarts Research Institute
Western University
London, Ontario, Canada

Ricardo Faingold, MD
Program Director of Pediatric Radiology
Assistant Professor of Radiology, McGill University
Montreal Children's Hospital
Montreal, Quebec, Canada

Jurgen J. Fütterer, MD, PhD
Department of Radiology and Nuclear Medicine
Radboud University Medical Center
Nijmegen, The Netherlands
MIRA Institute for Biomedical Technology and Technical Medicine
University of Twente
Enschede, The Netherlands

Byron Gaing, MD
Department of Radiology
NYU Langone Medical Center
New York, New York

Alexandros Georgakopoulos, MD
Clinical Fellow, PET-CT Department
Center for Experimental Surgery, Clinical & Translational Research
Biomedical Research Foundation of the Academy of Athens
Athens, Greece

Vicky Goh, MD, FRCR
Professor of Clinical Cancer Imaging
President, European Society of Oncologic Imaging
Division of Imaging Sciences and Biomedical Engineering
King's College London
Department of Radiology
Guy's and St. Thomas' NHS Foundation Trust
London, United Kingdom

Mayank Goyal, MD, FRCPC
Calgary Stroke Program
Department of Clinical Neurosciences
Department of Radiology
Hotchkiss Brain Institute
Diagnostic and Interventional Neuroradiology, Medical Director
Seaman Family MR Centre
University of Calgary
Calgary, Alberta, Canada

Edward G. Grant, MD, FACR
Professor and Chairman
Department of Radiology
Keck Hospital of USC
USC Norris Cancer Center
University of Southern California
Los Angeles, California

Thomas Fritz Hansen, MD
Consultant
Department of Cardiology
Gentofte Hospital
Copenhagen University
Hellerup, Denmark

Cameron Hassani, MD
Assistant Professor of Radiology
Department of Radiology
University of Southern California
USC University Hospital
Los Angeles, California

Thomas Henzler, MD
Section Chief of Cardiothoracic Imaging, Computed Tomography
Institute of Clinical Radiology and Nuclear Medicine
University Medical Center Mannheim
Medical Faculty Mannheim—Heidelberg University
Mannheim, Germany

Jiang Hsieh, PhD
GE Healthcare
Waukesha, Wisconsin

Javaid Iqbal, MRCP, PhD
Thoraxcenter
Erasmus Medical Centre
Rotterdam, The Netherlands
Sheffield Teaching Hospitals
University of Sheffield
Sheffield, United Kingdom

Ameera Ismail, MD
Staff Neuroradiologist
Imaging and Radiology Department
Long Beach Memorial Medical Center
Long Beach, California

Rolf Jager, MD
Consultant Neuroradiologist
UCL Institute of Neurology
The National Hospital for Neurology and Neurosurgery
University College Hospital
London, United Kingdom

Kay Jann, PhD
Laboratory of Functional MRI Technology
Ahmanson-Lovelace Brain Mapping Center
Department of Neurology
University of California Los Angeles
Los Angeles, California
Department of Psychiatric Neurophysiology
University Hospital of Psychiatry
University of Bern
Bern, Switzerland

Laurent Juillard, MD, PhD
Professor
Nephrology–Dialysis–Hypertension Unit
Édouard Herriot Hospital
Hospices Civils de Lyon
INSERM CARMEN 1060
University of Lyon
Lyon, France

Vasileios K. Katsaros, MD, PhD
Consultant Neuroradiologist
Director of MRI Department
St. Savvas Oncology Hospital
Scientific Associate
Department of Neurosurgery
University of Athens
Athens, Greece

Brian S. H. Ko, BSc, MBBS, PhD, FRACP
Monash Cardiovascular Research Centre
Department of Medicine (Monash Medical Centre)
Monash University and Monash Heart
Clayton, Victoria, Australia

Kohsuke Kudo, MD
Associate Professor
Department of Diagnostic and Interventional Radiology
Hokkaido University Hospital
Sapporo, Japan

Andrea Laghi, MD
Associate Professor of Radiology
Department of Radiological Sciences, Oncology and Pathology
University of Rome "SAPIENZA"
Latina, Italy

Simon A. Lambert, PhD
Centre de Recherche Biomédicale Bichat-Beaujon
Paris, France

Henrik Bo Wiberg Larsson, MD, PhD
Professor, Consultant
Head of Functional Imaging Unit
Diagnostic Department
Glostrup Hospital
Copenhagen University
Glostrup, Denmark

Ting-Yim Lee, PhD
Imaging Program
Lawson Health Research Institute
Imaging Research Lab
Robarts Research Institute
Medical Imaging and Medical Biophysics
Western University
London, Ontario, Canada

Sandrine Lemoine, MD, PhD
Nephrology–Dialysis–Hypertension Unit
Édouard Herriot Hospital
Hospices Civils de Lyon
INSERM CARMEN 1060
University of Lyon
Lyon, France

Benjamin Leporq, PhD
INSERM U1149
Centre de Recherche Biomédicale Bichat-Beaujon
Paris, France

Sebastian Ley, MD
Diagnostic and Interventional Radiology
Chirurgische Klinik Dr. Rinecker
Department of Clinical Radiology
Ludwig Maximilians University
Munich, Germany

Chia-Shang Jason Liu, MD, PhD
Assistant Professor of Radiology
Division of Neuroradiology
Department of Radiology
University of Southern California Keck School of Medicine
Los Angeles, California

Ervin L. Lowther, MD
Radiologist
Department of Radiology
Wake Forest School of Medicine
Winston Salem, North Carolina

Marco Maria Maceroni, MD
Department of Radiological Sciences, Oncology and Pathology
University of Rome "SAPIENZA"
Latina, Italy

Islam Z. Mahmoud, MD
Clinical Research Fellow in Cardiovascular Imaging
King's College London
Division of Imaging Sciences and Medical Engineering
Rayne Institute, St. Thomas' Hospital
London, United Kingdom

Joseph A. Maldjian, MD
Professor of Radiology
Department of Radiology
Wake Forest School of Medicine
Winston Salem, North Carolina

Harshawn Malhi, MD
Assistant Professor of Radiology
Keck Hospital of USC
University of Southern California
Los Angeles, California

George R. Matcuk Jr, MD
Assistant Professor of Clinical Radiology
Department of Radiology
University of Southern California
Keck Hospital of USC
Los Angeles, California

Hidenobu Matsuzaki, DDS
Assistant Professor of Oral Diagnosis and Dentomaxillofacial Radiology
Department of Oral Diagnosis and Dentomaxillofacial Radiology
Okayama University Hospital
Okayama, Japan

Bijoy K. Menon, MD
Calgary Stroke Program
Department of Clinical Neurosciences
Department of Radiology
Department of Community Health Sciences
University of Calgary
Hotchkiss Brain Institute
Seaman Family MR Centre
Calgary, Alberta, Canada

Karl Muchantef, MD
Residency Training Program Site Coordinator
Assistant Professor of Radiology, McGill University
Montreal Children's Hospital
Montreal, Quebec, Canada

Kenya Murase, PhD
Professor
Department of Medical Physics and Engineering
Division of Medical Technology and Science
Faculty of Health Science
Graduate School of Medicine, Osaka University
Osaka, Japan

Henri J. M. M. Mutsaerts, MD
Research Physician
Department of Radiology
Academic Medical Center
Amsterdam, The Netherlands

Eike Nagel, MD, PhD, FACC, FESC, MRCR
Professor
Head of the Department of Cardiovascular Imaging
King's College London
Division of Imaging Sciences and Medical Engineering
Rayne Institute, St. Thomas' Hospital
London, United Kingdom

Stephan G. Nekolla, FESC
Senior Physicist and Head Multimodal Cardiac Imaging
Nuklearmedizinische Klinik und Poliklinik
Klinikum rechts der Isar der Technischen Universitaet München
München, Germany

Nikolas Papanikolaou, PhD
CEO N. Papanikolaou & Associates LLC
Institute of Computer Science
Foundation for Research and Technology (FORTH)
Heraklion, Greece

Nicolleta Pianou, MD
Clinical Fellow
PET-CT Department
Center for Experimental Surgery, Clinical and Translational Research
Biomedical Research Foundation of the Academy of Athens
Athens, Greece

Francesca B. Pizzini, MD, PhD
Neuroradiology Unit
Department of Diagnostic and Pathology
University Hospital of Verona
Verona, Italy

Davide Prezzi, FRCR
Clinical Research Fellow
Division of Imaging Sciences and Biomedical Engineering
King's College London
Department of Radiology
Guy's and St Thomas' NHS Foundation Trust
London, United Kingdom

Emilio Quaia, MD
Assistant Professor of Radiology
Department of Radiology
Cattinara Hospital
Trieste, Italy

Marco Rengo, MD, PhD
Department of Radiological Sciences, Oncology and Pathology
University of Rome "SAPIENZA"
Latina, Italy

Maxime Ronot, MD, PhD
Department of Radiology
APHP
University Hospitals Paris Nord Val de Seine
Clichy, France
University Paris Diderot
INSERM U1149
Centre de Recherche Biomédicale Bichat-Beaujon
Paris, France

Henry Rusinek, PhD
Professor
Department of Radiology
NYU Langone Medical Center
New York, New York

Farhood Saremi, MD
Professor of Radiology and Medicine
Department of Radiology
USC University Hospital
University of Southern California
Los Angeles, California

Thomas Scholbach, Dr. med. Habil
Professor of Pediatrics, University of Dresden
Dresden, Germany
Head of the Hospital for Children and Adolescents
Chemnitz Clinics
Chemnitz, Germany

Sujith K. Seneviratne, MBBS, FRACP
Associate Professor of Medicine
Monash Cardiovascular Research Centre
Department of Medicine (Monash Medical Centre)
Monash University and Monash Heart
Clayton, Victoria, Australia

Patrick W. Serruys, MD, PhD
Thoraxcenter
Erasmus Medical Centre
Rotterdam, The Netherlands
International Centre for Circulatory Health
Imperial College London
London, United Kingdom

Marion Smits, MD, PhD
Associate Professor
Neuroradiology Section
Department of Radiology
Erasmus MC–University Medical Centre Rotterdam
Rotterdam, The Netherlands

Aaron So, PhD
Imaging Program
Lawson Health Research Institute
Imaging Research Lab
Robarts Research Institute
London, Ontario, Canada
GE Healthcare
Waukesha, Wisconsin

Stacul Fulvio, MD
Department of Radiology
Ospedale Maggiore
Trieste, Italy

Sonja Sudarski, MD
Institute for Clinical Radiology and Nuclear Medicine
University Medical Center Mannheim
Medical Faculty Mannheim—Heidelberg University
Mannheim, Germany

Juan Antonio Hernandez Tamames, MSc, PhD
Associate Professor
MRI Physicist
Head of Electronics Technology Department
Rey Juan Carlos University
Madrid, Spain

Henrik S. Thomsen, MD
Professor
Department of Diagnostic Radiology
Copenhagen University Hospital Herlev
Herlev, Denmark

Teruhisa Unetsubo, DDS
Assistant Professor of Oral and Maxillofacial Radiology
Department of Oral and Maxillofacial Radiology
Okayama University Graduate School of Medicine, Dentistry and Pharmaceutical Sciences
Okayama, Japan

Bernard E. Van Beers, MD, PhD
Department of Radiology
APHP
University Hospitals Paris Nord Val de Seine
Clichy, France
University Paris Diderot
INSERM U1149
Centre de Recherche Biomédicale Bichat-Beaujon
Paris, France

Vikas Veeranna, MD
Division of Nuclear Medicine and Molecular Imaging
Department of Radiology
Division of Cardiology
Department of Medicine
Noninvasive Cardiovascular Imaging Program
Departments of Medicine (Cardiology) and Radiology
Brigham and Women's Hospital
Boston, Massachusetts

Valérie Vilgrain, MD, PhD
Department of Radiology
APHP
University Hospitals Paris Nord Val de Seine
Clichy, France
University Paris Diderot
INSERM U1149
Centre de Recherche Biomédicale Bichat-Beaujon
Paris, France

Danny J. J. Wang, PhD, MSCE
Associate Professor
Department of Neurology
University of California Los Angeles
Ahmanson-Lovelace Brain Mapping Center
Los Angeles, California

Heidi Wassef, MD
Assistant Professor of Clinical Radiology
Department of Radiology
University of Southern California
Keck School of Medicine
Los Angeles, California

Kevin Wei, MD
Knight Cardiovascular Institute
Oregon Health & Science University
Portland, Oregon

Roman Wesolowski, PhD Eng
Research Fellow
King's College London
London, United Kingdom

Christopher T. Whitlow, MD, PhD
Associate Professor of Radiology/Neuroradiology
Department of Radiology
Wake Forest School of Medicine
Winston Salem, North Carolina

Dennis T. L. Wong, BSc, MBBS, PhD, FRACP
Monash Cardiovascular Research Centre
Department of Medicine (Monash Medical Centre)
Monash University and Monash Heart
Clayton, Victoria, Australia

Yoshinobu Yanagi, DDS
Senior Assistant Professor of Oral Diagnosis and Dentomaxillofacial Radiology
Department of Oral Diagnosis and Dentomaxillofacial Radiology
Okayama University Hospital
Okayama, Japan

PREFACE

The idea for this project formed out of the need for a textbook that describes various imaging approaches to both demonstrate and measure tissue perfusion in different organs. Although tissue perfusion is a common physiologic phenomenon in all organs, multiple mathematical models using different imaging techniques have been described. The clinical applications of these techniques are vast and broadly scattered throughout the literature, thus making it difficult for many radiologists and clinicians to understand the practical clinical implementations of these diagnostic methods.

Perfusion abnormalities due to microvascular dysfunction play an important role in the initiation and progression of several diseases. Depending on the severity and duration of tissue blood flow disturbances, alterations in the microvascular structure may take place causing permanent damage and organ failure. In the past, most of the scientific work on the morphology and function of the blood circulation has been focused on diagnosis and treatment of large vessel abnormalities. However, due to the limited spatial resolution of most diagnostic imaging techniques, direct visualization of microvasculature is not feasible in clinical practice and most imaging studies of the microvasculature depend upon indirect analysis of tissue perfusion.

Tissue perfusion imaging provides physiologic information unattainable from anatomic imaging. It has an established role in the early diagnosis of ischemia and functional and vascular abnormalities. The benefit of perfusion imaging for the prediction of tumor behavior and response to treatment has been established. With wide availability of noninvasive imaging technologies that includes nuclear perfusion imaging, magnetic resonance imaging (MRI), computed tomography (CT), and contrast sonography, microvascular dysfunction has been increasingly diagnosed. Using these diagnostic modalities, identification and characterization of both macro- and microvascular abnormalities is possible, even in the subclinical stages of vascular diseases. MRI and nuclear imaging have been the traditional methods in performing noninvasive perfusion studies, and both have immensely contributed to the ability to provide accurate diagnostic and prognostic information. Along with rapid technological development of CT scanners, perfusion studies using this modality have gained new interest. Introduction of 640-slice volume CT scanners and dual-source CT imagers, in conjunction with radiation dose–reduction strategies, have expanded the clinical applications of perfusion CT. With rapid advancement in both imaging hardware and software as well as development of newer analytical methods, tissue perfusion imaging can be routinely performed in most institutions, and many initial limitations such as poor anatomic coverage and low temporal resolution have already been compensated for. Perfusion imaging protocols are now readily incorporated into the existing diagnostic workstations, and postprocessing methods for perfusion analysis have been facilitated by the release of different commercial software packages.

One measurable aspect of the clinical application of perfusion imaging is the diversity and complexity of the topics that can be discussed using different imaging modalities and various mathematical models that can be used to solve the kinetic parameters. Compiled by authors with extensive experience in perfusion imaging, this textbook will address an unmet need in the existing literature by serving as a comprehensive resource for perfusion studies. It provides a practical yet detailed guide to the various analytical methods for qualitative and quantitative evaluation of tissue perfusion and a clinical text for studying organ-specific perfusion-related abnormalities.

This book is divided into two major parts. The length of each chapter and number of images vary in accordance with the complexity of the topic. In all instances, effort has been made to provide a concise yet comprehensive review of the topic. The first part primarily covers the technical aspect of perfusion imaging using CT, MRI, and ultrasound. Pertinent anatomy, microanatomy, and a brief description of physiology are discussed in Chapter 1. MR-related techniques including dynamic susceptibility contrast (DSC), dynamic contrast enhanced (DCE), and arterial spin labeling (ASL) are reviewed in separate chapters. Theoretical aspects of perfusion imaging with CT is described in the subsequent chapter, followed by methodology, imaging techniques, postprocessing, commercial software, and limitations of perfusion imaging. The principle of CT imaging, dose-reduction strategies, and fractional flow reserve imaging are also discussed in detail.

The second and larger part is mainly related to the clinical implementation of perfusion imaging. Each clinical chapter addresses the most common indications of perfusion imaging for a specific organ. The CT and MR imaging protocols, clinical examples, and limitations are then described and richly illustrated. The clinical use of contrast ultrasound, contrast echocardiography, and nuclear perfusion imaging are assigned to dedicated chapters.

As the editor of this textbook, I am fortunate to have colleagues in our facility who have shared their experience with me. Other contributors from high-ranking academic institutions have also provided substantial work and shared their expertise. Together we have worked to create a comprehensive reference textbook on perfusion imaging that will serve a broad spectrum of the medical community including radiologists, physicists, clinicians, and research scholars.

Finally, the work would have remained incomplete without the unreserved assistance of the product development editors of Wolters Kluwer Health, Amy Dinkel and Nicole Dernoski, editor Ryan Shaw, and medical illustrator Jonathan Dimes.

Farhood Saremi, MD
November 2014

CONTENTS

CHAPTER

1 Vascular Anatomy and Microanatomy

Farhood Saremi, MD, Cameron Hassani, MD, and Ameera Ismail, MD

Introduction

Normal function of every organ in the body depends on the integrity of macro- and microcirculation. The blood flow regulation is based on the specific needs of an organ as long as the arterial pressure is sufficient to maintain adequate tissue perfusion. In general, each artery entering an organ branches six to eight times before becoming arterioles (10 to 15 µm). To reach to the capillary level, with diameters of approximately 9 µm, two to five more branchings occur.[1] The term "microcirculation" is applied to the vessels less than 200 µm in diameter, including arterioles, capillaries, and venules, that are responsible for the distribution of blood, transportation of oxygen and nutrients, and removal of toxins within tissues. The abnormalities in the microcirculation play an important role in the start and progression of several diseases. Depending on the severity and duration of the tissue blood flow disturbances, alterations in the microcirculation structure may take place causing permanent modifications in the vessel morphology, a process known as "vascular remodeling."[1] It is shown that sustained vasoconstriction may lead to a decrease in the number and density of working small vessels. This phenomenon is called "functional rarefaction," which may promote permanent vascular regression and loss also termed "structural rarefaction." In turn, microvessel regression may further trigger the vicious circle of arterial remodeling, constriction, and rarefaction leading to further tissue injury.

Both CT and MR angiographies are great techniques to evaluate the macrovasculature of different organs. Given the limited spatial resolution of diagnostic imaging techniques, direct visualization of the microvasculature is not feasible in clinical practice, and most clinical imaging studies of the microvasculature revolve around indirect analysis of tissue perfusion. Microangiography using monochromatic synchrotron radiation has recently been used in animal studies for the assessment of the microvasculature in different organs such as the heart, brain, liver, kidneys, and lungs.[2–5] Although fluorescence microscopy has also been used to image small arteries for a long time, it does not show microvessels after they enter the parenchyma of an organ. High-resolution monochromatic synchrotron microimaging system allows simultaneous observations of up to four levels of branching of arteries/arterioles from approximately 30 to 400 µm in diameter and provides measurements of vascular diameters that are minimally affected by the relative distance or orientation of individual vessels to the camera or x-ray source. The vessel detection limit of the system is 10 µm.[4] However, synchrotron radiation technique is invasive and requires insertion of a catheter and injection of contrast media into the arterial system to achieve sufficient contrast of the blood vessels. New generation of micro-CT systems use a cone-beam x-ray source equipped with a multifocus x-ray tube allowing ultrafast in vivo CT angiography of small vessels at resolutions down to 16 µm.[6]

Brain Circulation

Brain perfusion imaging provides physiologic information, which goes beyond the anatomic imaging. It has an established role in acute stroke imaging, tumor staging, and its response to treatment, and developing role in demyelinating disorders and seizures. It is important to be familiar with the normal gross vascular and microvascular anatomy of the brain in order to master interpreting brain perfusion imaging. In this section, brain vascular anatomy, anastomotic network, and normal variations are briefly discussed.

Brain Arteries

The arterial supply of the brain is divided into anterior and posterior circulations, which have rich anastomosis together[7–10] (Fig. 1.1). The anterior circulation is derived from the internal carotid arteries and their branches. The posterior circulation is derived from the vertebrobasilar arteries and their branches. The arterial supply to the brain also anastomoses with external carotid, which supplies the scalp and calvarium. Anatomic variations are common and usually asymptomatic. Arterial fenestration is more common in the vertebrobasilar arteries. An association has been observed between fenestration and aneurysm formation.[10]

Anterior Circulation

Internal Carotid Artery

The internal carotid artery has six intracranial segments: the petrous segment (C2), lacerum segment (C3), cavernous segment (C4), clinoid segment (C5), supraclinoid segment "ophthalmic" (C6), and terminus segment (C7).

The internal carotid artery gives rise to the ophthalmic artery, the anterior choroidal artery, and the posterior communicating

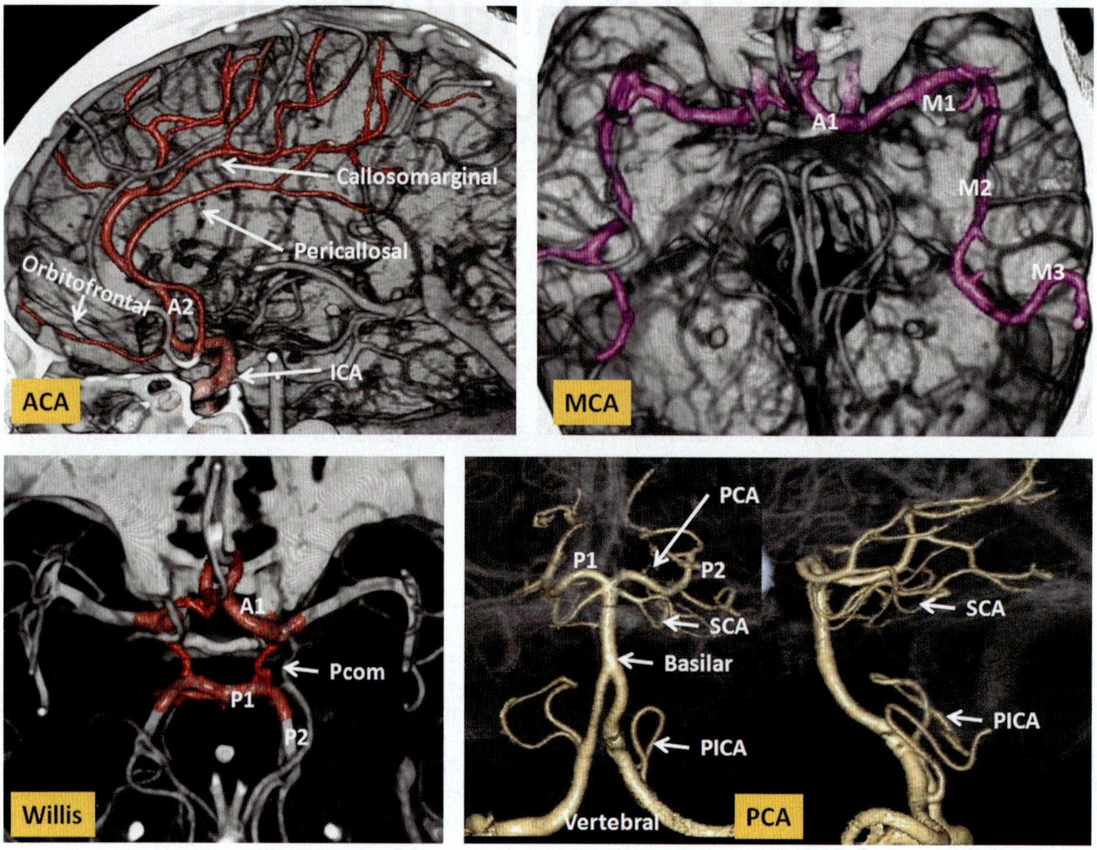

Figure 1-1. Color-coded brain CT angiography showing major arterial branches and segments of the anterior and posterior circulation arteries. The anterior cerebral artery (ACA) has three segments: horizontal (A1), vertical (A2), and distal (A3). The middle cerebral artery (MCA) has four segments: horizontal (M1), insular (M2), opercular (M3), and cortical (M4). The posterior cerebral artery (PCA) has four segments: precommunicating (P1), ambient (P2), quadrigeminal (P3), and calcarine (P4). Circle of Willis showing posterior communicating (Pcom) arteries. ICA, internal carotid artery; PICA, posterior inferior cerebellar artery; AICA, anterior inferior cerebellar artery; SCA, superior cerebellar artery.

artery before it terminates into its two terminal branches: the anterior cerebral artery (ACA) and the middle cerebral artery (MCA).

Anterior Cerebral Artery

The ACA has three segments: horizontal (A1), vertical (A2), and distal (A3). The anterior communicating artery connects the bilateral A1 segments. The ACA gives rise to perforating and cortical branches. The perforating arteries include the medial lenticulostriate arteries arising from the A1 segment and the anterior communicating artery, and the recurrent artery of Heubner arising from either the distal A1 or the proximal A2 segment.

The cortical branches include the orbitofrontal (proximal A2), frontopolar (mid A2), pericallosal, and callosomarginal (distal branches of A2).

Normal variants are seen in the ACA including (a) hypoplastic (10%) or aplastic (1% to 2%) A1 segment; (b) bihemispheric ACA, when the distal branches of an ACA supply the contralateral hemisphere; and (c) absent, fenestrated, or duplicated anterior communicating artery. Duplication of the anterior communicating artery is seen in 18%, whereas fenestration is present in 12% to 21% of the population.[11]

True vascular anomalies include (a) azygos ACA, a single ACA with absent anterior communicating artery, which is seen in 0.5% to 4%, and (b) infraoptic ACA, which is the A1 segment that passes under the optic chiasm instead of over it and is associated with aneurysms. Occlusion of an azygos ACA due to thromboembolic disease may result in ischemia/infarction of both hemispheres.

Middle Cerebral Artery

The MCA has four segments: horizontal (M1), insular (M2), opercular (M3), and cortical (M4).

The MCA gives rise to perforating branches and cortical branches. The perforating branches include the lateral lenticulostriate arteries and the anterior temporal artery, all arising from the M1.

The cortical branches arise from M4, including orbitofrontal artery, prefrontal artery, precentral (prerolandic) artery, central sulcus (rolandic) artery, postcentral (anterior parietal) artery, posterior parietal artery, angular artery, temporo-occipital artery, posterior temporal artery, and medial temporal artery.

There is high variability in the branching pattern of the MCA resulting in early bifurcation or early trifurcation of the artery. True vascular anomalies are rare and mainly include (a) hypoplastic or aplastic MCA; (b) duplicated MCA, arising from the distal ICA before its termination; (c) accessory MCA; and (d) fenestrated MCA. An accessory MCA arises from the ACA and runs parallel to M1. It is seen in less than 3% of cases and supplies the anteroinferior of the frontal lobe.[10]

Posterior Circulation

Posterior Cerebral Arteries

The two posterior cerebral arteries (PCAs) are the terminal branches of the basilar artery.

The PCA has four segments: precommunicating (P1), ambient (P2), quadrigeminal (P3), and calcarine (P4).

The PCA gives rise to perforating, choroidal, and cortical branches. The perforating branches include the posterior thalamoperforating arteries from P1, the thalamogeniculate arteries from P2, and the peduncular perforating branches from P2 as well.

The choroidal branches include the medial posterior choroidal and the lateral posterior choroidal arteries.

The cortical branches include the anterior and posterior temporal arteries arising from P2. Then, the distal PCA terminates into two trunks: (a) a medial trunk giving rise to the medial occipital artery, parietooccipital artery, calcarine artery, and posterior splenial arteries and (b) a lateral trunk giving rise to the lateral occipital artery and temporal arteries.

A normal variant of the PCA is a fetal origin of the PCA, where the PCA arises directly from the internal carotid artery as a large posterior communicating artery with hypoplastic or aplastic P1 segment. This variant is common and present in 10% of the population.[12]

A true vascular anomaly is persistent carotid–basilar anastomoses, where the PCA originates from persistent trigeminal artery or a proatlantal intersegmental artery.

Vertebrobasilar Arteries

The V4 segment is the intracranial segment of the vertebral artery starting after it enters the cranium through the foramen magnum, and both V4 segments unite to form the basilar artery. The V4 segment gives rise to the anterior and posterior spinal arteries, and the perforating branches give rise to the medulla and the posterior inferior cerebellar artery.

The basilar artery gives rise to the perforating pontine and midbrain branches, the anterior inferior cerebellar artery, and the superior cerebellar artery (SCA), and terminates in the PCA.

There are many variations in the dominance of the vertebral arteries and the branching pattern of the basilar artery. True vascular anomalies include fenestrated or duplicated basilar artery and persistent carotid–basilar anastomoses.

Arterial Vascular Territories

There is overlap between the vascular territories of the anterior, middle, and posterior cerebral arteries. Typically, vascular territories are as follows (Fig. 1.2):

Anterior Cerebral Artery

1. The perforating branches supply the caudate head, the anteromedial lenticular nucleus, the genu of the corpus callosum, and the anterior limb of the internal capsule.

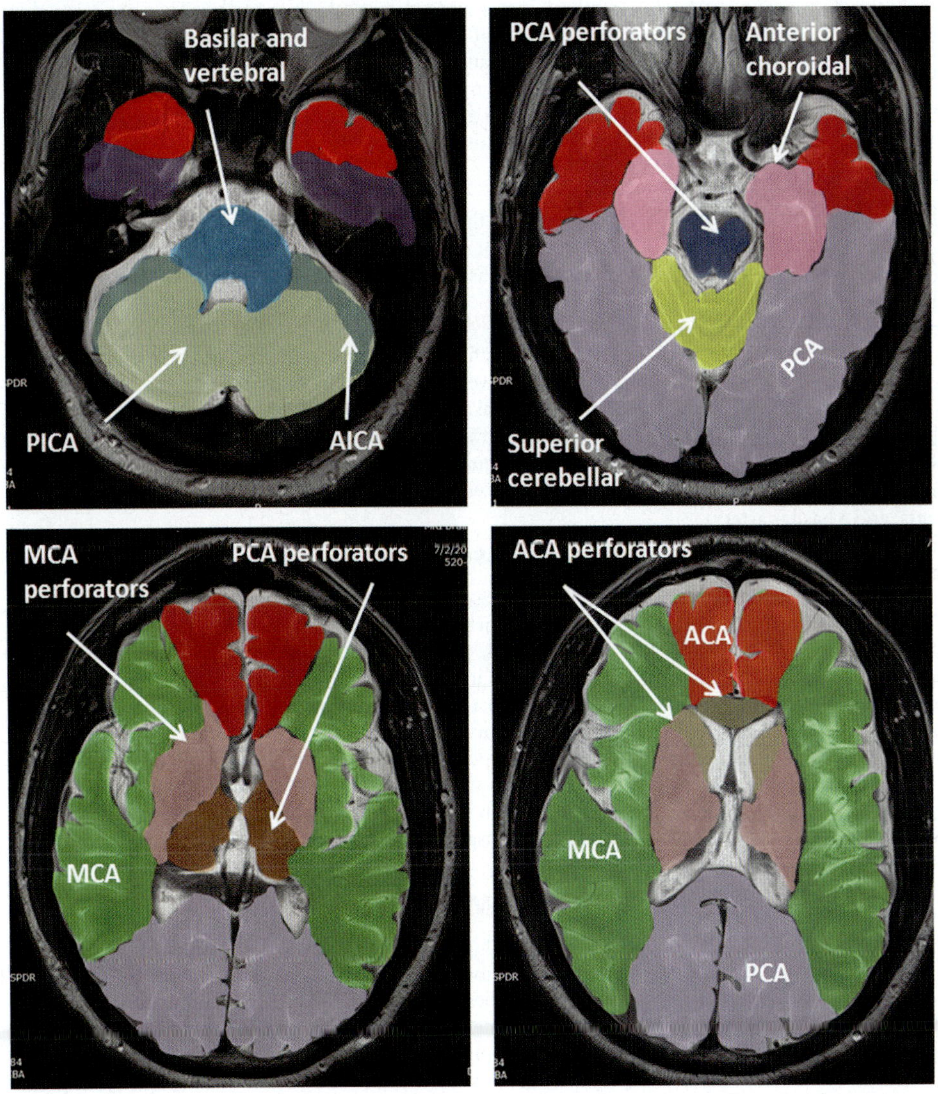

Figure 1-2. **Vascular territories of the carotid and vertebrobasilar circulation systems.** The perforator branches supply most of the lenticular nucleus (putamen and the globus pallidus), caudate nucleus, thalamus, and midbrain. ACA, anterior cerebral artery; MCA, middle cerebral artery; PCA, posterior cerebral artery; PICA, posterior inferior cerebellar artery; AICA, anterior inferior cerebellar artery.

2. The cortical branches supply the anterior two-thirds of the medial hemispheres, the inferomedial frontal lobes, and the medial 1 to 2 cm of the cerebral convexity.

Middle Cerebral Artery

1. The perforating branches supply most of the lenticular nucleus, most of the caudate nucleus, the superior internal capsule, and deep white matter.
2. The cortical branches supply the temporal poles and most of the lateral surface of the cerebral hemispheres.

Posterior Cerebral Artery

1. The perforating branches supply the thalamus, hypothalamus, midbrain, and choroid plexus.
2. The cortical branches supply most of the inferior temporal lobes, the occipital pole, and the posterolateral surface of the cerebral hemispheres.

Basilar Artery

It supplies the pons, superior vermis, and superior cerebellum and all the vascular territory of the PCA.

Vertebral Arteries

Supply the cerebellar tonsils, most of the medulla, and the inferior cerebellum and vermis.

Anterior Choroidal Artery

Supplies the posterior limb of the internal capsule and part of the hippocampus.

Arterial Watershed Areas

These are the border zones between arterial territories that become vulnerable to ischemia with hypoperfusion. There are two watershed zones:

- Cortical watershed zone, between the major cerebral arteries ACA, MCA, and PCA
- Deep white matter watershed zone, between the perforating branches and the cortical branches of the circle of Willis

Arterial Anastomosis

The circle of Willis forms the main anastomosis of the anterior and posterior circulation and is formed by 10 components: Two ICAs, two A1 segments, an anterior communicating artery, two posterior communicating arteries, two P1 segments, and a basilar artery.

The circle of Willis is more often found to be incomplete rather than complete. Absence of the anterior communicating artery is found in 5% of surgeries.[13]

Anastomosis also exists between the branches of the internal carotid and external carotid arteries.

In patients with intracranial arterial occlusion, sufficient blood supply may still be available via anastomotic collateral pathways. Demonstration of the extent of leptomeningeal collateral channels beyond the occlusion has important prognostic significance for patient outcome.[14] Collateral blood supply can be shown by digital subtraction angiography, MR angiography, or CTA. The effectiveness of collateral blood supply can be assessed by MR or CT perfusion techniques.[15,16] Overall poor collateral status is described as less than 50% collaterals and good collateral status as ≥50%.[16]

Brain Vein

The detailed anatomy of the brain venous system is beyond the scope of this chapter. It is grossly comprised of two groups that are interconnected:

1. Dural venous sinuses
2. Cerebral veins: superficial, deep, and brainstem and posterior fossa veins

The Dural Venous Sinuses

Dural venous sinuses are divided into the following:

Anteroinferior group including the cavernous sinus, the superior and inferior petrosal sinuses, the clival sinus, and the sphenoparietal sinuses.

Posterosuperior group including the superior sagittal sinus, the inferior sagittal sinus, the straight sinus, the transverse sinuses, the sigmoid sinuses, and the occipital sinus (Fig. 1.3).

Another way of classifying the dural venous sinuses is as paired and unpaired sinuses. Confluence of the sinuses or torcular herophili is usually defined as the confluence of the superior sagittal sinus, transverse sinus, and straight sinus (Fig. 1.3B). Confluence of all three sinuses is seen in less than 30% of patients. Common variants include branching of the straight sinus into the bilateral transverse sinuses and preferential drainage of the superior sagittal sinus draining into the right transverse sinus[17] (Fig. 1.3B).

Cerebral Veins

Superficial Veins

Superficial veins are located in the leptomeninges and drain the cerebral cortex and subcortical white matter. They are formed by three groups of veins: (a) superior group that includes the small cortical veins and vein of Trolard, (b) middle group that includes the superficial middle cerebral vein and the vein of Labbé, and (c) inferior group that includes the deep middle cerebral vein and the basal vein of Rosenthal.

Deep Veins

These include the subependymal veins, the internal cerebral veins, and the vein of Galen and drain the brain tissue around the ventricles or the basal cistern and connect with the cortical veins.

Brainstem and Posterior Fossa Veins

These are classified into superior, anterior, and posterior groups.

Emissary veins connect the veins outside the cranium with the intracranial venous sinuses. They are commonly found in CT or MR angiographies (Fig. 1.3A). These veins serve an important function of equalizing intracranial pressure and can act as safety valves during cerebral congestion.[18]

Venous Vascular Territories

The venous vascular territories are highly variable and not well known as the arterial vascular territories (Fig. 1.4).

In general, the basal ganglia and the deep white matter are drained by the internal cerebral veins.

While most of the superior and middle brain surfaces are drained by superficial cortical veins into the superior sagittal sinus, the temporoparietal lobes are drained by the vein of Labbé and transverse sinuses, and the insular cortex and the parenchyma around the sylvian fissure are drained by the sphenoparietal and cavernous sinuses.

Brain Microcirculation

The brain is a highly perfused organ, and in order to function normally, it consumes 20% of available oxygen delivered by carotid and vertebral arteries. The cerebral microcirculation comprises a network of terminal arterioles, capillaries, and postcapillary venules.[19] Its arterial supply is derived from recurrent branches of several cortical arteries penetrating into the Virchow-Robin spaces. Capillary

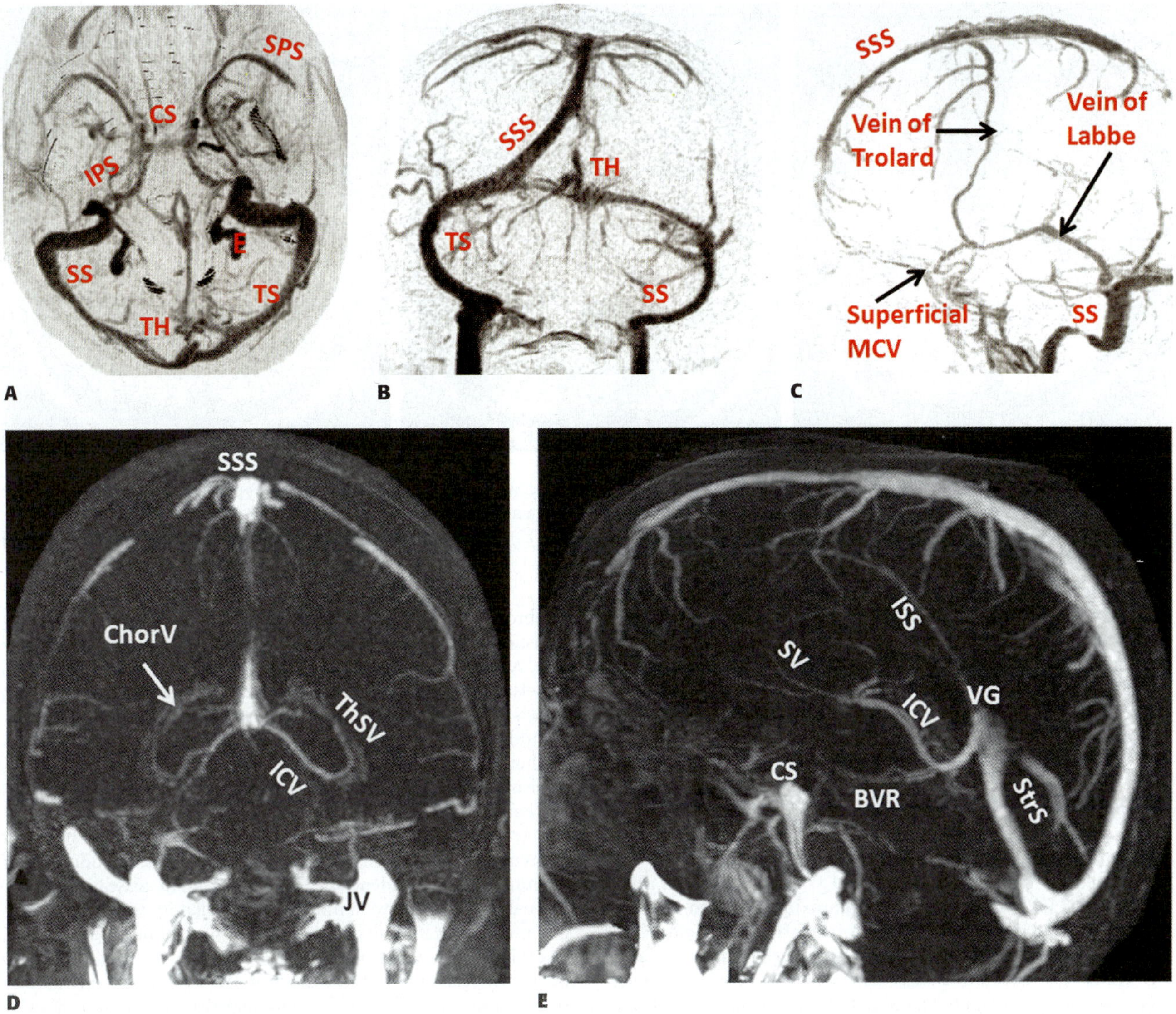

Figure 1-3. Brain veins. **A and B:** Dural venous sinuses. Note preferential drainage of the superior sagittal sinus (SSS) into the right transverse sinuses (TS). **C:** Superficial veins are shown including the vein of Labbé, vein of Trolard, and superficial middle cerebral vein (MCV). **D and E:** Deep veins are shown including the subependymal veins, internal cerebral veins (ICV), vein of Galen (VG), choroidal vein (ChorV), septal vein (SV), and thalamostriate vein (ThSV). CS, cavernous sinus; E, emissary vein (occipital); ISS, inferior sagittal sinus; BVR, basal vein of Rosenthal; SPS, sphenoparietal sinus; TH, torcular herophili; StrS, straight sinus; SS, sigmoid sinus.

density is about threefold higher in the cerebral gray matter than in the white matter. In contrast to other organs, both large arteries and small arterioles (<100 μm diameter) contribute significantly to vascular resistance. This is a protective mechanism that prevents vasogenic edema if the blood pressure is suddenly raised.

Distinguishing characteristics of the brain capillary circulation in the cortex compared to other organs are the existence of tortuous course of capillaries and a remarkably high velocity of red blood cells.[19–22] Other characteristics of the brain perfusion are continuous blood flow in the capillaries and that at rest greater than 90% of cortical capillaries are functional.[19] In spite of continuity of flow, transient regional variation in mean transit time (MTT) within the capillary network exists.[21] This variation in MTT is mainly due to differences in capillary path length and flow velocity and may change in response to various physiologic stimuli such as changes in arterial PCO_2 and perfusion pressure. For example, functional neuronal activation increases cerebral blood flow (CBF) and decreases the heterogeneity of capillary perfusion. The path length and velocity for red blood cells are important determinants of capillary gas and nutrient exchange.[19] In the brain, the tortuous course of capillaries tends to increase MTT, whereas the high velocity of flow has the opposite effect. The average capillary velocity is about 0.5 to 1.8 mm/s. At rest, red cells travel through the capillary network in 100 to 300 milliseconds along 150- to 500-μm-long paths.[21] MTT values of normal gray and white matter are not significantly different (5 to 6 seconds), but CBF of gray matter is higher than that of white matter (70 mL/100 g/min vs. 20 mL/100 g/min).[23]

Cerebral circulation time is an important parameter that provides information on cerebrovascular physiology and helps to define the perfusion status of the brain. It can be measured using CT perfusion techniques by measuring the times of contrast bolus arrival in the internal carotid artery and jugular bulb. The average value is 5.8 ± 1.4 seconds. The timing will be increased in arterial occlusion and is faster in arteriovenous malformations.[24]

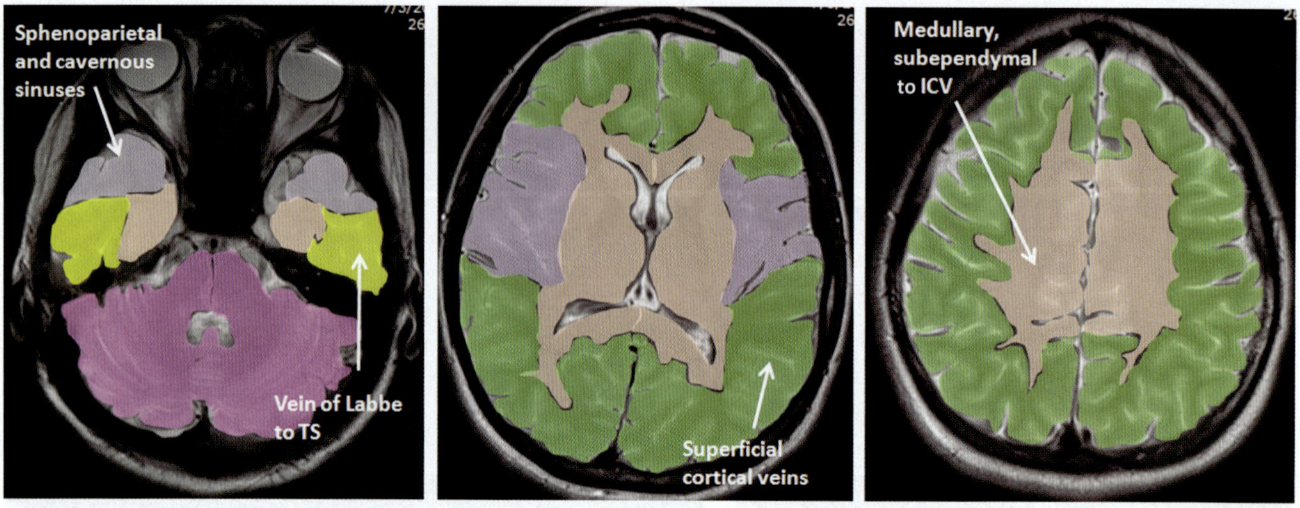

Figure 1-4. **Venous vascular territories.** In general, the basal ganglia and deep white matter (medullary and subependymal) are drained by the internal cerebral veins (ICV). Most of the superior and middle brain surfaces are drained by superficial cortical veins into the superior sagittal sinus. The temporoparietal lobes are drained by the vein of Labbé and transverse sinuses (TS), and the insular cortex and the parenchyma around the sylvian fissure are drained by the sphenoparietal and cavernous sinuses.

The response of capillary flow to decreased perfusion pressure reflects autoregulation of CBF (Fig. 1.5). Autoregulation is well developed in the brain to maintain a constant CBF despite changes in cerebral perfusion pressure (CPP).[22] The CPP is the difference between arterial and venous pressure. The brain venous pressure is proportional to intracranial pressure. According to Ohm law, CBF equals CPP divided by the vascular resistance, and according to Poiseuielle law, CBF is inversely related to vessel radius to the fourth power. Therefore, adjustment of vessels' diameter by autoregulatory mechanisms is the primary function to maintain vascular resistance hence CBF. In normotensive adults, CBF is maintained at approximately 50 mL/100 g of brain tissue per minute, provided CPP is in the range of approximately 60 to 160 mm Hg.[25] Above and below this limit, autoregulation is lost, and CBF becomes dependent on mean arterial pressure in a linear fashion[26] (Fig. 1.5). Cerebrovascular reserve (CVR) provides important information on hemodynamic status in patients with chronic

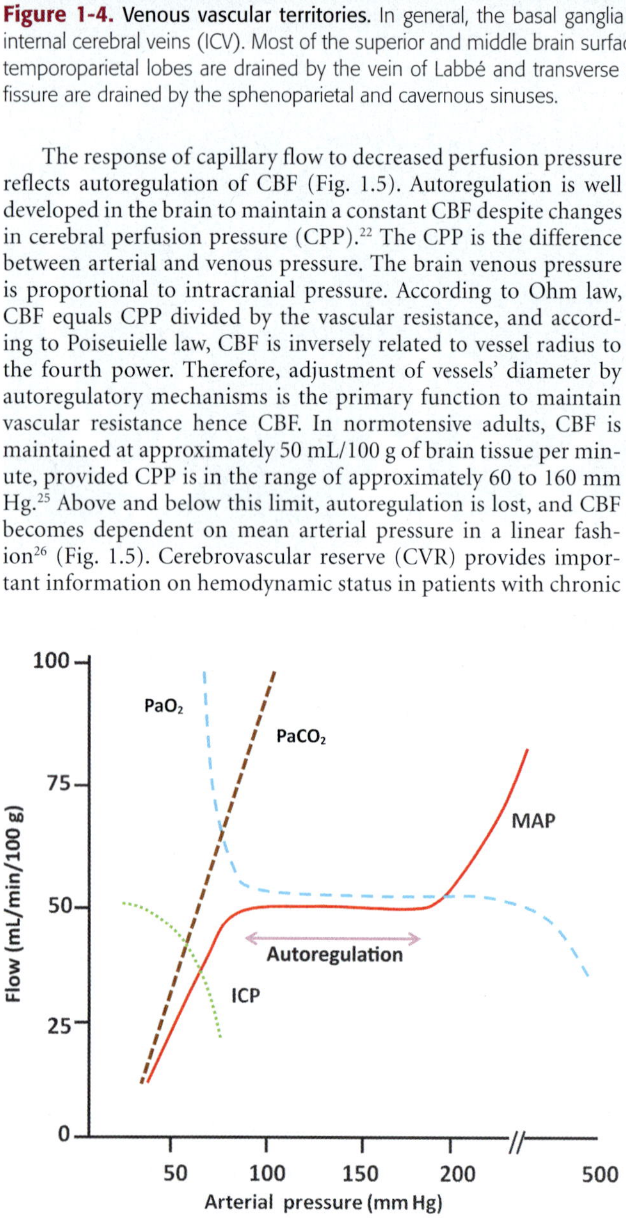

Figure 1-5. Brain circulation autoregulation.

cerebrovascular occlusive diseases.[27] CVR can be measured by measurement of CBF before and after acetazolamide administration. Acetazolamide is a carbonic anhydrase inhibitor that dilates vessels by increasing blood CO_2 levels. In patients with stenotic vessels and decreased CPP, the vessels are already maximally vasodilated by autoregulatory mechanisms and cannot respond further to acetazolamide. These patients are considered to be at increased risk of stroke and can be diagnosed with acetazolamide-challenged test.

Acute hypoxia causes vasodilation and increased CBF by direct effect on the arterial wall muscles, and increased local production of the nitric oxide and adenosine.[19] CBF does not increase until parenchymal PO_2 falls below 50 mm Hg.[21] Vasodilatory response of cerebral microcirculation to hypercapnia is also responsible for increase in capillary flow velocity and CBF, but the mechanism appears to be mainly related to a direct effect of extracellular H^+ on vascular smooth muscle.[28] It is seen that with hypercapnia, CBF increases by 54% and CBV increases by 41%.[29] CBV is the sum of arterial, capillary, and venous blood volumes with an arterial fraction of 30% in humans.[19] Changes in CBV during changes in PCO_2 are caused by changes in arterial blood volume without changes in venous blood volume.[30] Autoregulatory impairment in acute hypertension (e.g., eclampsia) occurs. Increased intravascular pressure in acute hypertension that is above the autoregulatory limit causes forced dilatation of cerebral vessels, decreased vascular resistance, increased CBF, and increased hydrostatic pressure resulting in brain edema.[31] Sustained hypertension above CBF autoregulation as seen in acute hypertensive encephalopathy causes cerebral vasospasm, ischemia, and edema.[32]

In acute tissue hypoxia such as within infarction core, cerebral autoregulation is severely disturbed in the early stages. Severe hypoxia leads to tissue lactate acidosis and local vascular paralysis, compromising the autoregulatory mechanism in both the ischemic core and periinfarct region.[33] Autoregulatory impairment tends to increase mainly in large infarction and involves the contralateral side during the first days after ischemic stroke.[34] A vicious cycle of reperfusion, production of inflammatory vasotoxic substances, impaired autoregulation, edema, and progression of ischemia has been described.[34] In acute brain infarction, both of the infarcted and ischemic (penumbra) zones show decreased CBF and increased MTT (Fig. 1.6). However, in the infarcted tissue, the cerebral blood volume (CBV) is markedly

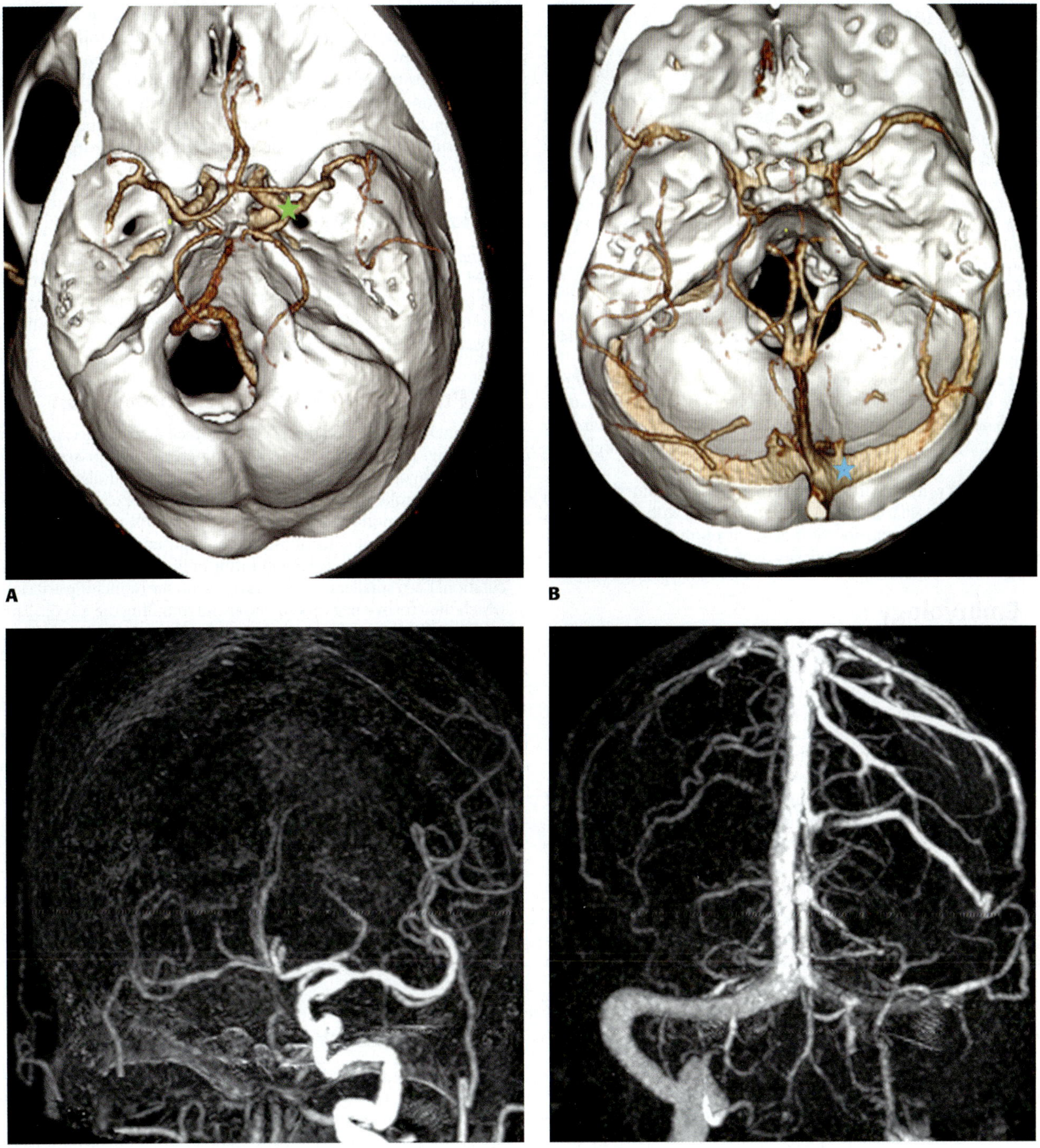

Figure 1-6. A and B: Color-coded brain CT angiography showing the skull base vasculature. **A**, arteries. **B**, veins. In perfusion imaging of the brain, knowledge of the anatomic location of major arteries and veins is essential for proper positioning of region of interests to analyze the arterial input or venous output functions. The best locations include middle cerebral artery (*green star*) or intracranial segment of the internal carotid artery for the arterial input function and the confluence of the venous sinuses (*blue star*) for the venous output function. This is preferentially done on the unaffected side in case of stroke. **C and D:** Right middle cerebral artery (MCA) infarction. **C**, arterial CT angiogram; **D**, venous phase. Note delayed visualization of the MCA and the superficial veins and incomplete arterial collaterals on the right side. Also note preferential emptying of the superior sagittal sinus into the right lateral sinus.

decreased, whereas in the penumbra, due to preserved autoregulatory mechanisms (vasodilatation and recruitment of collaterals), the CBV remains normal to slightly increased.[23] In ischemic gray matter, CBF values are close to normal white matter CBF values. Wintermark et al.[35] reported an MTT of greater than 145% as the threshold for the ischemic tissue at risk of infarction and absolute CBV of 2.0 mL/100 g as the most accurate parameter of the acute infarct core delineation and corresponds the restricted diffusion area in diffusion-weighted MR, indicating irreversible damage.[35]

Pulmonary Circulation

The flow of blood from the heart into the lungs and back to the heart is accomplished by two separate pathways, the pulmonary circulation and bronchial circulation. Pulmonary circulation represents the bulk of blood flow into the lungs for the primary goal of blood oxygenation, whereas the bronchial circulation nourishes the airways and lungs.

Pulmonary circulation arises directly from the right ventricle in a distinct, isolated circuit that runs in parallel to the systemic arterial circuit, from which bronchial blood supply originates. While the pulmonary vascular circuit runs in parallel to the systemic arterial circuit, there is an important difference, much lower pressure within the pulmonary circuit. Despite this low pressure, it is a high-flow circuit, receiving the entire volume of cardiac output with each stroke (5 to 6 L/min). The pulmonary circuit exists for the primary purpose of gas exchange and blood oxygenation.

The low overall pressure of the pulmonary circuit is the effect of low overall resistance from the pulmonary microcirculation. Pulmonary microcirculation is a smaller and shorter vascular network that is simultaneously more dense, offering a much larger surface area.

Pulmonary macrocirculation and microcirculatory arteries, arterioles, and capillaries are connected in series with one another, and their pathologic classification depends on their wall composition such as the degree of muscularity or presence of elastic lamina.[36]

Embryology

Pulmonary circulation arises in tandem to the development of the human cardiovascular system. By day 34, in embryogenesis, circulation exists between the primitive heart and the lung buds.[37]

There is a secondary system, which is present early in life, that exists to offer collateral circulation between the pulmonary and systemic circuits. This system seemingly recedes but remains a potential system for collateral flow between the higher pressure bronchial/systemic circuit and the much lower pressure pulmonary circuit if there is breakdown or disruption in either parent system.[37–39]

Pulmonary Artery Macrocirculation

Pulmonary arterial circulation passes deoxygenated blood from the right heart into the pulmonary capillary network throughout both lungs by way of a series of branching pulmonary arteries, which progressively decrease in caliber.

Normal Anatomy

From the right ventricular outflow tract of the heart arises the main pulmonary artery (MPA), a short conduit that arches from the anteriorly situated right ventricle to divide into the right pulmonary artery (RPA) and the left pulmonary artery (LPA).

The RPA has a longer course, having to cross the midline, coursing posterior to both the ascending aorta and the superior vena cava. The RPA simultaneously passes cranial to both the right atrium and the right superior pulmonary vein. At the level of the right hilum, the anterior-to-posterior relationship of vessels is vein, artery, and bronchus. RPA divides into three major trunks, the right upper, middle, and lower lobe arteries. The right upper artery subdivides into an apical, posterior, and anterior segmental artery. The right middle artery subdivides into medial and lateral segmental branches. Finally, the right lower artery subdivides into apical, anterior, posterior, medial, and lateral branches.[37]

The LPA is shorter and is a continuation of the curvature of the MPA. The LPA arches cranially over the left mainstem bronchus to ultimately hook over the left superior bronchus at the level of the pulmonary hilum. At the level of the left hilum, the anterior-to-posterior relationship of vessels is vein, bronchus, and artery. LPA divides into two major trunks, the upper and lower lobe pulmonary arteries. The upper lobe pulmonary artery subdivides into the apicoposterior, anterior, and lingular arteries, with superior and inferior branches of the lingular artery. The left lower lobe pulmonary artery subdivides into the superior as well as anteromedial, lateral, and posterior basal segmental arteries.[39,40]

Variant Anatomy

While the aforementioned pulmonary arterial relationships are the most commonly encountered, there is variability to this branching pattern encountered in 16.4% of patients.[41] The most common variants involve right middle lobe and lingular arteries, anomalously arising from the basal lower lobe arteries.

Pulmonary Artery Microcirculation

Pulmonary microcirculation consists of small arterioles and capillaries (Fig. 1.7). This microcirculation network comprises approximately 25% of lung volume[42] and is designed to handle the entirety of cardiac stroke volume, permitting proper gas exchange.

Small pulmonary arterioles contain smooth muscle fibers and thus have a level of control over blood distribution, acting as resistance vessels and allow for the shunting of blood within the microcirculation. Even smaller capillaries arise from the branching arterioles, which then form a network of vessels surrounding the alveoli. These capillaries have very thin walls, less than 0.1 μm thick, permitting gas exchange and oxygenation of blood. In addition to gas exchange, the capillaries play a vital role in chemical substance exchange, such as water and electrolytes, as well as biochemical destruction and synthesis. For example, the vasoconstrictive hormone angiotensin I is converted to the active angiotensin II form at the pulmonary capillary level. After gas exchange occurs, blood then continues within the pulmonary venous system for ultimate return to the heart.

Bronchial Artery Circulation

Bronchial circulation differs from pulmonary circulation in that it carries oxygenated blood on the arterial side, arising from the aorta. Bronchial circulation supplies the trachea and bronchia, bronchovascular bundles, pulmonary interstitium, lymph nodes, visceral pleura and the vasa vasorum of the aorta, pulmonary artery, and pulmonary vein.[43]

Normal Anatomy

Bronchial arteries arise directly from the aorta to supply both the right and left lung. There are four typical variations of bronchial artery anatomy, the most common variation (41% of people)[43,44] has one bronchial artery on the right and two on the left. In this variation, the bronchial arteries arise from the T5-6 level. The right bronchial artery arises from a crossing right intercostal artery. The left bronchial supply is, however, the result of two bronchial arteries (superior and inferior bronchial artery), arising directly from the aorta. The left superior bronchial artery directly branches from the anteromedial aorta, lateral to the carina and posterior to the left main bronchus. The left inferior bronchial artery has similar origin but inferior to the left main bronchus.

Variant Anatomy

There is a wide ranging distribution of variant bronchial anatomy; however, all variants ultimately arise from the aorta carrying oxygenated blood. Reported variants include right bronchial artery

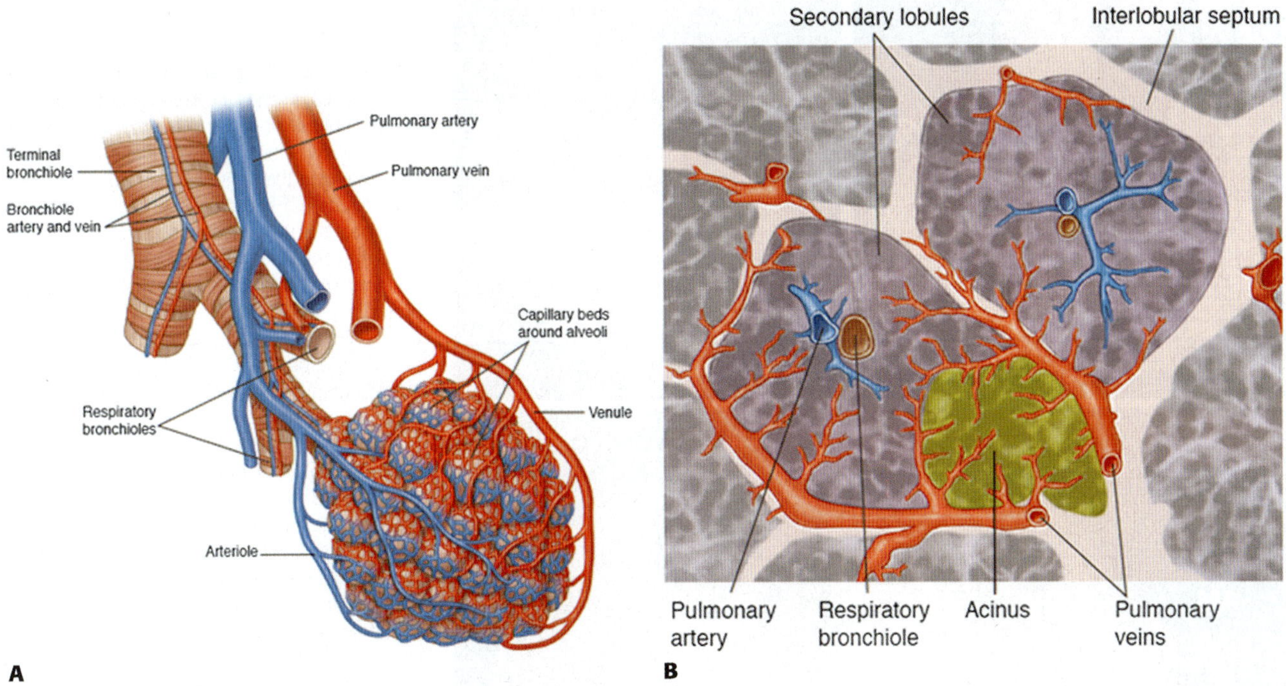

Figure 1-7. A and B: Pulmonary microvasculature and their relationship with the pulmonary lobules. Bronchial circulation contributes to the pulmonary microvasculature by supplying blood to the bronchovascular bundles, pulmonary interstitium, and the vasa vasorum of the pulmonary arteries and veins.

arising from the left superior bronchial artery, bronchial arteries arising from internal mammary arteries, and the thyrocervical trunk among some examples.

Bronchopulmonary Arterial Collateral Flow

Several studies have demonstrated the presence of collateral circulatory pathways between the pulmonary arterial system and bronchial arterial system early in life, but in the normal adult lung, this system recedes. While likely still present, there is no demonstrable flow within the collateral vessels.

However, anastomotic flow has been observed in cases of diseased lung, such as in cases of fibrotic interstitial lung disease,[42] atypical mycobacterial infection, or lung cancer. The result is much higher pressure systemic blood flow (bronchial) entering the lower pressure pulmonary circuit. The result of which is vascular breakdown and ultimate hemoptysis. In cases of pulmonary embolism, flow through these channels can compensate for lack of pulmonary flow and explains why pulmonary infarction is seen in only a minority of cases.

Cardiac Vessels

Knowledge of the anatomy and physiology of the coronary circulation including macro- and microcirculation is essential for understanding the mechanisms that lead to its dysfunction. Noninvasive techniques for evaluation of coronary artery anatomy include transthoracic echocardiography, transesophageal echocardiography, coronary magnetic resonance angiography (MRA), and coronary computed tomography angiography (CTA). Coronary MRA and CTA have emerged in recent years as recommended noninvasive imaging of epicardial coronary arteries. Although CTA is the best technique for demonstration of medium-sized epicardial coronary vessels, none of the imaging tests listed above has adequate spatial and temporal resolutions to directly demonstrate microvessels in clinical practice.

Coronary Arteries

Recent histologic analysis in mouse and cardiac organ culture have shown that coronary vessels arise from the angiogenic sprouts of the sinus venosus, the major vein that returns circulating blood to the embryonic heart.[45] Some sprouting venous endothelial cells dedifferentiate into arteries and capillaries as they invade the myocardium and some remain on the surface and differentiate into veins.[45] Coronary arteries are variable in anatomic origin, course, and branching. In the majority of hearts, two coronary arteries exist, the right coronary artery (RCA) and the left main coronary artery bifurcating into the left anterior descending (LAD) and the left circumflex (LCx) arteries (Figs. 1.8 and 1.9). In 10% to 15%, the left main coronary artery trifurcates into the LAD, LCx, and ramus intermedius arteries. The main coronary vessels are considered arteries, and the smaller, more distal vessels are generally termed coronary branches. In spite of this generalization, it is not uncommon to call some small branches "artery," for example, sinoatrial node artery or posterior descending artery (PDA).

The relationship between the coronary artery branches at the crux cordis defines the type of coronary artery dominance and is determined by the artery giving rise to the posterior interventricular branch (PDA)[46–49] (Fig. 1.9). The PDA and posterolateral branches that supply the inferior wall can originate from the RCA only (right dominant, 65% to 85%), from the left circumflex artery (left dominant), or from both arteries (codominant). In another definition, coronary dominance describes the artery that gives rise to the atrioventricular node artery. In most patients, the PDA arises from the distal portion of the coronary artery, but some patients have early takeoff of the PDA from the mid RCA (split RCA), which then courses toward the apex along the diaphragmatic surface of the right ventricle. Dual

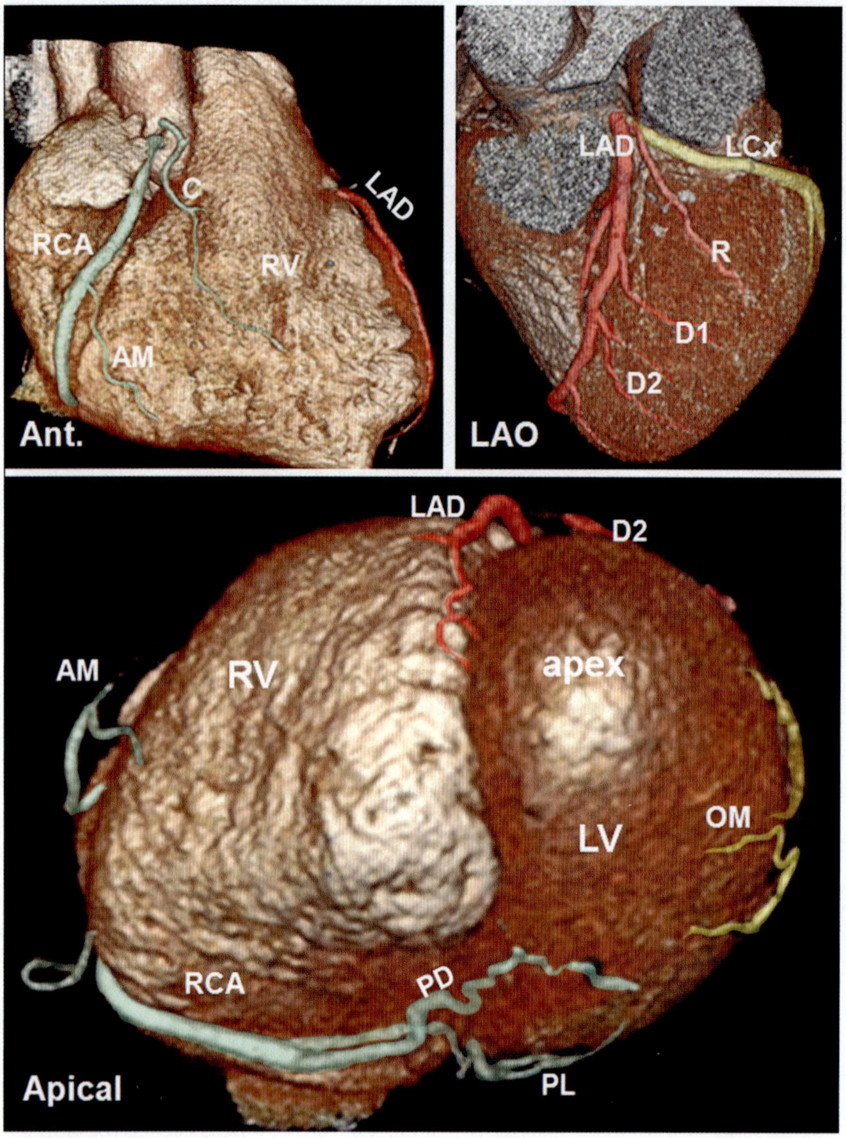

Figure 1-8. Coronary anatomy. Volume-rendered CT images in the anterior (Ant.), left anterior oblique (LAO), and apical projections. The anterior view shows right coronary artery (RCA) descending in the right atrioventricular groove. A large conus (C) branch is seen arising from the aorta near the RCA ostium and is directed toward the right ventricular free wall. Marginal and acute marginal (AM) branches are usually seen in this projection. The distal RCA usually descends into the inferior (posterior) interventricular groove to provide the posterior descending (PD) branch. The PD branch can reach the apex and provides posterior septal branches. If the RCA extends beyond the crux, the branches are called right posterolateral (PL) branches. LAO view shows trifurcation of the left main coronary artery into the left anterior descending (LAD), the left circumflex (LCx), and ramus intermedius arteries. The ramus intermedius, also known as the intermediate branch, or ramus, varies in length and size. It typically supplies the lateral wall of the left ventricle in a territory similar to that supplied by the diagonal or obtuse marginal branches. The LAD descends in the anterior interventricular groove. It will usually reach the apex, and in some cases, it extends beyond the apex to the inferior wall. During its entire course, the LAD gives rise to septal branches that penetrate into the interventricular septum; the first septal branch is often large. The diagonal (D) branches are variable in size and number. The LCX enters the left atrioventricular groove and usually gives rise to one or several obtuse marginal (OM) branches and may continue to end in several left posterolateral branches (LCx dominant or codominant). The OM branch is usually larger than the segment of the LCX that continues beyond its origin.

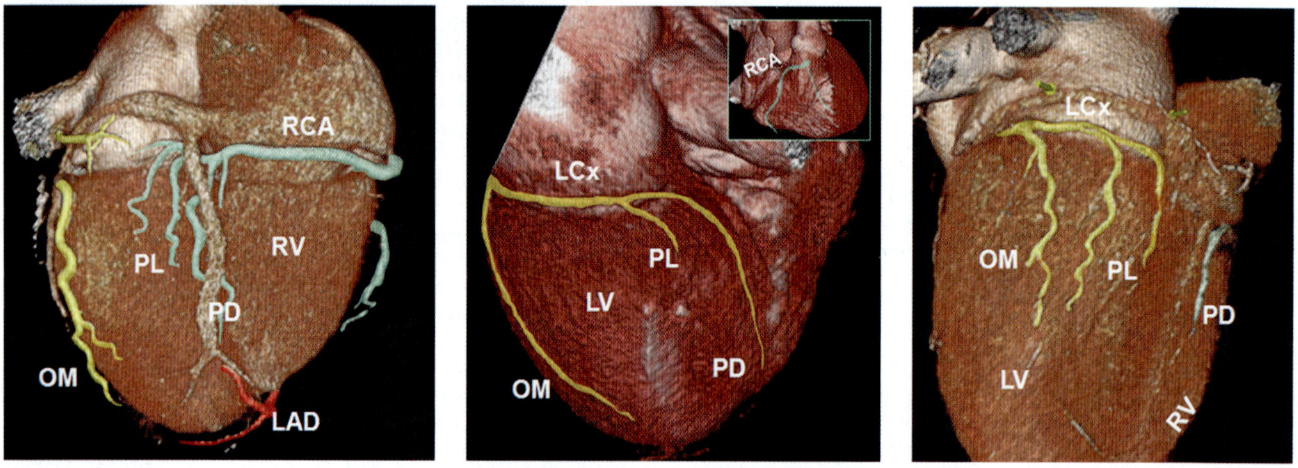

Figure 1-9. Coronary dominance. Posterior view of volume-rendered CT angiographies. **A**, right dominant; **B**, left dominant; **C**, codominant. In right dominant system, the right coronary artery (RCA) gives rise to the posterior descending (PD) branch and at least one right posterolateral (PL) branch. In left dominant, the left circumflex coronary (LCx) artery is large and provides a PD branch. The RCA is small and does not extend beyond the acute margin of the heart (shown in *inlay image*). In codominant system, most PL branches are provided by the LCx and PD branch by the RCA. OM, obtuse marginal; LV, left ventricle; RV, right ventricle.

origin of the PDA is not uncommon, one from the mid RCA (marginal branch) and the second from the distal RCA. This variant has been reported in up to 30% of individuals.[50] In patients presenting with an acute coronary syndrome, left coronary dominance appears to be independently associated with increased long-term mortality, especially with involvement of the inferior wall of the heart.[51] In most individuals with left coronary dominance, the RCA is usually small and an unreliable source of left myocardial perfusion.[52]

Segmental Blood Supply

The standard 17-myocardial segment model of the left ventricle is suggested by the American Heart Association for all cardiac imaging modalities to facilitate a more detailed analysis of regional left ventricular function and perfusion[53] (Fig. 1.10). However, the adopted model shows significant variability and overlap of the segments assigned to a specific territory that makes it difficult to generalize data among different studies (Fig. 1.11).

The vascular supply to the inferior wall of the left ventricle has a spectrum of variations. This part is mainly supplied by the RCA and the LCx. The LAD artery that wraps around the apex can supply some of the apical inferior wall. The lateral wall territory is supplied by the LCx in vast majority of individual but can be shared with a large diagonal from the LAD or the ramus branch. Myocardial blood supply in the inferolateral region corresponds to the LCx or RCA distribution, and the inferoseptal region can be supplied by the LAD or RCA.[54] In a correlative MR study, the presence of hyperenhancement in the basal and mid anterior and anteroseptal or apical anterior wall has been 100% specific for LAD artery occlusion.[55] The LAD infarcts frequently involve the midanterolateral, apical lateral, and apical inferior walls. No segment is 100% specific for the RCA occlusion. Combination of hyperenhancement in the anterolateral and inferolateral walls is 100% specific for the LCx occlusion, and when extended to the inferior wall, is also 100% specific for a dominant or codominant LCx occlusion. Hybrid imaging combined with the anatomic

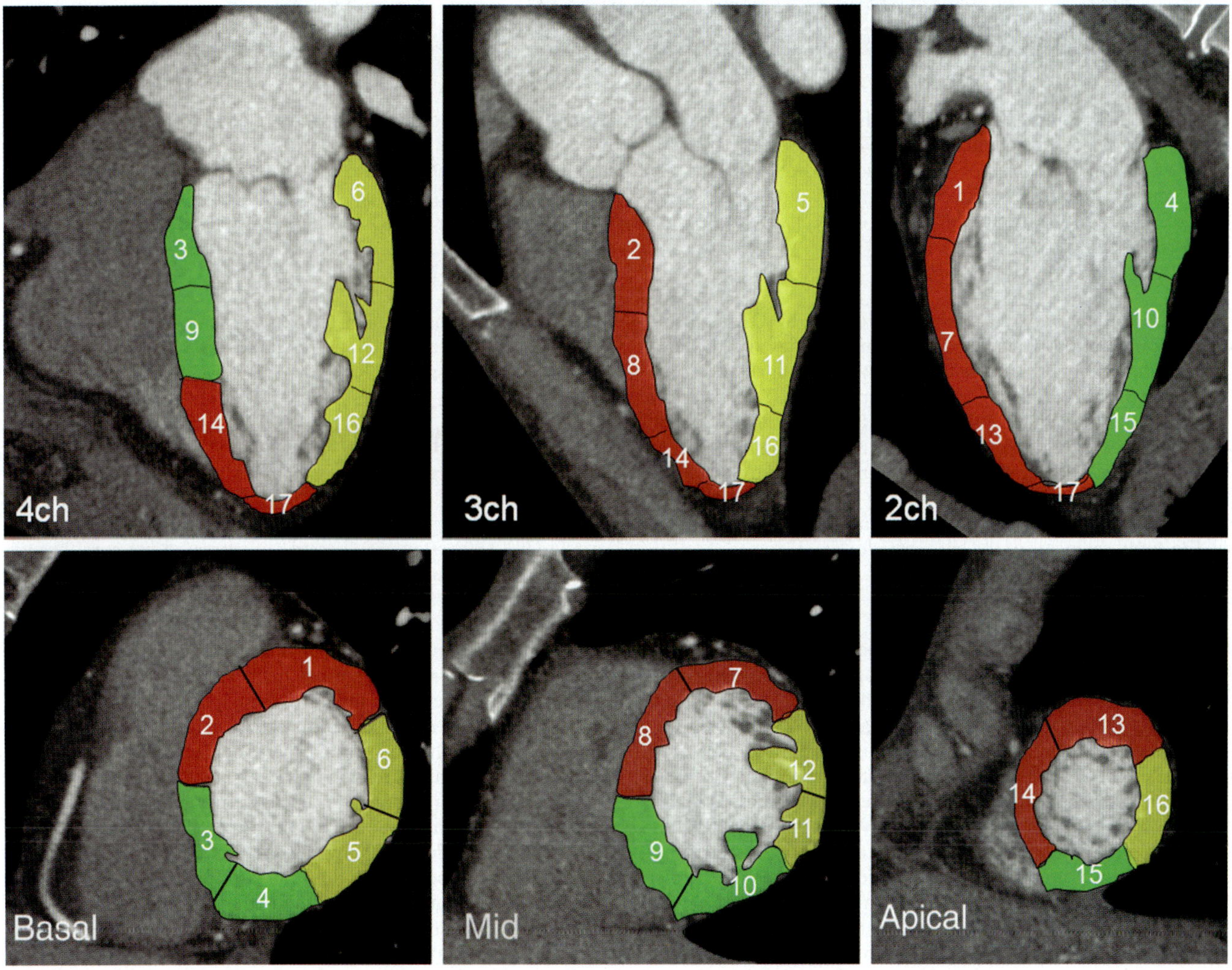

Figure 1-10. Long- and short-axis CT angiography images show distribution of left ventricular 17 myocardial segments based on AHA model: basal anterior (*1*), basal anteroseptal (*2*), midanterior (*7*), midanteroseptal (*8*), apical anterior (*13*), apical septal (*14*), and apex (*17*) segments corresponded to LAD (*red*). Basal anterolateral (*6*), basal inferolateral (*5*), midanterolateral (*12*), midinferolateral (*11*), and apical lateral (*16*) segments correspond to LCX (*yellow*). Basal inferoseptal (*3*), basal inferior (*4*), midinferoseptal (*9*), midinferior (*10*), and apical inferior (*15*) segments correspond to RCA (*green*) distribution. LAD, left anterior descending; RCA, right coronary artery; LCx, left circumflex artery; ch, chamber. (From Gupta T, Saini A, Sahni D. Terminal branching pattern of the right coronary artery in left-dominant hearts: a cadaveric study. *Cardiovasc Pathol* 2013;22(3):179–182.)

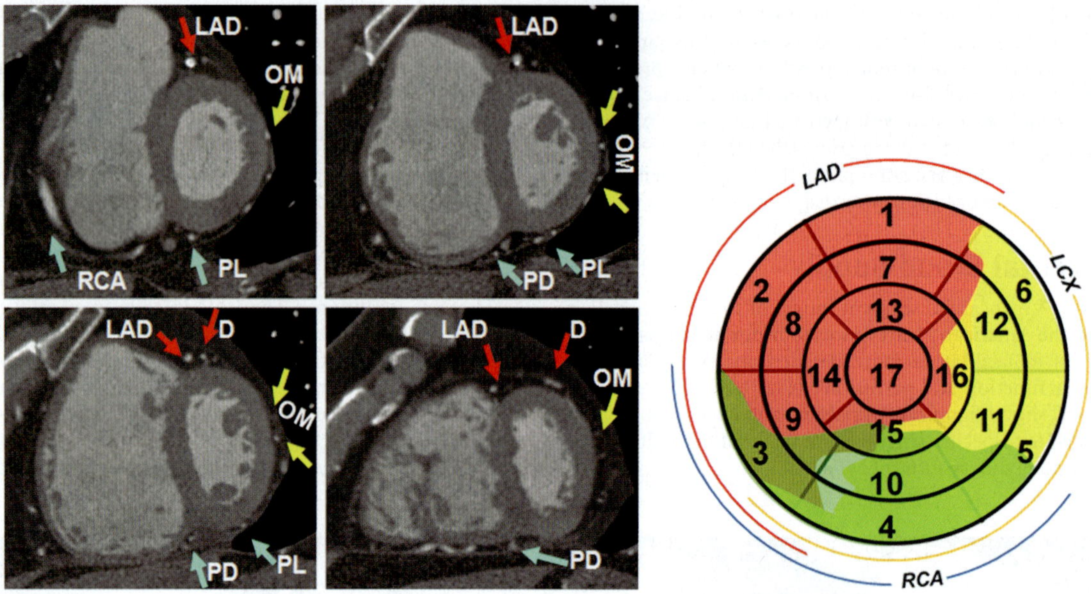

A B

Figure 1-11. A: Short-axis CT angiography images show anatomical distribution of the coronary arteries in relation to left ventricular segments. *Arrows* show territories of the LAD (*red*), RCA (*blue*), and LCx (*yellow*). LAD, left anterior descending; D, diagonal branch; RCA, right coronary artery; PL, posterolateral branch; PD, posterior descending branch; OM, obtuse marginal branch of left circumflex artery (LCx). **B:** Maximal extent of myocardium perfusion for LAD (*red*), RCA (*green/blue*), and LCX (*yellow*) and overlapped regions in the polar map of 17 segments based on Pereztol-Valdés O, Candell-Riera J, Santana-Boado C, et al. Correspondence between left ventricular 17 myocardial segments and coronary arteries. *Eur Heart J* 2005;26(24):2637–2643.

information of vascular distribution provided by CTA is useful to study myocardial tissue perfusion abnormalities and the coronary anatomy for more accurate assignment to culprit vessels and to improve monitoring of targeted therapy.[56,57] CT studies have shown common overlap between the LAD and the RCA perfusion territories at the inferoseptal region and between the LAD and the LCx territories at the anterolateral region. It is important to realize that the LAD territory can be larger than the AHA-proposed 17-segment model, due to the involvement of the anterolateral and all the apical segments of the left ventricle.[54]

Coronary Veins

Modern anatomical classification divides the cardiac veins into two main groups including tributaries of the greater cardiac vascular system (CVS) and tributaries of the smaller CVS, consisting of the thebesian vessels.[58,59] The greater CVS is subdivided into two groups including coronary sinus and noncoronary sinus tributaries. In ventricular myocardium, the external two-thirds are drained by the greater CVS, and the internal third is mainly drained by tributaries of the smaller CVS. The left ventricle and part of the right ventricle and the left atrium are drained by the coronary sinus tributaries, and the majority of the right ventricle and both atria are drained by the noncoronary sinus tributaries (Fig. 1.12). Almost all veins of the greater CVS are finally drained into the right atrium. The coronary sinus tributaries include the coronary sinus, the great cardiac vein, the left marginal vein, the posterolateral vein of the left ventricle, and the inferior interventricular vein (middle cardiac vein). In 30%, it receives the right marginal vein blood through the small cardiac vein. The thebesian valve demarcates the distal end of coronary sinus. Variants of the coronary sinus and coronary veins morphology are common. The coronary sinus length is between 30 and 50 mm in 75% of the anatomic sections and can be easily recognized in most CTAs. Coronary sinus flow can be measured with phase-contrast MRI at stress and rest, and the ratio equals coronary flow reserve (CRF).

Coronary Artery Collaterals

It is suggested that vessels less than 200 μm in diameter serve as the precursor of the collateral circulation.[60] These vessels are not visible angiographically, but in case a major artery becomes occluded (>90% stenosis), because of increased pressure through these small anastomotic vessels, they dilate and become visible by imaging methods. Collaterals may be protective against myocardial ischemia when abundant. In patients with occluded coronary artery and "adequate" coronary collaterals, regional myocardial contraction can remain normal in 43%.[60] Animal studies have shown that differences in myocardial infarct size and shape may be secondary to the extent of coronary collateral vessel formation.[61] For example, high subepicardial perfusion in dogs leads to nontransmural, subendocardial infarcts with acute coronary occlusion, whereas transmural infarction in pig hearts owing to the lack of collateral perfusion in both subepicardium and subendocardium. Generally, subendocardial flow decreases as a function of time after occlusion and subepicardial flow increase, but this is not the case in every situation, and transmural infarct can develop due to lack of collateral flow in some cases. Ischemic myocardium triggers near-maximal vasodilation of collateral blood vessels. The amount of collateral blood flow depends on the extent of infarct, transmural pressure of left myocardium, arterial blood pressure, and hydraulic resistance of the collaterals. During maximal dilation, overall collateral resistance is 3.5 resistance units. In other words, a perfusion pressure of 350 mm Hg is needed to drive 100 mL of blood per minute through 100 g of tissue. Overall, small ischemic areas receive a relatively larger amount of collateral flow that delays or prevents necrosis following epicardial arterial occlusion.[62] The

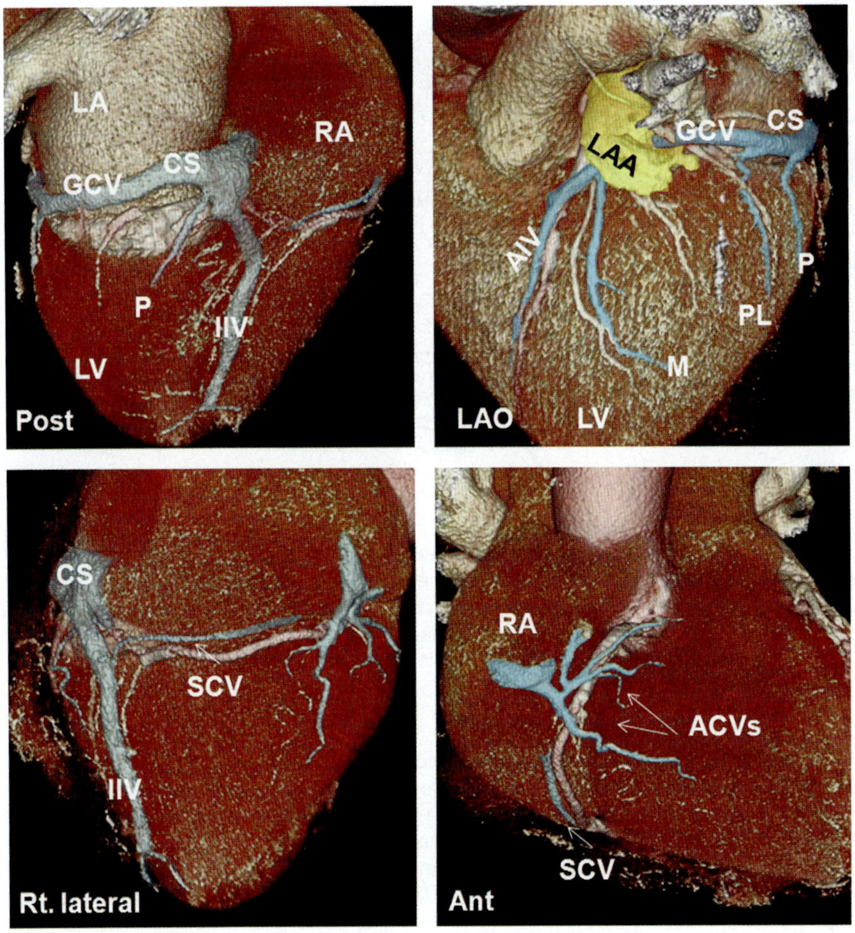

Figure 1-12. **Normal coronary veins in CT angiography shown in *blue*.** Posterior (Post), left anterior oblique (LAO), right (Rt) lateral, and anterior (Ant) views are shown. Approximately 80% of venous blood return is achieved via coronary veins on the surface of the heart. The remaining 20% of drainage is into the thebesian veins (venae cordis minimae), which drain directly into the cardiac chambers. Several small "anterior" cardiac veins (ACVs) may drain directly into the right atrium (RA). The remaining blood drainage is achieved via the anterior interventricular vein/great cardiac vein (AIV/GCV) that runs parallel to the left anterior descending coronary artery. Close to the left main bifurcation, it enters the atrioventricular groove and runs parallel to the left circumflex coronary artery. The left marginal (M), posterolateral (PL), and posterior (P) veins of the left ventricle (LV) enter the GCV, which is then referred to as the coronary sinus (CS). The CS enters the RA. Immediately before the ostium, the inferior interventricular (middle cardiac) vein (IIV) (which has a course alongside the posterior descending artery) and the small cardiac vein (SCV) (parallel to the right coronary artery) also drain into the coronary sinus. SCV may directly drain into the RA as shown in this case.

underlying mechanism of the "natural process" of coronary collateral formation is a complex participation of several growth factors. Vascular endothelial growth factor (VEGF) is a potent angiogenic factor for collateral growth that can be blocked when nitric oxide (NO) production is inhibited (Fig. 1.13). X-ray micro-CT analysis by Toyota et al.[63] showed a threefold increase in the number of arterial–arterial anastomoses in rats after repetitive episodes of myocardial ischemia, which was prevented by administration of anti-VEGF.

Coronary Microvasculature

In the past, most of the scientific work on morphology and function of the coronary circulation has been focused on diagnosis and treatment of the obstructive atherosclerosis of the major epicardial coronary arteries visible on conventional imaging. In recent years, attention has been shifted to the fact that microvascular component of the coronary circulatory system may be the source of coronary dysfunction and increased vascular resistance. Microcirculation is responsible for the CRF, which allows up to four- to fivefold increase in maximal flow rate. Endothelial dysfunction and loss of vasodilatory capacity of the microcirculation (microvascular dysfunction) is an early manifestation of vascular disease and plays a role in the development of coronary artery disease.[64,65]

The coronary arterial system is composed of three compartments.[64–69] These three compartments include epicardial arteries, prearterioles, and arterioles, although the anatomical borders of each compartment cannot be clearly defined (Fig. 1.14).

1. Epicardial (conductant) coronary arteries are relatively large (>500 μm) extramyocardial vessels that are visible by conventional imaging techniques such as coronary angiography and CT scan. They function as capacitance with little resistance to coronary blood flow. During systole, blood content of the epicardial coronary arteries increases up to 25%. As a result of this dilation, elastic energy accumulates, which prompts reopening of intramyocardial vessels in early diastole that are compressed by systolic myocardial contraction.
2. Prearterioles (100 to 500 μm) are also extramyocardial and therefore are not under direct vasomotor control by diffusible myocardial metabolites. Their specific function is to maintain flow and pressure at the origin of arterioles within a narrow range when coronary perfusion flow or pressure changes. Proximal prearterioles are more responsive to changes in flow, whereas distal prearterioles are more responsive to changes in pressure. Flow-mediated vasoreactivity in proximal prearterioles is endothelium dependent. Release of vasodilators by endothelial cells results in vasodilation and increase in flow. Distal prearterioles react predominantly to intraluminal pressure changes sensed by stretch receptors located in smooth muscle cells of the vessel (myogenic control). When aortic pressure increases, distal prearterioles undergo myogenic constriction in order to maintain a constant pressure at the origin of the arterioles. Distal prearterioles dilate when the pressure decreases.
3. Arterioles (<100 μm) are intramyocardial, and their tone is influenced by myocardial metabolism. They are characterized by a considerable pressure drop along their length, and their specific function is to match the myocardial blood supply with

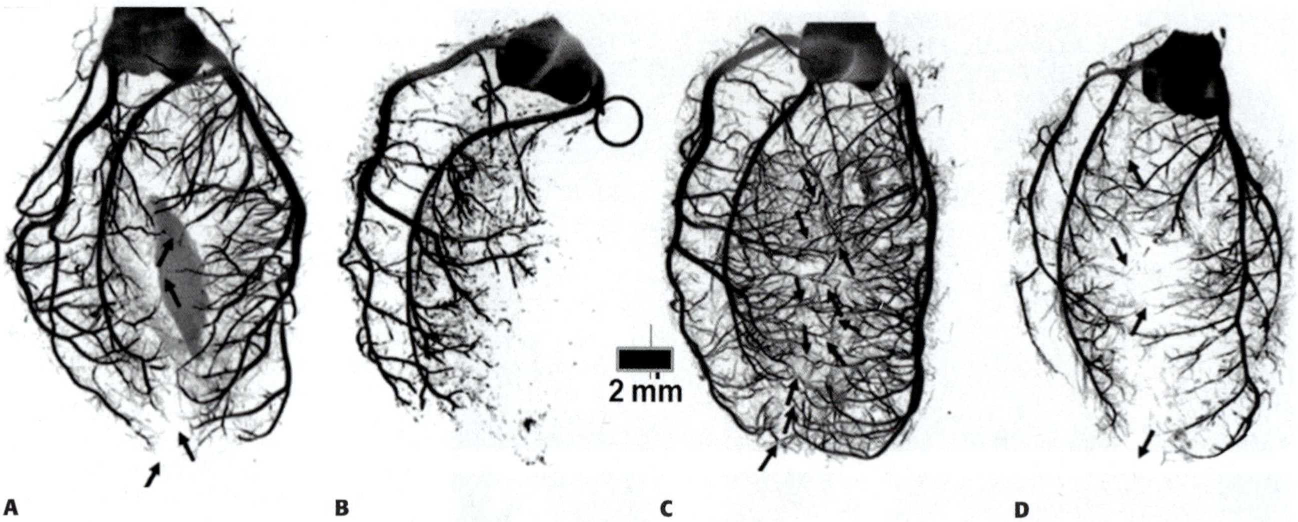

Figure 1-13. **Coronary artery collaterals.** Representative micro-CT images of coronary microvasculature in rats. **A:** Sham heart with balloon implantation but no occlusion reveals four collaterals (*arrows*). **B:** An intact heart with complete ligation of the proximal left anterior descending (LAD) shows no collateral perfusion into the LAD region. **C:** Visualization of collaterals after repeated arterial occlusion reveals multiple anastomoses compared with the sham (**A**). **D:** Heart after anti-vascular endothelial growth factor administration shows inhibited collateral growth. (Reproduced from Toyota E, Warltier DC, Brock T, et al. Vascular endothelial growth factor is required for coronary collateral growth in the rat. *Circulation* 2005;112(14):2108–2113, with permission.)

the myocardial oxygen demand. Arterioles have a fundamental role in the metabolic regulation of coronary blood flow. Their resting tone is high and dilates in response to the release of metabolites by the myocardium when myocardial oxygen consumption increases. Arteriolar dilatation decreases both resistance, in the overall network, and pressure, in the distal prearterioles, causing their myogenic dilatation. Furthermore, dilatation of the distal prearterioles and arterioles results in an increase in shear stress, which triggers flow-dependent dilatation in proximal prearterioles and conductance arteries. Flow-mediated dilatation in response to increased shear stress is achieved through endothelial release of vasodilators, in particular NO, endothelium-derived hyperpolarizing factor (EDHF), and prostacyclin. NO appears to play a key role in flow-mediated relaxation of large epicardial vessels. NO synthesis can be prevented by NG monomethyl-L-arginine (L-NMMA). The endothelium-dependent relaxation of EDHF is more apparent in resistance vessels and might play an important role in prearteriolar flow–mediated dilatation. The contribution of prostacyclin-mediated relaxation is limited to a compensatory response when bioavailability of NO is reduced as a result of endothelial dysfunction.[70]

Since the microvascular compartment is the site of major resistance (approximately 70% with normal vasomotor tone), pressure mainly drops in this compartment. About 30% of the pressure drops is in prearterioles and 40% in arterioles. Pressure drop along conductant vessels is minimal and less than 10%. Capillaries and

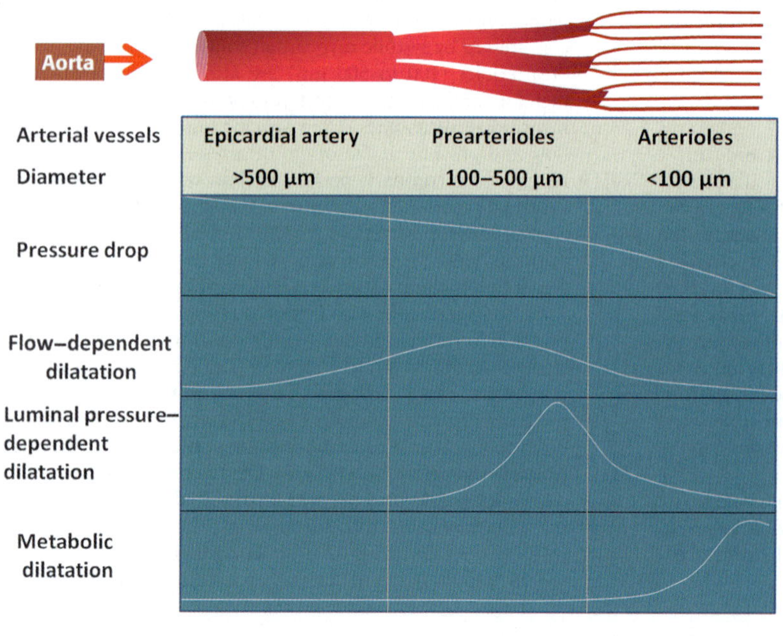

Figure 1-14. **Functional subdivisions of the coronary arterial system include conductive epicardial arteries, prearterioles, and arterioles.** Coronary blood flow is driven by the pressure difference between the aorta and the capillary bed and modulated further by various physical and neural factors, which affect the microcirculation. The pressure drop in conductive arteries is minimal, moderate in prearterioles, and large through the arterioles. Conductive arteries and proximal prearterioles are both responsive to flow-dependent dilatation. Distal prearterioles are more responsive than are the other types of vessels to changes in intravascular pressure and are mainly responsible for autoregulation of coronary blood flow. Arterioles are responsive to changes in the intramyocardial concentration of metabolites and are mainly responsible for the metabolic regulation of coronary blood flow. Prearterioles, by definition, are not exposed to myocardial metabolites because of their extramyocardial position and their wall thickness. (From Camici PG, Crea F. Coronary microvascular dysfunction. *N Engl J Med* 2007;356:830–840.)

venules are likewise responsible for only 10% to 20% of coronary blood flow resistance and mainly function as capacitance vessels, holding 90% of the total myocardial blood volume.[65,71]

Coronary Blood Flow and Myocardial Perfusion

The coronary circulation is distinguished from other vascular networks by its phasic flow pattern, which is mainly related to the mutual interaction of coronary flow with cardiac contraction called "mechanical cross talk."[72] Most of the coronary arterial flow occurs in diastole, while during systole, the arterial flow may slow down or even reverse, while the venous flow accelerates (Fig. 1.15). Capillaries are relatively resistant to the systolic myocardial compression compared with pre- and postcapillary microvessels.[73,74] This is beneficial for the myocardial oxygen delivery throughout a cardiac cycle. During systole, subepicardial arterial flow remains anterograde, while flow in subendocardial arteries is reverse.[74] However, it should be noticed that the effect of powerful cardiac contraction on deeper myocardial perfusion is compensated for by a sufficiently high perfusion pressure and long diastole in normal hearts, which makes the perfusion fairly uniform over the myocardium.[74–76]

It a recent myocardial perfusion study for evaluation of transmural perfusion comparing systole and diastole, it is shown that under adenosine-induced hyperemia (not at rest), myocardial blood flow and myocardial perfusion reserve were significantly higher in diastole than in systole and a reversal of the typical subendocardial to subepicardial myocardial blood flow gradient occurs in systole but not in diastole under stress.[77]

Coronary perfusion is regulated in a number of ways. These can be divided into extrinsic, such as the humoral–nervous regulation, and intrinsic, such as autoregulation. Autoregulation is the intrinsic tendency of the vascular system to maintain a constant flow in the setting of variation in perfusion pressure (i.e., pressure fluctuation between 70 and 120 mm Hg).[78]

In heart muscle, autoregulation is mainly due to a myogenic change in diameter of distal prearteriolar vessels in response to changes in perfusion pressure. The tone of the coronary resistive vessels (arterioles and prearterioles) is high at resting state. This intrinsically high resting tone allows the coronary circulation to increase flow by dilating small vessels when myocardial oxygen consumption increases. Autoregulation is better maintained in the subepicardial myocardium compared with the subendocardium. When perfusion pressure at the origin of the arteriolar vessels, compared with that of the aorta, is reduced, perfusion becomes jeopardized earlier in the subendocardial than in the subepicardial layers of the left ventricle. In addition, the subendocardium becomes even more susceptible to underperfusion if diastolic time is short[76] and myocardial hypertrophy is present.[68,69]

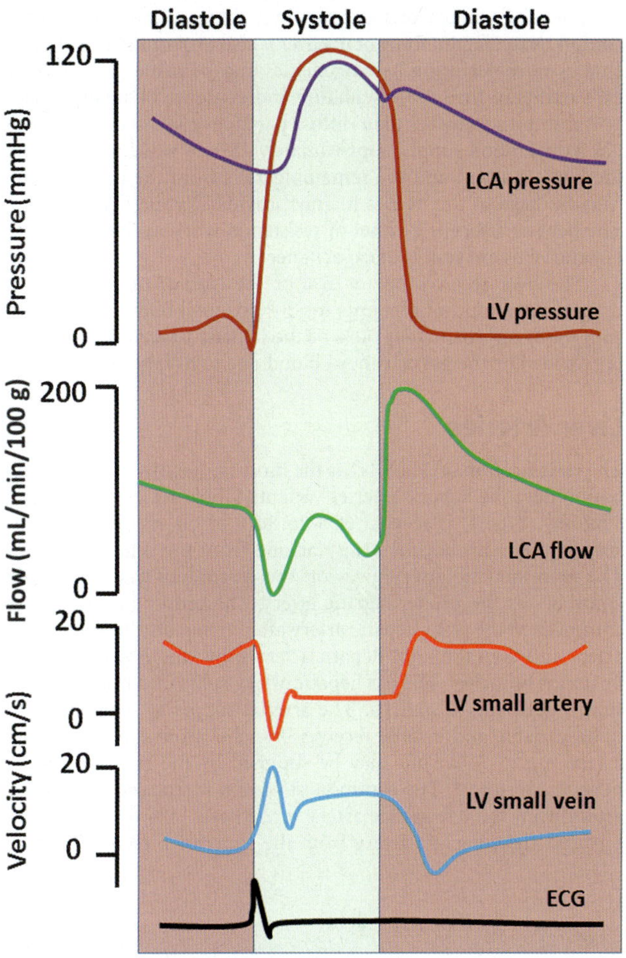

Figure 1-15. Wiggers diagram of a typical human heart. Pressure and flow in the left coronary artery (LCA) along with the left ventricular (LV) pressure are shown. The LCA flow is impeded during systolic phases due to contraction of the myocytes and the transmitted pressure from LV. The pressure in the LCA is maintained into diastole, when most arterial flow occurs, and depends primarily on the systemic afterload rather than the LV pressure since the aortic valve is closed. Also shown are typical examples of the blood flow and velocity in epicardial small arteries just before their entrance into myocardium and small veins just after their exit from myocardium. Note the phase difference between arterial inflow and venous outflow. A reverse flow is frequently recognized in artery in early systole possibly due to abrupt increase in intramyocardial pressure and fiber deformation. A flow reversal is also observed in the vein in early diastole, which may be related to diastolic myocardial suction. (From Kaufmann PA, Camici PG. Myocardial blood flow by PET: technical aspects and clinical applications. *J Nucl Med* 2005;46:75–88; Lee J, Smith NP. The multi-scale modelling of coronary blood flow. *Ann Biomed Eng* 2012;40(11):2399–2413.)

Liver Vasculature and Microcirculation

There are two major indications for studying perfusion in the liver. The most common indication is study of perfusion in tumoral processes followed by analysis of perfusion alterations in diffuse parenchymal diseases. Perfusion study of the liver abnormalities can be very challenging. Liver perfusion can be examined by ultrasound, CT, or MRI. Each imaging technique has its limitations and specific mathematical models for perfusion analysis. Common problems in perfusion assessment of the liver include dual blood supply, parasitic and aberrant vascular supply, arteriovenous shunting, and respiratory motions. The liver is a large organ, and its complete perfusion assessment can be difficult.[79] One important question that may be raised in perfusion imaging of the liver is whether the detected perfusion abnormality is real or simply a pseudolesion due to vascular territorial variants in tissue perfusion. It is therefore crucial to learn about liver vascular anatomy, anatomical variants, microcirculation, and physiology.

Macrovasculature and Anatomical Variants

The study of hepatic vasculature is important in several clinical situations, in particular, before or after liver surgeries such as liver transplantation and segmentectomy procedures and in chemotherapy treatment of primary or secondary liver tumors. Knowledge of the complex vascular anatomy of the liver is also important in perfusion studies since perfusion heterogeneities may be related to anatomical variants in the liver vasculature and existence of small arterioportal shuntings rather than diffuse parenchymal disease. The liver has a dual blood supply, approximately 25% of which comes from the hepatic artery and the remaining 75% from the portal vein.[79] The drainage of the liver is mainly provided by the hepatic veins. The hepatic artery is a vessel of resistance, whereas the portal and hepatic veins are vessels of capacitance.

The liver receives up to 25% of the cardiac output, and its oxygen consumption accounts for 20% of total body oxygen consumption. Approximately 50% of the hepatic oxygen requirement is provided by the portal venous blood due to its high flow rate.

Liver Arteries

The classification of Michels[80] is the most frequently employed system to describe hepatic arteries variants (Table 1.1). Conventional anatomy (type I) is seen in 60% to 80% of CT studies and consists of the main hepatic artery arising from the celiac trunk.[81–84] The main hepatic artery gives off the gastroduodenal artery and continues as the proper hepatic artery. The proper hepatic artery continues as the right hepatic artery after giving off the left hepatic artery and then the right hepatic artery splits into its anterior and posterior branches. The left hepatic artery splits into branches that supply segments II and III. The arterial supply to segment IV is quite variable and usually receives branches from the left hepatic artery (up to 75%) but may be supplied by the right or proper hepatic arteries.[85,86] The commonest variant is replaced left hepatic artery from the left gastric artery in 2.5% to 14% of cases and a replaced right hepatic artery from the superior mesenteric artery that is seen in 8% to 9% of cases.[81–83] Nonclassified variants such as direct origin of the right or proper hepatic arteries from the aorta are rare but may be seen (Fig. 1.16). From a surgical point of view, replaced arteries must be always preserved in reconstructive surgeries. In contrast, accessory arteries do not necessarily need to be reconstructed if adequate flow is established after the anastomosis of the major branches.[87]

TABLE 1.1 **Michaels Classification of Hepatic Arterial Anomalies**

Classification	Pattern	Percentage
I	Normal anatomy	61–79
II	Repl. LHA from LGA	2.5–14
III	Repl. RHA from SMA	8.0–9.0
IV	Repl. LHA from LGA and repl. RHA from SMA	1.0–2.0
V	Acc. LHA from LGA	5.0–11
VI	Acc. RHA from SMA	1.5–4.0
VII	Acc. LHA from LGA and acc. RHA from SMA	1.0–2.0
VIII	Acc. LHA from LGA and RHA from SMA	0.2–3.0
IX	CHA from SMA	2.0–3.0
X	CHA from LGA	0
NC	Variable	2.0–12.5

LHA, left hepatic artery; LGA, left gastric artery; RHA, right hepatic artery; SMA, superior mesenteric artery; CHA, common hepatic artery; Repl., replaced; Acc., accessory; LHA, left hepatic artery; LGA, left gastric artery; RHA, right hepatic artery.

Portal Veins

The portal vein is a valveless afferent vessel that drains the blood from the capillary system of the intestine, spleen, pancreas, omentum, and gallbladder. Variations in the portal vein branching and configuration are common.[88–90] The conventional pattern is for the main portal vein to divide into the left and right portal branches.[90] The right portal vein is formed by the anterior and posterior branches. Conventional pattern is present in 64% to 80% of the patients. Venous anomalies in the form of early connection of the right posterior branch or trifurcation of the portal vein can make surgery difficult, as more vascular anastomosis is then required with the recipient portal vein. Trifurcation of the main portal vein into the left portal, right anterior, and right posterior branches is seen in 9% to 11% of the cases (Fig. 1.17). Split living related liver transplantation of segments V to VIII can be challenging when portal trifurcation exists. In 10% to 23% of the patients, the main portal vein is formed by the right posterior portal vein as the first branch, which then connects to a common trunk of the left and right anterior portal veins. The later variant may have important surgical implications. For example, if the left portal vein is resected at the bifurcation, the right anterior portal vein may be sacrificed resulting in devascularization of segments IV, V, and VIII. Therefore, the resection has to be distal to the origin of the right anterior portal vein. In case of liver transplant, if a portal vein branch is too short for anastomosis to the recipient portal vein, an interposition graft of greater saphenous vein may be required. Another common variant is the absence of right posterior branch but the immediate bifurcation in two branches for segments VI and VII. A further variation is the origin of the segment V branch from the right posterior portal vein or directly from the right portal vein. It is shown by CT scan that portal vein variants are associated with a significantly higher number of biliary hilar variations. Conventional biliary branching pattern with a right posterior biliary duct joining the right anterior branch is seen in 74% of cases in patients without portal variant and in only 32% of cases with portal vein variation.[91]

Hepatic Veins

Preoperative mapping of the hepatic venous system is also important prior to liver transplantation surgery, as the transection plane is determined by the anatomic distribution of the hepatic veins.[92] Analysis of patency of all hepatic veins is helpful before interpretation of perfusion imaging since absence or thrombosis may affect the results. The hepatic venous system usually consists of three major hepatic veins. Veins of the caudate lobe are directly connected to the inferior vena cava (IVC). Of particular clinical concern is the site of drainage of the middle hepatic vein. The middle and left hepatic veins form a common trunk in 65% to 85% and are separate in 15% to 35% of cases.[93] The draining veins of segment IV can be highly variable. If the patency of the segment IV vein in a left lobe graft is not preserved, venous congestion will occur, leading to atrophy of this segment. In a recent study by Scatton et al.,[94] drainage of segment IV into the middle hepatic vein occurred in 39% and into the left hepatic vein in 61% of individuals. In 50% of cases with drainage of the segment IV into the left hepatic vein, an accessory umbilical (scissural) vein was seen in the umbilical fissure draining

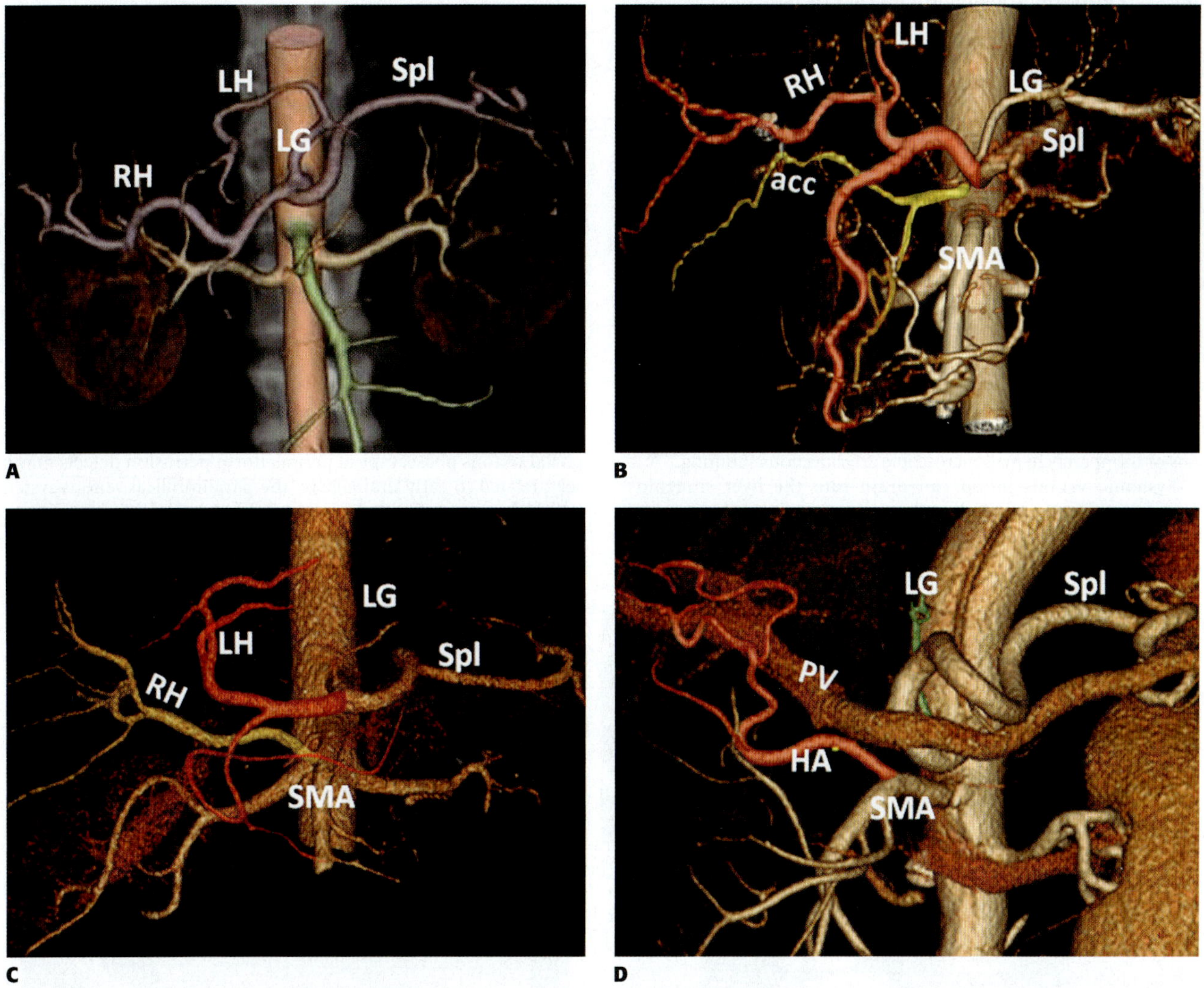

Figure 1-16. **Anatomical variants of the hepatic arteries. A:** Left hepatic (LH) artery arising from the left gastric (LG) artery is seen in 10%. **B:** Accessory (acc) right hepatic artery arising directly from the aorta. Accessory right hepatic artery is seen in 8%, supplying the posterior right liver, and usually arises from the superior mesenteric artery (SMA) but rarely from the aorta. **C:** Replaced right hepatic artery from the SMA is seen in 3%. **D:** Replaced hepatic artery from the SMA is seen in 2.5% based on Parmar H, Sitoh YY, Hui F. Normal variants of the intracranial circulation demonstrated by MR angiography at 3T. *Eur J Radiol* 2005;56:220–228. Spl, splenic artery; PV, portal vein.

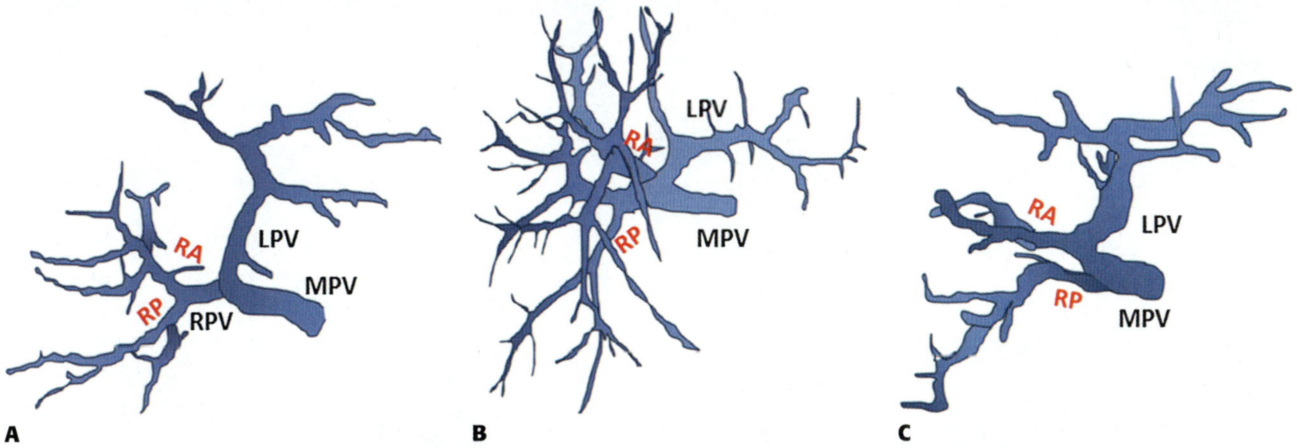

Figure 1-17. **Main types of portal vein division. A:** Conventional pattern (64% to 80%) is defined by bifurcation of the main portal vein (MPV) into the left portal vein (LPV) and the right portal vein (RPV) branches. The RPV is formed by the right anterior (RA) and the right posterior (RP) branches. **B:** Anterior view of the MPA with trifurcation that is formed directly by three branches, the LPV, RA, and RP. This form is seen in 10% of individuals. **C:** Anterior view of a portal system with the early origin of the RP branch from the MPV seen in 10% to 23% of the patients. (From Schmidt S, Demartines N, Soler L, et al. Portal vein normal anatomy and variants: implication for liver surgery and portal vein embolization. *Semin Intervent Radiol* 2008;25(2):86–91.)

a portion of segment IV. In 18% of cases, an accessory/replaced inferior right hepatic vein is seen draining segment VI of the liver into the IVC. Information on the location of accessory hepatic veins and their distance from the main hepatic veins is crucial before surgery as their inadvertent transection can cause bleeding and atrophy of the supplied segment of the liver.

Aberrant Blood Supply and Arterioportal Shunting

In perfusion study of the liver and especially during arterial phase, it is common to find areas of hyperenhancement in different locations and configurations in normal and abnormal liver tissue. These pseudolesions may be secondary to aberrant venous drainage into systemic veins or intraparenchymal microscopic arteriovenous shunting.[95,96]

Systemic venous blood can drain into the liver sinusoids through small veins of the liver capsule, accessory cystic vein, or aberrant right gastric vein. Focal enhancing areas are seen on arterial phase images due to the early inflow of contrast material through these systemic veins compared with the inflow into the surrounding parenchyma provided by the portal system tributaries. Common locations are around the gallbladder and falciform ligament and in the subcapsular region.[12,30,31] Pseudolesions at the periphery of the left liver lobe (segments I, II, and IV) are secondary to aberrant right gastric venous drainage from the gastric antrum[97] (Fig. 1.18). Nodular subcapsular enhancing foci similar to small angioma or hepatocellular carcinoma (HCC) are common normal or cirrhotic liver[98] and mainly are due to small capsular venous inflow. These hyperattenuation foci should not be mistaken with hyperemia of liver parenchyma surrounding cholangitic biliary ducts, abscesses, cellulitis, and metastatic foci.[99] Hepatic arterial supply derived from the cystic artery branches can produce a peripheral rim of hyperattenuation around the gallbladder fossa in arterial liver imaging. At portal venous phase, typical perifalciform perfusion defects may be seen related to early drainage by the paraumbilical venous system, which also connect with the internal thoracic and inferior epigastric veins through veins of Sappey. These veins become more apparent

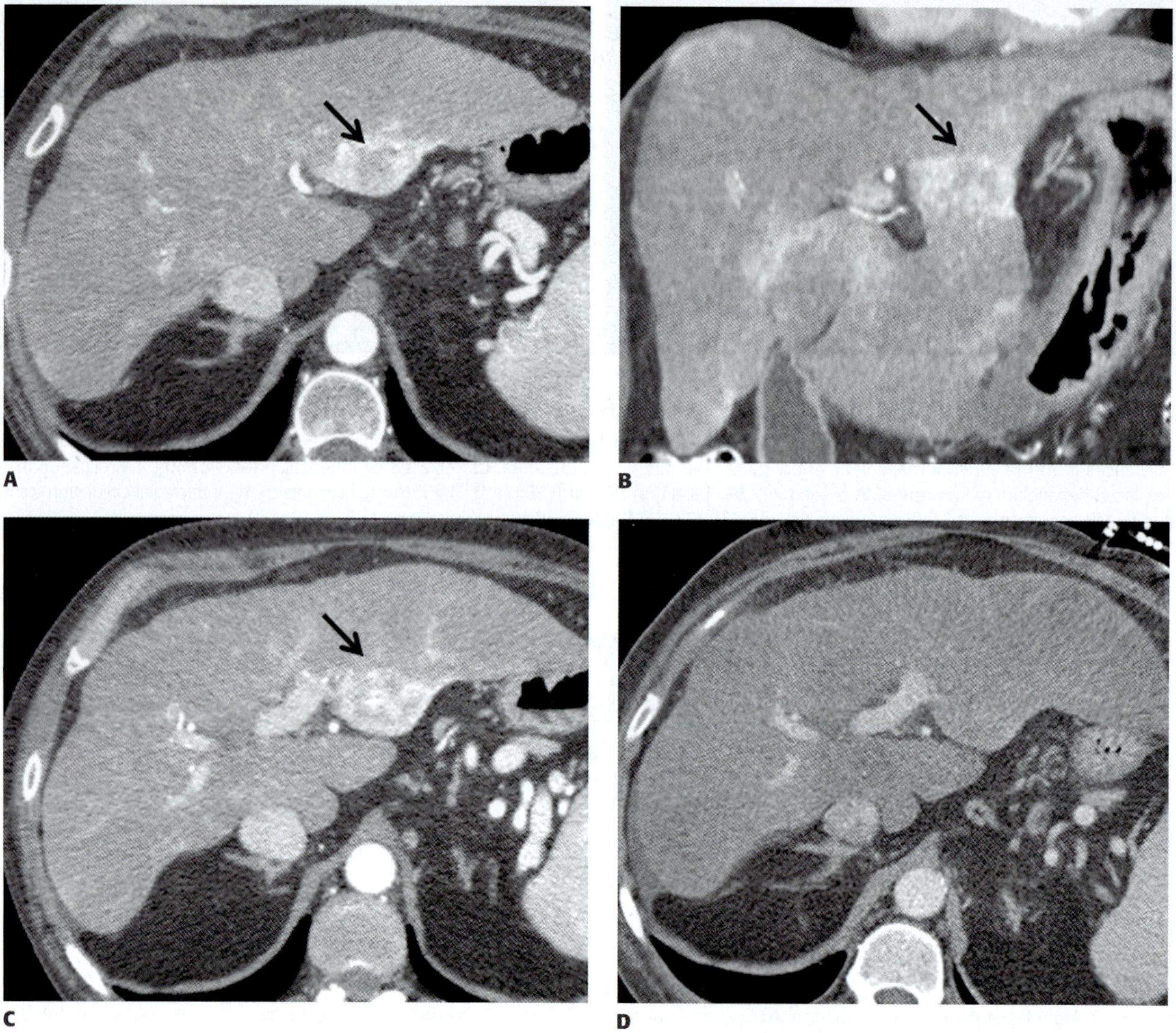

Figure 1-18. Axial and coronal (**A and B**) early arterial phase and axial late arterial phase (**C**) images in a 52-year-old female with cirrhosis show transient hepatic enhancement (*arrows*) in posterior margin of segment 3 that disappears in axial portal phase image (**D**). This perfusion disorder probably corresponds to the third hepatic inflow tracts (aberrant gastric venous drainage or parabiliary venous system).

in the setting of portal hypertension or superior vena cava obstruction.[99] Parabiliary venous plexus drainage also causes small defects in the portal venous perfusion of the perihilar liver and frequently seen at the dorsal aspect of segment IV and around the gallbladder fossa.

Another reason of benign focal enhancing areas in the liver is transsinusoidal or peribiliary plexus communications between microscopic interlobular arterioles and portal venules, resulting in redistribution of arterial flow into a focal region of portal venous flow. Cirrhosis is a known cause of transsinusoidal arterioportal shunting and is believed to be secondary to thrombosis of the small hepatic venules and retrograde hepatofugal flow filling of the small portal vein branches.[100] Similar shunting can occur after liver biopsy, postradiofrequency ablation, and in the presence of hypervascular tumors. These shunts may be significant when the portal vein is thrombosed or compressed. Image findings include transient, wedge-shaped peripheral parenchymal enhancement, and early visualization of the peripheral portal vein branches. Early-phase portal vein opacification is more common in macroscopic arterioportal fistulas and transtumoral shunts, whereas transient parenchymal enhancement occurs in cases of transsinusoidal shunts.

Pseudolesions are sometimes seen on nonenhanced CT scans as focal spared areas in a fatty liver or as areas of focal fatty infiltration. In the setting of arterioportal shunting, the hepatocytes in that region are subject to less portal and more arterial blood and therefore being protected from fatty changes compared to the rest of the liver.

Intrahepatic Circulation

Approximately 80% of the blood entering the liver is poorly oxygenated venous blood supplied by the portal vein, whereas the remainder is well oxygenated and supplied by the hepatic artery.

Intrahepatic branches of the portal vein and hepatic artery run in parallel. In the liver, there is no hepatic capillary network. Instead, terminal branches of the afferent vasculature (portal venules and hepatic arterioles) supply blood to the fenestrated sinusoids contained within hepatic lobules (Fig. 1.19). The hepatic sinusoids represent the segment of the microcirculation in which supply of nutrients and removal of metabolic products takes place. Sinusoids are lined by unique endothelial cells fenestrated by clusters of pores known as "sieve plates." The diameter of sinusoids increases in the pericentral area. Sinusoids lining cells are separated from hepatocytes by the interstitial space of Disse.[101] Sinusoid is also composed of nonparenchymal cells, such as hepatic stellate cells and Kupffer cells, which are involved in the regulation of blood flow through sinusoids. Both afferent vessels interconnect with each other through sinusoidal spaces (Fig. 1.4). Other forms of anastomosis between afferent vessels are transversal (arterioportal) and through the peribiliary plexus.[102] Branches of hepatic arterioles also supply blood to the liver capsule and the capillaries of the peribiliary plexus, which finally drains into the sinusoids. Hepatic arterioles also send branches to the portal venules causing direct arteriolo-portal anastomoses. Flowing blood in the sinusoids collects in the central venules, which in turn drain into hepatic veins.

The dual blood supply of the liver is a unique feature of the hepatic vasculature, and there is an intimate relationship between the two vascular systems, termed the "hepatic arterial buffer response" (HABR).[101] HABR describes the ability of the hepatic artery to produce compensatory flow changes in response to changes in portal venous flow. With this adenosine-mediated arterial autoregulation, hepatic arterial blood flow can increase diameter to buffer approximately 25% to 60% of the decreased portal flow. However, there is no reciprocity of the HABR, and the portal vein cannot control its blood flow. In other word, changes in hepatic arterial perfusion do not induce compensatory alteration of the portal flow.

Lymphatic vessels originate as blind-ending capillaries in the portal tracts. The lymph primarily comes from the hepatic sinusoids. Fluid filtered out of the sinusoids into the space of Disse flows through the lymphatic channels and then toward the hepatic hilum and eventually into the cisterna chyli. The liver produces a large amount of lymph, which is estimated to be 25% to 50% of lymph flowing through the thoracic duct.[103] Approximately 80% of the hepatic lymph drains into the portal lymphatic vessels, and the remainder drains through the sublobular and capsular lymphatic vessels. The area of the portal lymphatic vessels increases in liver fibrosis and cirrhosis and in idiopathic portal hypertension. Lymphatic vessels are abundant in the immediate vicinity of the HCC. Increasing lymphangiogenesis may be associated with increasing metastasis in HCC.[103]

Microvascular Functional Units

Several models of the organization of the liver into structural or functional units have been proposed. These include the classic lobule, the acinus, and the portal lobule (Fig. 1.20). Overall, the hepatic microcirculatory subunit is the "primary lobule," also known as "hepatic microvascular subunits (HMS)." It is a cone-shaped area consisting of the two terminal afferent vessels, the associated cholangioles and canaliculi, the network of sinusoids, and the efferent terminal hepatic venule.[101] This functional subunit is in line with the proposed zonal gradient in hepatocellular metabolic activity and the mount of tissue oxygenation.

The "classic lobule" comprising several cone-shaped primary lobules is a polygonal structure with ill-defined margin separated from adjacent lobules by variable amount of connective tissue. A hepatic venule is seen in the center of a classic lobule, and portal tracts are distributed along its periphery. The blood collected by each central venule is supplied by several portal venules. Additionally, intersinusoidal anastomoses occur between adjacent lobules. The hepatic "acinus" is formed by the port tract in the middle and the neighboring central hepatic venules in the periphery. Three zones exist within the acinus depending on the levels of oxygenation and metabolic function. The term "portal lobules" is defined as a unit with the portal tract in the center and the central veins around it.

Sinusoidal pressure is relatively low and will be maintained by sphincter-like structures at the entrance and exit zones of the sinusoids, in particular where the hepatic arteriolar system join the sinusoids. It is also documented that stellate cells and endothelial cells within the sinusoids can actively control the functions of the microvasculature by various endothelial mediators such as nitrous oxide (NO) as an endothelium-derived relaxing factor and endothelin (ET) as an endothelium-constricting factor. Along with Kupffer cells, the sinusoidal endothelium participates in host defense mechanisms and blood flow regulation and represents a major target for injury in the early phase of inflammation. Hepatic injury is caused by several mechanisms, including inflammation and microcirculatory dysfunction. Sinusoidal perfusion failure is a major factor in the pathogenesis of tissue injury, which is most pronounced in the periportal zone of the sinusoids. Loss of balance of vasomotor control due to injury results in contraction of sinusoidal endothelium, which reduces the diameters of the hepatic sinusoids, causing an increase in vascular resistance and a decrease in blood flow. The development of liver fibrosis and progression of fibrosis to cirrhosis is associated with vasomotor disturbances, increased intrahepatic resistance, and microarchitectural perfusion changes causing portal hypertension. Increased vascular resistance and diminished portal perfusion will be in part compensated by an increase in arterial perfusion, but later an overall fall in perfusion occurs. With imaging studies, information about hepatic hemodynamic changes in accordance with severity of liver fibrosis can be shown. In a recent study, liver microbubble contrast imaging with

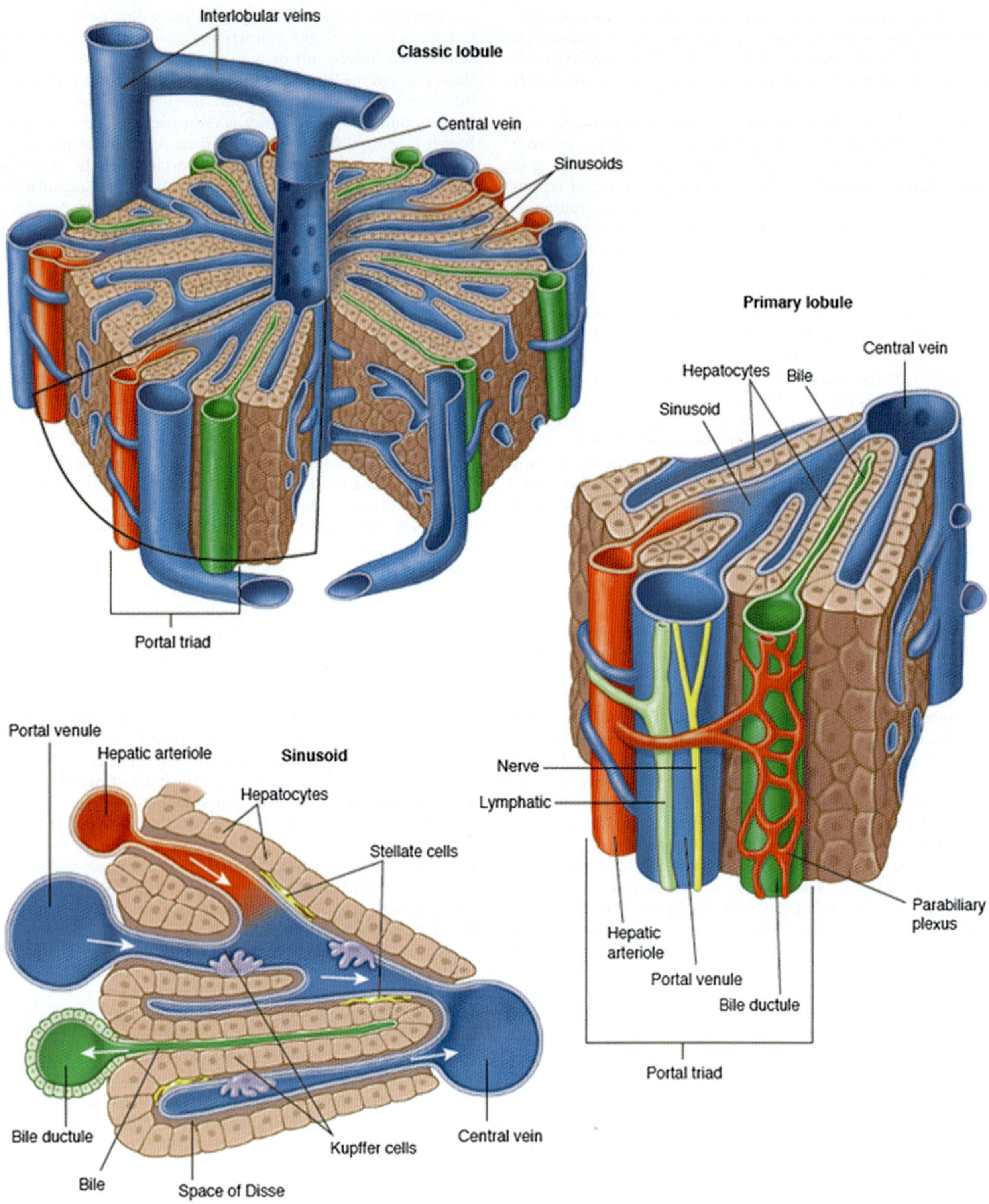

Figure 1-19. Liver microvascular anatomy and vascular communications around the portal triad. *Arrows* in sinusoids (S) indicate direction of flow. (From Breen DJ, Rutherford EE, Stedman B, et al. Intrahepatic arterioportal shunting and anomalous venous drainage: understanding the CT features in the liver. *Eur Radiol* 2004;14(12):2249–2260.)

ultrasound showed a decreased hepatic vein transit arrival time (<24 seconds) in cirrhosis, with a left shift in the time intensity curve due to the increased arterial supply and intrahepatic shunts.[104] Liver MR and CT perfusion imaging studies have confirmed a reduction in portal perfusion and an increase in arterial perfusion and the MTT of the liver in established cirrhosis.[105,106] TIPS placement is shown to improve the total hepatic perfusion significantly.[107] In addition to perfusion changes, inflammation-mediated

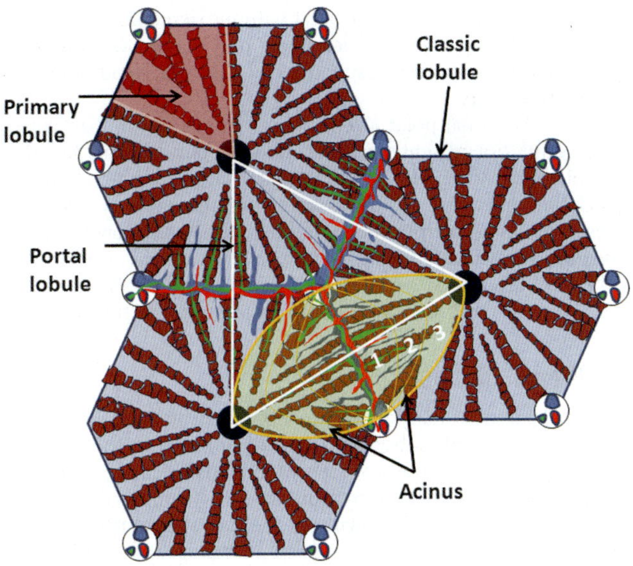

Figure 1-20. **Functional units of the liver.** The "primary lobule" represents a slice (*red region*) of the hexagonal "classic lobule" with the central hepatic vein at its apex and portal triad vessels at the outer margin. The "acinus" borders (*oval-shaped yellow line*) are formed by the penetrating vessels at the bases where inflow blood from the portal vein and hepatic artery enters sinusoids and ends in the central hepatic vein. Three zones (1, 2, and 3) of the acinus represent metabolic regions that are increasingly distant from the inflow vessels. The *white triangle* represents the "portal lobule."

adherence of leukocytes in outflow venules and sluggish blood flow due to increased viscosity may cause perfusion failure in sinusoids. Additional structural lesions have been described as important factors of sinusoidal narrowing, including fibrosis, sinusoidal collapse, defenestration of sinusoidal cells (capillarization), hepatocyte enlargement, and formation of a basement membrane in the space of Disse. These alterations in the sinusoids and extravascular Disse spaces increase the transit time and the distribution volume of small and large molecules (e.g., gadolinium contrast). Steatosis is the most common form of liver disease and mainly related to alcohol, obesity, diabetes, and metabolic syndrome. Hepatocellular injury in fatty liver disease and fibrosing steatohepatitis are secondary to a combination of impaired sinusoidal circulation narrowing and distortion of sinusoid lumens due to lipid accumulation in hepatocytes and collagen deposition in the space of Disse that will be exacerbated by a microvascular inflammatory response of leukocytes trapped in the sinusoids.[108]

Renal Vessels

Renal macrovasculature including arteries and vein varies in distribution and numbers (Fig. 1.21). These common anatomical variations are mainly related to embryonic development of the kidneys and systemic veins.[109,110] Around 5 weeks of development, the mesonephros is supplied by the various numbers of lateral branches of dorsal aorta, and the drainage occurs into the subcardinal veins. With embryonic development, some arteries disappear and the ones between the 10th thoracic and the 3rd lumbar segments (between the two mesenteric arteries) persist as gonadal, suprarenal glands, metanephros, and inferior diaphragmatic arteries. During superior migration of the metanephros or "future kidney" to the lumbar region, the kidneys

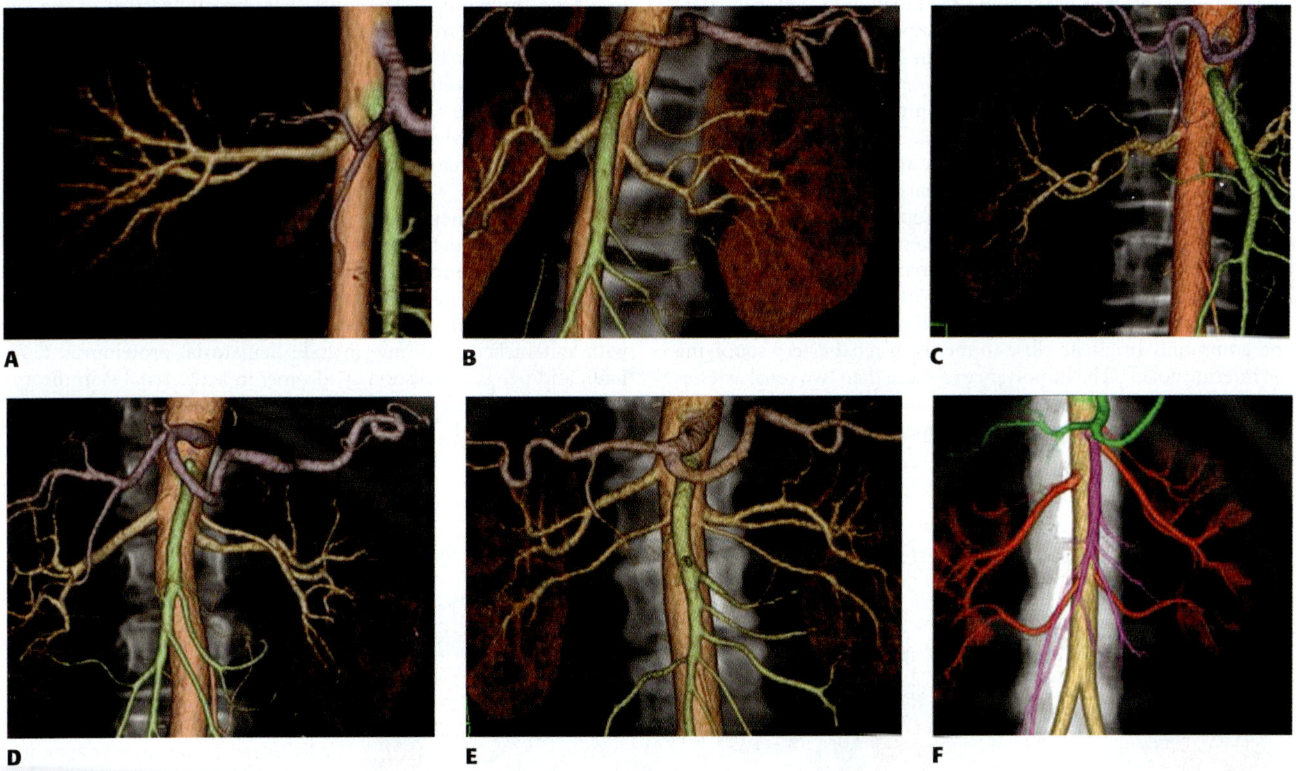

Figure 1-21. **Anatomical variation of renal arteries. A:** Classic pattern of the right kidney with two segmental branches. The anterior segment supplies apical, upper, middle, and lower segments while the posterior segment is mainly feeding the posterior segment. **B:** Accessory polar branch, arising above the left main renal, supplies the left apical segment. **C:** Polar artery arises from the main renal artery. **D:** Similar to (**B**), but the accessory branch supplies the inferior pole. **E:** Accessory branches on both sides to lower poles. **F:** Two branches for the right and three branches for the left kidney.

are supplied by various arteries. One of these arteries remains as the main renal artery while the rest either disappear or persist as accessory renal arteries. The development of the renal veins and their primitive origin are also complex. The mesonephros drains in the subcardinal veins that develop during the 5th week. The two subcardinal veins connect together in the middle and with the supracardinal veins as well, to form the future IVC. They also develop a venous network that connects with the posterior cardinal veins. Major portions of the posterior cardinal veins regress, and the supracardinal veins transform into the lower IVC and lumbar and azygos/hemiazygos venous systems. Persistence of some of these anastomotic channels explains many of the variants we can find.

Renal Arteries

Variations in number, source, and course of renal arteries are very common especially in malpositioned, malrotated, fused, or horseshoe kidneys[111–113] (Fig. 1.21). Renal arteries enter the kidney at three locations: (a) hilar artery enters at the hilum, (b) polar artery enters the kidney at the renal poles and may be an accessory or a branch of main renal artery, and (c) capsular artery may enter from the periphery of the kidney.[114]

The kidneys are usually supplied by single hilar arteries arising from the abdominal aorta below the origin of the mesenteric artery at the level of the L1 to L2 vertebral bodies. The main renal artery divides into the anterior and posterior presegmental and then into four or more segmental branches[109] (Fig. 1.22). There is no collateral arterial circulation between the segments, and each renal segment is supplied by its own segmental artery. The first segmental division is the posterior branch, which exits the main renal artery before it enters the renal hilum. The four anterior segmental divisions include the apical, upper, middle, and lower segmental branches. The segmental arteries branch into the lobar and interlobar arteries. The renal vascular anatomy is an important consideration for partial nephrectomy and renal transplant surgery.

Early branching of the renal arteries (<2 cm from the aorta or retrocaval on the right side) is a common anatomical variant, which is more common on the right side (20%) than on the left side (15%).[111,115] Expert surgeons require at least 1 cm of main renal artery in order to clamp and properly anastomose it.

In multiple renal arteries with a separate origin, the largest vessel is considered the "main" renal artery, and the rest are called accessory or supernumerary. Accessory renal arteries can be seen in 25% to 30% of individuals. In less than 5%, more than two arteries exist on same side. Accessory renal arteries are usually polar arteries and commonly originate close to the main renal artery supplying the inferior pole.[113] The importance of more than two renal arteries is mainly for renal transplant surgery and a contraindication for donation. If the third artery is a small superior polar artery less than 2 mm in diameter, it can be ligated without significant parenchymal loss.[112,115] The inferior polar artery may supply the collecting system, and its ligation can cause ureteral ischemia, stenosis, or urinary tract leakage.

Accessory renal polar arteries may arise from the iliac, superior and inferior mesenteric, celiac, middle colic, lumbar, gonadal, and middle sacral arteries.[109,114] Capsular arteries are generally small but can be large when serving as collaterals in renal artery stenosis. These arteries arise from the main renal artery but may originate from the segmental branches or the retroperitoneal arteries. The right renal arteries pass posterior to the IVC, but in 5%, the main and accessory right renal arteries can pass anterior to the IVC.[116]

Renal Veins

The renal parenchyma is drained consecutively by the stellate veins, the arcuate, and interlobar veins, and as opposed to the segmental arrangement of intrarenal arteries, there is extensive intrarenal anastomoses between venous tributaries. In turn, ligation of the venous branches is possible without the risk of parenchymal loss. The renal veins have a more uniform anatomical pattern and are single in 92% of individuals.[113] The renal vein is typically located anterior to the renal artery at the renal hilum. The right renal vein is less than 2.5 cm and does not receive extrarenal tributaries. The left renal vein is 8 cm in length and receives the left adrenal vein superiorly and the left gonadal vein inferiorly.[117] In 75% of cases, it may connect with the ascending lumbar and hemiazygos veins. Lumbar veins are much more common in the left side and may be the source of bleeding after left nephrectomy. These veins are also a major route of retroperitoneal splenorenal shunt development in portal hypertension. Supernumerary renal veins are the most common renal venous variant that can be seen in approximately 15% to 30% of individuals. The most characteristic variant of the left renal vein is the circumaortic renal vein (5% to 7% of patients), with one vein coursing anterior and the other posterior to the aorta. Retroaortic renal vein is a less common venous anomaly with a frequency of 3% to 5%.[117] Direct drainage of the right gonadal veins and retroperitoneal veins into the right renal vein is seen in 5% of individuals. The right adrenal vein drains into the right renal vein in 30% of cases.

Nutcracker phenomenon refers to morphologic compression of the left renal vein between the superior mesenteric artery and the aorta. This is a common finding that is seen in 27% of asymptomatic population. Dilated gonadal and lumbar veins are seen in 50% of cases.[118] Clinical and laboratory findings reported in association with nutcracker syndrome include hematuria, proteinuria, flank pain, and pelvic congestion syndrome. In acute renal vein thrombosis, renal perfusion can be disturbed involving both the cortex and renal pyramids.[119]

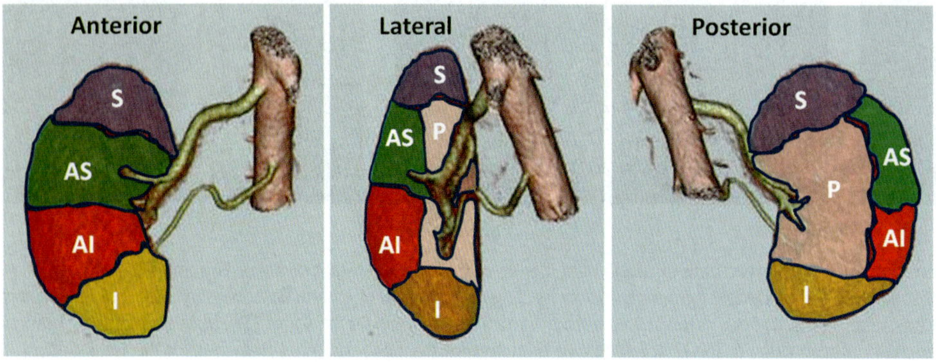

Figure 1-22. Segmental anatomy of the kidney. The size of each segment may vary depending on the blood supply. Posterior (p) segment may extend to the superior apex. It is supplied by the posterior segmental artery or a separate accessory artery. S, superior (apical); AS, anterosuperior (upper); AI, anteroinferior (middle); I, inferior (lower); P, posterior.

Renal Microvasculature

Like other organs, microvasculature in kidneys refers to vessels less than 150 to 200 μm in diameter including arterioles, capillary, and venules.[120–122] Afferent arterioles originate from interlobular arteries and lead to the glomerular capillaries, and the distal ends of the capillaries of each glomerulus join together to form the efferent arterioles, followed by a second capillary network constituted by the peritubular capillaries surrounding renal tubules (Fig. 1.23). A distinct feature of the renal circulation is the dual capillary bed in the glomerulus and around the tubules, which is a key component to efficient filtration, secretion, and reabsorption of minerals and removal of unwanted substances from the filtrate. The peritubular capillaries are followed by the venous system that runs in parallel to the arteriolar vessels and progressively forms the interlobular, arcuate, interlobar, and renal vein.

Using high-resolution microimaging system with synchrotron radiation, it is possible to demonstrate small vessels.[123] However, this technique does not have the required resolution for quantification of afferent and efferent arteriolar caliber unless contrast agents with better radiopacity are introduced and ultra-high-resolution x-ray camera systems are available.[124] The classical anatomical classification of renal arterial elements into interlobar, arcuate, and interlobular arteries is not a great model for microvascular study using microangiography system. Instead, classification of renal vessels according to Strahler order might be a more acceptable form of data collection. Afferent arterioles having lumen diameters ranging from approximately 10 to 14 μm are defined as Strahler orders 0 and 1, respectively. Vessels of Strahler orders 2 to 6 (approximately 20 to 55 μm) are considered interlobular arteries. The arcuate arteries (approximately 55 to 85 μm) are Strahler orders 6 to 7, interlobar vessels (approximately 140 to 190 μm) are considered Strahler orders 8 and 9, and feeding renal arteries (approximately 190 to 215 μm) are marked as Strahler orders 9 and 10.[123]

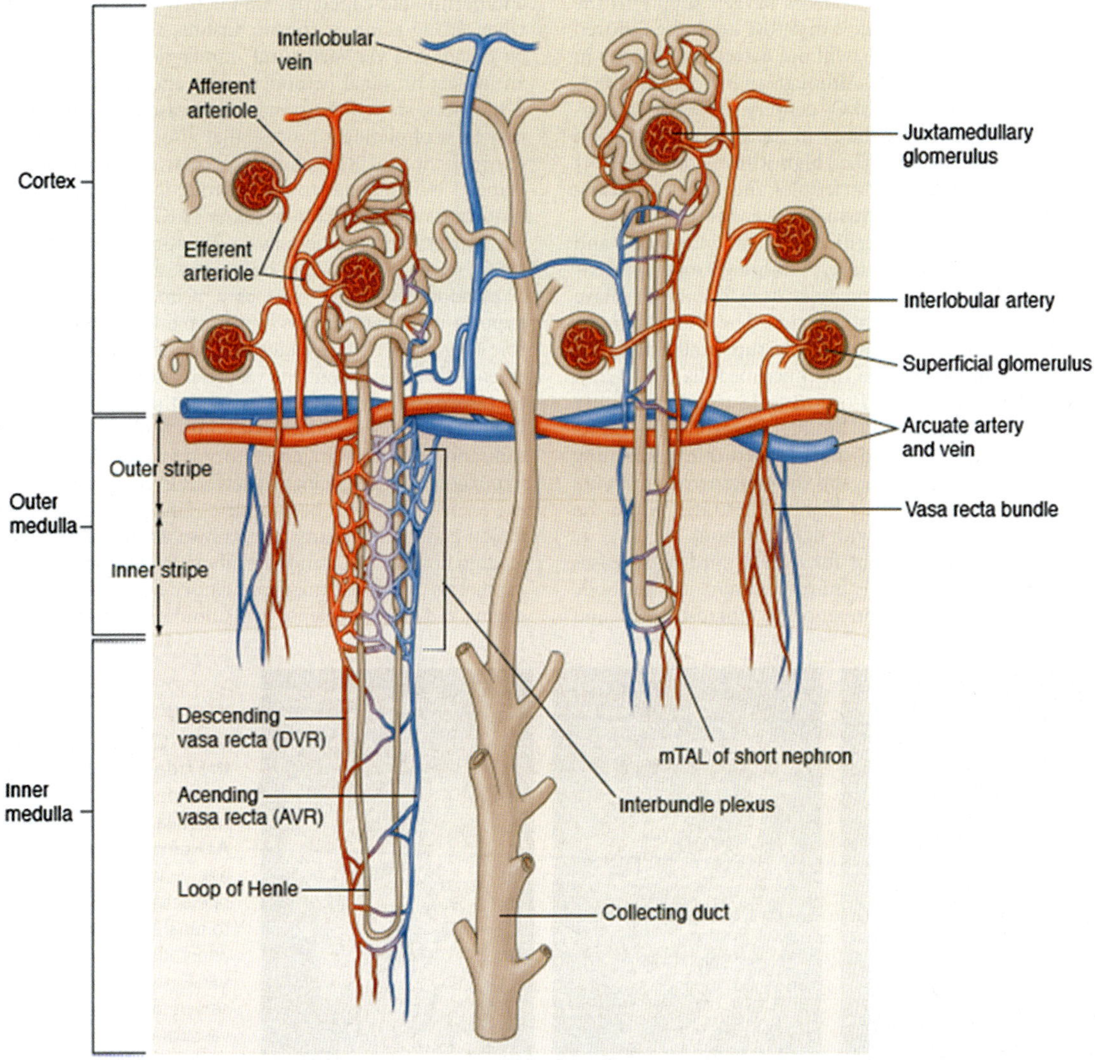

Figure 1-23. Microcirculation of the renal cortex and medulla. The interlobular arteries, arising from the arcuate artery, ascend toward the cortical surface. The majority of blood flow to the medulla arises from juxtamedullary efferent arterioles. In the outer medulla, juxtamedullary efferent arterioles give rise to descending vasa recta (DVR) that coalesce with ascending vasa recta (AVR) and, sometimes, thin descending limbs of Henle, to form vascular bundles. Vascular bundles are prominent in the inner stripe of the outer medulla. Peripheral DVRs form the interbundle capillary plexus that supplies the nephrons, and central DVRs perfuse the inner medulla. In the inner medulla, vascular bundles disappear and vasa recta become dispersed. (From Pallone TL, Edwards A, Mattson DL. Renal medullary circulation. *Compr Physiol* 2012;2:97–140.)

The kidneys are relatively small organs and accounts for 0.5% of total body weight. In contrast, renal blood flow (RBF) is high and involves 1 L/min, which is 20% to 22% of the cardiac output.[120] This high blood flow is necessary for the kidneys to maintain their function in order to meet the metabolic requirements. Renal perfusion is very heterogeneous ranging from 7 mL/min/g tissue in the cortex to approximately 3 mL/min/g tissue at the corticomedullary junction, 2 mL/min/g in the outer medulla, and 0.5 mL/min/g tissue in the inner medulla. In spite of high blood flow, the kidneys are very sensitive to hypoxia, especially the medulla. This is because of unique microvasculature architecture of the kidney. The oxygen tensions in the kidney are varies from 70 mm Hg in the cortex to 20 mm Hg in the medulla.[122] The reason for this remarkable discrepancy between blood supply and oxygenation is the regionally specialized renal microvasculature. The cortex receives a large amount of blood for the filtration function, but 80% of renal oxygen consumption is used to drive Na-K-ATPase to reabsorb most of the NaCl filtered into the proximal tubule. This in combination with arteriovenous shuntings between the descending vasa recta (DVR) and ascending vasa recta (AVR) further compromises oxygen supply to the medulla. It is shown by Leong et al.[125] that RBF could be reduced or increased by approximately 30%, without detectable changes in tissue PO_2 in the cortex or medulla. Although an increase in RBF is accompanied by an increase in renal O_2 delivery, the renal O_2 consumption remains stable. This stability in renal O_2 consumption despite an increase in O_2 delivery (i.e., high RBF) is due to direct shunting between the precapillary arterioles and venules causing dynamic regulation of renal parenchymal oxygenation.[125]

Renal medullary circulation is critical in maintaining water and fluid balance as well as blood pressure.[126] Although only approximately 10% of total RBF enters the medulla, its deficiency may have a significant impact on normal renal function. The DVR, originating from the juxtamedullary efferent arteriole, supply all blood flow to the renal medulla and extends to the inner medulla (Fig. 1.23). The diameter of the DVRs ranges from 12 to 18 μm. In the inner stripe of the outer medulla, vascular bundles formed by the DVRs move in parallel with the AVR and short-looped thin descending limbs of Henle. The AVR are larger and more numerous than are the DVR, and their endothelium is highly fenestrated while the DVR's endothelium is continuous with tight junctions.[127]

Vascular nephropathies account for over a third of all cases of end-stage renal disease and are more common in metabolic syndrome, diabetes, and in the presence of atherosclerosis and hypertension.[122] Renal artery stenosis may progressively induce renal tissue injury, ischemic nephropathy, and end-stage renal disease by promoting microvascular endothelial dysfunction, damage, and loss.[128] In chronic renal disease (CKD), there are extensive vascular intimal and medial calcifications, leading to an increased vascular stiffening, loss of compliance, and increased peripheral resistance. Microvascular disease is also a prominent causal factor of tubulointerstitial and glomerular fibrosis in CKD. Renal microvessel damage and their eventual loss have important roles in the progression of renal injury. This microvessel regression process, also known as microvascular rarefaction, results from endothelial dysfunction (functional rarefaction) and direct vascular loss (structural rarefaction) (Fig. 1.24). It is proven that renal microvascular "rarefaction" is a key pathologic event in most renal diseases.[129] Imbalance between the angiogenic factors (such as VEGF and angiopoietins) and the endogenous angiogenic inhibitors (such as thrombospondin-1, angiostatin, and endostatin) negatively influence the capillary formation as compared to the capillary regression, resulting in capillary rarefaction[129] (Fig. 1.25). Smaller arterioles and peritubular capillaries are the first to suffer a vascular dropout when facing acute or chronic insults, and the loss of microvascular circulation via "structural" rarefaction has been shown to have an impact on renal hemodynamics and function.[124] Furthermore, it has been shown that renal microvascular structural rarefaction may be a physiologic process that also plays an important role in the reduction of RBF and glomerular filtration rate with normal aging.[130] Ischemia due to severe reductions in RBF is the most common cause of acute kidney injury (AKI) after cardiac surgery and renal artery reconstructions, contrast-agent nephropathy, cardiac arrest, sepsis, and shock in both native and transplanted organs.[122]

Endothelial injury acts as a primary event leading to renal hypoxia with disturbances in nitric oxide pathways playing a major role (Fig. 1.25). With endothelial injury, there is the impairment of endothelium-dependent vasorelaxation and increased reactivity to vasoconstrictive agents (i.e., endothelin-1) causing hypoperfusion. Furthermore, endothelial injury leads to leukocyte accumulation and secondary inflammatory response that exacerbates renal hypoxia at a microcirculatory level.[122] Even after reperfusion in AKI, the recovery may not be complete. This process of ischemia–reperfusion endothelial injury, also known as "no-reflow" phenomenon, leads to flow cessation and thrombosis of peritubular and glomerular capillaries, increased microcirculatory permeability, and interstitial edema.[122] There is evidence that stimulation of vascular proliferation

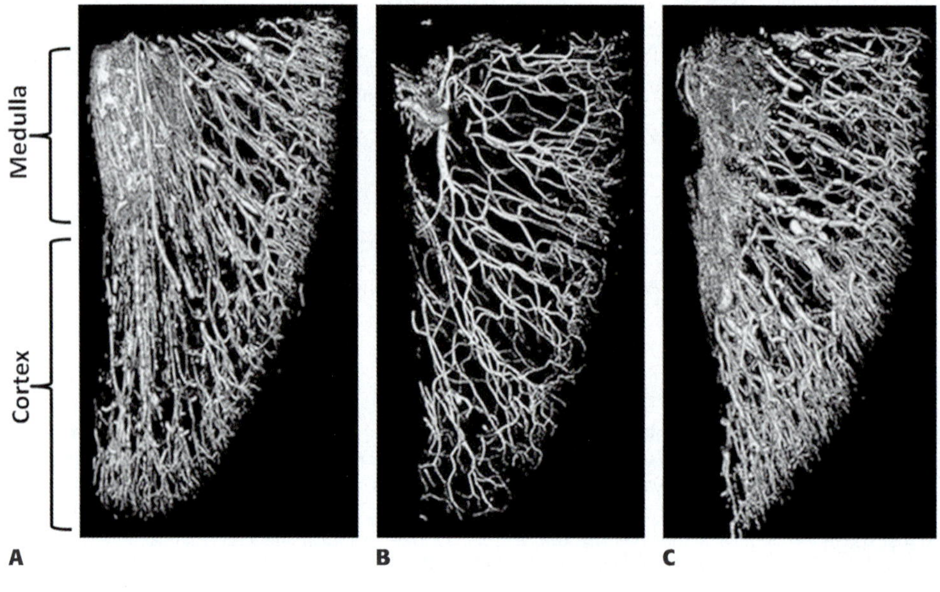

Figure 1-24. Representative 3D-micro-CT angiography images of the kidney demonstrating microvascular density of the renal cortex and medulla in three different conditions. **A:** Normal kidney. **B:** Kidney after renal artery stenosis showing microvascular rarefaction and increased vascular due to renal scarrings. **C:** Kidney with renal artery stenosis treated with intrarenal VEGF. Intrarenal VEGF distinctly preserved cortical and medullary microvascular density of those microvessels under 80 μm, partly by promoting MV proliferation. (From Iliescu R, Fernandez SR, Kelsen S, et al. Role of renal microcirculation in experimental renovascular disease. *Nephrol Dial Transplant* 2010;25(4):1079–1087, with permission.)

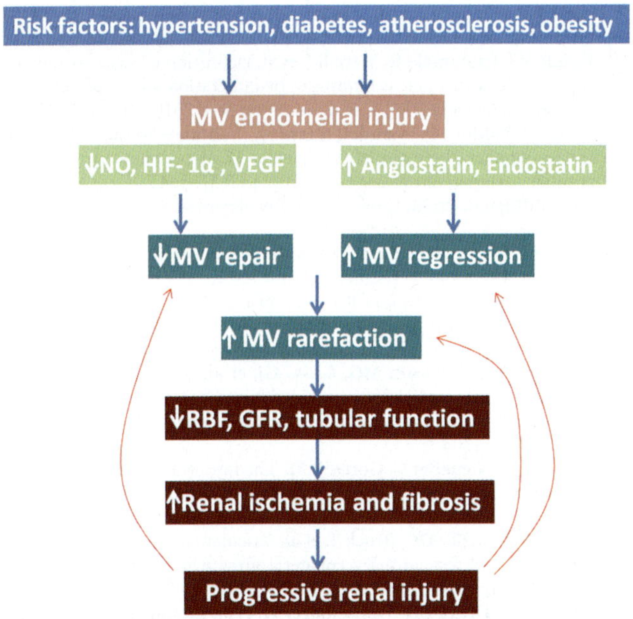

Figure 1-25. **Potential mechanisms of renal microvascular (MV) rarefaction and consequences on renal function and structure.** Sustained MV endothelial injury can lead to an imbalance between factors involved in MV repair, proliferation, and regression, leading to a progressive MV rarefaction that can deteriorate renal hemodynamics, function, and tissue damage. Progression of the renal damage may further stimulate MV damage and loss (*reverse arrows*) resulting in a vicious circle. NO, nitric oxide; VEGF, vascular endothelial growth factor; HIF-1α, hypoxia-induced factor-1α. (From Chade AR. Renal vascular structure and rarefaction. *Compr Physiol* 2013;3(2):817–831.)

and repair may stabilize renal function and slow the progression of renal disease.[120] Targeted interventions to enhance endogenous renoprotective mechanisms focused on the microcirculation, such as cell-based therapy or the use of angiogenic cytokines, have shown promising results in some experimental and clinical settings.

Acknowledgment

We would like to thank Arvin Saremi, BS, and Shahriar Shahriarian, MD, for their assistance in reconstructing the anatomic images of this chapter.

REFERENCES

1. **Chade AR.** Renal vascular structure and rarefaction. *Compr Physiol* 2013;3(2):817–831.
2. **Iwasaki H, Fukushima K, Kawamoto A, et al.** Synchrotron radiation coronary microangiography for morphometric and physiological evaluation of myocardial neovascularization induced by endothelial progenitor cell transplantation. *Arterioscler Thromb Vasc Biol* 2007;27:1326–1333.
3. **Kobayashi S, Hori M, Dono K, et al.** In vivo real-time microangiography of the liver in mice using synchrotron radiation. *J Hepatol* 2004;40:405–408.
4. **Myojin K, Taguchi A, Umetani K, et al.** Visualization of intracerebral arteries by synchrotron radiation microangiography. *AJNR Am J Neuroradiol.* 2007;28(5):953–957.
5. **Figueiredo G, Brockmann C, Boll H, et al.** Comparison of digital subtraction angiography, micro-computed tomography angiography and magnetic resonance angiography in the assessment of the cerebrovascular system in live mice. *Clin Neuroradiol* 2012;22(1):21–28.
6. **Schambach SJ, Bag S, Steil V, et al.** Ultrafast high-resolution in vivo volume-CTA of mice cerebral vessels. *Stroke* 2009;40(4):1444–1450.
7. **Katz DA, Marks MP, Napel SA, et al.** Circle of Willis: evaluation with spiral CT angiography, MR angiography, and conventional angiography. *Radiology* 1995;195:445–449.
8. **Harnsberger H, Osborn A, Ross J, et al.** Diagnostic and surgical imaging anatomy: brain, head and neck, spine. Salt Lake City, USA: Amirsys; 2006. ISBN-13: 978-1931884297.
9. **Parmar H, Sitoh YY, Hui F.** Normal variants of the intracranial circulation demonstrated by MR angiography at 3T. *Eur J Radiol* 2005;56:220–228.
10. **Dimmick SJ, Faulder KC.** Normal variants of the cerebral circulation at multidetector CT angiography. *Radiographics* 2009;29(4):1027–1043.
11. **Perlmutter D, Rhoton AL Jr.** Microsurgical anatomy of the anterior cerebral–anterior communicating–recurrent artery complex. *J Neurosurg* 1976;45:259–272.
12. **Caldemeyer KS, Carrico JB, Mathews VP.** The radiology and embryology of anomalous arteries of the head and neck. *AJR Am J Roentgenol* 1998;170:197–203.
13. **Rhoton AL Jr, Saeki N, Perlmutter D, et al.** Microsurgical anatomy of common aneurysm sites. *Clin Neurosurg* 1979;26:248–306.
14. **Smit EJ, Vonken EJ, van Seeters T, et al.** Timing-invariant imaging of collateral vessels in acute ischemic stroke. *Stroke* 2013;44(8):2194–2199. doi: 10.1161/STROKEAHA.
15. **Christoforidis GA, Mohammad Y, Kehagias D, et al.** Angiographic assessment of pial collaterals as a prognostic indicator following intra-arterial thrombolysis for acute ischemic stroke. *AJNR Am J Neuroradiol* 2005;26:1789–1797.
16. **Kim JJ, Fischbein NJ, Lu Y, et al.** Regional angiographic grading system for collateral flow: correlation with cerebral infarction in patients with middle cerebral artery occlusion. *Stroke* 2004;35:1340–1344.
17. **Kobayashi K, Matsui O, Suzuki M, et al.** Anatomical study of the confluence of the sinuses with contrast-enhanced magnetic resonance venography. *Neuroradiology* 2006;48:307–311.
18. **Braun JP, Tournade A.** Venous drainage in the craniocervical region. *Neuroradiology* 1977;13(3):155–158.
19. **Hudetz AG.** Blood flow in the cerebral capillary network: a review emphasizing observations with intravital microscopy. *Microcirculation* 1997;4(2):233–252.
20. **Hudetz AG, Fehér G, Knuese DE, et al.** Erythrocyte flow heterogeneity in the cerebrocortical capillary network. *Adv Exp Med Biol* 1994;345:633–642.
21. **Ivanov KP, Kalinina MK, Levkovich YI.** Blood flow velocity in capillaries of brain and muscles and its physiological significance. *Microvasc Res* 1981;22:143–155.
22. **Cipolla MJ.** The cerebral circulation. San Rafael, CA: Morgan & Claypool Life Sciences; 2009. Chapter 5, Control of Cerebral Blood Flow. Available from: http://www.ncbi.nlm.nih.gov/books/NBK53082/
23. **Wintermark M, Fischbein NJ, Smith WS, et al.** Accuracy of dynamic perfusion CT with deconvolution in detecting acute hemispheric stroke. *AJNR Am J Neuroradiol* 2005;26:104–112.
24. **Siebert E, Diekmann S, Masuhr F et al.** Measurement of cerebral circulation times using dynamic whole-brain CT-angiography: feasibility and initial experience. *Neurol Sci* 2012;33(4):741–747. doi: 10.1007/s10072-011-0785-z.
25. **Phillips SJ, Whisnant JP.** Hypertension and the brain. *Arch Intern Med* 1992;152:938–945.
26. **Paulson OB, Strandgaard S, Edvinsson L.** Cerebral autoregulation. *Cerebrovasc Brain Metab Rev* 1990;2:161–192.
27. **Yamamoto S, Watanabe M, Uematsu T, et al.** Correlation of angiographic circulation time and cerebrovascular reserve by acetazolamide-challenged single photon emission CT. *AJNR Am J Neuroradiol* 2004;25:242–247.
28. **Johansson BB, Auer LM, Sayama I.** Reaction of pial arterioles and veins to hypercapnia in hypertensive and normotensive rats. *Stroke* 1985;16:320–323.
29. **Olsen AK, Keiding S, Munk OL.** Effect of hypercapnia on cerebral blood flow and blood volume in pigs studied by positron emission tomography. *Comp Med* 2006;56(5):416–420.
30. **Ito H, Kanno I, Fukuda H.** Human cerebral circulation: positron emission tomography studies. *Ann Nucl Med* 2005;19(2):65–74.

31. **Euser AG, Cipolla MJ.** Cerebral blood flow autoregulation and edema formation during pregnancy in anesthetized rats. *Hypertension* 2007;49: 334–340.
32. **Skinhøj E, Strandgaard S.** Pathogenesis of hypertensive encephalopathy. *Lancet* 1973;1:461–462.
33. **Dohmen C, Bosche B, Graf R, et al.** Identification and clinical impact of impaired cerebrovascular autoregulation in patients with malignant middle cerebral artery infarction. *Stroke* 2007;38:56–61.
34. **Reinhard M, Rutsch S, Lambeck J, et al.** Dynamic cerebral autoregulation associates with infarct size and outcome after ischemic stroke. *Acta Neurol Scand* 2012;125(3):156–162.
35. **Wintermark M, Flanders AE, Velthuis B, et al.** Perfusion-CT assessment of infarct core and penumbra: receiver operating characteristic curve analysis in 130 patients suspected of acute hemispheric stroke. *Stroke* 2006;37:979–985.
36. **Townsley MI.** Structure and composition of pulmonary arteries, capillaries, and veins. *Compr Physiol* 2012;2(1):675–709.
37. **Murillo H, Cutalo MJ, Jones RP, et al.** Pulmonary circulation imaging: embryology and normal anatomy. *Semin Ultrasound CT MR* 2012;33(6): 473–484.
38. **Van Der Spuy JC.** The surgical anatomy of the pulmonary vessels. *Thorax* 1953;8(3):189–194.
39. **Hasegawa I, Kobayashi K, Kohda E, et al.** Bronchopulmonary arterial anastomosis at the precapillary level in human lung. Visualization using CT angiography compared with microangiography of autopsied lung. *Acta Radiol* 1999;40(6):578–584.
40. **Matsumoto K, Yamasaki N, Tsuchiya T, et al.** Three-dimensional computed tomography for a mediastinal basal pulmonary artery. *Ann Thorac Surg* 2012;94(5):e115–e116.
41. **Subotich D, Mandarich D, Milisavljevich M, et al.** Variations of pulmonary vessels: some practical implications for lung resections. *Clin Anat* 2009;22:698–705.
42. **Ivanov KP.** Circulation in the lungs and microcirculation in the alveoli. *Respir Physiol Neurobiol* 2013;187(1):26–30.
43. **Cauldwell EW, Siekert RG, Lininger RE, et al.** The bronchial arteries: an anatomic study of 105 human cadavers. *Surg Gynecol Obstet* 1948;86:395–412.
44. **Yoon W, Kim JK, Kim YH, et al.** Bronchial and nonbronchial systemic artery embolization for life-threatening hemoptysis: a comprehensive review. *Radiographics* 2002;22(6):1395–1409.
45. **Mark-Paul FM, Peeters V, Gittenberger-de Groot AC, et al.** Differences in development of coronary arteries and veins. *Cardiovasc Res* 1997;36: 101–110.
46. **Schlessinger MJ.** Significant variations in the anatomic pattern of coronary vessels. *Blood Heart Circ* 1940;13:93–97.
47. **Vasko JS, Gutelius J, Sabiston DC Jr.** A study of predominance of human coronary arteries determined by arteriographic and perfusion technics. *Am J Cardiol* 1961;8:379–384.
48. **Abuchaim DC, Spera CA, Faraco DL, et al.** Coronary dominance patterns in the human heart investigated by corrosion casting. *Rev Bras Cir Cardiovasc* 2009;24(4):514–518.
49. **Ortale JR, Keiralla LC, Sacilotto L.** The posterior ventricular branches of the coronary arteries in the human heart. *Arq Bras Cardiol* 2004;82(5):468–472; 463–467.
50. **Adams J, Treasure T.** Variable anatomy of the right coronary artery supply to the left ventricle. *Thorax* 1985;40:618–620.
51. **Goldberg A, Southern DA, Galbraith PD, et al.** Alberta Provincial Project for Outcome Assessment in Coronary Heart Disease (APPROACH) Investigators. *Am Heart J* 2007;154(6):1116–1122.
52. **Gupta T, Saini A, Sahni D.** Terminal branching pattern of the right coronary artery in left-dominant hearts: a cadaveric study. *Cardiovasc Pathol* 2013;22(3):179–182.
53. **Cerqueira MD, Weissman NJ, Dilsizian V, et al.** Standardized myocardial segmentation and nomenclature for tomographic imaging of the heart. A Statement for Healthcare Professionals from the Cardiac Imaging Committee of the Council on Clinical Cardiology of the American Heart Association. *Circulation* 2002;105:539–542.
54. **Donato P, Coelho P, Santos C, et al.** Correspondence between left ventricular 17 myocardial segments and coronary anatomy obtained by multi-detector computed tomography: an ex vivo contribution. *Surg Radiol Anat* 2012;34(9):805–810.
55. **Ortiz-Pérez JT, Rodríguez J, Meyers SN, et al.** Correspondence between the 17-segment model and coronary arterial anatomy using contrast-enhanced cardiac magnetic resonance imaging. *JACC Cardiovasc Imaging* 2008;1(3):282–293.
56. **Javadi MS, Lautamäki R, Merrill J, et al.** Definition of vascular territories on myocardial perfusion images by integration with true coronary anatomy: a hybrid PET/CT analysis. *J Nucl Med* 2010;51(2):198–203.
57. **Pereztol-Valdés O, Candell-Riera J, Santana-Boado C, et al.** Correspondence between left ventricular 17 myocardial segments and coronary arteries. *Eur Heart J* 2005;26(24):2637–2643.
58. **von Lüdinghausen M.** Clinical anatomy of cardiac veins. Vv. cardiacae. *Surg Radiol Anat* 1987;9:159–168.
59. **Saremi F, Muresian H, Sánchez-Quintana D.** Coronary veins: comprehensive CT-anatomic classification and review of variants and clinical implications. *Radiographics* 2012;32(1):E1–E32.
60. **Levin DC.** Pathways and functional significance of the coronary collateral circulation. *Circulation* 1974;50:831–837.
61. **Warltier DC, Zyvoloski MG, Gross GJ, et al.** Subendocardial versus transmural myocardial infarction: relationship to the collateral circulation in canine and porcine hearts. *Can J Physiol Pharmacol* 1982; 60(12):1700–1706.
62. **Schaper W, Nienaber C, Gottwik M.** The importance of the collateral circulation for myocardial survival. *Acta Med Scand Suppl* 1981;651: 29–35.
63. **Toyota E, Warltier DC, Brock T, et al.** Vascular endothelial growth factor is required for coronary collateral growth in the rat. *Circulation* 2005;112(14):2108–2113.
64. **Zeiher AM, Drexler H, Wollschlager H, et al.** Endothelial dysfunction of the coronary microvasculature is associated with coronary blood flow regulation in patients with early atherosclerosis. *Circulation* 1991;84: 1984–1992.
65. **Camici PG, Crea F.** Coronary microvascular dysfunction. *N Engl J Med* 2007;356:830–840.
66. **Cecchi F, Olivotto I, Gistri R, et al.** Coronary microvascular dysfunction and prognosis in hypertrophic cardiomyopathy. *N Engl J Med* 2003;349:1027–1035.
67. **Chilian WM.** Coronary microcirculation in health and disease: summary of an NHLBI workshop. *Circulation* 1997;95:522–528.
68. **Duncker DJ, Bache RJ.** Regulation of coronary blood flow during exercise. *Physiol Rev* 2008;88:1009–1086.
69. **Rajappan K, Rimoldi OE, Dutka DP, et al.** Mechanisms of coronary microcirculatory dysfunction in patients with aortic stenosis and angiographically normal coronary arteries. *Circulation* 2002;105:470–476.
70. **Bassenge E, Heusch G.** Endothelial and neuro-humoral control of coronary blood flow in health and disease. *Rev Physiol Biochem Pharmacol* 1990;116:77–165.
71. **Kaufmann PA, Camici PG.** Myocardial blood flow by PET: technical aspects and clinical applications. *J Nucl Med* 2005;46:75–88.
72. **Lee J, Smith NP.**The multi-scale modelling of coronary blood flow. *Ann Biomed Eng* 2012;40(11):2399–2413.
73. **Kajiya M, Hiramatsu O, Yada T, et al.** Physiomic approach to biomechanics of coronary microcirculation. *J Mech Med Biol* 2005;5:1–9.
74. **Austin RE Jr, Smedira NG, Squiers TM, et al.** Influence of cardiac contraction and coronary vasomotor tone on regional myocardial blood flow. *Am J Physiol* 1994;266:H2542–H2553.
75. **Toyota E, Fujimoto K, Ogasawara Y, et al.** Dynamic changes in three-dimensional architecture and vascular volume of transmural coronary microvasculature between diastolic- and systolic-arrested rat hearts. *Circulation* 2002;105(5):621–626.
76. **Fokkema DS, VanTeeffelen JW, Dekker S, et al.** Diastolic time fraction as a determinant of subendocardial perfusion. *Am J Physiol Heart Circ Physiol* 2005;288(5):H2450–H2456.
77. **Radjenovic A, Biglands JD, Larghat A, et al.** Estimates of systolic and diastolic myocardial blood flow by dynamic contrast-enhanced MRI. *Magn Reson Med* 2010;64(6):1696–1703.
78. **DeFily DV, Chilian WM.** Coronary microcirculation: autoregulation and metabolic control. *Basic Res Cardiol* 1995;90:112–118.
79. **Ronot M, Lambert S, Daire JL, et al.** Can we justify not doing liver perfusion imaging in 2013? *Diagn Interv Imaging* 2013;94(12): 1323–1336.
80. **Michels NA.** Newer anatomy of the liver and its variant blood supply and collateral circulation. *Am J Surg* 1966;112:337–347.
81. **De Cecco CN, Ferrari R, Rengo M, et al.** Anatomic variations of the hepatic arteries in 250 patients studied with 64-row CT angiography. *Eur Radiol* 2009;19(11):2765–2770.

82. **Covey AM, Brody LA, Maluccio MA, et al.** Variant hepatic arterial anatomy revisited: digital subtraction angiography performed in 600 patients. *Radiology* 2002;224:542–547.
83. **Koops A, Wojciechowski B, Broering DC, et al.** Anatomic variations of the hepatic arteries in 604 selective celiac and superior mesenteric angiographies. *Surg Radiol Anat* 2004;26:239–244.
84. **Winston CB, Lee NA, Jarnagin WR, et al.** CT angiography for delineation of celiac and superior mesenteric artery variants in patients undergoing hepatobiliary and pancreatic surgery. *AJR Am J Roentgenol* 2007;188:W13–W19.
85. **Onishi H, Kawarada Y, Das BC, et al.** Surgical anatomy of the medial segment (S4) of the liver with special reference to bile ducts and vessels. *Hepatogastroenterology* 2000;47(31):143–150.
86. **Sahani D, D'souza R, Kadavigere R, et al.** Evaluation of living liver transplant donors: method for precise anatomic definition by using a dedicated contrast enhanced MR imaging protocol. *Radio Graphics* 2004;24:957–967.
87. **López-Andújar R, Moya A, Montalvá E, et al.** Lessons learned from anatomic variants of the hepatic artery in 1,081 transplanted livers. *Liver Transpl* 2007;13(10):1401–1404.
88. **Schmidt S, Demartines N, Soler L, et al.** Portal vein normal anatomy and variants: implication for liver surgery and portal vein embolization. *Semin Intervent Radiol* 2008;25(2):86–91.
89. **Koc Z, Oguzkurt L, Ulusan S.** Portal vein variations: clinical implications and frequencies in routine abdominal multidetector CT. *Diagn Interv Radiol* 2007;13(2):75–80.
90. **Atasoy C, Ozyurek E.** Prevalence and types of main and right portal vein branching variations on MDCT. *AJR Am J Roentgenol* 2006;187(3):676–681.
91. **Kitami M, Takase K, Murakami G, et al.** Types and frequencies of biliary tract variations associated with a major portal venous anomaly: analysis with multi-detector row CT cholangiography. *Radiology* 2006;238(1):156–166.
92. **Barbaro B, Soglia G, Alvaro G, et al.** Hepatic veins in presurgical planning of hepatic resection: what a radiologist should know. *Abdom Imaging.* 2013;38(3):442–460.
93. **Cheng YF, Huang TL, Chen CL, et al.** Variations of the middle and inferior right hepatic vein: application in hepatectomy. *J Clin Ultrasound* 1997;25(4):175–182.
94. **Scatton O, Plasse M, Dondero F, et al.** Impact of localized congestion related to venous deprivation after hepatectomy. *Surgery* 2008;143(4):483–489.
95. **Quiroga S, Sebastià C, Pallisa E, et al.** Improved diagnosis of hepatic perfusion disorders: value of hepatic arterial phase imaging during helical CT. *Radiographics* 2001;21(1):65–81.
96. **Kim TK, Choi BI, Han JK, et al.** Nontumorous arterioportal shunt mimicking hypervascular tumor in cirrhotic liver: two-phase spiral CT findings. *Radiology* 1998;208:597–603.
97. **Matsui O, Takahashi S, Kadoya M, et al.** Pseudolesion in segment IV of the liver at CT during arterial portography: correlation with aberrant gastric venous drainage. *Radiology* 1994;193:31–35.
98. **Matsui O, Kadoya M, Yoshikawa J, et al.** Aberrant gastric venous drainage in cirrhotic livers: imaging findings in focal areas of liver parenchyma. *Radiology* 1995;197(2):345–349.
99. **Breen DJ, Rutherford EE, Stedman B, et al.** Intrahepatic arterioportal shunting and anomalous venous drainage: understanding the CT features in the liver. *Eur Radiol* 2004;14(12):2249–2260.
100. **Brown JJ, Naylor MJ, Yagan N.** Imaging of hepatic cirrhosis. *Radiology* 1997;202:1–16.
101. **Vollmar B, Menger MD.** The hepatic microcirculation: mechanistic contributions and therapeutic targets in liver injury and repair. *Physiol Rev* 2009;89(4):1269–1339.
102. **McCuskey RS.** The hepatic microvascular system in health and its response to toxicants. *Anat Rec (Hoboken)* 2008;291(6):661–671.
103. **Ohtani S, Ohtani Y.** Lymph circulation in the liver. *Anat Rec* 2008;291:643–652.
104. **Blomley MJ, Lim AK, Harvey CJ, et al.** Liver microbubble transit time compared with histology and Child-Pugh score in diffuse liver disease: a cross sectional study. *Gut* 2003;52:1188–1193.
105. **Annet L, Materne R, Danse E, et al.** Hepatic flow parameters measured with MR imaging and Doppler US: correlations with degree of cirrhosis and portal hypertension. *Radiology* 2003;229(2):409–414.
106. **Van Beers BE, Leconte I, Materne R, et al.** Hepatic perfusion parameters in chronic liver disease: dynamic CT measurements correlated with disease severity. *AJR Am J Roentgenol* 2001;176(3):667–673.
107. **Weidekamm C, Cejna M, Kramer L, et al.** Effects of TIPS on liver perfusion measured by dynamic CT. *AJR Am J Roentgenol* 2005;184(2):505–510.
108. **Farrell GC, Teoh NC, McCuskey RS.** Hepatic microcirculation in fatty liver disease. *Anat Rec (Hoboken)* 2008;291(6):684–692.
109. **Arévalo Pérez J, Gragera Torres F, et al.** Angio CT assessment of anatomical variants in renal vasculature: its importance in the living donor. *Insights Imaging* 2013;4(2):199–211.
110. **Cuttino JT, Clark RL.** The normal vasculature of the genitourinary tract: embryology, anatomy, and hemodynamics. In: Hillman BJ ed. *Clinical urography*, vol 3. Philadelphia, PA: Saunders; 1990: 2076–2091.
111. **Raman SS, Pojchamarnwiputh S, Muangsomboon K, et al.** Surgically relevant normal and variant renal parenchymal and vascular anatomy in preoperative 16-MDCT evaluation of potential laparoscopic renal donors. *AJR Am J Roentgenol* 2007;188(1):105–114.
112. **Türkvatan A, Akinci S, Yildiz S, et al.** MDCT for preoperative evaluation of vascular anatomy in living renal donors. *Surg Radiol Anat* 2009;31(4):227–235.
113. **Pollak R, Prusak BF, Mozes MF.** Anatomic abnormalities of cadaver kidneys procured for purposes of transplantation. *Am Surg* 1986;52:233–235.
114. **Sebastià C, Peri L, Salvador R, et al.** Multidetector CT of living renal donors: lessons learned from surgeons. *Radiographics* 2010;30(7): 1875–1890.
115. **Kawamoto S, Montgomery RA, Lawler LP, et al.** Multidetector CT angiography for preoperative evaluation of living laparoscopic kidney donors. *AJR Am J Roentgenol* 2003;180(6):1633–1638.
116. **Yeh BM, Coakley FV, Meng MV, et al.** Precaval right renal arteries: prevalence and morphologic associations at spiral CT. *Radiology* 2004;230(2):429–433.
117. **Koc Z, Ulusan S, Oguzkurt L, et al.** Venous variants and anomalies on routine abdominal multi-detector row CT. *Eur J Radiol* 2007; 61(2):267–278.
118. **Grimm LJ, Engstrom BI, Nelson RC, et al.** Incidental detection of nutcracker phenomenon on multidetector CT in an asymptomatic population: prevalence and associated findings. *J Comput Assist Tomogr* 2013;37(3):415–418.
119. **Grzelak P, Kurnatowska I, Sapieha M, et al.** Disturbances of kidney graft perfusion as indicators of acute renal vein thrombosis in contrast-enhanced ultrasonography. *Transplant Proc* 2011;43(8): 3018–3020.
120. **Chade AR.** Renovascular disease, microcirculation, and the progression of renal injury: role of angiogenesis. *Am J Physiol Regul Integr Comp Physiol* 2011;300:R783–R790.
121. **Nordsletten DA, Blackett S, Bentley MD, et al.** Structural morphology of renal vasculature. *Am J Physiol Heart Circ Physiol* 2006; 291:H296–H309.
122. **Le Dorze M, Legrand M, Payen D, et al.** The role of the microcirculation in acute kidney injury. *Curr Opin Crit Care* 2009;15(6): 503–508.
123. **Eppel GA, Jacono DL, Shirai M, et al.** Contrast angiography of the rat renal microcirculation in vivo using synchrotron radiation. *Am J Physiol Renal Physiol* 2009;296:F1023–F1031.
124. **Tanaka T, Nangaku M.** Angiogenesis and hypoxia in the kidney. *Nat Rev Nephrol* 2013;9(4):211–222.
125. **Leong CL, Anderson PW, O'Connor PM, et al.** Evidence that renal arteriovenous shunting contributes to dynamic regulation of renal oxygenation. *Am J Physiol Renal Physiol* 2007;292:1726–1733.
126. **Pallone TL, Turner MR, Edwards A, et al.** Countercurrent exchange in the renal medulla. *Am J Physiol Regul Integr Comp Physiol* 2003;284:R1153–R1175.
127. **Pallone TL, Edwards A, Mattson DL.** Renal medullary circulation. *Compr Physiol* 2012;2:97–140.
128. **Thang OH, Serné EH, Grooteman MP, et al.** Premature aging of the microcirculation in patients with advanced chronic kidney disease. *Nephron Extra* 2012;2(1):283–292.
129. **Ilicscu R, Fernandez SR, Kelsen S, et al.** Role of renal microcirculation in experimental renovascular disease. *Nephrol Dial Transplant* 2010;25(4):1079–1087.
130. **Futrakul N, Futrakul P.** Renal microvascular disease in an aging population: a reversible process? *Ren Fail* 2008;30(4):353–356.

CHAPTER

2 CT Perfusion Imaging Principles

Farhood Saremi, MD and Erin Angel, PhD

Introduction

In 1980, Leon Axel[1] introduced a method for assessing regional cerebral blood flow (CBF) using dynamic contrast–enhanced CT data. He applied the principles of indicator dilution analysis for nondiffusible indicators to the temporal changes of intravascular contrast concentration in order to measure blood volume, mean transit time (MTT) of the first passage of the bolus through the vessels, and the blood flow per unit of vascular volume. He described this method a few years after the first clinical introduction of CT for body imaging when clinical scanner's operation was very slow to obtain rapid sequence perfusion imaging and motion artifacts and high radiation dose were problematic.[2] Because of these limitations, most tissue perfusion imaging (TPI) studies in the 1980s were limited to a few research centers using electron beam CT scans, the only commercially available fast scanners, that could acquire a pair of adjacent, cross-sectional images in 50 milliseconds with spatial resolution of 1.5 mm.[3–5] The invention of multislice spiral scanners stimulated further interest and revolutionized perfusion imaging techniques.[6–8] More recently, 640-slice volume CT scanners and dual-source CT imagers, in conjunction with radiation dose reduction strategies, have expanded the clinical applications of perfusion CT from the assessment of brain ischemia to oncology perfusion and functional analysis of different organs.[9,10] Perfusion CT protocols are now readily incorporated into the existing CT workstations and postprocessing techniques for perfusion analysis and have been facilitated by the release of different commercial software packages.

In this chapter, a general overview of CT techniques is introduced and factors influencing TPI is discussed. Details of dose reduction strategies and tissue perfusion analysis models are presented in separate chapters.

State-of-the-Art Multidetector CT (MDCT) Scanners

With the introduction of spiral (helical) CT in the early 1990s, a fundamental evolutionary step was made toward the development of angiographic applications and modification of most dynamic contrast-enhanced CT imaging techniques.[11,12] One primary goal in dynamic CT imaging (including perfusion studies) of body organs is to obtain series of high-resolution images of a tissue volume over a short period of time. Although single-slice spiral CT scanners with 500-millisecond gantry rotation time were able to acquire images with temporal resolution of nearly 250 milliseconds, limitations exist to cover the entire volume of interest in a short period of time (i.e., a single breath-hold). Additionally, multiplanar reformations (MPRs) and three-dimensional (3D) reconstructions with the same spatial resolution of original axial images (isotropic resolution) were not technically feasible.[12,13] To surpass these limitations and in order to achieve the primary goals for high-quality dynamic CT imaging, several CT manufacturers introduced MDCT scanners around the beginning of the year 2000, which provided considerable improvement in scanning speed and multiplanar resolution.[14–16] These systems typically offered simultaneous acquisition of four sections at a gantry rotation time of 0.5 seconds. The increased performance of MDCT relative to older single-slice scanners allowed the optimization of a variety of clinical protocols especially in cardiac imaging.[16,17] Simultaneous acquisition of multiple slices and increasing body coverage in a short period of time just by recruiting more detectors were strong motivators for all CT manufactures to try to upgrade their scanners with larger detector span. Production of new detector designs and development of more efficient reconstruction algorithms including cone-beam reconstructions allowed the release of 16, 32, and 64 MDCTs by different manufacturers, which made possible the routine acquisition of substantial anatomic coverage in a short time and with submillimeter isotropic spatial resolution. With the addition of electrocardiographic (ECG)-gating capability and faster rotation times (i.e., 275 ms) and dedicated image reconstruction approaches, the temporal resolution for motion-free volume acquisitions of the heart became feasible.[18,19]

320-Detector Row/640-Slice Volume CT

Initially, vendors introduced scanners with greater and greater z-axis coverage in order to shorten scan time and minimize patient motion. In 2007, Toshiba released the first volume CT scanner, which substantially increased the detector coverage to 16 cm in the z-direction (Fig. 2.1). The main driving factor for this innovation was functional imaging (such as perfusion CT). With 16 cm of coverage, the Aquilion ONE Dynamic Volume CT (Toshiba Medical Systems, Otawara, Japan) can image an entire organ in a single rotation with a rotation time as fast as 0.275 seconds. With this capability, all

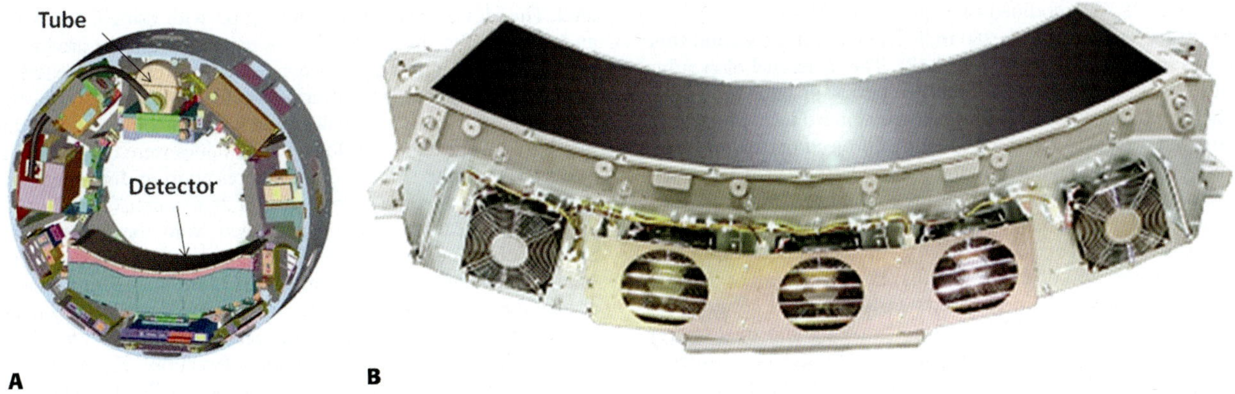

Figure 2-1. **A:** Tube–detector system configuration for volume scanner. **B:** A 16-cm detector panel. (Courtesy of Toshiba Medical System.)

iodinated contrast within a large organ (e.g., brain, heart) can be captured at the same instant in time; this is called isotemporal imaging. Isotemporal imaging is a key feature for accurate CT perfusion analysis in which contrast uptake and washout are imaged at multiple time points. As one could imagine, without isotemporal imaging, it is nearly impossible to separate the change in contrast due to the difference in acquisition time from the change in contrast due to physiologic processes. CT perfusion applications using volume CT are vast and range from neuro applications to tumor or whole-organ perfusion in the body.[20–27] With isotemporal resolution, the contrast in the vessels and the surrounding tissues of an organ can be visualized at multiple time points to create a "movie" of the contrast uptake and wash out. This dynamic information can then be used to assess timing of contrast arrival and effect on surrounding tissues. Compared to the helical shuttle technique (see below), volume CT perfusion scanning is lower dose because there is no excess exposure from helical overranging. Helical overranging is the exposure at the beginning and end of a helical run.[28] Some of the overranging is necessary for helical reconstruction and some of it is excess. The excess exposure is often mediated with adaptive collimation, but the remaining overranging is unavoidable for helical reconstruction.

Dual-Source MDCT

Although the idea of a multitube scanner was formed by Franke in 1979, clinical dual-source CT scanners were introduced years later in 2005 with the main goal of increasing temporal resolution to improve quality of cardiac imaging.[29] The first generation of dual-source CT was introduced with two x-ray tubes and two corresponding detectors mounted onto the rotating gantry with an angular offset of 90 degrees capable of acquiring 2 × 32 slice readings by an alternating (dual) z-flying focal spot technique in a gantry rotation speed of 330 milliseconds (Fig. 2.2A). In this gantry, the first tube–detector system covers 50-cm field of view (FOV) and the second tube–detector covers a smaller measurement field of 26 cm, both with a minimum reconstructable slice width of 0.6 mm. The second-generation

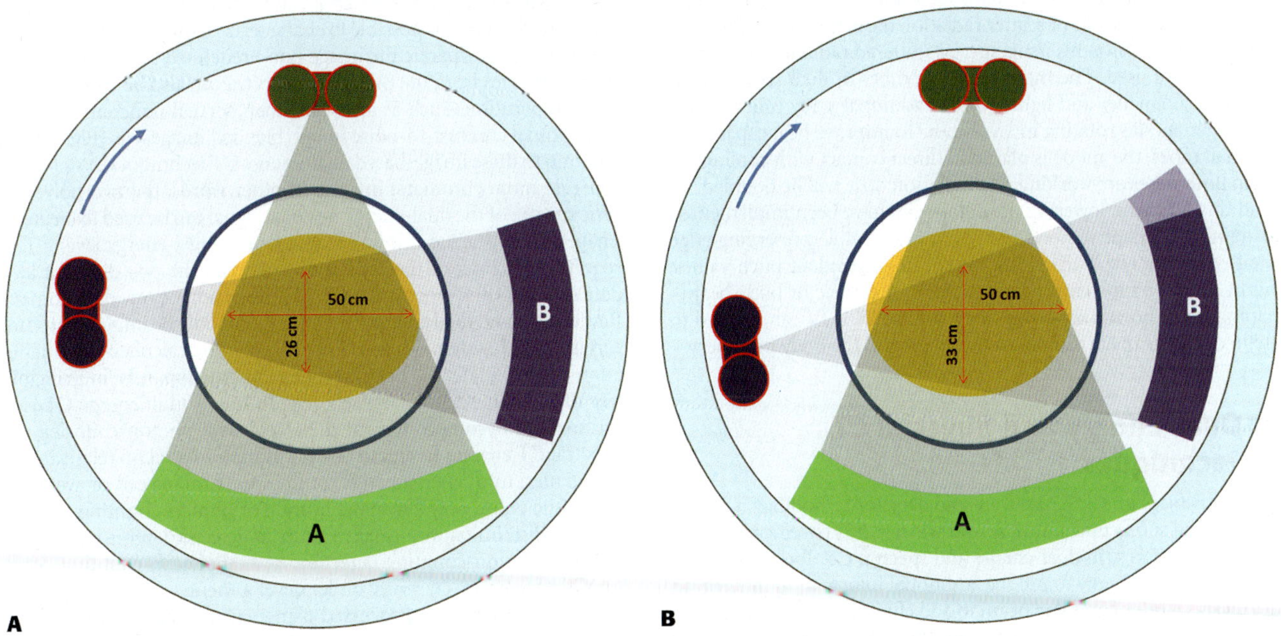

Figure 2-2. Dual-source CT system. **A:** First generation (Siemens SOMATOM Definition) with a 50-cm FOV for *detector A* and a smaller (26-cm) FOV for *detector B*, due to space limitations. **B:** Second generation (Siemens SOMATOM Definition Flash) increases the FOV for *detector B* to 33 cm by increasing the angle between the two tubes from 90 to 94 degrees.

dual-source CT was modified to acquire 2 × 128 slices, the gantry rotation time was reduced to 280 milliseconds, and the second tube FOV was increased to 33 cm (Fig. 2.2B). The main goal of creating this scanner was to improve the quality of cardiac imaging by increasing the temporal resolution.[30] This construction led to a reduction of the rotation needed to acquire the required projection data for image reconstruction from half of a rotation in single-source CT to a quarter of a rotation in dual-source CT using a monosegment reconstruction mode that is consistent throughout various heart rates owing to individual adaptation of the table pitch.[31] Another desirable approach in the new generation of the scanner has been widening of the scan field for the second tube/detector system to improve coverage for other applications, especially perfusion imaging and dual-energy scanning. This required decreasing gantry rotation speed in order to maintain the temporal resolution for cardiac scanning and a system angle of slightly larger than 90 degrees between the two tube–detector systems (Fig. 2.2B). With this new geometry, the two separate x-ray tube and detector array systems are arranged 94 degrees apart, which also allows helical data acquisition at a high pitch. In contrast to the single-source multidetector CT (MDCT), where the maximum pitch is roughly 1.5 in order to reconstruct gapless images, the second-generation dual-source CT can achieve gapless *z*-axis sampling even at a pitch value of up to 3.2.[32] Therefore, it enables coverage of the entire heart in a single heartbeat. However, slow and regular heart rates are required for this single-heartbeat acquisition, which uses prospectively triggered ECG gating. For heart rates greater than 55 or 60 beats per minute, multiphase acquisition is used, which requires pitch ranges from 0.2 to 0.5 (depending on the heart rate), and a retrospective ECG gating will be used for data acquisition.[33,34] Due to the high temporal resolution, the scanner has been commonly used for the assessment of coronary artery stenosis and is currently being assessed for myocardial perfusion.[35,36] Another application of dual-source CT is tissue characterization when both detector systems are operated at different kilovolts, so-called "dual-energy CT."[37] One limitation of this scanner particularly in perfusion studies has been small detector span to cover the entire anatomy of interest in one pass. This limitation has been partially solved using dynamic spiral scanning with variable pitch ("toggling table" technique).[38] One problem with the anatomic configuration of dual-source scanners is image degradation due to the presence of scatter radiation induction in the presence of two tubes. To solve this issue, special scattered radiation correction algorithms are used. The mounted x-ray tubes in dual-source scanners are also smaller and lighter than traditional x-ray tubes, which have larger anodes rotating in a vacuum. To improve heat capacity of the small tubes, the anode is placed in direct contact with cooling oil. When both tubes are working, the radiation dose will be doubled. To avoid this problem, lowering dose strategies have been implemented including, 3D adaptive noise reduction filter (while preserving edge detail), iterative reconstructions, heart rate–dependent pitch values, and ECG-based tube current modulation. A cardiac or body beam–shaping filter (bowtie or wedge filter) and small FOV can be used to attenuate or eliminate unnecessary radiation to the body periphery.

Dual-Energy and Spectral CT Techniques

Recent advances in MDT hardware and detector technology have not only enabled subsecond scanning and wider *z*-axis coverage but have also revived interest in dual-energy and spectral CT. Today investigators are examining how to use the additional information inherent in the full spectrum of an x-ray beam to add clinical value. Clinical work on the extraction of information from the full spectrum of an x-ray beam has opened new venues for the diagnostic capability of CT by combining x-ray beams acquired at different energy levels or separating of the x-ray beam into multiple energy windows at the detector level. The idea of dual-energy subtraction with using CT is not new and goes back to the 1970s.[39] Two separate scans were used in early investigations, but the results were not very promising due to technical limitations causing spatial misregistration, noisy images, and increased radiation exposure. In the 1980s, rapid kVp switching was introduced in which data at high- and low-voltage values were obtained during one scan.[29] A rapid surge in clinical application of dual-energy technique occurred after the introduction of dual-source CT in 2000s.[30]

The dual-energy concept originated from the fact that tissue attenuation values represented by CT numbers are dependent not only on the material and electron density of the attenuating object but also on the energy spectrum of the x-ray beam. At the energy levels of CT, the attenuation mechanism is generally caused by a combination of photoelectric and Compton photon interactions. The photoelectric effect predominates at lower photon energies and has higher probability of occurrence for elements with high atomic numbers (Z), whereas the Compton scattering almost independently depends on the electron density of the material. It should be mentioned that for most tissues in the body, there is a higher probability of Compton interactions than photoelectric interactions in CT. Since Compton interaction probability is fairly constant at CT energy levels, these interactions do not contribute to the dual-energy signal. Nevertheless, when the net effects of all photon interactions are combined, there is a clear energy dependence for the mass attenuation coefficient of high Z materials. Taking advantage of this energy dependence, the dual-energy technique is able to distinguish structures with large differences in atomic numbers.[40,41] For example, the iodine signal of a 140-kVp beam (with an effective energy of approximately 60 keV) is approximately twice as strong as a 80-kVp beam (with an effective energy of 40 keV), while the bone signal does not fall as quickly (Fig. 2.3). CT attenuation value of iodine with $Z = 53$ is much higher for a low-energy beam (i.e., 40 kVp) compared to a high-energy x-ray (140 kVp). This difference is less apparent for calcium with $Z = 20$. Therefore, in a low-kVp image, the contrast between iodine and calcium is much higher than a high-kVp CT image. Although traditional Hounsfield unit (HU) allows discrimination of many general categories (air, water, soft tissue, bone, etc.), there is considerable overlap in HU for many common anatomic materials. For example, HU values of a calcified structure ($Z = 20$) and a contrast-enhanced material can measure the same. With dual-energy technique, it is possible to characterize tissues by using different energy levels to separate the image into predefined basis material categories. Images from the two energy spectra can also be combined for other applications such as an iodine map, virtual noncontrast imaging, optimal contrast-to-noise image, blended image, etc. (Fig. 2.4). In addition to these image-based dual-energy CT techniques, systems can generate monochromatic images. In other words, the two polyenergetic spectra of the dual-energy raw data signal can be used to create an image that appears as if it was acquired at a single-energy level.[38] This requires matching of the projections between the two different kVp data sets and thus is performed in the projection or raw data domain. Raw data–based dual energy CT (DECT) can only be implemented for certain DECT system designs. Since this method calculates the attenuation of base materials prior to the reconstruction, it is, in principle, free of beam-hardening artifacts. The future of multienergy CT is in the spectral decomposition of the signal with photon-counting CT. Spectral CT enables tissues to be discriminated based on relative x-ray attenuation into "energy bands" of the spectrum instead of averaging across the entire polychromatic beam. For photon-counting systems, spectral discrimination usually occurs at detector level using energy-sensitive photon-counting detectors. Several photon-counting detector CT systems are currently under development.

DECT images are processed using various techniques that can be categorized as either raw data–based or image-based methods. For raw data–based methods, the dual-energy data processing is performed before images are reconstructed from high- and low-energy sinograms (projection domain). Projection data from the

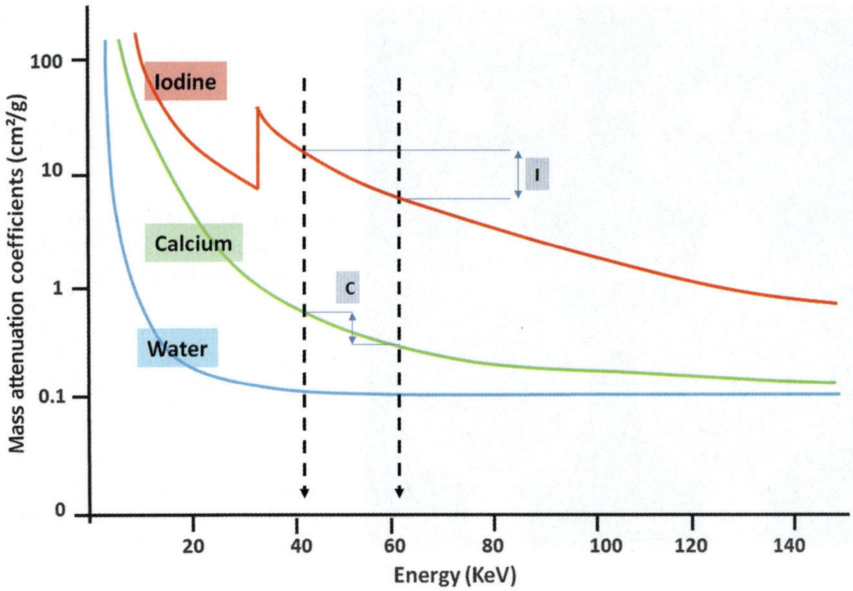

Figure 2-3. **Attenuation curves for iodine, calcium, and water plotted versus photon energy.** The *dotted lines* represent a typical effective energy for 80- and 140-kVp beams. The difference in attenuation between the effective energies of the spectra at two different energies of 40 and 60 keV (*vertical dashed lines*) shows that iodine (I) demonstrates a greater decrease in attenuation than calcium (C) in the specified kVp range, whereas the attenuation of water remains almost constant.

low- and high-energy spectra (e.g., 80 and 140 kVp) will be decomposed into two basis materials such as water and iodine to form the material density pair. Alternatively, DECT data can be decomposed into energy functions and can be used to generate monochromatic images through sophisticated reconstruction algorithms[42] (Fig. 2.5). For image-based methods, the dual-energy data processing is performed after the reconstruction of high- and low-energy images (image-based domain). DECT images are created through various mathematical combinations of the low-energy and high-energy images such as subtraction and blending. Monochromatic spectral image processing is not possible with image-based dual-energy methods, only with raw data–based methods. Currently, CT systems from most vendors are capable of dual-energy material decomposition. Some of these systems are also capable of raw data–based

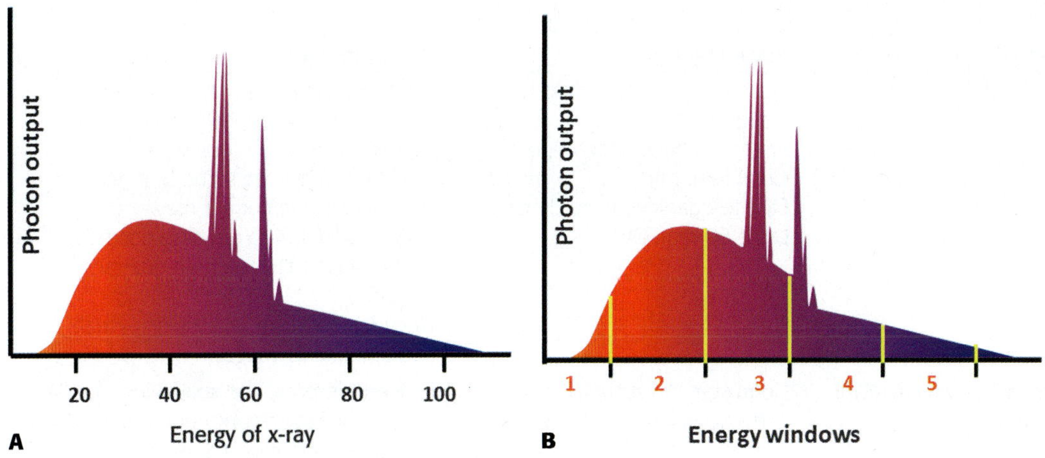

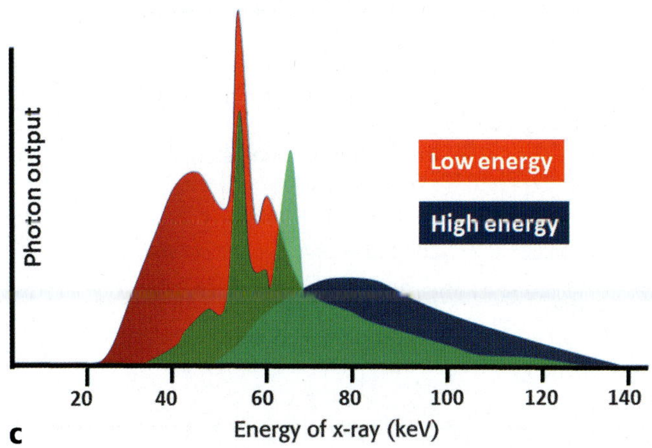

Figure 2-4. **A:** Polychromatic x-ray energy spectrum. **B:** Dual-energy separation of high (140 kVp) and low energy (80 kVp). **C:** Photon-counting detectors image the spectrum of x-ray radiation in "energy bands" in order to form images based on the analysis of the spectral signature of tissues. Overlap between both spectra is quite broad, limiting spectral contrast (green spectrum).

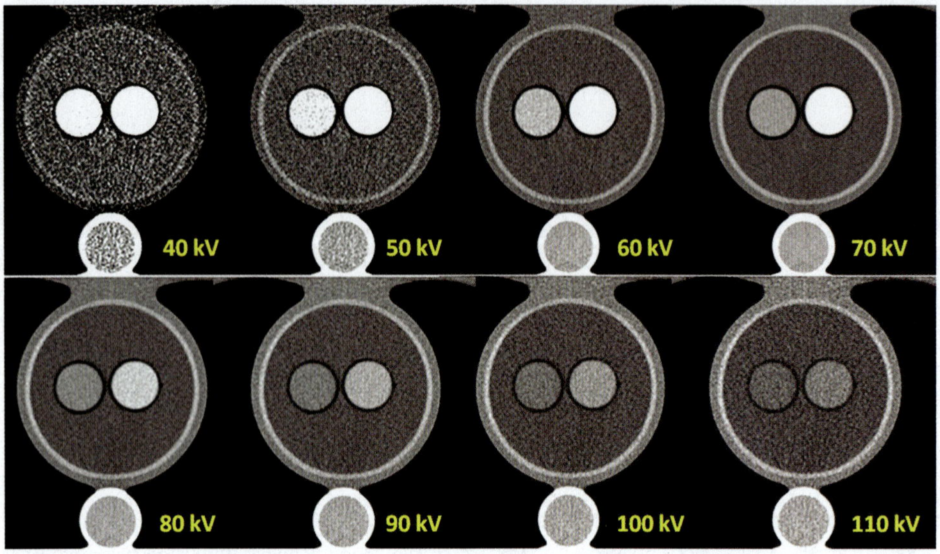

Figure 2-5. An example of monochromatic images from 40 to 110 kV created from a dual-energy scan. Display window level and width are 40 and 400 HU, respectively. Optimal level of contrast and minimal noise are seen at 70 to 80 kV. (From Yu L, Christner JA, Leng S, et al. Virtual monochromatic imaging in dual-source dual-energy CT: radiation dose and image quality. *Med Phys* 2011;38(12):6371–6379, with permission.)

monoenergetic CT image reconstruction. There are three different CT designs to perform dual-energy decomposition (Table 2.1):

1. Single source with rapid kVp switching (Fig. 2.6A and B).
2. Dual-source scan in that high- and low-energy beams are produced during one scan (Fig. 2.7).
3. Single source using sandwich detectors or energy-discriminating photon-counting detectors (Fig. 2.6C). The latter method uses one kVp setting and detects radiation using innovative, spectral CT detectors that separate the x-ray beam into its spectral components (i.e., polychromatic x-ray detection).

TABLE 2.1 **Dual-Energy CT Techniques**

Scanner Type	Tube Detector	Advantages	Disadvantages
Single tube with fast KVp switching	Single tube, single detector array	Good temporal and spatial registration Projection-based decomposition Great flexibility Easy to quantify iodine density Large 50-cm FOV	Limited spectral separation between high- and low-energy scans Higher image noise for lower-voltage image for some scanner designs (tube current may not be modulated to equalize dose and noise between both energy levels) Uncertain reliability of HUs on virtual unenhanced images
Dual-source CT	Two tubes, two detector arrays	Good spectral separation between high- and low-energy scans Easy to modulate each tube current to equalize dose and noise between both energy levels HUs can be measured on virtual unenhanced images	Limited temporal and spatial registration (i.e., cardiac imaging) due to time lag between the two acquisitions. Small FOV for dual-energy acquisition (33 cm) Cross scatter artifacts Low-energy image can be limited by higher noise levels Image domain dual-energy decomposition Increased radiation dose
Multilayered detector or photon counting	Single tube, dual-detector layers	Perfect temporal and spatial registration Reasonable radiation dose Large FOV Projection-based dual-energy decomposition	Limited energy separation with substantial spectral overlap. Longer scanning times with current detector technology

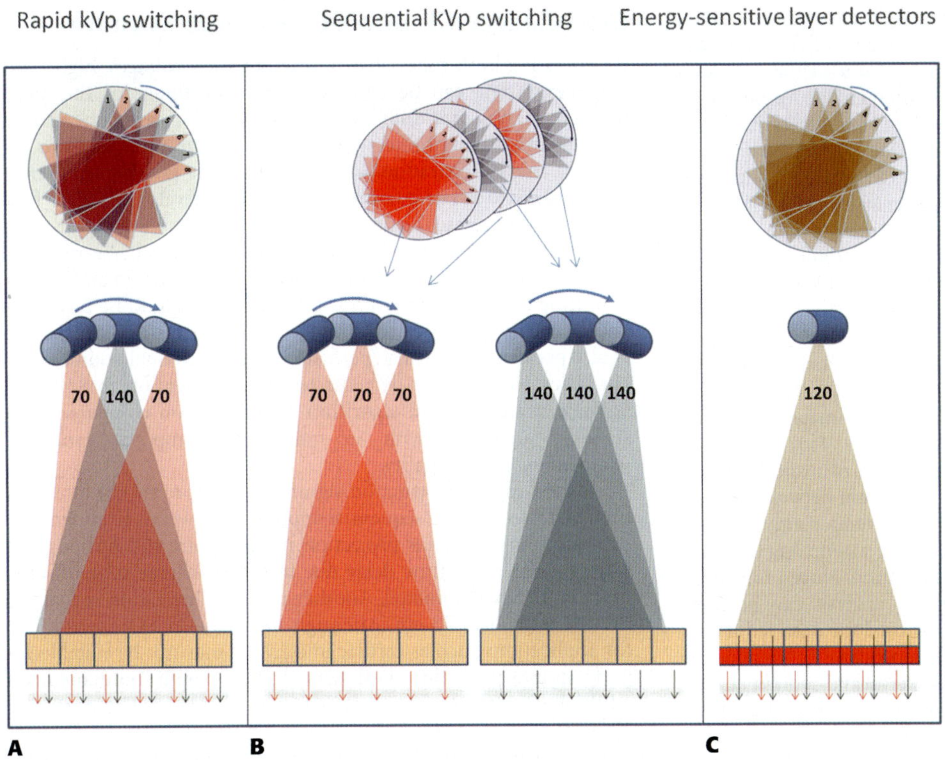

Figure 2-6. Illustration of different hardware approaches to dual-energy CT imaging for single-tube scanners. **A, B:** Show sequential kVp switching. **A:** The x-ray tube voltage is rapidly modulated to different kVp (140 and 70 kVp) levels during single tube rotation, producing spectra of lower and higher energies. For cardiac imaging, switching is done alternatively at 0.2-millisecond intervals during middiastole for every other heartbeat. **B:** kVp switching to 140 kVp is performed after finishing all projections at 70 kVp in the first rotation. The switching can be performed slice by slice or volume by volume. **C:** In energy-sensitive layer detectors technique, the top-layer detector absorbs lower-energy x-ray photons, whereas the bottom-layer detector detects higher-energy x-ray photons. Projections are acquired at 120 kVp only throughout the entire gantry rotation.

The basis material analysis of dual-energy CT images obtained with fast kVp switching can be processed in projection domain. The basis material decomposition for dual-source or dual-layer dual-energy CT scanners is performed only in the image domain.[43] Projection domain decomposition is preferred because it enables greater flexibility in material decomposition and permits the preprocessing correction of data to minimize beam-hardening artifacts.[43] Although beam-hardening correction techniques are usually applied before image reconstruction, it is not always perfect, and residual artifacts in low kVp especially for dense bones and iodine can be disturbing. The image domain decomposition allows for more readily derived HU measurements.

Rapid kVp Switching with a Single-Source Scanner

There are three types of rapid kVp switching implementations. The first, which will be referred to as "in-plane rapid kVp switching," uses a conventional MDCT scanner (e.g., 64 detector helical scanner) with a unique x-ray tube and detector system that enables near-simultaneous acquisition of high- (140 kVp) and low-energy (70 kVp) projection data. The x-ray source undergoes rapid kV switching (0.5 milliseconds), which allows for a high degree of coregistration of the two energy acquisitions (Fig. 2.6A). This type of single-source dual-energy CT, introduced by GE (Discovery CT 750 High definition CT (HDCT), GE Healthcare, Milwaukee, WI), utilizes a garnet-based scintillator detector with low afterglow allowing fast sampling rate. The scan allows for a large FOV of 50 cm that covers the whole body. In dual-energy mode, a collimation of 64 × 0.625 mm can be used. The gantry rotation time is slower than single-energy mode (0.8 seconds). While previously limited to a single selection of 600 mA in dual-energy mode, new scanners provide for different selections (600, 375, and 260 mA), thus allowing for patient-optimized technique and dose reduction. This type of in-plane DECT fast kVp switching allows for good matching of the projection data thus permitting raw data–spaced dual-energy analysis. Within the axial plane, there is minimal time for patient motion

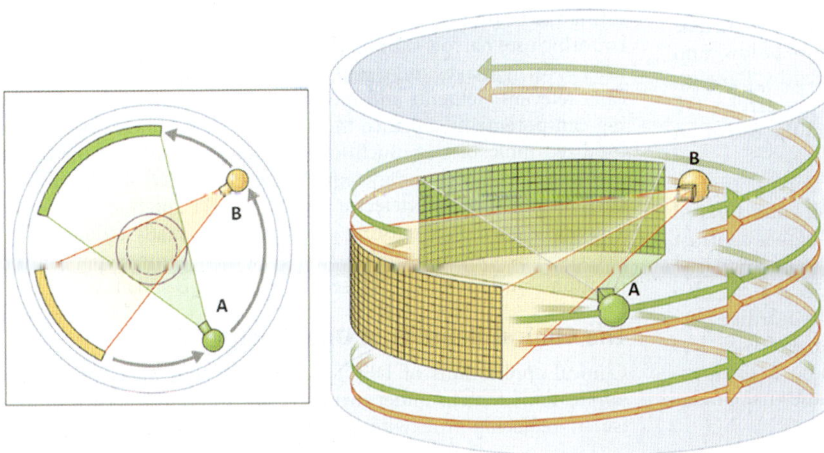

Figure 2-7. In dual-source CT approach for dual-energy technique separate, x-ray tubes are operated at different kVp levels, allowing simultaneous dual-energy data acquisition. A double-helix trajectory is formed by a helical scan in a dual-source geometry. Because the projection data from *source A* and *source B* are never coincident with each other during the helical scan, it is difficult to perform a dual-energy processing in projection data domain. This is one of the reasons why the monochromatic images are currently generated in image space for dual-source CT. (From Yu L, Christner JA, Leng S, et al. Virtual monochromatic imaging in dual-source dual-energy CT: radiation dose and image quality. *Med Phys* 2011;38(12):6371–6379, with permission.)

between kVps, which is optimal for reducing patient motion between kVp settings. No tube current modulation can be used (limiting dose reduction options), and the same mA must be used for both kVp levels. Since the mA is maintained at a constant value for both kVp levels, it is necessary to run the DECT mode at an mA level that is low enough to minimize excess exposure from the 140-kVp beam while ensuring it is high enough to obtain the necessary image quality from the 80 kVp. As a result, the 80-kVp images may be too noisy, or the 140-kVp images may be generated with unnecessarily high dose.

The second type of fast kVp switching is "volume rapid kVp switching." In this implementation, the entire low-kVp image series is acquired in a single rotation, the high-kVp image series is then acquired with a subsequent single rotation. This DECT implementation requires a volume CT scanner such as the Toshiba Aquilion ONE scanner (Toshiba Medical Systems, Otawara, Japan). With 16 cm of detector coverage, volume CT enables image acquisition of whole organs in a single rotation (Fig. 2.6B). This implementation of DECT provides a nearly exact match of projection data with the only mismatch due to patient movement between the volume scans (subsecond interval). As a result, dual-energy mode is used only for noncardiac applications. The kVp switching takes less than 1 second, and scan starts are synchronized. Since projections are matched, raw data–based dual-energy analysis can be used. In-plane tube current modulation can be used for dose reduction. The mA levels for each kVp can be set independently, thus allowing for optimization of image quality for each level and avoiding excess dose. Two volume scans with different kVps are acquired, and mA can be set independently.

The third type of rapid kVp switching is "helical rapid kVp switching." This implementation, found in Toshiba's Aquilion PRIME and Aquilion ONE models, uses a different kVp with each rotation during a helical acquisition. When greater than 16 cm needs to be imaged, this scan mode is used in place of the volume rapid kVp switching mode. This implementation allows only for image-based dual-energy analysis because the projections are not matched to allow for raw data–based analysis. There is a fourth category of kVp switching that does not fall under the umbrella of "rapid kVp switching" because it requires separate helical runs for the low- and high-energy acquisitions. Siemens Somatom Definition Edge and Somatom Definition AS models are single-source scanners and dual-energy mode consists of two successive spiral scans at different kVp and mA levels. This implementation can allow for projection matching and raw data dual-energy analysis, but the long time between scans warrants patient motion considerations.

The main benefit of kVp switching is a more accurate beam hardening correction when raw data–based DECT analysis is available, which becomes clinically apparent in brain, cardiac, and abdominal studies. The disadvantages of the fast kVp switching methods are that the energy separation is currently not as good as using two separate tubes with different filters, and automated tube current modulation techniques can be difficult to implement. The switching time delay precludes the direct combination of low- and high-energy images voxel by voxel to form a standard CT image. The time lag limits application to dynamic events like cardiac CT and suffers the same penalty of higher dose due to the use of an additional low-dose beam.

Pinho et al.[42] assessed the image quality of virtual monochromatic spectral angiography images obtained with a rapid kVp switching scanner and showed less noise and higher contrast enhancement at a virtual 70-kV monochromatic beam compared with 120-kVp images of a single-source scanner. So et al.[44,45] also used rapid kVp switching technique to assess myocardial perfusion. They were able to obtain high-quality images with less beam-hardening artifact and radiation dose using a prospective ECG-gated technique compared with the traditional single-energy CT protocol.

Dual-Energy CT with Dual-Source Scanner

By operating both tubes at two different tube voltages, high- and low-energy data can be obtained.[37] The advantage of the dual-source design is that different tube currents for each tube can be selected and different filters can be used for the x-ray tubes to get the best energy separation. Increasing mAs for low-kVp tube may be necessary to lower quantum mottle noise levels (Fig. 2.7). This strategy will increase the dose when both tubes are working.

In dual-energy mode, the rotation speed should be reduced, and larger number of subvolumes (slabs) is required. Therefore, the scan time can extend to over 5 seconds, which could be problematic for cardiac perfusion imaging. Using a hybrid algorithm, Nance et al.[46] performed a cardiac perfusion study with dual-source scanner. They were able to decrease temporal resolution to 83 milliseconds using a hybrid algorithm reconstruction compared with standard algorithm with 165-millisecond temporal resolution while saving image quality.

Dual-source construction significantly improves the interscan time delay seen in the sequential approach. However, simultaneous data sampling and thus projection matching are still not possible since the interscan time delay due to the 90-degree tube offset is not completely eliminated. Another practical limitation is that the FOV is limited to 33 cm. Although this reduced FOV works fine for applications such as cardiac imaging, it may not be suitable for body applications. Since both x-ray tubes operate simultaneously, additional scatter generated artifacts may be created. These artifacts along with excess noise of low-energy tube could result in decreasing conspicuity of small objects. As mentioned earlier, the material separation in dual source is performed in image domain, because the raw data are not perfectly registered (they are acquired at different times, due to the angular offset of the tube/detector systems). As a result, beam-hardening artifacts may be more noticeable.

Single-Source, Dual-Layer Detector CT

In a single-source, dual-layer detector scanner configuration, one x-ray tube is used to expose a detector consisting of two layers (Fig. 2.6C). The first layer on the top absorbs most (approximately 50% of the beam) of the low-energy spectrum, and the layer on the bottom absorbs the remaining higher-energy photons.[40,41,43] An advantage to this form of spectral energy separation system is the elimination of the time lag that exists with other dual-energy CT approaches, making it ideal for imaging moving tissue. The use of a single source also obviates the potential scatter limitation of dual-source techniques. Furthermore, if required, this approach allows a full 50-cm FOV without adding the radiation dose levels.

Photon counting represents the most advanced form of spectral CT. Photon-counting detectors count each individual incident x-ray, measuring the energy of each photon.[47,48] Rather than separating the beam into merely high- and low-energy ranges, photon counting uses narrow subranges or bins of the spectrum that can be used to form images and classify spectral "k-edge" patterns of clinically relevant elements and molecules (Fig. 2.4C). Photon counting can potentially enhance the ability to detect these specifically localized molecules at much lower concentrations than the other methods.[41] This technology requires very fast detectors. Because of current limitations in detector design, the CT rotation speed and x-ray tube current of existing prototypes are greatly reduced. The net effect is longer scanning times—several seconds per gantry rotation—and the goal of subsecond scanning is still elusive.

The Clinical Benefits of Dual-Energy CT

Clinical applications of DECT vary widely and many promising applications remain under investigation. DECT has shown promise in replacing true with synthesized unenhanced imaging to save radiation, improving lesion conspicuity, iodine extraction, and improving tissue/material characterization (e.g., renal stone composition).[49–51] In angiographic studies, higher intravascular attenuation on 50- and 70-keV monochromatic images can potentially enable high-quality CT angiography (CTA) studies at lower doses of contrast media.[52–54] The use of colored iodine overlay to improve the detection of endoleaks and the subtraction of heavily calcified plaques to improve visualization of vessel stenosis are additional clinical applications. While it is relatively easy to separate iodine in well-opacified vessels from dense calcium in cortical bone or large calcified atherosclerotic plaques, this may not be the case when the density of contrast and calcium is in the same range. It is also technically challenging to separate calcified plaques in small coronary arteries.

Iodine distribution maps obtained by dual-energy techniques allow for accurate assessment of cardiac "perfusion" defects compared with single photon emission CT.[37] Cardiac CT perfusion images can be obtained with minimal beam-hardening artifact. This could have important clinical application in order to measure perfusion parameters accurately. The diagnosis of pulmonary embolism can be improved by displaying the iodine distribution in the lung parenchyma.[55] Regional variation of lung perfusion can be mapped by dual-energy CT in patients suffering from emphysema.[56] In a recent animal study for liver tumors in rabbits, contrast-enhanced dual-energy CT and perfusion CT were compared.[57] It was shown that viable tumor enhancement values in iodine maps correlated well with tumor perfusion CT parameters and that the radiation dose was less in dual-energy CT.

Influencing Factors in CT Perfusion Imaging

The ideal CT scanner for perfusion imaging is the one with the best possible temporal and spatial resolution that is capable of reconstructing high-quality images of the entire anatomy of interest at multiple time points while delivering the smallest radiation dose to the patient. Current technology allows up to 16 cm of body coverage in less than 300 milliseconds with 0.35-mm isotropic spatial resolution. In addition, a CT perfusion study is not complete without availability of a robust postprocessing method to quantify perfusion parameters with good interoperator reproducibility and great interscan repeatability when follow-up comparisons are required.

Spatial Resolution

One of the greatest challenges in CT imaging is the detailed evaluation of small anatomic structures and visualization of small vessels that requires high-resolution imaging. To achieve this goal, thinner collimation, smaller detector size, and special reconstruction algorithms are required. Spatial resolution is a measure of the accuracy of an imaging system to discriminate between two adjacent high-contrast objects and is usually expressed as line pairs per millimeter.[58] In CT, voxel size is the major determinant of spatial resolution. A CT scanner with 0.4-mm^3 isotropic voxels will depict a 2.2-mm contrast-enhanced vessel on approximately 8 voxels. Typical fluoroscopy tubes have a spatial resolution of approximately 0.16 mm, and the same vessel will be depicted on roughly 20 pixels. With large voxels volume, averaging artifacts occur due to thicker slice thickness. In CT, in-plane spatial resolution describes pixel dimensions in the x–y plane, which depends on the size of reconstruction matrix and on the reconstructed FOV and will be selected by the CT technologist at the time of image reconstruction. This is different from scan FOV, which is the total body area scanned at the time of image acquisition. Currently, CT images by convention have a 512 × 512 matrix size regardless of the reconstructed FOV. A quick way to think about in-plane resolution and pixel size in a reconstructed 2D axial CT image is to divide the reconstructed FOV (in millimeters) by 512 for the matrix dimensions. For example, reconstructed FOV = 300 mm/512 provides pixel of roughly 0.6 × 0.6 mm, and reconstructed FOV = 250 mm/512 provides pixel of roughly 0.5 × 0.5 mm.[32]

On the other hand, longitudinal (out-of-plane) spatial resolution describes the size of image voxel in z-axis and is related to x-ray collimation chosen and longitudinal dimension of the detectors. Since for most MDCT applications, the smallest collimation is essentially always chosen (i.e., 0.5 mm for cardiac imaging), the main limiting factor for the z-axis of a voxel is determined by the detector thickness. Longitudinal spatial resolution determines the minimum achievable slice thickness. In an ideal volumetric data reconstruction, true isotropic voxels can be reconstructed. That means that a voxel has the same size in all dimensions. Isotropic voxels are required to reconstruct images in all planes at the same high quality. Current CT systems provide an isotropic spatial resolution of up to 0.3 mm. The effect of detector size in the longitudinal spatial resolution is very significant and has become one of the driving forces in the advancement of MDCT technology. Further improvement of spatial resolution for detection of small structures may require a different detector design (i.e., flat panel) and a higher radiation exposure to maintain sufficient signal-to-noise ratio (SNR).[59] Overall, increasing spatial resolution is not a simple task and necessities improvement in all three dimensions. For detailed recording of moving structures as in cardiac imaging, improving the fourth dimension of time or temporal resolution also is required (governed by gantry rotation time, number of x-ray sources, and segmented reconstruction techniques). With the continued evolution of detector technology and increasing z-axis resolution, now seen with some flat panel detectors in development, we are very near a time when maintaining isotropic voxels in reconstructed images may require a 1,024 × 1,024 matrix.

Contrast Resolution and Noise

Contrast resolution in CT is the ability of system to distinguish low-contrast anatomic or pathologic structures in an image.[60–62] For example, relative attenuation differences (HU) between gray and white matter in the brain or detectability of cirrhotic nodules relative to the normal liver tissue. Obviously, enhancement of one structure relative to another after intravenous contrast injection will increase soft tissue contrast resolution in post–contrast-enhanced images. The most important parameter influencing contrast resolution is noise. Image noise impairs the detection of lesions. Higher noise levels can be better tolerated in physiologic high-contrast area (e.g., bone–soft tissue interface) than in low-contrast region (e.g., liver). The SNR and contrast-to-noise ratio (CNR) are useful descriptors of CT image quality with respect to the noise. In general, noise in CT depends on the quantum noise (statistical fluctuation in the number of x-ray photons), patient size, quality of the detector system, and the reconstruction kernel (sharper algorithm gives noisier images).[60] Quantum noise is probably the most influential factor.[60] Accurate measurement of noise is difficult because noise on CT images is not mathematically uniform and does not follow a defined statistical distribution.[61] Relative background noise in the image can be estimated in the air outside the image by placing a large area of interest (2 cm) in an artifact-free region. Thinner CT slice thickness decreases SNR unless exposure factors such as tube potential and current are increased. This results in an increased radiation dose to the patient. An increase in the SNR by a factor of 1.4 results in doubling of the radiation dose. Alternatively, less noisy images can be obtained by increasing the slice thickness. In perfusion studies of low-contrast regions (e.g., soft tissue tumors), it is suggested to use a slice thickness of not less than 5 mm, which guarantees a correct balance between optimal spatial resolution and acceptable SNR in perfusion scans.[63] It is important to realize that larger patients have a higher total x-ray CT attenuation and increasing exposure factors may be necessary to compensate for photon starvation and decreased SNR. In MDCT, noise increases if pitch is greater than 1 (assuming technique factors are held constant). When pitch is greater than 1, photon-deficient zones can occur in the z-direction causing increasing noise. This phenomenon is less apparent for studies using pitch less than 1 (e.g., cardiac).[60] In most scanners, tube current–time product is automatically increased in proportion to increasing pitch to keep noise level low. The term "effective" mAs is used by Siemens and equals to mAs/pitch in noncardiac scan modes, and in cardiac mode, the term total mAs delivered per gantry rotation is used, which is defined as mAs/rotation.

High-quality images with clear depiction of low-contrast objects and minimal noise level are necessary for both qualitative and quantitative tissue perfusion analysis. However, radiation dose control in accordance with the ALARA (as low as reasonably achievable) principle demands careful adjustment of the perfusion acquisition protocols to limit the volume of scan to answer the specific clinical question. During image data reconstruction, a "soft" reconstruction kernel may be used to increase visual low-contrast lesion detectability. Thin-cut scanning to minimize partial volume averaging (PVA) effects, along with sliding-thin-slab averaging and adjustment of the window and level settings during image review may be applied to optimize the depiction of low-contrast lesions.[61]

CT perfusion studies have been performed at a range of x-ray energies and beam intensities, from 80 to 120 kVp and 80 to 210 mAs, respectively. In most of the recently published studies, in order to reduce the x-ray dose, it is recommended to use relatively low tube voltage (80 to 100 kVp) and current (120 to 200 mA) for perfusion scans.[63] In perfusion studies that demand higher image sampling frequency, the tube current may need to be reduced to lower radiation dose. Wintermark et al.[64] compared the use of 80 and 120 kVp at 200 mAs on quality of brain perfusion images. At 80 kVp, greater contrast between white and gray material was shown and the radiation dose was lower by a factor of 2.8 compared with 120 kVp. The difference in noise between 80- and 120-kVp images was not significant. The 80 kVp setting would also increase the conspicuity of intravenous contrast due to greater participation of the photoelectric effect for 80-kV photons, which are closer to the "k-edge" of iodine.[65]

Murase et al.[66] studied the effect of x-ray tube current on the accuracy of cerebral perfusion parameters. MDCT scanner with a tube voltage of 80 kVp and a tube current of 200 mA was used. Using a noise simulation software, simulated images were generated with tube currents of 50, 100, and 150 mA. They found a significant difference between 50 and 100 mA for all perfusion parameters. Deconvolution perfusion analysis is less sensitive to noise and can therefore tolerate a lower tube current condition and allows a higher image frequency. On the other hand, protocols that can be done at lower sampling frequency (tumor capillary permeability) but require higher tube current are appropriate for compartmental analysis methods.[67] Generally, perfusion CT imaging protocol can be modified depending on the organs or tissues imaged and the physiologic parameters of interest in the study.

Temporal Resolution

The temporal resolution refers to the time needed to acquire a complete data set for image reconstruction. It is different from temporal (frequency of) sampling, which refers to the rate of sampling of images for dynamic CT acquisitions such as perfusion. Temporal resolution is a term mainly used in cardiac imaging and relates to the ability of a system to capture images of the moving structure. Superior temporal resolution improves the ability to freeze cardiac motion. Therefore, in myocardial perfusion imaging, a high temporal resolution is the prerequisite in order to compensate for the rapid and continuous cardiac motions. High attenuation of left ventricle intraluminal contrast can create artifacts at the interface with the myocardium due to beam hardening that can be mistaken with hypoperfused myocardium. This artifact is even more severe by superimposed motion when the CT data acquisition is not fast enough to compensate for it in systole and near the base of left ventricle where longitudinal and circumferential contractions are dominant.

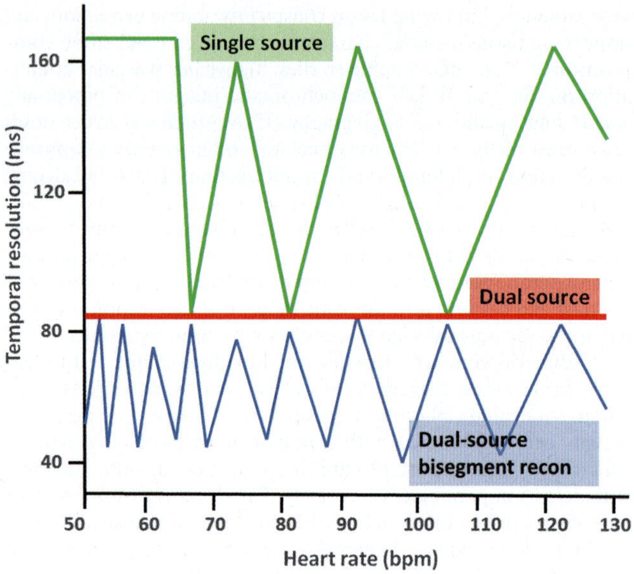

Figure 2.8. **Temporal resolution as a function of the heart rate for single-source (*green line*) and dual-source (*red line*) CT scans, both with a rotation time of 330 ms.** The single-source CT reaches a temporal resolution of less than 100 ms only by means of a multisegment reconstruction approach at specific heart rates. The dual-source system (first generation) shows a constant temporal resolution of 83 ms for all heart rates. Utilizing bisegment techniques for a dual source further improves the temporal resolution (*blue line*). An average temporal resolution of 60 ms can be achieved. (From Scheffel H, Alkadhi H, Plass A, et al. Accuracy of dual-source CT coronary angiography: first experience in a high pre-test probability population without heart rate control. *Eur Radiol* 2006;16(12):2739–2747, with permission.)

There are a number of factors that influence the temporal resolution achieved with MDCT scanners including gantry rotation time, number of x-ray tubes, acquisition mode, image reconstruction, heart rate in cardiac imaging, and pitch[58,68] (Fig. 2.8). Temporal resolution is often defined in the x/y plane (axial in-plane temporal resolution). The z-axis resolution is also very important for ensuring isotropic imaging and uniform contrast timing. But z-axis temporal resolution is a by-product of z-axis coverage and is often discussed in that context.

The rotation time is the major factor that determines the temporal resolution of a scanner. It is the time required for the gantry to complete 360-degree revolution. Since image reconstruction requires approximately 50% (180 degrees) of the gantry rotation, the temporal resolution of a single x-ray CT tube and detector system is one half of the gantry rotation time. The minimum amount of projection data required to construct a complete image in MDCT is a little longer and equals 180 degrees plus the fan angle of the CT detectors in the axial plane.

In order to increase the temporal resolution, faster rotation times are required. Manufacturers have been able to lower the gantry rotation time to as low as 250 to 280 milliseconds.[68] Therefore, minimum achievable temporal resolution with single-tube MDCT scanners using current technology is around 140 milliseconds (7 frames per second). Although this temporal resolution is enough to record high-quality diastolic images, it may not be enough to clearly demonstrate artifact-free phases of systole, which may require a temporal resolution of 50 milliseconds (i.e., isovolumic contraction). In comparison, temporal resolution of conventional angiography is around 33 to 40 milliseconds (25 to 30 frames per second) and with echocardiography is 33 to 66 milliseconds (15 to 30 frames per second), adequate for motion-free cardiac imaging. With MRI using current technology, temporal resolution of 50 to 100 milliseconds can be achieved. Electron beam CT provided a temporal resolution in the range of 50 to 100 milliseconds, by magnetically steering an electron beam around a 210-degree stationary tungsten target. Temporal resolution can also be improved by increasing the number of x-ray tubes, each with an independent detector system. A dual-source CT with two x-ray tubes and gantry rotation time of 280 milliseconds can provide a temporal resolution of 75 milliseconds, because only one-quarter of a gantry rotation is needed for reconstruction.[32] A new dual-source scanner introduced by Siemens (SOMATOM Force) enables rotation speed of 250 milliseconds in combination with a full FOV of 50 cm and a temporal resolution of 66 milliseconds.

In cardiac imaging using single-tube spiral MDCT scanners, faster gantry rotation requires a slower pitch to avoid discontinuities in the anatomic coverage of the heart between images reconstructed from consecutive cardiac cycles. Therefore, decreasing the heart rate to less than 65 beats per minute using beta-blockers is essential to improve temporal resolution. Faster gantry rotation also necessitates increasing tube current value in order to save image quality. It is important to know that increasing gantry rotation time beyond a certain limit is very difficult demanding special engineering designs. This is mainly due to higher G forces created by rapid movement of heavy mechanical components inside the CT gantry. For a 640-volume scanner, this may reach up to 40 G for 280-millisecond rotation time. It should be noted that the 640-slice volume CT scanner has optimal z-axis temporal resolution because the entire heart can be imaged in a single rotation. Thus, the contrast is not moving through the anatomy much during the time of acquisition.

Almost all cardiac CT acquisitions require ECG gating using either a retrospective gating or a prospective triggering. During retrospective gating, the image data from the entire cardiac cycle are collected. The collected data are retrospectively assigned to different phases of cardiac cycle during image reconstruction, hence the name retrospective gating. With this form of acquisition, most cardiac phases (depending of temporal resolution of the scanner) can be demonstrated. This technique is now mainly used for the assessment of cardiac and valve functions. The disadvantage of retrospective gating is increased radiation dose, because the data are acquired throughout the heart cycle. The tube can be modulated down during the phases of the heart's cycle that do not require high-quality images. In prospective ECG triggering, only a preselected temporal window (phase window) of the cardiac cycle is scanned, and radiation can be limited to that window. Scan starts at a preset point in the cardiac cycle, for example, between 50% and 80% of the R-R interval. Alternatively, the phase window can also be described as a "center" phase and a surrounding "pad," for example, 100 milliseconds centered on 75% of the R-R interval. Prospective ECG triggering technique was originally described as "step-and-shoot" technique using 64-slice scanners (3-cm detector width), which required at least three steps to cover the entire heart. In a typical prospective cardiac imaging over seven heartbeats, four beats will be used to acquire scans (the "shoot") and the intervening three beats will be used to move the patient to a new location between the scans (the "step"). With 640 scanners, 16 cm of the chest (entire heart) can be scanned in a single heartbeat using either a retrospective or prospective gating, and the concept of "step-and-shoot" does not apply to this group of scanners. The main benefits of this type of imaging are that all images come from the same heart cycle and the images are captured with isotemporal resolution (same time point in all directions). When using isotemporal imaging, there is no risk of misregistration artifacts being mistaken as lesions. When viewing the length of a vessel, if different regions of the heart are imaged over different heartbeats, there may be slight differences in position between the locations, which can be mistaken as narrowing of the coronary arteries. With isotemporal resolution, the entire coronary artery was captured at the same time, so the reviewer can be confident that any visible narrowing in the image is, in fact, narrowing and not artifact. This concept of isotemporal imaging becomes especially important when doing any sort of CT perfusion imaging. Since perfusion imaging involves calculation of the blood flow and uptake acquired at intervals of time, it is important that the blood within the organ was captured at a single instant in time for each interval. Otherwise, it becomes very challenging to decouple the effects of physiologic blood flow differences and blood flow timing differences due to the acquisition.

Temporal resolution is also affected by the type of data reconstruction. Multisegment reconstruction improves the effective temporal resolution by using CT data from more than one R-R interval to reconstruct a volume. For example, in two-segment reconstruction, the scanned volume is reconstructed from CT data obtained over two R-R intervals. Therefore, only half the data are necessary for each R-R interval, and the effective temporal resolution is halved (or in other words, the total temporal resolution is ¼ rotation for a two-segment, acquisition mode). Multisegment acquisition can be used to mitigate higher heart rates for helical MDCT or for 640-slice volume CT. One major limitation of multisegment reconstruction is increasing radiation exposure as the number of reconstructed segments increases (more R-R intervals).

Pitch

The concept of pitch was introduced with the advent of spiral CT. The pitch is defined by the International Electrotechnical Commission specifications as the ratio of table feed per gantry rotation to the total x-ray beam width. This definition applies to both single-section and MDCT. For example, with 64 sections at 0.5-mm collimation and a table feed of 32 mm per rotation, the pitch is 1.0 [$32/(64 \times 0.5) = 1.0$].

The need for gating the study to the cardiac cycle, and the need for high spatial and temporal resolutions in diagnostic cardiac imaging, mandates using small pitch values (<0.4). This results in increasing radiation dose up to a factor of five times in a pitch of 0.2 (80% radiation beam overlap) compared to a pitch of 1. In cardiac imaging using ECG-gated single-segment reconstruction, the pitch factor is proportional to heart rate. For heart rate of 45 to 100, pitch may vary between 0.4 and 0.9. Therefore, it is important to lower heart rate in order to obtain high-quality images. In multiple-segment reconstruction, along with increasing number of segments, smaller pitch is required.

The demand for reducing radiation dose and faster scans especially for perfusion imaging derived manufacturers to introduce wider detector panels (320 detector rows) and newer flat panel technologies to cover the entire heart region without the need to overlap radiation beams. The introduction of high-pitch imaging has reduced doses below 3 mSv for static coronary CT angiography in a small to average size patient.[32,69] This seems to be a reasonable dose number compared to earlier MDCT generations, which was around 12 mSv.[70] For perfusion imaging, depending on the tube current and frequency of image sampling, the total radiation exposure is much higher. Future optimization techniques and the adoption of iterative reconstruction methods may substantially reduce radiation exposure at similar image quality.[71] An innovative alternative solution for high radiation exposure in perfusion studies has been the introduction of high pitch technique using alternating table positions in dual-source scanner.[72,73] In an experimental adenosine stress myocardial perfusion imaging by Bamberg et al.,[72] ECG-triggered end-systolic images were acquired timed by a dual-source CT system (128 detector, 0.28-second rotation time) with sequential forward and backward table positions and a temporal sampling of 2.5 to 3.0 seconds to cover a scan range of 73 mm. Dynamic imaging started 4 seconds before the arrival of the bolus (50 mL at 5 mL/s) in the ascending aorta. Data were acquired for 30 seconds (100 kV, 300 mAs), and the average radiation dose was measured at 9.6 mSv.

Reconstruction Interval

Reconstruction interval is defined as the amount of overlap between consecutive axial images. It does not change the scan time or patient exposure because it is simply a postprocessing step. Increasing overlap will improve longitudinal resolution, especially for 3D volume rendering and MPR images. This is especially the case for cardiac CT that requires 0.5-mm slice thickness with 0.25- to 0.3-mm (50% to 60%) overlaps. Overlapping may help detect small lesions that otherwise would have fallen between contiguous slices and missed. Overlapping also helps avoid partial voluming effects. For perfusion imaging, a diagnosis can be made based on only axial images and reconstruction interval may not be required. It should be noted that increasing overlap results in longer reconstruction time and a large number of images to view.

A different option to increase the number of images that can be reconstructed for a given interval is the use of alternating x-ray CT source focal spot, which doubles the number of slices with respect to the number of detector rows. It is important to know that this technique does not double the volume coverage. For example, a 128-detector rows with two focal spot positions and 0.625-mm detector diameter can obtain 256 (128 × 2) slices per gantry rotation while the z-axis coverage is 80 mm (128 × 0.625 mm).

Anatomic Coverage

The most dramatic advances in CT technology came from the increasing in number of detectors from single-detector slip ring CT to 2-, to 8-, to 64-, and eventually to 320-detector row CT.[74] Along with faster gantry rotation times, increasing coverage in the z-axis direction has further reduced acquisition time. This facilitates shorter breath-hold time of scan, which may be important in scanning patients who have difficulty holding their breath for long time.

A major limitation of most perfusion imaging studies is narrow scan coverage, which is typically limited to less than 4 cm for most spiral scanners used in the reported studies. Wide detector area technology can solve this problem. The largest volume coverage to date is the 640-slice CT (Toshiba Aquilion One Dynamic Volume CT) that features a 320 × 0.5 mm configuration or 16 cm of craniocaudal coverage per gantry rotation. In cardiac imaging, this large coverage permits to obtain single heartbeat myocardial perfusion images that span the entire heart in one rotation (275 ms) and eliminates banding artifacts related to irregular cardiac rhythm and "stair-step" inherent to spiral acquisition in which cardiac subvolumes over multiple gantry rotations are subsequently stacked to create a cardiac volume (Please see Misregistration Artifacts). In noncardiac applications, increased coverage lets perfusion examination of regions such as the brain, kidney, and upper abdomen to have a temporal uniformity throughout the organ, which allows comparing different parts of an organ at the same time. As previously discussed, this is referred to as isotemporal resolution. Most 64-slice spiral scanners require approximately eight heartbeats to cover the heart span; therefore, the iodinated contrast opacification would be different for each slab. It is likely that accurate delineation of either small or subtle perfusion defects will require that images of the entire organ volume are obtained at a single point of iodinated contrast opacification.

Another potential advantage of wide area detector coverage scanners is less radiation exposure by avoiding the oversampling related to helical scanning. In addition, by using volume mode, the volume CT scanner avoids overranging, which is the excess exposure at the beginning and end of a helical run. Note that overranging is lessened by adaptive collimation, but some overranging excess exposure is always necessary for helical reconstruction. As mentioned earlier, in perfusion CT imaging of the moving structures, dual-source CT has the advantage of higher temporal resolution around 83 milliseconds. In a 640 scanner with a rotation time of 275 milliseconds using a two-segment reconstruction, a temporal resolution of 70 milliseconds can be achieved. To achieve this temporal resolution, two R-R intervals instead of one are required to complete the two-segment reconstruction, and the radiation exposure will be increased.

Although ideal for perfusion studies, 640-slice scanner technology is not always available, and the cost of scanner can be high compared to basic MDCT systems.[75,76] To solve this limitation and increase the scan coverage of MDCT scanners, new approaches have been introduced. One approach is the "toggling table" technique. In this technique, the table rapidly alternates between two scan positions with temporal sampling rates of 3 to 4 seconds to cover 8 cm (4 × 2 cm). In a modification of this technique, also known as periodic spiral (Helical Shuttle [GE], Adaptive 4D Spiral [Siemens]), the table moves back and forth periodically between the two end positions with variable pitch, fast table acceleration (up to 200 mm/s^2), and two (average pitch 0.5) full rotations at every z-position (Fig. 2.9). Therefore, the scan range depends not only on the detector width but also on table acceleration/deceleration

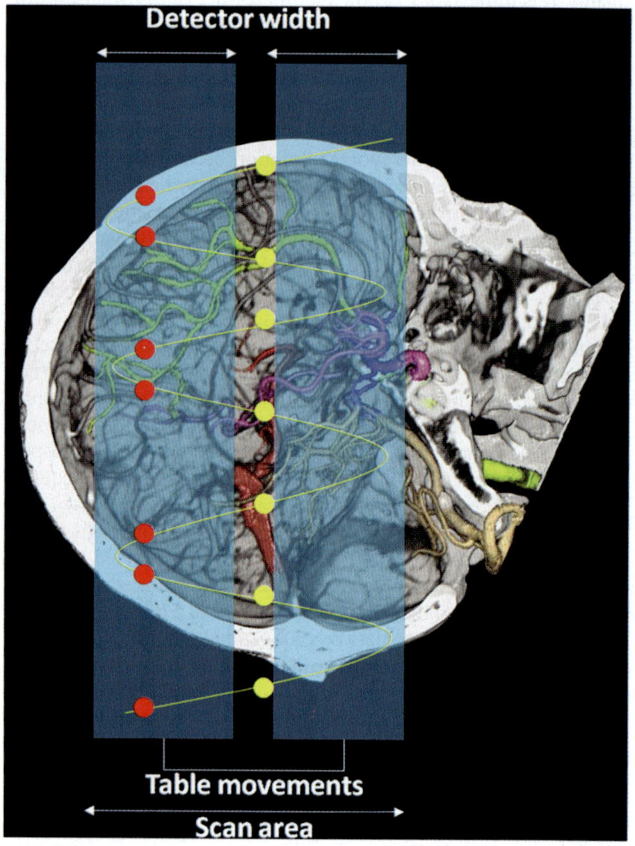

Figure 2-9. Adaptive 4D spiral mode technique. Using this technique, time-resolved scanning of areas larger than the detector width is feasible by continuous periodic table movement. The temporal sampling of the scan is therefore equidistant in the center of the scan range (*yellow circles*) and nonequidistant in peripheral slices (*red circles*). Travel path of the 100 mm is covered in 1.5 seconds. (From Haberland U, Klotz E, Abolmaali N. Performance assessment of dynamic spiral scan modes with variable pitch for quantitative perfusion computed tomography. *Invest Radiol* 2010;45(7):378–386, with permission.)

(210 mm/s^2) and the gantry rotation time (0.28 seconds). Using this modification, scan sampling rate has been reduced to 1.5 seconds for 10-cm coverage, and good reproducibility of the tissue flow determination has been shown compared with standard dynamic mode.[38,77]

To implement periodic spiral technique in clinical practice, Reiner et al.[78] used a dual-source 128-slice CT system with a detector width of 3.84 cm (Siemens 64 detector row with two focal spot positions) for renal tumor perfusion analysis. A range of 10 cm was scanned using a cycle time of 1.5 seconds with an alternating craniocaudal and caudocranial scan direction. During the total examination time of 40 seconds, 26 scans were obtained. Scanning parameters were 100-kV tube voltage and 100 mAs per rotation, and the estimated effective dose was 16.3 mSv for 10-cm coverage.[78]

In comparison to the method described above, similar results have been reported by Motosugi et al.[79] using a 640 scanner (Aquilion ONE; Toshiba Medical Systems). The authors suggest that the nonhelical scan used in their study would be advantageous for reducing incorrect registration of the multiphase images. In this report, a volumetric scan mode was used for upper abdominal imaging, and the perfusion was calculated on a pixel-by-pixel basis by using the maximum slope model. In this study, 24 scans were obtained (every 2 seconds for 28 seconds, every 4 seconds for 24 seconds, and every 8 seconds for 32 seconds), the average dose length product (DLP) was 1,070 mGy cm, and the calculated effective radiation dose was 16.1 mSv for 16-cm coverage.

Scan Duration and Frequency of Sampling

During the first pass of contrast material through the vascular system (typically 45 to 60 seconds), the contrast material is predominantly intravascular. During this period, optimum tissue perfusion analysis requires rapid sequence images and higher sampling frequency to improve perfusion parameters measurements (i.e., blood volume). An average sampling frequency of 1 second is suggested for perfusion analysis using the deconvolution kinetic model and 3 to 5 seconds for protocols defined for perfusion analysis using the single- or double-compartmental kinetic models.[63] As time progresses, passage of intravascular contrast into the extravascular space continues until equilibrium is reached. In the presence of tumors, the equilibrium takes longer and significant return of contrast material into the intravascular space can be observed within 2 minutes. Therefore, for the assessment of tumor vascular permeability, longer acquisition (2 to 6 minutes) is required.[67] The perfusion scans performed during the interstitial phase, after analysis of the first pass of contrast agent, have to be performed every 10 seconds for less than 2 minutes after the administration of contrast agent using deconvolution kinetic model for data analysis and every 10 to 20 seconds for 2 to 10 minutes using the single- or double-compartmental kinetic models.[63] This strategy increases the exposure dose unless the frequency of sampling is reduced.[80]

Modifications of perfusion protocols in order to lower radiation risks and yet provide optimal assessment of tissue vascularity are important. Increasing sampling interval to 2 seconds and reducing cine phase duration to less than 30 seconds have been shown to substantially reduce dose (31% to 65%) and data processing time and provide comparable perfusion parameter values.[80] Multiphasic sequences are a great solution to this problem and provide reliable estimations of the blood flow and volume as well as permeability surface area product without additional radiation burden. In the first phase (including noncontrast mask images), images can be acquired every second for 40 seconds. In the second phase, images can be acquired every 2 to 3 seconds for an additional 35 to 45 seconds, and in third phase (only when permeability measurements are required), images are acquired every 10 to 15 seconds for an additional 2 minutes.

In a contrast-enhanced MR perfusion study for breast cancer, Henderson et al.[81] showed that for optimum measurement of perfusion parameters, a rapid bolus injection of contrast is necessary and that the arterial input function (AIF) be sampled every second and the tissue residue function be sampled every 4 seconds. The effect of sampling frequency on lung tumor perfusion parameters is shown in a recent study, and a sampling interval of 0.5 seconds is suggested for optimum result.[82]

Examining the effect of acquisition time in permeability imaging, Goh et al.[83] showed interestingly that there are significant changes in permeability values between 45-, 65-, and 130-second examination protocols in colorectal cancer imaging. However, in perfusion imaging of the brain to estimate CBF and transit time, it is commonly believed that duration of about 50 seconds could be adequate. In brain ischemia perfusion study, scanning until the end time of the first pass of contrast in a venous output is necessary and sufficient for reliable measurement. It is observed that the end of exam equals to the end time of the first pass (mean, 38.6±5 seconds; range, 32 to 48 seconds), which is the same as the end time–attenuation curve (TAC) of the venous output (superior sagittal sinus).[84] Kämena et al.[85] performed a study to evaluate the influence of different temporal sampling rates on the accuracy of the results from cerebral perfusion CT in acute stroke patients. Parametric perfusion maps were calculated for sampling intervals of 0.5, 1, 2, 3, and 4 seconds. Significant variations in perfusion parameters were found depending on the sampling frequency. Ischemic lesions were best differentiated from normal tissue with sampling intervals of 0.5 and 1 seconds. Other studies have shown[86,87] that the image interval can be increased to 2 to 3 seconds for both normal and ischemic tissue without substantial variance (<10%) in perfusion parameter measurements. The benefit of this technique is significant reduction in the radiation dose of the patient. Increasing image interval is somehow mandatory when using periodic spiral technique to increase z-direction coverage in small detector span scanners as explained above. In a typical brain perfusion in our institution using a 640 scanner (0.5 mm thickness, 16-cm coverage, 80 kVp, 300 mA), 50 mL of nonionic iodinated contrast media (350 mg/mL of iodine), followed by saline at the rate of 5 mL/s will be injected intravenously. Three seconds after injection, a total of 13 volumes will be acquired every 2 seconds followed by 5 more volumes every 5 seconds covering the whole brain.[88]

Contrast Material Factors

Most perfusion techniques require at least one noncontrast image in the image series for subtraction. Cardiac output and contrast transit times can change, depending on heart rate, contractility, and peripheral vascular resistance. To measure the exact timing to contrast arrival in the target artery, an initial test bolus scan can be performed. Knowing the timing for contrast arrival may be important in order to save radiation dose by not starting too early. Most scanners have a scan delay of at least 2 seconds after the "start scan" button is pressed. This delay needs to be measured for each scanner selected for perfusion imaging purposes.

Scans can be triggered by real-time bolus tracking in the target artery for qualitative perfusion scans. This technique is not practical when noncontrast images are necessary to obtain. Scan triggering thresholds must be adjusted for various scanners. The 64-detector row scanners are generally slower compared to newer 640 scanners, and a longer delay between bolus tracking threshold detection and the onset of scan is necessary.

Contrast factors in perfusion imaging are mainly related to the amount of contrast, iodine concentration, injection rate, and number of injections. These parameters may affect the estimation of kinetic parameters in perfusion CT. Saline flush seems to be essential to maintain contrast flow. With monophasic bolus injection without saline flush (20 to 30 mL), about one-third of the contrast agent does not contribute to the first pass.[89] The optimum contrast volume and injection rates have not been carefully studied in perfusion CT. The slope of the TAC is dependent on the bolus volume, the rate of injection, and the patient's cardiac output.[67] Significant reduction of perfusion parameters are shown when contrast bolus is injected manually. Since most scanners are fast enough to acquire data for perfusion imaging, most investigators believe that contrast should be injected as fast as possible to create a rapidly passing bolus in order to obtain correct arterial input measurements. Optimal values of injection rate are 5 to 7 mL/s. However, the rate of injection may be modified depending on the rotation time of scanner and frequency of data sampling. In perfusion studies for brain ischemia, the maximum slope of tissue TAC in organs must be reached before the peak enhancement time of the venous output (sagittal sinus). To reach this goal and obtain reliable data, if the data acquisition time is 1 second for each scan, and the time interval between scans is also 1 second, it is suggested to inject 30-mL contrast at a rate of 9 mL/s.[90] Goh et al.[91] performed a study to compare the effect of contrast volume on tumor perfusion assessment. They showed similar results for quantitative parameters including tumor blood volume, blood flow, and permeability surface area product comparing 100-mL with 50-mL contrast injection protocols. Tumor peak enhancement and time to peak (TTP) were significantly greater with larger contrast volume.

To evaluate the impact of iodine concentrations on CT perfusion image quality, König et al.[92] compared 300 to 400 mg/mL iodine concentrations. Factors including the maximum tissue enhancement and SNR were found to be improved resulting in better image quality in low perfusion brain areas, but no significant differences were found for the cerebral blood volume (CBV), blood flow, and TTP. Overall, for a brain ischemia study, 35 to 45 mL of contrast at concentration of 350 to 370 g/dL of iodine will be power injected at a rate of 7 mL/s followed by with a saline "chaser" of 20 to 40 mL at the same injection rate to provide optimum peak enhancement and SNR for perfusion analysis.[93]

The speed of contrast injection is important to obtain good TAC for AIF, but contrast volume is the main factor to correctly measure tissue function. It is shown that biphasic injection of two boluses improves the precision in the estimation of blood flow and MTT, by 36.9% and 38.4%, respectively, compared to the standard uniphasic injection protocol using deconvolution-based analysis incorporating an adiabatic approximation of tissue homogeneity (ATH) model.[94] However, measurement of the permeability surface area product and extravascular extracellular space volume favors a single fast bolus of the same contrast amount. The two-compartment model and the modified Kety model benefited more from the single fast bolus.[94]

Modified bolus techniques with gradually decreasing injection rates (32 mL at 4 mL/s, 16 mL at 2 mL/s, and 60 mL at 1 mL/s) followed by a saline flush (20 mL at 1 mL/s) have been introduced in CT perfusion analysis of lung tumors.[95,96] The rationale for the contrast material infusion protocol was to maintain a more constant intravascular concentration of contrast material, to minimize the concentration gradient between the intravascular and extravascular spaces, to optimize conditions for Patlak analysis, and to improve the SNR.

The compartmental analysis (slope method) is generally more sensitive to variations in contrast injection parameters than the deconvolution method.[97] When using slope method to obtain perfusion values, a relative small bolus (40 to 50 mL) and fast injection rates (5 to 10 mL/s) are necessary because the validity of the method requires that peak arterial concentration occurs prior to the time of maximal increase in tissue enhancement.[67] Deconvolution analysis is relatively resistant to slower injection rates, but higher rates may still be beneficial by increasing tissue enhancement and SNR.[67]

Partial Volume Averaging

PVA is a universal phenomenon in CT imaging and results from the limited spatial resolution of the scanner. PVA is directly proportional to the slice thickness. Because of PVA, the enhancement in small blood vessels cannot be accurately measured with CT, since their volume is averaged together with that of surrounding tissue.[1] This may impact accurate measurements of the arterial input or venous output functions (VOFs). Since attenuation coefficient of the extravascular tissue is much lower than the intravascular contrast, volume averaging of the two structures can lower the mean CT number of the region of interest selected for arterial function. Therefore, a falsely lower arterial enhancement (and wider) curve would be measured, which would lead to overestimation of regional volume and flow and an underestimation of the MTT.[98]

Most methods quantifying tissue perfusion from CT images measure temporal changes in attenuation values during the first pass of a bolus of an iodinated contrast agent. Temporal changes in attenuation are linearly related to the concentration of the contrast agent in that voxel. TACs for arterial and tissue functions will be drawn, and blood volume can be calculated as the ratio of the area under the curve (AUC) of the tissue to AUC of the feeding artery. Both blood volume and flow are inversely proportional to the AUC of the feeding artery or draining vein. In brain perfusion study, because the AUC of the first passage of contrast agent through a vein is equal to the AUC of an artery when the blood–brain barrier is intact, a larger vein may be preferred for vascular function measurement. Therefore, correct measurement of CBV requires knowledge of contrast enhancement in an arterial (or venous) pixel devoid of PVAs. In perfusion estimates, the MTT is calculated by means of deconvolution analysis. In practice, the MTT can be thought of as the difference between the width of the tissue curve and the width of the AIF.

In an experimental study by van der Schaaf et al.,[99] the authors compared arterial input and VOFs in 3-, 6-, and 12-mm-thick sections. They showed that with the use of thinner sections, the AUC of the VOF and especially the AIF increased significantly and the width of the AIF decreased slightly. They concluded that thick slices (>6 mm) may result in an overestimation of the blood volume and flow. The MTT was hardly influenced by section thickness. It was recommended that the VOF measurement would better be performed on thin sections (3 mm) and tissue function would be more correct if performed on thicker sections (e.g., 10 mm).

Arterial Input and Venous Output Functions

The determination of tissue perfusion using CT is based on examining the relationships between the arterial, tissue, and potentially the venous enhancement after the injection of a bolus of contrast material along with repeated rapid CT scans at the same location.[100,101] In the simplified three-compartment model, blood flow passes from a single arterial inflow, through the capillary bed, and then through the venous outlet, and the AIF is assumed to represents the exact arterial inflow to the capillary bed without any delay due to stenosis or dispersion due to collateral flow.[102] Inaccuracies in the input function propagate through the estimated tissue parameters (Figs. 2.10 to 2.12). In semiautomated techniques, the detection of AIF is based on the triggering of an early rise of attenuation in an area that is typically 4 pixels in size and a small half width at half maximum of the peak enhancement of TAC.[102] As explained earlier, selection of smaller arteries as the AIF is hampered by PVA effects, potentially underestimating the arterial AUC and therefore overestimation of the tissue blood volume. To correct for these partial volume effects, a VOF is selected. Therefore, the tissue blood volume (i.e., CBV) is also inversely related to the AUC VOF. This correction

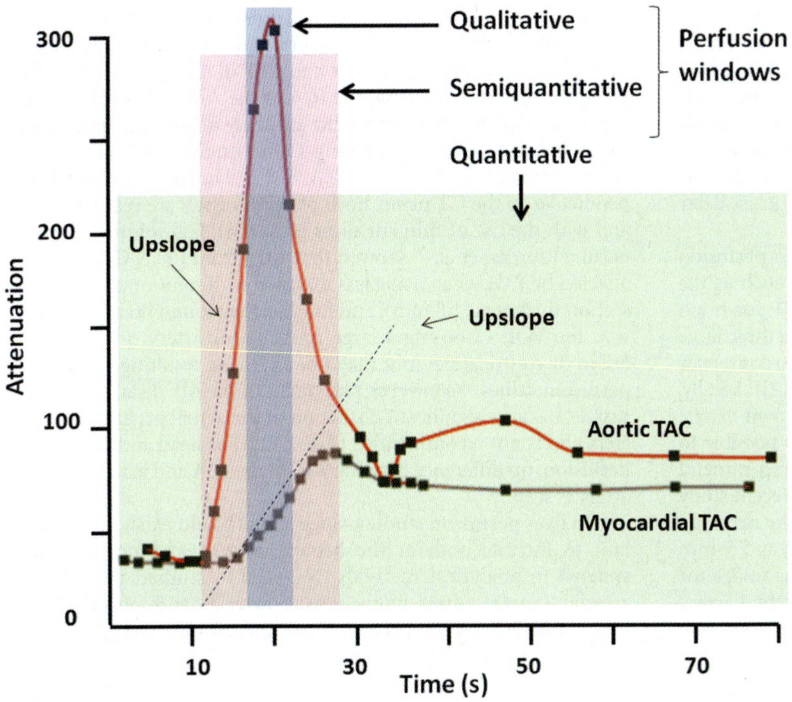

Figure 2-10. **Myocardial CT perfusion protocol.** The *color boxes* represent qualitative (*blue*), semiquantitative (*pink*), and quantitative (*light green*) data acquisition windows with respect to the aortic and myocardial time attenuation curves (TAC). The *dashed lines* denote the upslope of each TAC. Quantitative myocardial CTP requires measurement of the entire TAC causing highest radiation dose. For dose saving, a two-phase acquisition protocol can be used. The second phase acquisition can be performed at a much lower frequency (every 15 seconds) than the first phase (every 1 second). This is justified because change in contrast concentration in myocardium and its supply arteries toward the end of first pass is significantly slower than that in the beginning of first pass.

assumes that without PVA, all AIFs and VOFs should have equal AUCs and that a VOF selected in a large vein like the superior sagittal sinus or the straight sinus is unaffected by PVA. By comparing the areas of the venous and arterial TACs, one can correct for the PVA of the arterial TAC.

Arteries larger than 2 mm are generally less susceptible to volume averaging especially within thin cut slices (<1 mm).[98] In brain studies, most vessels are small, and it is important to select a vessel with a relative perpendicular course to the imaging plane to minimize PVA. Veins are generally larger and less subject to PVA. That is why measuring VOF is suggested in the brain, but outside brain arteries are large enough, and there is no need to find a vein for VOF. There are additional benefits for the measurement of VOF, since deconvolution analysis based on singular (arterial) value decomposition is susceptible to dispersion (multiple vascular routes) or delay in the arrival of contrast material, leading

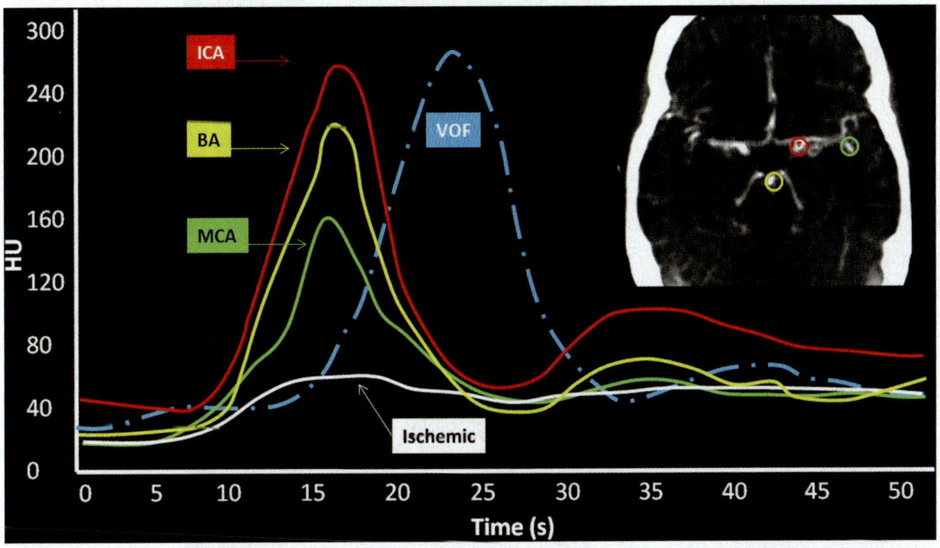

Figure 2-11. **Effect of partial volume averaging and vessel size on the shape of arterial input function (AIF) curve.** AIF curves for normal internal carotid artery (ICA), middle cerebral artery (MCA), and basilar artery (BA) are shown for slice thickness of 0.5 mm in a brain CT perfusion study. Venous output function (VOF) and the AIF of a vessel in an ischemic zone are shown for comparison. The accuracy of the quantitative perfusion maps can be improved by selecting an artery with the least partial volume effects. Partial volume averaging (especially for small-sized arteries) on the AIF results in a decreased signal-to-noise ratio. As a result, the time–attenuation curves become less precise, leading to an underestimation of the MTT, an overestimation of the CBF, and finally underestimation of the ischemic zone. To correct for these partial volume effects, a VOF is selected.

to underestimation of blood flow and overestimation of MTT.[99] These miscalculations may have clinical implications; for example, in the brain, underestimated blood flow (longer MTT) could lead to an overestimation of the ischemic area and inappropriate treatment. Other factors that contribute to delay contrast arrival include proximal arterial occlusion or severe narrowing with poor collaterals, small venous access cannula, and low cardiac output.[103] Techniques are developed to correct for the effect of contrast delay on measurements.[104]

Scanners with 256 or 320 detector rows provide wider perfusion slab coverage that can include larger supplying arteries such as the internal carotid artery (ICA) or basilar artery as the AIF for brain study and include more anatomy. The influence of PVA in these large and perpendicular arteries will be a lot smaller. Overall, no consensus has been reached as to which artery would be ideal for the AIF. Ideally, each perfusion territory should be deconvolved by its own artery. Some investigators advise to select the artery as close as possible to the region of interest of the tissue, whereas other studies recommend to use a nearby larger vessel. Niesten et al.[105] performed a recent study to evaluate the optimal artery for the AIF and to assess the necessity of the VOF. They used a 256-slice (128 × 0.625) scanner, and 5-mm images were acquired at a temporal sampling rate of one image for every 2 seconds at 80 kVp and 150 mAs. The anterior cerebral artery (ACA), middle cerebral artery (MCA), ICA, and basilar artery were selected as the AIF. The ICA had the largest AUC and resulted in the highest MTT and lowest CBF. Including the VOF in measurements showed significantly higher CBV and CBF in 66% of patients. It was recommended that selecting the ICA as the AIF and continuing the use of the VOF would improve the accuracy of absolute quantitative values in brain perfusion mapping. Other studies have found no difference between the ACA and MCA.[103,106,107] The ACA is relatively perpendicular to the CT plane. Both of these vessels are relatively large, and with the use of thin cut slices (0.5 mm), less volume averaging occurs. Riordan et al.[108] showed that AIFs from the MCAs were not affected by PVA when using less than 1-mm resolution and medium section thickness (1.8 mm), and for this, they found no need to measure the VOF. Choosing a large proximal or artery on the side of lesion or contralateral to it may not affect the resulting quantitative perfusion values.[109] However, placement of the AIF distal to occluded vessel can cause significant distortion of the actual perfusion parameters and is not recommended (Fig. 2.12). For head and neck tumor perfusion, no difference between AIF of the ICA and external carotid artery is seen.[110]

In liver perfusion studies, since a dual blood exists, it is important to include both of the hepatic arterial and portal venous systems in analytical methods. Ng et al.[111] studied the effect of arterial (aorta) input alone versus arterial and portal venous inputs together on the perfusion parameters of liver tumors using

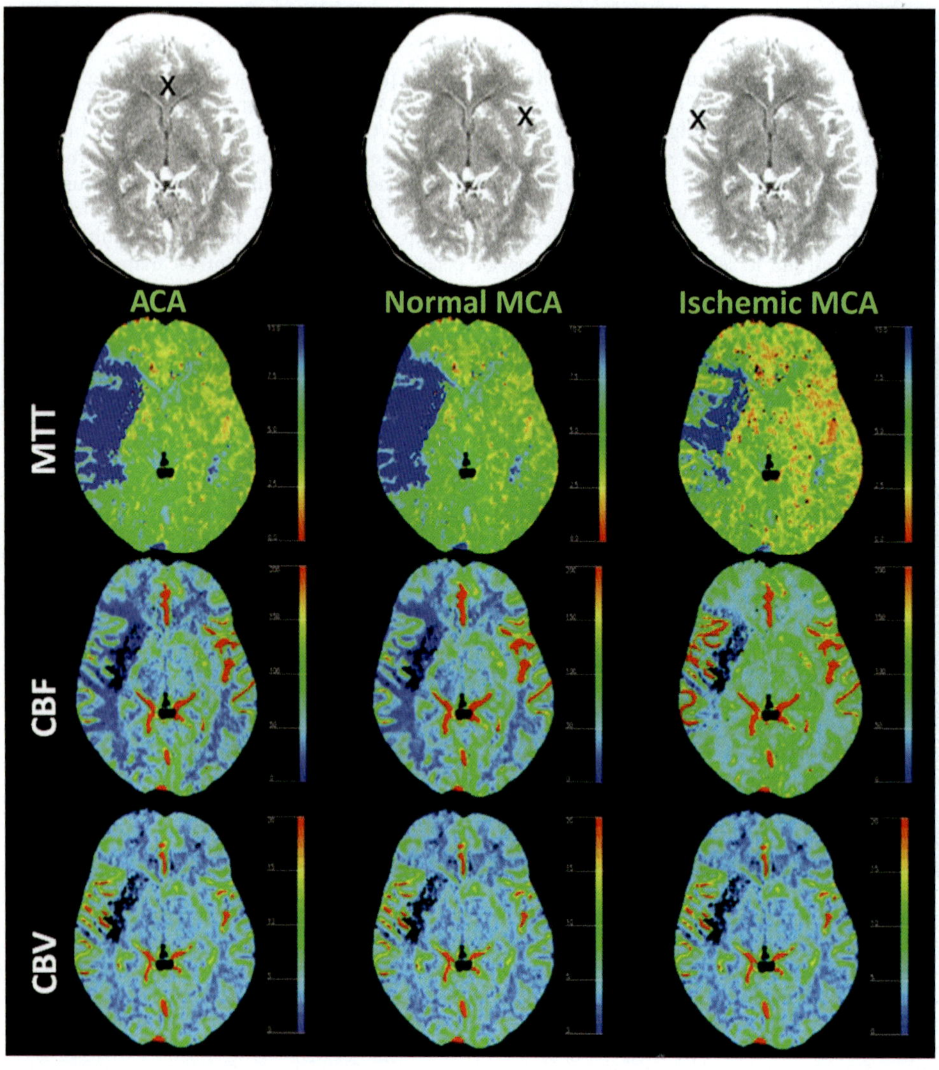

Figure 2-12. **Mean transit time (MTT), cerebral blood flow (CBF), and cerebral blood volume (CBV) maps obtained using three typical AIFs (shown by *X*) in a patient with a right M1–M2 junction occlusion.** MTT values are shorter, and CBF values are greater, when using the "ischemic" right AIF compared to the anterior cerebral artery (ACA) and "nonischemic" left middle cerebral artery (MCA) AIFs. CBV maps are mainly determined by the reference "vein" and are not influenced by the selection of the AIF. (From Wintermark M, Lau BC, Chien J, et al. The anterior cerebral artery is an appropriate arterial input function for perfusion CT processing in patients with acute stroke. *Neuroradiology* 2008;50:227–236, with permission.)

deconvolution modeling. Scan (16 slice, 20-mm z-coverage) started 5 seconds after intravenous injection of 50 mL of contrast agent (7 mL/s). Thirty-second cine acquisitions were obtained during a breath-hold and followed by six scans at every 3 seconds. For liver tumor and normal liver, median flow, volume, and permeability values were significantly higher when both arterial and venous inputs were included in analysis. For example, blood flow for normal liver was approximately 40 mL/min/100 g for single vascular versus 170 mL/min/100 g for dual vascular inputs. Large z-coverage is required to include portal vein in the image. Software to perform dual vascular input deconvolution modeling algorithm is now commercially available.

Dual-input perfusion concept may be used for analysis of lung tumor perfusion. Malignant tumors, especially larger ones, may be supplied by both systemic circulation (bronchial artery) and pulmonary circulation. It is therefore suggested that including both arterial flow in perfusion measurements may be more accurate.[112] Whatever method is used, the result may be affected by the post-processing model used. In perfusion study of lung nodules by Ohno et al.,[25] the authors showed improved accuracy of perfusion parameters obtained by a dual-input maximum slope method (Fig. 2.13) compared with single-input maximum slope and Patlak plot methods using a 320-volume scanner at 80 kVp.[25,26] In another study of lung tumors, Shi et al.[113] used a dual-source scanner for dynamic

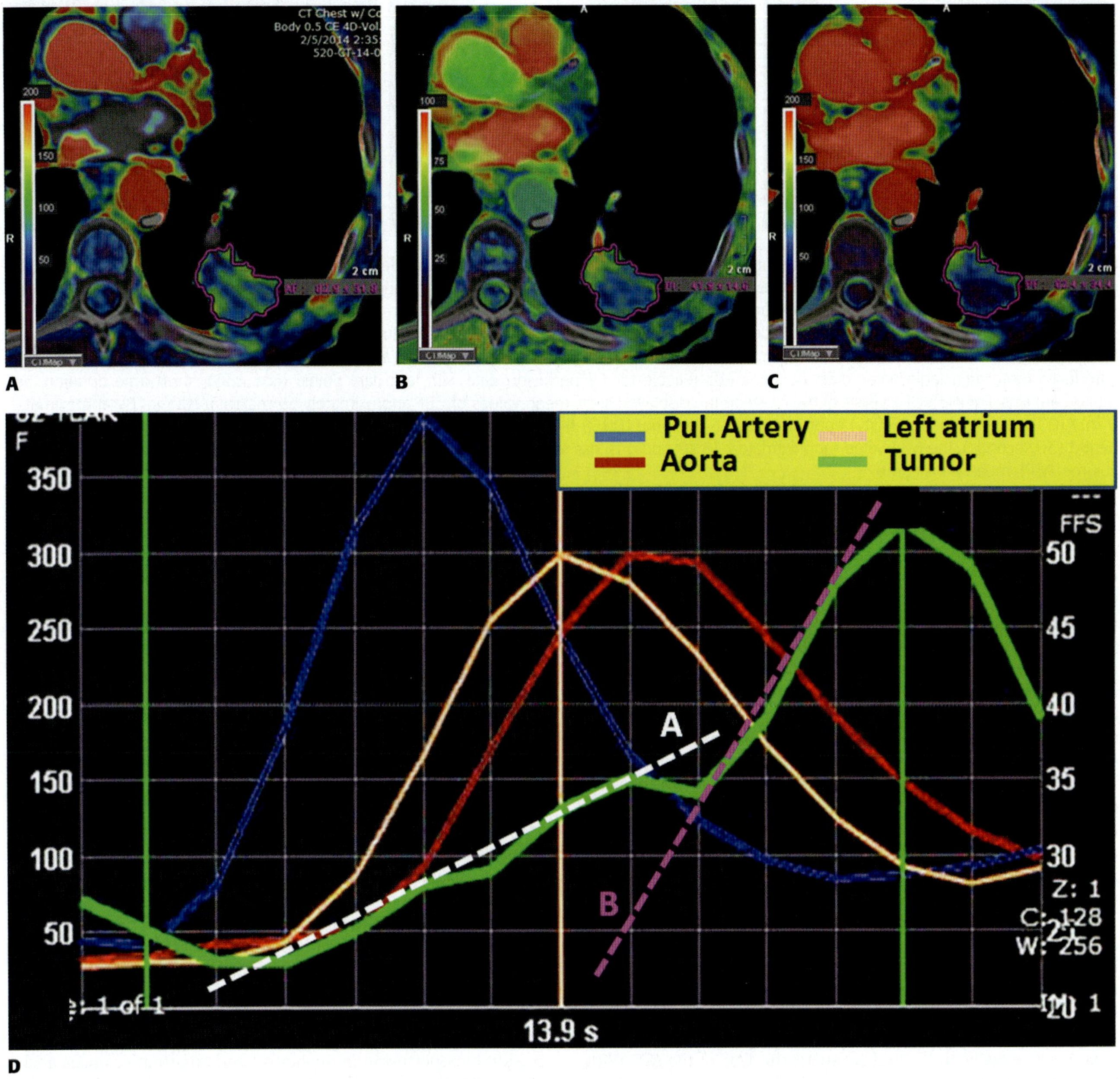

Figure 2-13. Pulmonary CT perfusion technique using dual-input maximum slope analysis in an 82-year-old female with a malignant left lower lobe tumor using a 320-volume scanner. Serial volume data were obtained over 30 seconds with 2 seconds temporal frequency. On the top, color-coded maps at peak pulmonary artery **(A)**, peak left atrium **(B)**, and peak aortic **(C)** enhancement are shown. **D:** Bottom image shows TACs of the pulmonary (pul.) artery, left atrium, descending aorta, and tumor. The peak time of the left atrium TDC is used to differentiate pulmonary circulation (before the peak time point) and aortic/bronchial circulation (after the peak time point). *White dotted line* (*A*) represents maximum slope of the lung cancer TDC for pulmonary arterial phase, and *pink dotted line* (*B*) represents maximum slope of lung cancer TDC for bronchial (aortic) arterial phase.

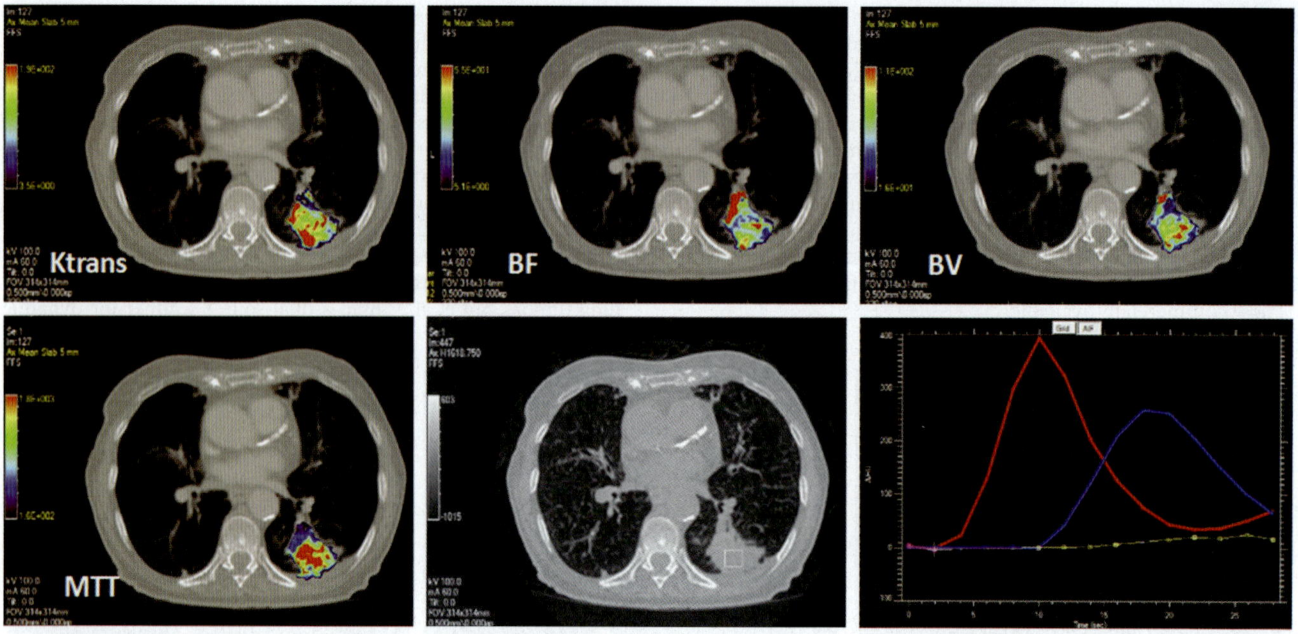

Figure 2-14. Pulmonary CT perfusion technique using single-input deconvolution model with delay and dispersion correction in the same patient shown in Figure. Serial volume data were obtained over 30 seconds with 2-second temporal frequency. A global AIF was measured from the pulmonary artery, a vascular transport model involving delay and dispersion can actually model the contrast profile at each downstream site (e.g., left atrium, ascending aorta, descending aorta). Therefore, it is equivalent to dual inputs without differentiating from which input. Dual-input deconvolution model is based on model above extended for two blood supplies (aorta and pulmonary artery). However, this mode introduces more adjustable parameters hence is less reliable for CT perfusion data with less data points (i.e., <30), short time duration, and motion artifacts. For the ROI analysis of the mass on the displayed slice, mean values of CBF approximately 55 mL/min/100 g, CBV approximately 8 mL/100 g, Ktrans (permeability) approximately 16 mL/min/100 g, MTT approximately 15 seconds. Since this protocol covered a short time period (30 seconds), the MTT value (approximately 15 seconds) is less reliable since the tail part of the bolus is missed. BF, blood flow; BV, blood volume; MTT, mean transit time.

scanning at 80 kVp and a deconvolution method for data processing (Fig. 2.14). The AIF was measured in the descending aorta and entire tumor (excluding large intratumoral vessels). They reported encouraging result to distinguish lung cancer subtypes. Tumor permeability was significantly different between adenocarcinoma, squamous cell carcinoma, and small cell lung cancer, but MTT did not differ between these tumor.[113] For such lung perfusion CT data, motion artifacts are inevitable. Although image registration can be applied, it is not always easy to get perfect alignment. Although some software could perform nonlinear (deformable) registration to align the lesion shape, the density variations still remain a major problem since perfusion quantification is dependent on the signal intensity or density rather than on the shape of lesion. Therefore, deconvolution method has a great advantage since it uses all time points minimizing motion/streak artifact. On the other hand, the slope method is more sensitive to motion/streak artifacts since it only uses a few time points at the corresponding maximum slope period.

In cardiac examination, selection of the AIF is different. The ascending aorta or left ventricle cavity are usually used for this purpose. Again, choosing a coronary artery branch may cause underestimation of the arterial TAC due to PVA effect.[114,115] In a limited semiquantitative dynamic contrast-enhanced CT and by combining bolus-tracking and time-registered helical CT image data sets, George et al.[116] could construct the TAC of the AIF. With this technique, radiation dose was reasonable because only the rising portion of TACs was sampled (Fig. 2.15); however, myocardial perfusion value was underestimated compared to the gold standard microspheres technique.[117] The quantitative approach requires a more complicated mathematical model (deconvolution) and can quantify absolute myocardial perfusion in units of milliliters per minute per gram of tissue. A bolus of iodinated contrast is injected intravenously while dynamic scanning (1 scan every 1 to 2 heartbeats) initiated 3 to 5 seconds after contrast injection, using breath-hold prospective ECG triggering technique, and continued for 30 seconds to monitor the first pass of contrast through the heart.

Artifacts

Artifacts are major sources of diagnostic problem in perfusion imaging of different organs. Artifacts may be related to patient, scan parameters, reconstruction algorithm, or postprocessing models.

Patient-Related Artifacts

Artifacts due to motion are one of the most common reasons for poor image quality. Although motion can be less problematic in brain perfusion examinations, in stroke patients, severe image degradation is not uncommon due to rapid head movements during examination.

In cardiac imaging, breath-holding and ECG gating are usually sufficient to account for motions during a typical image acquisition time. Unfortunately, problems with poor breath-holding or poor gating are not uncommon. The image degradation that can result from poor gating can sometimes be quite subtle but be sufficient to suggest hypoperfusion in qualitative and quantitative image analysis. Cardiac motion can lead to the appearance of focal areas of low attenuation, alternating with areas of high attenuation mimicking or masking a perfusion deficit. The strategy used to overcome motion artifacts includes the use of beta-blockers, maximizing temporal resolution with appropriate acquisition and reconstruction, and the examination of multiple phases to confirm persistence of

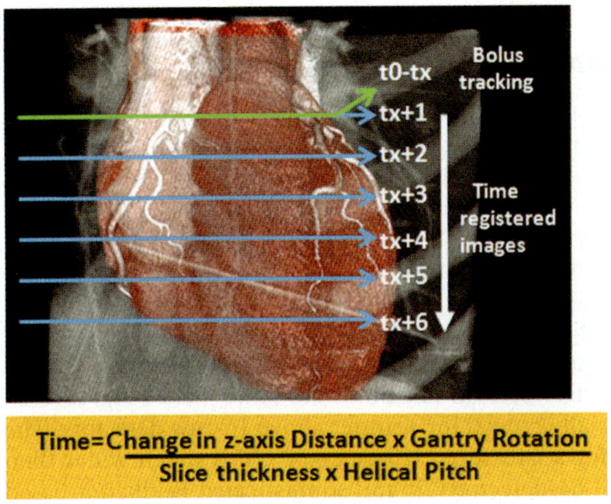

A

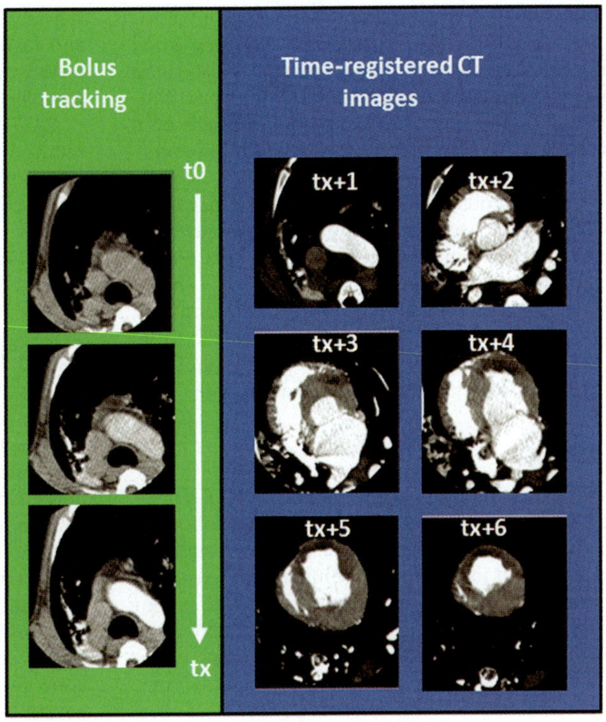

B

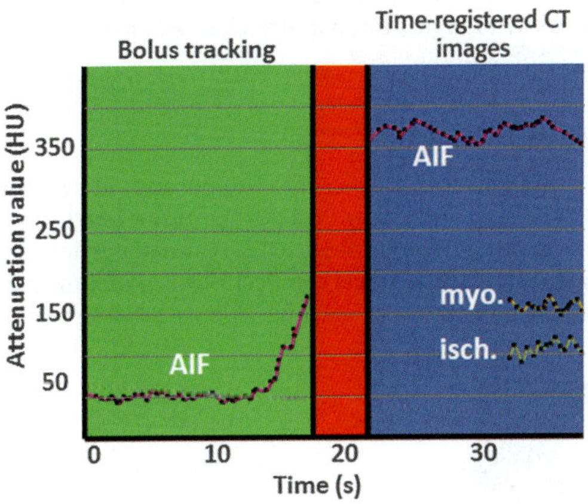

C

Figure 2-15. Arterial input function (AIF) simulated by using combined dynamic bolus tracking and time-registered helical CT. **A:** Bolus tracking is performed at the aortic root (*green line*) until threshold of 180 HU is reached. This is followed by 3.6-second pause and onset of helical imaging (*blue lines*). Each helical CT–acquired section is registered in time (t0 – tx in **A** and **B**) according to equation shown, where change in z-axis distance is change in distance on z-axis with respect to most cranial acquired axial sections. **B,C:** Bolus tracking and helical CT image data are reconstructed in axial plane **(B)**, and arterial blood pool attenuation is measured during bolus-tracking imaging (**left**, *green panel*) and on each helical CT image (**right**, *blue panel*). **C:** Attenuation values (HU) are plotted over time, and AIF is reconstructed by using bolus-tracking and time-registered CT data (*red dotted line*). Horizontal lines are designated by values on the y-axis. Time-registered myocardial HUs in ischemic myocardium (isch.) and normal myocardium (Myo.) are also plotted. HU, Hounsfield units. (Modified from So A, Wisenberg G, Islam A, et al. Non-invasive assessment of functionally relevant coronary artery stenoses with quantitative CT perfusion: preliminary clinical experiences. *Eur Radiol* 2012;22(1):39–50.)

a perfusion deficit. The persistence of an area of hypoattenuation in all phases suggests a true perfusion deficit unlike a motion artifact that usually moves or disappears by reviewing multiphase images. The use of metoprolol is mandatory to slow the heart rate in patients with heart rate of greater than 65 beats per minutes. Likewise, the solution to a gating problem in a patient with atrial fibrillation or frequent ventricular ectopy is different than in a patient with rapid heart rate. In the former, prospective ECG triggering in "target mode" to scan at a specific time period (i.e., 600 to 800 milliseconds) after the R wave may be helpful. Increased heart rate at the time of scan can cause motion artifacts, which can be removed by editing and adjustment of the R-R interval before data reconstruction.

Respiratory motion is also a major issue in perfusion CT imaging causing image misregistration that leads to errors in perfusion measurements. The anatomical regions that are most subject to respiratory artifacts are the lower part of thorax and the upper part of the abdomen, due to diaphragmatic movements during breathing. In many cases, respiratory motions can be minimized by breath-holding instructions to patients for thoracic and upper abdominal applications. For perfusion studies lasting longer than a short breath-hold (i.e., tumor permeability), most patients will suspend respiration during the first part of the study but will resume breathing at the end of the study, leading to motion artifacts. Therefore, patients should be trained by breath-hold exercising and educated about the length of breath-holding and that to resume shallow breathing when breath-holding is no longer possible. Good quality perfusion images can be obtained using quiet respiration. In some patients, the problem is not the inability to breath-hold for a few seconds, but the fact that "straining" occurs during breath-holding, which leads to small motions that degrade image quality. The solution in this case is to coach the patient to relax during breath-holding, which should usually take place after a normal expiration rather than after forced inspiration or expiration. Anterior abdominal wall motion during breathing movements can be reduced by using abdominal straps.

Bowel peristalsis can also cause motion artifacts during abdominal perfusion scans. These artifacts can be reduced by administering motility-inhibiting agents such as hyoscine butylbromide or glucagon, immediately before scanning, to reduce bowel peristalsis during perfusion scanning.[63] Swallowing can also cause significant artifacts in perfusion scans performed on the upper thorax and lower neck. It is possible to correct motion artifacts even after the perfusion scans have been performed using motion correction software.

Noise is a common problem with large patients. Increasing exposure parameters may be necessary to improve image quality at the expense of increasing radiation dose. Virtual monochromatic reconstruction of dual-energy CT processed at 70 kVp is shown to be effective in decreasing noise and improving CNR compared to conventional polychromatic CT.[118] Noise can be reduced using iterative reconstruction compared to filtered back projection. These techniques also have the potential to decrease radiation dose.

Beam Hardening

This artifact occurs when x-rays pass through a bone, metal, or high-density contrast, leading to absorption of low-energy photons, which results in a hypoattenuated shadowing artifact. Although CT software can correct for soft tissue during the initial reconstruction process, beam hardening related to high-density material cannot be effectively eliminated. Beam-hardening artifact is usually characterized by a triangular area of hypoattenuation adjacent to the high-density structures, which does not represent a specific anatomic territory.

Uncorrected beam hardening can significantly affect the accuracy of perfusion measurement. In the process of analysis for perfusion, it would be important to avoid areas close to metallic stents, prosthesis, or surgical implant, which result in distorted values of perfusion parameters. Filling of air-containing structures such as the colorectum and stomach with saline and water prior to imaging help reduce artifacts.[80]

In cardiac CT, one of the obstacles for optimum perfusion analysis is the beam hardening arising from high-density iodinated contrast in the left ventricle or aorta.[114,119] The inferobasal wall of the left ventricle is most commonly affected. Less commonly the anterior wall of the left ventricle may be affected in the presence of sternal wires. Beam hardening leads to distortion of both arterial and myocardial input functions, and deconvolution of their distorted values will lead to inaccurate estimation of absolute myocardial perfusion.

As stated earlier in this chapter, beam-hardening artifact can be reduced by dual-energy CT.[43,120] Using this technique, low-energy (70 kVp) virtual monochromatic (single energy) spectral images will be generated with the potential of providing high-quality images with better soft tissue contrast. This technique has been tested for cardiac, brain, and abdominal imaging with encouraging results.[115,142]

Cone-Beam Artifact

In MDCT systems, the measurement rays are tilted by the so-called "cone angle" with respect to the center plane. Cone angle denotes the widening of the measurement rays in the z-direction and should not be mistaken with "fan angle" in x/y plane, which determines the size of the FOV. Along with increasing beam angle (in proportion to the number of detector row), the reconstruction algorithm needs to be modified to account for the cone-beam geometry of the x-ray beam. This artifact arises from the fact that the scanner isocenter and projections from the x-ray source on to the multiple detectors do not lie in the same plane (Fig. 2.16A). This is especially crucial for scanner above 16-row detectors. The cone angle for a 640-slice, 320-detector CT is much wider than conventional 64-detector CT, and sophisticated Feldkamp-based cone-beam correction algorithms are required to avoid cone-beam artifact.[12,121] Cone-beam artifact presents as streaks and blurring and looks as though someone stretched and unstretched the image (Fig. 2.16B and C).

Misregistration Artifacts

Misregistration and banding artifacts are usually seen in cardiac imaging when a spiral scanner cannot cover the entire heart (e.g., 64 or 128-slice scanner). Because the heart is scanned partially in each single heartbeat, these artifacts can occur due to incomplete alignment of the scanned parts causing one or several bands

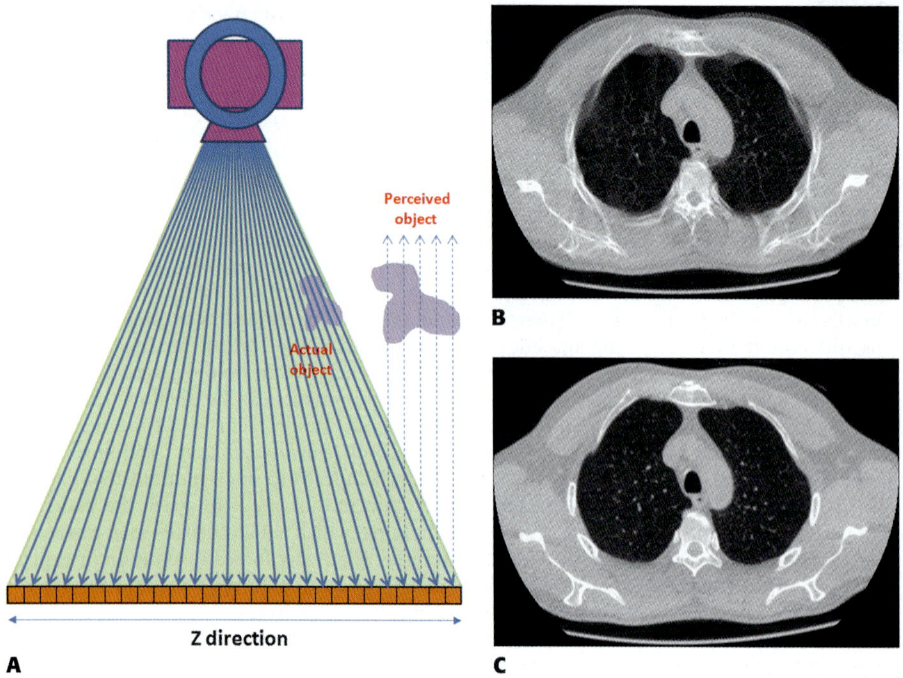

Figure 2-16. A: Misregistration of the actual object using routine axial filtered back projection reconstruction in a volume scanner because each detector row assumes all projections originated from directly above that Z-location. Cone-beam reconstruction is necessary to prevent this artifact. **B,C:** Cone-beam artifact in a chest CT. **B:** Reconstructed without correcting for the cone-beam geometry of the x-ray beam. Intrapulmonary vessels are blurred. Note *star-shaped* and streak artifacts around the vessels and bone sharp margins. **C:** CT at the same level and identical scan parameters following cone-beam reconstruction algorithm implementation. Image courtesy of Toshiba Medical Systems.

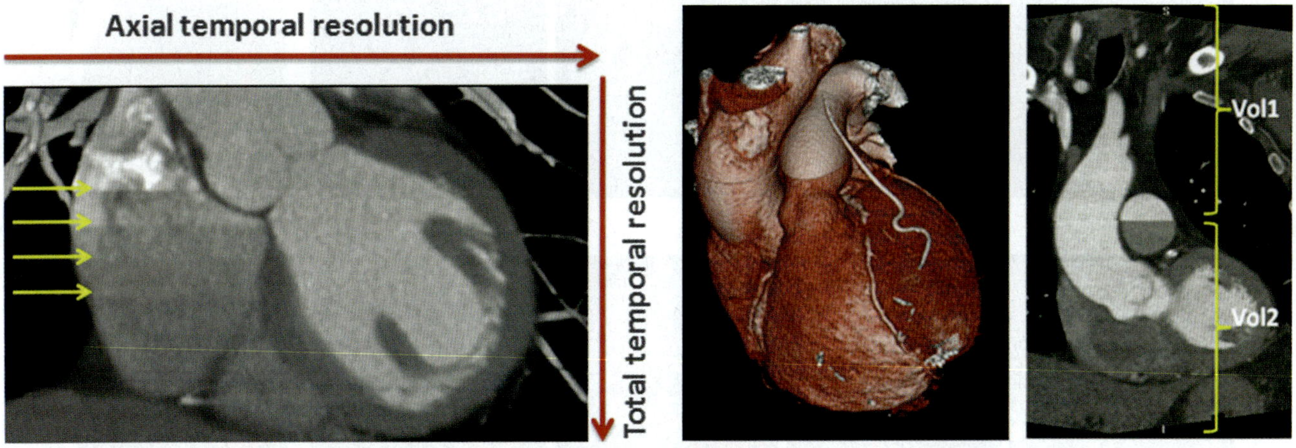

A B

Figure 2-17. A: Banding artifacts is shown on coronal reconstruction. Cardiac image acquired using helical acquisition with narrow collimation. Each *yellow arrow* points out a separate rotation. This is an example of poor total temporal resolution. **B:** Misregistration at the boundary of the two volume (Vol) scan to cover entire chest. No misregistration occurs inside the volume. Note contrast attenuation difference causing noncontrast–contrast level in the main pulmonary artery.

(Fig. 2.17A). In addition to misregistration, one part of the completed image (in z-axis) may have different attenuation values than the other part of it, depending on the direction of the scan acquisitions. Misalignment artifacts are avoided with 640 scanner in the area covered by the scan volume (16 cm), but it can occur when larger volume is scanned (e.g., entire thorax, head, and neck). In the latter condition, contrast differences between the two volumes may also be apparent (Fig. 2.17B).

Partial Scan Artifacts

In cardiac imaging, improving temporal resolution can be achieved by lowering the scan range from 360 to 180 degrees plus fan angle (partial scan).[122] This, however, may introduce CT attenuation value variations in the range of a few HU due to inconsistencies in the angular data range used to reconstruct images and prevent correct quantitative evaluation of perfusion measurements. Newer partial scan algorithms are designed to decrease partial scan artifact.[123]

Postprocessing and Data Analysis

In visual assessment of perfusion images, adjustment of window level and width help to reduce the appearance of noise level and improve detectability of perfusion defects. Almost all commercial multimodality and Picture Archiving and Communication System workstations have preset windows to review the images and at the same time allow interactive adjustment of the window width and level settings for optimal display and interpretation of a particular image data set. Postprocessing filters are also available to reduce image noise level and enhance low-contrast lesion visualization. Filters should be used cautiously since they may degrade image quality. One way to improve low-contrast delectability is to reconstruct thicker slices using thin cut source images without an increase in patient dose. The major drawback of increasing the slice thickness is PVA effects and higher likelihood of missing small perfusion defects. Sliding-thin-slab averaging during image post-processing and review is suggested as a technique to overcome this limitation by reconstructing thicker sections with lower noise levels from thin-section data obtained with dose-saving protocols.[124]

Most manufacturers provide commercial software in their scanner for quantitative analysis of CT perfusion images. Although quantitative perfusion analysis has many advantages over qualitative image review, it has not yet gained widespread acceptance as a reliable method owing to substantial variability in analytical methods that lead to considerable differences in the blood volume and flow thresholds used to differentiate normal from abnormal tissue. This variability may be related to the scan protocol parameters, including injections method, tube voltage, tube current, spatial resolution, and temporal resolution. Variations may also be secondary to postprocessing factors, such as the definition of AIF and VOF and deconvolution algorithms[98,100,109,125–127] (Fig. 2.18).

Two common methods of analysis are compartmental (slope method) and deconvolution methods.[100] In both methods, rapid sequence CT scans are acquired at the same location and following intravenous administration of contrast. In these tracer-based techniques, changes in attenuation numbers are directly proportional to the concentration of the injected contrast material, which allows demonstration of TACs. Compartmental technique is based on single-compartment or double (or three)-compartment models. The single-compartment model is based on Fick principle, and both of the intravascular and extravascular spaces are assumed to be one single unit. It estimates the perfusion either from the maximal slope or from the peak height of the same tissue concentration curve normalized to the AIF. In two-compartmental model, intravascular and extravascular spaces are separate compartments, and data are analyzed by Patlak method, which is mainly used for evaluation of tumor vasculature permeability, to quantify the passage of contrast from the intravascular into the extravascular space.[128]

The slope method requires good contrast material enhancement with minimum noise in those images used to calculate perfusion.[67,100] This mandates higher radiation dose per image, but the technique generally needs a shorter acquisition time for image analysis. The blood volume value is obtained from the ratio of peak tissue enhancement to the peak arterial enhancement. Deconvolution method is not as sensitive to noise in any particular image but in general requires more images. Therefore, optimum acquisition parameters may have a lower dose per image but lead to a similar radiation dose due to a greater number of images. The slope of the tissue enhancement curve, the time taken to reach the maximum slope, and maximum arterial enhancement are dependent on the bolus volume, the rate of injection, and the patient's cardiac output. While variations in these parameters have little impact on the deconvolution method, they can affect the slope method.

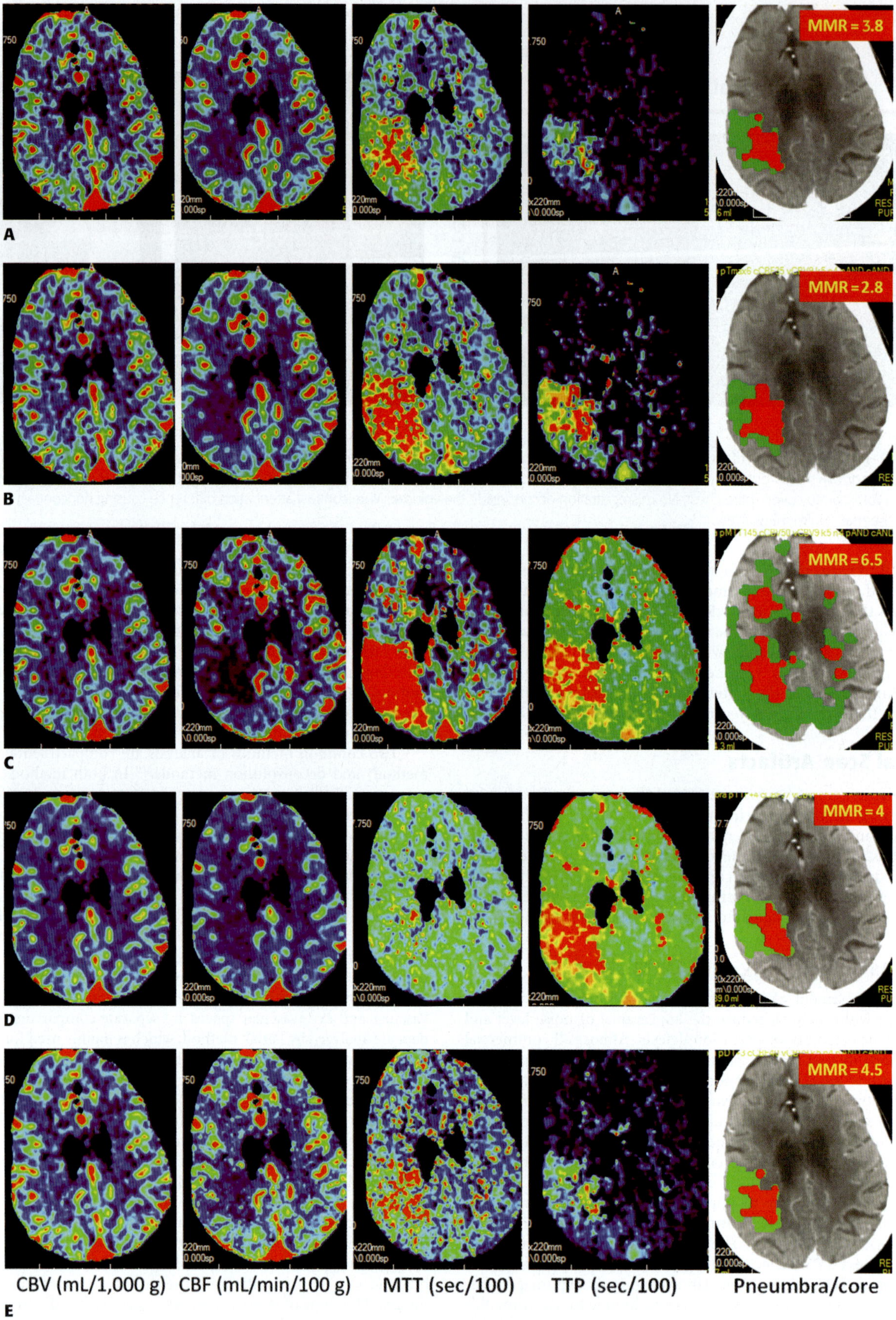

Figure 2-18. **Comparison of result of five different methods of deconvolution using CT perfusion images in a 45-year-old man with acute infarct core confirmed by MRI and occluded right internal carotid artery.** Images show cerebral blood volume (CBV), cerebral blood flow (CBF), mean transit time (MTT), time to peak (TTP), and mismatch ratio (MMR) with optimal thresholds describing acute infarct core (*red*) and penumbra (*green*). Note the variability in the extent of the infarct core and perfusion lesion with differing methods including **(A)** SVD with delay and dispersion correction, **(B)** SVD, **(C)** partial deconvolution, **(D)** maximum slope, and **(E)** stroke–stenosis model.

Deconvolution is a common method employed for postprocessing CT (and MR) perfusion images. This technique is based on the analysis of arterial and tissue TACs to calculate the impulse response (residue) function for the tissue. In order to measure absolute blood flow values, the calculation of the MTT is necessary. The MTT calculation requires simultaneous acquisition of the AIF and tissue input function curves, and deconvolution between these two curves gives the MTT value. With old scanners, due to slow sampling frequency and PVA effects, deconvolution method of calculating MTT was of low accuracy. With new scanners and introduction of new software packages, deconvolution algorithm provides better result but still can be a source of error.

Different commercial software packages can be used for neuro perfusion, each of which has a different algorithm[127] including singular value decomposition (SVD, GE Healthcare), maximum slope and partial deconvolution (Siemens Medical Systems MS), inverse filter (Hitachi Medical Systems, IF), block-circulant deconvolution (Toshiba and Philips), and box modulation transfer function based on the standard SVD (Toshiba Medical Systems, bMTF), delay-insensitive SVD and nonparametric deconvolution (Vital Images, Toshiba Medical Systems), a stroke–stenosis model (MIStar, Apollo Medical Imaging Technology), or custom-made software with standard (sSVD) and block-circulant (bSVD) SVD methods.[127] All postprocessing techniques generate quantitative maps of blood volume, blood flow, and MTT. In addition, maximum slope model produces a map of TTP, partial deconvolution, SVD, and block-circulant deconvolution, and stroke–stenosis models produce a map of TTP of the residual function (T_{max}), and SVD with delay correction produces a map of delay time. Vendors have also introduced several more perfusion algorithms for body and cardiac perfusion.

In a recent study, Kudo et al.[125] reported that in spite of using identical source data, CT perfusion imaging maps can significantly differ among commercial software possibly due to differences in tracer delay sensitivity (Fig. 2.18). In their study, three SVD methods were compared. Among those tested, delay-insensitive, block-circulant type of SVD produced more reliable results compared with delay-sensitive algorithms, such as standard SVD, in CT perfusion map calculation.[125] Kanda et al.[129] compared three analytical methods of maximum slope, dual-input single-compartment model, and deconvolution for CT measurements of hepatic perfusion in metastatic liver tumors. Hepatic arterial and portal perfusions values (mL/min/100 mL) were higher for maximum slope compared with deconvolution. Bisdas et al.[130] studied the role of postprocessing in perfusion values in head and heck tumors. Two different analysis software were compared, including maximum-slope approach and Patlak analysis and deconvolution-based analysis using an adiabatic ATH model. All perfusion parameter (volume, flow, permeability) values were higher using the maximum-slope approach and Patlak analysis compared with deconvolution-based analysis.

Practical Considerations in the Application of Perfusion CT

Due to the heterogeneity of current perfusion-based studies, attempts have been made to form committees and publish consensus statements in regard to patient selection and to standardize the scan protocols.[131,132] CT perfusion for the assessment of brain viability and decision on reperfusion therapies in ischemic stroke patients is probably the most common clinical application of all kinds CT perfusion studies. In this effort, the Acute Stroke Research Imaging Roadmap consensus statement has recently encouraged adherence to common acquisition protocols.

With rapid development in technology, perfusion protocols have been modified, and it is difficult to directly compare various studies in order to find the best protocol for a particular organ study. In addition, protocols for moving organs such as the heart may be completely different from nonmoving structures. Clinical target also requires different protocol and acquisition parameters. Most tumor studies require increasing duration and frequency of data acquisition, and study can be limited to a portion of the organ while functional studies may necessitate to scan the entire organ. Other factors including injection methods, exposure factors, slice thickness, and postprocessing techniques may all affect the results. It is therefore quite obvious that the impact of heterogeneity in reported data and acquisition parameters can be complex and may explain, at least in part, the failure to replicate promising initial result. Consensus proposals in near future may give future authors the opportunity to state, at least in a generic manner. Improved homogeneity of acquisition parameters may aid clinical trial conduct as well as translation to clinical practice.

REFERENCES

1. **Axel L.** Cerebral blood flow determination by rapid-sequence computed tomography: theoretical analysis. *Radiology* 1980;137(3):679–686.
2. **Axel L.** Tissue mean transit time from dynamic computed tomography by a simple deconvolution technique. *Invest Radiol* 1983;18(1):94–99.
3. **Doherty PW, Skolderbrand CG, Redington RW, et al.** Measurement of regional myocardial perfusion using dynamic computed tomography and contrast medium. *Acta Radiol Diagn (Stockh)* 1983;24:297.
4. **Rumberger JA, Feiring AJ, Lipton MJ, et al.** Use of ultrafast computed tomography to quantitate regional myocardial perfusion: a preliminary report. *J Am Coll Cardiol* 1987;9:59.
5. **Blomley MJ, Coulden R, Bufkin C, et al.** Contrast bolus dynamic computed tomography for the measurement of solid organ perfusion. *Invest Radiol* 1993;28(Suppl 5):S72–S77.
6. **Gobbel GT, Cann CE, Fike JR.** Measurement of regional cerebral blood flow using ultrafast computed tomography. Theoretical aspects. *Stroke* 1991;22(6):768–771.
7. **Wu X, Latson LA, Wang T, et al.** Regional pulmonary perfusion estimated by high-speed volume scanning CT. *Am J Physiol Imaging* 1988;3(2):73–80.
8. **Miles KA, Hayball M, Dixon AK.** Colour perfusion imaging: a new application of computed tomography. *Lancet* 1991;337:643–645.
9. **Miles KA, Hayball MP, Dixon AK.** Functional images of hepatic perfusion obtained with dynamic CT. *Radiology* 1993;188:405–411.
10. **Miles KA.** Molecular imaging with dynamic contrast-enhanced computed tomography. *Clin Radiol* 2010;65(7):549–556.
11. **Kalender W, Seissler W, Klotz E, et al.** Spiral volumetric CT with single-breath-hold technique, continuous transport, and continuous scanner rotation. *Radiology* 1990;176:181–183.
12. **Flohr TG, Schaller S, Stierstorfer K, et al.** Multi-detector row CT systems and image-reconstruction techniques. *Radiology* 2005;235:756–773.
13. **Pannu HK, Flohr TG, Corl FM, et al.** Current concepts in multi-detector row CT evaluation of the coronary arteries: principles, techniques, and anatomy. *Radiographics* 2003;23(spec issue):S111–S125.
14. **Klingenbeck-Regn K, Schaller S, Flohr T, et al.** Subsecond multislice computed tomography: basics and applications. *Eur J Radiol* 1999;31:110–124.
15. **Hu H, He HD, Foley WD, et al.** Four multidetector- row helical CT: image quality and volume coverage speed. *Radiology* 2000;215:55–62.
16. **Ohnesorge B, Flohr T, Becker C, et al.** Cardiac imaging by means of electrocardiographically gated multisection spiral CT: initial experience. *Radiology* 2000;217:564–571.
17. **Achenbach S, Ulzheimer S, Baum U, et al.** Noninvasive coronary angiography by retrospectively ECG-gated multi-slice spiral CT. *Circulation* 2000;102:2823–2828.
18. **Leber AW, Knez A, von Ziegler F, et al.** Quantification of obstructive and nonobstructive coronary lesions by 64-slice computed tomography: a comparative study with quantitative coronary angiography and intravascular ultrasound. *J Am Coll Cardiol* 2005;46(1):147–154.
19. **Leschka S, Alkadhi H, Plass A, et al.** Accuracy of MSCT coronary angiography with 64-slice technology: first experience. *Eur Heart J* 2005;26(15):1482–1487.
20. **Hochberg AR, Young GS.** Cerebral perfusion imaging. *Semin Neurol* 2012;32(4):454–465.
21. **Mehta BK, Mustafa G, McMurtray A, et al.** Whole brain CT perfusion deficits using 320-detector-row CT scanner in TIA patients are associated with ABCD2 score. *Int J Neurosci* 2014;124(1):56–60.

22. **Kandel S, Kloeters C, Meyer H, et al.** Whole-organ perfusion of the pancreas using dynamic volume CT in patients with primary pancreas carcinoma: acquisition technique, post-processing and initial results. *Eur Radiol* 2009;19(11):2641–2646.
23. **Rochitte CE, George RT, Chen MY, et al.** Computed tomography angiography and perfusion to assess coronary artery stenosis causing perfusion defects by single photon emission computed tomography: the CORE320 study. *Eur Heart J* 2014;35:1120.
24. **Yuan X, Zhang J, Quan C, et al.** Differentiation of malignant and benign pulmonary nodules with first-pass dual-input perfusion CT. *Eur Radiol* 2013;23(9):2469–2474.
25. **Ohno Y, Nishio M, Koyama H, et al.** Comparison of quantitatively analyzed dynamic area-detector CT using various mathematic methods with FDG PET/CT in management of solitary pulmonary nodules. *AJR Am J Roentgenol* 2013;200(6):W593–W602.
26. **Ohno Y, Koyama H, Matsumoto K, et al.** Differentiation of malignant and benign pulmonary nodules with quantitative first-pass 320-detector row perfusion CT versus FDG PET/CT. *Radiology* 2011;258(2):599–609.
27. **George RT, Arbab-Zadeh A, Miller JM, et al.** Computed tomography myocardial perfusion imaging with 320-row detector computed tomography accurately detects myocardial ischemia in patients with obstructive coronary artery disease. *Circ Cardiovasc Imaging* 2012;5(3):333–340.
28. **Van der Molen AJ, Geleijns J.** Overranging in multisection CT: quantification and relative contribution to dose—comparison of four 16-section CT scanners. *Radiology* 2007;242(1):208–216.
29. **Fleischmann D, Boas FE.** Computed tomography—old ideas and new technology. *Eur Radiol* 2011;21(3):510–517.
30. **Flohr T, Mc Collough C, Bruder H, et al.** First performance evaluation of a dual source CT (DSCT) system. *Eur Radiol* 2006;16:256–268.
31. **Petersilka M, Bruder H, Krauss B, et al.** Technical principles of dual-source CT. *Eur J Radiol* 2008;68:362–368.
32. **Flohr TG, Leng S, Yu L, et al.** Dual-source spiral CT with pitch up to 3.2 and 75 ms temporal resolution: image reconstruction and assessment of image quality. *Med Phys* 2009;36(12):5641–5653.
33. **Scheffel H, Alkadhi H, Plass A, et al.** Accuracy of dual-source CT coronary angiography: first experience in a high pre-test probability population without heart rate control. *Eur Radiol* 2006;16(12):2739–2747.
34. **Lell M, Marwan M, Schepis T, et al.** Prospectively ECG-triggered high-pitch spiral acquisition for coronary CT angiography using dual source CT: technique and initial experience. *Eur Radiol* 2009;19(11):2576–2583.
35. **Neefjes LA, Dharampal AS, Rossi A, et al.** Image quality and radiation exposure using different low-dose scan protocols in dual-source CT coronary angiography: randomized study. *Radiology* 2011;261(3):779–786.
36. **Johnson TR, Nikolaou K, Busch S, et al.** Diagnostic accuracy of dual-source computed tomography in the diagnosis of coronary artery disease. *Invest Radiol* 2007;42(10):684–691.
37. **Ruzsics B, Lee H, Zwerner PL, et al.** Dual-energy CT of the heart for diagnosing coronary artery stenosis and myocardial ischemia-initial experience. *Eur Radiol* 2008;18(11):2414–2424.
38. **Goetti R, Leschka S, Desbiolles L, et al.** Quantitative computed tomography liver perfusion imaging using dynamic spiral scanning with variable pitch: feasibility and initial results in patients with cancer metastases. *Invest Radiol* 2010;45(7):419–426.
39. **Alvarez RE, Macovski A.** Energy-selective reconstructions in X-ray computerized tomography. *Phys Med Biol* 1976;21:733–744.
40. **Johnson TR.** Dual-energy CT: general principles. *AJR Am J Roentgenol* 2012;199(5 Suppl):S3–S8.
41. **Fornaro J, Leschka S, Hibbeln D.** Dual- and multi-energy CT: approach to functional imaging. *Insights Imaging* 2011;2:149–159.
42. **Pinho DF, Kulkarni NM, Krishnaraj A, et al.** Initial experience with single-source dual-energy CT abdominal angiography and comparison with single-energy CT angiography: image quality, enhancement, diagnosis and radiation dose. *Eur Radiol* 2013;23(2):351–359.
43. **Yu L, Christner JA, Leng S, et al.** Virtual monochromatic imaging in dual-source dual-energy CT: radiation dose and image quality. *Med Phys* 2011;38(12):6371–6379.
44. **So A, Hsieh J, Narayanan S, et al.** Dual-energy CT and its potential use for quantitative myocardial CT perfusion. *J Cardiovasc Comput Tomogr* 2012;6(5):308–317.
45. **So A, Hsieh J, Imai Y, et al.** Prospectively ECG-triggered rapid kV-switching dual-energy CT for quantitative imaging of myocardial perfusion. *JACC Cardiovasc Imaging* 2012;5(8):829–836.
46. **Nance JW Jr, Bastarrika G, Kang DK, et al.** High-temporal resolution dual-energy computed tomography of the heart using a novel hybrid image reconstruction algorithm: initial experience. *J Comput Assist Tomogr* 2011;35(1):119–125.
47. **Roessl E, Proksa, R.** K-edge imaging in X-ray computed tomography using multi-bin photon counting detectors. *Phys Med Biol* 2007;52(15):4679–4696.
48. **Roessl E, Brendel B, Engel KJ, et al.** Sensitivity of photon-counting based K-edge imaging in X-ray computed tomography. *IEEE Trans Med Imaging* 2011;30(9):1678–1690.
49. **Chae EJ, Seo JB, Goo HW, et al.** Noninvasive differentiation of uric acid versus nonuric acid kidney stones using dual-energy CT. *Acad Radiol* 2007;14:1441–1447.
50. **Heye T, Nelson RC, Ho LM, et al.** Dual-energy CT applications in the abdomen. *AJR Am J Roentgenol* 2012;199(5 Suppl):S64–S70.
51. **Uotani K, Watanabe Y, Higashi M, et al.** Dual-energy CT head bone and hard plaque removal for quantification of calcified carotid stenosis: utility and comparison with digital subtraction angiography. *Eur Radiol* 2009;19:2060–2065.
52. **Chandarana H, Godoy MCB, Vlahos I, et al.** Abdominal aorta: evaluation with dual-source dual-energy multidetector CT after endovascular repair of aneurysms–initial observations. *Radiology* 2008;249:692–700.
53. **Wang Q, Shi G, Liu X, et al.** Optimal contrast of computed tomography portal venography using dual-energy computed tomography. *J Comput Assist Tomogr* 2013;37(2):142–148.
54. **Schwarz F, Ruzsics B, Schoepf UJ, et al.** Dual-energy CT of the heart—principles and protocols. *Eur J Radiol* 2008;68:423–433.
55. **Thieme SF, Graute V, Nikolaou K, et al.** Dual energy CT lung perfusion imaging—correlation with SPECT/CT. *Eur J Radiol* 2012;81(2):360–365.
56. **Pansini V, Remy-Jardin M, Faivre JB, et al.** Assessment of lobar perfusion in smokers according to the presence and severity of emphysema: preliminary experience with dual-energy CT angiography. *Eur Radiol* 2009;19:2834–2843.
57. **Zhang LJ, Wu S, Wang M, et al.** Quantitative dual energy CT measurements in rabbit VX2 liver tumors: comparison to perfusion CT measurements and histopathological findings. *Eur J Radiol* 2012;81(8):1766–1775.
58. **Mahesh M, Cody DD.** Physics of cardiac imaging with multiple-row detector CT. *Radiographics* 2007;27(5):1495–1509. Review.
59. **Entrikin DW.** True high-definition in cardiac imaging will require 4 dimensions of technologic innovation. *J Cardiovasc Comput Tomogr* 2009;3(4):252–256.
60. **Primak AN, McCollough CH, Bruesewitz MR, et al.** Relationship between noise, dose, and pitch in cardiac multi-detector row CT. *Radiographics* 2006;26(6):1785–1794.
61. **von Falck C, Galanski M, Shin HO.** Informatics in radiology: sliding-thin-slab averaging for improved depiction of low-contrast lesions with radiation dose savings at thin-section CT. *Radiographics* 2010;30(2):317–326.
62. **Shin HO, Falck CV, Galanski M.** Low-contrast detectability in volume rendering: a phantom study on multidetector-row spiral CT data. *Eur Radiol* 2004;14(2):341–349.
63. **Petralia G, Bonello L, Viotti S, et al.** CT perfusion in oncology: how to do it. *Cancer Imaging* 2010;10:8–19.
64. **Wintermark M, Maeder P, Verdun FR, et al.** Using 80 kVp versus 120 kVp in perfusion CT measurement of regional cerebral blood flow. *AJNR Am J Neuroradiol* 2000;21:1881–1884.
65. **Nabavi DG, Cenic A, Dool J, et al.** Quantitative assessment of cerebral hemodynamics using CT: stability, accuracy, and precision studies in dogs. *J Comput Assist Tomogr* 1999;23:506–515.
66. **Murase K, Nanjo T, Ii S, et al.** Effect of x-ray tube current on the accuracy of cerebral perfusion parameters obtained by CT perfusion studies. *Phys Med Biol* 2005;50(21):5019–5029.
67. **Miles KA.** Perfusion CT for the assessment of tumour vascularity: which protocol? *Br J Radiol* 2003;76(Spec No 1):S36–S42.
68. **Hsiao EM, Rybicki FJ, Steigner M.** CT coronary angiography: 256-slice and 320-detector row scanners. *Curr Cardiol Rep* 2010;12(1):68–75.
69. **Feuchtner G, Goetti R, Plass A, et al.** Adenosine stress high-pitch 128-slice dual-source myocardial computed tomography perfusion for imaging of reversible myocardial ischemia: comparison with magnetic resonance imaging. *Circ Cardiovasc Imaging* 2011;4:540–549.
70. **Blankstein R, Shturman LD, Rogers IS, et al.** Adenosine-induced stress myocardial perfusion imaging using dual-source cardiac computed tomography. *J Am Coll Cardiol* 2009;54:1072–1084.

71. **Gramer BM, Muenzel D, Leber V, et al.** Impact of iterative reconstruction on CNR and SNR in dynamic myocardial perfusion imaging in an animal model. *Eur Radiol* 2012;22:2654–2661.
72. **Bamberg F, Klotz E, Flohr T, et al.** Dynamic myocardial stress perfusion imaging using fast dual-source CT with alternating table positions: initial experience. *Eur Radiol* 2010;20:1168–1173.
73. **Schwarz F, Hinkel R, Baloch E, et al.** Myocardial CT perfusion imaging in a large animal model: comparison of dynamic versus single-phase acquisitions. *JACC Cardiovasc Imaging* 2013;6(12):1229–1238.
74. **Otero HJ, Steigner ML, Rybicki FJ.** The "post-64" era of coronary CT angiography: understanding new technology from physical principles. *Radiol Clin North Am* 2009;47(1):79–90.
75. **Kanda T, Yoshikawa T, Ohno Y, et al.** Perfusion measurement of the whole upper abdomen of patients with and without liver diseases: initial experience with 320-detector row CT. *Eur J Radiol* 2012;81(10):2470–2475.
76. **Goshima S, Kanematsu M, Nishibori H, et al.** CT of the pancreas: comparison of anatomic structure depiction, image quality, and radiation exposure between 320-detector volumetric images and 64-detector helical images. *Radiology* 2011;260(1):139–147.
77. **Haberland U, Klotz E, Abolmaali N.** Performance assessment of dynamic spiral scan modes with variable pitch for quantitative perfusion computed tomography. *Invest Radiol* 2010;45(7):378–386.
78. **Reiner CS, Goetti R, Eberli D, et al.** CT perfusion of renal cell carcinoma: impact of volume coverage on quantitative analysis. *Invest Radiol* 2012;47(1):33–40.
79. **Motosugi U, Ichikawa T, Sou H, et al.** Multi-organ perfusion CT in the abdomen using a 320-detector row CT scanner: preliminary results of perfusion changes in the liver, spleen, and pancreas of cirrhotic patients. *Eur J Radiol* 2012;81(10):2533–2537.
80. **Kambadakone AR, Sharma A, Catalano OA, et al.** Protocol modifications for CT perfusion (CTp) examinations of abdomen-pelvic tumors: impact on radiation dose and data processing time. *Eur Radiol* 2011;21(6):1293–1300.
81. **Henderson E, Rutt BK, Lee TY.** Temporal sampling requirements for the tracer kinetics modeling of breast disease. *Magn Reson Imaging* 1998;16(9):1057–1073.
82. **Ng CS, Chandler AG, Wei W, et al.** Effect of sampling frequency on perfusion values in perfusion CT of lung tumors. *AJR Am J Roentgenol* 2013;200(2):W155–W162.
83. **Goh V, Halligan S, Hugill JA, et al.** Quantitative colorectal cancer perfusion measurement using dynamic contrast-enhanced, multidetector-row computed tomography: effect of acquisition time and implications for protocols. *J Comput Assist Tomogr* 2005;29:59–63.
84. **Hirata M, Sugawara Y, Murase K, et al.** Evaluation of optimal scan duration and end time in cerebral CT perfusion study. *Radiat Med* 2005;23(5):351–363.
85. **Kämena A, Streitparth F, Grieser C, et al.** Dynamic perfusion CT: optimizing the temporal resolution for the calculation of perfusion CT parameters in stroke patients. *Eur J Radiol* 2007;64(1):111–118.
86. **Wintermark M, Smith WS, Ko NU, et al.** Dynamic perfusion CT: optimizing the temporal resolution and contrast volume for calculation of perfusion CT parameters in stroke patients. *AJNR Am J Neuroradiol* 2004;25:720–729.
87. **Wiesmann M, Berg S, Bohner G, et al.** Dose reduction in dynamic perfusion CT of the brain: effects of the scan frequency on measurements of cerebral blood flow, cerebral blood volume, and mean transit time. *Eur Radiol* 2008;18(12):2967–2974.
88. **Shankar JJ, Lum C.** Whole brain CT perfusion on a 320-slice CT scanner. *Indian J Radiol Imaging* 2011;21(3):209–214.
89. **Schramm P, Huang Y, Erb G, et al.** How does the injection protocol influence the attenuation-time curve in CT perfusion measurements: comparison of measured and simulated data. *Med Phys* 2009;36(8):3487–3494.
90. **Machida K, Oohashi N, Nakano H.** Method of injection of contrast medium for brain perfusion CT. *Nihon Hoshasen Gijutsu Gakkai Zasshi* 2002;58(7):962–966.
91. **Goh V, Bartram C, Halligan S.** Effect of intravenous contrast agent volume on colorectal cancer vascular parameters as measured by perfusion computed tomography. *Clin Radiol* 2009;64(4):368–372.
92. **König M, Bültmann E, Bode-Schnurbus L, et al.** Image quality in CT perfusion imaging of the brain. The role of iodine concentration. *Eur Radiol* 2007;17(1):39–47.
93. **Konstas AA, Goldmakher GV, Lee TY, et al.** Theoretic basis and technical implementations of CT perfusion in acute ischemic stroke, part 2: technical implementations. *AJNR Am J Neuroradiol* 2009;30(5):885–892.
94. **Kim SM, Cho YB, Haider MA, et al.** Multiphasic contrast injection for improved precision of parameter estimates in functional CT. *Med Phys* 2008;35(12):5921–5933.
95. **Ng QS, Goh V, Milner J, et al.** Acute tumor vascular effects following fractionated radiotherapy in human lung cancer: in vivo whole tumor assessment using volumetric perfusion computed tomography. *Int J Radiat Oncol Biol Phys* 2007;67:417–424.
96. **Ng QS, Goh V, Fichte H, et al.** Lung cancer perfusion at multidetector row CT: reproducibility of whole tumor quantitative measurements. *Radiology* 2006;239:547–553.
97. Bell SD, Peters AM. Measurement of blood flow from first-pass radionuclide angiography: influence of bolus volume. *Eur J Nucl Med* 1991;18:885–888.
98. **Cenic A, Nabavi DG, Craen RA, et al.** Dynamic CT measurement of cerebral blood flow: a validation study. *AJNR Am J Neuroradiol* 1999;20(1):63–73.
99. **van der Schaaf I, Vonken EJ, Waaijer A, et al.** Influence of partial volume on venous output and arterial input function. *AJNR Am J Neuroradiol* 2006;27(1):46–50.
100. **Miles KA, Griffiths MR.** Perfusion CT: a worthwhile enhancement? *Br J Radiol* 2003;76(904):220–231.
101. **Eastwood JD, Lev MH, Azhari T, et al.** CT perfusion scanning with deconvolution analysis: pilot study in patients with acute MCA stroke. *Radiology* 2002;222:227–236.
102. **Ferreira RM, Lev MH, Goldmakher GV, et al.** Arterial input function placement for accurate CT perfusion map construction in acute stroke. *AJR Am J Roentgenol* 2010;194(5):1330–1336.
103. **Wintermark M, Lau BC, Chien J, et al.** The anterior cerebral artery is an appropriate arterial input function for perfusion-CT processing in patients with acute stroke. *Neuroradiology* 2008;50:227–236.
104. **Wittsack HJ, Wohlschlager AM, Ritzl EK, et al.** CT-perfusion imaging of the human brain: advanced deconvolution analysis using circulant singular value decomposition. *Comput Med Imaging Graph* 2008;32:67–77.
105. **Niesten JM, van der Schaaf IC, Riordan AJ, et al.** Optimisation of vascular input and output functions in CT-perfusion imaging using 256(or more)-slice multidetector CT. *Eur Radiol* 2013;23(5):1242–1249.
106. **Bisdas S, Konstantinou GN, Gurung J, et al.** Effect of the arterial input function on the measured perfusion values and infarct volumetric in acute cerebral ischemia evaluated by perfusion computed tomography. *Invest Radiol* 2007;42:147–156.
107. **Chiu FY, Teng MM, Kao YH, et al.** Selection of arterial input function for postprocessing of cerebral ct perfusion in chronic unilateral high-grade stenosis or occlusion of the carotid or middle cerebral artery. *Acad Radiol* 2012;19:8–16.
108. **Riordan AJ, Bennink E, Viergever MA, et al.** CT brain perfusion protocol to eliminate the need for selecting a venous output function. *AJNR Am J Neuroradiol* 2013;34(7):1353–1358.
109. **Sanelli PC, Lev MH, Eastwood JD, et al.** The effect of varying user-selected input parameters on quantitative values in CT perfusion maps. *Acad Radiol* 2004;11:1085–1092.
110. **Tawfik AM, Razek AA, Elsorogy LG, et al.** Perfusion CT of head and neck cancer: effect of arterial input selection. *AJR Am J Roentgenol* 2011;196(6):1374–1380.
111. **Ng CS, Chandler AG, Wei W, et al.** Effect of dual vascular input functions on CT perfusion parameter values and reproducibility in liver tumors and normal liver. *J Comput Assist Tomogr* 2012;36(4):388–393.
112. **Nakano S, Gibo J, Fukushima Y, et al.** Perfusion evaluation of lung cancer: assessment using dual-input perfusion computed tomography. *J Thorac Imaging* 2013;28(4):253–262.
113. **Shi J, Schmid-Bindert G, Fink C, et al.** Dynamic volume perfusion CT in patients with lung cancer: baseline perfusion characteristics of different histological subtypes. *Eur J Radiol* 2013;82(12):e894–e900.
114. **So A, Lee TY.** Quantitative myocardial CT perfusion: a pictorial review and the current state of technology development. *J Cardiovasc Comput Tomogr* 2011;5(6):467–481.
115. **So A, Wisenberg G, Islam A, et al.** Non-invasive assessment of functionally relevant coronary artery stenoses with quantitative CT perfusion: preliminary clinical experiences. *Eur Radiol* 2012;22(1):39–50.

116. **George RT, Jerosch-Herold M, Silva C, et al.** Quantification of myocardial perfusion using dynamic 64-detector computed tomography. *Invest Radiol* 2007;42:815–822.
117. **George RT, Ichihara T, Lima JA, et al.** A method for reconstructing the arterial input function during helical CT: implications for myocardial perfusion distribution imaging. *Radiology* 2010;255(2):396–404.
118. **Matsumoto K, Jinzaki M, Tanami Y, et al,** Virtual monochromatic spectral imaging with fast kilovoltage switching: improved image quality as compared with that obtained with conventional 120-kVp CT. *Radiology* 2011;259:257–262.
119. **Mehra VC, Valdiviezo C, Arbab-Zadeh A, et al.** A stepwise approach to the visual interpretation of CT-based myocardial perfusion. *J Cardiovasc Comput Tomogr* 2011;5(6):357–369.
120. **Pomerantz SR, Kamalian S, Zhang D, et al.** Virtual monochromatic reconstruction of dual-energy unenhanced head CT at 65–75 keV maximizes image quality compared with conventional polychromatic CT. *Radiology* 2013;266(1):318–325.
121. **Feldkamp L, Davis L, Kress J.** Practical cone beam algorithm. *J Opt Soc Am* 1984;1(6):612–619.
122. **Stenner P, Schmidt B, Bruder H, et al.** Partial scan artifact reduction (PSAR) for the assessment of cardiac perfusion in dynamic phase-correlated CT. *Med Phys* 2009;36(12):5683–5694.
123. **Ramirez-Giraldo JC, Yu L, Kantor B, et al.** A strategy to decrease partial scan reconstruction artifacts in myocardial perfusion CT: phantom and in vivo evaluation. *Med Phys* 2012;39(1):214–223.
124. **von Falck C, Hartung A, Berndzen F, et al.** Optimization of low-contrast detectability in thin-collimated modern multidetector CT using an interactive sliding-thin-slab averaging algorithm. *Invest Radiol* 2008;43(4):229–235.
125. **Kudo K, Sasaki M, Ogasawara K, et al.** Difference in tracer delay-induced effect among deconvolution algorithms in CT perfusion analysis: quantitative evaluation with digital phantoms. *Radiology* 2009;251:241–249.
126. **Kudo K, Sasaki M, Yamada K, et al.** Differences in CT perfusion maps generated by different commercial software: quantitative analysis by using identical source data of acute stroke patients. *Radiology* 2010;254(1):200–209.
127. **Bivard A, Levi C, Spratt N, et al.** Perfusion CT in acute stroke: a comprehensive analysis of infarct and penumbra. *Radiology* 2013;267(2):543–550.
128. **Patlak CS, Blasberg RG, Fenstermacher JD.** Graphical evaluation of blood-to-brain transfer constants from multiple-time uptake data. *J Cereb Blood Flow Metab* 1983;3:1–7.
129. **Kanda T, Yoshikawa T, Ohno Y, et al.** CT hepatic perfusion measurement: comparison of three analytic methods. *Eur J Radiol* 2012;81(9):2075–2079.
130. **Bisdas S, Konstantinou G, Surlan-Popovic K, et al.** Dynamic contrast-enhanced CT of head and neck tumors: comparison of first-pass and permeability perfusion measurements using two different commercially available tracer kinetics models. *Acad Radiol* 2008;15(12):1580–1589.
131. **Wintermark M, Albers GW, Alexandrov AV, et al.** Acute stroke imaging research roadmap. *Stroke* 2008;39:1621–1628.
132. **Dani KA, Thomas RG, Chappell FM, et al.** Systematic review of perfusion imaging with computed tomography and magnetic resonance in acute ischemic stroke: heterogeneity of acquisition and postprocessing parameters. *Stroke* 2012;43(2):563–566.

CHAPTER

3 New Dose Reduction Strategies in CT Myocardial Perfusion Imaging

Ting-Yim Lee, PhD, Aaron So, PhD, Esmaeil Enjilela, PhD, and Jiang Hsieh, PhD

Introduction

With the advent of fast scanning capability through the development of slip-ring technology, CT has become the imaging modality of choice in the assessment of coronary artery disease (CAD), particularly in the emergent situation of acute chest pain. Coronary computed tomography angiography (CCTA) is now widely used to image the morphology of coronary vessels to detect severe stenosis that requires revascularization.[1–3] Even with its prevalence in the diagnostic armamentarium, CCTA remains an anatomical technique rather than a functional/physiologic technique for the sensitive detection of functional myocardial ischemia downstream to a stenosis.[4–6] To address this shortcoming of CCTA, myocardial perfusion imaging (MPI) lately has become a focus of research for cardiac CT. In the triage of acute chest pain, the combination of CCTA and MPI promises to be the ideal one-stop shop for the comprehensive anatomical and physiologic evaluation of CAD[6] before directing the appropriate patient to revascularization.

However, one main limitation of MPI with CT is the high radiation dose (approximately 20 mSv) from the necessity of repeatedly scanning the heart following injection of contrast (see next section). As such, recently a variety of methods have been developed to reduce the radiation dose of CT MPI. This chapter discusses these methods and illustrates them with examples.

CT Myocardial Perfusion Imaging

To understand better how the new radiation dose reduction methods work, it is useful to describe the three different scanning protocols/methods for CT MPI. First, perfusion in ischemic myocardium is visually assessed from source CCTA images as the relative contrast enhancement with respect to normal myocardium[7,8] (Fig. 3-1). Hypoattenuation relative to other parts of the myocardium is taken as ischemia. It is a qualitative assessment and depends on the time of arrival of contrast in the ischemic relative to that in the normal myocardium as well as the timing of the CCTA acquisition relative to the arterial (aorta) concentration. Second, the initial phase of time–density curves (TDCs) is acquired by scanning the heart with prospective ECG gating[9,10] (Fig. 3-2). Myocardial perfusion is calculated as the front slope of the myocardial TDC normalized by the maximum value of the aortic TDC.[10] Figure 3-2A–C shows an example of MPI in a dog model of acute heart attack. As shown, the method is able to detect stress- (adenosine) induced ischemia. One fundamental assumption of the upslope method is that during the time interval (10 seconds in Fig. 3-2) of its measurement, there is no outflow of contrast from the myocardium—no venous outflow. This is a rather stringent condition, and in general, it is not known whether it will be satisfied in all ischemic conditions. Third, entire TDCs are acquired by either cine-retrospective[11] or prospective ECG gating,[10,12] and kinetics modeling is applied to derive myocardial perfusion as shown in Figure 3-3. The application of kinetics modeling obviates the need of the no venous outflow assumption, and myocardial perfusion measurements obtained with this last method are the most accurate resulting in one-to-one correspondence with the gold standard microsphere measurements.[13] The main disadvantage is the high radiation dose imparted.

As a comparison, the effective dose for a prospectively gated CCTA is about 3.7 mSv,[14] while the effective dose of the kinetics modeling method for MPI of the whole heart using either cine-retrospective gating[11] or prospective gating[10] is 19.4 and 6 to 17.7 mSv, respectively. The upslope method, because of its shorter acquisition window compared to the kinetics modeling method (Fig. 3-2 vs. Fig. 3-3), has an effective dose that is 40% to 50% less. Given the clinical utility of accurate MPI,[6] there is an impetus to develop methods to reduce the higher effective dose required by the kinetics modeling. In the following sections, a number of recently developed methods for reduction of radiation dose are presented.

Current Methods for Reducing Radiation Dose in Myocardial Perfusion Imaging

Besides prospective gating that can reduce the radiation dose of MPI by two to three times relative to retrospective gating, and currently, there are three methods under investigation: (a) iterative image reconstruction; (b) principal component analysis (PCA) of TDCs; and (c) compressed sensing (CS) image reconstruction.

Iterative Image Reconstruction

The concept of iterative reconstruction (IR) as embodied in the algebraic reconstruction technique (ART)[15] predates filtered back projection (FBP) for the reconstruction of CT images.[16] However,

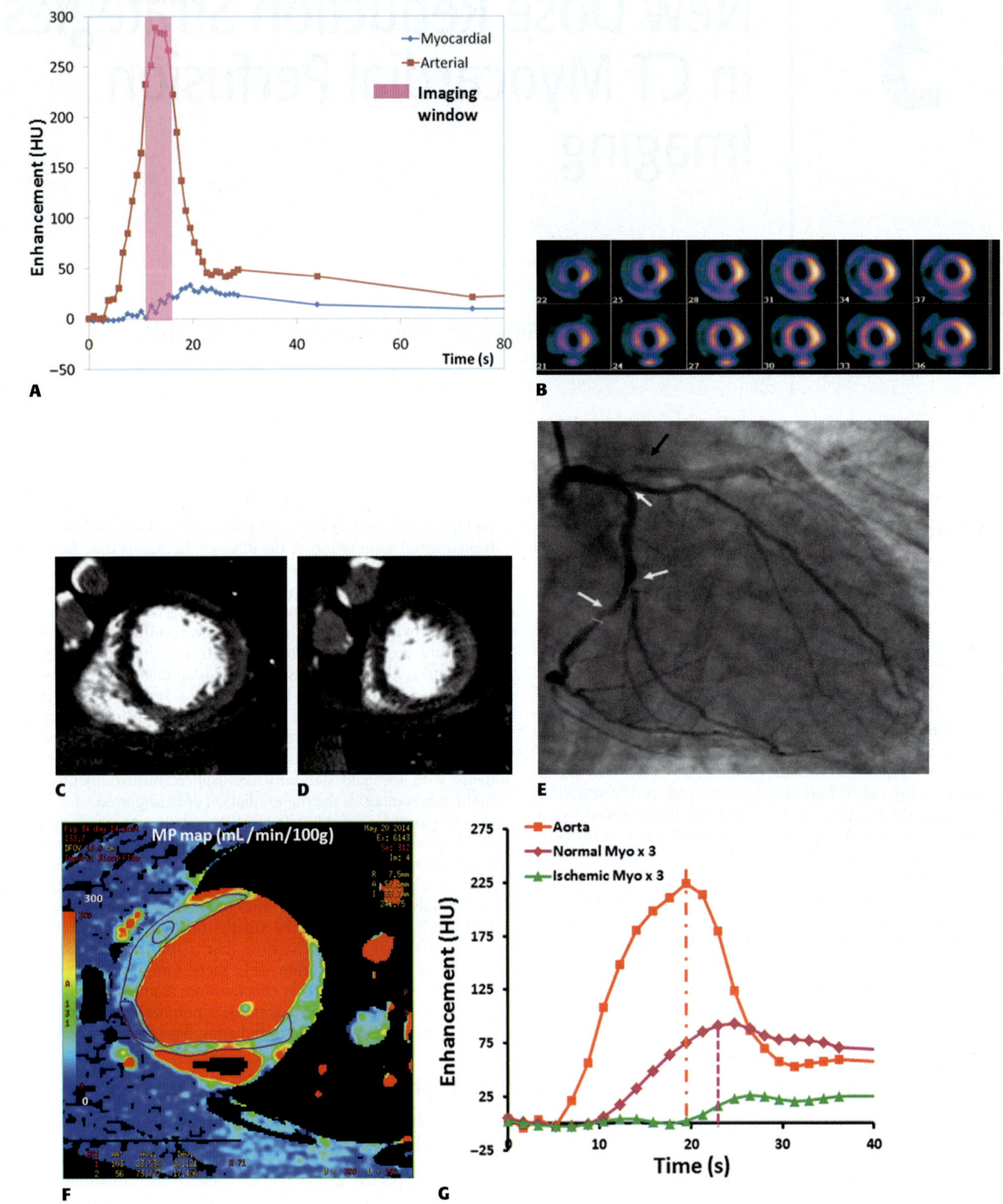

Figure 3-1. A: Time–density curves measured in the aorta and myocardium following intravenous contrast injection. Coronary CTA (CCTA) acquires images of the heart (vessels and myocardium) at the maximum of arterial contrast concentration. **B:** SPECT myocardial perfusion imaging shows ischemia in the left anterior descending (LAD) and right coronary artery (RCA) territories. **C, D:** Source CCTA images show corresponding hypoattenuation in the same territories. **E:** Catheter-based coronary angiogram shows stenosis in both LAD and RCA arteries. **F:** Myocardial perfusion map of a pig obtained 3 days after its LAD had been occluded for 1 hour and then reperfused. Two small regions of interest (ROIs) one in the ischemic apical region and one in the distant lateral wall of the LV are shown. **G:** Time–density curves of the normal and ischemic myocardium from the two ROIs in **(F)** as well as that of the aorta. The relative enhancements of normal versus ischemic ROI at peak (*red dashed line*) and after peak (*pink dashed line*) aortic enhancement are shown. (Courtesy of Dr. Jonathan Leipsic, St. Paul's Hospital, Vancouver, British Columbia, Canada.)

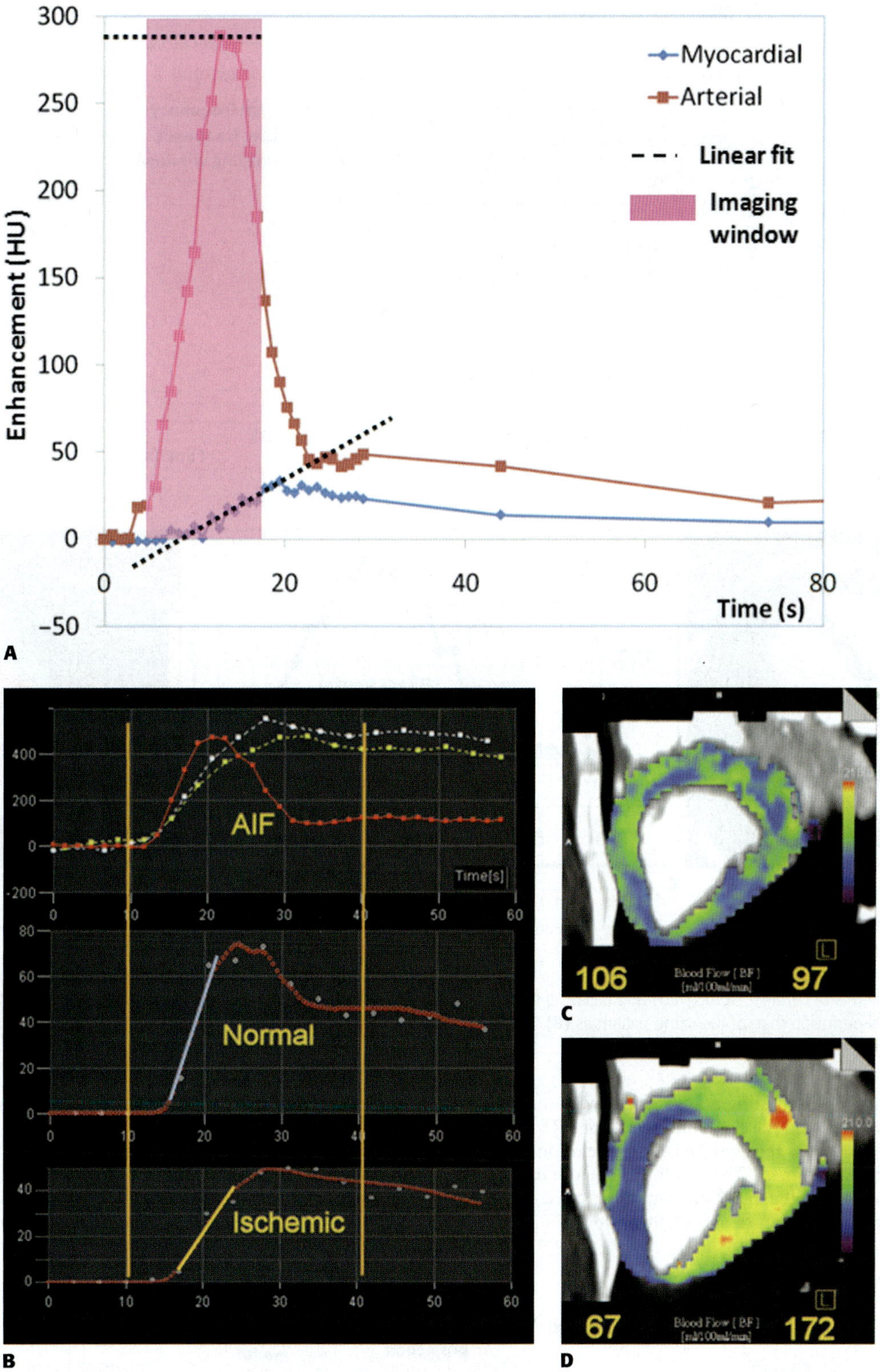

Figure 3-2. A: Time–density curves measured in the aorta and myocardium following intravenous contrast injection. For the implementation of the upslope method for the calculation of myocardial perfusion, the image acquisition window (*pink box*) centers around the peak of the aortic (*arterial*) curve. **B:** Aortic (AIF), normal, and ischemic myocardium time–density curves (TDCs) obtained in a dog 15 minutes after occluding 80% diameter of a distal segment of LAD. As shown, the upslope of the ischemic TDC is significantly less than that of the normal TDC. **C, D:** Myocardial perfusion map of the same dog as **(B)** in a sagittal reformat before **(C)** and after **(D)** adenosine stress. The numbers in **(C)** and **(D)** are the perfusion in the anterior and posterior wall of the LV. Under stress, perfusion in the anterior wall within the LAD territory decreased from 106 to 67 mL/min/100 g, while perfusion in the remaining unaffected (normal) myocardium increased from 97 to 172 mL/min/100 g. (Modified from Mahnken AH, Klotz E, Pietsch H, et al. Quantitative whole heart stress perfusion CT imaging as noninvasive assessment of hemodynamics in coronary artery stenosis: preliminary animal experience. *Invest Radiol* 2010;45:298–305.)

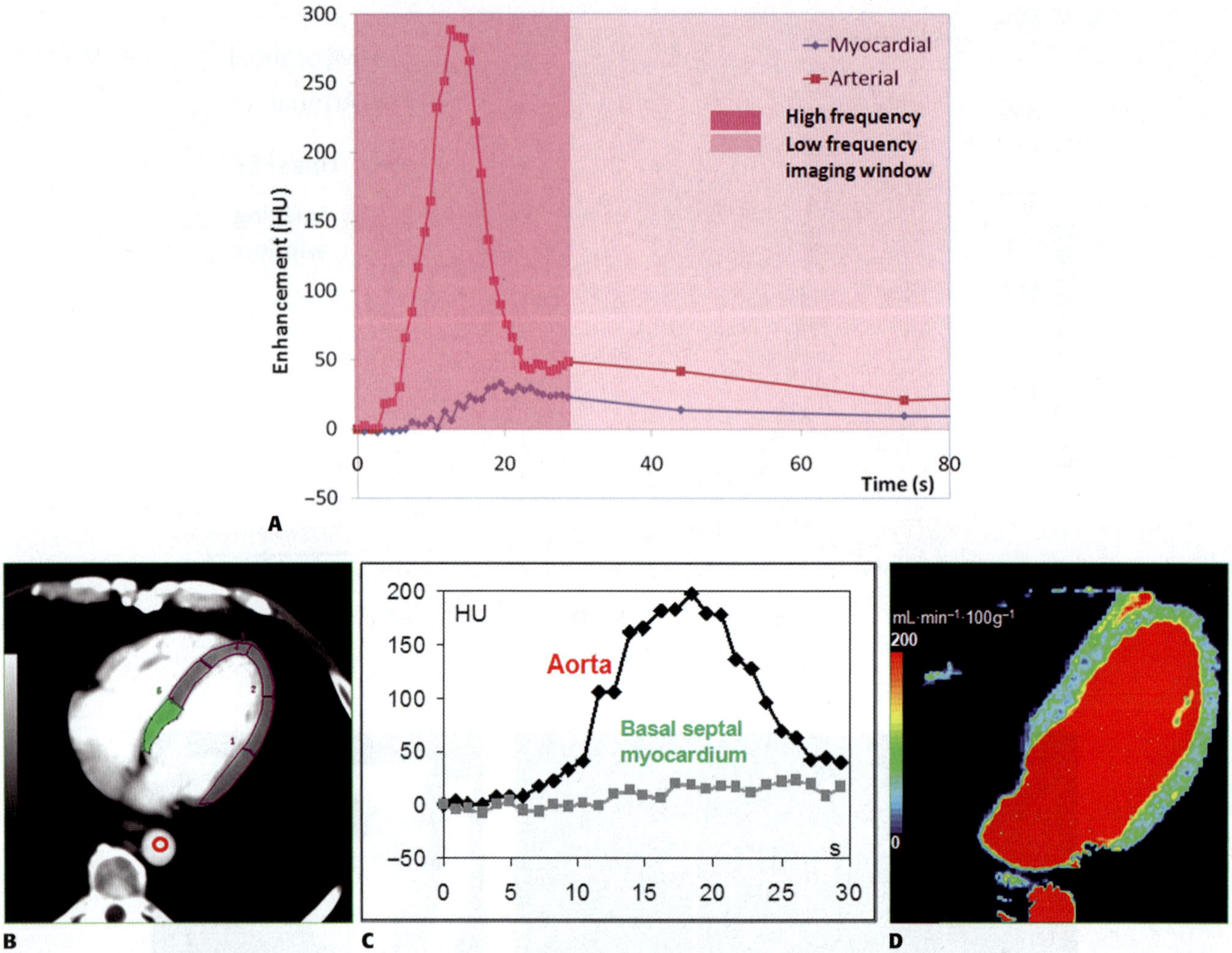

Figure 3-3. A: Time–density curves measured in the aorta and myocardium following intravenous contrast injection. For the implementation of kinetics modeling for the calculation of myocardial perfusion, the image acquisition window (dark and light pink box) has to cover both the first pass and recirculation phases of the TDC at different image frequencies being higher for the first-pass phase. **B:** Four chamber view of a patient's heart when all chambers were filled with contrast. Aortic (red) and basal septal wall (green) ROIs to generate TDCs are shown. **C:** Aorta and basal septal wall TDCs. **D:** Rest myocardial perfusion map of the same patient as **(B)**. Perfusion values are displayed in a rainbow color scale from 0 to 200 mL/min/100 g.

because of the limited computing power of image reconstruction computer workstations and the slow convergence of ART for noisy data, until recently FBP has replaced ART for image reconstruction in all commercial CT scanners. The current resurgence of interest in IR not only stems from the increased computing speed of reconstruction workstations but, more importantly, allows CT scanning at lower radiation dose with similar noise levels and image quality as routine dose FBP.[17–20]

The core of IR consists of a loop of backward and forward projection steps that can be iterated a number of times to improve image quality as shown in Figure 3-4. To start the IR, the first step is a normal FBP of the measured (raw) projection data to reconstruct

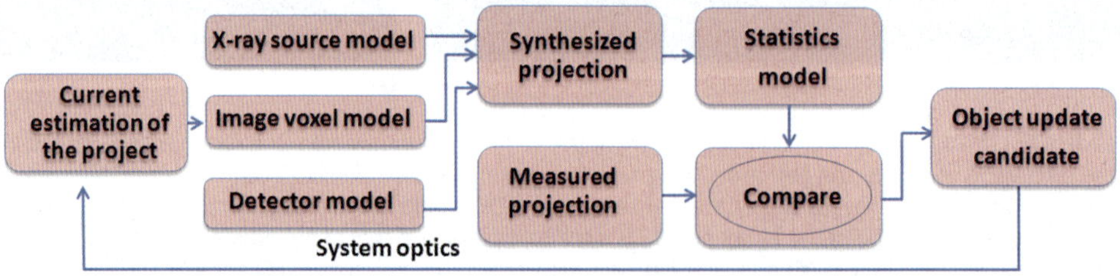

Figure 3-4. The generic algorithm for modeled-based iterative image reconstruction. Details of the algorithm are discussed in the text.

a CT image of the object. Then, the CT image is forward-projected while simulating CT acquisition by using a priori knowledge of the characteristics of the CT system (e.g., machine geometry, size of detector, and voxel) to obtain synthesized projections. These projections are further modified by the statistics model, which accounts for photon noise, efficiency of individual detector elements, and electronic noise, before they are compared with the measured projections. The differences between the synthesized and measured projections are backward projected to generate an object update candidate (image), which is used to correct the current object estimate (image). Forward and backward projection steps are repeated a fixed number of times or until corrections become very small. GE Healthcare has implemented the full IR algorithm as described above in their Modeled Based Iterative Reconstruction (MBIR) algorithm.[21] However, even with current computing speed of a multiprocessor computer (Veo), the reconstruction time for each heart volume is about 10 minutes. For now, this long reconstruction time will limit the use of MBIR for dose reduction in MPI since multiple (approximately 20 to 25) volumes of the heart following contrast injection have to be reconstructed.

To avoid the computation burden of a fully fledged MBIR, most vendors instead have concentrated on statistical modeling, which can be implemented in the raw projection domain alone, in the image domain alone, or in both domains. The projection domain methods denoise the raw projections with an adaptive or iterative 2D edge-preserving filter,[22,23] which adaptively denoise more strongly regions with higher attenuation. The noise-reduced data are then used for image reconstruction with either FBP or an iterative method resulting in reduced noise in the reconstructed images. The image domain methods denoise the images after FBP reconstruction by image processing designed to reduce noise but preserve spatial resolution.[24] The combined image and projection domains methods use postreconstruction image processing as the image domain method, but in addition, use photon statistics information derived from raw projection data to guide selective smoothing of the reconstructed image.[25,26] The statistical IR algorithms from different vendors are summarized in Table 3.1.

Principal Component Analysis

While IR methods, particularly statistical iterative methods, can reduce noise in the spatial domain, temporal noise filtering of the acquired dynamic images in MPI could be equally important in MPI. They could reduce noise (fluctuations) in the derived TDCs resulting in more robust estimates of myocardial perfusion via kinetics modeling and ultimately better quality MPI. There are many temporal noise filtering techniques, but PCA could be best suited for MPI applications because it is not model dependent and is entirely data driven.[31] This would customize the noise filtering on an individual patient basis. PCA finds common temporal patterns (principal components) in all TDCs from the entire myocardium by analyzing the variations of each TDC from the mean curve of all TDCs. These variations will reflect the temporal behavior of TDCs following contrast injection and random noise. Each principal component accounts for, in order, the largest remaining variations from the mean curve. Each TDC can be reconstituted by summation of the principal components found. By retaining only components that reproduce variations in keeping with the expected rapid wash-in and wash-out of contrast and discarding those that do not, random noise in the reconstituted TDC can be effectively minimized.

Compressed Sensing

The dose reduction from statistical IR in the projection domain alone or in both image, and projection domain arise from noise filtering of the projections as discussed above. In CT scanning, photons measured by the detectors are assumed to be Poisson distributed, which may be valid in the case when the mAs, hence radiation dose, used in acquiring projections is high. With the successful application of statistical IR to reduce mAs (dose) in the acquisition of projections, a situation will be reached when electronic noise in the detector will dominate over photon (Poisson) noise. At that point, it will not be possible to reduce radiation dose further. Current CT image reconstruction, using FBP or IR, uses a large number of projections (approximately 1,000). One method to maintain a high mAs to avoid overwhelming detector electronic noise in acquiring projections, while reducing radiation dose is to decrease the number of projections required. Assuming the same mAs is used to acquire a projection, by reducing the number of acquired projections from 1,000 to 250 to 330, the radiation dose will be decreased by three to four times.

The feasibility of reconstructing images from sparse noisy projections is based on the theory of signal recovery from CS (i.e., few inaccurate data samples or measurements).[32,33] The basis of CS is that

TABLE 3.1 **Statistical Iterative Reconstruction Algorithms from Different CT Vendors**

Algorithm	Domain of Iteration: Projection only	Image only	Projection and Image	Vendor
IRIS—Iterative Reconstruction in Image Space[27]	—	✓	—	Siemens Healthcare
SAFIRE—Sinogram Affirmed Iterative Reconstruction[28]	—	—	✓	Siemens Healthcare
AIDR 3D—Adaptive Iterative Dose Reduction 3D[29]	—	—	✓	Toshiba Medical Systems
iDose[4](Ref. 30)	—	—	✓	Philips Healthcare
ASIR—Adaptive Statistical Iterative Reconstruction[31]	—	—	✓	GE Healthcare

compressible signals (i.e., having few nonzero significant values) can be fully recovered from a small number of linear measurements that satisfy an incoherence property.[33] CT images that usually are made up of few regions of more or less homogenous attenuation qualified as compressible signals, because they can be sparsified to a limit number of distinct edges by calculating their derivatives. Thus, CS can be used for reconstructing CT images via the derivative domain from fewer numbers (approximately 100 to 300) of projections compared to what the Nyquist-Shannon theorem dictates for FBP.[34,35]

CS solves the image reconstruction problem using nonlinear optimization to minimize an objective function, which exploits the sparsity of the transformed image. A popular sparsifying function is total variation (TV), which is the magnitude of the local gradient vector in the image.[36] As discussed before, CT images generally consist of a small number of significant pixels, usually at the boundaries between homogeneous internal structures; thus, the TV function is a suitable sparsifying transform for CS. One of the CS-based image reconstruction algorithms, applicable to MPI, which acquires a sequence of dynamic contrast-enhanced (DCE) images as a prerequisite, is prior image constrained compressed sensing (PICCS).[37] PICCS uses an average image of all DCE images reconstructed with FBP from sparse projections as the constraint during CS image reconstruction. This approach is effective in preserving image edges (anatomical information) but may lead to systematic error in the reconstructed DCE images from which TDC curves are derived for kinetics modeling. The average DCE image represents the mean enhancement level during the first-pass (circulation) phase of contrast. By constraining the TV optimization to minimize difference between the reconstructed and the average image, pixel value in the reconstructed image can be shifted closer to that of the average image (Fig. 3-5). This will result in significant distortion of the myocardial TDCs and hence inaccurate perfusion estimates. The findings of Lauzier et al.[37] suggested that the shift in pixel values (measured in Hounsfield Unit or HU) from the reference FBP method could be more than 10 HU. Given the maximal change in myocardial pixel values (enhancement) in a DCE CT study is roughly 30 HU, this effect of PICSS could significantly affect the accuracy of CT MPI studies.

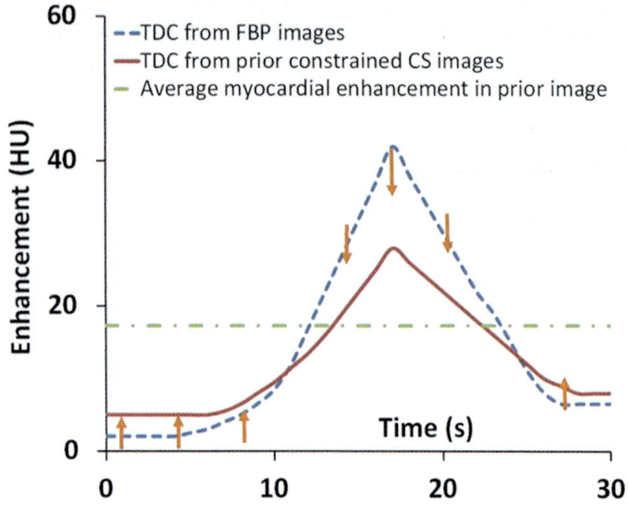

Figure 3-5. Schematic to illustrate the effect of constraining the reconstructed image to be close to the prior (average) image in prior image constrained compressed sensing (PICCS), which shifts the myocardial time–density curve (TDC) toward the mean myocardial enhancement in the prior image.

Applications in Myocardial Perfusion Imaging

Radiation Dose Reduction with Joint Application of Statistical Iterative Reconstruction and Principal Component Analysis of Time–Density Curves

As discussed above joint application of Statistical IR and PCA afford independent spatial and temporal noise filtering of TDCs, it is expected to reduce radiation dose more than either Statistical IR or PCA alone while maintaining the same image quality of MPI. To demonstrate this effect, we studied five pigs weighing 30 ± 12 kg with two scanning protocols and injection of contrast at concentration of 225 mgL/mL, dosage of 0.7 mL/kg, and rate of 2.5 mL/s via an ear vein. One protocol used cine (continuous) scanning at 140 kV, 80 mA, and 0.4 second per scan (rotation) for 30 seconds, and used retrospective ECG gating to select middiastole images after image reconstruction. The second scan protocol was prospectively ECG gated to middiastole and scan at 140 kV, either 40 or 20 mA, and 0.35 second per scan (rotation) for 20 scans every two to three heartbeats. All scans (cine or prospectively gated) were performed on a CT 750 HD scanner (GE Healthcare) and covered 4-cm section of the heart in eight 5-mm-thick slices. Images from the cine acquisition were reconstructed with FBP, while the two (40 and 20 mA) ECG-gated acquisitions were reconstructed with FBP and ASIR, and the 20 mA images were further denoised with PCA. Each set of dynamic images were then processed with CT Perfusion (GE Healthcare) to generate myocardial perfusion (MP) maps. The maps were compared both in quantitative values of MP as well as figure of merit (FOM) defined as the ratio of standard deviation to mean myocardial perfusion in the lateral wall. Since perfusion is expected to be homogeneous in the myocardium under normal conditions, FOM is an indicator of how photon noise in the processed images affects the quality of MP maps. A smaller value of FOM suggests a better quality MP map than one with a larger FOM. Finally, the effective dose of the 80 mA cine scan and 40 and 20 mA ECG-gated scans are compared.

Figure 3-6A compares one image at the same time after contrast injection from the following four sets of dynamic images: (a) cine 80 mA FBP; (b) gated 20 mA FBP; (c) gated 20 mA ASIR; and (d) gated mA ASIR + PCA. The MP maps derived from the same four sets of dynamic images are also shown in Figure 3-7B. Both CT images and MP maps show that ASIR + PCA performs the best with increased noise from four times reduction in radiation dose (80 vs. 20 mA), ASIR is next while FBP is the last in performance. Figure 3-7A shows that compared to 80 mA FBP, both 40 and 20 mA FBP have higher MP and lower MP FOM because of the increased noise, but ASIR and ASIR + PCA were able to restore MP and MP FOM to those of 80 mA FBP even at two and four times less mA (radiation dose), respectively. The effective doses for cine 80 mA, gated 40 mA, and gated 20 mA were 16, 2, and 1 mSv, respectively (Fig. 3-7B). Taken the results in Figures 3-6 and 3-7 together, it can be concluded that prospectively gated scan and ASIR + PCA can reduce the radiation dose required for MPI by 16 times from a cine retrospectively gated scan, and FBP without sacrificing accuracy and FOM of MP measurement. If we assume that prospectively gated scan has a dose reduction of two to three times compared to cine scan, then the dose reduction from the application of ASIR + PCA is five to eight times that of FBP.

Radiation Dose Reduction with Compressed Sensing

As discussed above, by requiring a prior (average) image to constraint the optimization of TV in the reconstructed images, PICCS applied to MPI may lead to inaccurate perfusion measurements.

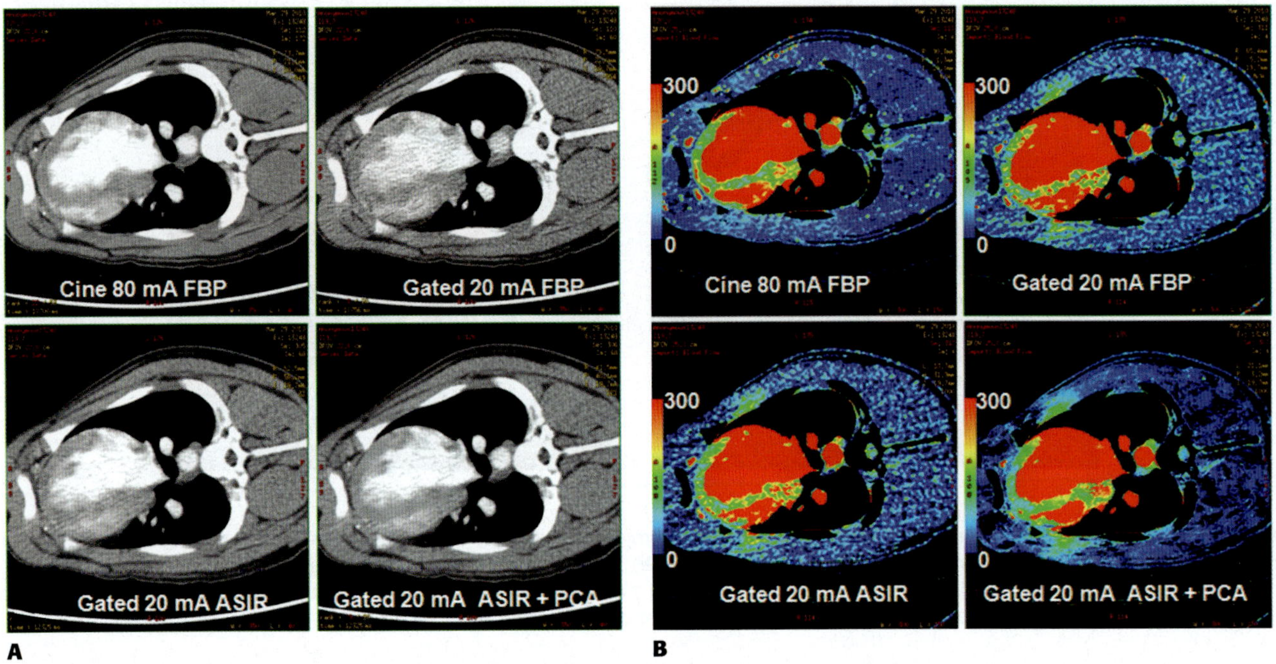

Figure 3-6. A: CT images at the same time after contrast injection from the following four sets of dynamic images: (a) cine 80 mA FBP; (b) gated 20 mA FBP; (c) gated 20 mA ASIR; and (d) gated mA ASIR + PCA. **B:** Myocardial perfusion (MP) maps derived from the same four sets of dynamic image.

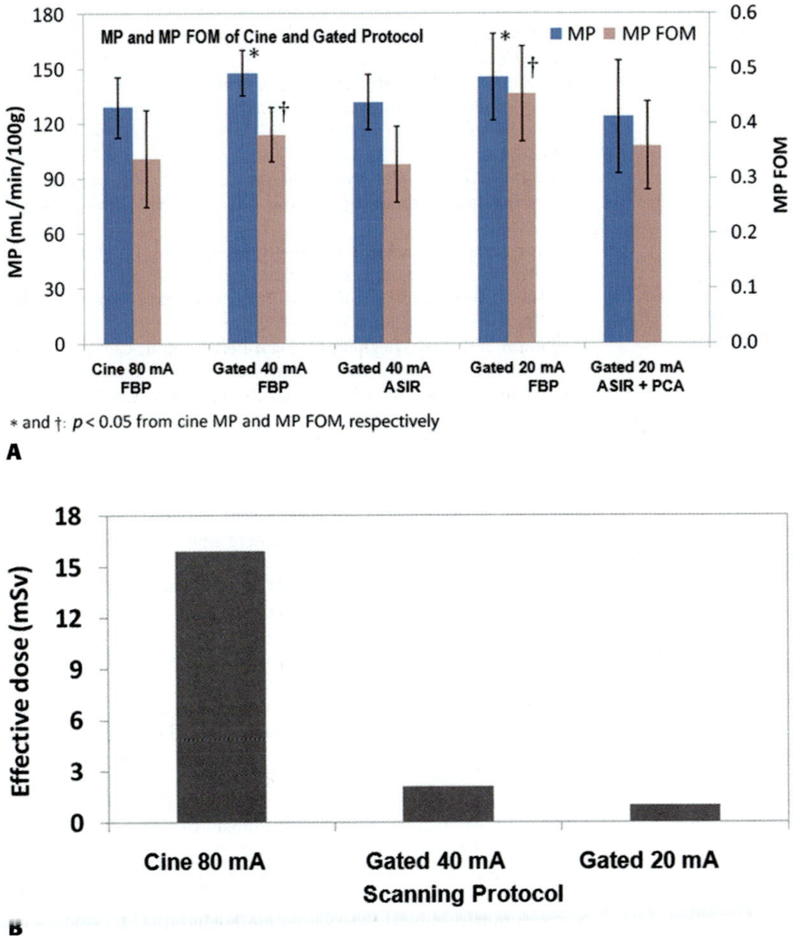

Figure 3-7. A: Comparison of myocardial perfusion (MP) and MP figure of merit (FOM) among different scanning protocols and image reconstruction methods. **B:** Effective dose of different scanning protocols.

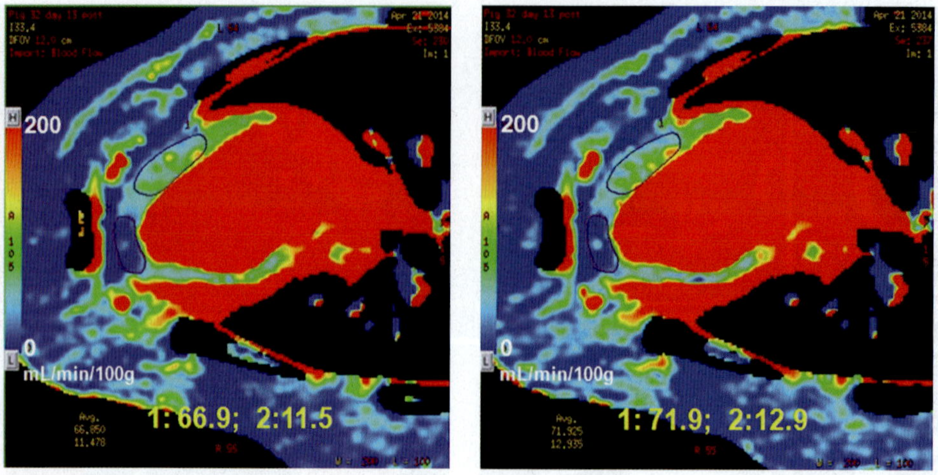

A B

Figure 3-8. **Comparison of (A) filtered back projection (FBP) (984 projections) and (B) compressed sensing (CS) (328 projections) myocardial perfusion (MP) maps from a myocardial perfusion imaging (MPI) study on a pig with an apical infarct.** Each map was displayed using a rainbow color scale from 0 to 200 mL/min/100 g. ROI #1 was defined in the lateral wall which was free of ischemia, while ROI #2 was defined in the apical infarct. The two numbers on each map give the mean MP in ROI #1 and #2, respectively.

To investigate whether prior image constraint is required, we have implemented TV optimization without constraint for image reconstruction with sparse projections and compared the MP maps obtained with those from FBP of a full set of projections. Figure 3-8 shows that the CS image reconstruction from a sparse set of 328 projections without prior image constraint produces MP map that is comparable in accuracy to that from FBP with a full set of 928 projections. Since the number of projections required for CS is three times less than FBP, radiation dose for MPI will also be reduced by the same factor.

Conclusions

Until now CT MPI has been limited by the high radiation dose required. The introduction of statistical IR and CS reconstruction as well as temporal noise filtering technique, like PCA, holds the promise to significantly reduce the radiation dose for whole heart MPI from approximately 20 to 1 to 2 mSv without compromising the quality of the MP maps. This development will lead to the increased clinical acceptance of CT-based MPI. The combination of CCTA and MPI will afford accurate morphologic and functional assessment of coronary stenosis in higher spatial resolution than MRI and help to propel cardiac CT as the one-stop shop for the triage of acute chest pain.

Acknowledgments

This work was partially supported by the Canadian Foundation of Innovation, Canadian Institutes of Health Research, Heart and Stroke Foundation of Canada and Ontario Innovation Trust. Figure 3-1A–D was contributed by Dr. Jonathan Leipsic, St. Paul's Hospital, Vancouver, British Columbia, Canada. Figure 3-2A–C was modified from Mahnken et al. publication in *Investigative Radiology*.[10]

Financial Disclosure

T-Y Lee licenses the software CT Perfusion to GE Healthcare and receives royalties from the licensing.

REFERENCES

1. **Budoff MJ, Dowe D, Jollis JG, et al.** Diagnostic performance of 64-multidetector row coronary computed tomographic angiography for evaluation of coronary artery stenosis in individuals without known coronary artery disease: results from the prospective multicenter accuracy (assessment by coronary computed tomographic angiography of individuals undergoing invasive coronary angiography) trial. *J Am Coll Cardiol* 2008;52:1724–1732.
2. **Meijboom WB, Meijs MF, Schuijf JD, et al.** Diagnostic accuracy of 64-slice computed tomography coronary angiography: a prospective, multicenter, multivendor study. *J Am Coll Cardiol* 2008;52:2135–2144.
3. **Miller JM, Rochitte CE, Dewey M, et al.** Diagnostic performance of coronary angiography by 64-row CT. *N Engl J Med* 2008;359:2324–2336.
4. **van Werkhoven JM, Schuijf JD, Gaemperli O, et al.** Prognostic value of multislice computed tomography and gated single-photon emission computed tomography in patients with suspected coronary artery disease. *J Am Coll Cardiol* 2009;53:623–632.
5. **Meijboom WB, Van Mieghem CA, van Pelt N, et al.** Comprehensive assessment of coronary artery stenoses: computed tomography coronary angiography versus conventional coronary angiography and correlation with fractional flow reserve in patients with stable angina. *J Am Coll Cardiol* 2008;52:636–643.
6. **Gould KL.** Does coronary flow trump coronary anatomy? *JACC Cardiovasc Imaging* 2009;2:1009–1023.
7. **Blankstein R, Shturman LD, Rogers IS, et al.** Adenosine-induced stress myocardial perfusion imaging using dual-source cardiac computed tomography. *J Am Coll Cardiol* 2009;54:1072–1084.
8. **George RT, Arbab-Zadeh A, Miller JM, et al.** Adenosine stress 64- and 256-row detector computed tomography angiography and perfusion imaging: a pilot study evaluating the transmural extent of perfusion abnormalities to predict atherosclerosis causing myocardial ischemia. *Circ Cardiovasc Imaging* 2009;2:174–182.
9. **Bastarrika G, Ramos-Duran L, Rosenblum MA, et al.** Adenosine-stress dynamic myocardial CT perfusion imaging: initial clinical experience. *Invest Radiol* 2010;45:306–313.
10. **Mahnken AH, Klotz E, Pietsch H, et al.** Quantitative whole heart stress perfusion CT imaging as noninvasive assessment of hemodynamics in coronary artery stenosis: preliminary animal experience. *Invest Radiol* 2010;45:298–305.
11. **So A, Wisenberg G, Islam A, et al.** Non-invasive assessment of functionally relevant coronary artery stenoses with quantitative CT perfusion: preliminary clinical experiences. *Eur Radiol* 2012;22:39–50.

12. **So A, Hsieh J, Imai Y, et al.** Prospectively ECG-triggered rapid kV-switching dual-energy CT for quantitative imaging of myocardial perfusion. *JACC Cardiovasc Imaging* 2012;5:829–836.
13. **So A, Hsieh J, Li J-Y, et al.** Quantitative myocardial perfusion measurement using CT Perfusion: a validation study in a porcine model of reperfused acute myocardial infarction. *Int J Cardiovasc Imaging* 2012;28: 1237–1248.
14. **Huang B, Li J, Law MW, et al.** Radiation dose and cancer risk in retrospectively and prospectively ECG-gated coronary angiography using 64-slice multidetector CT. *Br J Radiol* 2010;83:152–158.
15. **Gordon R, Bender R, Herman GT.** Algebraic reconstruction techniques (ART) for three-dimensional electron microscopy and x-ray photography. *J Theor Biol* 1970;29:471–481.
16. **Fleischmann D, Boas FE.** Computed tomography—old ideas and new technology. *Eur Radiol* 2011;21:510–517.
17. **Hara AK, Paden RG, Silva AC, et al.** Iterative reconstruction technique for reducing body radiation dose at CT: feasibility study. *AJR Am J Roentgenol* 2009;193:764–771.
18. **Funama Y, Taguchi K, Utsunomiya D, et al.** Combination of a low-tube-voltage technique with hybrid iterative reconstruction (iDose) algorithm at coronary computed tomographic angiography. *J Comput Assist Tomogr* 2011;35:480–485.
19. **Ghetti C, Palleri F, Serreli G, et al.** Physical characterization of a new CT iterative reconstruction method operating in sinogram space. *J Appl Clin Med Phys* 2013;14:4347.
20. **Blobel J, Mews J, Schuijf JD, et al.** Determining the radiation dose reduction potential for coronary calcium scanning with computed tomography: an anthropomorphic phantom study comparing filtered backprojection and the adaptive iterative dose reduction algorithm for image reconstruction. *Invest Radiol* 2013;48:857–862.
21. **Thibault JB, Sauer KD, Bouman CA, et al.** A three-dimensional statistical approach to improved image quality for multislice helical CT. *Med Phys* 2007;34:4526–4544.
22. **Hsieh J.** Adaptive streak artifact reduction in computed tomography resulting from excessive x-ray photon noise. *Med Phys* 1998;25:2139–2347.
23. **Rivière PJL.** Penalized-likelihood sinogram smoothing for low-dose CT. *Med Phys* 2005;32:1676–1683.
24. **Nelson RC, Feuerlein S, Boll DT.** New iterative reconstruction techniques for cardiovascular computed tomography: how do they work, and what are the advantages and disadvantages? *J Cardiovasc Comput Tomogr* 2011;5:286–292.
25. **Moscariello A, Takx RAP, Schoepf UJ, et al.** Coronary CT angiography: image quality, diagnostic accuracy, and potential for radiation dose reduction using a novel iterative image reconstruction technique comparison with traditional filtered back projection. *Eur Radiol* 2011;21:2130–2138.
26. **Winklehner A, Karlo C, Puippe G, et al.** Raw data-based iterative reconstruction in body CTA: evaluation of radiation dose saving potential. *Eur Radiol* 2011;21:2521–2526.
27. **Anonymous.** Iterative Reconstruction in Image Space (IRIS). Siemens Healthcare Whitepaper; 2009.
28. **Grant K, Raupach R.** SAFIRE: Sinogram Affirmed Iterative Reconstruction. Siemens Healthcare Whitepaper; 2012.
29. **Anonymous.** AIDR 3D Iterative Reconstruction: Integrated, Automated and Adaptive Dose Reduction. Toshiba Medical Systems Whitepaper; 2012.
30. **Anonymous.** iDose[4] iterative reconstruction technique. Philips Healthcare Whitepaper; 2011.
31. **Jolliffe IT.** *Principal component analysis*. 2nd ed. Springer Science, New York; 2004.
32. **Donoho D.** Compressed sensing. *IEEE Trans Inf Theory* 2006;52: 1289–1306.
33. **Candés E, Romberg J, Tao T.** Stable signal recovery from incomplete and inaccurate measurements. *Commun Pure Appl Math* 2006;59:1207–1223.
34. **Kak AC, Slaney M.** Chapter 5. Aliasing artifacts and noise in CT images. In: *Principles of computerized tomographic imaging*. Society of Industrial and Applied Mathematics; 2001.
35. **Joseph PM, Schulz RA.** View sampling requirements in fan beam computed tomography. *Med Phys* 1980;7:692–702.
36. **Yu G, Li L, Gu J, et al.** *Total variation based iterative image reconstruction, computer vision for biomedical image applications*. Berlin, Heidelberg: Springer; 2005:526–534.
37. **Lauzier PT, Tang J, Chen GH.** Prior image constrained compressed sensing: implementation and performance evaluation. *Med Phys* 2012;39:66–80.

CHAPTER

4 Dynamic Contrast-Enhanced Perfusion CT: Basics of Mathematical Tracer Kinetic Models and Applications

Kenya Murase, PhD

Introduction

Dynamic contrast-enhanced CT (DCE-CT) acquires CT images serially after the administration of intravenous contrast agent. Recently, DCE-CT has become a major imaging technique and has been widely used for diagnosing normal tissue and benign and malignant tumors as well as for monitoring treatment effectiveness during and after therapy.[1] In addition to its easy accessibility in most clinical facilities, DCE-CT can provide quantification of the hemodynamics of lesions, if combined with appropriate tracer kinetic analysis.[2]

One of the advantages of using CT for tracer kinetic analysis is that the relationship between the concentration of the administered iodinated contrast agent in the tissue and the attenuation of x-rays is almost always linear.[2] This results in simpler analysis and fewer errors than dynamic contrast-enhanced magnetic resonance imaging (DCE-MRI). On the other hand, the major disadvantages of using CT are its potentially high radiation exposure due to repetitive scanning and the need for iodinated contrast agent that can be nephrotoxic and allergenic.[3] Recently, however, several studies have been performed to reduce these drawbacks in DCE-CT.[4]

In this chapter, the basic theory of tracer kinetic analysis and the practical methods for estimating kinetic parameters using DCE-CT will be described. The factors affecting the accuracy of the kinetic parameters obtained using DCE-CT and their correction methods will also be described.

Relationship between CT Number and Concentration of Contrast Agent

Image contrast in CT is determined by differences in the attenuation of x-rays in different tissues. The CT number (in Hounsfield units) of tissues in the reconstructed images (CT_t) is given by

$$CT_t = \frac{\mu_t - \mu_w}{\mu_w} \times 1{,}000, \quad (1)$$

where μ_t and μ_w denote the linear attenuation coefficients of the tissue and water, respectively. After administration of contrast agent, the linear attenuation coefficient of the tissue at time t ($\mu_t(t)$) is given by[2]

$$\mu_t(t) = \mu_t(0) + \Delta\mu_t(t), \quad (2)$$

where $\mu_t(0)$ is the linear attenuation coefficient of the tissue immediately before administration of contrast agent and $\Delta\mu_t(t)$ is an increase of the linear attenuation coefficient at time t due to administration of contrast agent. $\Delta\mu_t(t)$ is related to the amount of the administered contrast agent and is directly proportional to the concentration of the contrast agent at time t ($C_{CA}(t)$), thus yielding

$$\Delta\mu_t(t) = k \cdot C_{CA}(t), \quad (3)$$

where k is a constant of proportionality that depends on the energy spectrum of the x-ray beam passing through the tissue and the atomic constituents of the contrast agent.[2] Since beam-hardening effects are usually corrected in most CT systems, it appears to be a good approximation that k does not vary among different tissues.[2] Finally, an increase in CT number in tissue after administration of contrast agent ($\Delta CT_t(t)$) can be obtained from Eqs. (1), (2), and (3) as

$$\Delta CT_t(t) = CT_t(t) - CT_t(0) = K \cdot C_{CA}(t), \quad (4)$$

where $CT_t(t)$ and $CT_t(0)$ denote the CT numbers in tissue at time t and before administration of contrast agent, respectively, and $K = 1{,}000.k/\mu_w$. Therefore, the concentration of the administered contrast agent is proportional to an increase of CT number, that is, contrast enhancement.

In DCE-CT studies, the first time points of the concentration–time curves are generated and subtracted from the subsequent time points to ensure that the initial baseline concentration of the contrast agent is zero. After this normalization, the postcontrast density measurement using CT is directly proportional to the concentration of contrast agent, as given by Eq. (4). Since K in Eq. (4) is the same for the blood and tissues, the constant K cancels out in DCE-CT studies and thus does not need to be calculated or known.

Basics of Tracer Kinetic Analysis

Vascular System

When a contrast agent is injected and enters a vascular system with a single inlet and a single outlet as a bolus as shown in Figure 4.1, the concentration–time curve measured at the exit of the vascular system is dispersed as the molecules in contrast agent may have different transit times through the system. Furthermore, there is a

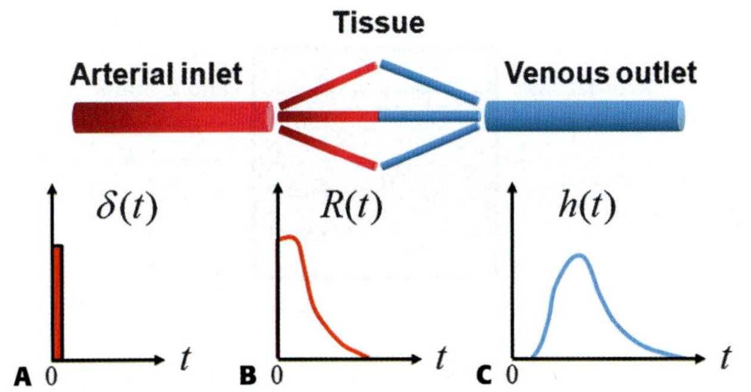

Figure 4-1. Single-inlet, single-outlet vascular system. **A:** Ideal input function represented by Dirac delta function ($\delta(t)$). **B:** Impulse residue (retention) function ($R(t)$) showing the fraction of contrast agent remaining in the vascular system. **C:** Impulse response function ($h(t)$) showing the distribution of transit times of contrast agent at the venous outlet through the vascular system.

delay time before they can be detected at the exit, because a specific time is necessary for traversing the system.

Figure 4.1A shows an ideal bolus input at time 0. Mathematically, this is represented by Dirac delta function defined by

$$\delta(t)=\begin{cases}\infty & t=0\\ 0 & t\neq 0\end{cases} \quad \text{and} \quad \int_{-\infty}^{\infty}\delta(t)\mathrm{d}t=1. \tag{5}$$

Figure 4.1B shows the corresponding tissue response function ($R(t)$), which shows the fraction of contrast agent remaining in the vascular system and is referred to as the "impulse residue (retention) function." Figure 4.1C shows the distribution of transit times of contrast agent at the venous outlet through the vascular system, which is denoted by $h(t)$ and is referred to as the "impulse response function."

When we analyze the kinetic behavior of contrast agent in the vascular system (Fig. 4.1), a relationship between the inflow and outflow is based on the fundamental assumption that the system is both linear and stationary. This means that the response to an influx is assumed to be proportional to the injected dose and that the distribution of transit times through the system is constant in time.[5]

Concept of Convolution

Mathematical solutions are represented for simple models under the condition of an ideal bolus, that is, the tracer appears for one capillary transit without recirculation. Actually, however, the input to the tissue is represented by a continuous concentration–time curve. In other words, the tissue response is a sum of the individual responses scaled in magnitude and shifted in time to match each bolus input, which is mathematically represented by convolution integral.

Figure 4.2 illustrates the concept of convolution integral. Figure 4.2A shows an ideal bolus input of contrast agent injected at time 0, that is, $\delta(t)$ defined by Eq. (5), and Figure 4.2B shows the corresponding impulse residue (retention) function ($R(t)$). Figure 4.2C shows an ideal bolus input injected at time τ, that is, $\delta(t-\tau)$, and Figure 4.2D shows the corresponding tissue response to this bolus input, which is represented by $R(t-\tau)$. When the arterial

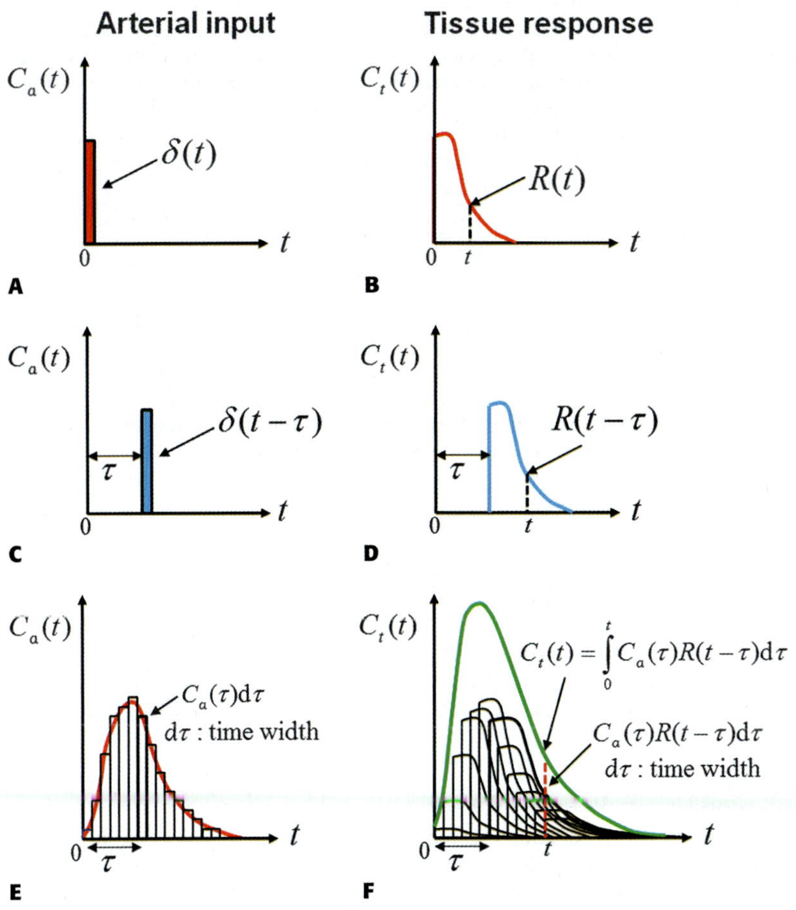

Figure 4-2. Concept of convolution integral. **(A) and (B)** show the AIF obtained by an ideal bolus injection at time 0 and the corresponding tissue response (impulse residue [retention] function), respectively. **(C) and (D)** show the AIF obtained by an ideal bolus injection at time τ and the corresponding tissue response, respectively. **(E)** shows a continuous AIF (*red line*), which can be interpreted as a series of bolus injections of varying magnitudes (*thin columns*). **(F)** shows the tissue response to **(E)** (*green line*), which can be interpreted as the sum of the tissue responses to each bolus (*thin lines*).

input function (AIF) is not bolus (ideal) but continuous (real) as shown in Figure 4.2E, it can be interpreted as a series of bolus inputs with an area of $C_a(\tau)d\tau$ (black square in Fig. 4.2E). In this case, the tissue response to the continuous input function can be interpreted as the sum of the responses to each bolus input given by $C_a(\tau)R(t-\tau)d\tau$ (Fig. 4.2F). Mathematically, this can be expressed as

$$C_t(t) = \int_0^t C_a(\tau)R(t-\tau)d\tau = C_a(t)\otimes R(t), \qquad (6)$$

where the symbol ⊗ denotes convolution integral and τ is a dummy integration variable. When $R(t) = 0$ for $t < 0$, the following equation holds

$$\int_0^\infty C_t(t)dt = \int_0^\infty C_a(t)\otimes R(t)dt = \int_0^\infty C_a(t)dt \cdot \int_0^\infty R(t)dt, \qquad (7)$$

because the area of the convolution of two functions is equal to the product of the areas of the functions. If all tracers that enter the system leave it eventually, the principle of conservation of mass, that is, $\int_0^\infty C_t(t)dt = \int_0^\infty C_a(t)dt$, holds (see Eq. (16)). Substituting this relation into Eq. (7) yields

$$\int_0^\infty R(t)dt = 1. \qquad (8)$$

The idea of a system's impulse response is commonly used in systems theory.[6] When we consider a hypothetical tracer experiment with an ideal bolus input of tracer at the arterial inlet of the vascular system (Fig. 4.1A), the injected tracer would not appear all at once at the venous outlet[6] and the transit times of tracer (contrast agent) through the vascular system are dispersed, as previously described. The distribution of transit times of tracer (contrast agent) at the venous outlet through the vascular system is described by the impulse response function ($h(t)$) (Fig. 4.1C). The relationship between $h(t)$ and $R(t)$ can be given by[6]

$$R(t) = 1 - \int_0^t h(\tau)d\tau. \qquad (9)$$

Differentiating Eq. (9) yields the alternative relation

$$h(t) = -\frac{dR(t)}{dt}. \qquad (10)$$

Because $h(t)$ is the probability density function of transit times of tracer through the vascular system, the first moment of $h(t)$ gives the mean transit time (MTT) of the tracer, that is,

$$\text{MTT} = \int_0^\infty th(t)dt. \qquad (11)$$

Substituting Eq. (10) into Eq. (11) and using the formula for integration by parts yield

$$\text{MTT} = \int_0^\infty R(t)dt. \qquad (12)$$

Fick Principle

When a contrast agent is injected and enters a vascular system as shown in Figure 4.1, the concentration of contrast agent at the venous outlet of the system cannot be measured using DCE-CT, but only the average concentration within the distribution space of contrast agent in the tissue can be measured. Thus, we consider the vascular system consisting of the tissue region including the distribution space of contrast agent as illustrated in Figure 4.3. If the administered tracer enters and leaves the system with blood flow F as illustrated in Figure 4.3, then the temporal change of the tracer mass (concentration × volume) inside the tissue distribution space at time t is described by Fick principle as

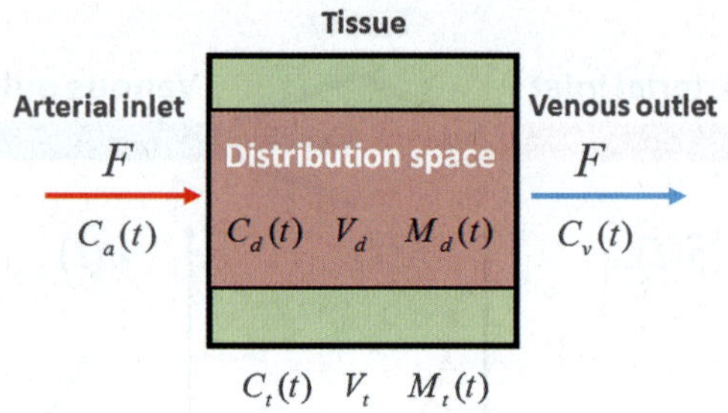

Figure 4-3. Model for Fick principle (single-compartment model). V_t and V_d are the volumes of the tissue and distribution space, respectively. V_d is equal to the sum of the volumes of the intravascular and interstitial distribution space and is generally smaller than V_t. When using the intravascular tracer, V_d is equal to the volume of the intravascular space. $C_d(t)$ and $C_t(t)$ represent the concentrations in the distribution space and the tissue, respectively. $M_d(t)$ and $M_t(t)$ represent the mass (concentration × volume) in the distribution space and the tissue, respectively.

$$\frac{dM_d(t)}{dt} = V_d\frac{dC_d(t)}{dt} = F[C_a(t) - C_v(t)], \qquad (13)$$

where $C_d(t)$, $C_a(t)$, and $C_v(t)$ are the concentrations of the tracer in the tissue distribution space, arterial blood, and venous blood at time t, respectively, and $M_d(t)$ is the mass of tracer inside the tissue distribution space with a volume of V_d, that is, $M_d(t) = C_d(t)V_d$. If we use the concentration of contrast agent in whole blood ($C_b(t)$) for $C_a(t)$, F represents whole blood flow. If the concentration of contrast agent in arterial plasma ($C_p(t)$) is used for $C_a(t)$, F represents plasma flow and $C_p(t)$ is given by $C_p(t) = C_b(t)/(1 - \text{Hct})$, where Hct denotes hematocrit.

The extraction fraction (E) is defined by dividing both sides of Eq. (13) by the influx ($FC_a(t)$) as

$$E = \frac{F[C_a(t) - C_v(t)]}{FC_a(t)} = \frac{C_a(t) - C_v(t)}{C_a(t)}. \qquad (14)$$

E is the fraction of the inflowing tracer that does not leave the system via outflow. Note that E is usually given in the form of $E = (C_a(\infty) - C_v(\infty))/C_a(\infty)$. The complement of E is also sometimes used, that is, $T = 1 - E$. Correspondingly, T is defined as the fraction of the inflowing tracer that leaves the system via outflow and is called the "throughput" or "transmission."

Integrating both sides of Eq. (13) from $t = 0$ to ∞ with an assumption of $C_d(0) = 0$ yields

$$\frac{F}{V_d} = \frac{C_d(\infty)}{\int_0^\infty C_a(t)dt - \int_0^\infty C_v(t)dt}. \qquad (15)$$

Equation (15) is known as "Kety-Schmidt equation."[7] When $C_d(0) = 0$ and $C_d(\infty) = 0$, that is, all tracers entering the tissue leave it eventually, we obtain the following relation from Eq. (13):

$$\int_0^\infty C_a(t)dt = \int_0^\infty C_v(t)dt. \qquad (16)$$

Equation (16) represents the principle of conservation of mass.

It should be noted that blood flow is the amount of blood flowing through an organ, tissue, or vessel at a given time, whereas perfusion is the flow per given volume or mass of tissue. Thus, a large organ could have greater blood flow but less perfusion.

Central Volume Principle

The concentration of the tracer in venous blood ($C_v(t)$) in Eq. (13) can be given by convolution integral between $C_a(t)$ and $h(t)$ as $C_v(t) = C_a(t) \otimes h(t)$. Substituting this relation into Eq. (13) and integrating both sides of Eq. (13) yield[2]

$$C_d(t) = \frac{F}{V_d}\int_0^t [C_a(\tau) - C_a(\tau)\otimes h(\tau)]d\tau = C_a(t)\otimes R_d(t), \quad (17)$$

where

$$R_d(t) = \frac{F}{V_d}\left[1 - \int_0^t h(\tau)d\tau\right] = \frac{F}{V_d}R(t). \quad (18)$$

$R_d(t)$ is referred to as the "tissue response function." When we integrate both sides of Eq. (17) and use the principle of conservation of mass in a similar manner to that in Eq. (8), we obtain $\int_0^\infty R_d(t)dt = 1$. Furthermore, integrating both sides of Eq. (18) and using this relation yield $\int_0^\infty R(t)dt = \frac{V_d}{F}$. Therefore, from Eq. (12), we obtain the MTT of tracer in the tissue distribution space (MTT_d) as

$$MTT_d = \frac{V_d}{F}. \quad (19)$$

Equation (19) is the basic equation of "central volume principle," stating that the MTT of tracer in the tissue distribution space can be given by the quotient of distribution volume and blood flow, and it is equal to the reciprocal of perfusion.

The MTT of tracer in the tissue (MTT_t) is given by replacing V_d by V_t as[2]

$$MTT_t = \frac{V_t}{F} = \frac{V_t}{V_d}MTT_d. \quad (20)$$

As illustrated in Figure 4.4, the following relation holds:

$$R_d(0)\times MTT_d = \int_0^\infty R_d(t)dt = 1. \quad (21)$$

Thus, we obtain

$$R_d(0) = \frac{1}{MTT_d} = \frac{F}{V_d}. \quad (22)$$

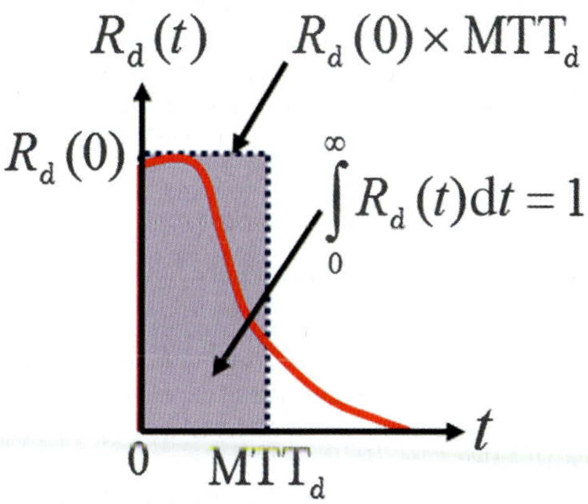

Figure 4-4. Relationship between the tissue response function ($R_d(t)$) and the MTT of tracer in the tissue distribution space (MTT_d), from which the relation $R_d(0) = 1/MTT_d$ is obtained.

Equation (22) implies that the initial height of the tissue response function is equal to F/V_d, that is, perfusion.

Tracer Kinetic Analysis

Model-Independent Method and Model-Dependent Method

A tracer kinetic model is a mathematical description of the transport processes of the tracer within the tissue.[6] Recently, various methods have been proposed for the quantification of kinetic parameters including perfusion.[8,9] These methods can be roughly classified into two groups; one is a model-independent method and the other is a model-dependent method.

The model-independent method yields kinetic parameters for a tissue region described as a "black box" and thus does not provide insight into its internal structure.[2] For quantification of perfusion using a model-independent method, deconvolution between the measured tissue residue curve and the AIF is needed to obtain the tissue response function, from which the perfusion can be quantified based on the central volume principle (Eq. (19)).[10] Thus, the model-independent method is also called "deconvolution analysis."

For a model-dependent method, compartment models are usually employed as tracer kinetic models, and kinetic parameters are quantified using compartment analysis based on the assumption that tissues can be kinetically represented by a set of interacting subcompartments that represent distinguishable states of an administered tracer.[2]

The kinetic models employed in compartment analysis can be classified as lumped parameter or distributed parameter models. The compartments are used to describe the physical distribution spaces of the tracer in the tissue. Conventionally, these compartments are assumed to be well mixed, that is, tracer movement is sufficiently fast and distributes evenly throughout the compartments, such that tracer concentration is only a function of time, but not space. Thus, conventional compartment models are called lumped parameter models. On the other hand, a distributed parameter model attempts to account for tracer concentration gradient within the compartments, such that concentration can be a function of both time and space.[6]

In contrast to the model-independent method, the model-dependent method generally requires specific knowledge about the vascular and compartmental architecture, the volumes of the compartments comprising the model, and the tracer-dependent permeability of compartment barriers. The assumptions in these models are generally valid under normal conditions, but for pathologic conditions, it is often difficult to independently verify which model parameters changed significantly, in particular when the model involves a large number of parameters or if the sensitivity ranges for the different parameters overlap significantly.[11]

Generally, model-independent deconvolution analysis has been applied to the data obtained by intravascular tracers.[12] Recently, the accuracy of model-independent deconvolution analysis when applied to the data obtained by extravascular contrast agents, that is, the effect of the leakage of contrast agent from the intravascular space to the extravascular space, has been studied in Ref. [13]

To investigate the effect of the leakage of contrast agent from the intravascular space to the extravascular space, it is necessary to use a model in which the concentration of contrast agent within the tissue is treated as a function of both time and position, that is, distributed parameter models.[9] The distributed parameter models describe tracer concentration in the vascular compartment as a function of both time and position along the capillary and are generally believed to be more realistic than the lumped parameter models. One of the simple distributed parameter models is the tissue homogeneity model, which was initially developed by Johnson and Wilson.[14] This model is based on both convective and diffusive transport of contrast agent in capillaries represented together as a single cylinder and is composed of the intravascular space surrounded by the extravascular space. The two spaces are separated by a permeable barrier. St. Lawrence and Lee[15] derived an approximate closed-form solution to the tissue homogeneity model using the adiabatic approximation. The details of the adiabatic approximation to the tissue homogeneity model will be described afterwards.

Model-Independent Method

With a model-independent method, perfusion is quantified from the tissue response function obtained by deconvolution between the measured tissue concentration–time curve and the AIF.

The relationship between the concentration–time curve of contrast agent in tissue ($C_t(t)$) and that in a feeding artery, that is, the AIF ($C_a(t)$), can be described as convolution integral in a similar manner to Eq. (17):

$$C_t(t) = \frac{F}{V_t}\int_0^t C_a(\tau)R(t-\tau)\mathrm{d}\tau = C_a(t)\otimes R_t(t). \tag{23}$$

In Eq. (23), $R_t(t) = FR(t)/V_t$ is the tissue response function, which is the amount of the contrast agent in the tissue in an idealized perfusion experiment, where a unit area bolus is instantaneously injected ($R(0) = 1$) and subsequently washed out by perfusion ($R(\infty) = 0$). The procedure of finding a solution for the tissue response function that satisfies Eq. (23) is called "deconvolution analysis." It is known from Eq. (22) that the initial height of the deconvolved tissue response function equals F/V_t, that is, perfusion.

Because the model-independent method only requires minimal user interaction or expertise in modeling, this approach appears to be easier to implement than the model-dependent method. Thus, the model-independent method has been applied to the quantification of perfusion in various organs such as the brain,[16] the heart,[17] and the lungs.[18] Furthermore, this method has been applied to the evaluation of the hemodynamic change due to angiogenesis in tumors[19] and monitoring the effect of therapeutic strategies on tumor vascular activity.[20]

Quantification of Perfusion Using Truncated Singular Value Decomposition

If it is assumed that the functions $C_a(t)$ and $R(t)$ in Eq. (23) are constant over small time intervals, Δt, Eq. (23) is reduced to

$$C_t(t_j) = \frac{F}{V_t}\sum_{i=1}^{n} C_a(t_i)R(t_j - t_i)\Delta t, \tag{24}$$

where t_i and n denote the time of the ith frame and the total number of frames, respectively. It should be noted that it was assumed that $t_1 = 0$ and the duration of each frame (Δt) is equal when converting Eq. (23) to Eq. (24). Equation (24) can then be formulated as a matrix equation

$$\mathbf{c} = \mathbf{A}\cdot\mathbf{b}, \tag{25}$$

where

$$\mathbf{A} = \begin{pmatrix} C_a(t_1) & 0 & \cdots & 0 \\ C_a(t_2) & C_a(t_1) & \cdots & 0 \\ \cdots & \cdots & \cdots & \cdots \\ C_a(t_n) & C_a(t_{n-1}) & \cdots & C_a(t_1) \end{pmatrix},\quad \mathbf{b} = \frac{F}{V_t}\begin{pmatrix} R(t_1) \\ R(t_2) \\ \cdots \\ R(t_n) \end{pmatrix}\Delta t, \text{ and}$$

$\mathbf{c} = \begin{pmatrix} C_t(t_1) \\ C_t(t_2) \\ \cdots \\ C_t(t_n) \end{pmatrix}$. To solve Eq. (25) for **b** is called "deconvolution," which is an inverse problem and is a well-known ill-posed problem especially when there exists statistical noise. Thus, it is necessary to convert an ill-posed problem to a well-posed one to solve Eq. (25). The procedure of modifying an ill-posed problem to obtain a robust solution is called "regularization." Of the regularization methods, the truncated singular value decomposition (TSVD) is a popular method for computing regularized solutions for ill-posed inverse problems.[12,21]

With singular value decomposition, the matrix **A** in Eq. (25) can be expressed as the product of an $n \times n$ column orthogonal matrix **U**, an $n \times n$ diagonal matrix **W**, and the transpose of an $n \times n$ orthogonal matrix **V**,[17] that is,

$$\mathbf{A} = \mathbf{U}\mathbf{W}\mathbf{V}^T = \mathbf{U}\left[\mathrm{diag}(w_i)\right]\mathbf{V}^T, \tag{26}$$

where w_i ($i = 1, 2, \ldots, n$) are the diagonal elements of **W** (singular values), which are nonnegative and can be ordered such that

$$w_1 \geq w_2 \geq \cdots \geq w_n \geq 0. \tag{27}$$

The singular value decomposition constructs the matrices so that the inverse of **A** can be written as

$$\mathbf{A}^{-1} = \mathbf{V}\left[\mathrm{diag}(1/w_i)\right]\mathbf{U}^T, \tag{28}$$

where $\mathbf{U}^T$ is the transpose of **U**. The matrix **b** can then be calculated as

$$\mathbf{b} = \mathbf{V}\left[\mathrm{diag}(1/w_i)\right](\mathbf{U}^T\mathbf{c}). \tag{29}$$

That is, Eq. (29) is used to solve for **b**, which contains the elements of $R(t)$.

With TSVD, if w_i was smaller than the maximal value of w_i multiplied by a threshold value, $1/w_i$ in Eq. (29) was replaced by zero. This threshold value can be thought of as a regularization parameter. The F/V_t value is obtained from the initial height (or maximum value) of **b** calculated from Eq. (29).[12,21]

Figure 4.5 shows an example of the tissue response functions obtained from $C_a(t)$ and $C_t(t)$ shown in Figure 4.5A by deconvolution using the TSVD with various threshold values (0.01, 0.2, and 0.5).

As shown in Figure 4.5, the tissue response function obtained by deconvolution using the TSVD depends largely on the threshold value. When the threshold value is small, the tissue response function oscillates largely. On the other hand, the oscillation of the response function decreases with increasing threshold value, but the initial height of the tissue response function decreases. The choice of a suitable regularization parameter is generally important, but can be difficult without auxiliary information about the problem being solved. The threshold value used in the TSVD is usually determined empirically by inspection of the results. Several methods, however, have been proposed to determine the optimal threshold value for TSVD automatically. These methods include a method using generalized cross-validation[22] and L-curve method.[23]

Model-Dependent Method

As previously described, compartment models are usually employed in the model-dependent method, and the kinetic parameters are quantified using compartment analysis based on the assumption that tissues can be kinetically represented by a set of interacting subcompartments.[2]

Many investigators have proposed various kinetic models for the quantification of physiologic parameters using DCE-CT or DCE-MRI. The models originally proposed by Tofts and Kermode,[24] Larsson et al.,[25] and Brix et al.[26] are known to be the three major

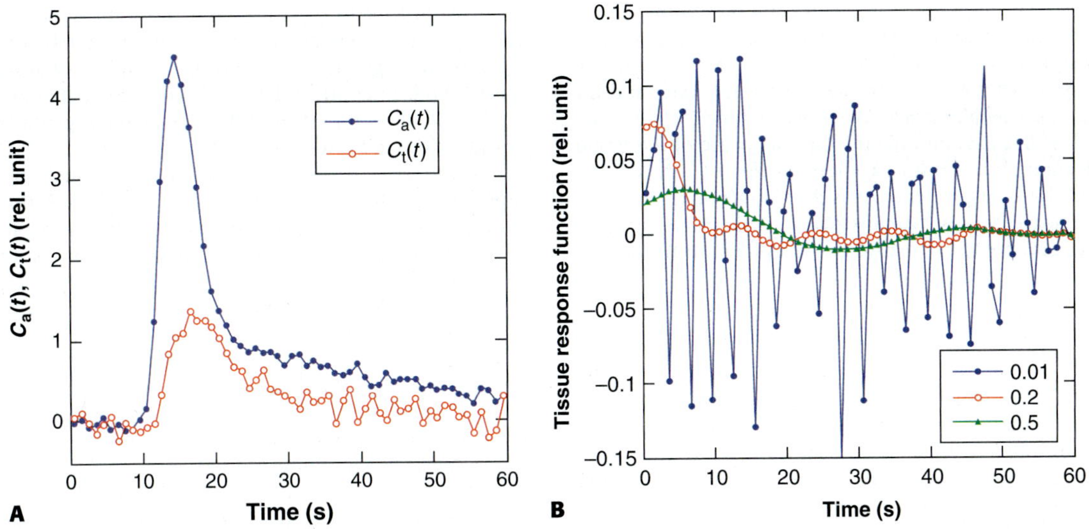

Figure 4-5. Example of deconvolution analysis using TSVD. **(A)** shows an example of arterial input function ($C_a(t)$) and the concentration–time curve in tissue ($C_t(t)$), and **(B)** shows the tissue response functions obtained from $C_a(t)$ and $C_t(t)$ by deconvolution using TSVD with various threshold values (0.01, 0.2, and 0.5).

models. For the quantification of physiologic parameters in terms of absolute values, the AIF of the contrast agent entering the tissue has to be determined.[27] When AIF is not directly assessed, the models proposed by Tofts and Kermode[24] and Brix et al.[26] have proved useful. However, when an artery runs through the imaged slices, the AIF can be obtained noninvasively from the arterial pixels.[27] Although techniques to achieve this are not yet in common use, an increasing number of investigators are developing practical methods for doing so.[27]

In the model proposed by Tofts and Kermode[24], the plasma concentration after the injection of a bolus of contrast agent was assumed to be the same as that measured in normal control subjects, which was fitted to a biexponential decay. Without AIF and with limited temporal resolution, this model has proved useful. However, the use of a fixed AIF is known to introduce considerable error into the estimate of physiologic parameters.[27] The model proposed by Brix et al.[26] is also one of the several models that deal with the situation in which AIF is not directly assessed. Instead, the vascular space is assumed to be a perfect mixing chamber with uniform concentration and a constant clearance rate (k_{el}).[26] The vascular concentration curve is assumed to be the result of a constant infusion of contrast agent of known duration into the vascular space. This results in a mathematical expression for the extravascular–extracellular concentration in terms of three parameters: an amplitude parameter (A), k_{el}, and a rate constant for transfer of contrast agent from peripheral to central compartment (k_{21}).

To consider a more realistic nature, a physiologic model incorporating multiple parallel pathways and heterogeneous flow should be realized.[28] Recently, St. Lawrence and Lee[15] have derived an equation describing the kinetic behavior of the tracer in a more realistic model. Their model offers the possibility of assessing the blood flow and extraction fraction or permeability–surface area product simultaneously, but may require carefully constrained supervised data fitting, additional measurements, or multiple tracers to overcome problems with parameter correlation.[28] The choice of this model for data analysis requires a sampling interval less than the MTT of the tracer in the vascular space. When the sampling interval is equal to or greater than the MTT (the order of a few seconds), this model may be simplified to a form similar to the model described by Eq. (33).[15]

Two-Compartment Model

The majority of clinical studies have used a simple two-compartment model illustrated in Figure 4.6. This model is known as "extended Tofts model."[29] Unless an independent estimate of blood flow or capillary permeability is essential, this model may be an appropriate choice for the analysis of DCE-CT or DCE-MRI data.[28] This model assumes that the contrast agent resides in and exchanges between two compartments in the tissue: an intravascular plasma space and an extravascular–extracellular space (Fig. 4.6). When using this model, the differential equation describing the kinetic behavior of the contrast agent in the tissue of interest is given by

$$v_e \frac{\mathrm{d}C_e(t)}{\mathrm{d}t} = K^{\mathrm{trans}} \cdot \left[C_p(t) - C_e(t)\right], \quad (30)$$

where $C_e(t)$ and $C_p(t)$ are the concentrations of the contrast agent at time t in the extravascular–extracellular space and the intravascular

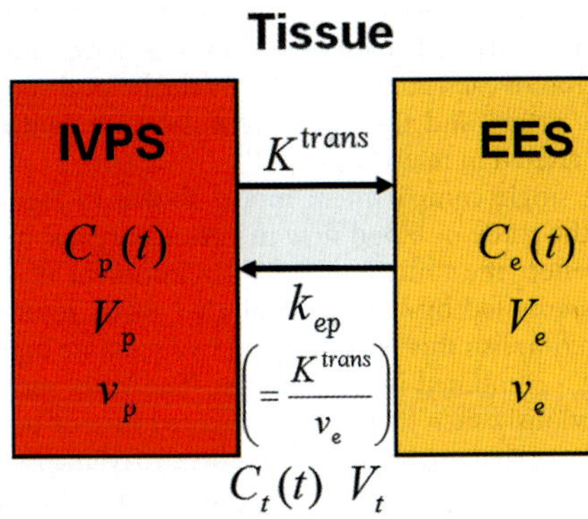

Figure 4-6. Extended Tofts model consisting of two compartments (intravascular plasma space [IVPS] and extravascular–extracellular space [EES]). K^{trans} and k_{ep} ($=K^{trans}/v_e$) denote the volume transfer constant and the rate constant between the IVPS and the EES, respectively, and $C_t(t)$, $C_p(t)$, and $C_e(t)$ are the concentrations of contrast agent in the tissue, IVPS, and EES, respectively. V_t, V_p, and V_e are the volumes of the tissue, IVS, and EES, respectively. $v_p = V_p/V_t$ and $v_e = V_e/V_t$.

plasma space, respectively, and v_e is the distribution volume of contrast agent in the extravascular–extracellular space per unit volume of tissue; that is, $v_e = V_e/V_t$. K^{trans} is the volume transfer constant of contrast agent between the intravascular plasma space and the extravascular–extracellular space. When we assume that the contrast agent does not pass into the intracellular space of the tissue, the concentration of the contrast agent in the tissue ($C_t(t)$) is given by $C_t(t) = v_pC_p(t) + v_eC_e(t)$, where v_p is the volume of the intravascular plasma space per unit volume of tissue, that is, $v_p = V_p/V_t$. Using this equation and by rearrangement of Eq. (30), we then obtain the following differential equation:

$$\frac{d\left[C_t(t)-v_pC_p(t)\right]}{dt} = K^{trans}C_p(t) - k_{ep}\cdot\left[C_t(t)-v_pC_p(t)\right], \quad (31)$$

where $k_{ep} = K^{trans}/v_e$, which represents the rate constant between the intravascular plasma space and the extravascular–extracellular space. In accord with recent standardization[30], K^{trans} is given by $K^{trans} = EF_p/V_t = EF_b(1 - \text{Hct})/V_t$, where F_p and F_b are plasma and whole blood flow, respectively, V_t is the volume of tissue, and Hct is hematocrit. E is the extraction fraction given by

$$E = 1-\exp\left(-\frac{PS}{F_p/V_t}\right) = 1-\exp\left(-\frac{PS}{F_b(1-Hc)/V_t}\right), \quad (32)$$

where PS is the capillary permeability–surface area product per unit volume of tissue. Equation (32) is called "Renkin-Crone equation."[31,32]

Solving Eq. (31) with the assumption that the initial conditions are zero yields

$$C_t(t) = K^{trans}\cdot\int_0^t C_p(\tau)\cdot e^{-k_{ep}\cdot(t-\tau)}d\tau + v_p\cdot C_p(t). \quad (33)$$

This equation has been used to analyze DCE-CT or DCE-MRI data in a number of studies.

Dual-Input Single-Compartment Model

Quantitative measurement of hepatic perfusion has the potential to provide important information in the assessment and management of various liver diseases and in the determination of their outcome.[33,34] Liver metastases play a major role in the morbidity and mortality associated with many cancers. The noninvasive measurement of regional blood flow within the liver is of particular clinical interest, since changes in tumor blood flow have been recognized as an important factor for assessing the treatment response of hepatic cancers.[35,36] The utility of hepatic perfusion characterization relies on the resolution of each component of its dual blood supply, that is, the hepatic artery and the portal vein, because contributions from each are altered in many diseases.[37]

While the single-compartment model shown in Figure 4.3 is applicable to the study of blood flow in various organs, it must be modified to reflect the unique delivery environment of the liver, where the tissue is fed by both arterial and portal inputs.[36] Two methods to accomplish this include using two separate input functions or using a combined input function. The latter method has been used previously such that a flow-weighted sum of both input functions was applied to hepatic ^{18}F-fluorodeoxyglucose uptake, assuming a constant arterial-to-portal ratio across all regions of the liver.[38] However, such a fixed ratio system does not allow for the measurement of independent regional arterial and portal flow fluctuations. A more flexible approach is to incorporate the two separate input functions into the single-compartment model (dual-input single-compartment model), whereby the second input function reflects the tracer supplied by the portal vein. In this case, the model complexity increases and a third parameter for the local portal venous blood flow has to be estimated from the data.[36]

It is difficult to measure the dual vascular input of the liver via the hepatic artery and the portal vein separately using positron emission tomography, because of the limited spatial resolution of the method. In contrast, DCE-CT has high spatial and temporal resolution, allowing for separate measurement of the arterial and portal venous input functions.[34,39]

In the early 1970s, it was discovered through necropsy that lung tumors also have a dual vascular supply[1], indicating that lung tumors can also become the target for tracer kinetic analysis using a dual-input single-compartment model. Recent advances in CT technology, particularly the development of a CT scanner with a large detector system composed of 320-detector row, enabled one temporally uniform acquisition of the pulmonary artery, the aorta, the left atrium, and the lesion studied, which makes it possible to quantify the dual blood supply (pulmonary artery and bronchial artery) in lung cancer. The quantification of the dual blood supply to lung tumors and the relative portions of each can potentially aid in the management of lung cancer.[1]

The compartment model used to describe the kinetic behavior of the contrast agent in the liver is illustrated in Figure 4.7. This model consists of a single compartment with two inputs. When using this model, the differential equation describing the kinetic behavior of contrast agent in the liver region of interest is given by

$$\frac{dC_L(t)}{dt} = K_{1a}\cdot C_{ha}(t) + K_{1p}\cdot C_{pv}(t) - k_2\cdot C_L(t), \quad (34)$$

where $C_L(t)$, $C_{ha}(t)$, and $C_{pv}(t)$ are the concentrations of the contrast agent at time t in the liver region of interest, hepatic artery or aorta, and portal vein, respectively. K_{1a}, K_{1p}, and k_2 are the rate constants for the exchanges of contrast agent from the hepatic artery or aorta to the liver, from the portal vein to the liver, and from the liver to plasma, respectively. It should be noted that whole-blood perfusion is obtained by dividing plasma perfusion by 1 minus the small vessel hematocrit, as in Eq. (32). When deriving Eq. (34), the transit times of the contrast agent from the hepatic artery (alternatively aorta) and portal vein regions of interest to the liver region of interest were assumed to be negligible for simplicity. When these transit times are not negligible, they can be taken into account by replacing $C_{ha}(t)$ and $C_{pv}(t)$ in Eq. (34) by $C_{ha}(t - \tau_a)$ and $C_{pv}(t - \tau_p)$, respectively, where τ_a and τ_p denote the transit time of the contrast agent from the hepatic artery or aorta and portal vein to the liver, respectively.[40] Note that when analyzing the kinetic behavior of the contrast agent in lung tumors, $C_L(t)$, $C_{ha}(t)$, and $C_{pv}(t)$ in Eq. (34)

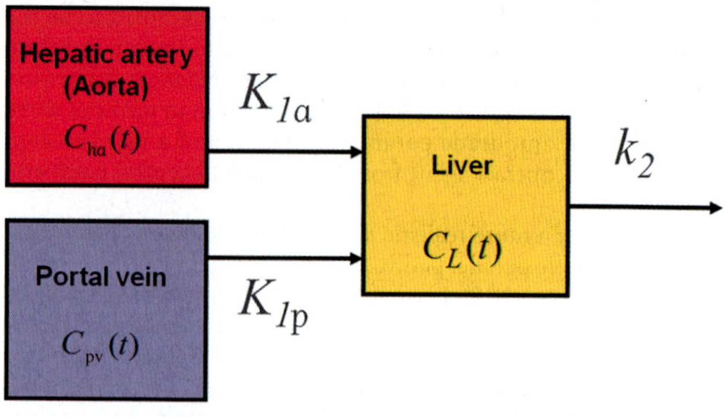

Figure 4-7. Illustration of a dual-input single-compartment model for analysis of liver perfusion. $C_{ha}(t)$, $C_{pv}(t)$, and $C_L(t)$ represent the concentrations of contrast agent at time t in the hepatic artery or aorta, the portal vein, and the liver region of interest, respectively. K_{1a}, K_{1p}, and k_2 are the rate constants for the exchanges of contrast agent from the hepatic artery or aorta to the liver, from the portal vein to the liver, and from the liver to plasma, respectively.

correspond to the concentrations of the contrast agent in the lung tumor, pulmonary artery, and bronchial artery, respectively, and K_{1a}, K_{1p}, and k_2 correspond to the rate constants for the exchanges of contrast agent from the pulmonary artery to the lung tumor, from the bronchial artery to the lung tumor, and from the lung tumor to plasma, respectively.

When the kinetic model includes a vascular term, Eq. (34) becomes

$$\frac{d\{C_L(t)-v_0\cdot[C_{ha}(t)+C_{pv}(t)]\}}{dt} = K_{1a}\cdot C_{ha}(t)+K_{1p}\cdot C_{pv}(t)-k_2\cdot \{C_L(t)-v_0\cdot[C_{ha}(t)+C_{pv}(t)]\}, \tag{35}$$

where v_0 is the capillary plasma volume per unit volume of tissue. v_0 is given by a weighted average of v_{ha} and v_{pv} as[41]

$$v_0 = \frac{v_{ha}\cdot C_{ha}(t)+v_{pv}\cdot C_{pv}(t)}{C_{ha}(t)+C_{pv}(t)}, \tag{36}$$

where v_{ha} and v_{pv} denote the relative volume fractions of the hepatic arterial plasma and the portal venous plasma, respectively. Solving Eq. (35) with the assumption that the initial conditions are zero yields

$$C_L(t)=\int_0^t [K_{1a}\cdot C_{ha}(\tau)+K_{1p}\cdot C_{pv}(\tau)]\cdot e^{-k_2(t-\tau)}d\tau+v_0\cdot[C_{ha}(t)+C_{pv}(t)]. \tag{37}$$

Methods for Kinetic Parameter Estimation

Nonlinear Least-Squares Method

In the case of a two-compartment model (Fig. 4.6), fitting Eq. (33) to the concentration–time curve in the tissue obtained by DCE-CT allows the estimation of K^{trans}, k_{ep}, and v_p. In the case of a dual-input single-compartment model (Fig. 4.7), fitting Eq. (37) to the concentration–time curve in the liver allows the estimation of K_{1a}, K_{1p}, k_2, and v_0. In general, these estimations can be performed by minimizing the sum of the squares of the differences between the data points and the model-estimated points, that is, a merit function, using the nonlinear least-squares (NLSQ) method. For minimization of the merit function, there are several methods such as the Levenberg-Marquardt method[42] and the simplex method.[43] They are classified into two categories.[44] One is the method that requires both function evaluations and derivatives, and the other is the method that requires only function evaluations, not derivatives.[44] The Levenberg-Marquardt method belongs to the former category, whereas the simplex method belongs to the latter category. Algorithms using the derivative are somewhat more powerful than those using the only function, but not always enough so as to compensate for the additional calculations of derivatives.[44]

The above methods search for the best combination of unknown parameters in a hypothetical model that predicts the measured data. These methods, however, are prone to estimating erroneous values. This is probably due to the noise intrinsic in the data and the inability of any search algorithm to find a global minimum of the merit function; that is, the algorithm falls into a localized minimum of the merit function.[42] A strategy to avoid the selection of the localized minimum is to repeat the NLSQ fitting for a variety of initial guesses and to select the solution with the smallest value of the merit function.

When using a model-dependent method, it is often unclear which combination of unknown parameters best approximates the measured data. A commonly used means to decide which model is the best is the corrected Akaike information criterion (cAIC).[45] This criterion penalizes the goodness of the fit, based on not only the merit function (*SSR*) but also the number of estimated parameters (*K*) and sample size (*N*).[45] That is, cAIC is given by

$$\text{cAIC} = N\ln\left(\frac{\text{SSR}}{N}\right)+\frac{2N(K+1)}{N-K-2}. \tag{38}$$

The value of the cAIC itself for a given data set has no meaning, and it can only be interpreted comparing the cAIC of a series of models based on the same data set. Then, the model with the lowest cAIC is the best model among all considered models.[45]

Although the NLSQ method is a powerful tool for estimating kinetic parameters, it is not always suitable for generating parametric images of physiologic parameters, because it is not efficient in terms of computation time. Furthermore, appropriate choices of initial guesses of the parameters are important in the NLSQ method; poor initial guesses result in long computation times or occasionally failure to converge on a good fit. Thus, to generate parametric images of physiologic parameters using DCE-CT, an efficient method for estimating kinetic parameters is necessary, which is computationally efficient and does not need initial guesses of the parameters.

Linear Least-Squares Method

Two-Compartment Model

Integrating both sides of Eq. (31) with the assumption that the initial conditions are zero and expressing the result in a discrete form yield[46]

$$C_t(t_k) = (K^{trans}+k_{ep}\cdot v_p)\cdot\int_0^{t_k} C_p(\tau)d\tau - k_{ep}\cdot \int_0^{t_k} C_t(\tau)d\tau + v_p\cdot C_p(t_k)\quad (k=1,2,\cdots,n). \tag{39}$$

Equation (39) can be given in a matrix form as

$$\mathbf{C}=\mathbf{A}\cdot\mathbf{B}, \tag{40}$$

where

$$\mathbf{A}=\begin{pmatrix} \int_0^{t_1} C_p(\tau)d\tau & -\int_0^{t_1} C_t(\tau)d\tau & C_p(t_1)\\ \int_0^{t_2} C_p(\tau)d\tau & -\int_0^{t_2} C_t(\tau)d\tau & C_p(t_2)\\ \vdots & \vdots & \vdots \\ \int_0^{t_n} C_p(\tau)d\tau & -\int_0^{t_n} C_t(\tau)d\tau & C_p(t_n) \end{pmatrix},$$

$$\mathbf{B}=\begin{pmatrix} K^{trans}+k_{ep}\cdot v_p \\ k_{ep} \\ v_p \end{pmatrix}, \text{ and } \mathbf{C}=\begin{pmatrix} C_t(t_1)\\ C_t(t_2)\\ \vdots \\ C_t(t_n)\end{pmatrix}.$$ When $C_t(t_k)$ and $C_p(t_k)$ ($k = 1, 2, \ldots, n$) are measured, Eq. (40) can be easily solved for the elements of **B** using the conventional linear least-squares (LLSQ) method,[44] and finally, K^{trans}, k_{ep}, and v_p can be easily obtained from the elements.[46] We call this method the "LLSQ method." The elements of **A** can be generated by numerical integration using trapezoidal rule.[44]

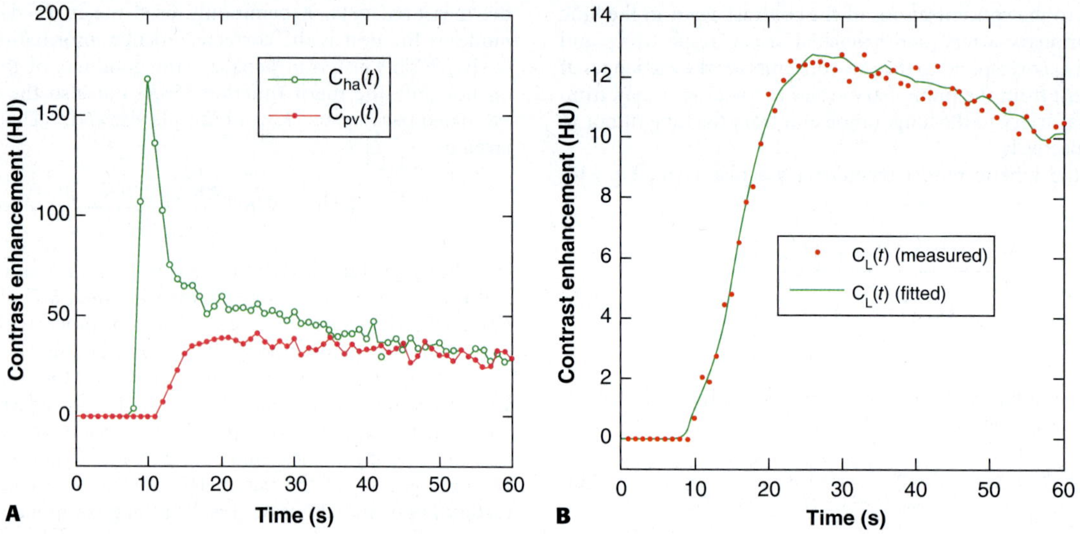

Figure 4-8. Example of the LLSQ method for the dual-input single-compartment model applied to the DCE-CT data in the liver. The open and closed circles in **(A)** represent the concentration–time curves in the hepatic artery ($C_{ha}(t)$) and portal vein ($C_{pv}(t)$), respectively. The *closed circles* and *solid line* in **(B)** represent the concentration–time curve in the liver measured using DCE-CT and that estimated from $C_{ha}(t)$ and $C_{pv}(t)$ using the LLSQ method, respectively.

It has been demonstrated that the LLSQ method can estimate the kinetic parameters faster and more accurately than the NLSQ method especially at low signal-to-noise ratio.[46] Furthermore, the LLSQ method does not need initial guesses of the parameters unlike the NLSQ method.[46] These results suggest that the LLSQ method is useful for kinetic analysis of contrast agent in the tissue using DCE-CT or DCE-MRI and especially for generating the parametric images of kinetic parameters by applying it pixel by pixel.

Dual-Input Single-Compartment Model

Integrating both sides of Eq. (35) with the assumption that the initial conditions are zero and expressing the result in a discrete form yield

$$C_L(t_k) = (K_{1a} + k_2 \cdot v_0) \cdot \int_0^{t_k} C_{ha}(\tau)d\tau + (K_{1p} + k_2 \cdot v_0) \cdot \int_0^{t_k} C_{pv}(\tau)d\tau - k_2 \cdot \int_0^{t_k} C_L(\tau)d\tau + v_0 \cdot \left[C_{ha}(t_k) + C_{pv}(t_k)\right] (k = 1, 2, \cdots, n). \quad (41)$$

Equation (41) can be given in a matrix form as

$$\mathbf{C} = \mathbf{A} \cdot \mathbf{B} \quad (42)$$

where

$$\mathbf{A} = \begin{pmatrix} \int_0^{t_1} C_{ha}(\tau)d\tau & \int_0^{t_1} C_{pv}(\tau)d\tau & -\int_0^{t_1} C_L(\tau)d\tau & C_{ha}(t_1)+C_{pv}(t_1) \\ \int_0^{t_2} C_{ha}(\tau)d\tau & \int_0^{t_2} C_{pv}(\tau)d\tau & -\int_0^{t_2} C_L(\tau)d\tau & C_{ha}(t_2)+C_{pv}(t_2) \\ \vdots & \vdots & \vdots & \vdots \\ \int_0^{t_n} C_{ha}(\tau)d\tau & \int_0^{t_n} C_{pv}(\tau)d\tau & -\int_0^{t_n} C_L(\tau)d\tau & C_{ha}(t_n)+C_{pv}(t_n) \end{pmatrix},$$

$$\mathbf{B} = \begin{pmatrix} K_{1a} + k_2 \cdot v_0 \\ K_{1p} + k_2 \cdot v_0 \\ k_2 \\ V_0 \end{pmatrix}, \text{ and } \mathbf{C} = \begin{pmatrix} C_L(t_1) \\ C_L(t_2) \\ \vdots \\ C_L(t_n) \end{pmatrix}.$$

When $C_L(t_k)$, $C_{ha}(t_k)$, and $C_{pv}(t_k)$ $(k = 1, 2, \ldots, n)$ are measured, Eq. (42) can be easily solved for the elements of **B** using the LLSQ method as in Eq. (40), and finally, K_{1a}, K_{1p}, k_2, and v_0 can be easily obtained from the elements.[41] The elements of **A** can be generated by numerical integration using the trapezoidal rule[44] as in Eq. (40).

Figure 4.8 shows an example of the LLSQ method for the dual-input single-compartment model applied to the DCE-CT data in the liver. As shown in Figure 4.8B, the concentration–time curve in the liver estimated by the LLSQ method (solid line) is well fitted to that actually measured (closed circles).

It has been demonstrated by computer simulations that the LLSQ method can estimate the kinetic parameters in the liver with almost the same accuracy as the NLSQ method.[41] Furthermore, the LLSQ method can estimate them faster than the NLSQ method by a factor of approximately 10.[41] These results suggest that the LLSQ method is useful for analyzing the kinetic behavior of contrast agent in the organ or tissue having a dual blood supply such as the liver and lung tumor, especially when generating the parametric images of kinetic parameters by applying it pixel by pixel.

Graphical Method

When using a two-compartment model illustrated in Figure 4.6, the differential equation describing the kinetic behavior of the contrast agent in the tissue is given by Eq. (31).[46] Solving Eq. (31) for $C_t(t)$ with the assumption that the initial conditions are zero and k_{ep} is negligible during the sampling period yields

$$C_t(t) = K^{\text{trans}} \cdot \int_0^t C_p(\tau)d\tau + v_p \cdot C_p(t). \quad (43)$$

Dividing both sides of Eq. (43) by $C_p(t)$ yields

$$\frac{C_t(t)}{C_p(t)} = K^{\text{trans}} \cdot \frac{\int_0^t C_p(\tau)d\tau}{C_p(t)} + v_p. \quad (44)$$

K^{trans} and v_p can be estimated from Eq. (44) using the Patlak graphical method.[47] In the Patlak graphical method, the normalized time given by $\int_0^t C_p(\tau)d\tau / C_p(t)$ is taken as the x-axis and $C_t(t)/C_p(t)$ is taken as the y-axis. K^{trans} and v_p can be obtained from the slope and y-intercept of the regression line fitted to the Patlak plot, respectively.

Figures 4.9A and B show an example of $C_p(t)$ and $C_t(t)$ obtained by DCE-CT and the Patlak plot obtained from these data, respectively. In Figure 4.9B, the regression line fitted to the Patlak plot is also shown by solid line, whose slope and y-intercept correspond to K^{trans} and v_p, respectively.

The graphical method is superior to other methods in terms of the simplicity and easiness to implement, but attention should be paid to setting the range of linear regression for calculating the slope and y-intercept, because the resultant K^{trans} and v_p values may vary depending on this range.

Maximum Slope Method

When we assume that there is no tracer in venous blood during the initial uptake phase, that is, $C_v(t) \cong 0$ in Eq. (13), Eq. (13) for the tissue (not for the distribution space) is reduced to

$$\frac{dC_t(t)}{dt} \cong \frac{F}{V_t} C_a(t). \quad (45)$$

It is known from Eq. (45) that the slope of the tissue concentration–time curve, that is, $dC_t(t)/dt$, reaches a maximum ($[dC_t(t)/dt]_{max}$) when $C_a(t)$ is at its maximum ($[C_a(t)]_{max}$). At this time point, the tissue perfusion, F/V_t is given by

$$\frac{F}{V_t} \cong \frac{\left[\frac{dC_t(t)}{dt}\right]_{max}}{[C_a(t)]_{max}}. \quad (46)$$

Actually, $[dC_t(t)/dt]_{max}$ and $[C_a(t)]_{max}$ do not always occur at the same time point as illustrated in Figure 4.10, because there is a time delay between the AIF measured over a large artery such as aorta and the input function at the inlet of the tissue being studied. Even when $[dC_t(t)/dt]_{max}$ and $[C_a(t)]_{max}$ do not occur at the same time point, Eq. (46) holds true.[48] With the maximum slope method, tissue perfusion is estimated by the maximum slope of the tissue concentration–time curve divided by the maximum value of the measured AIF.

The maximum slope method can also be applied to the dual-input single-compartment model (Fig. 4.7) to obtain K_{1a} and K_{1p} in Eq. (34).[49] First, the peak upslope of the liver curve, in the time period before peak splenic enhancement occurs, is recorded and K_{1a} is calculated from the ratio of this upslope to the peak $C_{ha}(t)$. The peak upslope of the splenic curve is then obtained. The ratio of the early liver upslope to the splenic upslope is found. This represents the ratio of hepatic arterial to splenic arterial perfusion. The splenic curve is multiplied by this ratio, and this is subtracted from the raw liver curve. Finally, K_{1p} is estimated from the ratio of the upslope of the curve thus obtained to the peak $C_{pv}(t)$.

Adiabatic Approximation to the Tissue Homogeneity Model

When we consider the effect of the leakage of contrast agent from the intravascular space to the extravascular space, it is necessary to use the distributed parameter model, which describes the concentration of contrast agent within the tissue as a function of both time and position. As previously described, one of the models describing the tracer concentration in the vascular space as a function of both time and position along the capillary is the tissue homogeneity model, and St. Lawrence and Lee[15] derived an approximate closed-form solution to the tissue homogeneity model using the adiabatic approximation.

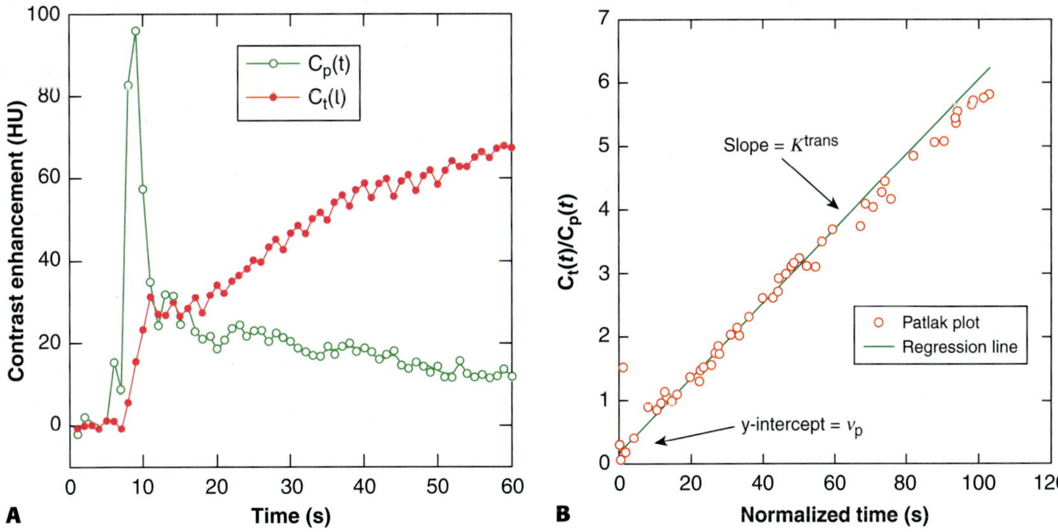

Figure 4-9. Example of the Patlak plot obtained by the graphical method. **(A) and (B):** show an example of $C_p(t)$ and $C_t(t)$ and the Patlak plot obtained from $C_p(t)$ and $C_t(t)$, respectively. The K^{trans} and v_p values can be obtained from the slope and y-intercept of the regression line fitted to the Patlak plot, respectively. Note that the normalized time in **(B)** is defined by $\int_0^t C_p(\tau)d\tau / C_p(t)$.

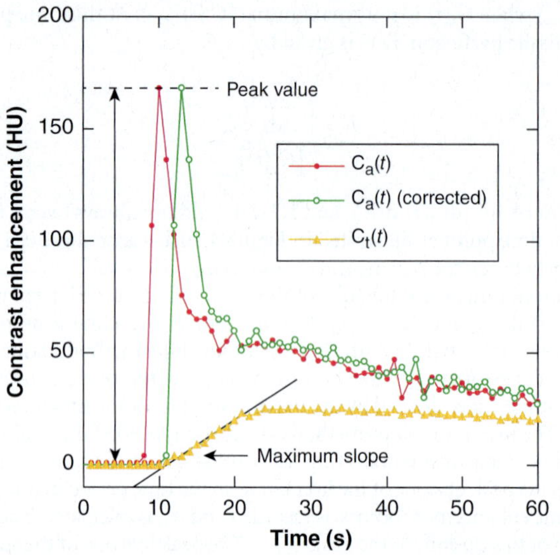

Figure 4-10. Example of the maximum slope method applied to DCE-CT data, in which tissue perfusion is estimated by the maximum slope of the tissue concentration–time curve ($C_t(t)$) divided by the maximum value of the arterial input function ($C_a(t)$). Although the peak of $C_a(t)$ and the maximum slope of $C_t(t)$ do not always occur at the same time point, they do when the arrival time of $C_a(t)$ is corrected.

In adiabatic approximation to the tissue homogeneity model, the impulse residue (retention) function ($R(t)$) is given by[15]

$$R(t) = \begin{cases} 1 & \text{for} \quad 0 \le t < t_c \\ E \cdot \exp\left(-\dfrac{EF}{V_e}(t - t_c)\right) & \text{for} \quad t \ge t_c \end{cases}, \tag{47}$$

where V_e is the distribution volume of contrast agent in the extravascular–extracellular space and t_c is the transit time through the capillary, which is equal to the distribution volume of contrast agent in the intravascular space (V_i) divided by blood flow (F), that is, $t_c = V_i/F$. E is the extraction fraction defined by Eq. (32). Figure 4.11 illustrates $R(t)$ given by Eq. (47). Inserting Eq. (47) into Eq. (23) yields[15]

$$C_t(t) = \frac{F}{V_t}\int_0^{t_c} C_a(t-\tau)\mathrm{d}\tau + \frac{EF}{V_t}\int_{t_c}^{t} C_a(t-\tau) \exp\left(\frac{-EF(\tau - t_c)}{V_e}\right)\mathrm{d}\tau. \tag{48}$$

Figure 4.12 shows an example of the results obtained by applying the adiabatic approximation to the tissue homogeneity model to DCE-CT data acquired from a patient with meningioma. Six parameters (F/V_t, K_1 (= EF), PS, k_2 (= EF/V_e), t_c, and E) were estimated by fitting Eq. (48) to the DCE-CT data using the NLSQ method. E was calculated from F/V_t and PS using Eq. (32). In Figure 4.12, solid lines show the fitted curves using Eq. (48). In this case, F/V_t, K_1 (= EF), PS, k_2 (= EF/V_e), t_c, and E were 40.1 mL/100 mL/min, 1.7 mL/100 mL/min, 1.6 mL/100 mL/min, 0.8 min^{-1}, 4.8 seconds, and 0.04, respectively, for a normal region (open circles), whereas they were 82.6 mL/100 mL/min, 54.1 mL/100 mL/min, 88.0 mL/100 mL/min, 2.2 min^{-1}, 8.4 seconds, and 0.7, respectively, for a tumor region (closed circles), indicating that both the blood flow and permeability are considerably increased compared to those in a normal region. These results suggest that this method will be useful for evaluating perfusion and capillary permeability simultaneously and separately.

Factors Affecting the Accuracy of Kinetic Parameters and Their Corrections

Extraction of Arterial Input Function

The kinetic models used in analysis of DCE-CT data usually require the knowledge of the concentration–time curve of contrast agent in arterial blood, that is, AIF. The traditional method for determination of the AIF is a manual region-of-interest method, which

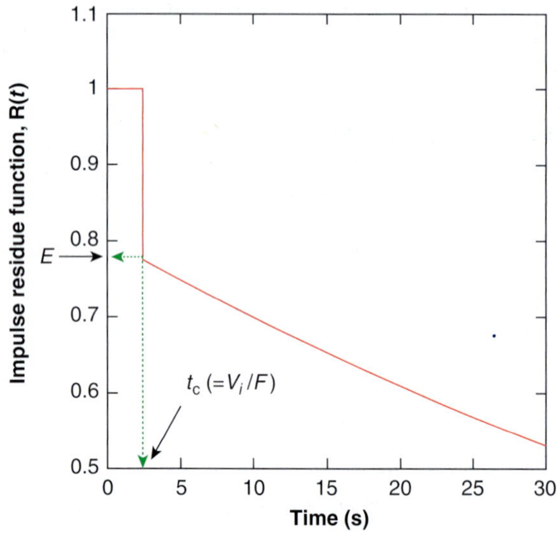

Figure 4-11. Impulse residue (retention) function derived from adiabatic approximation to the tissue homogeneity model. t_c is the transit time through the capillary, which is equal to the distribution volume of contrast agent in the intravascular space (V_i) divided by blood flow (F), that is, $t_c = V_i/F$.

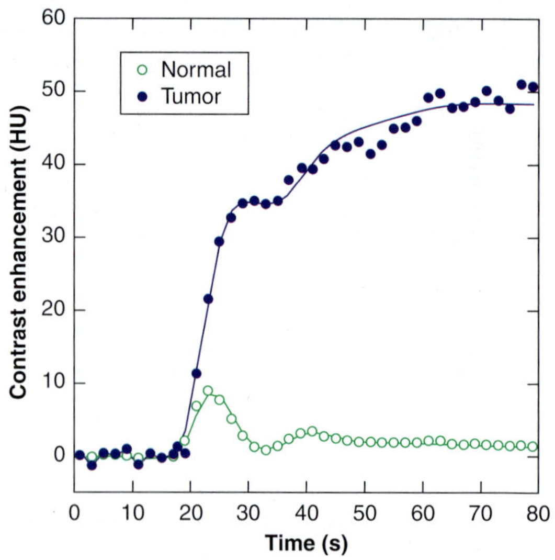

Figure 4-12. Example of the adiabatic approximation to the tissue homogeneity model applied to the DCE-CT data acquired from a patient with meningioma. The *open* and *closed circles* represent the contrast enhancement in the normal and tumor regions, respectively. The *solid lines* show the concentration–time curves estimated using the adiabatic approximation to the tissue homogeneity model.

requires a manual drawing of the region of interest according to the operator's experience and subjective judgment. However, the time-consuming and operator-dependent procedures in this method would reduce the reproducibility of AIF, leading to a serious effect on the resultant estimation of kinetic parameters.[50] Recently, many researchers have paid attention to developing semi- or full-automatic methods to determine AIF. These methods include c-means and K-means clustering approaches[27,51] and independent component analysis.[52] Accurate measurements of AIF, however, are generally difficult, largely because of rather limited temporal resolution, especially in a standard clinical setting. The use of population-averaged AIF has also been proposed.[53] This approach may be useful especially when the feeding artery is not imaged in the field of view. It is known, however, that patient-specific physical factors such as cardiac output, blood flow distribution, and renal function affect the dynamics of AIF.[54] Therefore, the use of population-averaged AIF may cause large systematic errors in resultant kinetic parameters.

Recently, methods have been proposed in the literature that eliminate the need to directly measure the AIF, including reference region models[55] and blind estimation.[56] Although the reference region methods have shown some promise, they are fundamentally limited by the need for inclusion of a region of normal tissue within the field of view. The blind estimation can simultaneously extract AIF and kinetic parameters from DCE-CT or DCE-MRI data sets. This blind estimation process, however, has relatively high noise sensitivity and is often ill conditioned owing to large number of unknown parameters.[50]

Accurate quantification of the true AIF still remains a major challenge to tracer kinetic analysis using DCE-CT or DCE-MRI.

Delay and Dispersion in Arterial Input Function

Since it is not practically possible to measure the true AIF for each pixel of the targeted tissue, it is usually estimated from a major blood vessel such as the aorta, internal carotid artery, or middle cerebral artery.[57] Therefore, the estimated AIF may undergo delay and/or dispersion during its passage from the point of measurement to the particular pixel of tissue.

To illustrate the effects of delay and dispersion in AIF, the simulation results are shown in Figure 4.13. In the simulation, a delay was taken into account by adding a delay time to the AIF ($C_a(t)$), and the effect of dispersion was taken into account by convolving $C_a(t)$ with a vascular transport function $h_v(t)$ from the site of measurement to the given pixel, which is given by

$$h_v(t) = \frac{1}{\tau} e^{-t/\tau}, \tag{49}$$

where τ denotes a dispersion constant.[21] The solid, dotted, and dashed lines in Figure 4.13 show an example of the AIF without delay and dispersion, that with delay with a delay time of 5 seconds, and that with dispersion with a dispersion constant of 5 seconds, respectively. In these cases, statistical noise was neglected to focus on the effects of delay and dispersion in AIF.

Calamante et al.[57] investigated the effect of delay and dispersion in AIF on the accuracy of the cerebral blood flow (CBF) obtained by deconvolution analysis based on singular value decomposition. They reported that the CBF value was underestimated until a delay time of approximately 1.5 to 2.0 seconds and then oscillated around a 35% underestimation. The maximum CBF underestimation obtained with the simulated delayed data was approximately 40% for a delay of approximately 2 seconds. An equivalent underestimation is very quickly reached with a dispersion constant of approximately 1.5 to 2 seconds, but in the case of dispersion, this

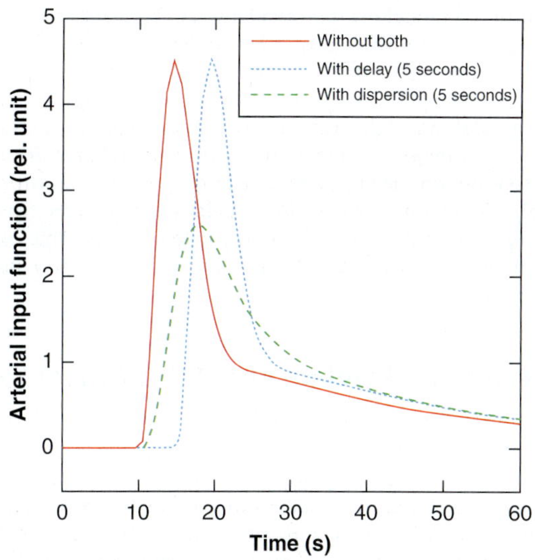

Figure 4-13. Effects of delay and dispersion on the shape of arterial input function. The *solid*, *dotted*, and *dashed lines* represent the arterial input function without delay and dispersion, that with delay with a delay time of 5 seconds, and that with dispersion with a dispersion constant of 5 seconds, respectively.

continues to increase further thereafter as dispersion increases. Murase et al.[21] also investigated the effect of delay and dispersion in AIF on the CBF estimation (Fig. 4.14). Their results were similar to those reported by Calamante et al.,[57] and the effect of dispersion was much larger than that of delay when the threshold value in the TSVD was fixed at a constant (0.2).

As pointed out by Calamante et al.,[57] while the error introduced by the delay can be corrected using information on the arrival time of the bolus, the correction for the dispersion is less straightforward

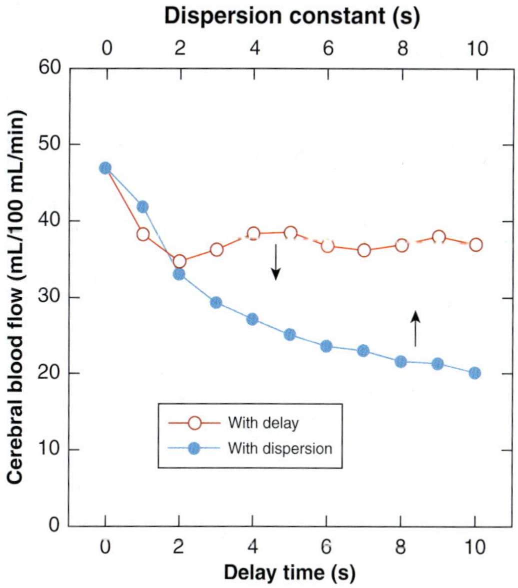

Figure 4-14. Effects of delay (*open circles*) and dispersion (*closed circles*) in arterial input function on the CBF estimated using TSVD (Eq. (29)) with a threshold value of 0.2. In these cases, the CBF and cerebral blood volume were assumed to 60 mL/100 mL/min and 4 mL/100 mL, respectively.

and requires a model for the vasculature. Ostergaard et al.[58] incorporated a more complicated vascular model into a dynamic susceptibility contrast MRI study to try to account for the effect of delay and dispersion in AIF. In that study, they applied a modified version of the vascular model described by Kroll et al.[59] The vasculature was modeled as a major feeding artery (with fixed relative dispersion and a delay determined by its volume fraction) in a series with small parallel vessels (considered as simple delay lines) with relative flows and weights according to a given flow heterogeneity. This method could be used to correct for the dispersion, but further validation will be necessary.

Correction of Baseline and Bolus Arrival Time

Along with AIF, the tracer kinetic models also require the estimation of bolus arrival time, that is, the time instance of arrival of contrast agent.[60] Erroneous estimate of the bolus arrival time leads to increased uncertainty in the estimated kinetic parameters. The estimation of bolus arrival time has generally been performed by manual trimming or realignment of precontrast points in the data sets.[61] This may not be practical for a large-scale data processing such as the generation of parametric images.

Cheong et al.[61] developed an automated approach for estimating bolus arrival time using piecewise continuous regression models, in which the portion of the concentration–time curve in the vicinity of bolus arrival time is approximated by a linear–linear (L-L) or linear–quadratic (L-Q) continuous function. Figure 4.15 shows an example of estimating bolus arrival time using the L-Q model approach. In this approach, the bolus arrival time is estimated by finding a point that best separates the concentration–time data by an L-Q piecewise continuous function connected at this point. To find such a separation point, the sum of squared error between the concentration–time data and the L-Q continuous function is calculated. With this method, the baseline can also be estimated simultaneously as the linear function, which can be used for the correction of the initial baseline concentration of contrast agent.

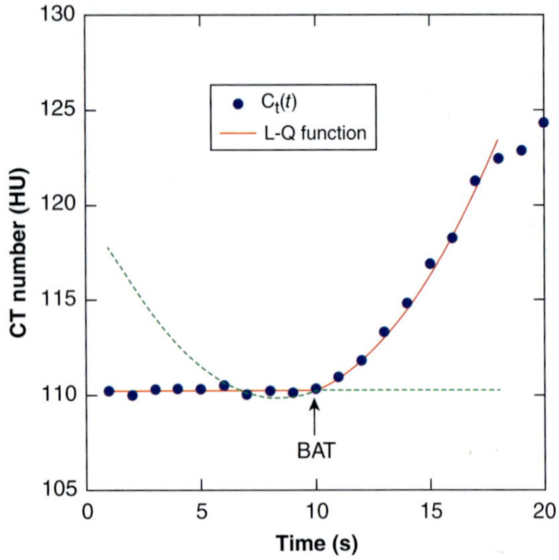

Figure 4-15. Example of the determination of baseline and bolus arrival time (BAT) using a linear–quadratic (L-Q) piecewise continuous regression model. The *closed circles* and *solid line* represent the concentration–time curve in the tissue and the L-Q continuous function, respectively.

Correction of Partial Volume Effect

The partial volume effect on AIF is also an important issue in tracer kinetic analysis using DCE-CT. The partial volume effect should be taken into account especially when the AIF is obtained using a manual region-of-interest method, because the partial volume effect depends on the region-of-interest size and increases at the larger region-of-interest size.[62] Cenic et al.[63] devised a method for correcting for the partial volume effect in DCE-CT. Briefly, a calibration curve is first generated by phantom experiments containing background and contrast tubes with various diameters.[63,64] From the calibration curve, the recovery coefficient value is then determined, knowing the standard deviation of the gaussian fit to the background-subtracted image profile of the artery from which the AIF is obtained. Finally, the AIF corrected for the partial volume effect is obtained by multiplying the AIF by the recovery coefficient value obtained above.[63,64]

Radiation Dose Reduction Techniques

It is known that to obtain reliable kinetic parameters, scanning with high temporal resolution and a long scanning time is required, which leads to relatively high patient radiation dose. Radiation dose is an important issue for CT studies and is most important in young patients due to their increased radiation susceptibility. In recent years, several studies have addressed this issue and several radiation dose reduction techniques have been developed, which are roughly classified into tube current modulation, tube voltage modulation, scan length adjustment, use of iterative image reconstruction method, and use of dual-energy CT.[4,65] Thakur et al.[4] reviewed these strategies for radiation dose optimization and suggested that tube current modulation should be used in all cases in younger and physically smaller individuals. The iterative image reconstruction method with associated radiation dose adjustment is recommended for younger patients but may be used in all patients once familiarity has been achieved with the new look of the images.[4] Patients requiring contrast-enhanced CT examinations with impaired renal function may benefit from dual-energy CT acquisition with an approximately 50% reduction in iodine load.[4]

Conclusion

In this chapter, we described the basics of tracer kinetic analysis for quantifying perfusion using DCE-CT and various methods for estimating kinetic parameters, which include NLSQ method, LLSQ method, graphical method, and maximum slope method. We also described the factors affecting the accuracy of the kinetic parameters obtained using DCE-CT and their correction methods. Finally, we touched on radiation dose reduction techniques. We hope that these will be useful and helpful for clinical practice.

REFERENCES

1. **Yuan X, Zhang J, Ao G, et al.** Lung cancer perfusion: can we measure pulmonary and bronchial circulation simultaneously? *Eur Radiol* 2012;22:1665–1671.
2. **Brix G, Griebel J, Kiessling F, et al.** Tracer kinetic modelling of tumour angiogenesis based on dynamic contrast-enhanced CT and MRI measurements. *Eur J Nucl Med Mol Imaging* 2010;37:S30–S51.
3. **Morcos SK, Thomsen HS.** Adverse reactions to iodinated contrast media. *Eur Radiol* 2001;11:1267–1275.
4. **Thakur Y, McLaughlin PD, Mayo JR.** Strategies for radiation dose optimization. *Curr Radiol Rep* 2013;1:1–10.
5. **Zierler KL.** Equations for measuring blood flow by external monitoring of radioisotopes. *Circ Res* 1965;16:309–321.
6. **Koh TS, Bisdas S, Koh DM, et al.** Fundamentals of tracer kinetics for dynamic contrast-enhanced MRI. *J Magn Reson Imaging* 2011;34:1262–1276.

7. **Kety SS, Schmidt CF.** The determination of cerebral blood flow in man by the use of nitrous oxide in low concentrations. *Am J Physiol* 1945;143:53–66.
8. **Lee TY.** Functional CT: physiological models. *Trends Biotechnol* 2002;20:S3–S10.
9. **Koh TS, Tan CKM, Cheong LHD, et al.** Cerebral perfusion mapping using a robust and efficient method for deconvolution analysis of dynamic contrast-enhanced images. *Neuroimage* 2006;32:643–653.
10. **Meier P, Zierler KL.** On the theory of the indicator-dilution method for measurement of blood flow and volume. *J Appl Physiol* 1954;6:731–744.
11. **Kershaw LE, Buckley DL.** Precision in measurements of perfusion and microvascular permeability with T1-weighted dynamic contrast-enhanced MRI. *Magn Reson Med* 2006;56:986–992.
12. **Ostergaard L, Weisskoff RM, Chesler DA, et al.** High resolution measurement of cerebral blood flow using intravascular tracer bolus passages. part 1: mathematical approach and statistical approach. *Magn Reson Med* 1996;36:715–725.
13. **Murase K, Miyazaki S.** Error analysis of tumor blood flow measurement using dynamic contrast-enhanced data and model-independent deconvolution analysis. *Phys Med Biol* 2007;52:2791–2805.
14. **Johnson JA, Wilson TA.** A model for capillary exchange. *Am J Physiol* 1966;210:1299–1303.
15. **St. Lawrence KS, Lee TY.** An adiabatic approximation to the tissue homogeneity model for water exchange in the brain. I. theoretical derivation. *J Cereb Blood Flow Metab* 1998;18:1365–1377.
16. **Eastwood JD, Lev MH, Azhari T, et al.** CT perfusion scanning with deconvolution analysis: pilot study in patients with acute middle cerebral artery stroke. *Radiology* 2002;222:227–236.
17. **George RT, Jerosch-Herold M, Silva C, et al.** Quantification of myocardial perfusion using dynamic 64-detector computed tomography. *Invest Radiol* 2007;42:815–822.
18. **Won C, Chon D, Tajik J, et al.** CT-based assessment of regional pulmonary microvascular blood flow parameters. *J Appl Physiol* 2003;94:2483–2493.
19. **Miles KA, Lee TY, Goh V, et al.** Current status and guidelines for the assessment of tumor vascular support with dynamic contrast-enhanced computed tomography. *Eur Radiol* 2012;22:1430–1441.
20. **Kusakabe Y, Miyazaki S, Tachibana A, et al.** Development of a method to quantitatively monitor the effect of inhibition of nitric oxide synthase on tumor vascular activity using dynamic contrast-enhanced computed tomography. *J Med Eng Technol* 2009;33:460–469.
21. **Murase K, Shinohara M, Yamazaki Y.** Accuracy of deconvolution analysis based on singular value decomposition for quantification of cerebral blood flow using dynamic susceptibility contrast-enhanced magnetic resonance imaging. *Phys Med Biol* 2001;46:3147–3159.
22. **Murase K, Yamazaki Y, Miyazaki S.** Deconvolution analysis of dynamic contrast-enhanced data based on singular value decomposition optimized by generalized cross validation. *Magn Reson Med Sci* 2004;3:165–175.
23. **Hansen PC.** Analysis of discrete ill-posed problems by means of the L-curve. *SIAM Rev* 1992;34:561–580.
24. **Tofts PS, Kermode AG.** Measurement of the blood–brain barrier permeability and leakage space using dynamic MR imaging. I fundamental concepts. *Magn Reson Med* 1991;17:357–367.
25. **Larsson HBW, Stubgaard M, Frederiksen JL, et al.** Quantitation of blood–brain barrier defect by magnetic resonance imaging and gadolinium-DTPA in patients with multiple sclerosis and brain tumors. *Magn Reson Med* 1990;16:117–131.
26. **Brix G, Semmler W, Port R, et al.** Pharmacokinetic parameters in CNS Gd-DTPA enhanced MR imaging. *J Comput Assist Tomogr* 1991;15:621–628.
27. **Murase K, Kikuchi K, Miki H, et al.** Determination of arterial input function using fuzzy clustering for quantification of cerebral blood flow with dynamic susceptibility contrast-enhanced MR imaging. *J Magn Reson Imaging* 2001;13:797–806.
28. **Buckley DL.** Uncertainty in the analysis of tracer kinetics using dynamic contrast-enhanced T_1-weighted MRI. *Magn Reson Med* 2002;47:601–606.
29. **Tofts PS.** Modeling tracer kinetics in dynamic Gd-DTPA MR imaging. *J Magn Reson Imaging* 1997;7:91–101.
30. **Tofts PS, Brix G, Buckley DL, et al.** Estimating kinetic parameters from dynamic contrast-enhanced T_1-weighted MRI of a diffusible tracer: standardized quantities and symbols. *J Magn Reson Imaging* 1999;10:223–232.
31. **Renkin EM.** Capillary permeability to lipid-soluble molecule. *Am J Physiol* 1952;168:538–545.
32. **Crone C.** The permeability of capillaries in various organs as determined by use of the "indicator diffusion" method. *Acta Physiol Scand* 1963;58:292–305.
33. **Miles KA, Hayball MP, Dixon AK.** Functional images of hepatic perfusion obtained with dynamic CT. *Radiology* 1993;188:405–411.
34. **Materne R, Van Beers BE, Smith AM, et al.** Non-invasive quantification of liver perfusion with dynamic computed tomography and a dual input one-compartmental model. *Clin Sci* 2000;99:517–525.
35. **Leggett DA, Kelley BB, Bunce IH, et al.** Colorectal cancer: diagnostic potential of CT measurements of hepatic perfusion and implications for contrast enhancement protocols. *Radiology* 1997;205: 716–720.
36. **Becker GA, Muller-Schauenburg W, Spilker ME, et al.** A priori identifiability of a one-compartment model with two input functions for liver blood flow measurements. *Phys Med Biol* 2005;50:1393–1404.
37. **Pandharipande PV, Krinsky GA, Rusinek H, et al.** Perfusion imaging of the liver: current challenges and future goals. *Radiology* 2005;234:661–673.
38. **Munk OL, Bass L, Roelsgaard K, et al.** Liver kinetics of glucose analogs measured in pigs by PET: importance of dual-input blood sampling. *J Nucl Med* 2001;42:795–801.
39. **Van Beers BE, Leconte I, Materne R, et al.** Hepatic perfusion parameters in chronic liver disease: dynamic CT measurements correlated with disease severity. *Am J Roentgenol* 2001;176:667–673.
40. **Miyazaki S, Murase K, Yoshikawa T, et al.** A quantitative method for estimating hepatic blood flow using a dual-input single-compartment model. *Br J Radiol* 2008;81:790–800.
41. **Murase K, Miyazaki S, Yang X.** An efficient method for calculating kinetic parameters in a dual-input single-compartment model. *Br J Radiol* 2007;80:371–375.
42. **Ahearn TS, Staff RT, Redpath TW, et al.** The use of the Levenberg-Marquardt curve-fitting algorithm in pharmacokinetic modelling of DCE-MRI data. *Phys Med Biol* 2005;50:N85–N92.
43. **Nelder JA, Mead R.** A simplex method for function minimization. *Comput J* 1965;7:308–313.
44. **Press WH, Teukolsky SA, Vetterling WT, et al, ed.** *Numerical recipes in C.* New York: Cambridge University Press; 1992.
45. **Glatting G, Kletting P, Reske SN, et al.** Choosing the optimal fit function: comparison of the Akaike information criterion and the F-test. *Med Phys* 2007;34:4285–4292.
46. **Murase K.** Efficient method for calculating kinetic parameters using T1-weighted dynamic contrast-enhanced magnetic resonance imaging. *Magn Reson Med* 2004;51:858–862.
47. **Patlak CS, Blasberg RG.** Graphical evaluation of blood-to-brain transfer constants from multiple-time uptake data. generalizations. *J Cereb Blood Flow Metab* 1985;5:584–590.
48. **Brix G, Zwick S, Griebel J, et al.** Estimation of tissue perfusion by dynamic contrast-enhanced imaging: simulation-based evaluation of the steepest slope method. *Eur Radiol* 2010;20:2166–2175.
49. **Blomley MJK, Coulden R, Dawson P, et al.** Liver perfusion studied with ultrafast CT. *J Comput Assist Tomogr* 1995;19:424–433.
50. **Shi L, Wang D, Liu W, et al.** Automatic detection of arterial input function in dynamic contrast enhanced MRI based on affinity propagation clustering. *J Magn Reson Imaging* 2014;39:1327–1337.
51. **Mouridsen K, Christensen S, Gyldensted L, et al.** Automatic selection of arterial input function using cluster analysis. *Magn Reson Med* 2006;55:524–531.
52. **Calamante F, Morup M, Hansen LK.** Defining a local arterial input function for perfusion MRI using independent component analysis. *Magn Reson Med* 2004;52:789–797.
53. **Parker GJ, Roberts C, MacDonald A, et al.** Experimentally-derived functional form for a population-averaged high-temporal-resolution arterial input function for dynamic contrast enhanced MRI. *Magn Reson Med* 2006;56:993–1000.
54. **Fedorov A, Fluckiger J, Ayers GD, et al.** A comparison of two methods for estimating DCE-MRI parameters via individual and cohort based AIFs in prostate cancer: a step towards practical implementation. *Magn Reson Imaging* 2014;32:321–329.
55. **Yang C, Karczmar GS, Medved M, et al.** Reproducibility assessment of a multiple reference tissue method for quantitative dynamic contrast enhanced-MRI analysis. *Magn Reson Med* 2009;61:851–859.

56. **Fluckiger JU, Schabel MC, Dibella EV.** Model-based blind estimation of kinetic parameters in dynamic contrast enhanced (DCE)-MRI. *Magn Reson Med* 2009;62:1477–1486.
57. **Calamante F, Gadian DG, Connelly A.** Delay and dispersion effects in dynamic susceptibility contrast MRI: simulations using singular value decomposition. *Magn Reson Med* 2000;44:466–473.
58. **Ostergaard L, Chesler DA, Weisskoff RM, et al.** Modeling cerebral blood flow and flow heterogeneity from magnetic resonance residue data. *J Cereb Blood Flow Metab* 1999;19:690–699.
59. **Kroll K, Wilke N, Jerosch HM, et al.** Modeling regional flows from residue functions of an intravascular indicator. *Am J Physiol* 1996;271:H1643–H1655.
60. **Singh A, Rathore RKS, Haris M, et al.** Improved bolus arrival time and arterial input function estimation for tracer kinetic analysis in DCE-MRI. *J Magn Reson Imaging* 2009;29:166–176.
61. **Cheong LH, Koh TS, Hou Z.** An automatic approach for estimating bolus arrival time in dynamic contrast MRI using piecewise continuous regression models. *Phys Med Biol* 2003;48:N83–N88.
62. **Driscoll B, Keller H, Coolens C.** Development of a dynamic flow imaging phantom for dynamic contrast-enhanced CT. *Med Phys* 2011;38:4866–4880.
63. **Cenic A, Nabavi DG, Craen RA, et al.** Dynamic CT measurement of cerebral blood flow: a validation study. *AJNR Am J Neuroradiol* 1999;20:63–73.
64. **Murase K, Tachibana A, Kusakabe Y, et al.** A method for quantitative assessment of renal function using dynamic contrast-enhanced computed tomography: evaluation of drug-induced nephrotoxicity in rats. *Med Phys* 2008;35:5768–5776.
65. **Kim SM, Haider MA, Milosevic M, et al.** A method for patient dose reduction in dynamic contrast enhanced CT study. *Med Phys* 2011;38:5094–5103.

CHAPTER

5 CT and MR Contrast-Enhanced Tissue Perfusion Imaging: Basic Methodology, Postprocessing, Reliability Testing

Kohsuke Kudo, MD

Introduction

Tissue perfusion can be measured using several methods, such as positron emission tomography (PET),[1,2] single photon emission computed tomography (SPECT),[3,4] computed tomography (CT),[5,6] and magnetic resonance (MR) imaging.[7,8] Among these techniques, PET and SPECT are the current standards of reference for in vivo assessment of the cerebral blood flow (CBF) and metabolism. However, high costs and limited accessibility have restricted the widespread clinical use of these modalities.

Compared to nuclear medicine methods, dynamic CT and MR perfusion techniques using bolus injection of contrast material have a number of practical advantages. First, these techniques can be applied immediately after unenhanced brain CT or MRI, which are performed to evaluate acute ischemic change, hemorrhage, and occlusion of arteries; CT and MRI are the choice modalities when acute stroke is suspected. Second, the examination time is considerably shorter for CT and MR perfusion (acquisition times typically range from 60 to 90 seconds). Third, the spatial resolution is much higher in these techniques compared with PET or SPECT. Finally, no special equipment is needed, except for a power injector, which is usually available in the scanner room in most hospitals. The potential limitation of short scan range in CT perfusion has now been overcome with advances in multidetector row CT (MDCT) including moving table techniques (toggling table or shuttle mode)[9,10] and area detector CT (ADCT).[11] Another drawback of CT perfusion is the radiation exposure. Attempts have been made to reduce the radiation dose, and the use of lower tube voltages (i.e., 80 kVp) and currents has become standard in many protocols.[12,13] Quantitative analysis with both CT and MR perfusion is a common practice now, and there are several reports that have confirmed good correlations with PET or SPECT.[14–17] Accuracy and reliability tests have been conducted using digital phantoms,[18,19] and extensive refinement of analysis algorithms has been carried out.

CT perfusion imaging is also performed using cold Xe (Xe-CT),[20,21] in which Xe acts as a diffusible tracer. However, it has several disadvantages such as the sedative effect of Xe and the requirement for special equipment (an inhalation system for Xe). Therefore, the clinical use of this technique is limited. MR perfusion is also known as perfusion-weighted imaging (PWI), and there are two types of MR perfusion that use dynamic contrast injection, that is, dynamic susceptibility contrast (DSC)[7,8] and dynamic contrast-enhanced (DCE) PWI.[22] DSC uses T2 or T2* contrast and is mainly used for blood flow measurement, while DCE uses T1 contrast and its main application is permeability analysis. In addition, arterial spin labeling (ASL) is now available in most clinical MR scanners.[23,24] As ASL uses an intrinsic tracer of labeled blood, it is completely noninvasive and does not require contrast injection.

This chapter discusses basic principles, methods, and postprocessing issues for dynamic contrast-enhanced CT and DSC-MR perfusion. These techniques share the same methods for analysis as they use the same principles. Therefore, there are many common characteristics including behavior of the tracer, analysis algorithms, and limitations, albeit several differences also exist. CT perfusion has several advantages over MR perfusion, including more reliable quantitative results, higher spatial resolution, less image distortion, and better suitability for emergency scans. In contrast, MR perfusion has higher image contrast and wider scan coverage than has CT, and involves no radiation exposure (Table 5.1).

Methodology

In order to measure blood flow dynamics, a "tracer" that flows in the bloodstream is required. Iodine and gadolinium (Gd) contrast materials are used in CT and MR perfusions, respectively, as these are commonly used in clinical practices. These contrast materials are macromolecules that do not pass through the blood–brain barrier (BBB). Therefore, they act as nondiffusible intravascular tracers (remaining in the blood) in normal brain tissue in which the BBB is intact, while diffusible tracers (freely diffuse across vascular wall into extravascular space) are used in PET and SPECT. As the kinetics of these tracers are different, so are the principles and analysis method.

When an intravascular tracer is used, rapid injection of the tracer and repetitive scans during its first passage are required for measuring the hemodynamics; this is based on the indicator dilution theory.[25,26] Many hemodynamic parameters are derived from the measured dynamic curve. For quantitative analysis, the concentration of the tracer should be used, rather than the CT number or the MR signal itself. Therefore, CT numbers and MR signals are converted into tracer concentrations. In contrast to the linear relationship between CT number and iodine concentration, the concentration of Gd contrast is related to $\Delta R2^*$.[7,27] Therefore, the following equation is used for the conversion.

TABLE 5.1 **Characteristics of CT and MR Perfusion**

	CT Perfusion	MR Perfusion
Available scanner	Helical or volume scanners	Higher field preferred (≧1.5T)
Radiation exposure	Yes	No
Image contrast and SNR	Low	High
Scan range	Narrow	Wide
Spatial resolution	High	Low
Image distortion	No	Yes
Linearity of contrast concentration	High	Low
Quantitative results	Better	Limited
Manual selection of AIF	Easy	Difficult
Potential Risk of Metallic Objects	No	Yes
Emergency Scan	Easy	Difficult

SNR, signal-to-noise ratio; AIF, arterial input function.

$$C(t) = k \times \Delta R2^{*} = -\frac{k}{\mathrm{TE}}\ln\left(\frac{S(t)}{S(0)}\right) \quad (1)$$

where $C(t)$ is tracer (contrast) concentration at a given time t, k is a constant, and $S(t)$ is the MR signal. This constant value, k, depends on the scan sequence, parameters, magnetic field strength, and tissue properties.[27] Therefore, MR perfusion has potential difficulties in the accurate quantification of hemodynamic parameters. After this conversion, the time–concentration curve (TCC), $C(t)$, is derived, and TCC is further used for quantitative analysis. TCC is recommended for semiquantitative analysis, but the time signal curve, $S(t)$, can be also be used, especially for time-related parameters (see below), because such parameters are not affected by this conversion of contrast.

Semiquantitative Parameters

Semiquantitative parameters are derived directly from the TCC of tissue without any complex calculations (Fig. 5.1).[28] The time-related parameters are bolus arrival time (BAT), time to peak (TTP), first moment (FMT), and the full width at half maximum (FWHM), and these are sensitive to hemodynamic delay due to ischemia. Maximum slope (MS) and area under the curve (AUC) reflect CBF and cerebral blood volume (CBV), respectively, but not quantitatively. Maximum concentration (C_{max}) also reflects CBV. All these parameters are affected by injection speed, amount of contrast material and saline chase, cardiac output, carotid stenosis, etc. For example, when the injection speed is low, BAT, TTP, and FMT become larger, and MS becomes smaller. AUC and C_{max} are directly related to the amount of contrast. Therefore, they cannot be compared among subjects and even for studies on the same subject. The absolute values of these parameters are less meaningful, and relative values should be used for comparison.

Quantitative Parameters

Quantitative analysis is performed by using the TCC of both tissues and arteries ($C(t)$ and $C_a(t)$, respectively). For both CT and MR perfusion, deconvolution is the most common method for quantitative analysis (Fig. 5.1).[8,29,30] The following relationship has been shown for $C(t)$ and $C_a(t)$.

$$C(t) = C_a(t) \otimes R(t) \quad (2)$$

where $R(t)$ is the tissue residue function and ⊗ denotes the convolution operation. $R(t)$ represents the fraction of the injected tracer remaining in the vasculature at time t, and is calculated through deconvolution. If the contrast bolus remains in the artery for an infinitely short time, the shape of $C_a(t)$ would be an impulse. In such an ideal situation, the observed $C(t)$ becomes equal to $R(t)$ (Fig. 5.2). However, in a practical situation, $C_a(t)$ becomes a curve owing to the finite duration of the venous injection of contrast and mixture in the lungs and heart. Therefore, deconvolution is needed to obtain $R(t)$ from measured $C_a(t)$ and $C(t)$, even with relatively low injection rates (3 to 5 mL/s), which are clinically possible.[30] After deconvolution, CBF, CBV, and mean transit time (MTT) are derived from $R(t)$. In practice, $C_a(t)$ is called the arterial input function (AIF), which is determined by measuring the TCC of a large artery such as the middle cerebral artery (MCA) or the anterior cerebral artery (ACA), by the region of interest (ROI). However, the ROI usually has partial volume averaging, which causes the underestimation of AIF.[27,31] Therefore, correction for partial volume averaging should be carried out before deconvolution with a scaling factor, which is determined by AIF and the venous output function (VOF).[32] In brain, the VOF, $C_v(t)$, is usually determined by the ROI of the superior sagittal sinus (SSS), which is sufficiently large to avoid partial volume averaging.

$$\text{Correction Factor} = \frac{\int C_v(t)}{\int C_a(t)} = \frac{\mathrm{AUC[VOF]}}{\mathrm{AUC[AIF]}} \quad (3)$$

$$C_a(t)\_\text{corrected} = \text{Correction factor} \times C_a(t)\_\text{measured} \quad (4)$$

CBF refers to the blood volume flowing through a unit tissue volume for a unit of time (mL/100 g/min) and is one of the most important physiologic parameters, which is closely related to maintaining electronic functions and cellular metabolisms.[33–35] For example, a study of monkeys showed that reversible motor dysfunction (paralysis) occurs for CBF below 23 mL/100 g/min, and complete hemiplegia occurs for CBF less than 8 to 9 mL/100 g/min. Furthermore, an electroencephalogram showed decreased action potential below 20 mL/100 g/min and electronic failure at 15 to 16 mL/100 g/min.[34] In addition to these electronic failures, morphologic damage is also induced by failure of the integrity of the cell membrane due to depletion of adenosine triphosphate. This membrane failure is time dependent, as it occurs at 6 to 8 mL/100 g/min for 1-hour ischemia[36] and at 12 mL/100 g/min for 2-hour.[37] Therefore, quantification of CBF is theoretically important for the evaluation of tissue viabilities in acute stroke.

In a deconvolution method, CBF is determined as the peak height of $R(t)$; however, CBF is also quantified by a MS model that assumes no venous output during the contrast bolus.[5,38]

$$\mathrm{CBF} = \frac{\mathrm{MaxSlope}[C(t)]}{\mathrm{Max}[C_a(t)]} \quad (5)$$

CBV refers to the blood volume in a unit tissue volume, which is independent of flow (mL/100 g), and, thereby, is related to the vascular bed. When cerebral perfusion pressure (CPP) decreases due to stenosis or occlusion of a proximal artery, an increase in CBV occurs as the first compensation mechanism to maintain

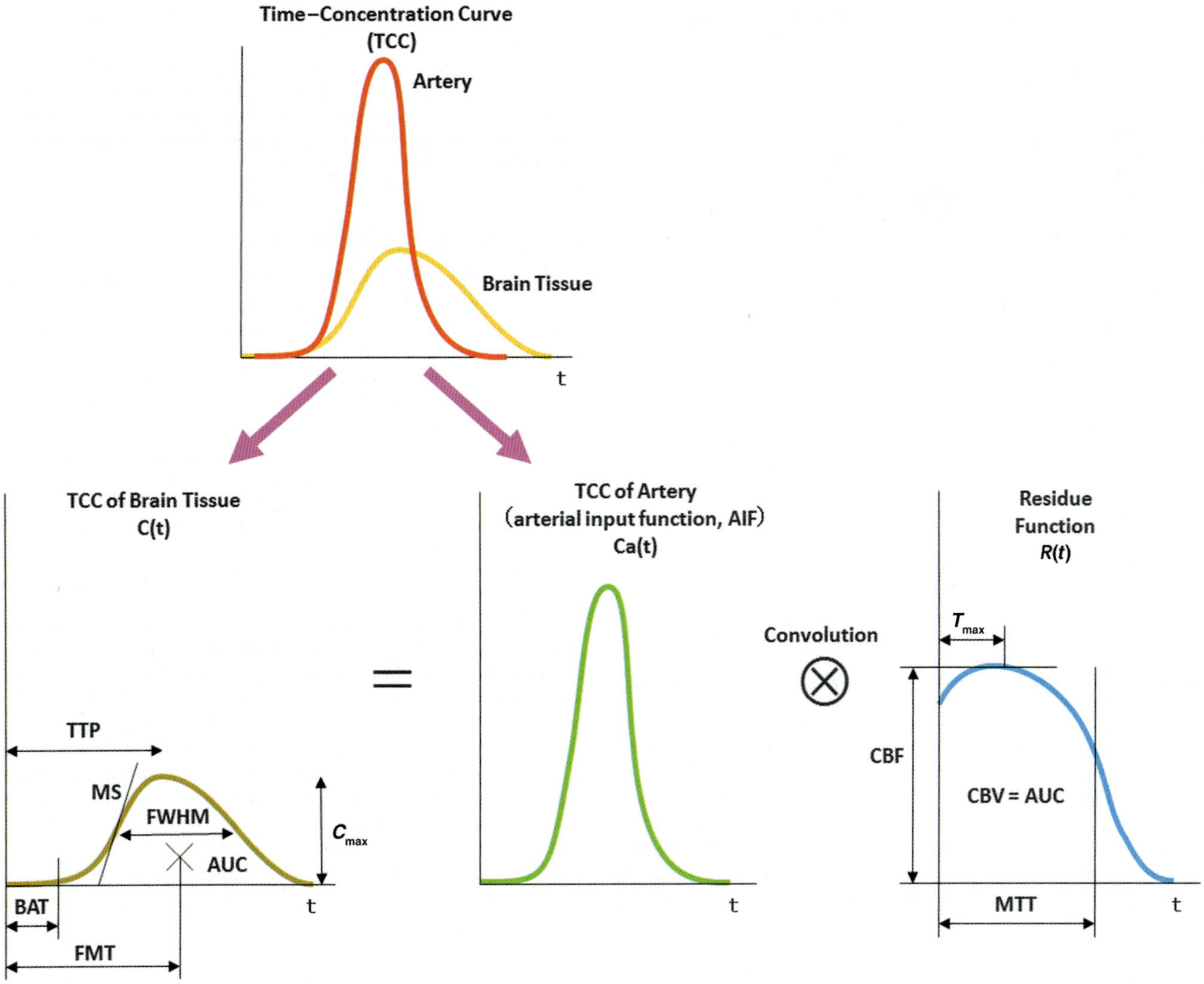

Figure 5-1. Semiquantitative and quantitative curve analysis. TCCs are measured by CT or MR perfusion scans. Semiquantitative parameters such as bolus arrival time (BAT), time to peak (TTP), first moment (FMT), and full width half maximum (FWHM), maximum slope (MS), area under the curve (AUC), and C_{max} are calculated from the tissue TCC. BAT, TTP, FMT, and FWHM are time-related parameters that are sensitive to ischemia. MS and AUC are related to CBF and CBV, respectively, and C_{max} is related to both. Quantitative analysis is achieved by adding TCC of artery (arterial input function, AIF) to the analysis. Residue function, $R(t)$, is derived from deconvolution of AIF and tissue TCC. Quantitative parameters such as cerebral blood flow (CBF), cerebral blood volume (CBV), and mean transit time (MTT) are calculated from $R(t)$, and these three parameters have the following relationship: CBF = CBV/MTT. T_{max} is also calculated as the TTP of $R(t)$.

CBF in ischemic tissue, and this mechanism is called "vascular reserve" (Figs. 5.3 and 5.4).[34] After maximum dilatation of the vascular bed, CBF decreases by a further reduction in CPP. In the infarct core, a severe decrease of CBV is observed. In tumor cases, CBV is used for the estimation of vascular bed, which sometimes reflects malignancy (neovascularity).[39] CBV is quantified as the AUC of $R(t)$, but it is also estimated as the ratio of AUC of tissue and large vessel (VOF), which does not have partial volume averaging.[8]

$$\mathrm{CBV} = \frac{\kappa}{\rho} \times \frac{\int C(t)}{\int C_v(t)} \tag{6}$$

$$\kappa = \frac{1 - \mathrm{HCT_{LV}}}{1 - \mathrm{HCT_{SV}}} \tag{7}$$

where κ and ρ are correction factors for hematocrit (HCT) and brain density, respectively. κ is determined by the HCT of large vessels ($\mathrm{HCT_{LV}}$) and small vessels ($\mathrm{HCT_{SV}}$).

MTT is the average time for the transit of contrast bolus in a tissue volume (seconds). MTT is a sensitive marker to ischemic tissue because it increases at the very beginning of CPP decline and constantly increases as CPP decreases (Fig. 5.3).

From the central volume principle and indicator dilution theory, CBF, CBV, and MTT have the following relationship: CBF = CBV/MTT.[25] Therefore, determining any two of these three parameters yields the remaining one.

Another important parameter derived from $R(t)$ is T_{max}, which is the TTP of $R(t)$.[40] Although T_{max} is not a physiologic parameter, calculation is easy and reliable after deconvolution. It contains mixed information of delay, dispersion, and MTT,[19,41] and it provides additional information on hemodynamic status. Recently,

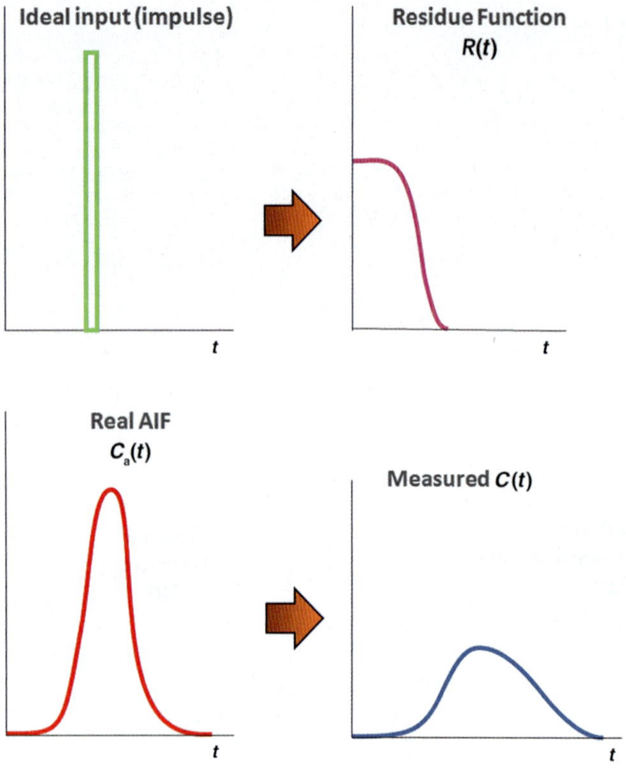

Figure 5-2. Residue function, *R*(*t*). In the ideal situation, arterial input (AIF) becomes impulse (an instantaneous, and infinitely short bolus of contrast), and measured response in tissue TCC becomes residue function, *R*(*t*), because the *R*(*t*) represents the fraction of the injected tracer remaining in the vasculature at time *t*. However, in the real situation, AIF becomes a brief but not instantaneous bolus, due to dispersion in the lung and heart. Then, measured tissue TCC becomes lower and more blurred.

several multicenter trials used T_{max} for the definition of perfusion abnormality in acute ischemic stroke.[42–44]

The advantage of quantitative analysis is that absolute values can be determined. Thus, inter- and intrasubject comparisons may be possible. However, care should be taken during the comparisons because of variation in the values between different software packages and versions.[45]

Imaging Techniques

Basic imaging methods are the same for CT and MR perfusion, as they share the same principles and theories. The essential points are dynamic infusion of the contrast material and repetitive scanning during the first passage of the contrast bolus. For dynamic injection, a power injector should be used, even in MR perfusion, to obtain a better shape of the contrast bolus. A higher injection rate is better; however, 3 to 5 mL/s is sufficient for clinical practice.[30] An infusion needle catheter (20 to 22 Gauge) should be placed in the right antecubital or forearm veins. The right side is better than the left, as blockage of the bolus sometimes occurs in the left brachiocephalic vein. In CT perfusion, the amount of contrast is around 35 to 50 mL, and a saline chase (20 to 40 mL) is recommended. In MR perfusion, a single dose (0.1 mmol/kg) is commonly used with a saline chase.

Before the scans, the head of the subject should be tightly restrained to avoid head motion during the scan. If a whole brain scan cannot be achieved, the scan range of CT or MR perfusion should be determined by the expected area of ischemia on the basis of the neurologic deficit or imaging findings. In CT perfusion, a hypodense area of early CT sign should be included,[46] and the occluded vessel is sometimes referred to as a hyperdense artery.[47] In MR perfusion, a diffusion-weighted image (DWI)-positive area, which represents irreversible infarct,[48] should be included, and vessel stenosis or occlusion is evaluated by MR angiography before the scan.

The recommendations for scan parameters have been reported as a consensus of experts of perfusion imaging.[13]

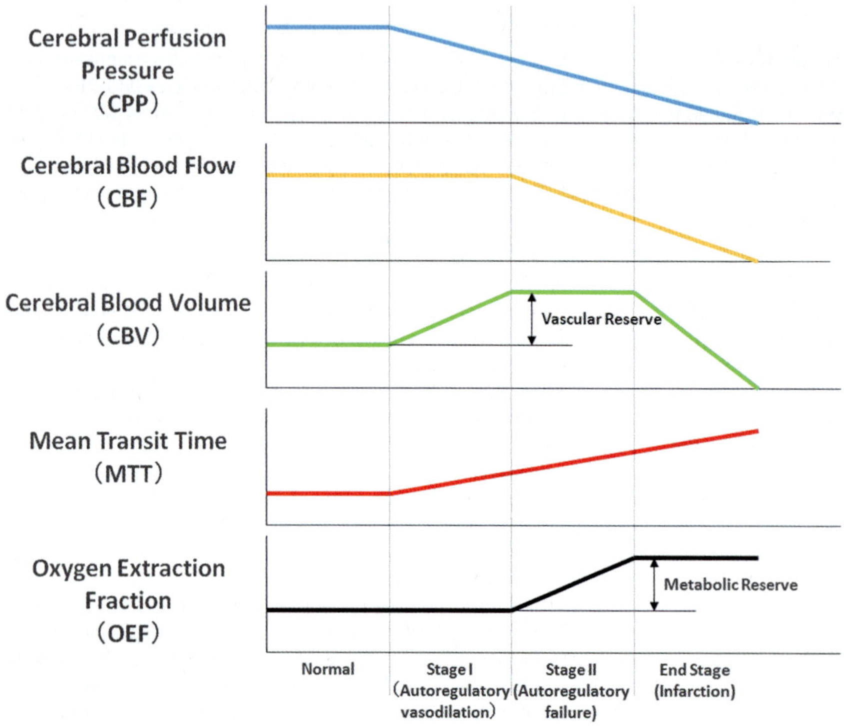

Figure 5.3. Hemodynamic parameters in ischemia. Against the decrease in CPP, CBV increases as the first compensation mechanism (vascular reserve, stage I), to maintain CBF. When CPP further decreases, OEF increases as the second compensation mechanism (metabolic reserve, stage II), to maintain tissue metabolism even with CBF decrease. Infarction occurs with severe CPP drop with CBV collapse. MTT constantly increases during these processes. Modified from Powers WJ, Grubb RL Jr, Raichle ME. Physiological responses to focal cerebral ischemia in humans. *Ann Neurol* 1984;16(5):546–552.

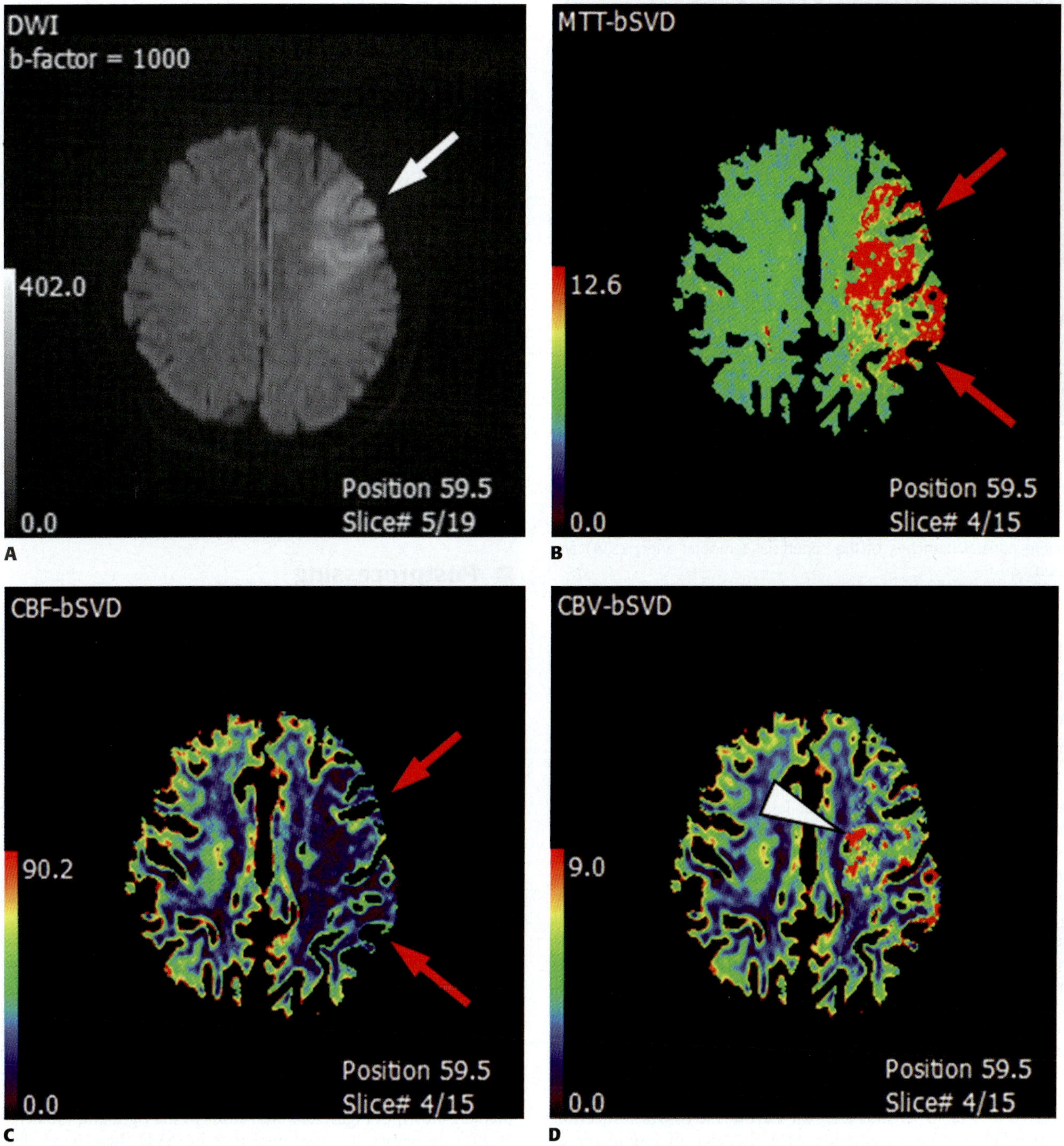

Figure 5-4. Diffusion-weighted image (DWI) and MR perfusion maps. On DWI **(A)**, high signal area is seen in the left frontal lobe (*white arrow*). Perfusion abnormality is noted in larger area on mean transit time (MTT) **(B)** and cerebral blood flow (CBF) **(C)** maps (*red arrows*), which means diffusion–perfusion mismatch (DPM). Cerebral blood volume (CBV) **(D)** increases in part of ischemic lesion (*white arrowhead*), which corresponds to vasodilation (vascular reserve, stage I). Note that vascular pixels are masked on the perfusion maps.

CT Perfusion

Recent advances in MDCT technology enable simultaneous multislice scans. The craniocaudal coverage is typically 32 to 40 mm, and it can be doubled by moving a table back and forth (shuttle mode or toggling table)[9,10] while temporal resolution increases. Two boluses are also used in scanners that do not use this technique to double the coverage, which also doubles the amount of contrast. Whole brain perfusion is possible with ADCT,[11] and CT angiography (CTA) and venography (CTV) can be performed simultaneously (Fig. 5.5).

For CT perfusion, it is very important to minimize radiation dose because the same location is continuously irradiated. To achieve a low-dose scan, the tube current and voltage should be

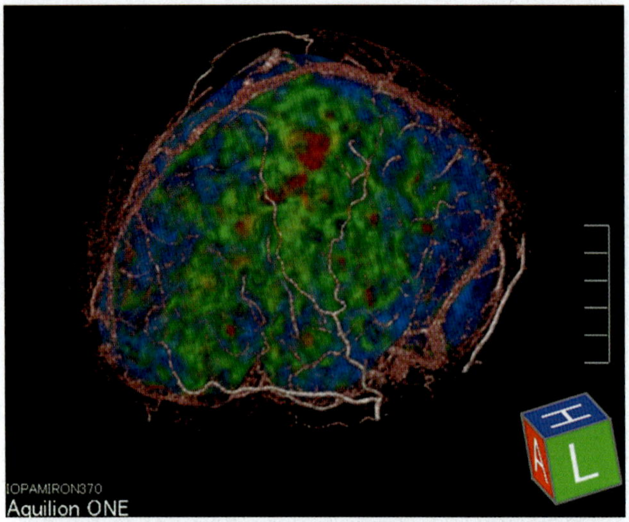

Figure 5-5. Fusion image of whole brain perfusion and CT angiography/venography. With ADCT, whole brain perfusion can be obtained with simultaneous acquisition of CTA and CT venography (CTV). In this case, TTP increase is noted in the vascular territory of the left MCA, where parietal branches of the superficial temporal artery (STA) are seen.

reduced. Specifically, a tube voltage of 80 kVp has the advantages of lower radiation dose and higher image contrast for iodine.[12] The tube current should be low, and it is typically chosen to be approximately 100 mAs in present scanners. Severe deterioration of image quality occurs with extremely low dose settings; therefore, appropriate image interpretation might be impossible. An intermittent scan is also an effective method to minimize the radiation dose; however, a temporal resolution of less than 2 seconds is recommended to maintain the accuracy of analysis.[49] A two-phase scan is also considered; the first phase has one image per second during bolus (up to 30 to 45 seconds), and the second phase has one image per 2 to 3 seconds.

Irradiation of the lens should be avoided. Recently, several techniques (such as imaging filter and iterative reconstruction) have been proposed to increase the signal-to-noise ratio (SNR) and reduce the radiation dose. As the SNR varies among scanners, even for those with the same scan parameters, the limit of dose reduction is carefully determined for each scanner by considering these techniques.

A higher iodine concentration (>350 mgI) is better for obtaining a stronger imaging contrast. The scan start should be delayed by 5 to 10 seconds after the start of the contrast injection to avoid unnecessary irradiation. An earlier start of scan increases radiation dose, but with a later start there is a risk that the contrast bolus has already reached the brain on the first image, which reduces the precision of analysis. The scan duration should be minimized as well. A total duration of 60 seconds is usually sufficient to cover the first passage of the contrast bolus; however, up to 70 to 90 seconds may be required for elderly patients with cardiac dysfunction.

CTA may be used to obtain information regarding the vessel status[50]; however, care should be taken regarding the total radiation dose and total amount of contrast, especially for young children and elderly patients with renal dysfunction. With the use of ADCT, CTA and CTV can be simultaneously obtained in one bolus of contrast for perfusion imaging. Three-dimensional fusion can be performed with this technique (Fig. 5.5).

MR Perfusion

Echo planar imaging (EPI) is used for DSC-MR perfusion, and the use of a higher magnetic field strength (>1.5 T) is recommended to obtain better image contrast. Generally, EPI of the gradient echo (GRE) is preferable, as its T2* contrast is larger than for the spin echo (SE) type EPI. SE-EPI is occasionally used for tumor imaging because it is more sensitive to smaller vessels than is GRE-EPI.[51] However, 3 T is recommended because the signal of SE-EPI is much smaller than GRE-EPI.

The echo time should be set to the smallest value to obtain a strong signal. The repetition time should be less than 2,000 milliseconds to maintain temporal resolution for the analysis. Whole brain coverage is possible with these parameters in present scanners. The use of parallel imaging is recommended to minimize image distortion. The same values of slice thickness, gap, and field of view as those used for DWI are preferred; this facilitates easy comparison with DWI abnormalities.

In MR perfusion, scan duration can be longer (90 to 120 seconds) as there is no radiation exposure. In order to stabilize the EPI signal, the scan start should precede the contrast injection. If repetitive exams for follow-up are required for patients with renal dysfunction, care should be taken to avoid nephrogenic systemic fibrosis.[52]

Postprocessing

All the CT and MR vendors have postprocessing software, and third party or academic software (such as Rapid,[53] Perfusion Mismatch Analyzer (http://asist.umin.jp/index-e.htm),[18,54] and stroketool (http://www.digitalimagesolutions.de/)[55]) can also be used. Recently, quantitative analysis has been implemented in most of these programs, and deconvolution has become the most common method. For quantification, AIF and VOF should be determined. In CT perfusion, it is simple to manually set ROI on MCA or ACA (for AIF)[31] and SSS (for VOF). In contrast, manual determination of AIF in MR perfusion is usually difficult because of the distortion of the curve shape due to the partial volume effect of AIF.[27] Therefore, automated AIF detection is recommended.[56] Underestimation of AIF and VOF is another problem that causes overestimation of CBF and CBV, and VOF is not necessarily used in MR perfusion.

There are several variations in deconvolution processes, such as singular value decomposition (SVD)[8,57] and fast Fourier transform (FFT).[53,58] Among these, the standard SVD (sSVD) is one of the most popular methods and is easily implemented. However, delay and dispersion issues have been reported that cause underestimation of CBF and overestimation of MTT.[59] These occur when the AIF and measured tissue are spatially distant or there is stenosis among them. Once the arrival of tracer is delayed in the tissue, then, as shown in Figure 5.6, $R(t)$ shifts to the right and the height of $R(t)$ decreases. It is assumed that in sSVD there is no delay between AIF and tissue curves. A proposed solution for the delay effect is the use of delay-insensitive algorithms, such as the circular type of deconvolution[60] (oscillation index SVD [oSVD] or block-circulant SVD [bSVD]) and FFT-based methods.[53] By using these algorithms, the quantification of CBF and MTT becomes more accurate, irrespective of the amount of delay (Figs. 5.6 and 5.7). Delay-compensated SVD[61] has also been proposed; however, it has a potential limitation because the estimation of the delay is sometimes difficult if the SNR is too small or the delay is too long. The solution for dispersion is to use local AIF,[62] that is, use of AIF near the measured tissue. This also compensates for the delay; however, the implementation of local AIF is not straightforward. Therefore, the current standard for analysis is one global AIF with delay-insensitive deconvolution.

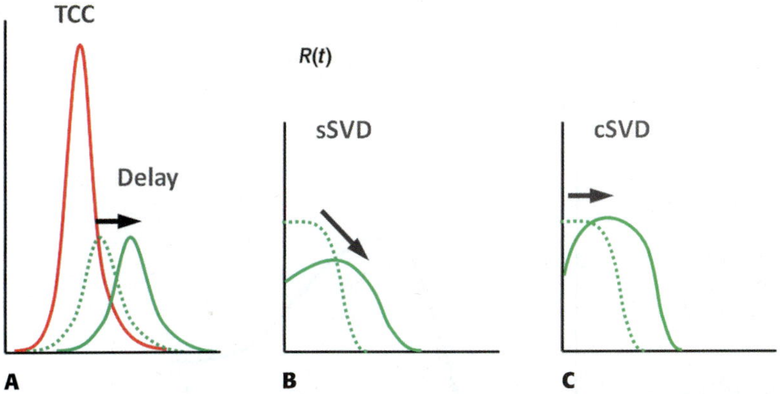

Figure 5-6. Delay effect. Time concentration curves (TCC) of the artery (*red*) and tissue (*green*) are shown **(A)**. Delay of contrast arrival in tissue is represented as rightward shift of TCC. In the deconvolution of standard SVD (sSVD), $R(t)$ shifts to the right and its height becomes lower **(B)**. Since CBF is determined as the peak height of $R(t)$, CBF underestimation occurs. In the circular types of SVD (cSVD), rightward shift of $R(t)$ occurs but the height is the same **(C)**. Therefore, CBF decrease is not seen.

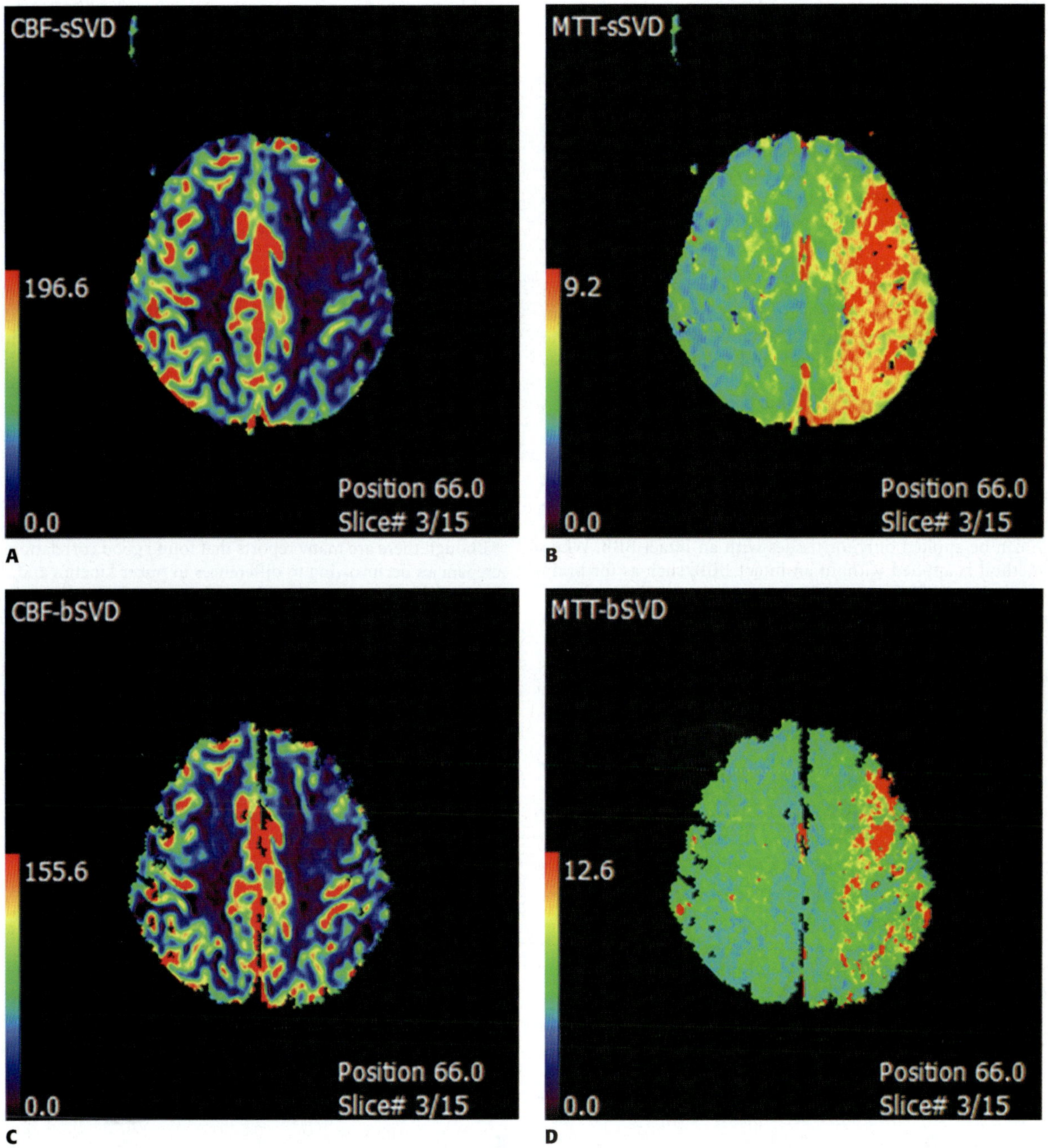

Figure 5-7. Delay-sensitive and delay-insensitive analysis. In delay-sensitive, standard SVD (sSVD), decrease in cerebral blood flow (CBF) **(A)** and increase in mean transit time (MTT) **(B)** are shown in the area of left middle cerebral artery (MCA). However, in delay-insensitive type of SVD (in this case, block-circulant SVD [bSVD]), the area of CBF decrease and MTT increase **(C** and **D)** are smaller than in sSVD. These discrepancies are derived from sensitivity of delay effect, that is, most of perfusion abnormalities seen in sSVD are calculation errors due to delay effect (erroneous CBF decrease and MTT increase).

Reliability Testing

During the early stages of perfusion imaging, a classical method, such as microspheres in animals, was used for validating the technique.[6,63] However, it would be preferable in clinical validation to compare perfusion imaging with other established methods such as PET, SPECT, and XeCT, all of which use a diffusible tracer and are considered to be the current standards of reference in hemodynamic measurement. There are numerous reports that discuss the good correlation between CT or MR perfusion and these standard techniques.[14–16,64,65]

These comparisons with other techniques are reliable; however, they cannot be carried out frequently, as the subjects undergo additional examinations with radiation exposure and contrast injection. Furthermore, differences in the implementations of analysis algorithms are evident among commercial software packages.[45] Recently, digital phantoms have been introduced to evaluate the accuracy and reliability of the software.[18,66] The digital phantom contains simulated curves that have true values of CBF, CBV, MTT, and delay. As the data format is DICOM, any software can load the data, and exported results can be compared with true values for the validation. As expected, these studies revealed that delay-sensitive algorithms are less accurate than are delay-insensitive ones. However, more interestingly, the degree of accuracy varies among different programs that implement the same delay-insensitive algorithm. Some software vendors claim that their software is delay insensitive, but the digital phantom reveals delay-dependent results.[18] Therefore, the use of a digital phantom is effective for improving and validating the analysis algorithm.

Limitations

One of the major limitations of CT and MR perfusion imaging is that these methods use intravascular, nondiffusible tracers. Therefore, kinetic models are based on the intravascular model, which can be applied only for tissues with an intact BBB. When this method is applied without an intact BBB, such as for brain tumors and outside the central nervous system (CNS), overestimation of CBV occurs owing to extravasation and retention

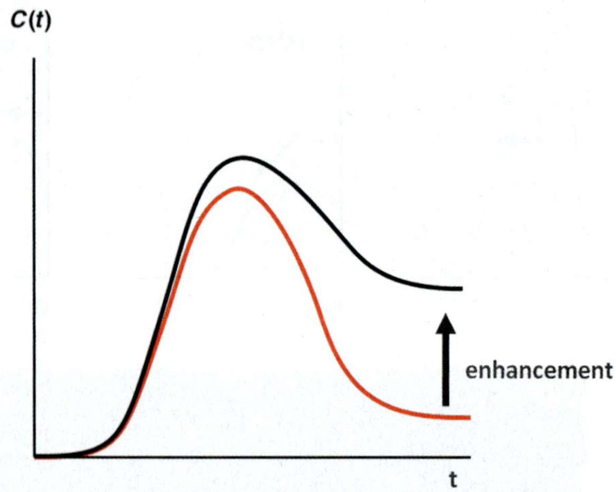

Figure 5-8. **Effect of extravasation of contrast (CT perfusion).** Even in the first passage of contrast bolus, extravasation of contrast occurs in the area where the BBB) breaks down (e.g., in the brain tumors) or BBB does not exist (outside of the CNS). Due to contrast enhancement, the AUC increases causing overestimation of the CBV.

contrast in CT perfusion (Fig. 5.8) or underestimation occurs owing to the T1 effect for Gd contrast in MR perfusion (Fig. 5.9).[39] To compensate for these possibilities, a baseline correction or predose of Gd-contrast in MR should be considered. Special postprocessing techniques after deconvolution have also been reported.[67] Another potential solution is the use of models other than deconvolution, such as the MS[38] and two-compartment model[22]; however, the former theoretically requires very rapid injection of contrast.

Moreover, comparison of quantitative results with other established techniques, such as PET and SPECT, is not straightforward. Although there are many reports that found good correlations, discrepancies occur owing to differences in tracer kinetics and analysis models. Thus, care should be taken when comparing absolute values among different modalities. Alternatively, the use of relative

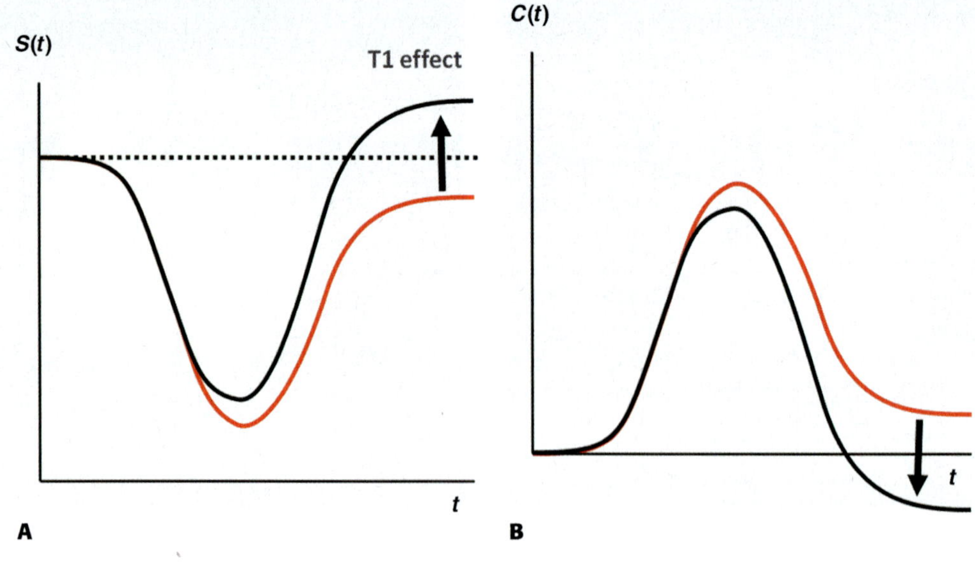

Figure 5-9. **Effect of extravasation of contrast (MR perfusion).** When extravasation of contrast occurs in MR perfusion, signal increase is seen due to T1 enhancement effect **(A)**. After the conversion of signal to concentration, decrease in concentration is noted **(B)**. Therefore, decreases in AUC and underestimation of CBV occur. In contrast, if T2* effect is dominant, signal decrease occurs and AUC increases similar to CT perfusion.

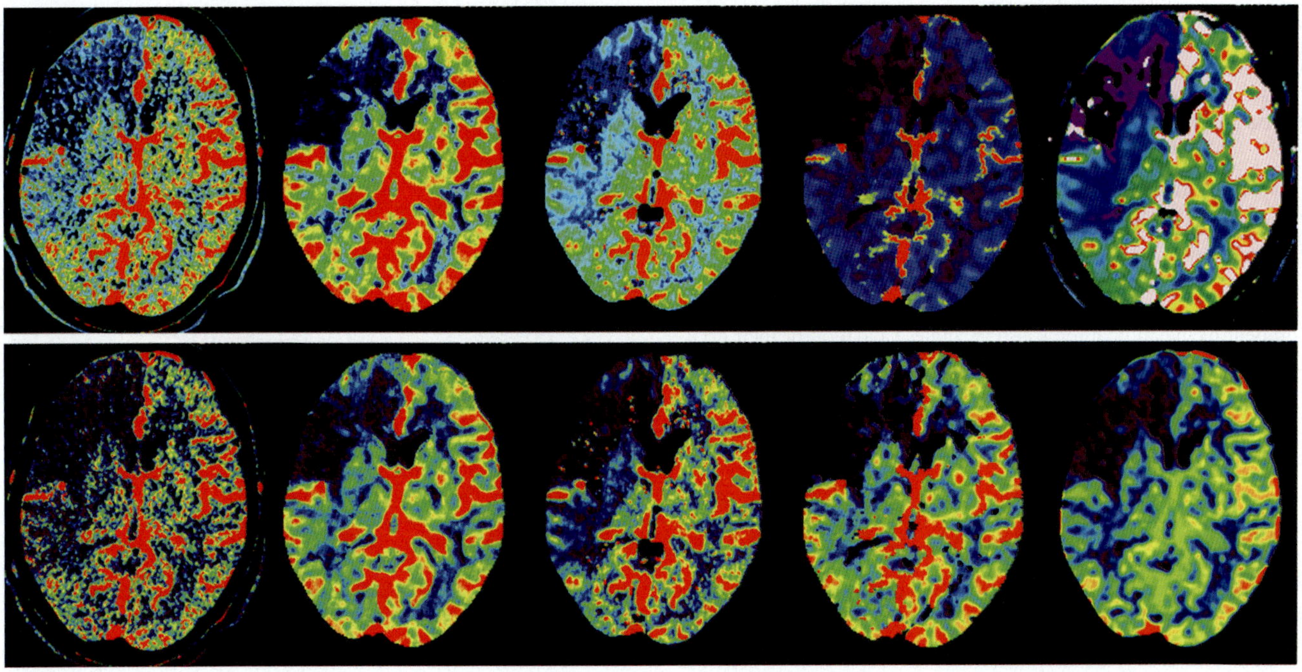

Figure 5-10. Difference in CT perfusion maps with identical source data. In the **upper row**, five different CBF maps are shown, in which identical source data are analyzed by five different software packages (commercial software of CT vendors). The color scales and quantitative values are quite different. The same data are shown with identical color scale in **lower row**, and the differences become smaller.

values (such as the contralateral ratio) is recommended to minimize such discrepancies.

In addition, there are still variations in results from different software packages, even with the same source data (Fig. 5.10).[45] These variations result from different analysis algorithms or different implementations of the same algorithm. User-dependent selection of parameters or AIF/VOF locations is another source of difference (Fig. 5.11).[68] These discrepancies have been reduced

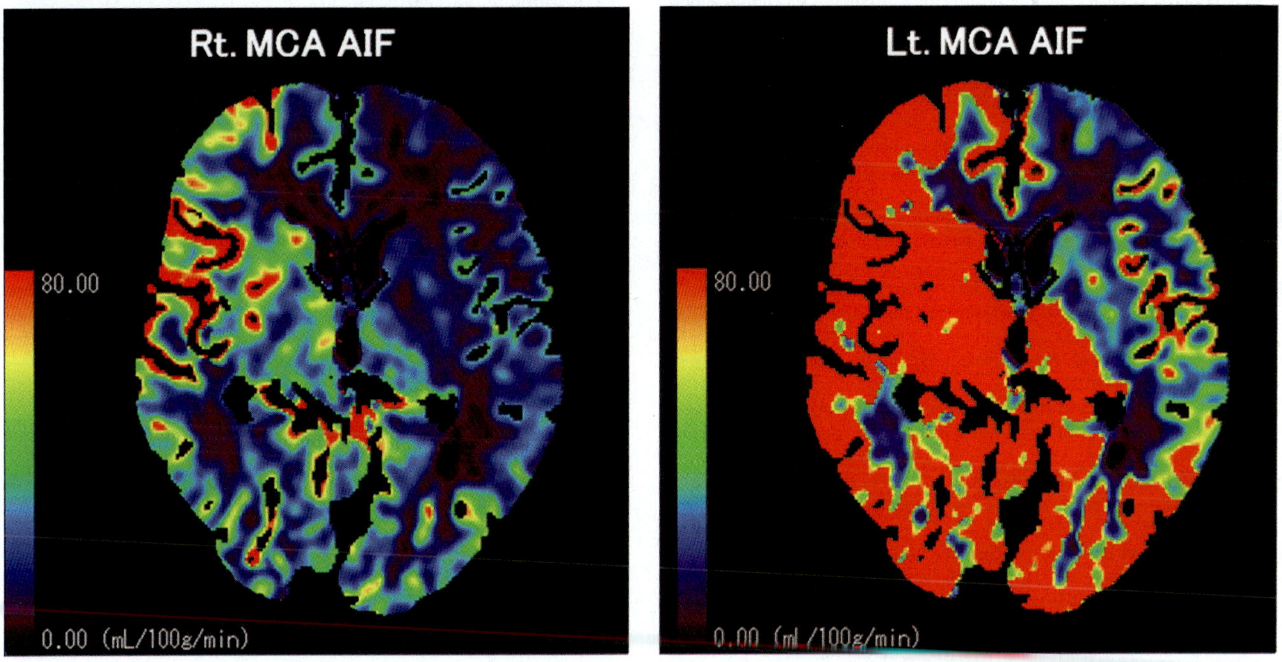

A B

Figure 5-11. Difference in CBF maps with different AIF. These two CBF maps are analyzed with AIF of MCA in the right side **(A)** and left side **(B)**. Due to the difference in the height and shape of the two AIFs, quantitative values are quite different (please note that these maps are shown in the same color scale).

by using validation processes such as digital phantoms[18]; however, improving and producing new versions of software packages usually takes months or years, especially for commercial software. Once a new version is released, differences between the versions may also cause problems.

Conclusions

The methods of CT and MR perfusion have been well established, and are readily available in clinical settings. Improvements of scans and analyses have been achieved because of developments in software and hardware and many basic and clinical studies. The recent development of digital phantoms also facilitates validation of their accuracy and reliability. Therefore, these techniques have become available for reliable hemodynamic measurements with short scan times.

REFERENCES

1. **Frackowiak RS, et al.** Quantitative measurement of regional cerebral blood flow and oxygen metabolism in man using 15O and positron emission tomography: theory, procedure, and normal values. *J Comput Assist Tomogr* 1980;4(6):727–736.
2. **Kanno I, et al.** A system for cerebral blood flow measurement using an H215O autoradiographic method and positron emission tomography. *J Cereb Blood Flow Metab* 1987;7(2):143–153.
3. **Baird AE, et al.** Preliminary experience with 99mTc-HMPAO SPECT in cerebral ischaemia. *Clin Exp Neurol* 1991;28(6-7):43–49.
4. **Yoon BW, et al.** Assessment of regional cerebral blood flow (rCBF) in ischemic stroke using Tc-99m HMPAO SPECT–comparison with CT and MR findings. *J Korean Med Sci* 1991;6(1):21–29.
5. **Koenig M, et al.** Perfusion CT of the brain: diagnostic approach for early detection of ischemic stroke. *Radiology* 1998;209(1):85–93.
6. **Cenic A, et al.** A CT method to measure hemodynamics in brain tumors: validation and application of cerebral blood flow maps. *AJNR Am J Neuroradiol* 2000;21(3):462–470.
7. **Ostergaard L, et al.** High resolution measurement of cerebral blood flow using intravascular tracer bolus passages. Part II: experimental comparison and preliminary results. *Magn Reson Med* 1996;36(5):726–736.
8. **Ostergaard L, et al.** High resolution measurement of cerebral blood flow using intravascular tracer bolus passages. Part I: mathematical approach and statistical analysis. *Magn Reson Med* 1996;36(5):715–725.
9. **Roberts HC, et al.** Multisection dynamic CT perfusion for acute cerebral ischemia: the "toggling-table" technique. *AJNR Am J Neuroradiol* 2001;22(6):1077–1080.
10. **Youn SW, et al.** Perfusion CT of the brain using 40-mm-wide detector and toggling table technique for initial imaging of acute stroke. *AJR Am J Roentgenol* 2008;191(3):W120–W126.
11. **Murayama K, et al.** Whole-brain perfusion CT performed with a prototype 256-detector row CT system: initial experience. *Radiology* 2009;250(1):202–211.
12. **Wintermark M, et al.** Using 80 kVp versus 120 kVp in perfusion CT measurement of regional cerebral blood flow. *AJNR Am J Neuroradiol* 2000;21(10):1881–1884.
13. **Wintermark M, et al.** Acute stroke imaging research roadmap. *Stroke* 2008;39(5):1621–1628.
14. **Ernst T, et al.** Correlation of regional cerebral blood flow from perfusion MRI and SPECT in normal subjects. *Magn Reson Imaging* 1999;17(3):349–354.
15. **Hagen T, Bartylla K, Piepgras U.** Correlation of regional cerebral blood flow measured by stable xenon CT and perfusion MRI. *J Comput Assist Tomogr* 1999;23(2):257–264.
16. **Yoshiura T, et al.** MR relative cerebral blood flow mapping of Alzheimer disease: correlation with Tc-99m HMPAO SPECT. *Acad Radiol* 2002;9(12):1383–1387.
17. **Kudo K, et al.** Quantitative cerebral blood flow measurement with dynamic perfusion CT using the vascular-pixel elimination method: comparison with H2(15)O positron emission tomography. *AJNR Am J Neuroradiol* 2003;24(3):419–426.
18. **Kudo K, et al.** Accuracy and reliability assessment of CT and MR perfusion analysis software using a digital phantom. *Radiology* 2013;267(1): 201–211.
19. **Kudo K, et al.** Susceptibility of T(max) to tracer delay on perfusion analysis: quantitative evaluation of various deconvolution algorithms using digital phantoms. *J Cereb Blood Flow Metab* 2011;31(3):908–912.
20. **Drayer BP, et al.** Xenon enhanced CT for analysis of cerebral integrity, perfusion, and blood flow. *Stroke* 1978;9(2):123–130.
21. **Kaufmann AM, et al.** Ischemic core and penumbra in human stroke. *Stroke* 1999;30(1):93–99.
22. **Tofts PS, et al.** Estimating kinetic parameters from dynamic contrast-enhanced T(1)-weighted MRI of a diffusible tracer: standardized quantities and symbols. *J Magn Reson Imaging* 1999;10(3):223–232.
23. **Luh WM, et al.** QUIPSS II with thin-slice TI1 periodic saturation: a method for improving accuracy of quantitative perfusion imaging using pulsed arterial spin labeling. *Magn Reson Med* 1999;41(6):1246–1254.
24. **Zaharchuk G, et al.** Arterial spin-label imaging in patients with normal bolus perfusion-weighted MR imaging findings: pilot identification of the borderzone sign. *Radiology* 2009;252(3):797–807.
25. **Meier P, Zierler KL.** On the theory of the indicator-dilution method for measurement of blood flow and volume. *J Appl Physiol* 1954;6(12):731–744.
26. **Axel L.** Cerebral blood flow determination by rapid-sequence computed tomography: theoretical analysis. *Radiology* 1980;137(3):679–686.
27. **van Osch MJ, van der Grond J, Bakker CJ.** Partial volume effects on arterial input functions: shape and amplitude distortions and their correction. *J Magn Reson Imaging* 2005;22(6):704–709.
28. **Leiva-Salinas, C., et al.** The alphabet soup of perfusion CT and MR imaging: terminology revisited and clarified in five questions. *Neuroradiology* 2012;54(9):907–918.
29. **Gobbel GT, Fike JR.** A deconvolution method for evaluating indicator-dilution curves. *Phys Med Biol* 1994;39(11):1833–1854.
30. **Eastwood JD, et al.** Practical injection-rate CT perfusion imaging: deconvolution-derived hemodynamics in a case of stroke. *Neuroradiology* 2001;43(3):223–226.
31. **Wintermark M, et al.** The anterior cerebral artery is an appropriate arterial input function for perfusion-CT processing in patients with acute stroke. *Neuroradiology* 2008;50(3):227–236.
32. **van der Schaaf I, et al.** Influence of partial volume on venous output and arterial input function. *AJNR Am J Neuroradiol* 2006;27(1):46–50.
33. **Astrup J, Siesjo BK, Symon L.** Thresholds in cerebral ischemia—the ischemic penumbra. *Stroke* 1981;12(6):723–725.
34. **Jones TH, et al.** Thresholds of focal cerebral ischemia in awake monkeys. *J Neurosurg* 1981;54(6):773–782.
35. **Heiss WD.** Flow thresholds of functional and morphological damage of brain tissue. *Stroke* 1983;14(3):329–331.
36. **Morawetz RB, et al.** Cerebral blood flow determined by hydrogen clearance during middle cerebral artery occlusion in unanesthetized monkeys. *Stroke* 1978;9(2):143–149.
37. **Tamura A, Asano T, Sano K.** Correlation between rCBF and histological changes following temporary middle cerebral artery occlusion. *Stroke* 1980;11(5):487–493.
38. **Klotz E, Konig M.** Perfusion measurements of the brain: using dynamic CT for the quantitative assessment of cerebral ischemia in acute stroke. *Eur J Radiol* 1999;30(3):170–184.
39. **Boxerman JL, Schmainda KM, Weisskoff RM.** Relative cerebral blood volume maps corrected for contrast agent extravasation significantly correlate with glioma tumor grade, whereas uncorrected maps do not. *AJNR Am J Neuroradiol* 2006;27(4):859–867.
40. **Olivot JM, et al.** Optimal Tmax threshold for predicting penumbral tissue in acute stroke. *Stroke* 2009;40(2):469–475.
41. **Calamante F, et al.** The physiological significance of the time-to-maximum (Tmax) parameter in perfusion MRI. *Stroke* 2010;41(6):1169–1174.
42. **Davis SM, et al.** Effects of alteplase beyond 3 h after stroke in the Echoplanar Imaging Thrombolytic Evaluation Trial (EPITHET): a placebo-controlled randomised trial. *Lancet Neurol* 2008;7(4):299–309.
43. **Mlynash M, et al.** Refining the definition of the malignant profile: insights from the DEFUSE-EPITHET pooled data set. *Stroke* 2011;42 (5):1270–1275.
44. **Albers GW, et al.** Magnetic resonance imaging profiles predict clinical response to early reperfusion: the diffusion and perfusion imaging evaluation for understanding stroke evolution (DEFUSE) study. *Ann Neurol* 2006;60(5):508–517.
45. **Kudo K, et al.** Differences in CT perfusion maps generated by different commercial software: quantitative analysis by using identical source data of acute stroke patients. *Radiology* 2010;254(1):200–209.

46. **Jaillard A, et al.** Significance of early CT signs in acute stroke. A CT scan-diffusion MRI study. *Cerebrovasc Dis* 2002;13(1):47–56.
47. **Pressman BD, Tourje EJ, Thompson JR.** An early CT sign of ischemic infarction: increased density in a cerebral artery. *AJR Am J Roentgenol* 1987;149(3):583–586.
48. **Neumann-Haefelin T, et al.** Diffusion- and perfusion-weighted MRI. The DWI/PWI mismatch region in acute stroke. *Stroke* 1999;30(8): 1591–1597.
49. **Wintermark M, et al.** Dynamic perfusion CT: optimizing the temporal resolution and contrast volume for calculation of perfusion CT parameters in stroke patients. *AJNR Am J Neuroradiol* 2004;25(5):720–729.
50. **Morhard D, et al.** Optimal sequence timing of CT angiography and perfusion CT in patients with stroke. *Eur J Radiol* 2013;82(6): e286–e289.
51. **Boxerman JL, et al.** MR contrast due to intravascular magnetic susceptibility perturbations. *Magn Reson Med* 1995;34(4):555–566.
52. **Abujudeh HH, et al.** Retrospective assessment of prevalence of nephrogenic systemic fibrosis (NSF) after implementation of a new guideline for the use of gadobenate dimeglumine as a sole contrast agent for magnetic resonance examination in renally impaired patients. *J Magn Reson Imaging* 2009;30(6):1335–1340.
53. **Straka M, Albers GW, Bammer R.** Real-time diffusion-perfusion mismatch analysis in acute stroke. *J Magn Reson Imaging* 2010;32(5): 1024–1037.
54. **Kudo K, et al.** Development of perfusion mismatch analyzer (PMA): fully automated, operator-independent and standardized PWI-DWI analysis software. 93rd Annual Meetings of RSNA, Educational Exhibit; 2007. LL-NR3212.
55. **Wittsack HJ, Ritzl A, Modder U.** User friendly analysis of MR investigations of the cerebral perfusion: Windows(R)-based image processing. *Röfo* 2002;174(6):742–746.
56. **Mlynash M, et al.** Automated method for generating the arterial input function on perfusion-weighted MR imaging: validation in patients with stroke. *AJNR Am J Neuroradiol* 2005;26(6):1479–1486.
57. **Liu HL, et al.** Cerebral blood flow measurement by dynamic contrast MRI using singular value decomposition with an adaptive threshold. *Magn Reson Med* 1999;42(1):167–172.
58. **Gall P, et al.** On the design of filters for Fourier and oSVD-based deconvolution in bolus tracking perfusion MRI. *MAGMA* 2010;23(3):187–195.
59. **Calamante F, Gadian DG, Connelly A.** Delay and dispersion effects in dynamic susceptibility contrast MRI: simulations using singular value decomposition. *Magn Reson Med* 2000;44(3):466–473.
60. **Wu O, et al.** Tracer arrival timing-insensitive technique for estimating flow in MR perfusion-weighted imaging using singular value decomposition with a block-circulant deconvolution matrix. *Magn Reson Med* 2003;50(1):164–174.
61. **Ibaraki M, et al.** Tracer delay correction of cerebral blood flow with dynamic susceptibility contrast-enhanced MRI. *J Cereb Blood Flow Metab* 2005;25(3):378–390.
62. **Calamante F, Morup M, Hansen LK.** Defining a local arterial input function for perfusion MRI using independent component analysis. *Magn Reson Med* 2004;52(4):789–797.
63. **Heymann MA, et al.** Blood flow measurements with radionuclide-labeled particles. *Prog Cardiovasc Dis* 1977;20(1):55–79.
64. **Karonen JO, et al.** Combined diffusion and perfusion MRI with correlation to single-photon emission CT in acute ischemic stroke. Ischemic penumbra predicts infarct growth. *Stroke* 1999;30(8):1583–1590.
65. **Olivot JM, et al.** Perfusion MRI (Tmax and MTT) correlation with xenon CT cerebral blood flow in stroke patients. *Neurology* 2009;72(13): 1140–1145.
66. **Kudo K, et al.** Susceptibility of Tmax to tracer delay on perfusion analysis: quantitative evaluation of various deconvolution algorithms using digital phantoms. *J Cereb Blood Flow Metab* 2011;31(3):908–912.
67. **Nabavi DG, et al.** CT assessment of cerebral perfusion: experimental validation and initial clinical experience. *Radiology* 1999;213(1):141–149.
68. **Bisdas S, et al.** Effect of the arterial input function on the measured perfusion values and infarct volumetric in acute cerebral ischemia evaluated by perfusion computed tomography. *Invest Radiol* 2007;42(3):147–156.

CHAPTER

6 Coronary Fractional Flow Reserve Based on Computed Tomography

Javaid Iqbal, MRCP, PhD and Patrick W. Serruys, MD, PhD

Introduction

Coronary angiography is the standard imaging modality for diagnosis and management of coronary artery disease in contemporary practice. However, its invasive nature and potential limitations have led to the development of noninvasive imaging modalities to investigate the extent and significance of coronary artery disease. Recent advancements in image processing, modeling, and computational fluid dynamics offer calculation of coronary artery pressure and flow from conventional coronary computed tomography (CT) scans. Computed fractional flow reserve (FFR_{CT}) is the ratio of mean coronary artery pressure divided by mean aortic pressure under conditions of simulated maximal coronary hyperemia, thus providing a noninvasive estimate of fractional flow reserve (FFR). Clinical trials have shown that FFR_{CT} improves diagnostic accuracy and discrimination compared to CT angiography alone for the diagnosis of hemodynamically significant coronary artery disease, when compared to invasive FFR as the reference gold standard. This promising new technology provides a combined anatomic and physiologic assessment of coronary artery disease in a single noninvasive test that can help select patients for invasive angiography and revascularization or optimal medical therapy. This chapter will discuss the rationale, technique, clinical application, limitations, and future of noninvasive FFR_{CT}.

Invasive Assessment of Coronary Artery Disease

Coronary Angiography

Sones performed the first selective coronary angiogram in 1957, enabling physicians to visualize the extent and severity of atherosclerotic coronary disease.[1] Coronary angiography completely revolutionized cardiovascular medicine and has remained the gold standard for defining coronary anatomy during the last 50 years. It has made a substantial impact on the diagnosis and management of ischemic heart disease. Patients with significant lesions seen on angiography can undergo mechanical revascularization, either coronary artery bypass grafting or percutaneous coronary intervention.[2]

Limitations of Invasive Angiography

Although the utility of coronary angiography in contemporary clinical practice remains undisputed, it can often underestimate or overestimate the severity of a lesion. Angiography displays coronary cross-sectional anatomy from a planar two-dimensional silhouette of the contrast-filled vessel lumen. However, coronary lesions are often complex, with markedly distorted or eccentric luminal shapes, and angiography can misrepresent the severity of luminal narrowing.[3] Additionally, visual interpretation of coronary angiography has a significant intra- and interobserver variability.[4,5] The angiographic severity of a lesion poorly correlates to postmortem histology.[6,7] More importantly, the relationship between stenosis and myocardial ischemia is complex, and whether the lesion is hemodynamically or functionally significant often cannot be reliably assessed by coronary angiography.[8] The nuclear substudy of COURAGE (Clinical Outcomes Utilizing Revascularization and Aggressive Drug Evaluation) trial showed that among patients with ≥70% stenosis, only 32% exhibited severe ischemia and 40% manifested no or mild ischemia according to myocardial perfusion scintigraphy.[9]

Potential Solutions

The main limitations of coronary angiography, that is, invasive nature and lack of hemodynamic significance, can be solved by noninvasive testing for coronary artery disease and assessment of FFR (Table 6.1). FFR is traditionally assessed invasively, but noninvasive FFR assessment can solve both limitations. A multitude of noninvasive imaging modalities offer functional assessment of coronary artery disease by identifying regional differences in coronary flow reserve or wall motion abnormalities.[10,11] Dobutamine stress echocardiography, adenosine stress first-pass perfusion magnetic resonance imaging, and myocardial single photon emission tomography (SPECT) are well-established modalities. While these serve as useful surrogate for ischemia, they do not directly visualize coronary stenoses or assess the hemodynamic significance of individual coronary lesions. Furthermore, these noninvasive stress tests have significant false-positive and false-negative rates when compared with coronary angiography.[12] This may result in either unnecessary referral for invasive tests or falsely misclassifying the

TABLE 6.1 **Limitation of Coronary Angiography and Potential Solutions**

Limitation	Solution	Unifying Solution
Intra- and interobserver variability	Computer software–based automated quantitative coronary angiography	Computed tomography to provide angiography as well as computed fractional flow reserve to provide noninvasive anatomical and functional assessment of coronary lesions
Invasive procedure	Noninvasive tests including nuclear imaging, computed tomography, or magnetic resonance imaging	
Lack of hemodynamic significance of stenotic lesions	Invasive functional flow reserve or computed flow reserve from invasive coronary angiography or computed flow reserve from computed tomography	

patient as low risk. Accordingly, some experts advocate for hybrid imaging with physiologic and anatomic evaluation of CAD by stress testing and CT.[13,14] However, this approach requires two tests and is associated with higher costs, time delay, and a greater radiation burden for the patient.[14] A long-standing goal of noninvasive coronary imaging has been to develop a single test that identifies high-grade stenosis and determines its functional significance.[15,16] The recent developments in CT-derived FFR assessment combined with the anatomic imaging capabilities of CT provide such a combined anatomic–physiologic assessment of coronary artery disease from a single imaging test.[17]

Fractional Flow Reserve

FFR measurement is based on the relationship between coronary artery pressure and blood flow. This relationship is quite variable at rest; however, it is almost linear during maximal hyperemia as the peripheral resistance is minimal and constant.[18] FFR is thus defined as the ratio of maximal blood flow on either side of a coronary artery stenosis (distal vessel flow divided by proximal vessel flow during maximal coronary hyperemia).[19,20] FFR is conventionally measured during invasive angiography by using a guide wire with a pressure-sensing transducer that is placed across the stenotic lesion. After induction of maximal hyperemia by using a vasodilator agent such as intravenous or intra-arterial adenosine, the pressure gradient across the lesion is recorded, and FFR is calculated as the mean distal coronary pressure divided by mean aortic pressure. Coronary stenoses with FFR less than 0.75 are almost always functionally significant, whereas lesions with FFR greater than 0.80 are rarely associated with inducible ischemia.[20] Prospective, multicenter, randomized clinical trials have shown that FFR-guided revascularization provides a sustained clinical benefit with improved event-free survival and reduced health care expenditures compared with the traditional strategy of angiographic stenosis guidance.[21–23] FFR has demonstrated its clinical utility in safely deferring coronary revascularization procedures for non–flow-limiting stenoses.[24] A subanalysis of the FAME (Fractional Flow Reserve vs. Angiography for Multivessel Evaluation) trial demonstrated that two-thirds of coronary lesions with a diameter stenosis more than 50% were not ischemia producing. Routine measurement of FFR in patients with multivessel coronary artery disease who are undergoing PCI with drug-eluting stents significantly reduces the rate of the composite end point of death, nonfatal myocardial infarction, and repeat revascularization at 1 year.[25] Patients with ischemia-causing stenoses benefit from revascularization[25], whereas patients with hemodynamically insignificant stenoses require no intervention and experience favorable outcomes on medical therapy alone, with myocardial infarction and mortality rates of less than 1% per year.[21,24] FFR is now considered to be the standard of care for guiding percutaneous coronary revascularization in both European and American guidelines.[26,27] Despite the solid data for the utility of FFR to guide clinical decision making, adoption into daily clinical practice has been limited, and FFR is currently used in only a minority of coronary revascularization procedures. This may be due in part to the invasive nature of the procedure, the need for pharmacologic vasodilation, an expensive coronary pressure wire, and risks related to instrumentation of the coronary arteries. It has been proposed in the recent years that FFR can be derived from coronary angiography alone without the need for pressure wire or vasodilatation[28,29]; however, it still requires invasive coronary angiography. Hence, there is a definite need for a noninvasive method to determine the functional significance of individual coronary lesions.

Computed Tomography to Assess Coronary Artery Disease

Noninvasive evaluation of coronary artery disease can be readily performed using CT scanning.

CT Angiography

Computed tomography angiography (CTA) can provide high-resolution anatomic imaging of the coronary arteries.[30,31] CTA is emerging as noninvasive tool of choice for the detection, characterization, and quantification of coronary atherosclerotic plaques.[32–34] It is commonly employed for exclusion of coronary artery disease and demonstration of the extent of coronary artery disease. Accuracy of quantitative measurements for lumen, vessel, and plaque volume derived from multislice computed tomography (MSCT) scans in comparison with intravascular ultrasound (IVUS) gray scale was assessed in a cohort of 47 patients: An excellent correlation and a relatively acceptable agreement were shown.[33] In another study, Voros et al.[34] analyzed the relationship between MSCT- and IVUS-derived measures for lumen and plaque area. They concluded that for lumen and vessel areas, good correlations exist with a coefficient higher than 0.7 and a systematic error of about 20%, MSCT values being consistently overestimated. Regarding percentage of

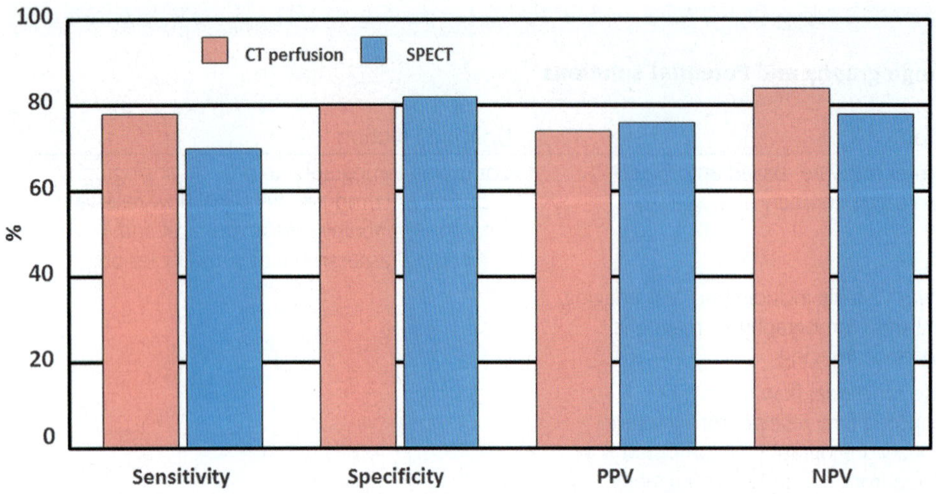

Figure 6-1. **Diagnostic accuracy of CT perfusion and SPECT for the detection of stenosis.** (Adapted from Blankstein R, Shturman LD, Rogers IS, et al. Adenosine-induced stress myocardial perfusion imaging using dual-source cardiac computed tomography. *J Am Coll Cardiol* 2009;54:1072–1084.)

atheroma volume, the correlation was only modest with a coefficient of correlation close to 0.5, and in general, the Bland-Altman plot showed an acceptable mean difference though with relatively wide limits of agreement. The same authors also reviewed the capability of MSCT to characterize tissues, using the classical threshold of more than 150 Hounsfield units (HU) for calcified plaque, 30 to 149 HU for high-density noncalcified plaque, and −100 to 30 HU for low-density noncalcified plaque. Only a modest correlation was found for both calcified and noncalcified plaque areas, and both components were excessively overestimated by CTA with rather poor overall agreement. A number of other prospective, multicenter studies have demonstrated high diagnostic performance for the identification and exclusion of anatomically obstructive coronary artery disease compared to ICA.[35–37] One of the intrinsic limitations of CTA in assessing plaque characteristics is the fact that the contrast density of the lumen impacts on the plaque density in the surroundings of the lumen.[38,39] Despite this limitation, computer algorithms have been developed, which can differentiate between diverse types of tissue based on MSCT.[34,40–42]

Beyond luminography and plaque characterization, MSCT has so far been unable to provide a functional assessment of the severity of coronary stenosis. Even among severe stenoses identified by CT and confirmed by angiography, less than half are functionally significant when compared to FFR.[17,43] This unreliable relationship between severity of stenosis and functional significance has raised concerns that the use of coronary CTA may lead to unnecessary invasive angiography and unneeded revascularization procedures.[17,44]

CT Myocardial Perfusion Imaging

To overcome the limitation of CTA, one potential strategy is to combine CTA with CT perfusion imaging. Experimental work has validated multidetector CT-based estimates of myocardial perfusion against microsphere-derived measurement of myocardial blood flow in a canine model.[45] Recently, several clinical trials have shown the feasibility and diagnostic accuracy of adenosine stress CT perfusion imaging for the detection of perfusion abnormalities, which is comparable to those of SPECT.[46–48] George et al. studied 40 patients with abnormal SPECT perfusion imaging who underwent adenosine stress CT perfusion and coronary CTA.[48] In a subset of 27 patients who underwent invasive coronary angiography, CT perfusion imaging, when combined with coronary CTA, accurately predicted coronary stenosis causing perfusion deficits as compared to the combination of quantitative coronary angiography and SPECT as a reference standard with sensitivity, specificity, positive predictive value, and negative predictive value of 86%, 92%, 92%, and 85%, respectively. Blankstein et al. reported the diagnostic accuracy of adenosine stress CT perfusion for the identification of hemodynamically significant stenosis as compared with that of SPECT.[47] The study included 34 patients who underwent SPECT and invasive coronary angiography. On a per-vessel basis, CT perfusion alone had a sensitivity of 79% and a specificity of 80% for the detection of stenosis ≥50%, while those for SPECT perfusion imaging were 67% and 83%, respectively (Fig. 6.1). For the detection of vessels with ≥50% stenosis with a corresponding SPECT perfusion abnormality, CT perfusion had a sensitivity of 93% and a specificity of 74%. A distinct benefit of CT perfusion imaging is the ability to simultaneously visualize both anatomical stenosis and its physiologic consequences. However, there are several limitations that are pertinent to CT perfusion imaging. First, although the radiation exposure of comprehensive cardiac CT examination was equivalent to that of SPECT,[47] it is still high. Second, in comparison to conventional coronary CTA, a larger volume of iodinated contrast is required as both rest and stress images are acquired. Third, CT perfusion imaging performed during adenosine infusion increases heart rate and thus the likelihood of artifactual reduction in CT attenuation densities caused by cardiac movement, partial volume effects, and beam-hardening artifacts, which can be mistaken for myocardial perfusion deficits. Finally, CT perfusion imaging does not provide lesion-specific ischemia data and cannot distinguish between diffuse disease and stenoses, which may be targets for revascularization.[49]

CT Fractional Flow Reserve

Over the last decade, research in the field has made major progress and some landmark discoveries, such as the introduction and validation of patient-specific 3D blood flow analysis, the development of adaptive finite element models for simulating cardiovascular blood flow, the definition of physiologically realistic inflow and outflow boundary conditions, as well as the coupled description of blood flow and vessel wall dynamics.[50] The recent introduction of a novel computational method has enabled the calculation of FFR_{CT} without the need for additional imaging, medication, or modification of CT acquisition protocols.[51]

Computed Fractional Flow Reserve

Computational fluid dynamics, as applied to coronary CTA images, represents a novel noninvasive method that quantitates coronary blood flow, flow velocity, and pressure in the major epicardial coronary arteries to calculate FFR_{CT}.[49]

Principles

FFR_{CT} technology is based on three key underlying principles for the generation of physiologic models of coronary blood flow. The first principle is that baseline coronary blood flow is proportional to myocardial oxygen demand at rest. This enables calculation of total resting coronary blood flow relative to patient-specific myocardial mass that can be quantified on the MSCT scan. Naturally, this assumption does not apply to patients with angina at rest and thus would prohibit analysis with FFR_{CT} technology in them. The second principle is that the resistance of the microcirculatory vascular bed at rest is inversely, but not linearly, proportional to the size of the feeding vessel, as has been demonstrated in prior morphometry, shear stress autoregulation, and compensatory remodeling research.[52–57] The third principle states that the coronary microcirculation has a predictable vasodilatory response to adenosine.[58] When the myocardium lacks oxygen, ATP breaks down with a resulting release of endogenous adenosine. Exogenous administration of adenosine elicits the maximum hyperemic responses by producing complete relaxation of the smooth muscle cells lining the resistance arterioles. Coronary flow reserve (ratio of flow during maximum hyperemia to resting flow) is modulated by both epicardial and microcirculatory resistance.[58] This is based upon a prior landmark study that identified a predictable response of the total coronary resistance to hyperemia induction by intravenous or intracoronary administration of adenosine. Thus, FFR is computed by applying a dynamic physiologic model of coronary flow to patient-specific coronary anatomy as revealed by the coronary CTA. This coronary CTA can be performed in the usual manner, using standard acquisition protocols, with no need for additional imaging or radiation exposure and no need for adenosine administration.

Technique

Computation of FFR from coronary CT involves three basic elements[50]:

1. Constructing an accurate patient-specific anatomic model of the epicardial coronary arteries.
2. Specifying inflow and outflow boundary conditions reflecting patient-specific coronary physiology during maximal hyperemia.
3. Performing a numerical solution of the laws of physics governing fluid dynamics. This combination of anatomy, physiology, and computational fluid dynamics enables the calculation of coronary artery blood flow and pressure under conditions of maximum hyperemia.

Computation of coronary flow and pressure is based on "Navier-Stokes equations" of fluid dynamics, which are founded in the relationship between conservation of mass and momentum balance.[17] The equations are solved for coronary flow and pressure as a function of three spatial coordinates and time. The physical properties of blood (fluid density and fluid viscosity) are assumed, and blood is treated as a noncompressible Newtonian fluid with a constant viscosity in the coronary arteries. Since the governing equations of blood flow are nonlinear partial differential equations, which can only be solved analytically under highly idealized circumstances, solutions for realistic patient-specific models of the coronary tree require a numerical approximation for velocity and pressure at a finite, but very large, number of points.[59] This requires the computation of millions of nonlinear equations simultaneously and repeating this process for thousands of time intervals in a single cardiac cycle.[17] In addition, it is necessary to define the boundary conditions that interface the modeled domain to the remainder of the circulation; this represents the biggest challenge in blood flow modeling.[17] Realistic modeling of coronary flow requires coupling of lumped parameter models of the heart, systemic circulation, and coronary circulation to a patient-specific model of the root of the aorta and epicardial coronary arteries extracted from coronary CTA data.[50] These lumped parameter models combine peripheral resistance, blood vessel compliance, and other factors into distinct elements dependent on the specific parameters of each circulatory bed. Importantly, neither pressure nor flow rate is directly specified at the boundaries of the 3D model, but instead arises naturally from the interaction between the 3D model and the lumped parameter models representing cardiac output, aortic pressure, and microcirculatory resistance.[50] As a final step, the boundary condition of maximum coronary hyperemia is modeled by simulating the effect that adenosine has on reducing the peripheral resistance of the downstream microcirculatory coronary bed.[17]

HeartFlow

Based upon the above-mentioned principles, a dedicated algorithm using cardiovascular computational flow dynamics was created (HeartFlow; HeartFlow, Inc., Redwood City, CA, USA) for noninvasive FFR derivation. The anatomy of the coronary arterial bed of a particular patient is not known a priori and has to be extracted from a patient-specific medical imaging data set. MSCT can provide an accurate coronary geometric model, including branching and pathology specific to a patient. Based upon this geometric information, a volumetric finite element mesh with anisotropic refinement and boundary layers is generated in order to compute numerical results (Fig. 6.2).

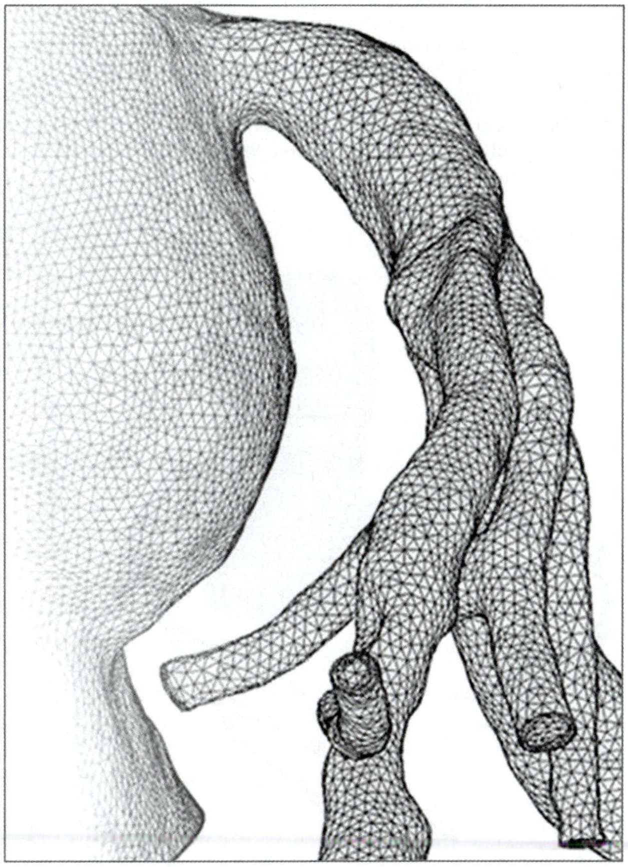

Figure 6-2. Finite element model of a left coronary artery. The distribution of element size and density can be iteratively adapted to computation requirements. (Reproduced from Serruys, et al. *EuroIntervention* 2012;8:511–519, with permission.)

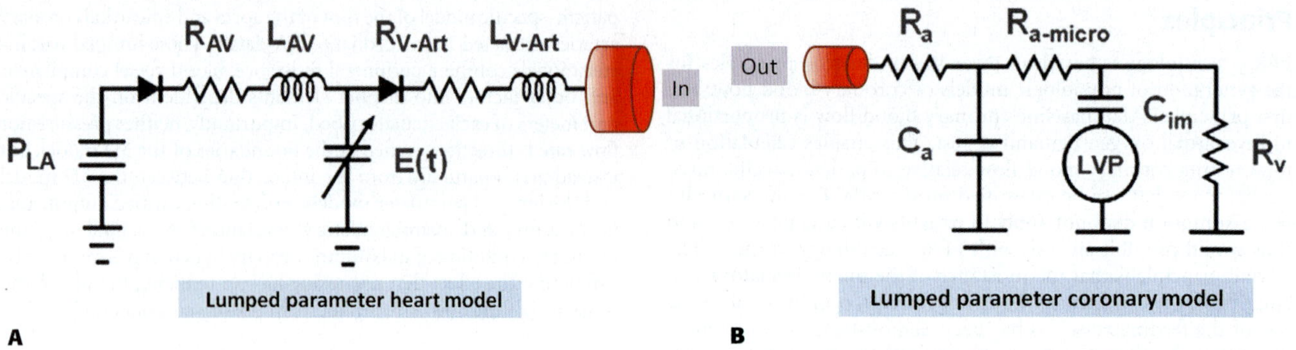

Figure 6-3. Lumped (zero-dimensional) parameter models used in cardiovascular blood flow simulations. **A:** Lumped parameter heart model coupling the left heart side to the aortic inlet (In) of a closed loop system comprising the systemic and pulmonary circulation. The left heart side model consists of left atrial pressure PLA, mitral valve, atrioventricular valvular resistance RAV, atrioventricular inductance LAV, aortic valve, ventriculoarterial valvular resistance RV-Art, ventriculoarterial inductance LV-Art, and left ventricular (LV) pressure. The LV pressure is modeled with time-varying LV elastance *E*(*t*). **B**: Lumped parameter coronary vascular bed model coupled to a coronary branch outlet (Out). This model consists of coronary arterial and venous resistance (Ra and Rv, respectively), coronary arterial microcirculation resistance Ra-micro, coronary arterial capacitance Ca, intramyocardial vascular capacitance Cim, and LV pressure; LV pressure stands for intramyocardial pressure for branches perfusing the left ventricle and septum. (Reproduced from Serruys, et al. *EuroIntervention* 2012;8:511–519, with permission.)

Using a proprietary algorithm, the heart–vessel interaction can be defined, whereas time-varying coronary resistance for each coronary branch can be determined relative to intramyocardial pressure and microvasculature impedance. This latter component can be represented by a so-called lumped (zero-dimensional) parameter model, which resembles an electric circuit, including resistive and capacitive elements (Fig. 6.3).[60] Finally, the complex fluid properties of the blood are entered into the model, in order to refine the computations. Examples of FFR calculated for the vessel tree with and without stenosis are shown in Figure 6.4.

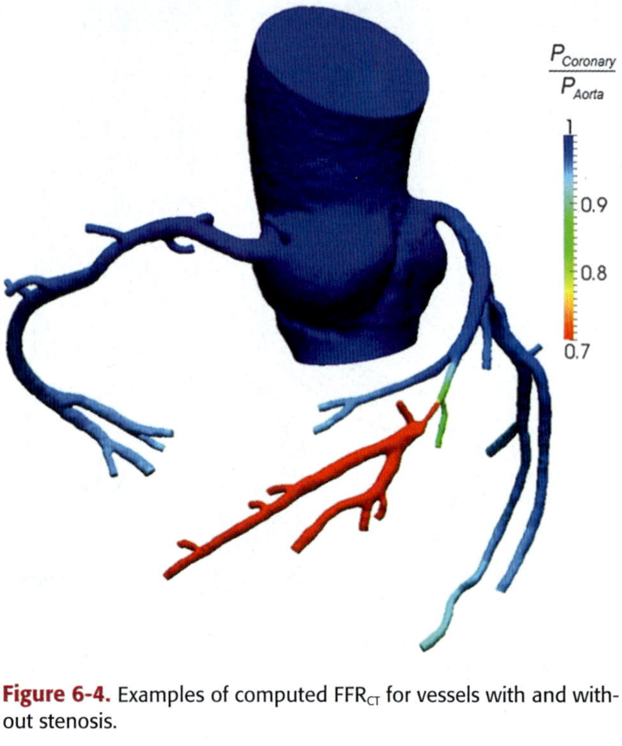

Figure 6-4. Examples of computed FFR_{CT} for vessels with and without stenosis.

Clinical Cases of FFR_{CT}

Case 1

The first clinical example concerns a patient who 5 years ago received a bioresorbable everolimus-eluting scaffold in the proximal right coronary artery (RCA). At 6-month and 24-month follow-up, the conventional angiography did not show any significant stenosis in the scaffolded segment. At 5-year follow-up, the MSCT scan showed a patent, nonstenotic scaffolded area demarcated by the two radiopaque platinum markers (*black arrows*, Fig. 6.5). On the maximum intensity projection, two small calcified plaques are visible distal to the scaffold. Noninvasive functional assessment showed that all three vessels exhibited distally FFR_{CT} values above a threshold of 0.80: specifically, there was no gradient in FFR_{CT} along the scaffolded segment.

Case 2

The second case concerns a patient with obstructive disease in the proximal left anterior descending (LAD) coronary artery, causing ischemia in both LAD and the first diagonal branch (D1). Disease extends from the proximal LAD to the takeoff of the first septal branch. Using the computer models based on noninvasive FFR derivation (Fig. 6.6), one could describe this anatomy as a Medina (1,0,0) lesion at the LAD-D1 bifurcation plus one separate distal LAD lesion just proximal to the takeoff of the septal branch. Alternatively, one could describe two sequential (1,0,0) bifurcation lesions, if the septal is considered to be a major vessel and therefore warrants protection. Following these diagnostic considerations, the treatment strategy with percutaneous coronary intervention can be planned upfront.

Case 3

The last case concerns a 65-year-old male patient with stable angina: His coronary risk factors were hypertension and hypercholesterolemia. MSCT angiography disclosed two stenotic lesions, one in the ostium of the LAD and one in the midportion of the RCA, respectively (not shown). The mid- to distal LAD had an FFR_{CT} of 0.71 versus 0.74 with the invasive approach (Fig. 6.7). Left main stem (LM) anatomy could be interpreted as either a trifurcation with one

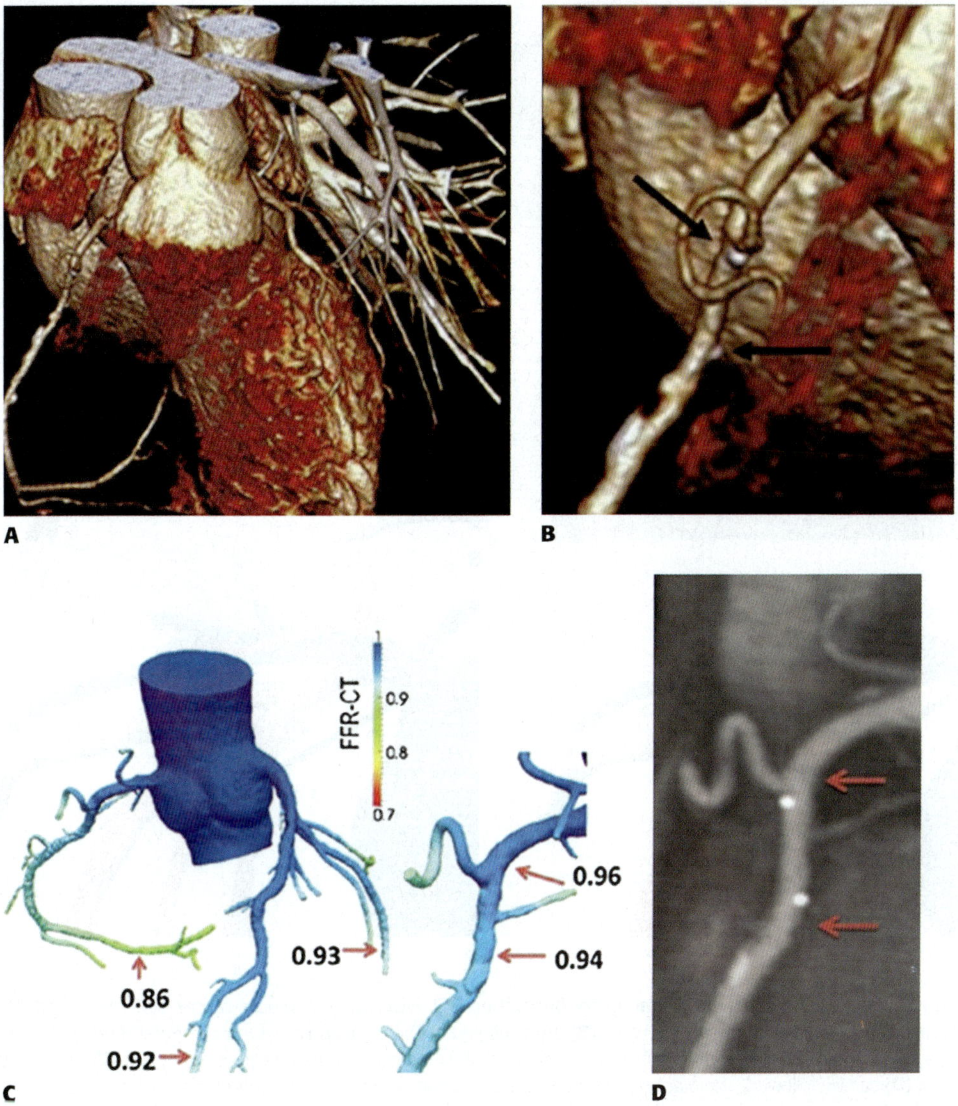

Figure 6-5. Use of noninvasive FFR for follow-up of a bioresorbable scaffold. **A:** Three-dimensional volume-rendered CT angiogram of a right coronary artery. Magnification of the proximal artery segment **(B)** shows the platinum markers of the resorbed scaffold (*black arrows*). **C:** Noninvasive FFR derivation did not show ischemia in any coronary artery. Specifically, FFR_{CT} measured 0.96 and 0.94 at the inflow and outflow of the scaffolded segment (*red arrows* on the curved multiplanar CT image) **(D)**. The color scale of the CCTA-derived computer models is based on the FFR_{CT} values. CCTA, coronary CT angiography; FFR, fractional flow reserve. (Reproduced from Serruys, et al. *EuroIntervention* 2012;8:511–519, with permission.)

vessel segment diseased (LAD ostium), hence a Medina (0,1,0,0) lesion, or as a trifurcation with two diseased vessel segments (also involving the LM), therefore a (1,1,0,0) lesion. Irrespective of diagnostic interpretation, one would consider stenting the midintermediate branch lesion without touching the trifurcation. Nevertheless, according to interpretation, one could consider treating the LAD ostium alone, or alternatively place a stent from the LM into the proximal LAD with a provisional 2 to 3 stent strategy. Virtual PCI[61] of the LAD ostium alone resulted in a limited improvement, FFR_{CT} slightly increasing from 0.77 to 0.80. The most striking observation was a drop in FFR_{CT} along the LM measuring 0.81 in its midportion. Virtual treatment of LM alone already normalized FFR_{CT} in the mid-LAD ($FFR_{CT} = 0.90$). The combined treatment of LM and LAD ostium resulted in further improvement of the FFR_{CT} up to a value of 0.93.

Clinical Data of FFR_{CT}

Clinical validation of FFR_{CT} is based on a direct comparison to measured FFR during invasive coronary angiography. Currently, there are three multicenter trials, namely, DISCOVER-FLOW (Diagnosis of Ischemia-Causing Coronary Stenoses by Noninvasive FFR Computed from Coronary Computed Tomographic Angiograms), DeFACTO (Determination of Fractional Flow Reserve by Anatomic Computed Tomographic Angiography), and NXT (Analysis of Coronary Blood Flow Using CT Angiography: Next Steps), investigating the diagnostic value of FFR_{CT}. A summary of published clinical studies reporting diagnostic performance of FFR_{CT} is shown in Table 6.2. The diagnostic sensitivity and specificity of FFR_{CT} ranged from 81% to 90% and 54% to 82%, respectively.

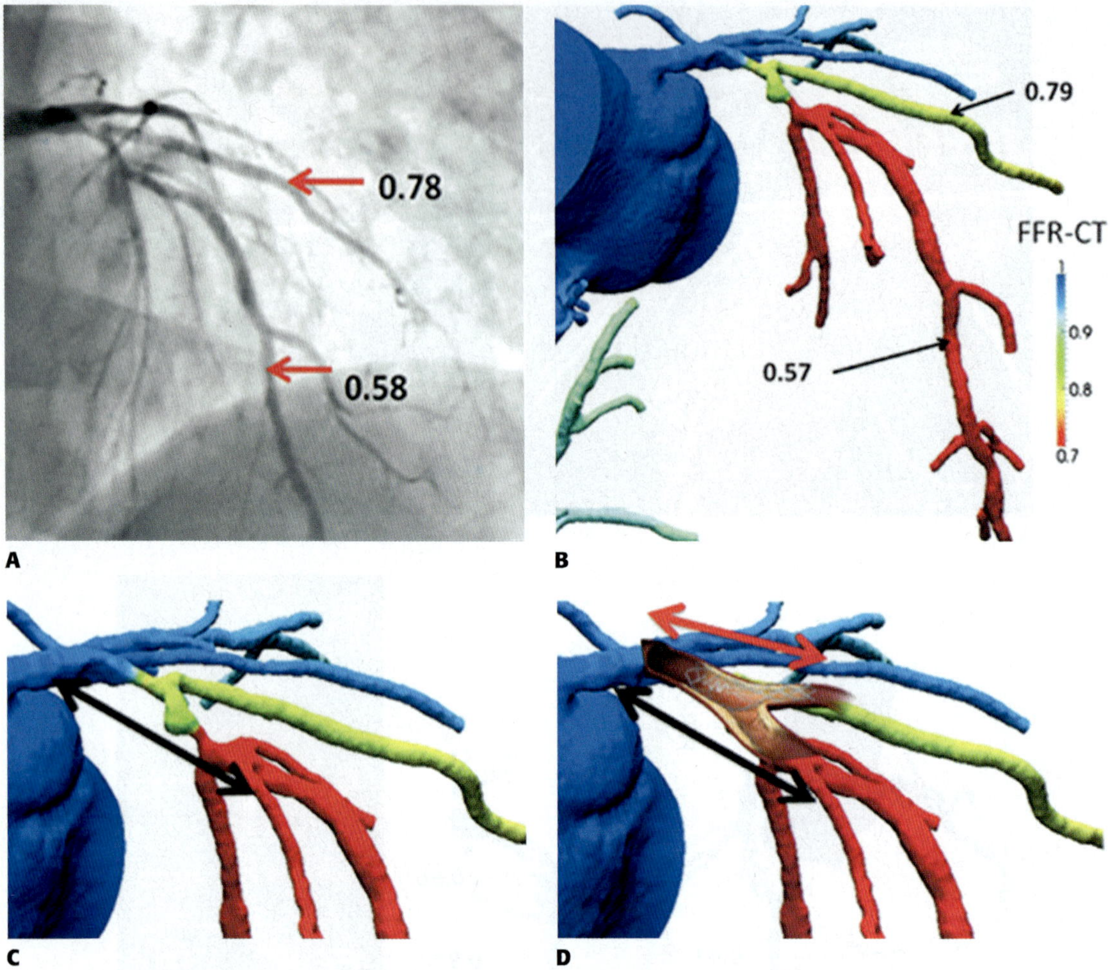

Figure 6-6. Use of noninvasive FFR in procedural strategy for bifurcation PCI. Proximal LAD disease causes ischemia in both the distal LAD and first diagonal branch (D1); invasive **(A)** and noninvasive estimates **(B)** are concordant. The color coding of the computer models facilitates ischemia localization. Dependent on diagnostic interpretation (including the size of the first septal branch), either a provisional T-stent **(C)** or a culotte approach using a Tryton Side-Branch Stent **(D)** can be followed. The *black arrows* indicate the position where the drug-eluting stent will be placed in the proximal LAD. FFR, fractional flow reserve; LAD, left anterior descending coronary artery. (Reproduced from Serruys, et al. *EuroIntervention* 2012;8:511–519, with permission.)

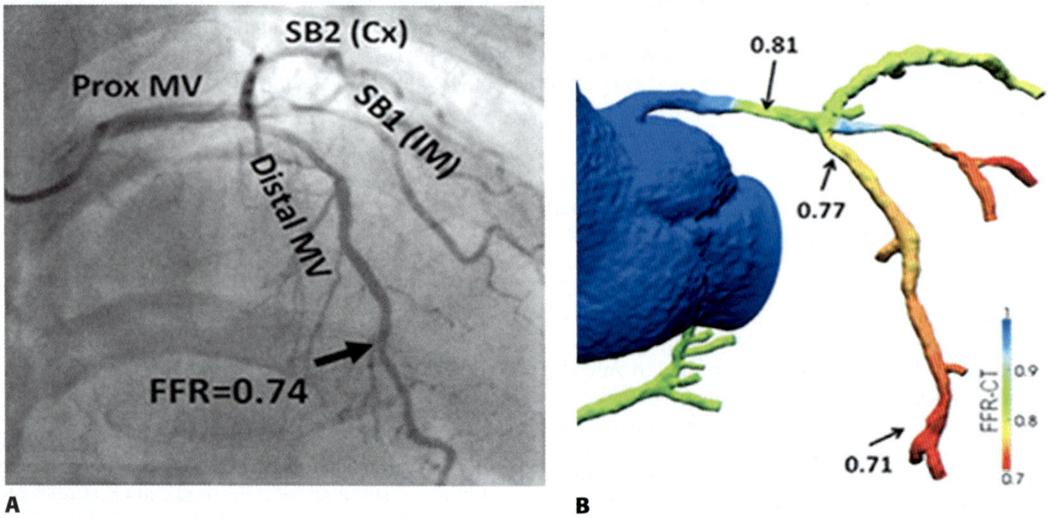

Figure 6-7. The yield of virtual treatment planning with noninvasive FFR measurements in an ambiguous left main (LM) stem anatomy. Both invasive **(A)** and noninvasive FFR estimates **(B)** showed ischemia in the middistal LAD. According to diagnostic interpretation (see case description)

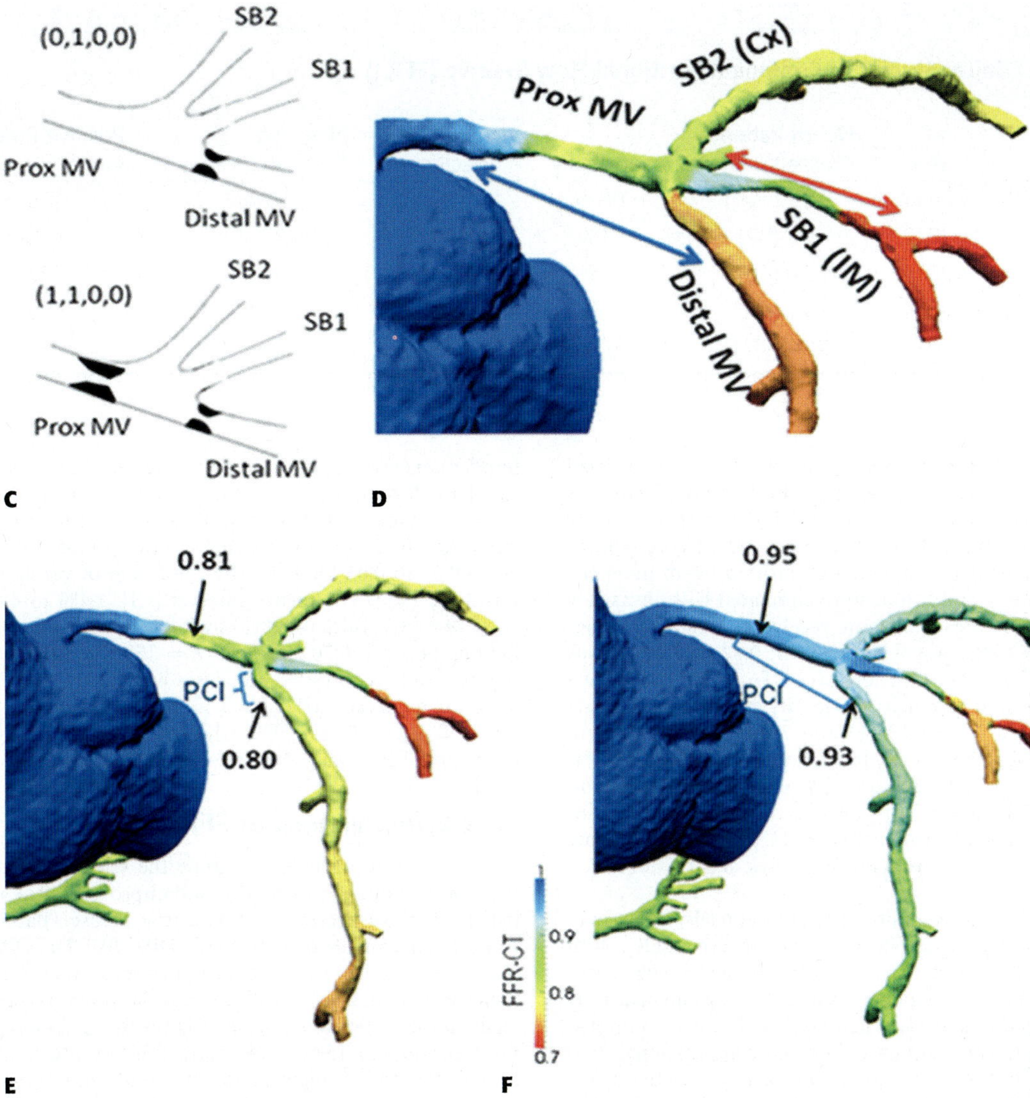

Figure 6-7. (*Continued*) **(C)**, one can opt for treating the LAD ostium alone or place a stent from the LM into the proximal LAD (*blue arrow*) **(D)**. The former option does not fully alleviate ischemia **(E)**, whereas the latter one does **(F)**. Cx, (left) circumflex coronary artery; FFR, fractional flow reserve; IM, intermediate (branch); LAD, left anterior descending coronary artery; MV, main vessel; PCI, percutaneous coronary intervention; SB, side branch. (Reproduced from Serruys, et al. *EuroIntervention* 2012;8:511–519, with permission.)

DISCOVER-FLOW study included 103 patients (159 arteries) with suspected or known coronary artery disease who underwent coronary CTA and coronary angiography and invasive FFR measurement.[51] Per-vessel analysis demonstrated a good correlation between FFR_{CT} and invasive FFR ($R = 0.7$; $p < 0.0001$). Fifty-six percent of patients had ≥1 vessel with FFR ≤0.80. On a per-vessel basis, the accuracy, sensitivity, specificity, positive predictive value, and negative predictive value were 84.3%, 87.9%, 82.2%, 73.9%, and 92.2%, respectively, for FFR_{CT} and were 58.5%, 91.4%, 39.6%, 46.5%, and 88.9%, respectively, for CTA stenosis (Table 6.2). The area under the receiver–operator characteristics curve was 0.90 for FFR_{CT} and 0.75 for CTA ($p = 0.001$). The FFR_{CT} and FFR were well correlated ($r = 0.717$, $p < 0.001$) with a slight underestimation by FFR_{CT} (0.022 ± 0.116, $p = 0.016$).[51]

The DeFACTO study included 252 patients (407 vessels) at 17 centers who underwent CT, FFR_{CT}, invasive coronary angiography, and invasive FFR.[62] Accuracy of FFR_{CT} for diagnosis of ischemia was compared with an invasive FFR reference standard. Ischemia was defined by an FFR or FFR_{CT} of 0.80 or less, while anatomically obstructive CAD was defined by a stenosis of 50% or larger on CTA and invasive coronary angiography. Among study participants, 137 (54.4%) had an abnormal invasive FFR. On a per-patient basis, diagnostic accuracy, sensitivity, specificity, positive predictive value, and negative predictive value of FFR_{CT} were 73% (95% CI, 67% to 78%), 90% (95% CI, 84% to 95%), 54% (95% CI, 46% to 83%), 67% (95% CI, 60% to 74%), and 84% (95% CI, 74% to 90%), respectively. Compared with CTA alone, FFR_{CT} was associated with improved discrimination.[62] For lesions of intermediate stenosis (defined as 30% to 69% stenosis), severity, accuracy, sensitivity, specificity, positive predictive value, and negative predictive value of FFR_{CT} were 71%, 74%, 67%, 41%, and 90%, whereas accuracy, sensitivity, specificity, positive predictive value, and negative predictive value of CTA stenosis were 63%, 34%, 72%, 27%, and 78%.

The NXT trial (Analysis of Coronary Blood Flow Using CT Angiography: Next Steps)[63] included 254 patients scheduled to undergo clinically indicated invasive coronary angiography for

TABLE 6.2 Main Clinical Studies of Computed Fractional Flow Reserve (FFR_{CT})

Study	Year	No. of Patients (Vessels)	Sensitivity	Specificity	Negative Predictive Value	Positive Predictive Value
DISCOVER-FLOW	2011	103 (159)	88%	82%	92%	74%
Yoon et al.	2012	53 (82)	81%	94%	89%	90%
DeFACTO	2013	252 (407)	90%	54%	84%	67%
Kim et al.	2014	44 (48)	85%	57%	62%	83%
NXT	2014	254 (484)	86%	79%	92%	65%

suspected coronary artery disease. Coronary CTA was performed before invasive coronary angiography. Evaluation of stenosis (>50% lumen reduction) in coronary CTA was performed by local investigators and in ICA by an independent core laboratory. FFR_{CT} was calculated in a blinded fashion by an independent core laboratory, and results were compared with invasively measured FFR. The area under the receiver–operating characteristic curve for FFR_{CT} was 0.90 (95% CI: 0.87 to 0.94) versus 0.81 (95% CI: 0.76 to 0.87) for coronary CTA ($p = 0.0008$). Per-patient sensitivity and specificity to identify myocardial ischemia were 86% (95% CI: 77% to 92%) and 79% (95% CI: 72% to 84%) for FFR_{CT} versus 94% (86 to 97) and 34% (95% CI: 27% to 41%) for coronary CTA and 64% (95% CI: 53% to 74%) and 83% (95% CI: 77% to 88%) for invasive coronary angiography, respectively (Fig. 6.8). In patients (n = 235) with intermediate stenosis (95% CI: 30% to 70%), the diagnostic accuracy of FFR_{CT} remained high.[63]

Apart from these three multicentre clinical trials, a few small studies have also investigated the use of noninvasive FFR_{CT}. Kim et al. prospectively enrolled 44 patients (48 lesions) who had coronary CTA before invasive angiography and stenting and invasively measured FFR before and after stenting.[61] FFR_{CT} was computed in blinded fashion using coronary CTA and computational fluid dynamics before and after virtual coronary stenting. Virtual stenting was performed by modification of the computational model to restore the area of the target lesion according to the proximal and distal reference areas. Before intervention, invasive FFR was 0.70 ± 0.14, and noninvasive FFR_{CT} was 0.70 ± 0.15. FFR after stenting and FFR_{CT} after virtual stenting were 0.90 ± 0.05 and 0.88 ± 0.05, respectively ($R = 0.55$, $p < 0.001$). The mean difference between FFR_{CT} and FFR was 0.006 for preintervention (95% limit of agreement: −0.27 to 0.28) and 0.024 for postintervention (95% limit of agreement: −0.08 to 0.13). Diagnostic accuracy of FFR_{CT} to predict ischemia (FFR ≤ 0.8) prior to stenting was 77% (sensitivity: 85.3%, specificity: 57.1%, positive predictive value: 83%, and negative predictive value: 62%) and after stenting was 96% (sensitivity: 100%, specificity: 96% positive predictive value: 50%, and negative predictive value: 100%).[61] Yoon et al. enrolled 53 consecutive patients who underwent invasive coronary angiography and FFR as well as CTA and FFR_{CT}. Among 82 vessels, 32 lesions (39%) had ischemia by invasive FFR (FFR ≤0.80). Sensitivity, specificity, positive and negative predictive values, and positive and negative likelihood ratio of FFRCT were 81%, 94%, 90%, 89%, 13.54, and 0.20, respectively.[64] A recent study has also shown good reproducibility of FFR_{CT} measurements.[65] Coronary CTA and invasive coronary angiography with repeated FFR measurements were performed in 28 patients (58 vessels) with suspected stable coronary artery disease. Based on the coronary CTA data set, FFR_{CT} analyses were performed twice by two independent blinded analysts. In 12 of 58 (21%) vessels, FFR was ≤0.80. The standard deviation for the difference between first and second FFR_{CT} analyses was 0.034 versus 0.033 for FFR repeated measurements ($p = 0.72$). Limits of agreement were −0.06 to 0.08 for FFR_{CT} and −0.07 to 0.06 for FFR. The coefficient of variation of FFR_{CT} was 3.4% (95% confidence interval [CI], 1.4% to 4.6%) versus 2.7% (95% CI, 1.8% to 3.3%) for FFR. In vessels with mean FFR ranging between 0.70 and 0.90 (n = 25), the difference between the first and second FFR_{CT} analyses was 0.035 and FFR repeated measurements was 0.043 ($p = 0.357$), whereas coefficient of variation of FFR_{CT} was 3.3% (95% CI, 1.5% to 4.3%) and coefficient of variation for FFR was 3.6% (95% CI, 2.3% to 4.6%).[65]

Cost-Effectiveness of FFR_{CT}

A strategy of using FFR_{CT} to guide the selection of patients for ICA and PCI might reduce costs and improve clinical outcomes in patients with suspected coronary artery disease. Hlatky et al. used clinical data from 96 patients in the DISCOVER-FLOW study and outcomes data from the literature to project the initial management costs and 1-year death/myocardial infarction rates associated with five clinical strategies: (1) invasive angiography-guided intervention, (2) invasive FFR-guided intervention, (3) CTA followed by invasive angiography and intervention, (4) CTA followed by invasive angiography and FFR-guided intervention, and (5) FFR_{CT} and invasive angiography and intervention of lesions with FFR_{CT} ≤0.80.[66] The projected initial management costs were highest for the invasive angiography-guided strategy ($10,702) and lowest for the FFR_{CT}-guided invasive angiography and intervention strategy ($7,674). The use of FFR_{CT} to select patients for invasive coronary angiography and intervention would result in 30% lower costs and 12% fewer events at 1 year compared with the most commonly used invasive coronary angiography-guided strategy.[66] Another study from Japan used clinical data from 254 patients in the NXT trial, costs of goods and services in Japan, and clinical outcome data from the literature to estimate the costs and outcomes of four clinical pathways: (1) invasive angiography-guided intervention, (2) invasive FFR-guided intervention, (3) CTA followed by invasive angiography-guided intervention, and (4) FFR_{CT}-guided intervention.[67] The invasive angiography-guided strategy demonstrated the highest projected cost ($10,360) and highest projected 1-year death/myocardial infarction rate (2.4%). An assumed price for FFR_{CT} of US $2,000 produced equivalent clinical outcomes (death/MI rate: 1.9%) and health care costs ($7,222) for the FFR-CT–guided strategy and the invasive FFR-guided intervention strategy. Use of the FFR_{CT} strategy to select patients for intervention would result in 32% lower costs and 19% fewer cardiac events at 1 year compared to the most commonly used invasive angiography-guided strategy.[67]

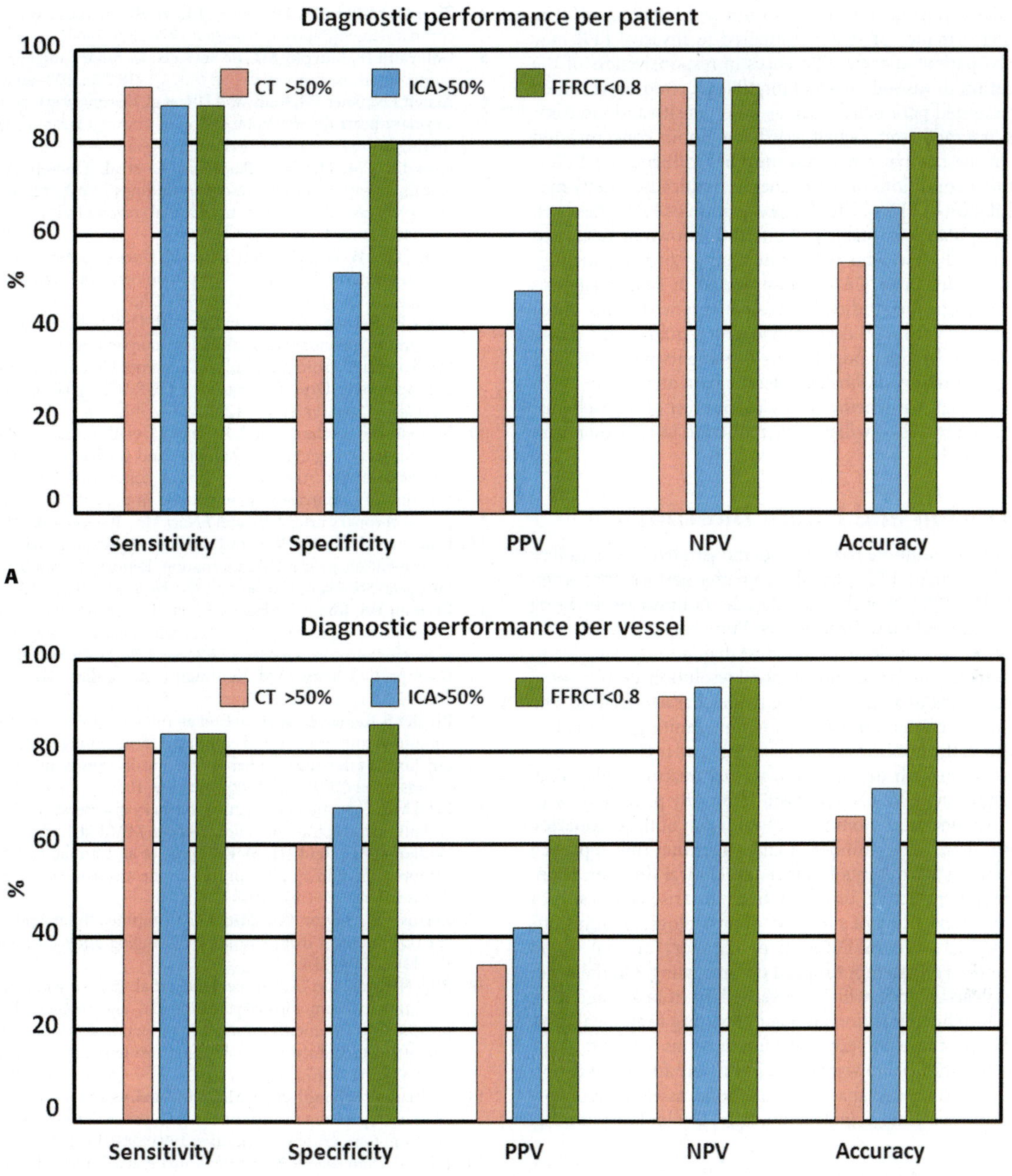

Figure 6-8. Diagnostic performance of FFR_{CT} in NXT trial presented as per-patient analysis (**A**, n = 254) and per-vessel analysis (**B**, n = 484). CT, computer tomography; ICA, invasive coronary angiography; FFR, fractional flow reserve; PPV, positive predictive value; NPV, negative predictive value. (Adapted from Norgaard BL, Leipsic J, Gaur S, et al. Diagnostic performance of noninvasive fractional flow reserve derived from coronary computed tomography angiography in suspected coronary artery disease: the NXT trial [Analysis of Coronary Blood Flow Using CT Angiography: Next Steps]. *J Am Coll Cardiol* 2014;63:1145–1155.)

Limitations and Challenges

A number of potential limitations exist that may influence the diagnostic performance of FFR_{CT}, most notably impaired coronary CT image quality. Significant CT imaging artifacts include misalignment, motion, beam hardening from coronary calcification, and increased image noise.[17] These issues can be minimized by close adherence to CCTA image acquisition guidelines, in particular by the use of beta blockers to reduce heart rate and heart rate variability as well as administration of sublingual nitrates to dilate the coronary arteries. In the clinical studies of FFR_{CT}, CT image quality was evaluated by independent core laboratories, and all patients judged to have evaluable images were included for FFR_{CT} analysis. In the DeFACTO study, 11% of patients were judged by the core laboratory to have nonevaluable CT images and were excluded from the study. Given the dependence of FFR_{CT} on accurate coronary segmentation for proper image-based modeling, excellent image quality should remain a primary goal of cardiac CT imaging. Another potential drawback of FFR_{CT} relates to the fact that

FFR is calculated during simulated and not real hyperemia.[68] The diagnostic performance of FFR_{CT} compared to invasive FFR may be affected by patient-specific differences in responsiveness of the microcirculation to vasodilators and physiologic conditions, which may affect assumed parameters such as fluid density and viscosity. Viscosity is assumed from hematocrit/hemoglobin concentration and, when in the normal range, has minimal influence on FFR_{CT}. However, under conditions of severe anemia, reduced viscosity may impact calculation of FFR_{CT}.[17] To date, evaluation of FFR_{CT} has been limited to a population of stable patients with known or suspected coronary artery disease who were undergoing coronary angiography. Patients with prior CABG or suspected in-stent restenosis were excluded from the studies as were patients with acute coronary syndrome or within 30 days of myocardial infarction.[69] Thus, generalizability to broader populations of patients with coronary artery disease is unknown. Finally, outcome data are not yet available, and it is unknown whether revascularization of the ischemic lesions identified by FFR_{CT} will achieve reduction in ischemia from revascularization.[17]

Conclusion and Future Directions

Clinical data from multiple trials have demonstrated the feasibility of FFR_{CT} measurement. FFR_{CT} has shown better performance when compared with CTA. Over the past decade, noninvasive imaging using MSCT has lived up to its promises: Luminography and tissue characterization have made major progress in quantification, due to continuous increase in spatial and temporal resolution, despite some inherent limitations of x-ray regarding tissue characterization. The adjunction of functional assessment for flow-limiting lesions is a quantum leap in the noninvasive evaluation of patients prior to coronary intervention with the option of virtual treatment planning. Consequently, a single MSCT study will ultimately provide us with comprehensive "one-stop" noninvasive evaluation of the coronaries.

However, there are a number of challenges that this approach is likely to face as it attempts to enter the clinical domain. From an engineering perspective, issues are likely to arise as a result of the necessary introduction of a number of physiologic assumptions and the potential oversimplification of coronary arterial blood flow mechanics in an attempt to speed up processing. On the other hand, clinical acceptance will be governed by robust validation studies, a well-defined position among preexisting functional tests, and an analysis of the health economic implications that FFR_{CT} may entail.[70] Further studies are warranted, but future for this technology to provide a combined anatomic–functional assessment of coronary artery disease using a single noninvasive test looks promising.

Acknowledgments

The authors would like to acknowledge the contribution of Christopher Zarin and Campbell Rogers (HeartFlow, Inc., Redwood City, CA, USA) regarding the description of HeartFlow Technology. We are also thankful to Bon Kwon Koo (Seoul National University Hospital, Seoul, South Korea) and James K. Min (Cedars-Sinai Heart Institute, Los Angeles, CA, USA) for providing case examples from the DISCOVER-FLOW study.

REFERENCES

1. **Sones FM Jr, Shirey EK.** Cine coronary arteriography. *Mod Concepts Cardiovasc Dis* 1962;31:735–738.
2. **Iqbal J, Serruys PW.** Revascularization strategies for patients with stable coronary artery disease. *J Intern Med* 2014;276(4):336–351.
3. **Topol EJ, Nissen SE.** Our preoccupation with coronary luminology. The dissociation between clinical and angiographic findings in ischemic heart disease. *Circulation* 1995;92:2333–2342.
4. **Zir LM, Miller SW, Dinsmore RE, et al.** Interobserver variability in coronary angiography. *Circulation* 1976;53:627–632.
5. **Galbraith JE, Murphy ML, de Soyza N.** Coronary angiogram interpretation. Interobserver variability. *JAMA* 1978;240:2053–2056.
6. **Arnett EN, Isner JM, Redwood DR, et al.** Coronary artery narrowing in coronary heart disease: comparison of cineangiographic and necropsy findings. *Ann Intern Med* 1979;91:350–356.
7. **Grondin CM, Dyrda I, Pasternac A, et al.** Discrepancies between cineangiographic and postmortem findings in patients with coronary artery disease and recent myocardial revascularization. *Circulation* 1974;49:703–708.
8. **White CW, Wright CB, Doty DB, et al.** Does visual interpretation of the coronary arteriogram predict the physiologic importance of a coronary stenosis? *N Engl J Med* 1984;310:819–824.
9. **Shaw LJ, Berman DS, Maron DJ, et al.** Optimal medical therapy with or without percutaneous coronary intervention to reduce ischemic burden: results from the Clinical Outcomes Utilizing Revascularization and Aggressive Drug Evaluation (COURAGE) trial nuclear substudy. *Circulation* 2008;117:1283–1291.
10. **Berman DS, Hachamovitch R, Shaw LJ, et al.** Roles of nuclear cardiology, cardiac computed tomography, and cardiac magnetic resonance: noninvasive risk stratification and a conceptual framework for the selection of noninvasive imaging tests in patients with known or suspected coronary artery disease. *J Nucl Med* 2006;47:1107–1118.
11. **Underwood SR, Bax JJ, vom Dahl J, et al.** Imaging techniques for the assessment of myocardial hibernation. Report of a Study Group of the European Society of Cardiology. *Eur Heart J* 2004;25:815–836.
12. **Berman DS, Kang X, Slomka PJ, et al.** Underestimation of extent of ischemia by gated SPECT myocardial perfusion imaging in patients with left main coronary artery disease. *J Nucl Cardiol* 2007;14:521–528.
13. **Gaemperli O, Bengel FM, Kaufmann PA.** Cardiac hybrid imaging. *Eur Heart J* 2011;32:2100–2108.
14. **Rispler S, Keidar Z, Ghersin E, et al.** Integrated single-photon emission computed tomography and computed tomography coronary angiography for the assessment of hemodynamically significant coronary artery lesions. *J Am Coll Cardiol* 2007;49:1059–1067.
15. **Patel MR.** Detecting obstructive coronary disease with CT angiography and noninvasive fractional flow reserve. *JAMA* 2012;308:1269–1270.
16. **Williams MC, Reid JH, McKillop G, et al.** Cardiac and coronary CT comprehensive imaging approach in the assessment of coronary heart disease. *Heart* 2011;97:1198–1205.
17. **Zarins CK, Taylor CA, Min JK.** Computed fractional flow reserve (FFTCT) derived from coronary CT angiography. *J Cardiovasc Transl Res* 2013;6:708–714.
18. **Pijls NH, van Son JA, Kirkeeide RL, et al.** Experimental basis of determining maximum coronary, myocardial, and collateral blood flow by pressure measurements for assessing functional stenosis severity before and after percutaneous transluminal coronary angioplasty. *Circulation* 1993;87:1354–1367.
19. **De Bruyne B, Baudhuin T, Melin JA, et al.** Coronary flow reserve calculated from pressure measurements in humans. Validation with positron emission tomography. *Circulation* 1994;89:1013–1022.
20. **Pijls NH, Van Gelder B, Van der Voort P, et al.** Fractional flow reserve. A useful index to evaluate the influence of an epicardial coronary stenosis on myocardial blood flow. *Circulation* 1995;92:3183–3193.
21. **Pijls NH, Fearon WF, Tonino PA, et al.** Fractional flow reserve versus angiography for guiding percutaneous coronary intervention in patients with multivessel coronary artery disease: 2-year follow-up of the FAME (Fractional Flow Reserve Versus Angiography for Multivessel Evaluation) study. *J Am Coll Cardiol* 2010;56:177–184.
22. **De Bruyne B, Pijls NH, Kalesan B, et al.** Fractional flow reserve-guided PCI versus medical therapy in stable coronary disease. *N Engl J Med* 2012;367:991–1001.
23. **Fearon WF, Bornschein B, Tonino PA, et al.** Economic evaluation of fractional flow reserve-guided percutaneous coronary intervention in patients with multivessel disease. *Circulation* 2010;122:2545–2550.
24. **Pijls NH, van Schaardenburgh P, Manoharan G, et al.** Percutaneous coronary intervention of functionally nonsignificant stenosis: 5-year follow-up of the DEFER Study. *J Am Coll Cardiol* 2007;49:2105–2111.
25. **Tonino PA, De Bruyne B, Pijls NH, et al.** Fractional flow reserve versus angiography for guiding percutaneous coronary intervention. *N Engl J Med* 2009;360:213–224.

26. **Wijns W, Kolh P, Danchin N, et al.** Guidelines on myocardial revascularization. *Eur Heart J* 2010;31:2501–2555.
27. **Levine GN, Bates ER, Blankenship JC, et al.** 2011 ACCF/AHA/SCAI Guideline for Percutaneous Coronary Intervention: a report of the American College of Cardiology Foundation/American Heart Association Task Force on Practice Guidelines and the Society for Cardiovascular Angiography and Interventions. *Circulation* 2011;124:e574–e651.
28. **Morris PD, Ryan D, Morton AC, et al.** Virtual fractional flow reserve from coronary angiography: modeling the significance of coronary lesions: results from the VIRTU-1 (VIRTUal Fractional Flow Reserve From Coronary Angiography) study. *JACC Cardiovasc Interv* 2013;6:149–157.
29. **Papafaklis MI, Muramatsu T, Ishibashi Y, et al.** Fast virtual functional assessment of intermediate coronary lesions using routine angiographic data and blood flow simulation in humans: comparison with pressure wire—fractional flow reserve. *EuroIntervention* 2014;10(5):574–583.
30. **Min JK, Shaw LJ, Berman DS.** The present state of coronary computed tomography angiography a process in evolution. *J Am Coll Cardiol* 2010;55:957–965.
31. **Mowatt G, Cook JA, Hillis GS, et al.** 64-Slice computed tomography angiography in the diagnosis and assessment of coronary artery disease: systematic review and meta-analysis. *Heart* 2008;94:1386–1393.
32. **Leber AW, Knez A, Becker A, et al.** Accuracy of multidetector spiral computed tomography in identifying and differentiating the composition of coronary atherosclerotic plaques: a comparative study with intracoronary ultrasound. *J Am Coll Cardiol* 2004;43:1241–1247.
33. **Otsuka M, Bruining N, Van Pelt NC, et al.** Quantification of coronary plaque by 64-slice computed tomography: a comparison with quantitative intracoronary ultrasound. *Invest Radiol* 2008;43:314–321.
34. **Voros S, Rinehart S, Qian Z, et al.** Prospective validation of standardized, 3-dimensional, quantitative coronary computed tomographic plaque measurements using radiofrequency backscatter intravascular ultrasound as reference standard in intermediate coronary arterial lesions: results from the ATLANTA (assessment of tissue characteristics, lesion morphology, and hemodynamics by angiography with fractional flow reserve, intravascular ultrasound and virtual histology, and noninvasive computed tomography in atherosclerotic plaques) I study. *JACC Cardiovasc Interv* 2011;4:198–208.
35. **Budoff MJ, Dowe D, Jollis JG, et al.** Diagnostic performance of 64-multidetector row coronary computed tomographic angiography for evaluation of coronary artery stenosis in individuals without known coronary artery disease: results from the prospective multicenter ACCURACY (Assessment by Coronary Computed Tomographic Angiography of Individuals Undergoing Invasive Coronary Angiography) trial. *J Am Coll Cardiol* 2008;52:1724–1732.
36. **Miller JM, Rochitte CE, Dewey M, et al.** Diagnostic performance of coronary angiography by 64-row CT. *N Engl J Med* 2008;359:2324–2336.
37. **Meijboom WB, Meijs MF, Schuijf JD, et al.** Diagnostic accuracy of 64-slice computed tomography coronary angiography: a prospective, multicenter, multivendor study. *J Am Coll Cardiol* 2008;52:2135–2144.
38. **Cademartiri F, Mollet NR, Runza G, et al.** Influence of intracoronary attenuation on coronary plaque measurements using multislice computed tomography: observations in an ex vivo model of coronary computed tomography angiography. *Eur Radiol* 2005;15:1426–1431.
39. **Cademartiri F, Runza G, Palumbo A, et al.** Lumen enhancement influences absolute noncalcific plaque density on multislice computed tomography coronary angiography: ex-vivo validation and in-vivo demonstration. *J Cardiovasc Med (Hagerstown)* 2010;11:337–344.
40. **Sun J, Zhang Z, Lu B, et al.** Identification and quantification of coronary atherosclerotic plaques: a comparison of 64-MDCT and intravascular ultrasound. *AJR Am J Roentgenol* 2008;190:748–754.
41. **Motoyama S, Sarai M, Harigaya H, et al.** Computed tomographic angiography characteristics of atherosclerotic plaques subsequently resulting in acute coronary syndrome. *J Am Coll Cardiol* 2009;54:49–57.
42. **Rinehart S, Vazquez G, Qian Z, et al.** Quantitative measurements of coronary arterial stenosis, plaque geometry, and composition are highly reproducible with a standardized coronary arterial computed tomographic approach in high-quality CT datasets. *J Cardiovasc Comput Tomogr* 2011;5:35–43.
43. **Meijboom WB, Van Mieghem CA, van Pelt N, et al.** Comprehensive assessment of coronary artery stenoses: computed tomography coronary angiography versus conventional coronary angiography and correlation with fractional flow reserve in patients with stable angina. *J Am Coll Cardiol* 2008;52:636–643.
44. **Nissen SE.** Limitations of computed tomography coronary angiography. *J Am Coll Cardiol* 2008;52:2145–2147.
45. **George RT, Silva C, Cordeiro MA, et al.** Multidetector computed tomography myocardial perfusion imaging during adenosine stress. *J Am Coll Cardiol* 2006;48:153–160.
46. **Kurata A, Mochizuki T, Koyama Y, et al.** Myocardial perfusion imaging using adenosine triphosphate stress multi-slice spiral computed tomography: alternative to stress myocardial perfusion scintigraphy. *Circ J* 2005;69:550–557.
47. **Blankstein R, Shturman LD, Rogers IS, et al.** Adenosine-induced stress myocardial perfusion imaging using dual-source cardiac computed tomography. *J Am Coll Cardiol* 2009;54:1072–1084.
48. **George RT, Arbab-Zadeh A, Miller JM, et al.** Adenosine stress 64- and 256-row detector computed tomography angiography and perfusion imaging: a pilot study evaluating the transmural extent of perfusion abnormalities to predict atherosclerosis causing myocardial ischemia. *Circ Cardiovasc Imaging* 2009;2:174–182.
49. **Yoon YE, Koo BK.** Non-invasive functional assessment using computed tomography: when will they be ready for clinical use? *Cardiovasc Diagn Ther* 2012;2:106–112.
50. **Taylor CA, Fonte TA, Min JK.** Computational fluid dynamics applied to cardiac computed tomography for noninvasive quantification of fractional flow reserve: scientific basis. *J Am Coll Cardiol* 2013;61:2233–2241.
51. **Koo BK, Erglis A, Doh JH, et al.** Diagnosis of ischemia-causing coronary stenoses by noninvasive fractional flow reserve computed from coronary computed tomographic angiograms. Results from the prospective multicenter DISCOVER-FLOW (Diagnosis of Ischemia-Causing Stenoses Obtained Via Noninvasive Fractional Flow Reserve) study. *J Am Coll Cardiol* 2011;58:1989–1997.
52. **Murray CD.** The physiological principle of minimum work: I. The vascular system and the cost of blood volume. *Proc Natl Acad Sci U S A* 1926;12:207–214.
53. **Hutchins GM, Miner MM, Boitnott JK.** Vessel caliber and branch-angle of human coronary artery branch-points. *Circ Res* 1976;38:572–576.
54. **Kamiya A, Togawa T.** Adaptive regulation of wall shear stress to flow change in the canine carotid artery. *Am J Physiol* 1980;239:H14–H21.
55. **Zarins CK, Zatina MA, Giddens DP, et al.** Shear stress regulation of artery lumen diameter in experimental atherogenesis. *J Vasc Surg* 1987;5:413–420.
56. **Zhou Y, Kassab GS, Molloi S.** On the design of the coronary arterial tree: a generalization of Murray's law. *Phys Med Biol* 1999;44:2929–2945.
57. **Zhou Y, Kassab GS, Molloi S.** In vivo validation of the design rules of the coronary arteries and their application in the assessment of diffuse disease. *Phys Med Biol* 2002;47:977–993.
58. **Wilson RF, Wyche K, Christensen BV, et al.** Effects of adenosine on human coronary arterial circulation. *Circulation* 1990;82:1595–1606.
59. **Taylor CA, Hughes TJ, Zarins CK.** Finite element modeling of three-dimensional pulsatile flow in the abdominal aorta: relevance to atherosclerosis. *Ann Biomed Eng* 1998;26:975–987.
60. **Kim HJ, Vignon-Clementel IE, Coogan JS, et al.** Patient-specific modeling of blood flow and pressure in human coronary arteries. *Ann Biomed Eng* 2010;38:3195–3209.
61. **Kim KH, Doh JH, Koo BK, et al.** A novel noninvasive technology for treatment planning using virtual coronary stenting and computed tomography-derived computed fractional flow reserve. *JACC Cardiovasc Interv* 2014;7:72–78.
62. **Nakazato R, Park HB, Berman DS, et al.** Noninvasive fractional flow reserve derived from computed tomography angiography for coronary lesions of intermediate stenosis severity: results from the DeFACTO study. *Circ Cardiovasc Imaging* 2013;6:881–889.
63. **Norgaard BL, Leipsic J, Gaur S, et al.** Diagnostic performance of noninvasive fractional flow reserve derived from coronary computed tomography angiography in suspected coronary artery disease: the NXT trial (Analysis of Coronary Blood Flow Using CT Angiography: Next Steps). *J Am Coll Cardiol* 2014;63:1145–1155.
64. **Yoon YE, Choi JH, Kim JH, et al.** Noninvasive diagnosis of ischemia-causing coronary stenosis using CT angiography: diagnostic value of transluminal attenuation gradient and fractional flow reserve computed from coronary CT angiography compared to invasively measured fractional flow reserve. *JACC Cardiovasc Imaging* 2012;5:1088–1096.
65. **Gaur S, Bezerra HG, Lassen JF, et al.** Fractional flow reserve derived from coronary CT angiography: variation of repeated analyses. *J Cardiovasc Comput Tomogr* 2014;8:307–314.

66. **Hlatky MA, Saxena A, Koo BK, et al.** Projected costs and consequences of computed tomography-determined fractional flow reserve. *Clin Cardiol* 2013;36:743–748.
67. **Kimura T, Shiomi H, Kuribayashi S, et al.** Cost analysis of non-invasive fractional flow reserve derived from coronary computed tomographic angiography in Japan. *Cardiovasc Interv Ther* 2014.
68. **De Caterina AR, Leone AM, Crea F.** Limitations of noninvasive measurement of fractional flow reserve from coronary computed tomography angiography. *J Am Coll Cardiol* 2012;59:1408–1409; author reply 1409–1410.
69. **Min JK, Koo BK, Erglis A, et al.** Usefulness of noninvasive fractional flow reserve computed from coronary computed tomographic angiograms for intermediate stenoses confirmed by quantitative coronary angiography. *Am J Cardiol* 2012;110:971–976.
70. **Escaned J.** Imaging. Can FFRCT replace old indices of coronary stenosis severity? *Nat Rev Cardiol* 2014;11:252–254.

CHAPTER

7 Dynamic Susceptibility Contrast MRI: Technical Considerations and Practical Issues

Fernando Calamante, PhD

Introduction and Historical Background

Dynamic susceptibility contrast (DSC) MRI is an imaging technique that can be used to measure blood flow and other related hemodynamic parameters. It involves the intravenous injection of a paramagnetic MR contrast agent and relies on measuring and modeling the induced changes in T_2 and T_2* relaxation, brought about by the induced susceptibility effect (Fig. 7.1). These changes are amplified when the contrast agent remains compartmentalized[1]: the compartmentalization of the contrast agent leads to magnetic field perturbations that extend beyond the vascular space, thus creating long-range distortions to the magnetic field. These field inhomogeneities induce dephasing and therefore a shortening of T_2 and T_2*.[1] Due to this amplified effect related to compartmentalization, DSC-MRI is a technique that has primarily been used to assess *cerebral* perfusion: the blood vessels in the brain are surrounded by the so-called blood–brain barrier (BBB), which, when intact, makes the gadolinium-based contrast agents commonly used for DSC-MRI behave effectively as an intravascular contrast agent.[a] This chapter will therefore solely focus in DSC-MRI as a *brain* imaging tool.

From a historical point of view, DSC-MRI was first described by Arno Villringer, Bruce Rosen, and colleagues at Massachusetts General Hospital in the late 1980s,[1] using fast one-dimensional data in rat brains. This pioneering work was quickly followed by further imaging studies in dog and human brains, and the potential major clinical role of this technique was quickly recognized, with several major advances carried out in those early years,[2–6] which provided a very strong foundation for what this technique has now grown into.

Within the field of perfusion MRI, the terms cerebral perfusion, perfusion, cerebral blood flow, and its acronym CBF are all used indistinguishably. This same convention will be adopted throughout this chapter. Cerebral perfusion is arguably one of the key physiologic parameters in the brain, because it plays a central role to ensure tissue viability and function. Cerebral perfusion is responsible for the delivery of oxygen and nutrients and for the removal of waste products. It is therefore not surprising that numerous disease processes involve in one way or another disturbances to blood flow supply and that the development of robust methods to measure perfusion has been a major area of research in neuroimaging.

Some of the major attractions of DSC-MRI lie in its simple acquisition method [typically a single-shot echo-planar imaging (EPI) sequence], its short acquisition time (approximately 1 min), relative high signal-to-noise ratio (SNR) compared with other perfusion imaging methods (e.g., perfusion CT, arterial spin labeling, PET) (Fig. 7.2), and the wealth of information that can be obtained from the same acquired data set.

In the following sections, we will discuss the issues related to setting up a DSC-MRI protocol (both from the contrast agent, as well as from the MRI sequence points of view), introduce the concept of the arterial input function (AIF) and why its measurement is essential for CBF quantification, and describe the kinetic model used in DSC-MRI quantification and the role of the convolution and deconvolution mathematical steps. This will be followed by a description of the various parameters that can be calculated from DSC-MRI data, the practical factors to take into account to achieve quantification in absolute units, as well as the main technical limitations and errors that users must be aware of, including the modifications to the acquisition and analysis pipeline in order to deal with the presence of contrast agent extravasation (i.e., with BBB leakage). Finally, we will end the chapter with a brief description of the summary steps involved in a typical DSC-MRI study as well as a discussion regarding the current trend toward the use of fully automatic (black box) tools in DSC-MRI.

Contrast Agent and the DSC-MRI Protocol

Despite being a perfusion imaging method that involves no ionizing radiation (and therefore often referred to as a noninvasive perfusion imaging technique), DSC-MRI does require the bolus injection of an exogenous MR contrast agent. This bolus, typically injected in the antecubital vein,[7] most often involves a gadolinium-chelated contrast agent.[4]

The contrast dose, usually indicated as mL or mmol per kilogram of body weight, must be sufficient to induce a robustly measured transient signal drop (Fig. 7.1), and its optimal value depends on several factors such as the magnetic field strength, sequence parameters, injection rate, and type of contrast agent. In general,

[a]Modifications to the DSC-MRI kinetic model have been proposed to deal with disruption of the BBB, for example, as it is often observed in brain tumors. This case is discussed in the section DSC-MRI in the Presence of Contrast Leakage.

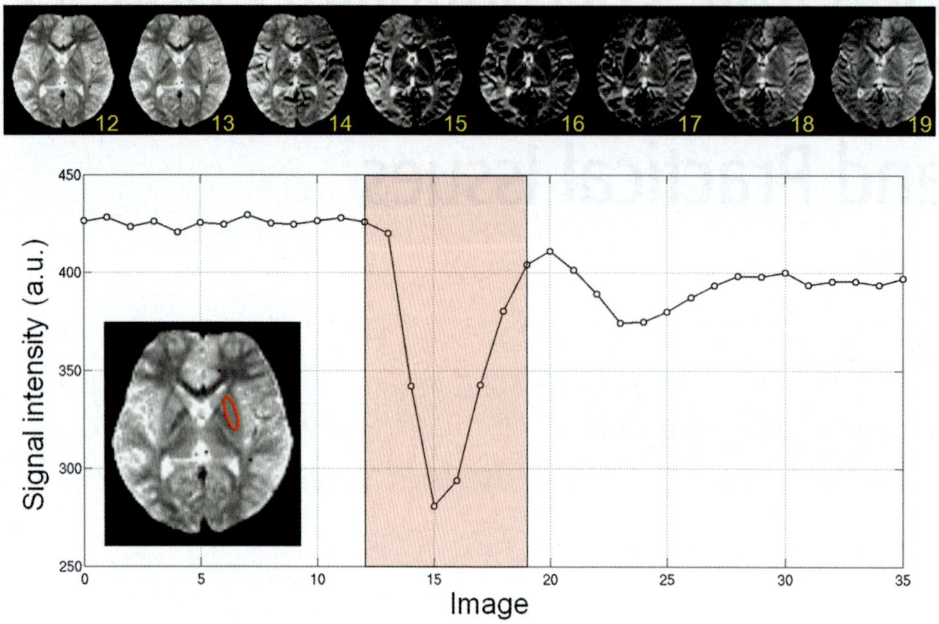

Figure 7-1. Effect of a bolus of contrast agent in the signal intensity data from a patient with right internal carotid artery stenosis (left side of the images). **Top row:** Eight images acquired during the first passage of the bolus through the brain; the number under each image indicates the image number (corresponding to the shaded time interval in the graph). **Bottom row:** Signal intensity time course for a contralateral region of interest (see insert). The images and the time course clearly show the transient decrease in signal intensity introduced by the contrast agent. (Figure previously published in Calamante F. Perfusion MRI using dynamic-susceptibility contrast MRI: quantification issues in patient studies. *Top Magn Reson Imaging* 2010;21(2):75–85, reprinted with permission of Lippincott Williams & Wilkins, © 2011.)

for a typical acquisition protocol at 3 T using one of the standard 0.5 M concentration contrast agents, a so-called single dose (equivalent to 0.1 mmol/kg or 0.2 mL/kg) is recommended.[7]

It is now a common practice to inject this bolus of contrast agent by using an MR-compatible power injector. This contributes to ensure a well-defined bolus, with relative good consistency between studies. However, it is important to emphasize that, even for a perfectly controlled injection protocol (i.e., injection volume, site, and rate), the bolus shape entering the brain cannot be ensured to be reproducible and consistent; this shape is primarily dominated

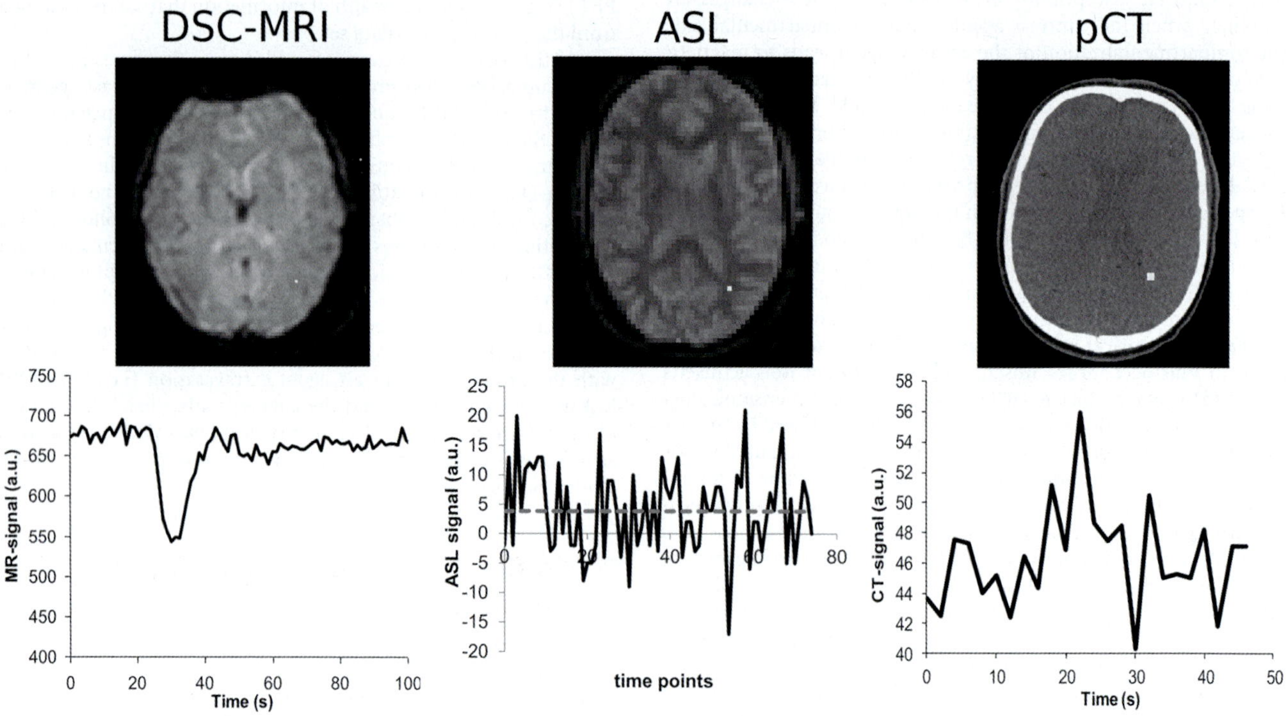

Figure 7-2. Figure illustrating the larger contrast-to-noise ratio (CNR) of DSC-MRI (left column) than arterial spin labeling (ASL, middle column) and perfusion CT (pCT, right column). The plots in the **bottom row** show data for a typical volume of interest (VOI), in white matter, as highlighted by the square region in each image shown in the **top row**. The VOIs are 39, 54, and 150 μL for the DSC-MRI, ASL, and pCT cases, respectively. Note that despite the smaller volume for the DSC-MRI region, the CNR is much higher, where the transient drop with the arrival of the bolus can be readily appreciated. On the other hand, both ASL and pCT methods are very noisy in white matter regions, and the non–zero offset for ASL (*dashed line*) or the transient signal increase for pCT is much more difficult to detect. (Figure previously published in Calamante F. Arterial input function in perfusion MRI: a comprehensive review. *Prog Nucl Magn Reson Spectrosc* 2013;74:1–32, reprinted with permission of Elsevier, © 2013.)

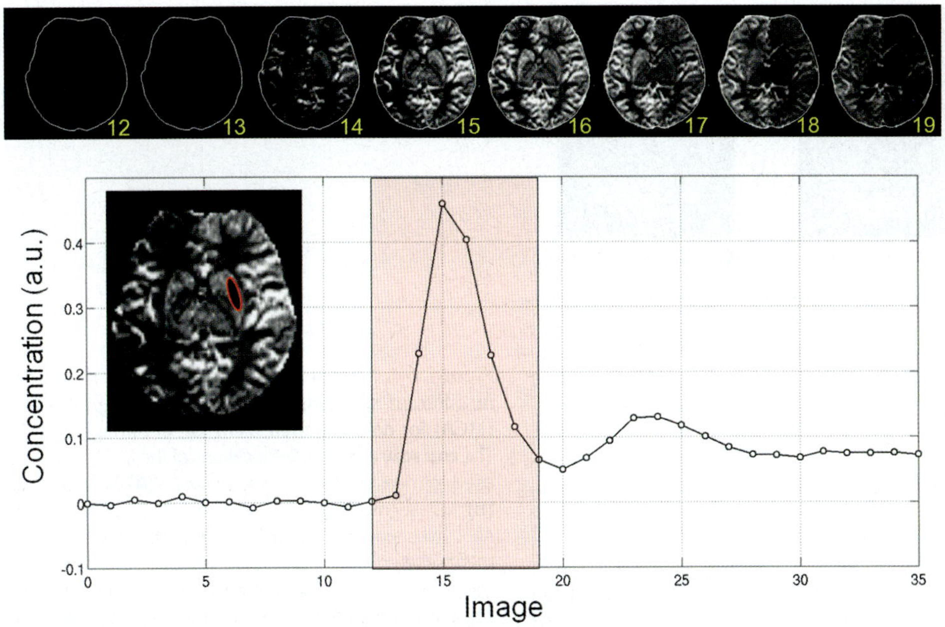

Figure 7-3. Contrast agent concentration corresponding to the data shown in Fig. 7.1. **Top row:** Contrast concentration images for eight time points during the first passage of the bolus; the number under each image indicates the image number (see *shaded* time interval in the graph). **Bottom row:** Time-dependent concentration for a contralateral region of interest (see insert); due to the shape of the curve, these data are usually referred to as the "peak." The data clearly show the transient increase in contrast agent concentration. (Figure previously published in Calamante F. Perfusion MRI using dynamic-susceptibility contrast MRI: quantification issues in patient studies. *Top Magn Reson Imaging* 2010;21(2):75–85, reprinted with permission of Lippincott Williams & Wilkins, © 2011.)

by the passage of the bolus from the site of injection, through the heart–lungs–heart system, and then through the arterial vasculature to the brain. Therefore, other factors such as the cardiac output and arterial status can play a major role in determining the shape. This is one of the main reasons why the measurement of the AIF (see next section) is essential for CBF quantification.

A safe injection rate, which is commonly used for DSC-MRI investigations in adult subjects, is 5 mL/s.[7] It is important that the injected bolus of contrast agent is immediately followed by a saline bolus (of about 20 to 30 mL and usually injected at the same rate as the contrast bolus), whose key role is to flush the contrast through the catheter and veins, to help maintain a well-defined bolus of contrast agent.

An important safety consideration when dealing with DSC-MRI studies relates to the small, but nonnegligible, risk of nephrogenic systemic fibrosis (NSF), a fibrosing disease, primarily involving the skin and subcutaneous tissues.[8] The risk of NSF is higher in patients with renal insufficiency, who have a glomerular filtration rate less than 30 mL/min/1.73 m^2.[9] In this high-risk patient group, the risk–benefit of a DSC-MRI investigation should be carefully considered.[10] Furthermore, the choice of contrast agent should be carefully selected given that some contrast agents are associated with increased risks,[9] and the dose should be kept to a minimum.

Given that DSC-MRI exploits the transient changes in T_2* and T_2 relaxation, the most commonly used MRI sequences in clinical investigations are based on a gradient-echo (GE) or a spin-echo (SE) EPI acquisition. While the SE-based sequence has low sensitivity to large vessels[11] (and, therefore, is more suited for measuring microvascular perfusion, i.e., at the capillary level), the much larger susceptibility effect in GE-based sequences makes them the sequence of choice in practice. This therefore comes at the expense of a significant macrovascular artifact (see section Macrovascular Artifacts below), where CBF is greatly overestimated in voxels containing partial volume effect (PVE) with large arteries and veins.

Apart from the sequence type (i.e., GE vs. SE), there are a number of sequence parameters that can have a major effect in the size of the detected DSC-MRI effect, including TE, TR, and flip angle. For example, the TE should be long enough to introduce a robust signal drop in the tissue, but not too long to completely null the arterial signal, which is needed to measure the AIF. Similarly, the TR must be short enough to allow for the sampling of a sufficient number of time points during the bolus passage, but not too short to make the SNR very low. In turn, the flip angle must be large enough to increase the SNR but not long enough to introduce a significant T_1 enhancement.[b] Based on the consensus of a group of experts in stroke imaging,[7] the following combination of parameters were recommended for a typical DSC-MRI investigation: TR approximately 1.5 seconds, TE approximately 30 ms (at 3 T) or 40 ms (at 1.5 T), and acquisition duration = 90 to 120 seconds (started 10 seconds before the contrast injection).

Once the changes in R_2* (=1/T_2*) are measured using a GE sequence, the time-dependent concentration of the contrast agent, $C(t)$, is usually estimated using a linear relationship[1,3,6,11]:

$$C(t) = \frac{1}{r}\Delta R_2{}^*(t) \tag{1}$$

where r is the relaxivity of the contrast agent (Fig. 7.3). While nonlinearities have been reported, particularly when measuring the concentration fully inside an artery,[12] the linear relationship is a reasonable approximation for the tissue measurements, particularly for longer TE, higher magnetic field, higher doses, or higher molar susceptibility.[13]

Given that a single-echo GE-EPI is most often used for DSC-MRI, the change in R_2* is calculated from the changes in signal intensity $S(t)$ from its baseline value (S_0), by neglecting the contribution from T_1 enhancement:

$$C(t) = -\frac{1}{r \times \mathrm{TE}}\ln\left(\frac{S(t)}{S_0}\right) \tag{2}$$

The Arterial Input Function

The shape of the concentration time course in Eq. (2) contains very useful hemodynamic information and, in the early years of DSC-MRI, quantification was carried out by measuring summary

[b]The contrast agent not only induces a change in T2* and T2 relaxation, but also a reduction in T1 relaxation. This effect leads to signal enhancement (i.e. the opposite effect to that associated with the susceptibility effect), which is usually neglected by the kinetic model used in DSC-MRI quantification.[3]

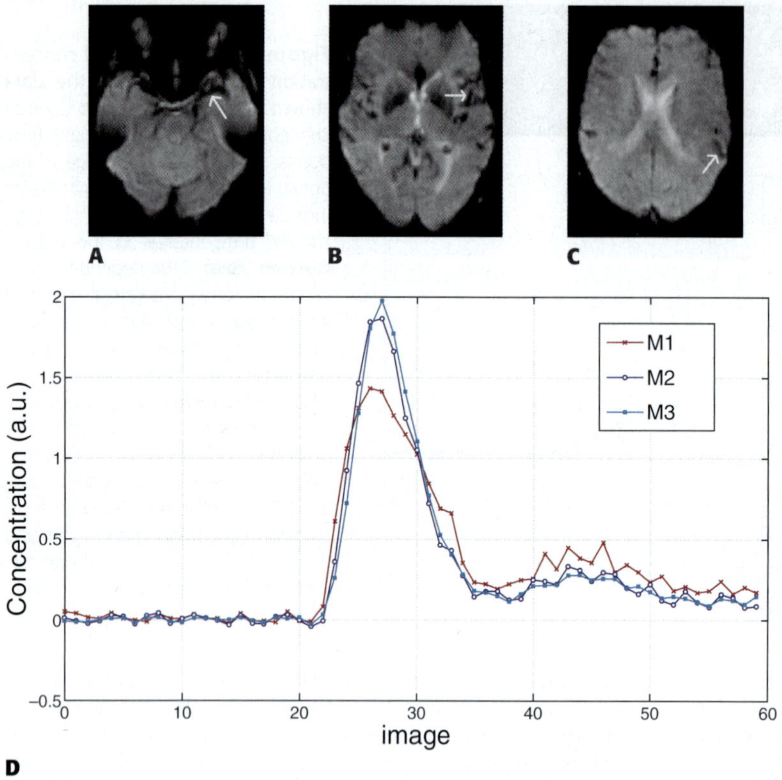

Figure 7-4. Arterial input functions (AIFs) measured in different segments of the middle cerebral artery (MCA) for data acquired using GE EPI imaging at 3T. The **top row** indicates the locations of the MCA segments used to measure the AIF (see *arrows*): **(A)** M1 segment, **(B)** M2 segment, **(C)** M3 segment. The corresponding AIF curves are shown in **(D)**, with the AIF for the M1 segment labeled with crosses, the M2 segment with *open circles*, and the M3 segment with *filled squares*. Note: for comparison purposes, all AIF curves were normalized to the same area. Due to signal truncation effects, the AIF is severely underestimated in the M1 segment location. (Figure previously published in Calamante F. Arterial input function in perfusion MRI: a comprehensive review. *Prog Nucl Magn Reson Spectrosc* 2013;74:1–32, reprinted with permission of Elsevier, © 2013.)

parameters directly from this curve,[14] such as the time to peak (TTP) or the maximum peak concentration (MPC). These parameters were often used as surrogate markers of perfusion, such that, for example, a brain area with increased TTP or decreased MPC was interpreted as an area with decreased tissue perfusion. However, it was later recognized that this was a very simplistic interpretation of the DSC-MRI data[15,16] and that a change in summary parameters could be not only due to a perfusion change but also due to a change in the injection protocol, the cardiac output, the presence of an arterial abnormality, etc. All these extra contributions can be taken into account by measuring the shape of the bolus *entering* the tissue of interest (given that this shape would contain information about all these other factors). This led to the concept of the AIF, which plays a central role in DSC-MRI quantification.[17] The AIF describes the time-dependent delivery of the contrast agent at the entrance of the tissue under study (i.e., it is the function describing the shape of the bolus input).

While a very simple concept in theory, the measurement of the AIF is in practice a very challenging task. It can be subject to a number of major sources of error for DSC-MRI quantification, including PVE, bolus delay and dispersion, nonlinearities, truncation effect, and voxel-shift signal artifacts, among others (see also section Sources of Error and Technical Limitations below). The reader is referred to a recent review article for a detailed description of all the main sources of error in the AIF.[17]

In practice, a single estimate of the AIF for the whole brain (the so-called *global* AIF) is obtained from measuring the changes in R_2* in and around a medium-size artery, such as the M1 or M2 segment of the middle cerebral artery (MCA) at 1.5T and the M2 or M3 segments at 3T (Fig. 7.4).[c] This provides a reasonable compromise between PVE, proximity to the tissue of interest, and saturation effects. In cases where there is an arterial abnormality to one side of the brain, the global AIF is commonly measured in the contralateral side. In particular, this avoids the unphysical situation of detecting a tissue passage that is narrower and/or earlier than the AIF.

In general, measurement of the AIF requires a reasonable level of expertise by the user and, given its central role in perfusion quantification, errors in the measured AIF can have major consequences.[17] Given that the AIF represents the input to the tissue, it is often identified by a searching criterion based on a combination of features of the concentration time course. For example, an AIF is expected to have an earlier arrival, a sharper rise, earlier TTP, higher MPC, and higher peak area than the tissue voxels. Performing this search in a manual way relies on highly trained local staff, and, even in that case, it is very subjective and can be very time consuming. It is for this reason that several automatic methods have been developed to measure the global AIF (Fig. 7.5).[18–22] These software tools search through the data set to identify voxels that satisfy a criteria similar to the one used for manual AIF measurement, that is, a criteria based on a combination of temporal and shape features of the measured bolus passage, in order to choose arterial-like curves. The use of these automatic methods is highly recommended because they help to improve reproducibility, remove subjectivity, ensure site quality consistency, and allow for advanced analysis methods to be widely applied, even in centers with limited specialist expertise.

From Convolution to Deconvolution

As expected, the shape of the bolus passage measured in the tissue is highly dependent on the input bolus, that is, on the AIF: the wider the input bolus, the wider the tissue concentration (for all other parameters unchanged). The tissue shape is, however, also influenced by the amount of blood delivered to the tissue (i.e., perfusion) and by other intrinsic tissue properties, which describe how the contrast agent is washed out from the capillary bed. For example, the wider the input bolus and/or the slower the washout

[c]The signal intensity measured at 3 T in the M1 segment often reaches the noise level during the maximum concentration of the bolus; this is due to complete signal dephasing for the typical contrast doses and TE used.

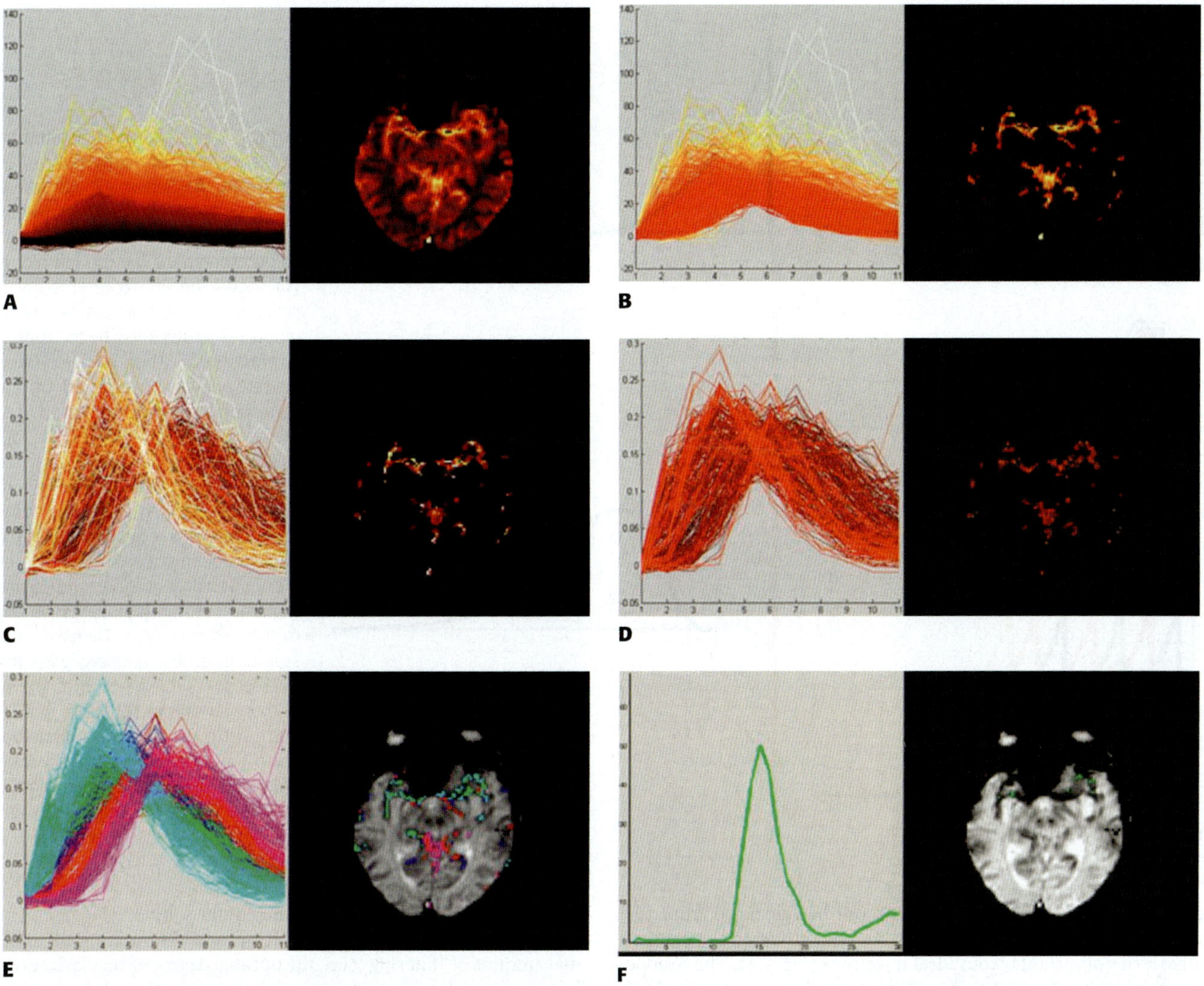

Figure 7-5. Illustration of the workflow in an automatic arterial input function (AIF) searching algorithm based on cluster analysis. In **(A)** and **(B)**, voxels and curves are color coded based on their area under the concentration time course. In **(A)**, all concentration time curves are shown, and in **(B)**, only 10% of the curves with the largest area are included. The set of curves in **(B)** standardized to unit area are displayed in **(C)** and colored according to roughness; in **(D)**, the 25% most irregular curves have been removed. The set of curves in **(D)** are then partitioned into five clusters such that the intracluster variance is minimized and the intercluster variation is maximized. The partition is indicated in **(E)**. The mean curve in the group of light blue curves had the lowest first moment and was, therefore, picked out by the algorithm and divided into five subclusters (not shown). The estimate of the AIF returned by the program was the mean curve with the lowest first moment, which is shown in **(F)** along with the anatomic location of the selected voxels. (Figure kindly provided by Dr. Kim Mouridsen, and reproduced from Mouridsen K, Christensen S, Gyldensted L, Ostergaard L. Automatic selection of arterial input function using cluster analysis. *Magn Reson Med* 2006;55(3):524–531, with permission of Wiley-Liss, Inc., © 2006.)

of contrast agent, the wider the shape of the bolus in the tissue. Similarly, the higher the blood flow rate, the larger the shape of the bolus.

Therefore, the shape of the tissue concentration is dependent on three main quantities: (i) the shape of the input bolus, (ii) the delivery rate of blood, and (iii) how fast/slow the contrast leaves the tissue through the veins. From a modeling point of view, DSC-MRI quantification is based on the principles of indicator dilution theory,[23] which relates these three quantities to the tissue concentration. Based on this theory, the concentration time course in the tissue is related to the AIF by a convolution equation:

$$C(t) = \text{CBF} \times \left(C_{\text{AIF}}(t) \otimes R(t)\right) \qquad (3)$$

where $C_{\text{AIF}}(t)$ is the AIF, $R(t)$ is the tissue residue function, and $\otimes$ is the mathematical convolution operator. The tissue residue function is an *idealized* mathematical concept, which describes the wash-out of the contrast agent from the tissue for the ideal case of an instantaneous bolus injection at time $t = 0$. In other words, for an ideal injection (i.e., an AIF corresponding to an instantaneous injection), the residue function (scaled by CBF) would correspond to the measured $C(t)$, which describes the amount of contrast agent remaining in the tissue at time t. For this reason, the CBF-scaled residue function is also known as the "impulse response function," that is, the function describing the response of the system to an instantaneous input bolus.

While the mathematical convolution can be a very obscure concept for nontechnical readers, it simply describes that the tissue

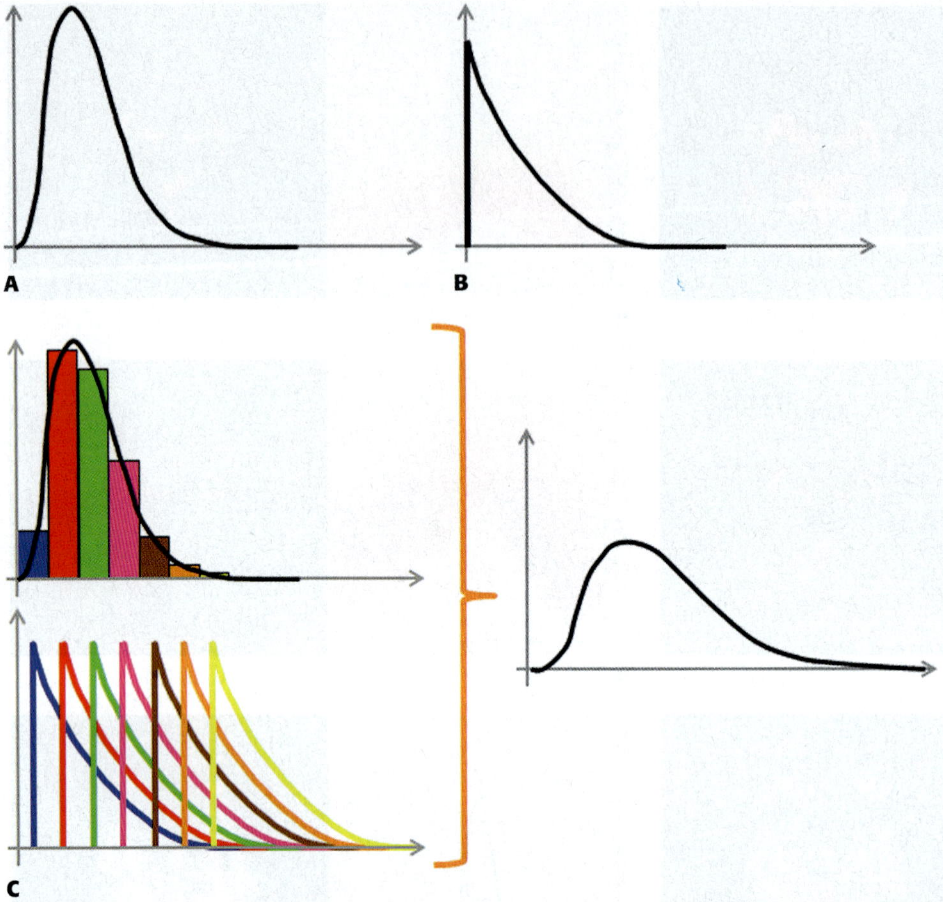

Figure 7-6. Schematic illustration of the role of convolution in DSC-MRI. **A:** Schematic AIF curve. **B:** Schematic tissue residue function curve. **C:** Discretization of the convolution expression. The top left plot in **(C)** shows the AIF represented as a series of consecutives discrete small inputs (as represented by the various *colored bars*). When each of these discrete inputs is multiplied by the corresponding residue function (i.e., the same residue function curve, but shifted to have the same delay, as shown by the curves in the bottom left plot in **(C)** with the colors corresponding to the colors of the discrete AIFs) and then scaled by CBF, it gives the tissue concentration time course (rightmost plot in **(C)**) corresponding to that discrete input. Therefore, the sum of these contributions gives the total tissue residue function, as shown in the right plot in **(C)**. Note that for the exact convolution, the discretization is done for an infinitesimally short time interval, with an infinite number of these inputs (cf. only seven discretized inputs are shown in **(C)**).

concentration at time t, that is, $C(t)$, can be calculated from the superposition of contributions from an AIF considered as a consecutive series of instantaneous ideal injections (Fig. 7.6). The residue function in the convolution Eq. (3) indicates how much of each of those consecutive ideal input functions remains in the tissue at time t, whose combination leads to the measured tissue concentration at time t. The reader is referred to Calamante et al.[24] for a detailed review of the deconvolution process in DSC-MRI.

Quantification of perfusion using DSC-MRI therefore requires inverting the expression in Eq. (3) to calculate CBF. From a mathematical point of view, inversion of a convolution expression is known as a "deconvolution" analysis. The concepts of convolution and deconvolution are, therefore, central to the model and analysis used in DSC-MRI, and a typical DSC-MRI experiment to quantify CBF always involves a measurement of an AIF and a deconvolution step.

Regularization

The major difficulty with inverting Eq. (3) is that deconvolution is an ill-posed problem,[24,25] in that even a very small amount of noise in the data makes the deconvolution step extremely unreliable. Therefore, deconvolution requires, in practice, special consideration to make the solution more physically meaningful. This process is known as "regularization" of the deconvolution.

There are many ways to implement the regularization, and in all cases, this involves discarding some of the high-frequency information, which has the highest noise sensitivity. From this point of view, regularization could be thought of as type of "filtering," but one that occurs during the deconvolution step. As with standard filtering, too little filtering leads to very unstable solutions, while too much filtering leads to oversmoothing of the solution (Fig. 7.7). The same applies to the deconvolution case, and determining the optimal amount of "filtering" (i.e., the optimal degree of regularization) is a very complex issue. In particular, the optimal level depends on many factors such as the SNR and the TR, and it even depends on tissue properties such as the CBF we are trying to quantify.[26–35]

In general, there are two main ways in which the degree of regularization is applied in practice. Either it is fixed, based on some previously optimized values,[26] or it is adapted to the data based on data quality (i.e., a data-driven approach).[30–32,34,36–39] An example of the former case is the traditional truncated singular value decomposition (SVD) approach,[26] where a fixed threshold is used for every voxel in the brain and for every patient (e.g., a 20% cutoff for the SVD expansion). An example of a data-driven approach is the so-called oSVD method,[31] a modification of the traditional SVD approach to make it delay insensitive, where a threshold for an oscillation index of the estimated residue function is used to determine the degree of regularization (i.e., the data are regularized until a certain level of smoothness is achieved based on an oscillation index). Data-driven approaches have the obvious advantage that regularization is more optimally adjusted to the available data quality (e.g., higher-quality data require less regularization than lower SNR data). However, this most often comes at the expense of larger processing times. For some applications, for example, acute stroke, the increased computation time is not a practical option (see also section DSC-MRI Analysis: Practical Implementation), which is the main reason why the faster fixed regularization approach has been more widely used.

The development of deconvolution algorithms for DSC-MRI has been a very active field of research. Most of the methods currently in

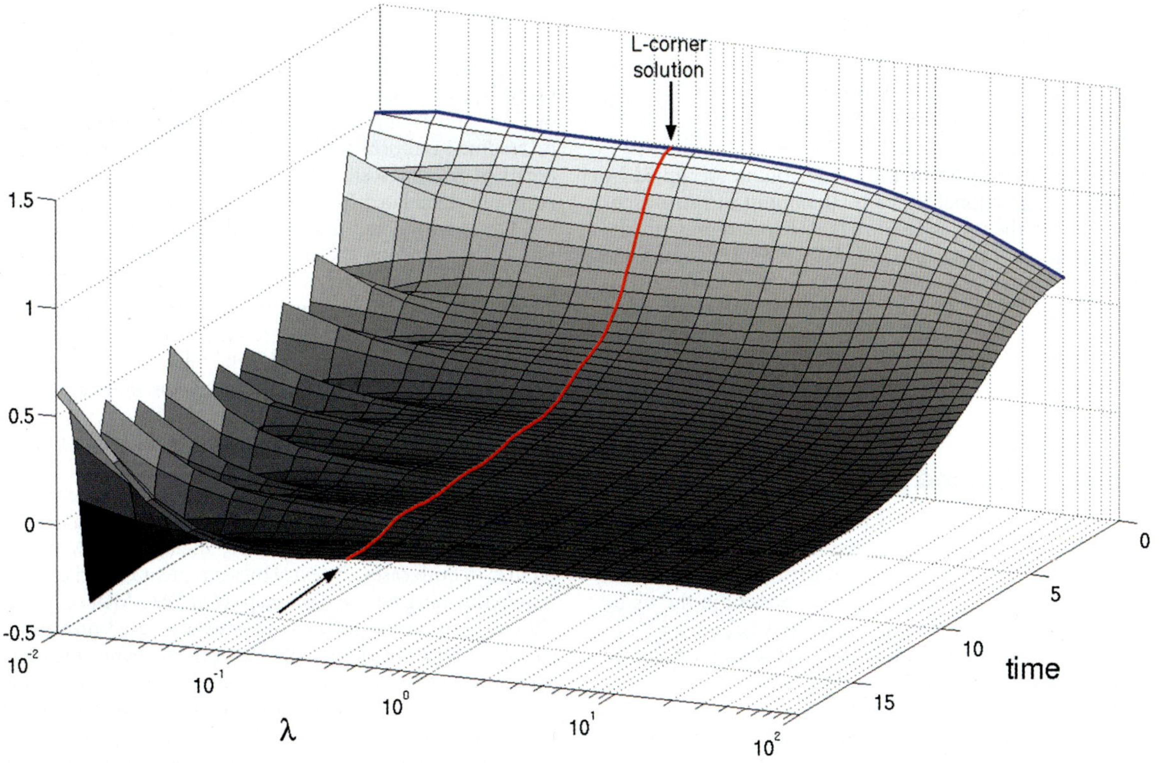

Figure 7-7. Example of regularization using Tikhonov for simulated data. The surface plot shows the Tikhonov solutions for the tissue residue function *R*(*t*) obtained for various regularization values (with increasing regularization for increasing value of the parameter λ). The vertical axis corresponds to the Tikhonov solution *R*(*t*) and its initial value (corresponding to the blue line at time = 0) to the estimated CBF. For this particular case, the optimal solution (as determined by the corner of the L curve criterion)[32] corresponds to the red curve, which is indicated by the *arrows*. Note that with low regularization (left side of the surface plot), there are large oscillations, and with high regularization (right side of the surface plot), the solution is oversmoothed, leading to reduced CBF estimate, as indicated by the decreasing values of the blue line with increasing regularization. (Modified from a Figure previously published in Calamante F, Gadian DG, Connelly A. Quantification of bolus-tracking MRI: Improved characterization of the tissue residue function using Tikhonov regularization. *Magn Reson Med* 2003;50(6):1237–1247, reprinted with permission of Wiley-Liss, Inc, © 2003.)

use are based on the so-called model-independent approach, where the shape of the residue function is also considered an unknown when performing the deconvolution. Model-independent methods include those based on SVD or its variants,[26,27,31,40] Fourier transform–based methods,[26,41] Tikhonov regularization,[32] iterative algorithms,[28,34,38] Bayesian-based methods,[30,39] among many others.[42–44] Each of these methods has some advantages and disadvantages regarding their accuracy, precision, processing speed, ease of implementation, sensitivity to the presence of bolus delay, etc. In fact, there is unfortunately no method currently available that is superior to all others in every single aspect, which is probably the reason why this field of research has been very active and there is no clear consensus as to what deconvolution method is preferable. In practice, the properties of the method that is given higher priority and, therefore, the actual choice of deconvolution algorithm are dependent on the specific circumstances and application. For example, if the patient population under study is likely to have considerable bolus delay (e.g., patients with severe carotid stenosis or occlusion),[45–47] then delay insensitivity should be among the highest priority for the criteria used to select a deconvolution method. Similarly, if data quality is very variable (e.g., in a multicenter study), then use of a data-driven regularization method should be essential.

DSC-MRI Parameters

There are a large number of hemodynamic parameters that have been calculated based on DSC-MRI data. These can be broadly divided into parameters that can only be calculated following a deconvolution analysis and those that can be calculated directly from the DSC-MRI data, often referred to as summary parameters.[14] It should be emphasized that all these parameters can be calculated from the same measured DSC-MRI data, just by varying the way the data are analyzed (i.e., different postprocessing methods). This represents one of the strengths of DSC-MRI and highlights the wealth of information that can be obtained from a relatively short MRI acquisition time.

Summary Parameters

These are the DSC-MRI parameters that can be calculated without requiring a deconvolution step. They represent properties of the measured signal time course or the concentration time curve. For example, there is a number of temporal summary parameters, including TTP, bolus arrival time, full width at half maximum, and the first moment of the curve. Apart from the bolus arrival time, all these temporal parameters reflect both macrovascular and microvascular properties and, therefore, cannot be interpreted as measures of perfusion status.[15,16]

There are also other summary parameters related to the size effect, such as MPC and the maximum signal drop, and others related to the peak area, such as the area under the curve (AUC) and the integral-to-peak area (i.e., the area of the initial part of the concentration time curve, until the maximum concentration has been reached). In particular, the area under the peak is related to an important physiologic parameter, the cerebral blood volume (CBV):

$$\mathrm{CBV} = \frac{\mathrm{AUC(C)}}{\mathrm{AUC(AIF)}}, \tag{4}$$

which represents the fraction of the tissue volume occupied by the blood and is proportional to the total amount of intravascular contrast agent in the tissue. In Eq. (4), AUC(C) represents the AUC of the tissue concentration and AUC(AIF) represents the corresponding AUC of the AIF. The normalization to the AIF is required to account for the amount of injected contrast agent. It should be noted that, for absolute quantification, the AUC ratio in Eq. (4) must be scaled by a factor describing the difference in hematocrit between arteries and capillaries and by the density of brain tissue.[14]

Deconvolution-Related Parameters

The main parameter in this case is CBF, which can be calculated, in principle, from the initial value of the impulse response function, CBF × $R(t)$. This follows from the fact that, by definition, $R(t = 0) = 1$, that is, all the contrast agent is present in the tissue at $t = 0$ following the injection of an ideal input bolus a $t = 0$. In practice, however, the shape of the impulse residue function can be subject to a number of artifacts,[48] including bolus dispersion and deconvolution errors (see section Sources of Error and Technical Limitations for more details). In particular, bolus dispersion makes the initial value of the impulse response function equal to zero.[49] It is for this reason that, in practice, CBF is most often estimated from the *maximum* of the impulse function rather than from its initial value.[26,49]

There are two further deconvolution-related parameters that are often calculated in DSC-MRI studies and that reflect temporal features: the mean transit time (MTT) and T_{max}. MTT corresponds to the average time it takes the blood (and therefore the contrast agent) to travel through the tissue capillary network following the injection of an ideal bolus. MTT can be calculated based on the central volume theorem[23] as the ratio of blood volume to blood flow:

$$\mathrm{MTT} = \frac{\mathrm{CBV}}{\mathrm{CBF}} \tag{5}$$

In turn, T_{max} represent the time to maximum of the impulse response function[50] and corresponds, in theory, to the bolus delay.[51] However, in practice, because a number of artifacts can distort the shape of the calculated impulse response function (see section Sources of Error and Technical Limitations for more details), T_{max} can be also influenced by bolus dispersion and, to a smaller extent, by MTT.[51] It should therefore be considered primarily a measure of macrovascular status. This parameter has increasingly being used in stroke imaging, and it has been one of the parameters of choice for several major stroke clinical trials.[52–55]

Absolute Quantification

DSC-MRI has been often criticized as a technique that can only measure CBF in *relative* units.[56,57] While this view was correct earlier on, technical developments in this field have made considerable progress in recent years, and DSC-MRI has now grown to be a perfusion imaging technique that can provide robust measurements in absolute units (e.g., in mL/100 g/min).

To obtain perfusion in absolute units, it is most often necessary to scale the results from the deconvolution analysis (which can be considered to be in arbitrary units, or "DSC units") to CBF measurements in absolute units.[d] It is essential, however, that this scaling is carried out using a *patient-specific* scaling factor. This scaling factor is aimed at compensating for scaling errors due to several factors, such as nonlinearities, and PVE (see section Sources of Error and Technical Limitations for more details), which cannot be assumed uniform across patients. Several methods that provide a patient-specific scaling have now been proposed.[58–63] The scaling is usually calculated from data obtained using an extra MR data set. For example, the first method proposed, the "bookend technique,"[58,59] calculates the scaling factor from a T_1-based CBV measurement obtained from two extra T_1 maps acquired just before and after DSCMRI (i.e., pre- and postcontrast agent T_1 measurements). This CBV map (which is in absolute units because it is based on T_1 data)[64] can be compared with the relative CBV map from DSC-MRI, to obtain a "bookend" scaling factor that can be applied to the CBF map.

Other alternative methods to obtain the patient-specific scaling relies, for example, on an extra regional CBF measurement from ASL data, with a method known as "combined ASL and DSC CBF" (CAD–CBF),[60] or on the total cerebral flow calculated from a complementary phase-contrast MR angiography (MRA) measurement.[61] In both cases, the extra measurement is used to calculate the required scaling for the CBF map from DSC-MRI on a patient-by-patient basis. Other further methods are based on scaling factors based on ratio measurements between the veins and the arteries, such as by using the venous output function (a function similar to the AIF but that characterizes the output of the bolus from the tissue, rather than the input)[62] or by using the pseudo–steady-state contrast concentration after the first pass (i.e., the measured concentration during the tail of the peak).[63]

These subject-specific scaling methods are in contrast to early attempts to convert to absolute units, using methods that relied in a uniform scaling factor for all patients.[41,42,65,66] The most common of these earlier methods was based on scaling the maps by fixing to 22 mL/100 g/min the CBF value of a reference region in contralateral white matter.[65] Any of these approaches that rely on a uniform scaling factor are strongly discouraged for clinical applications where absolute units are required.

Sources of Error and Technical Limitations

The vast majority of sources of error in DSC-MRI quantification relate to errors in the measurement of the AIF.[17] These errors are often related to the location where the AIF is measured from: there is practical compromise between measuring the AIF from a distal (and relatively large) artery, to minimize PVEs, and measuring it from a small artery close enough to the tissue of interest to minimize the possible presence of bolus delay and dispersion (Fig. 7.8). Ideally, the AIF should be measured from the small arteriole supplying the tissue of interest in the voxel, such that the true input to the tissue is obtained and bolus delay and dispersion are avoided. This requires a different specific AIF for each voxel in the brain, a concept known as the *local* AIF (see below). However, due to the relative coarse spatial resolution used in DSC-MRI (typically 2 × 2 × 5 mm^3) compared with the size of the arterioles in the brain (submillimeter in diameter), measurement of such a local AIF free from

[d]It should be noted that this scaling step to absolute units can be considered equivalent to the scaling required in other perfusion imaging methods, which despite this need of scaling are widely accepted as methods that can provide CBF measurements in absolute units. For example, for arterial spin labeling (ASL) measurements, the ASL perfusion-weighted signal must be scaled to convert it to mL/100 g/min, such as by using the blood equilibrium magnetization and the labeling efficiency.[14]

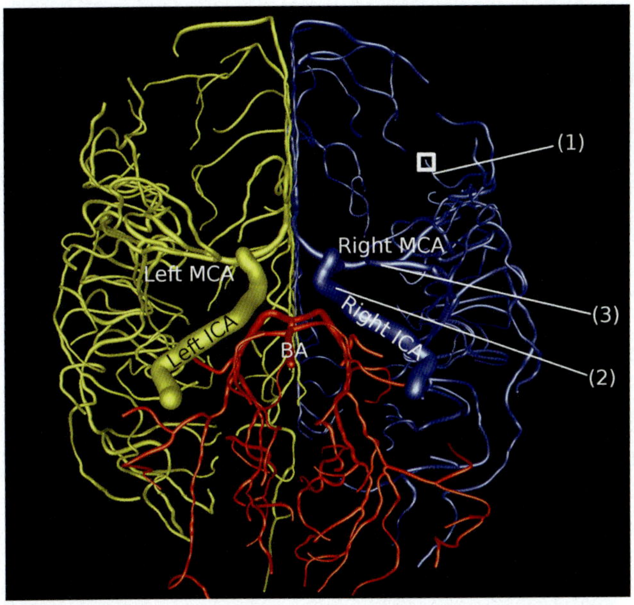

Figure 7-8. Typical locations for the measurement of the arterial input function (AIF). The figure shows a vascular tree in the brain (viewed from an inferior direction), with the three major arterial territories indicated by the *red* (basilar artery, BA), *green* (left internal carotid artery, ICA), and *blue* (right ICA) colors. To calculate cerebral blood flow (CBF) in a voxel located in the position indicated by the *white square*, the AIF should ideally be measured from small arteriole supplying the tissue in that voxel (location labeled (*1*) in the figure). However, this arteriole has a relatively small size and, therefore, the AIF would need to be measured from a much larger artery (e.g., location (*2*) in the ICA) to avoid PVE. In practice, a medium-sized artery (such as in the M1 or M2 segment of the MCA, e.g., location (*3*)) is commonly chosen as a compromise between minimizing PVE and reducing bolus delay and dispersion. (Based on an image kindly provided by Drs. Juan R. Cebral and Susan Wright.)

PVE with the surrounding tissue is a very complex (and, argued by some, an impossible) task. In the following paragraphs, the major sources of AIF error are described.

Partial Volume Effect

As mentioned before, the measure DSC-MRI signal in an AIF voxel is likely to contain a combination of arterial and tissue contributions. One of the complexities of this PVE in DSC-MRI relates to the angular dependency of these contributions: the magnitude of their contributions depends on the angle of the artery relative to the main magnetic field.[12] Furthermore, the MRI signal is a complex number, with a magnitude and phase. The total signal in the voxel is, therefore, the complex sum of the arterial and tissue contributions. In particular, the sum of a narrow arterial contribution and a wide tissue contribution can lead to both wider and narrower "partial-volumed" AIFs.[67] Therefore, it is not straightforward to identify AIFs that have been subjected to PVE: the wider curves can be easily identified and discarded, but the narrower curves would, in fact, be favored by most manual and automatic AIF searching methods, because they would actually satisfy the searching criteria of an earlier arrival, a sharper rise, earlier TTP, higher MPC, and higher peak area. In order to identify (and then discard) these narrower PVE AIFs, Bleeker et al.[68] recently proposed a further searching criterion based on the ratio of the (postpeak) pseudo–steady-state value to the area under the peak: the PVE in the narrower curves was shown to have a significantly reduced ratio (Fig. 7.9).

An elegant method to correct for PVE has been proposed for the specific case when the artery is parallel to the main magnetic field, which is often the case for measuring the AIF in the internal carotid artery.[12] This method relies on acquiring data with a double-echo sequence (to avoid complete dephasing from arterial signal) as well a relatively complex postprocessing analysis of the measured real/imaginary DSC-MRI data. This approach can be also very sensitive to delay and dispersion due to the relatively large distance to the tissue of interest. It is for all these reasons that this method, despite being the only robust method for correcting PVE, has not had widespread use.

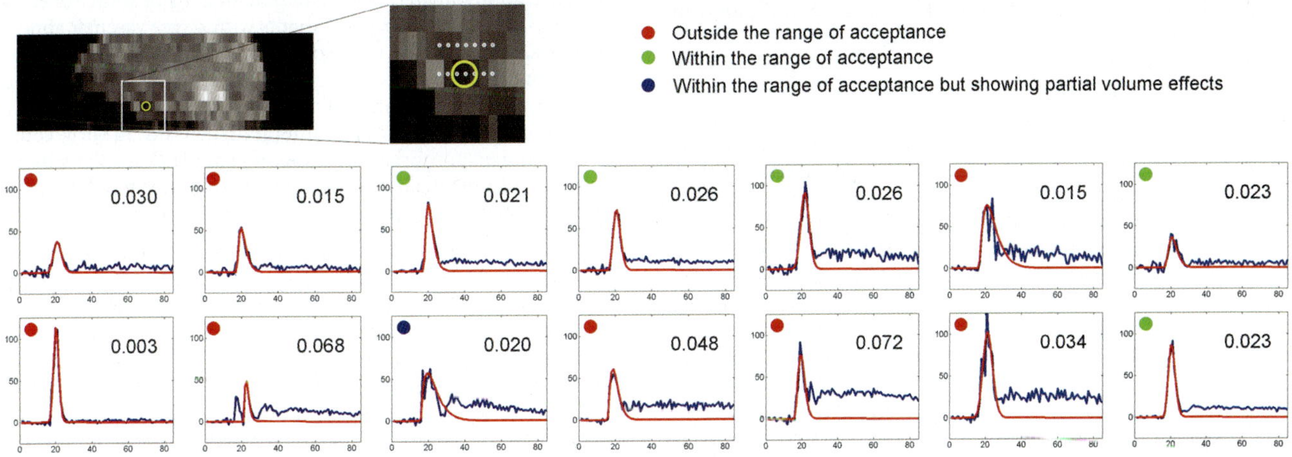

Figure 7-9. In vivo example of arterial input function (AIF) measurements in and around the middle cerebral artery (MCA, with its position labeled by the *yellow circle*). The profiles within the MCA, as well as the profile touching the artery, show PVEs. The range of acceptance for the ratio of the (postpeak) pseudo–steady-state value to the area under the peak for this subject is [0.019–0.028]. This metric can provide AIF measurements with minimal PVEs, which are located outside the MCA. In particular, note that the bottom left profile shows a narrow and sharp peak, which could have been picked by either a manual or an automatic method. However, this profile is heavily affected by PVE, as illustrated by its very low ratio (outside the range of acceptance). This metric can therefore be used to exclude these types of voxels from the AIF search, despite their apparent appropriate shape. (Figure previously published in Bleeker EJW, Van Osch MJP, Connelly A, Van Buchem MA, Webb AG, Calamante F. New criterion to aid manual and automatic selection of the arterial input function in dynamic susceptibility contrast MRI. *Magn Reson Med* 2011;65(2):448–456, reprinted with permission of Wiley-Liss, Inc., © 2010.)

Interestingly, it has been shown that despite the unavoidable presence of PVE, the contaminated AIF can still have a very good approximation to the correct *shape*, with the PVE primarily introducing a scaling.[69–71] In that case, the measured AIF can be used to quantify CBF in relative units, which can then be scaled to absolute units using one of the patient-specific scaling methods described in the section Absolute Quantification above. Somewhat surprisingly, these studies have shown that the locations where PVE leads to good approximations to the true AIF shape (albeit a scaled version) are actually measuring it from voxels in the vicinity of, but completely outside, an artery.[69–71] For example, extensive numerical simulations by van Osch et al.[70,71] have shown that various specific locations completely outside the M1 segment of the MCA (particularly posteriorly to this branch and, in some circumstances, in the slice immediately superior to the artery) provide good estimates for the AIF (e.g., see suitable locations identified in Figure 7.9, which are in locations superior and posterior relative to the M1 segment). However, they also found that the optimal locations depended on sequence type and parameters, as well as the diameter of the M1 segment.

It is therefore important to recognize that, while PVE is in general unavoidable in DSC-MRI, it does not imply that absolute quantification is not feasible, when special care is taken during data analysis.

Bolus Delay

As mentioned above, the AIF is most commonly measured from a somewhat distant place from the tissue of interest (to minimize PVE). This can introduce a delay between the arrival of the contrast agent to the place where the AIF was measured to the arrival of the bolus to the tissue, that is, a temporal shift between the start of the AIF and the start of tissue concentration. In patients with severe vascular abnormalities, this delay can be of several seconds,[45–47,72] particularly because the AIF is usually measured from a contralateral artery (see section The Arterial Input Function above).

The presence of delay is not, in principle, a problem. However, some deconvolution algorithms can be very sensitive to delay, due to their specific implementations. In particular, the popular SVD method[26] is one of these examples. Given the widespread use of this method, this source of error, which might otherwise remain insignificant, became a major problem in DSC-MRI quantification in stroke patients.[31,40,46,47,73–75]

Bolus delay can lead to either CBF underestimation or CBF overestimation (Fig. 7.10),[73,74] depending on whether the delay is positive (i.e., the measured AIF leading the tissue curve) or negative (tissue curve leading the measured AIF), respectively. In practice, since the AIF is measured in the contralateral side, negative delays are very uncommon and, therefore, bolus delays are more most often associated with underestimation of CBF.[73]

There are various approaches that can be used to deal with this source of delay. This include a preprocessing step, where the concentration time curves in each voxel are time shifted to have a common time origin, thus effectively removing the delay.[73,75,76] Alternatively, and more commonly in use, the deconvolution can be carried out using an algorithm either that is delay insensitive[31,40,41,77] or that explicitly models delay as an extra parameter.[28,34,37–39] It is important to note, however, that many of these deconvolution methods, despite their delay insensitivity, suffer from a number of other deconvolution-related errors (see below) and their CBF estimates are not, therefore, necessarily accurate (e.g., see Fig. 7.11)—they are just delay insensitive.[17]

Bolus Dispersion

In practice, any bolus delay due to the extra time taken for the bolus to transit to the tissue of interest (e.g., due to transit through a stenosis or to the presence of collateral flow) is highly likely to be associated also with a bolus dispersion, that is, a temporal spread, producing a wider bolus shape.[47,49,78]

There are three main differences between the effects of bolus delay and bolus dispersion and their effect on DSC-MRI data:

- *Ease of detectability*: while the presence of bolus delay can be very easily detected from the measured DSC-MRI data directly (e.g., by simply visually looking at the data on a cine loop),[72] bolus dispersion cannot be detected without first performing a deconvolution analysis.[32,34,38,49] Both dispersion and a prolonged MTT lead to a wider measured tissue concentration bolus, and therefore, they cannot be distinguished by a direct measurement of $C(t)$. In contrast, after performing the deconvolution, the presence of dispersion can be, in theory, detected by assessment of the measured impulse response function.[32,34,38] When there is no dispersion, this function should be a decreasing function of time; when there is dispersion, this function should have a peaked shape. However, in order to detect these shape differences robustly, it is essential to use a deconvolution method that provides an accurate characterization of the tissue residue function. This is, in fact, a very complex task, and only a few algorithms have been shown to be suitable to provide a good characterization of the full shape (e.g., references[32,34,38,79]), while others are well known to have limitations in this regard, including some of the SVD variants.[26,31]
- *Sensitivity of deconvolution algorithms*: while bolus delay only affects certain deconvolution algorithms (i.e., some of them are delay insensitive—see Bolus Delay section above), bolus dispersion affects *all* of them.[49] This originates on the fact that the standard kinetic model (see Eq. (3)) cannot distinguish between a *macro*vascular dispersion (i.e., widening during transit through arteries) from a *micro*vascular dispersion (i.e., widening associated with an increased MTT). Both of them are interpreted as microvascular dispersion, and therefore, the deconvolution step would lead to an overestimation of the MTT and, due to the central volume theory,[23] an underestimation of CBF.[49]
- *Effect on CBF*: it follows from the previous point that, while delay can lead to CBF underestimation and overestimation, bolus dispersion can only lead to CBF underestimation (e.g., see Fig. 7.12). Both numerical simulations[73,79] and in vivo data from patients with unilateral abnormalities of major arteries[38,47] have suggested that bolus dispersion can introduce CBF underestimation as much as approximately 70%. This potential major source of error in DSC-MRI, particularly in patients with severe vascular abnormalities, can lead to an overestimation of the severity of an ischemic abnormality. For example, a large CBF underestimation and MTT overestimation can lead to the erroneous classification of a benign oligemia tissue as penumbral tissue. This, in turn, could lead to the inappropriate selection of candidates for the administration of potentially risky treatments (e.g., thrombolytic therapy) in patients who might not benefit from such interventions.

One possible method to avoid bolus dispersion errors is the use of the so-called local AIF[80] (Fig. 7.13), that is, each tissue voxel is assigned to a locally measured AIF (ideally, from the arteriole supplying the tissue in the voxel). In theory, this input function close to the tissue should have minimal dispersion. Various methods to estimate a local AIF have been proposed.[38,43,80–88] For example, some of them rely on independent component analysis to isolate the arterial contribution to the measured voxel concentration, which is then used as the local AIF.[38,80] Other methods perform a search in the local neighborhood of each voxel to identify the voxel that has the most arterial-like features (e.g., the voxel with the smallest temporal first moment and largest AUC),[81–83] while others search the neighborhood based both on the spatial closeness to the voxel *and* temporal similarities.[88] The latter aims at addressing the fact that, near boundaries of arterial territories and in the periphery of ischemic lesions (where blood can be delivered by collaterals), the closest arterial-like input might not be the most appropriate.[72]

There is however still some controversy as to the validity of local AIF methods in DSC-MRI,[88,89] particularly related to

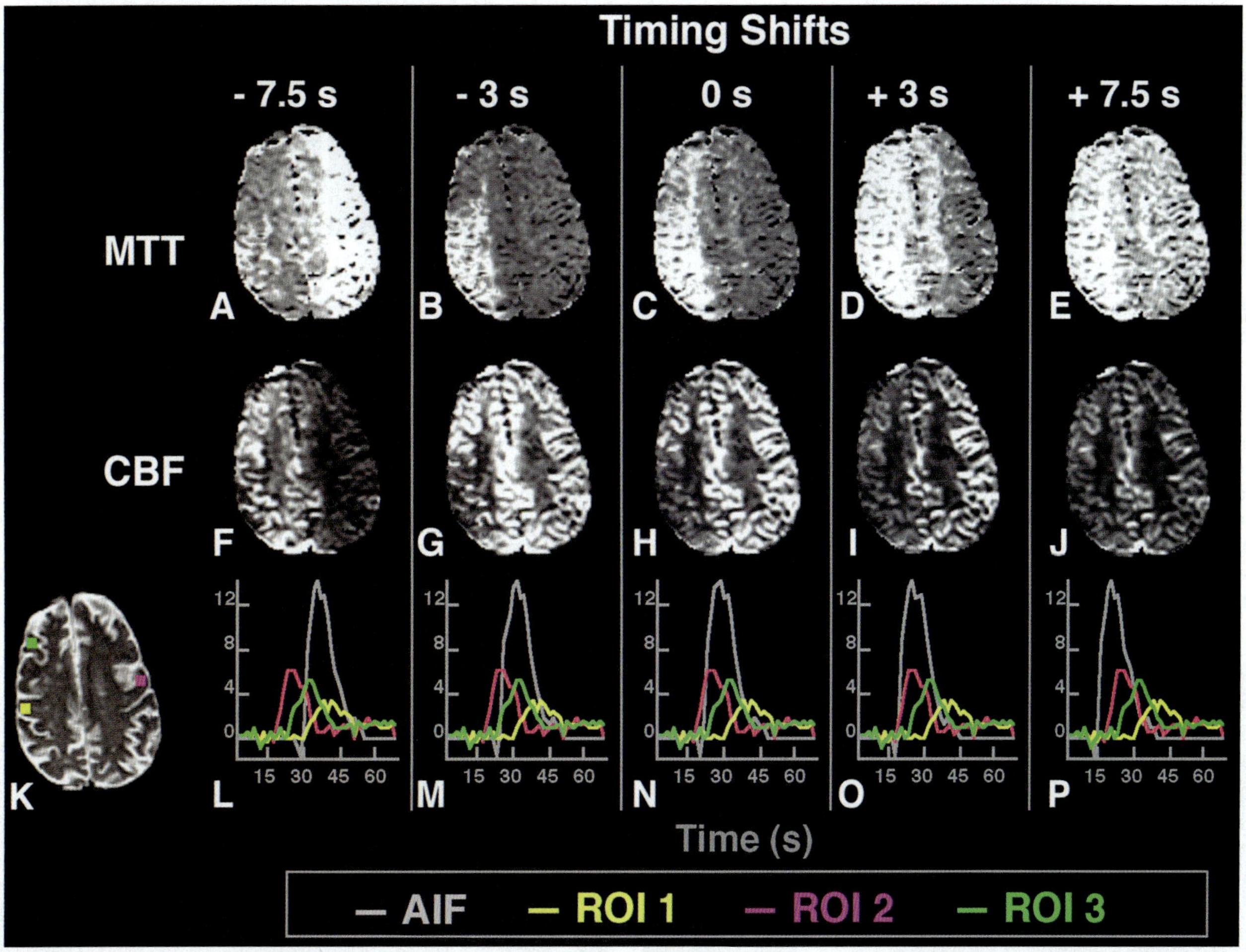

Figure 7-10. Example of delay-related errors for the standard singular value decomposition (SVD) method on a patient with right MCA stroke (left side of the images); the scan was carried out 5-hour post–symptom onset. The data were analyzed five times, with the arterial input function (AIF) artificially shifted forward and backward in time (as indicated by the amount of seconds in the top). The presence of AIF delays (shifts) leads to both over- and underestimation of cerebral blood flow (CBF). Each column represents the calculated **(A–E)** mean transit time (MTT) and **(F–J)** CBF for each shift. **(L–P): Bottom row** shows the change in relative timing of $\Delta R_2(t)$ in AIF selected ipsilaterally from the right MCA and in the three ROIs shown in **(K)**: one ROI in the ipsilateral hemisphere that is shown to infarct on follow-up imaging (*yellow*, ROI 1), one in the contralateral hemisphere (*magenta*, ROI 2), and one in the ipsilateral hemisphere that does not infarct (*green*, ROI 3). All CBF and MTT maps in a row are scaled using the same dynamic range for better comparison. This figure illustrates that the delay in the AIF can greatly affect the amount of tissue considered abnormal. In particular, note that the abnormality in the map (e.g., as seen by the area with increased MTT) can even change hemispheres. (Image kindly provided by Dr. Ona Wu, and modified from a figure previously published in Wu O, Østergaard L, Koroshetz WJ, et al. Effects of tracer arrival time on flow estimates in MR perfusion-weighted imaging. *Magn Reson Med* 2003;50(4):856–864, with permission of Wiley-Liss, Inc., © 2003.)

the contribution from PVE. Their use in practice is also limited due to the lack of local AIF software tools in general distribution. In fact, this DSC-MRI area of research is relatively in its infancy, and further validation and assessment work are urgently needed.

An alternative approach to correct for bolus dispersion errors is to include them within the tracer kinetic model used for quantification.[49] In particular, Eq. (3) can be modified to include the macrovascular contribution to the spread of the bolus by defining a vascular transport function (VTF, which describes the probability distribution of *vascular* transit times between the site of AIF measurement and the true input to the tissue)[17,49]:

$$C(t) = \text{CBF} \times \left(C_{\text{AIF}}(t) \otimes R(t) \otimes \text{VTF}(t)\right) \tag{6}$$

Recent studies have suggested that, with careful selection of the deconvolution algorithm and for low-to-medium levels of dispersion, it is possible to account for this confounding effect.[79]

Nonlinearities

As shown in Eq. (1), the tissue concentration can be reasonably assumed to be linearly related to the change in relaxation rate ΔR_2^*. This is actually not the case for the concentration time course measured inside an artery. It has been shown that, for the intravascular signal, a quadratic is a more appropriate model.[12,90] The situation is even more complex, because the quadratic coefficient in this relationship is hematocrit dependent,[90] such that a uniform value cannot be assumed for every case.[91]

A number of studies have now used a quadratic relationship to account for the nonlinearities in the AIF measurement.[22,60,91–93] Although most of these studies neglected the hematocrit dependency, it has been shown that a quadratic model should still produce more accurate AIF results than the linear model.[91]

A further possible solution to address the errors related with nonlinearities is to measure the AIF from the phase of the DSC-MRI signal[94–96]: it has been shown that phase changes are linearly

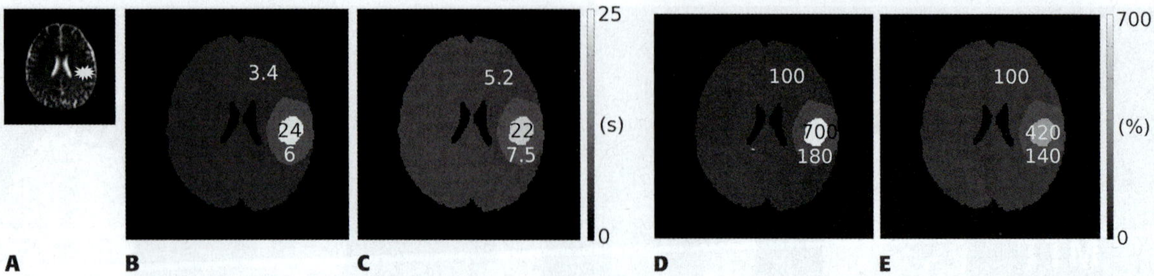

Figure 7-11. **Simulated example of the possible underestimation of the severity of a hypoperfusion abnormality by using delay-insensitive singular value decomposition (SVD), such as the oSVD method.[31]** **A:** Figure showing the location of a hypothetical vascular lesion (see region). As shown in ref.[31], deconvolution using oSVD will tend to underestimate the abnormality (since the degree of cerebral blood flow (CBF) underestimation decreases with increasing mean transit time (MTT); see Figure 2 in that article for more details). Based on the quantitative results shown in Figure 2 of ref.,[31] images **(B)** and **(C)** show the MTT for the true simulated case and for the measured MTT that would have been obtained using oSVD. Note: normal tissue was simulated with MTT = 3.4 seconds, the core of the lesion with 24 seconds, and the penumbra with 6 seconds—these values were chosen given that they were the values used for the simulation results shown in ref.[31]). The deconvolution-related errors associated with oSVD lead to loss of contrast (i.e., underestimation of the hypoperfusion abnormality)—cf. **(B)** and **(C)**. This loss of contrast is more easily appreciated when the MTT maps are displayed in relative units (relative to the normal contralateral side), as illustrated in **(D)** for the true simulated case and **(E)** for the measured relative MTT map using oSVD. For example, a 700% increase in MTT in the core of the lesion is only detected as just over half that severity. (Figure previously published in Calamante F. Arterial input function in perfusion MRI: a comprehensive review. *Prog Nucl Magn Reson Spectrosc* 2013;74:1–32, reprinted with permission of Elsevier, © 2013.)

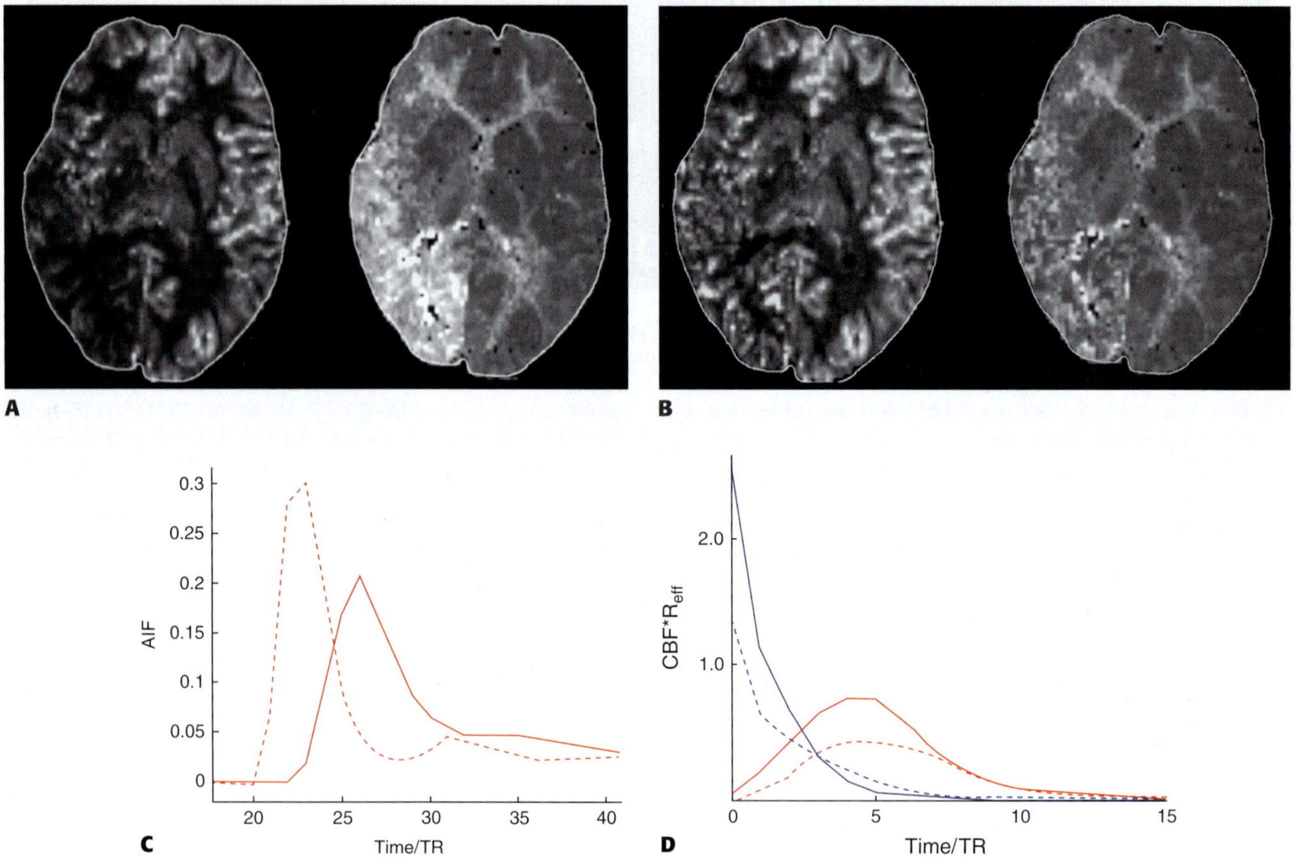

Figure 7-12. **Analysis of data from a patient with abnormalities in the right major arteries (left side of the images).** **A:** Cerebral blood flow (CBF, **left**) and mean transit time (MTT, **right**) maps calculated using a global arterial input function (AIF) taken from the left MCA. **B:** CBF **(left)** and MTT **(right)** maps calculated using a regionally defined AIF.[38] **C:** Global AIF (*dashed line*) and one of the regional AIF curves (*solid line*); there is clear delay and dispersion to the region supplied by this regional AIF. **D:** Two example impulse response functions (dashed and solid lines) extracted from the abnormal region deconvolved using the global (*red dispersed curves*) and regional (*blue nondispersed curves*) AIF. Blue curves show no dispersion, indicating that the regional AIF provides a more accurate CBF and MTT estimate, free from dispersion error. (Modified from a figure previously published in Willats L, Connelly A, Calamante F. Minimising the effects of bolus dispersion in bolus-tracking MRI. *NMR Biomed.* 2008;21(10):1126–1137, reprinted with permission of John Wiley & Sons, Ltd, © 2008.)

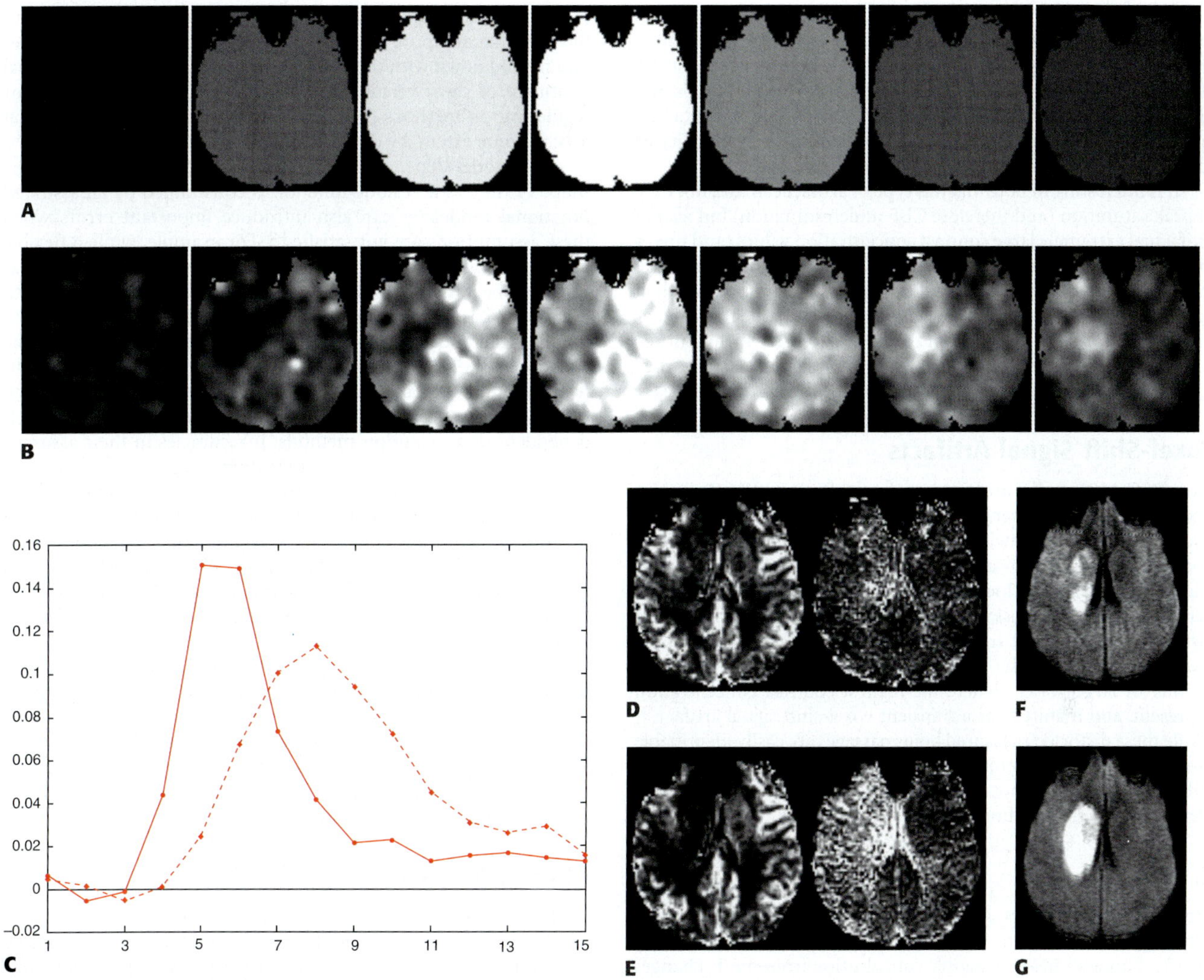

Figure 7-13. **Global arterial input function (AIF) and local AIF results for the data of a patient with right internal carotid dissection (left side of the images).** The set of images contains 7 time points of the global AIF **(A)** and local AIF **(B)** during the passage of the bolus. The local AIF data display heterogeneity throughout the slice, with bolus delay and dispersion in the right hemisphere. This is illustrated in the local AIF curves **(C)** obtained from a region in the contralateral hemisphere (*solid line*) and from an ipsilateral region (*dashed line*). Cerebral blood flow (CBF) and mean transit time (MTT) maps calculated by deconvolution using the local AIF **(D)** or global AIF data **(E)**. The global AIF methodology overestimates the extent and severity of the abnormality, with lower CBF and longer MTT (compared to the local AIF case) in regions where the local AIF was distorted. **(F)** Diffusion-weighted image acquired during the same examination; a region of abnormality (hyperintensity) can be readily appreciated. **(G)** Follow-up diffusion-weighted image, showing a small lesion expansion. (Figure previously published in Calamante F. Perfusion magnetic resonance imaging quantification in the brain. In: Badoer E, ed. *Visualization techniques. Vol 70. Neuromethods*. Humana Press; 2012:283–312, reprinted with kind permission of Springer Science+Business Media, © 2012.)

related to the concentration of the contrast agent and that they are hematocrit independent.[90] However, it should be noted that phase-based measurements from arteries are highly dependent on their relative orientation to the main magnetic field and are therefore usually carried out for the internal carotid artery (which is approximately parallel to the main magnetic field) or the M1 segment of the MCA (which is approximately perpendicular to the field).[12,70]

Signal Truncation

For the typical TEs used with GE EPI for DSC-MRI, particularly at 3 T, the relatively large contrast concentration in arteries can lead to a very large signal intensity decrease during the bolus passage. In fact, for some arterial voxels, the signal intensity can reach the noise floor level. This, in turn, leads to a truncation of the shape of the peak, when the concentration time course is calculated using the logarithm relationship from Eq. (2). This truncation of the peak can lead to CBF underestimation.

Various approaches have been proposed to address this source of error. Some involve modifications to the acquisition protocol, such as by using multiecho acquisitions with one of the TEs short enough to avoid saturation.[12,97,98] Other approaches simply identify (and then discard) the truncated AIF voxels by comparing the shape of the peak with that from the mean curve in a large region of interest in contralateral gray matter.[e] An alternative approach involves

[e]It should be noted that it is the characteristics of the candidate AIF voxels *relative* to the bolus passage in the rest of the brain that are of relevance when selecting an AIF.

correction of the shape of these truncated peaks.[62,99,100] For example, Brunecker et al.[100] proposed to discard the saturated time points and then to use transport–diffusion theory to reconstruct the shape of the peak. It should be noted, however, that all these methods that recover the shape of the peak from modeling part of the data rely on the validity of their assumed models and on the availability of sufficient unsaturated points for robust model fitting.

It is interesting to note that this type of artifact can lead not only to peak saturation (and therefore CBF underestimation) but also to artifactual extremely large contrast concentration values (and therefore CBF overestimation): for low SNR cases, the noise can make the measured signal intensity values very close to zero, which then produce very high measured concentration values, due to the logarithm relationship. Identification of these extremely high contrast concentration time courses is, however, very easy, given that they tend to have very unrealistic shapes, with a "spike" during the peak.

Voxel-Shift Signal Artifacts

Most DSC-MRI studies are based on the single-shot EPI acquisition. This sequence is very sensitive to magnetic field inhomogeneities due to its very low bandwidth per pixel in the phase-encoded direction.[101] This can lead to a special source of artifact in DSC-MRI, related to the transient local change in the magnetic field homogeneity induced by the passage of the bolus. This transient local field distortion can lead to a transient signal misregistration due to the low bandwidth per pixel. This artifact is mainly observed in the vicinity of large vessels, where the highest contrast concentration is present, and manifests as a transient voxel-shift signal artifact.[102] While these distorted measured bolus passages are easily identifiable (and the voxels are, therefore, unlikely to be selected as AIF candidates), it should be noted that DSC quantification will be completely meaningless in those voxels.

T_1 effects

Most DSC-MRI studies are currently carried out using a single-echo acquisition and the contrast concentration calculated using Eq. (2). This assumes a negligible contribution from the T_1 changes induced by the contrast agent. The validity of this assumption depends on many factors, including the sequence type and sequence parameters, field strength, and the status of the BBB. For most clinical studies, ensuring a negligible T_1 effect can be easily achieved by a careful selection of the flip angle,[103] due to the relatively long repetition time used to accommodate a large number of slices for brain coverage. Alternatively, the contribution from T_1 effects can be minimized by preinjecting a small dose of contrast agent,[104] although at the expense of an increased total volume of injected contrast agent.

Apart from sources of error related to the AIF measurement, there are a number of other possible important sources of error in DSC-MRI quantification. These are described below (for artifacts related to BBB leakage, see next section).

Deconvolution-Related Errors

As mentioned in section From Convolution to Deconvolution above, the deconvolution must be carried out with some form of regularization (e.g., the cutoff of the SVD expansion for the popular SVD algorithm).[26] Since regularization works by imposing some kind of constrain or "filtering" to the deconvolved solution, it can lead to errors in DSC-MRI quantification.

For example, most deconvolution methods have more difficulties deconvolving tissue concentration time courses with very short MTT, given that the corresponding tissue residue function decreases very fast, which in turn would require high-frequency components to characterize it properly; these high-frequency components are the ones that are more sensitive to the presence of noise and therefore filtered down with the regularization.[24,32,34,38,77] This differential treatment of short versus long MTT cases is more significant for regularization methods that are fixed[26] and can be ameliorated, at least to some extent, by data-driven regularization methods.[32,38,39]

The model-dependent deconvolution methods, for which the shape of the tissue residue function is constrained by an assumed functional model,[26,37] can also introduce important errors when these assumptions are not satisfied.[26] For example, while a flexible vascular model based on a gamma probability density function was shown to be a robust deconvolution method when combined with a Bayesian-based formalism,[37] the family of functions described by that model do not include peak-shaped curves required to describe a dispersed residue function (see Bolus Dispersion above). A modification to the vascular model to address this limitation has been proposed,[79] but it illustrates the general problem with model-dependent deconvolution methods: inaccuracies in their assumptions can lead to important quantification errors.

A further source of error related to the deconvolution is that associated with discretization errors. The calculated impulse response function is commonly obtained at a relatively coarse temporal resolution (approximately 1.5 to 2 seconds), which can therefore lead to errors in the estimate of its maximum (i.e., CBF) and the location of its peak (i.e., T_{max}). One approach to address this source of error involves interpolation of the calculated impulse response function.[51,105] Alternatively, a certain model can be assumed *after* performing the deconvolution[f] (e.g., for the tissue residue function), which is then fitted to the deconvolved solution to obtain a better estimate of the maximum of the impulse response function[106]; this method also attempts to minimize the underestimation introduce by regularization. Note, however, that this method relies on the validity of the assumed model used for the fitting.

Motion Artifacts

Although DSC-MRI is a relatively fast MRI method, with a total acquisition time of the order of 1 minute, it can be severely affected my motion due to its dynamic MRI nature. Motion is usually not a problem for the individual images that form the temporal dynamics, because a single-shot EPI is most often used. However, it can introduce major artifacts in the characterization of the concentration time course. The highest risk of motion can occur at the time of bolus injection, particularly with very ill or uncooperative patients. Due to the fast transit of the bolus from the site of injection to the brain, this motion can seriously affect the measurement of the baseline just before the arrival of the peak or, even more problematic, it can affect the measurement of the initial part of the peak, which is the one that has the most influence for DSC-MRI quantification.[17]

While motion correction can ameliorate these errors,[107] it is not always the solution, and through-slice motion can render a DSC-MRI study unusable. The main problem relates to the fact that DSC-MRI studies are commonly carried out using a multislice acquisition with a slice gap (to ensure whole brain coverage with a reasonable temporal resolution); artifacts related to spin history due to through-plane motion cannot be, therefore, corrected by standard rigid body motion correction methods.

For studies that involve very ill patients or very uncooperative subjects, the use of a three-dimensional acquisition method[108–110] can be a very useful acquisition alternative to EPI for DSC-MRI studies.

---

[f]Note that a model-independent deconvolution method can still be used. The assumed model is only used to fit the solution calculated after deconvolution, to recover its high-frequency components.[106]

Macrovascular Artifacts

The use of a GE sequence for most DSC-MRI studies, as it is the case with GE EPI, makes the acquisition sensitive to both microvasculature (i.e., the capillary bed) and macrovasculature (i.e., the medium-to-large vessels).[11,111] However, cerebral perfusion refers only to the blow flow at the capillary level, and the macrovascular contribution is, therefore, an artifact to CBF quantification.

In practice, this macrovascular contribution manifests as very bright foci in the calculated CBF maps in an around arteries, which can make interpretation of the perfusion status in cortical areas very complicated: the high arterial intensity dominates the contrast of the CBF maps. It can also lead to errors in CBF quantification, because the measured values will be highly influenced by the degree of partial volume with these bright foci. For example, it may lead to CBF underestimation in acute stroke patients when quantifying perfusion in relative units (e.g., relative to the homologous region in the contralateral side), given that the contralateral region often has more areas with macrovascular artifacts.

Various methods have been proposed to deal with this source of artifact, including the use of independent component analysis to try to identify (and then remove) the macrovascular contribution,[112,113] or to modify the kinetic model by explicitly including a macrovascular contribution within a Bayesian framework.[114] However, the accuracy of any of these methods remains to be established, and the methods are not in widespread use.

DSC-MRI in the Presence of Contrast Leakage

When the BBB is intact, the contrast agent injected during a DSC-MRI study can be considered as an intravascular bolus. This has two main advantages: (i) the compartmentalization of the contrast agent enhances the T_2^* effect, leading to a relatively large contrast-to-noise ratio, and (ii) the kinetic modeling is greatly simplified because it does not require a term describing the extravascular compartment or the exchange between the intra- and extravascular compartments.

However, when the BBB is compromised and there is leakage of the contrast agent outside the intravascular space, the induced susceptibility effect is modified and the kinetic model used for DSC-MRI quantification must be extended to include the extravascular effect.[64]

The leakage of the contrast agent can modify the susceptibility effect to such a degree that, depending on the sequence type and parameters and the DSC-MRI protocol,[115] the T_2^* relaxation effect may not be anymore the dominant effect, and the larger T_1 effect can lead to considerable signal enhancement (i.e., signal intensity higher than the baseline value) (e.g., see Fig. 7.14). In such cases, if the nonnegligible T_1 effect is not accounted for (e.g., if the relationship in Eq. (2) is used), quantification can lead to the nonphysical situation of negative contrast agent concentration values.

In order to account for the T_1 effect, several alternative approaches have been proposed, including a careful choice of the sequence parameters, the use of a prebolus of contrast agent to effectively "saturate" the T_1 effect, and/or the use of multiecho sequence to quantify the change in T_2^* directly and eliminating the T_1 term.[104,116–118]

It should be noted that, even when the T_1 effects are properly accounted for (e.g., by using a double-echo sequence),[117] the resulting measured ΔR_2^* time curve overestimates the true ΔR_2^* curve, leading to an overestimation of CBV.[117,119] Therefore, it should be emphasized that a protocol that properly accounts for the T_1 effect must be combined with a postprocessing correction of the modified T_2^* effects. The latter involves modifying the kinetic model to include the contribution from the exchange with the extravascular contrast agent.[117,119–122]

The most commonly used modified model was that proposed by Weisskoff et al.[123] in the 1994 meeting of the Society of Magnetic Resonance.[g] However, this leakage correction method assumes, among other things, that MTT in the BBB-compromised region is the same as that in the normal tissue; this can lead to CBV underestimation when MTT is significantly longer in the BBB-compromised area.[121,122] A modified approach was more recently proposed by Bjornerud et al.[121] to correct for this effect, which is independent of MTT of the affected tissue.

Interestingly, several studies have now shown that, while the CBV errors due to BBB leakage can be very substantial, the corresponding errors in CBF quantification are much less severe.[117,119]

Some of these modified kinetic models, which include the exchange with the extravascular compartment, not only provide also a means to estimate CBV, CBF, MTT, and the other hemodynamic parameters described in section DSC-MRI Parameters but also provide an estimate of the tissue permeability (or a parameter related to permeability).[117,119–121,123] However, although permeability measurements can indeed be carried out using DSC-MRI, they are more commonly obtained using dynamic contrast-enhanced MRI, which is based on T_1-based acquisition methods and a multicompartment modeling.[124–126] Furthermore, quantification of contrast agent concentration using T_1-based sequences has the further benefit of being better behaved, without many of the criticisms of susceptibility-based methods.[64]

DSC-MRI Analysis: Practical Implementation

As may have been appreciated from the description in the previous sections, a rigorous analysis of DSC-MRI data involves a certain degree of specialist expertise. This, in principle, can limit the widespread use of optimal advanced methods (e.g., AIF selection methods, deconvolution algorithms, BBB correction techniques) in nonspecialized centers. To address this issue, a number of automatic DSC-MRI tools have been recently developed,[22,63,127] which perform the various steps involved in the DSC-MRI analysis without requiring user input.

One of the disadvantages of these methods, however, is that they tend to be used as "black box" methods, where the user performs no quality control of the results from the intermediate steps, and only the final maps are assessed. Given that several artifacts can lead to major errors in DSC-MRI quantification (see section Sources of Error and Technical Limitations for more details), no automatic DSC-MRI method can be expected to be flawless. It is therefore highly recommended that, at least, a small degree of quality control is carried out by the user to assess the outcome of key steps in the DSC-MRI pipeline. For example, the user should assess the data quality of the input data (e.g., to determine the presence of severe motion or reduced contrast-to-noise ratio in the data), the shape and location of the automatically selected AIF, etc.

An issue to consider when implementing or when choosing an automatic algorithm is that of its processing time. This is particular the case for certain clinical applications, such as in acute stroke imaging, where there is very limited time available before a treatment decision must be done. In particular, in acute stroke, this is related to the "time is brain" concept, which has been elegantly quantified by Saver.[128] In this study, it was estimated that 1.9 million neurons, 14 billion synapses, and 12 km of myelinated

[g]A detailed description of this model, and the assumptions involved, was later included in an Appendix of a publication by the same authors.[120]

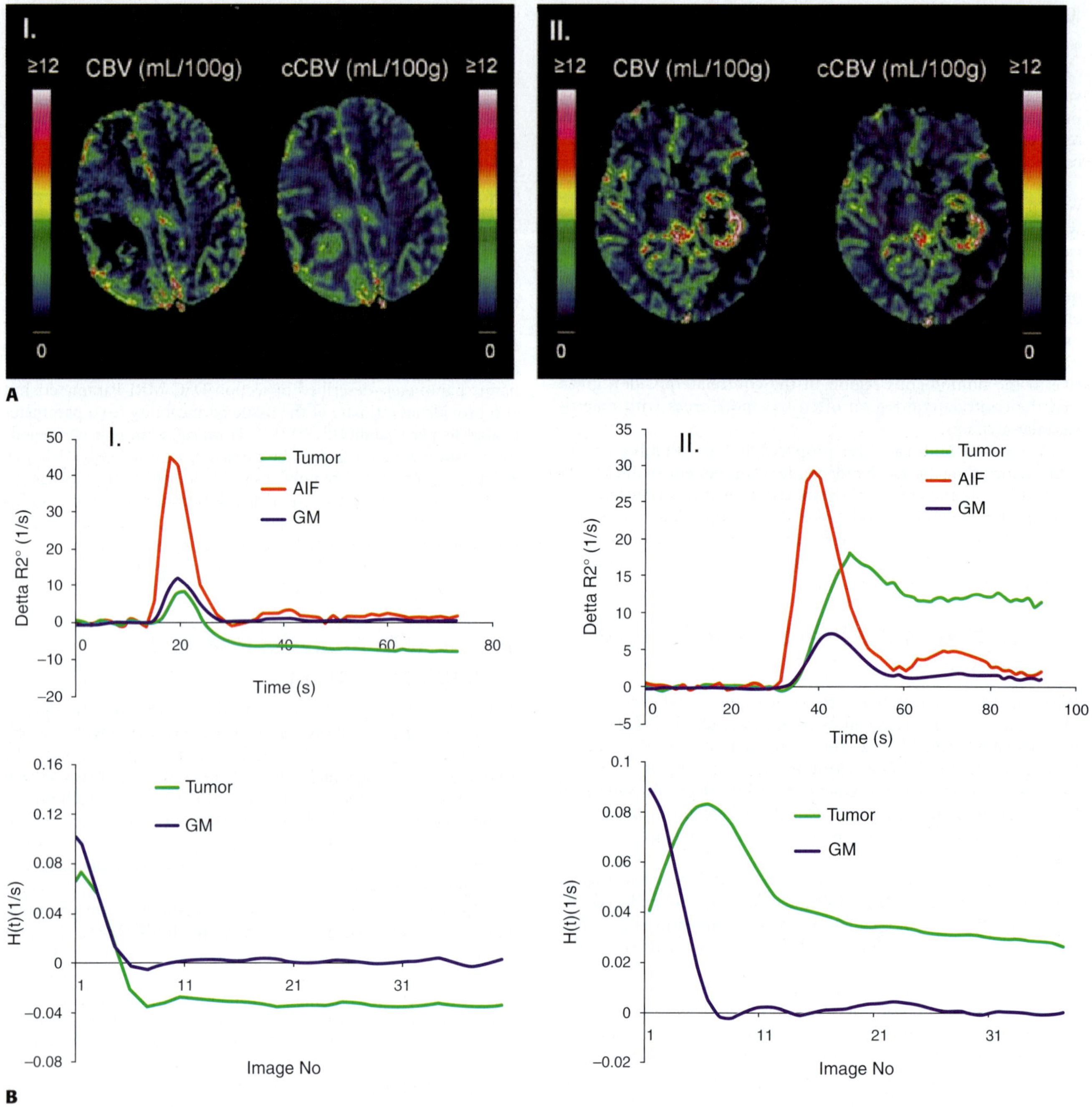

Figure 7-14. In vivo examples of T_1-dominated (case I, left column) and T_2*-dominated (case II, right column) extravasation effects. **A:** For each case, this figure shows the cerebral blood volume maps calculated without correction (CBV) and with leakage correction (cCBV). **B:** For each case, this figure shows the ΔR_2* profiles **(top row)** and residue functions **(bottom row)** obtained from tumor regions of interest. If left uncorrected, the CBV would be underestimated using the ΔR_2* profiles dominated by T_1 extravasation effects (case I) and overestimated using the ΔR_2* profiles dominated by T_2* extravasation effects (case II). AIF, arterial input function; GM, gray matter. (Image kindly provided by Dr. Atle Bjornerud, and modified from a figure previously published in Bjornerud A, Sorensen AG, Mouridsen K, Emblem KE. T1- and T2*-dominant extravasation correction in DSC-MRI: part I--theoretical considerations and implications for assessment of tumor hemodynamic properties. *J Cereb Blood Flow Metab* 2011;31(10):2041–2053, with permission of Macmillan Publishers Ltd., © 2011.)

fibers are lost each minute following a typical large vessel stroke. Interestingly, this corresponds to 720 km of myelinated fibers destroyed each hour, that is, 720 km/h; a typical stroke, therefore, destroys myelinated fibers at an effective speed of *twice* the top speed of a Formula One car! This illustrates the time constraints in acute stroke imaging.

DSC-MRI Pipeline: Typical Example

In this section, the various steps involved in the DSC-MRI analysis pipeline are described for a typical example study, for which it is assumed that suitable data have been acquired. For example, for a 80-kg adult subject, this usually involves data acquired using a GE

EPI sequence (with a temporal resolution of 1.5 seconds), following the injection in the right antecubital vein (using a power injector at a rate of 5 mL/s) of 16 mL of contrast agent (i.e., a dose of 0.2 mL/kg), immediately followed by the injection (at the same rate) of 20 mL of saline flush. The EPI data set consists of, for example, 80 volumes of 20 slices (covering the whole brain), where the contrast injection was carried out after acquisition of the 10th volume. For simplicity, in this example, we will assume that the BBB is intact. (Note: a simple way to determine the presence of contrast leakage is by assessing the presence of signal enhancement on a postcontrast T_1-weighted image[104]; for the case of BBB leakage, the data acquisition and analysis must be modified as described in section DSC-MRI in the Presence of Contrast Leakage.)

The initial step in the analysis pipeline is the assessment of data quality, which can include the following:

- *Determining the presence of image motion*: This can be easily assessed, for example, by playing the temporal image data as cine MRI. If significant image motion is detected, then motion correction should be carried out. Alternatively, if this is not possible (or if through-plane motion is present), then the actual temporal location of the motion should be identified, in order to determine whether part of the DSC-MRI data set can still be used. For example, if the motion occurs during the baseline and before the bolus arrives to the brain, then the baseline range could be restricted to those values after the motion has finished. A further case when the data can still be used is that when the motion occurs after the first passage of the bolus (i.e., during the "tail" of the concentration time course). In that case, the data can be truncated until before the motion occurs.[h] However, if the residual motion is very severe, or if it occurs during the first part of the bolus (before the arrival of the peak), the study may need to be discarded.
- *Ensuring a reasonable level of contrast-to-noise ratio*: This can be easily determined by evaluating the time course of a whole brain region of interest, which has relatively very high SNR and provides a general indication of the shape of the bolus in that subject. For example, the quality of the DSC-MRI data can be then determined by measuring the ratio of the maximum concentration relative to the noise in the baseline concentration (or similarly by the ratio of the maximum signal drop to the noise in the baseline signal). This approach can be used to identify cases where the peak is very broad and with very low concentration (e.g., due to a slow injection, low cardiac output, vascular abnormalities), for which the quality of the resulting deconvolution maps is expected to be much inferior. It should be also noted that such low-quality data should ideally be analyzed with a different degree of regularization in the deconvolution (see section From Convolution to Deconvolution for more details).
- *Assessing the presence of bolus delay*: This can also be easily determined by playing the data as cine MRI.[72] If significant delay is detected, then a delay-insensitive deconvolution algorithm should be selected to avoid introducing substantial errors.

The next step in the pipeline is the quantification of the contrast agent concentration, which is usually achieved by assuming a linear relationship (see Eq. (1)). This, in turn, requires measurement of the baseline signal intensity (see Eq. (2)), which involves averaging the signal intensity before the arrival of the bolus (but after a steady state has been achieved, i.e., usually having to discard the first two to three temporal volumes). It is important to ensure that there are no substantial residual motion artifacts when estimating the baseline intensity, given that, otherwise, the voxel-wise baseline values will not be appropriate.

Following this step, the AIF must be measured. For simplicity, we will assume here that a robust automatic AIF method is used (which searches for AIF candidates based on a combination of arterial-like features of the concentration time course). It is recommended that a number of voxels are averaged to calculate the AIF, to help increase the SNR. (Note that errors in the AIF can have major effect in CBF quantification.) Given that automatic AIF methods can be subjected to errors, it is important that the user checks both the shape of the selected AIF and the location of the chosen voxels.

Once the AIF has been measured, the deconvolution step in the pipeline can be carried out. If the degree of regularization is not determined by the data quality themselves (i.e., a data-driven method), then the user must select a suitable level of regularization based on their specific DSC-MRI protocol, data quality, and previously published recommendations/guidelines for that algorithm (e.g., this could include choosing a specific threshold for the truncation of the singular value expansion in the standard SVD method,[26] where, for example, a higher threshold is required for lower SNR data[27]).

The deconvolution step calculates the impulse response function for each voxel in the brain, which can be used to measure CBF (from its maximum value) and T_{max} (from its TTP). In order to measure MTT, we need a measure of CBV, which can be calculated by the area ratio from Eq. (4).

The computed CBF and CBV values can be reported as relative values (e.g., by referencing relative to the corresponding values in a manually drawn contralateral region of interest). Alternatively, the values can be scaled to absolute units by using a subject-specific scaling factor (see section Absolute Quantification for more details).

While this effectively ends the DSC analysis pipeline, the resulting maps are often used in combination with other MRI measures. For example, in acute stroke imaging (one of the most common applications for DSC-MRI), the DSC-MRI maps are used to calculate the so-called diffusion–perfusion mismatch (the spatial mismatch between the abnormality in the diffusion MRI data and the abnormality in the DSC-MRI data). This therefore requires two extra main steps for the DSC-MRI data:

- Defining the DSC-MRI abnormality: this is usually done either by manual delineation of the region of abnormality in the map (e.g., the area with increased MTT)[129] or by thresholding a DSC-MRI map (e.g., by using a T_{max} threshold[130]). More complex methods to define the mismatch area are also available, which combine the information of multiple DSC-MRI maps and diffusion MRI data in predictor models of infarction.[131,132] The means to define the DSC-MRI abnormality is in fact an area of active research in acute stroke imaging.[133]
- Coregistering the DSC-MRI data to the diffusion MRI data, to determine the mismatch. For simplicity, this step is often not carried out and the mismatch is estimated from the difference in volume between the perfusion MRI and diffusion MRI abnormalities.

Acknowledgments

I am grateful to the National Health and Medical Research Council (NHMRC) of Australia, the Australian Research Council (ARC), and the Victorian Government's Operational Infrastructure Support Grant for their support. I also thank Kim Mouridsen (Aarhus University, Denmark), Juan R. Cebral and Susan Wright (Krasnow Institute for Advanced Studies, George Mason University, USA), Ona Wu (Massachusetts General Hospital, USA), and Atle Bjornerud (Oslo University Hospital, Norway) for their contribution to materials used in the figures for this article.

[h]Note however that careful consideration should be made if there are areas with very large bolus delay and/or very prolonged MTT, because the peak in these areas could be truncated (in time) to a much larger extent than other areas, leading to errors in CBV and MTT.[73]

REFERENCES

1. **Villringer A, Rosen BR, Belliveau JW, et al.** Dynamic imaging with lanthanide chelates in normal brain: contrast due to magnetic susceptibility effects. *Magn Reson Med* 1988;6(2):164–174.
2. **Rosen BR, Belliveau JW, Chien D.** Perfusion imaging by nuclear magnetic resonance. *Magn Reson Q* 1989;5(4):263–281.
3. **Rosen BR, Belliveau JW, Vevea JM, et al.** Perfusion imaging with NMR contrast agents. *Magn Reson Med* 1990;14(2):249–265.
4. **Rosen BR, Belliveau JW, Buchbinder BR, et al.** Contrast agents and cerebral hemodynamics. *Magn Reson Med* 1991;19(2):285–292.
5. **Belliveau JW, Rosen BR, Kantor HL, et al.** Functional cerebral imaging by susceptibility-contrast NMR. *Magn Reson Med* 1990;14(3):538–546.
6. **Fisel CR, Ackerman JL, Buxton RB, et al.** MR contrast due to microscopically heterogeneous magnetic susceptibility: numerical simulations and applications to cerebral physiology. *Magn Reson Med* 1991;17(2): 336–347.
7. **Wintermark M, Albers GW, Alexandrov AV, et al.** Acute stroke imaging research roadmap. *Stroke* 2008;39(5):1621–1628.
8. **Kaewlai R, Abujudeh H.** Nephrogenic systemic fibrosis. *AJR Am J Roentgenol* 2012;199(1):W17–W23.
9. **ACR Committee on Drugs and Contrast Media.** *ACR manual on contrast media.* Version 9. American College of Radiology; 2013. Available at: http://www.acr.org/quality-safety/resources/contrast-manual
10. **Leiner T, Kucharczyk W.** NSF prevention in clinical practice: summary of recommendations and guidelines in the United States, Canada, and Europe. *J Magn Reson Imaging* 2009;30(6):1357–1363.
11. **Weisskoff RM, Zuo CS, Boxerman JL, et al.** Microscopic susceptibility variation and transverse relaxation: theory and experiment. *Magn Reson Med* 1994;31(6):601–610.
12. **Van Osch MJP, Vonken EPA, Viergever MA, et al.** Measuring the arterial input function with gradient echo sequences. *Magn Reson Med* 2003;49(6):1067–1076.
13. **Kiselev VG.** Transverse relaxation effect of MRI contrast agents: a crucial issue for quantitative measurements of cerebral perfusion. *J Magn Reson Imaging* 2005;22(6):693–696.
14. **Calamante F, Thomas DL, Pell GS, et al.** Measuring cerebral blood flow using magnetic resonance imaging techniques. *J Cereb Blood Flow Metab* 1999;19(7):701–735.
15. **Weisskoff RM, Chesler D, Boxerman JL, et al.** Pitfalls in MR measurement of tissue blood flow with intravascular tracers: which mean transit time? *Magn Reson Med* 1993;29(4):553–558.
16. **Perthen JE, Calamante F, Gadian DG, et al.** Is quantification of bolus tracking MRI reliable without deconvolution? *Magn Reson Med* 2002;47(1):61–67.
17. **Calamante F.** Arterial input function in perfusion MRI: a comprehensive review. *Prog Nucl Magn Reson Spectrosc* 2013;74:1–32.
18. **Murase K, Kikuchi K, Miki H, et al.** Determination of arterial input function using fuzzy clustering for quantification of cerebral blood flow with dynamic susceptibility contrast-enhanced MR imaging. *J Magn Reson Imaging* 2001;13(5):797–806.
19. **Carroll TJ, Rowley HA, Haughton VM.** Automatic calculation of the arterial input function for cerebral perfusion imaging with MR imaging. *Radiology* 2003;227(2):593–600.
20. **Mlynash M, Eyngorn I, Bammer R, et al.** Automated method for generating the arterial input function on perfusion-weighted MR imaging: validation in patients with stroke. *AJNR Am J Neuroradiol* 2005;26(6):1479–1486.
21. **Mouridsen K, Christensen S, Gyldensted L, et al.** Automatic selection of arterial input function using cluster analysis. *Magn Reson Med* 2006;55(3):524–531.
22. **Straka M, Albers GW, Bammer R.** Real-time diffusion-perfusion mismatch analysis in acute stroke. *J Magn Reson Imaging* 2010;32(5): 1024–1037.
23. **Meier P, Zierler KL.** On the theory of the indicator-dilution method for measurement of blood flow and volume. *J Appl Physiol* 1954;6(12):731–744.
24. **Calamante F, Straka M, Willats L.** Practical aspects of deconvolution. In: Bammer R, ed. *MR & CT perfusion imaging: clinical applications and theoretical principles.* 1st ed. Lippincott Williams & Wilkins; 2015: Chapter 36. Riverwoods, IL
25. **Hansen P.** Regularization tools: a MATLAB package for analysis and solution of discrete ill-posed problems. *Numerical Algorithms* 1994;6(1):1–35.
26. **Ostergaard L, Weisskoff RM, Chesler DA, et al.** High resolution measurement of cerebral blood flow using intravascular tracer bolus passages. Part I: Mathematical approach and statistical analysis. *Magn Reson Med* 1996;36(5):715–725.
27. **Liu HL, Pu Y, Liu Y, et al.** Cerebral blood flow measurement by dynamic contrast MRI using singular value decomposition with an adaptive threshold. *Magn Reson Med* 1999;42(1):167–172.
28. **Vonken EP, Beekman FJ, Bakker CJ, et al.** Maximum likelihood estimation of cerebral blood flow in dynamic susceptibility contrast MRI. *Magn Reson Med* 1999;41(2):343–350.
29. **Murase K, Shinohara M, Yamazaki Y.** Accuracy of deconvolution analysis based on singular value decomposition for quantification of cerebral blood flow using dynamic susceptibility contrast-enhanced magnetic resonance imaging. *Phys Med Biol* 2001;46(12):3147–3159.
30. **Andersen IK, Szymkowiak A, Rasmussen CE, et al.** Perfusion quantification using Gaussian process deconvolution. *Magn Reson Med* 2002; 48(2):351–361.
31. **Wu O, Østergaard L, Weisskoff RM, et al.** Tracer arrival timing-insensitive technique for estimating flow in MR perfusion-weighted imaging using singular value decomposition with a block-circulant deconvolution matrix. *Magn Reson Med* 2003;50(1):164–174.
32. **Calamante F, Gadian DG, Connelly A.** Quantification of bolus-tracking MRI: improved characterization of the tissue residue function using Tikhonov regularization. *Magn Reson Med* 2003;50(6):1237–1247.
33. **Knutsson L, Ståhlberg F, Wirestam R.** Aspects on the accuracy of cerebral perfusion parameters obtained by dynamic susceptibility contrast MRI: a simulation study. *Magn Reson Imaging* 2004;22(6):789–798.
34. **Willats L, Connelly A, Calamante F.** Improved deconvolution of perfusion MRI data in the presence of bolus delay and dispersion. *Magn Reson Med* 2006;56(1):146–156.
35. **Carpenter TK, Armitage PA, Bastin ME, et al.** DSC perfusion MRI-Quantification and reduction of systematic errors arising in areas of reduced cerebral blood flow. *Magn Reson Med* 2006;55(6): 1342–1349.
36. **Sourbron S, Luypaert R, Van Schuerbeek P, et al.** Deconvolution of dynamic contrast-enhanced MRI data by linear inversion: choice of the regularization parameter. *Magn Reson Med* 2004;52(1):209–213.
37. **Mouridsen K, Friston K, Hjort N, et al.** Bayesian estimation of cerebral perfusion using a physiological model of microvasculature. *Neuroimage* 2006;33(2):570–579.
38. **Willats L, Connelly A, Calamante F.** Minimising the effects of bolus dispersion in bolus-tracking MRI. *NMR Biomed* 2008;21(10): 1126–1137.
39. **Mehndiratta A, Macintosh BJ, Crane DE, et al.** A control point interpolation method for the non-parametric quantification of cerebral haemodynamics from dynamic susceptibility contrast MRI. *Neuroimage* 2012;64C:560–570.
40. **Smith MR, Lu H, Trochet S, et al.** Removing the effect of SVD algorithmic artifacts present in quantitative MR perfusion studies. *Magn Reson Med* 2004;51(3):631–634.
41. **Rempp KA, Brix G, Wenz F, et al.** Quantification of regional cerebral blood flow and volume with dynamic susceptibility contrast-enhanced MR imaging. *Radiology* 1994;193(3):637–641.
42. **Schreiber WG, Gückel F, Stritzke P, et al.** Cerebral blood flow and cerebrovascular reserve capacity: estimation by dynamic magnetic resonance imaging. *J Cereb Blood Flow Metab* 1998;18(10):1143–1156.
43. **Grüner R, Taxt T.** Iterative blind deconvolution in magnetic resonance brain perfusion imaging. *Magn Reson Med* 2006;55(4):805–815.
44. **Zanderigo F, Bertoldo A, Pillonetto G, et al.** Nonlinear stochastic regularization to characterize tissue residue function in bolus-tracking MRI: assessment and comparison with SVD, block-circulant SVD, and Tikhonov. *IEEE Trans Biomed Eng* 2009;56(5):1287–1297.
45. **Calamante F, Ganesan V, Kirkham FJ, et al.** MR perfusion imaging in Moyamoya Syndrome: potential implications for clinical evaluation of occlusive cerebrovascular disease. *Stroke* 2001;32(12):2810–2816.
46. **Calamante F, Gadian DG, Connelly A.** Quantification of perfusion using bolus tracking magnetic resonance imaging in stroke: assumptions, limitations, and potential implications for clinical use. *Stroke* 2002;33(4):1146–1151.
47. **Calamante F, Willats L, Gadian DG, et al.** Bolus delay and dispersion in perfusion MRI: implications for tissue predictor models in stroke. *Magn Reson Med* 2006;55(5):1180–1185.

48. **Willats L, Calamante F.** The 39 steps: evading error and deciphering the secrets for accurate dynamic susceptibility contrast MRI. *NMR Biomed* 2013;26(8):913–931.
49. **Calamante F.** Bolus dispersion issues related to the quantification of perfusion MRI data. *J Magn Reson Imaging* 2005;22(6):718–722.
50. **Kidwell CS, Saver JL, Mattiello J, et al.** Thrombolytic reversal of acute human cerebral ischemic injury shown by diffusion/perfusion magnetic resonance imaging. *Ann Neurol* 2000;47(4):462–469.
51. **Calamante F, Christensen S, Desmond PM, et al.** The physiological significance of the time-to-maximum (Tmax) parameter in perfusion MRI. *Stroke* 2010;41(6):1169–1174.
52. **Albers GW, Thijs VN, Wechsler L, et al.** Magnetic resonance imaging profiles predict clinical response to early reperfusion: the diffusion and perfusion imaging evaluation for understanding stroke evolution (DEFUSE) study. *Ann Neurol* 2006;60(5):508–517.
53. **Davis SM, Donnan GA, Parsons MW, et al.** Effects of alteplase beyond 3 h after stroke in the Echoplanar Imaging Thrombolytic Evaluation Trial (EPITHET): a placebo-controlled randomised trial. *Lancet Neurol* 2008;7(4):299–309.
54. **Lansberg MG, Straka M, Kemp S, et al.** MRI profile and response to endovascular reperfusion after stroke (DEFUSE 2): a prospective cohort study. *Lancet Neurol* 2012;11(10):860–867.
55. **Ma H, Parsons MW, Christensen S, et al.** A multicentre, randomized, double-blinded, placebo-controlled Phase III study to investigate EXtending the time for Thrombolysis in Emergency Neurological Deficits (EXTEND). *Int J Stroke* 2012;7(1):74–80.
56. **Wintermark M, Sesay M, Barbier E, et al.** Comparative overview of brain perfusion imaging techniques. *Stroke* 2005;36(9):e83–e99.
57. **Calamante F.** Artifacts and pitfalls in perfusion MR imaging. In: Gillard J, Waldman A, Barker PB, eds. *Clinical MR neuroimaging. Physiological and functional techniques*. 2nd ed. Cambridge University Press; 2009:137–155. Cambridge, UK
58. **Sakaie KE, Shin W, Curtin KR, et al.** Method for improving the accuracy of quantitative cerebral perfusion imaging. *J Magn Reson Imaging* 2005;21(5):512–519.
59. **Shin W, Horowitz S, Ragin A, et al.** Quantitative cerebral perfusion using dynamic susceptibility contrast MRI: evaluation of reproducibility and age- and gender-dependence with fully automatic image postprocessing algorithm. *Magn Reson Med* 2007;58(6):1232–1241.
60. **Zaharchuk G, Straka M, Marks MP, et al.** Combined arterial spin label and dynamic susceptibility contrast measurement of cerebral blood flow. *Magn Reson Med* 2010;63(6):1548–1556.
61. **Bonekamp D, Degaonkar M, Barker PB.** Quantitative cerebral blood flow in dynamic susceptibility contrast MRI using total cerebral flow from phase contrast magnetic resonance angiography. *Magn Reson Med* 2011;66(1):57–66.
62. **Knutsson L, Börjesson S, Larsson E-M, et al.** Absolute quantification of cerebral blood flow in normal volunteers: correlation between Xe-133 SPECT and dynamic susceptibility contrast MRI. *J Magn Reson Imaging* 2007;26(4):913–920.
63. **Bjørnerud A, Emblem KE.** A fully automated method for quantitative cerebral hemodynamic analysis using DSC-MRI. *J Cereb Blood Flow Metab* 2010;30(5):1066–1078.
64. **Jackson A, Buckley DL, Parker GJM, Baert AL.** *Dynamic contrast-enhanced magnetic resonance imaging in oncology*. Springer; 2005. Berlin, Germany.
65. **Ostergaard L, Sorensen AG, Kwong KK, et al.** High resolution measurement of cerebral blood flow using intravascular tracer bolus passages. Part II: Experimental comparison and preliminary results. *Magn Reson Med* 1996;36(5):726–736.
66. **Ostergaard L, Johannsen P, Høst-Poulsen P, et al.** Cerebral blood flow measurements by magnetic resonance imaging bolus tracking: comparison with [(15)O]H2O positron emission tomography in humans. *J Cereb Blood Flow Metab* 1998;18(9):935–940.
67. **Van Osch MJP, Van der Grond J, Bakker CJG.** Partial volume effects on arterial input functions: shape and amplitude distortions and their correction. *J Magn Reson Imaging* 2005;22(6):704–709.
68. **Bleeker EJW, Van Osch MJP, Connelly A, et al.** New criterion to aid manual and automatic selection of the arterial input function in dynamic susceptibility contrast MRI. *Magn Reson Med* 2011;65(2):448–456.
69. **Duhamel G, Schlaug G, Alsop DC.** Measurement of arterial input functions for dynamic susceptibility contrast magnetic resonance imaging using echoplanar images: comparison of physical simulations with in vivo results. *Magn Reson Med* 2006;55(3):514–523.
70. **Bleeker EJW, Van Buchem MA, Webb AG, et al.** Phase-based arterial input function measurements for dynamic susceptibility contrast MRI. *Magn Reson Med* 2010;64(2):358–368.
71. **Bleeker EJW, Van Buchem MA, Van Osch MJP.** Optimal location for arterial input function measurements near the middle cerebral artery in first-pass perfusion MRI. *J Cereb Blood Flow Metab* 2009;29(4):840–852.
72. **Christensen S, Calamante F, Hjort N, et al.** Inferring origin of vascular supply from tracer arrival timing patterns using bolus tracking MRI. *J Magn Reson Imaging* 2008;27(6):1371–1381.
73. **Calamante F, Gadian DG, Connelly A.** Delay and dispersion effects in dynamic susceptibility contrast MRI: simulations using singular value decomposition. *Magn Reson Med* 2000;44(3):466–473.
74. **Wu O, Østergaard L, Koroshetz WJ, et al.** Effects of tracer arrival time on flow estimates in MR perfusion-weighted imaging. *Magn Reson Med* 2003;50(4):856–864.
75. **Ibaraki M, Shimosegawa E, Toyoshima H, et al.** Effect of regional tracer delay on CBF in healthy subjects measured with dynamic susceptibility contrast-enhanced MRI: comparison with 15O-PET. *Magn Reson Med Sci* 2005;4(1):27–34.
76. **Rose SE, Janke AL, Griffin M, et al.** Improving the prediction of final infarct size in acute stroke with bolus delay-corrected perfusion MRI measures. *J Magn Reson Imaging* 2004;20(6):941–947.
77. **Salluzzi M, Frayne R, Smith MR.** An alternative viewpoint of the similarities and differences of SVD and FT deconvolution algorithms used for quantitative MR perfusion studies. *Magn Reson Imaging* 2005; 23(3):481–492.
78. **Calamante F, Yim PJ, Cebral JR.** Estimation of bolus dispersion effects in perfusion MRI using image-based computational fluid dynamics. *Neuroimage* 2003;19(2 Pt 1):341–353.
79. **Mehndiratta A, Calamante F, Macintosh BJ, et al.** Modeling and correction of bolus dispersion effects in dynamic susceptibility contrast MRI. *Magn Reson Med* 2014;72:1762–1764. doi:10.1002/mrm.25077.
80. **Calamante F, Mørup M, Hansen LK.** Defining a local arterial input function for perfusion MRI using independent component analysis. *Magn Reson Med.* 2004;52(4):789–797.
81. **Alsop DC, Wedmid A, Schlaug G.** Defining a local arterial input function for perfusion quantification with bolus contrast MRI. *Proceedings of International Society for Magnetic Resonance in Medicine (ISMRM), 10th Annual Meeting*, Honolulu, HI, USA, 18–24 May, 2002: 659.
82. **Lorenz C, Benner T, Chen PJ, et al.** Automated perfusion-weighted MRI using localized arterial input functions. *J Magn Reson Imaging* 2006;24(5):1133–1139.
83. **Lorenz C, Benner T, Lopez CJ, et al.** Effect of using local arterial input functions on cerebral blood flow estimation. *J Magn Reson Imaging* 2006;24(1):57–65.
84. **Knutsson L, Larsson E-M, Thilmann O, et al.** Calculation of cerebral perfusion parameters using regional arterial input functions identified by factor analysis. *J Magn Reson Imaging* 2006;23(4):444–453.
85. **Grüner R, Bjørnarå BT, Moen G, et al.** Magnetic resonance brain perfusion imaging with voxel-specific arterial input functions. *J Magn Reson Imaging* 2006;23(3):273–284.
86. **Grüner R, Taxt T.** Cepstral estimation of arterial input functions in brain perfusion imaging. *J Magn Reson Imaging* 2007;26(3):773–779.
87. **Lee JJ, Bretthorst GL, Derdeyn CP, et al.** Dynamic susceptibility contrast MRI with localized arterial input functions. *Magn Reson Med* 2010;63(5):1305–1314.
88. **Willats L, Christensen S, Ma HK, et al.** Validating a local Arterial Input Function method for improved perfusion quantification in stroke. *J Cereb Blood Flow Metab* 2011;31(11):2189–2198.
89. **Bleeker EJW, Webb AG, Van Walderveen MAA, et al.** Evaluation of signal formation in local arterial input function measurements of dynamic susceptibility contrast MRI. *Magn Reson Med* 2012;67(5):1324–1331.
90. **Akbudak E, Hsu RM, Li Y, et al.** DeltaR2* and Deltaphi contrast agent perfusion effects in blood: quantitation and linearity assessment. *Proceedings of the International Society for Magnetic Resonance in Medicine (ISMRM), 6th Annual Meeting, Sydney, Australia*, 18–24 April, 1998: 1197.
91. **Calamante F, Connelly A, Van Osch MJP.** Nonlinear DeltaR*2 effects in perfusion quantification using bolus-tracking MRI. *Magn Reson Med* 2009;61(2):486–492.

92. **Zaharchuk G, Bammer R, Straka M, et al.** Arterial spin-label imaging in patients with normal bolus perfusion-weighted MR imaging findings: pilot identification of the borderzone sign. *Radiology* 2009; 252(3):797–807.
93. **Knutsson L, Ståhlberg F, Wirestam R, et al.** Effects of blood ΔR2* nonlinearity on absolute perfusion quantification using DSC-MRI: comparison with Xe-133 SPECT. *Magn Reson Imaging* 2013;31(5):651–655.
94. **Conturo TE, Barker PB, Mathews VP, et al.** MR imaging of cerebral perfusion by phase-angle reconstruction of bolus paramagnetic-induced frequency shifts. *Magn Reson Med* 1992;27(2):375–390.
95. **Akbudak E, Conturo TE.** Arterial input functions from MR phase imaging. *Magn Reson Med* 1996;36(6):809–815.
96. **Akbudak E, Norberg RE, Conturo TE.** Contrast-agent phase effects: an experimental system for analysis of susceptibility, concentration, and bolus input function kinetics. *Magn Reson Med* 1997;38(6):990–1002.
97. **Newbould RD, Skare ST, Jochimsen TH, et al.** Perfusion mapping with multiecho multishot parallel imaging EPI. *Magn Reson Med* 2007; 58(1):70–81.
98. **Jochimsen TH, Newbould RD, Skare ST, et al.** Identifying systematic errors in quantitative dynamic-susceptibility contrast perfusion imaging by high-resolution multi-echo parallel EPI. *NMR Biomed* 2007; 20(4):429–438.
99. **Ellinger R, Kremser C, Schocke MF, et al.** The impact of peak saturation of the arterial input function on quantitative evaluation of dynamic susceptibility contrast-enhanced MR studies. *J Comput Assist Tomogr* 2000;24(6):942–948.
100. **Brunecker P, Villringer A, Schultze J, et al.** Correcting saturation effects of the arterial input function in dynamic susceptibility contrast-enhanced MRI: a Monte Carlo simulation. *Magn Reson Imaging* 2007;25(9):1300–1311.
101. **Schmitt F, Stehling K, Turner R.** *Echo-planar imaging: theory, technique and application.* Springer-Verlag GmbH; 1998. Berlin, Germany.
102. **Hou L, Yang Y, Mattay VS, et al.** Optimization of fast acquisition methods for whole-brain relative cerebral blood volume (rCBV) mapping with susceptibility contrast agents. *J Magn Reson Imaging* 1999;9(2):233–239.
103. **Calamante F, Vonken EPA, Van Osch MJP.** Contrast agent concentration measurements affecting quantification of bolus-tracking perfusion MRI. *Magn Reson Med* 2007;58(3):544–553.
104. **Sorensen AG, Reimer AGSP.** *Cerebral MR perfusion imaging: book + CD-ROM set: principles and current applications.* Thieme Medical Publisher; 2000. New York, NY
105. **Salluzzi M, Frayne R, Smith MR.** Is correction necessary when clinically determining quantitative cerebral perfusion parameters from multi-slice dynamic susceptibility contrast MR studies? *Phys Med Biol* 2006;51(2):407–424.
106. **Chen JJ, Smith MR, Frayne R.** Advantages of frequency-domain modeling in dynamic-susceptibility contrast magnetic resonance cerebral blood flow quantification. *Magn Reson Med* 2005;53(3):700–707.
107. **Kosior RK, Kosior JC, Frayne R.** Improved dynamic susceptibility contrast (DSC)-MR perfusion estimates by motion correction. *J Magn Reson Imaging* 2007;26(4):1167–1172.
108. **Flacke S, Urbach H, Folkers PJ, et al.** Ultra-fast three-dimensional MR perfusion imaging of the entire brain in acute stroke assessment. *J Magn Reson Imaging* 2000;11(3):250–259.
109. **Van Gelderen P, Grandin C, Petrella JR, et al.** Rapid three-dimensional MR imaging method for tracking a bolus of contrast agent through the brain. *Radiology* 2000;216(2):603–608.
110. **Manka C, Träber F, Gieseke J, et al.** Three-dimensional dynamic susceptibility-weighted perfusion MR imaging at 3.0 T: feasibility and contrast agent dose. *Radiology* 2005;234(3):869–877.
111. **Boxerman JL, Hamberg LM, Rosen BR, et al.** MR contrast due to intravascular magnetic susceptibility perturbations. *Magn Reson Med* 1995;34(4):555–566.
112. **Carroll TJ, Haughton VM, Rowley HA, et al.** Confounding effect of large vessels on MR perfusion images analyzed with independent component analysis. *AJNR Am J Neuroradiol.* 2002;23(6):1007–1012.
113. **Reishofer G, Koschutnig K, Enzinger C, et al.** Automated macrovessel artifact correction in dynamic susceptibility contrast magnetic resonance imaging using independent component analysis. *Magn Reson Med* 2011;65(3):848–857.
114. **Chappell MA, Mehndiratta A, Payne SJ, et al.** Correcting for large vessel contamination in dynamic susceptibility contrast perfusion MRI by extension to a physiological model of the vasculature. *Magn Reson Med.* 2014; doi: 10.1002/mrm.25390.
115. **Calamante F.** Perfusion MRI using dynamic-susceptibility contrast MRI: quantification issues in patient studies. *Top Magn Reson Imaging* 2010;21(2):75–85.
116. **Kassner A, Annesley DJ, Zhu XP, et al.** Abnormalities of the contrast re-circulation phase in cerebral tumors demonstrated using dynamic susceptibility contrast-enhanced imaging: a possible marker of vascular tortuosity. *J Magn Reson Imaging* 2000;11(2):103–113.
117. **Vonken EP, Van Osch MJ, Bakker CJ, et al.** Simultaneous quantitative cerebral perfusion and Gd-DTPA extravasation measurement with dual-echo dynamic susceptibility contrast MRI. *Magn Reson Med* 2000;43(6):820–827.
118. **Paulson ES, Schmainda KM.** Comparison of dynamic susceptibility-weighted contrast-enhanced MR methods: recommendations for measuring relative cerebral blood volume in brain tumors. *Radiology* 2008;249(2):601–613.
119. **Quarles CC, Ward BD, Schmainda KM.** Improving the reliability of obtaining tumor hemodynamic parameters in the presence of contrast agent extravasation. *Magn Reson Med* 2005;53(6):1307–1316.
120. **Boxerman JL, Schmainda KM, Weisskoff RM.** Relative Cerebral Blood Volume Maps Corrected for Contrast Agent Extravasation Significantly Correlate with Glioma Tumor Grade, Whereas Uncorrected Maps Do Not. *AJNR Am J Neuroradiol* 2006;27(4):859–867.
121. **Bjornerud A, Sorensen AG, Mouridsen K, et al.** T1- and T2*-dominant extravasation correction in DSC-MRI: part I—theoretical considerations and implications for assessment of tumor hemodynamic properties. *J Cereb Blood Flow Metab* 2011;31(10):2041–2053.
122. **Emblem KE, Bjornerud A, Mouridsen K, et al.** T(1)- and T(2)(*)-dominant extravasation correction in DSC-MRI: part II-predicting patient outcome after a single dose of cediranib in recurrent glioblastoma patients. *J Cereb Blood Flow Metab* 2011;31(10):2054–2064.
123. **Weisskoff RM, Boxerman JL, Sorensen AG,** Simultaneous blood volume and permeability mapping using a single Gd-based contrast injection. *Proceedings of the Society of Magnetic Resonance, 2nd Annual Meeting,* San Francisco, California, August 6–12, 1994: 279.
124. **Tofts PS.** Modeling tracer kinetics in dynamic Gd-DTPA MR imaging. *J Magn Reson Imaging* 1997;7(1):91–101.
125. **Sourbron SP, Buckley DL.** Tracer kinetic modelling in MRI: estimating perfusion and capillary permeability. *Phys Med Biol* 2012;57(2):R1–R33.
126. **Sourbron SP, Buckley DL.** Classic models for dynamic contrast-enhanced MRI. *NMR Biomed* 2013;26(8):1004–1027.
127. **Kim J, Leira EC, Callison RC, et al.** Toward fully automated processing of dynamic susceptibility contrast perfusion MRI for acute ischemic cerebral stroke. *Comput Methods Programs Biomed* 2010;98(2):204–213.
128. **Saver JL.** Time is brain—quantified. *Stroke* 2006;37(1):263–266.
129. **Geoffrey A, Donnan MD, Baron JC, et al,** *Sharp FR. The ischemic penumbra: pathophysiology, imaging and therapy* Taylor & Francis Group; 2007.
130. **Christensen S, Mouridsen K, Wu O, et al.** Comparison of 10 perfusion MRI parameters in 97 sub-6-hour stroke patients using voxel-based receiver operating characteristics analysis. *Stroke* 2009;40(6):2055–2061.
131. **Wu O, Koroshetz WJ, Ostergaard L, et al.** Predicting tissue outcome in acute human cerebral ischemia using combined diffusion- and perfusion-weighted MR imaging. *Stroke* 2001;32(4):933–942.
132. **Willats L, Connelly A, Christensen S, et al.** The role of bolus delay and dispersion in predictor models for stroke. *Stroke* 2012;43(4): 1025–1031.
133. **Wintermark M, Albers GW, Broderick JP, et al.** Acute Stroke Imaging Research Roadmap II. *Stroke* 2013;44(9):2628–2639.

CHAPTER

8

Dynamic Contrast-Enhanced T_1-Weighted MR Imaging: Theory, Quantitative Aspects, and Practical Implementation

Henrik Bo Wiberg Larsson, MD, PhD and Thomas Fritz Hansen, MD

Introduction

Dynamic contrast-enhanced T_1-weighted MRI (DCE-MRI) is relative easy to integrate in a conventional MRI setup, it is cheap, and it has the potential to provide important physiologic parameters. Large interest has focused on determination of the leakage, also called the permeability, of the capillary membranes. The reason is that the permeability can be associated with changes in the vascular structure seen in malign transformed tissue and in tissue inflammation. The reason why the DCE-MRI has this potential is the size of the contrast agent (CA) molecules we are using. Typically, MRI CA agents are not freely diffusible in tissue, and the capillary membrane normally imposes restriction of diffusivity through the capillary membrane in normal tissue. In the brain, the normal blood–brain barrier (BBB) is nearly impermeable for conventional MRI CA, but the barrier breaks down in a number of diseases such as acute multiple sclerosis, inflammation, tumors, stroke, and possible dementia and epilepsy.[1,2] Permeability is expressed as the permeability–surface area (PS) product, signifying that not only the permeability but also the available capillary surface area is determinant for the leakage. The PS product is ideally defined from a two-chamber experiment, the chamber having an initial concentration of C_1 and C_2 and J denoting the initial flux, that is, number of molecules moving from the first compartment to the second compartment per time unit. The relationship is

$$J_{1\to 2} = -\mathrm{PS}(C_2 - C_1) \qquad (1)$$

Note the transport is sign sensitive. The equation implies a first-order transport, that is, the flux out of a compartment is proportional to the concentration in that compartment, which is a reasonable assumption, because MRI CA are inert molecules and do not react with specific receptors. However, if the transport over the membrane is governed by a saturable transport system, the Michaelis-Menten kinetics is appropriate. This topic is outside the scope of this presentation. Using conventional MR CA, transport over the capillary membrane is driven by the concentration difference over the membrane as described by the equation. But this is not the whole story, because the blood flow through the capillary (the perfusion) will modify the actual flux over the membrane in a subtle way. Intuitively, the higher velocity of the blood through the capillary, the less likely is a passage over the capillary membrane. It turns out that the determining factor is the ratio PS/F, where F denotes the flow through the capillary. The dimension of the PS and F is mL/min or corresponding derivates. The relationship can be derived based on the following considerations: imaging a single capillary of length L and with radius R and having a specific PS product for the specific CA we are using. The flow is F, and the CA concentration at the inlet and outlet of the capillary is C_{in} and C_{o}, respectively (see Fig. 8.1). In order to simplify matters, these concentrations are constant in time, and we assume that the extravascular concentration is so small that it can be ignored, which also means no return to the blood, once the CA molecules have left the blood over the membrane. These assumptions can easily be modified later if needed and will not change the basic principle we are aiming at. The loss of CA from a short-segment dx centered at position x along the capillary using Eq. (1) is

$$\mathrm{d}J = -\frac{\mathrm{d}S}{S}\mathrm{PS}\left(C_{\text{e}} - C_{\text{p}}(x)\right) = \frac{2\pi r\,\mathrm{d}x}{2\pi rL}\mathrm{PS}C_{\text{p}}(x)$$

The CA change inside the capillary over this short segment where the concentrations in a thin layer at the entrance and exit of the short segment are $C(x_1)$ and $C(x_2)$, respectively, is

$$\mathrm{d}J = -F\left(C(x_2) - C(x_1)\right) = -F\,\mathrm{d}C(x)$$

Combining and integrate these equations gives

$$\int_{C_{\text{in}}}^{C_{\text{o}}} \frac{\mathrm{d}C(x)}{C(x)} = -\int_0^L \frac{\mathrm{PS}}{LF}\mathrm{d}x \Leftrightarrow \ln\frac{C_{\text{o}}}{C_{\text{in}}} = -\frac{\mathrm{PS}}{F} \Leftrightarrow C_{\text{o}} = C_{\text{in}}\exp\left(-\frac{\mathrm{PS}}{F}\right) \qquad (2)$$

Thus, the concentration at the outlet becomes smaller when the PS product is large relative to F and vice versa, verifying our initial intuition. In the same setup, we can define the extraction fraction as the ratio of the amount taken up by the tissue per unit time to the total amount entering the tissue per unit time:

$$E \equiv \frac{FC_{\text{in}} - FC_{\text{o}}}{FC_{\text{o}}} = \frac{C_{\text{in}} - C_{\text{o}}}{C_{\text{in}}} = 1 - \exp\left(-\frac{\mathrm{PS}}{F}\right) \qquad (3)$$

Renkin and Crone originally developed these equations.[3,4] A freely diffusible CA for which PS/F is very large has an extraction of nearly one and is called a flow limited tracer, because the amount

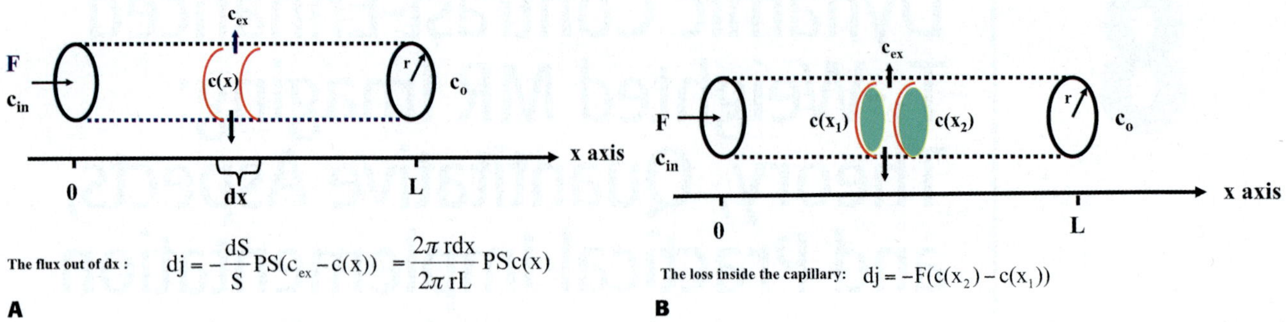

Figure 8-1. **The single-unit capillary model used to derive the Crone and Renkin equation.** Here, concentrations are only a function of position. Time dependence can be incorporated as well.

in tissue is determined by flow. If the CA is more or less confined to the vascular space, because it cannot easily diffuse over the capillary membrane, then PS/F is small and the extraction fraction approach zero. We then talk about a diffusion-limited CA, because the amount in the extravascular space is determined by the PS product. Note that the amount in the vascular space is of course determined by the delivery of the flowing blood entering the tissue. Because of the flow, Eq. (1) does not really describe the transport adequately. The transport is still linear meaning that the actual flux is proportional to the vascular concentration keeping F and PS the same. In order to deal with this situation, we define the clearance as the amount taken up by the tissue per unit time normalized to a reference concentration:

$$K_1 = \frac{J_{tis}}{C_{ref}} = \frac{FC_{in} - FC_o}{C_{ref}}$$

The dimension of the clearance is then volume per unit time. In words, the clearance is a (fictive) flow and is a measure of the volume of the reference solution containing the amount of the CA taken up or cleared by the tissue per unit time. Often, it is convenient to choose the reference concentration as the concentration of the CA at the inlet. In this case, we get

$$K_1 = \frac{J_{tis}}{C_{in}} = \frac{FC_{in} - FC_o}{C_{in}} = FE \tag{4}$$

and Eq. (1) can be replaced with

$$J_{1\to 2} = K_1C_1 - PSC_2$$

In order not to deal with too many physiologic constants, the last equation is replaced with

$$J_{1\to 2} = K_1C_1 - K_1C_2$$

using the argument of a membrane transport symmetry, although this may not be strictly correct. Note that K_1 approach F for E going towards 1 for a free diffusible CA (i.e., a flow-limited CA or tracer), while K_1 approaches the PS product for PS/F going towards zero (i.e., a diffusion-limited CA or tracer):

$$K_1 = FE = F\left(1 - \exp\left(-\frac{PS}{F}\right)\right) \approx F - F\left(1 - \frac{PS}{F}\right) = PS$$

It is often convenient to normalize flux, PS product, F, and K_1 to the tissue mass M_t or tissue volume V_t. In the following, relevant capital letters refer to no normalization, while small letters refer to a normalized metric, for example, F is in mL/min, while f is in mL blood/100 mL tissue/min. Strictly, this implies a dimension of f as 1/min, but it is important to keep the definition in mind. The choice between volume and mass is somewhat arbitrary, but strictly volume V_t and mass M_t are related as $M_t = \rho V_t$, where ρ is the tissue density, close to 1 g/mL.

DCE-MRI also allows determination of various compartment volumes, as the blood volume where V_p denotes the plasma volume, V_b denotes full blood volume, V_e denotes extravascular extracellular volume, and V_{tis} denotes extravascular intracellular tissue volume. Thus, $V_b + V_e + V_{tis} = V_t$, and $V_b/V_t + V_e/V_t + V_{tis}/V_t = v_b + v_e + v_{tis} = 1$, where, for example, v_e either is a fractional volume or has the dimension mL/100 mL or mL/100 g. The relationship-between V_b and V_p is given as $V_p = V_b(1\text{-}Hct_{sv})$, where Hct_{sv} is the small vessel hematocrit. More generally, in a given context, we talk about the volume of distribution (V_d) defined as $V_d = Q_t/C_{ref}$, where Q_t is the number of CA molecules in a piece of tissue and C_{ref} is the concentration of a reference solution of the CA, for example, plasma concentration. Ideally, V_d is defined in a situation where equilibration between a piece of tissue and the reference solution has been established. In words, V_d express the volume of the reference solution, which contains an amount equivalent to the amount in the tissue. If we normalize with the mass or volume of the tissue, we get the partition coefficient

$$\lambda = \frac{V_d}{M_t} = \frac{Q_t}{M_tC_{ref}} = \frac{C_t}{C_{ref}}[\text{mL/g}]$$

$$\text{or} \tag{5}$$

$$\lambda = \frac{V_d}{V_t} = \frac{Q_t}{V_tC_{ref}} = \frac{C_t}{C_{ref}}[\text{mL/mL}]$$

Note that the tissue concentration is then defined as $C_t = Q_t/V_t$ or $C_t = Q_t/M_t$.

DCE-MRI can also be used for assessing tissue perfusion, for example, myocardial perfusion,[5,6] and lately, it has been shown that when using a high scanner field strength of 3 T, brain perfusion can also be measured by DCE-MRI.[7,8] Tissue perfusion is vital for normal functionality of the tissue, and lack of adequate tissue perfusion in various organs is the cause of many diseases, and probably more than 50% of all human deaths is directly coursed by lack of perfusion, creating tissue starvation, hypoxia, and infarction. In that perspective, it is remarkable that the methodology of perfusion measurement is still a very dynamic research area, and many perfusion methods are based on Kety's pioneering work more than 60 years ago.[9,10] All perfusion methods have advantages and disadvantages with regard to accuracy, precision, invasiveness, and expensiveness. Accuracy is not necessarily the ultimate goal, but the applicability in clinical decision making may be more relevant.

Tissue perfusion (f) is ideally defined as the volume of blood that enters a distinct part of the vascular system such as the capillaries in one unit of tissue mass (or volume) per unit time. The dimension is therefore mL blood/100 mL tissue/min, which is equal with 1/min. Often, the dimension mL blood/100 g tissue/min is used and reminisces earlier studies of perfusion based on in vitro studies, where perfusion was normalized to mass of tissue. Keeping the older terminology helps keeping the correct interpretation of perfusion, which may become blurred if using 1/min. Because 1 mL of tissue nearly has a mass of 1 g, the number is unchanged.

Determination of perfusion, permeability, and distribution volumes is based on a mathematical framework, the tracer kinetic theory, which in essence are equations describing the mass balance, keeping track of the transport of the CA as a function of time.

Basic Tracer Kinetic Theory

The fundamental equation relating tissue concentration as a function of time, $C_t(t)$, the arterial concentration as a function of time, $C_a(t)$, perfusion f, and the residue impulse response function, RIF(t), is[11]

$$C_t(t) = C_a(t) \otimes f\,\mathrm{RIF}(t) = f\int_0^t C_a(\tau)\mathrm{RIF}(t-\tau)\mathrm{d}\tau \qquad (6)$$

The residue impulse response function is defined as the CA fraction remaining in the tissue, after a brief injected bolus, in principle as a $\delta(t)$ function, directly into the tissue (or voxel), as a function of time. Thus, RIF is dimensionless, and because the entire bolus by definition is injection at time zero, the first function value will be one: RIF(0) = 1. If the entire bolus has a minimum transit time through the tissue (the voxel), of several seconds, then the RIF holds a function value of one until some of the CA molecules begin to leave the tissue in focus. From now on, the RIF will show a monotone decrease until it becomes zero: the entire bolus has left the tissue, or if it happens that a fraction becomes bound irreversible to the tissue, the RIF ends at a corresponding value, that is, the fraction that remains in the tissue infinitively; this value may be related to the extraction fraction (if back-diffusion does not occur). The assumption related to this equation is that the system is linear: Doubling the dose or concentration, $C_a(t)$, results in a doubling of $C_t(t)$ (f remains the same as well as the RIF), and a delayed input of "a" seconds, $C_a(t-a)$, will result in a delayed output $(C_t(t-a))$ and that the CA is not being produced or metabolized inside the tissue. Such a system is called a linear and time-invariant system. This is correct for many of the MRI CA we are using. However, one important additional point is that the CA has to be equally "visible" irrespective of the location of CA, be it in the plasma, the interstitial space, or intracellularly. Due to the fact that MRI CA acts by changing the longitudinal relaxation rate, R_1, of adjacent water protons corresponding to the first hydration layer, the ability of water diffusion around the paramagnetic core of the CA can influence the level of visibility of the CA. As an example, if the CA becomes confined in a small compartment, without sufficient water exchange, then the CA loses its effect, because complete relaxation of the compartment is finite and therefore becomes invisible, that is, additional CA is without effect (see later).

Under these assumptions of linearity, ignoring the issue of water exchange, the convolution equation can be derived based on the following considerations. Imaging a short bolus $Q_{in}(0) = FC_a(0)\,dt = V_t f\,C_a(0)\,dt$ enters a tissue volume (V_t) at time zero. Using the definition of the RIF, the tissue "response" is simply

$$Q_t(t) = V_t f C_a(0)\Delta t\,\mathrm{RIF}(t)$$

If an additional input enters the tissue volume at a later time point, τ, the tissue response from this input is again

$$Q_t(t) = V_t f C_a(\tau)\Delta t\,\mathrm{RIF}(t-\tau)$$

Note the time shift of τ seconds of the RIF to the right. The total tissue response is the sum of all tissue response functions. Generally, if we imagine that the entire arterial input function is composed of short inputs (δ-functions), entering as a continuous function of τ (substituting Δt with $\mathrm{d}\tau$), and the tissue response is linear in the input, the total tissue response at time t will be the sum of all the tissue impulse responses corresponding to each τ, and we get

$$Q_t(t)/V_t = C_t(t) = C_a(t) \otimes f\,\mathrm{RIF}(t) = f\int_0^t C_a(\tau)\mathrm{RIF}(t-\tau)\mathrm{d}\tau$$

Tissue concentration is here defined as the total amount of CA molecules per unit volume of tissue (or unit mass of tissue).

The integration of two functions as in Eq. (6) is called a convolution integral and is described from an operational point of view in Figure 8.2.

It is remarkable that Eq. (6), under the above-mentioned restriction, is always correct. Obviously, the goal is to find the perfusion f and the RIF(t). The physiologic interpretation of the RIF(t) is that this function describes the destiny of the contrast molecule inside the tissue. The RIF(t) is related to the distribution of transit times through the tissue: $h(t)$. In words, $h(t)$ is the fraction of the CA, which leaves the tissue at time t, per unit time, after a bolus injection:

$$h(t) = \frac{\mathrm{d}N(t)}{N_0\,\mathrm{d}t}$$

where d$N(t)$ *is the number of CA molecules leaving the tissue at time t in the time interval dt* and N_0 is the entire bolus. Therefore, integrating over time in a time interval will give the fraction having left the tissue volume in that time interval, after a bolus injection. Specifically, in the time interval from zero (bolus injection) to time t_1, the fraction having left the tissue is

$$\int_0^{t_1} h(t)\mathrm{d}t = \frac{1}{N_0}\int_0^{t_1}\mathrm{d}N(t) = \frac{1}{N_0}[N(t)]_0^{t_1} = \frac{N(t_1) - N(0)}{N_0} = \frac{N(t_1)}{N_0}$$

Note $N(0) = 0$: nothing has left the tissue at time zero. The fraction remaining in the tissue at time t_1 is then

$$\frac{N_0 - N(t_1)}{N_0} = 1 - \int_0^{t_1} h(t)\mathrm{d}t = \mathrm{RIF}(t_1)$$

$h(t)$ is similar to a probability density function, known from statistic, and the expectation value of the time weighted distribution is the typical transit time, the mean transit time MTT, and is given as

$$\mathrm{MTT} = \int_0^\infty t h(t)\mathrm{d}t = -\int_0^\infty t\frac{\mathrm{dRIF}(t)}{\mathrm{d}t}\mathrm{d}t$$
$$= -[t\,\mathrm{RIF}(t)]_0^\infty + \int_0^\infty \mathrm{RIF}(t)\mathrm{d}t = \int_0^\infty \mathrm{RIF}(t)\mathrm{d}t$$

where we have used partial integration. Here, we assume that the RIF will be zero after sufficiently long time, that is, all CA molecules will leave the tissue eventually. Thus, MTT can be estimated either from the frequency function, $h(t)$, or from the RIF(t). In Figure 8.3, $h(t)$ is modeled as a gamma-variate function, and the corresponding RIF(t) and 1 − RIF(t) are also shown.

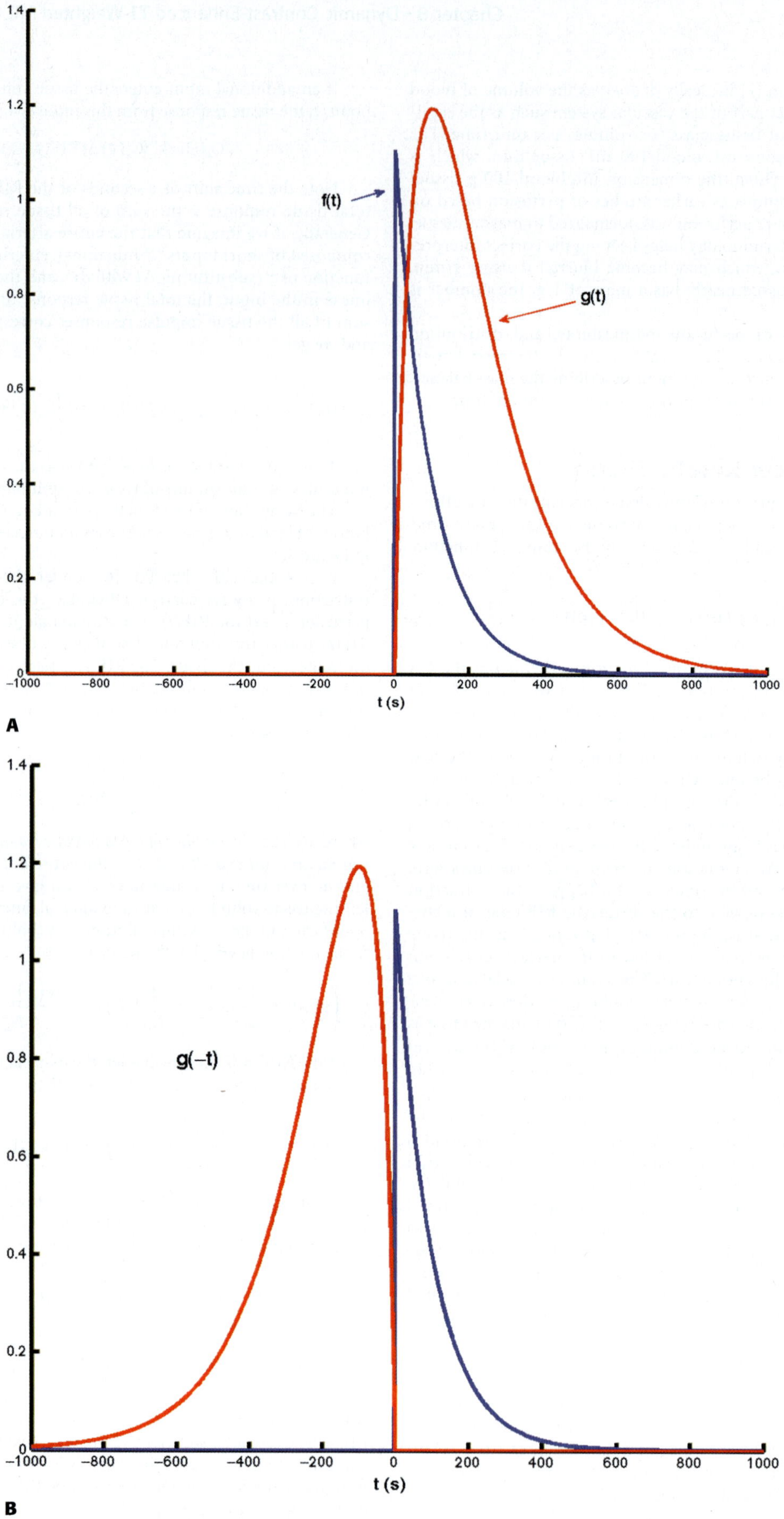

Figure 8-2. A: Convolution of two functions $f(t)$ and $g(t)$; the order of the functions is interchangeable. **B:** One of the functions is reflected by changing the sign of the argument, $g(-t)$.

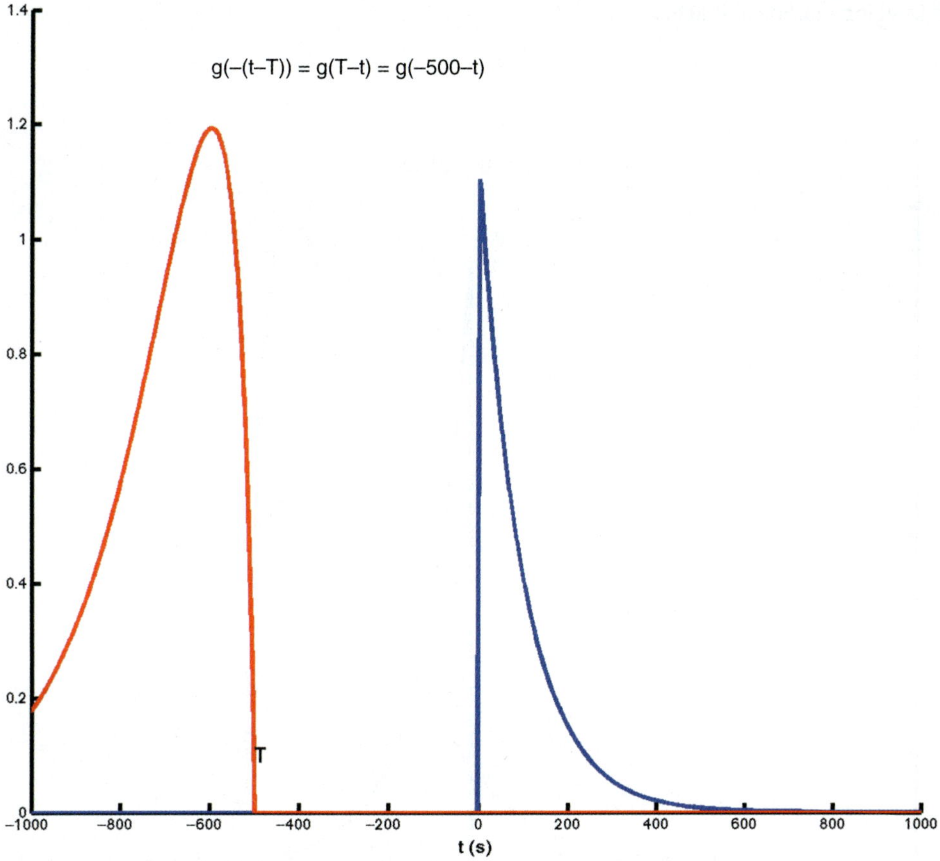

C

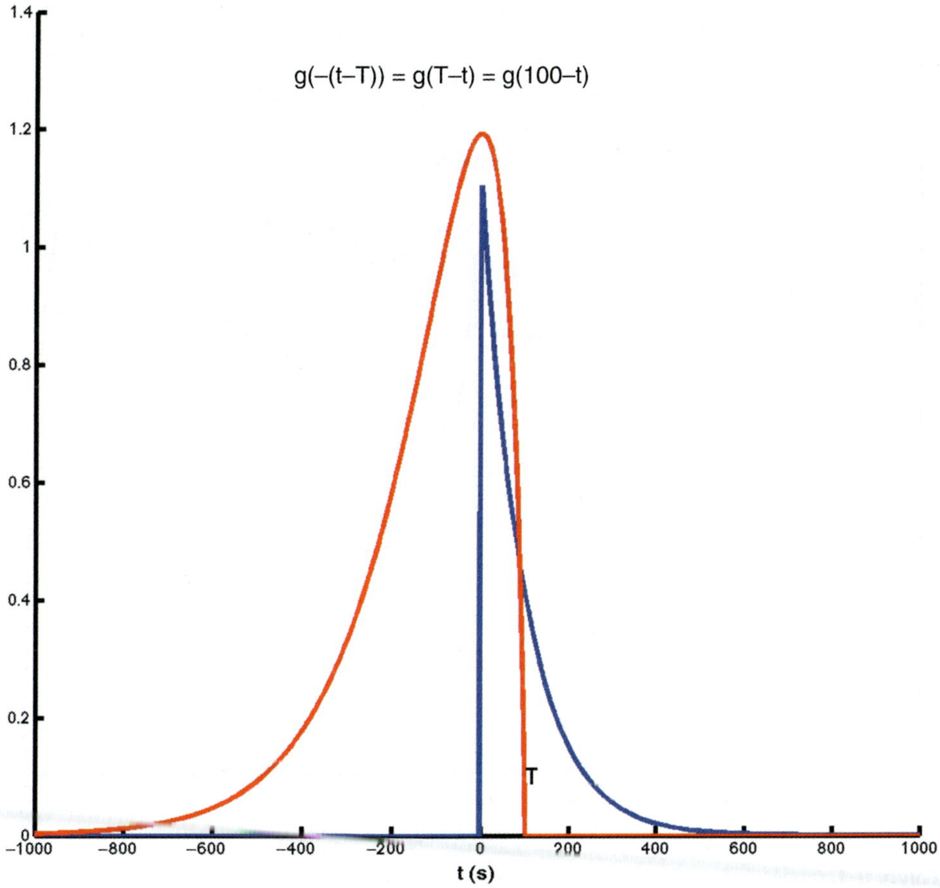

D

Figure 8-2. (*Continued*) **C–F:** The function $g(T - t)$ is created; T determines the exact position of this function.

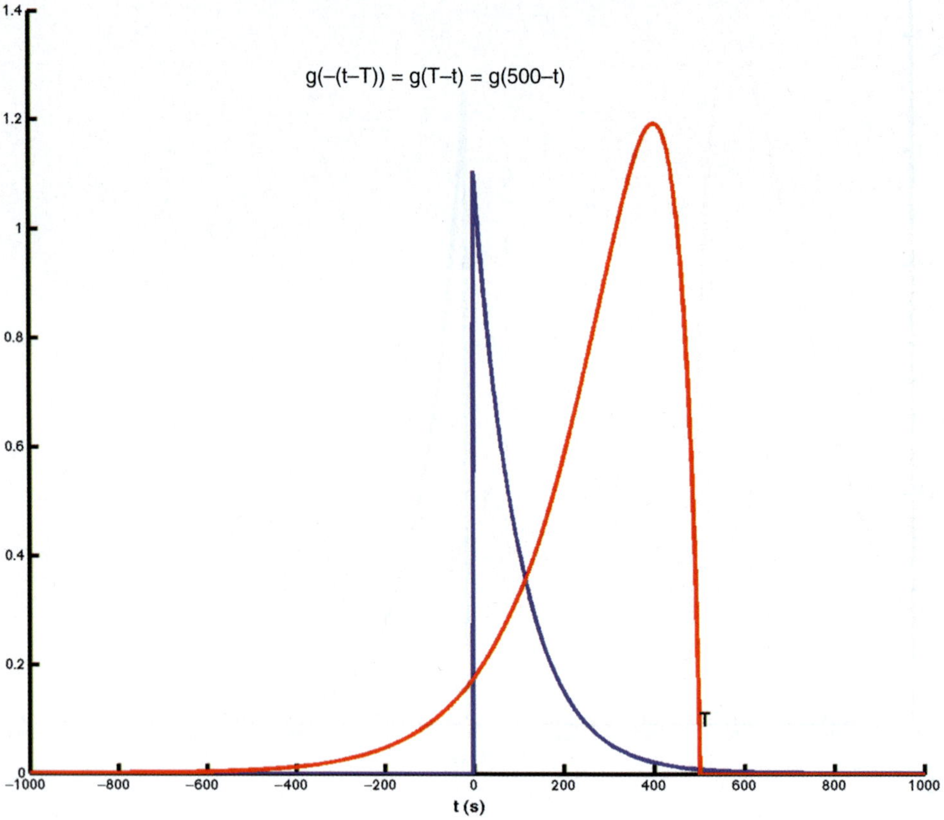

E

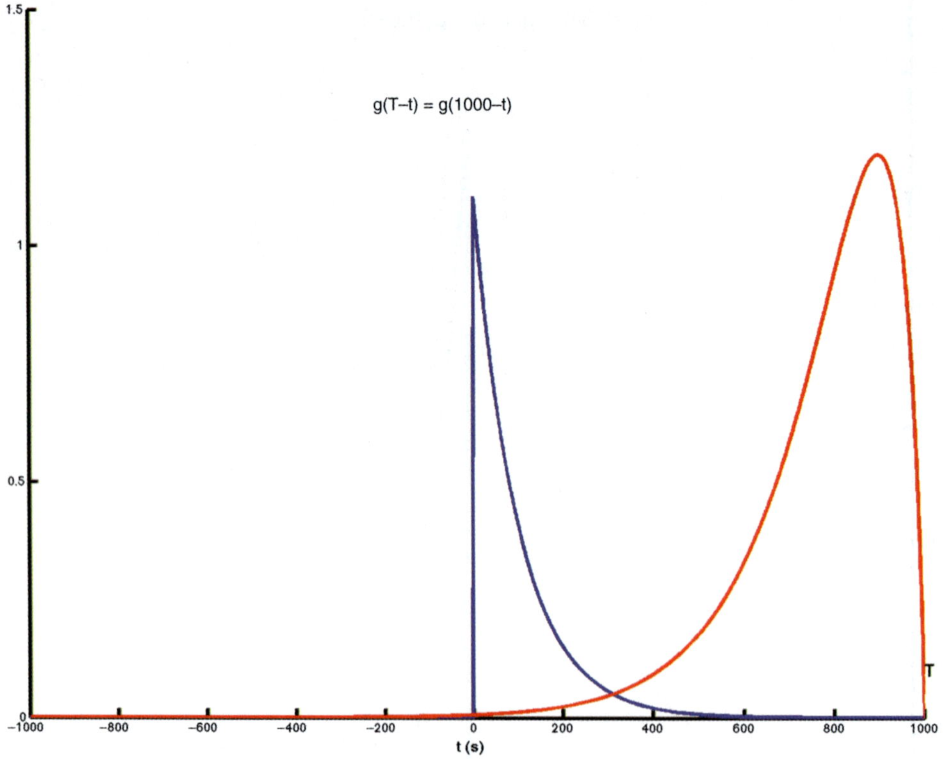

F

Figure 8-2. *(Continued)*

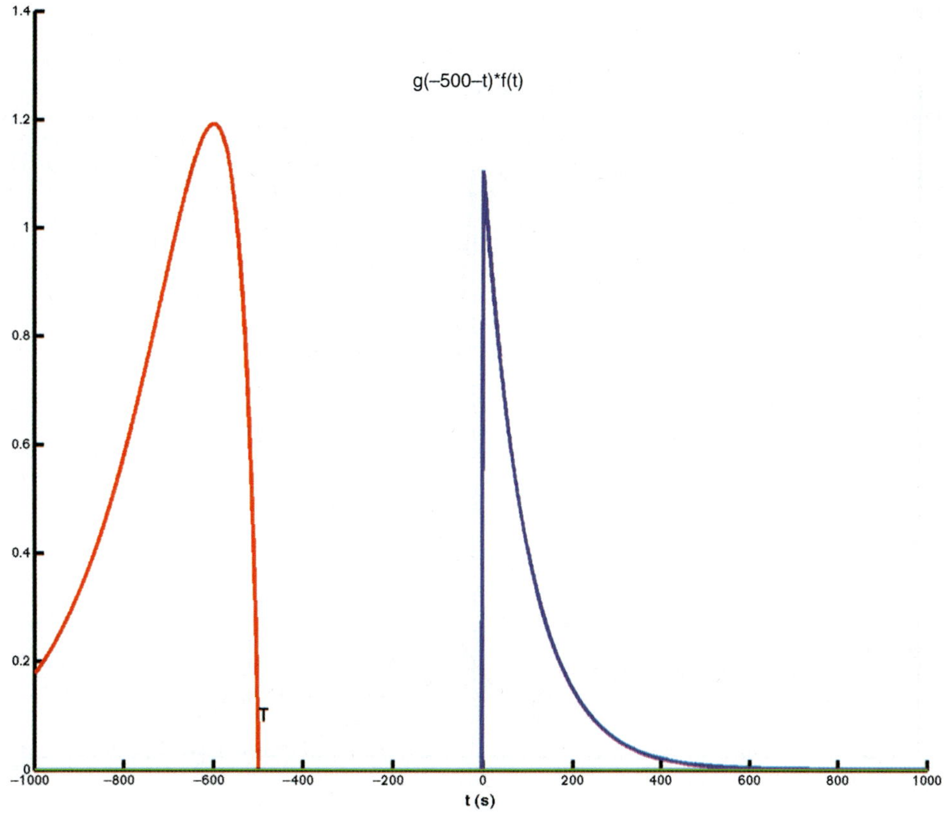

G

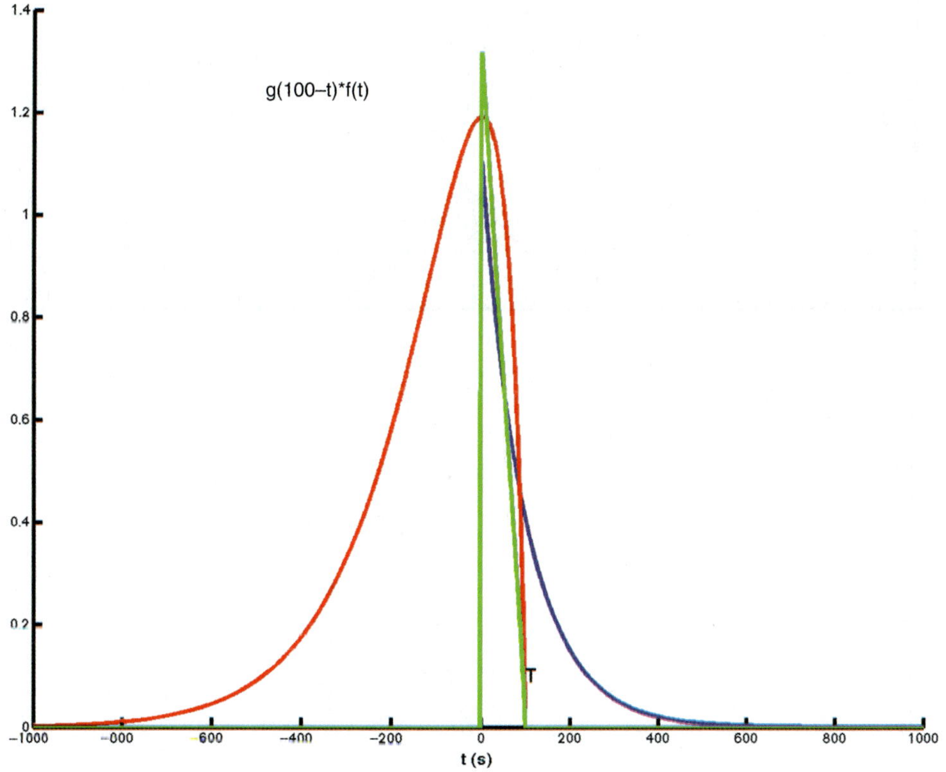

H

Figure 8-2. (*Continued*) **G–I:** For any given value of *T*, the function $g(T-t)$ is multiplied with $f(t)$ for all values of *t*, giving the green curve.

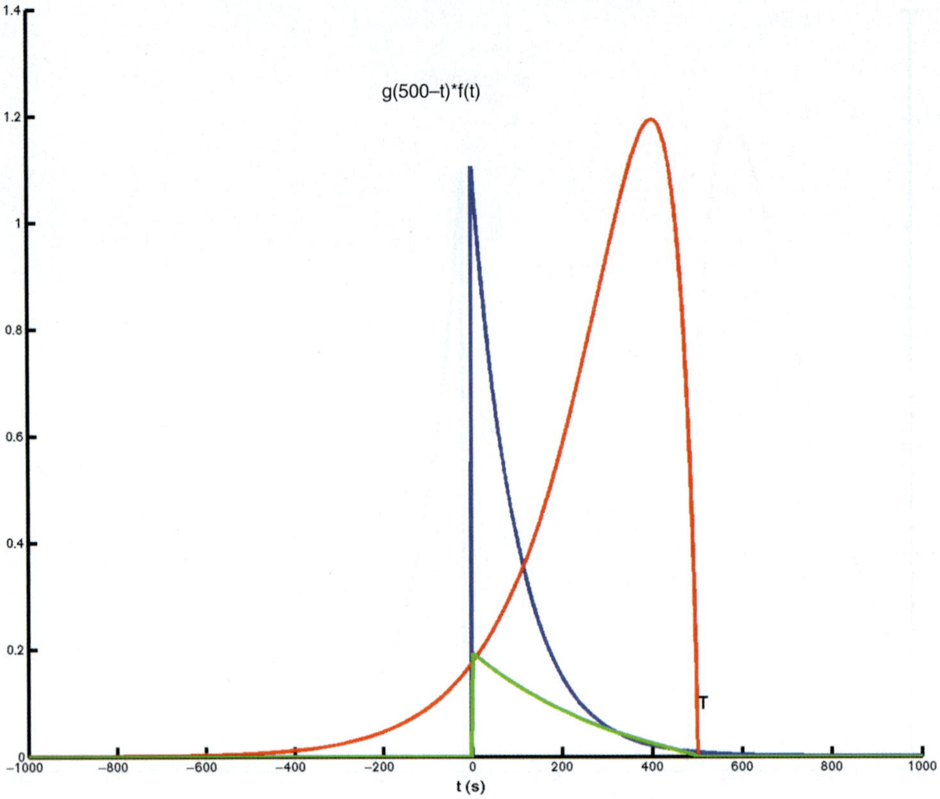

I

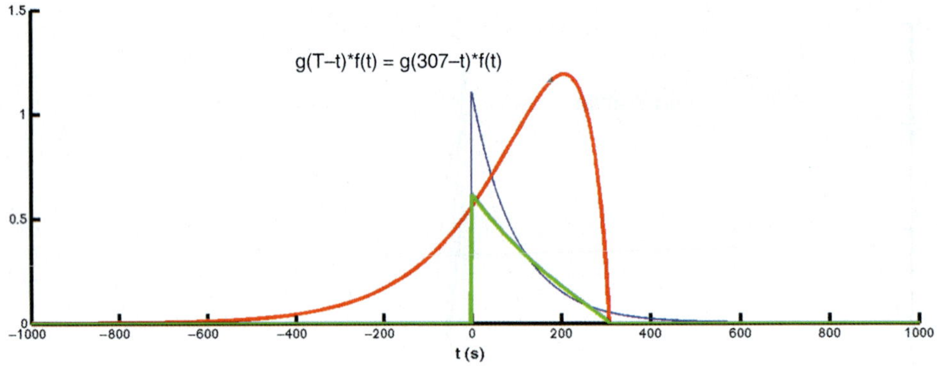

J

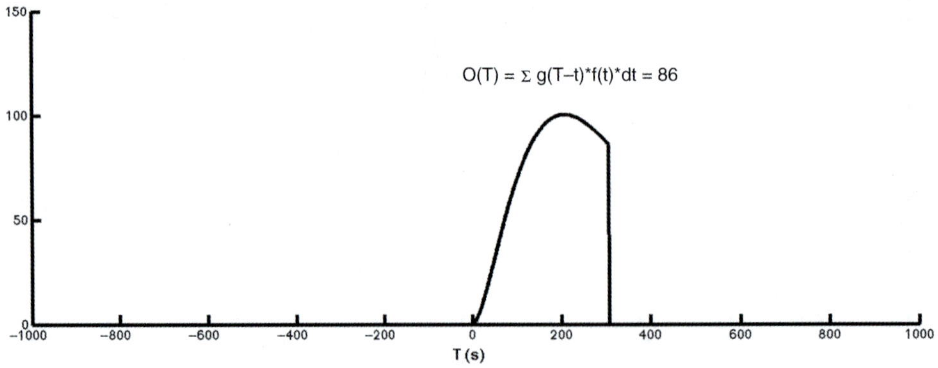

K

Figure 8-2. *(Continued)* **J and K:** For a given value of T, the result of the convolution at time T, $O(T)$, is the area under the green curve. At $T = 307$, $O(307) = 86$, which is the area under the green curve. By letting T go though all relevant values, $O(T)$ is calculated for all values of T in that interval. In the figure, $O(T)$ has been calculated up to $T = 307$.

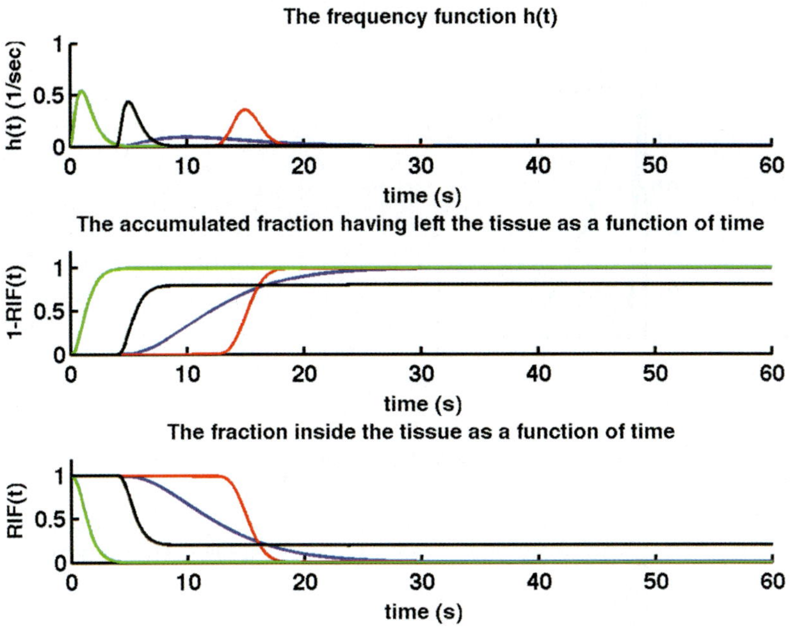

Figure 8-3. **Examples of frequency functions, *h*(*t*), all modeled as a gamma-variate function, and all but one normalized so area is 1.** The black gamma-variate function has an area of 0.8; that is, 20% of the CA is irreversible trapped in the tissue. Integration of *h*(*t*) gives the accumulated fraction, which has left the tissue as a function of time, 1 − RIF(*t*), while RIF(*t*) is the fraction remaining in the tissue as a function of time: The residue impulse response function. Note that 1 − RIF(*t*) + RIF(*t*) = 1 for all values of *t*, and the turning point (the point at which the first derivative change sign) of RIT(*t*) and 1 − RIT(*t*) occurs corresponding to the maximum of the frequency function: $\frac{\partial h(t)}{\partial t} = \frac{\partial^2 \mathrm{RIF}(t)}{\partial t^2} = 0.$

Is the frequency function $h(t)$ clinically interesting? In 1992, Kuschinsky and Paulson suggested that capillary perfusion heterogeneity had a significant impact on capillary diffusion capacity and that the capacity might be increased by homogenization of the perfusion pattern, a response elicited by neurovascular stimulation.[12] This has lately been theoretically substantiated in relation to brain oxygen extraction.[13] The variance of the frequency function, $h(t)$, is a measure of this kind of capillary heterogeneity.

The partition coefficient λ was mentioned above, and if we use the arterial full blood concentration as a reference concentration, the partition coefficient becomes $\lambda=C_t/C_a$. We could also choose the capillary concentration in the middle of the capillary or the concentration at the outlet (in a vein): $\lambda=C_t/C_o$. Ideally, the definition rests on an equilibrium experiment, but often one assumes instantaneous equilibration so $\lambda=C_t(t)/C_a(t)$. Using the relation

$$\lambda = \frac{\int_0^\infty C_t(t)\,dt}{\int_0^\infty C_a(t)\,dt} \tag{7}$$

the requirement of instantaneous equilibration can be relaxed. In the situation where the CA is confined to the vascular space, that is, no leakage, λ represents the blood volume, for example, in the brain, so λ becomes the cerebral blood volume, CBV. If the CA leaks easily through the capillary membrane, but does not enter the cells, then λ becomes the $v_e + v_b$. Finally, there exists an important relationship between MTT, λ, and f, called the central volume principle: MTT= λ/f.[11] It can be obtained from our basic tracer kinetic equation using the Laplace transformation

$$L(C_t(t)) = L(C_a(t) \otimes f\,\mathrm{RIF}(t)) = fL(C_a(t))L(\mathrm{RIF}(t))$$

using the fact that Laplace transformation of a convolution integral equals the product of the Laplace transformed functions itself, and we also get from Eq. (7)

$$\lambda \frac{L(C_a(t))}{s} = \frac{L(C_t(t))}{s}$$

which inserted in the former equation gives

$$\lambda \frac{L(C_a(t))}{s} = f\frac{L(C_a(t))L(\mathrm{RIF}(t))}{s} \Leftrightarrow \frac{\lambda}{s} = f\frac{L(\mathrm{RIF}(t))}{s}$$

where we have eliminated $L(C_a(t))$ on each side of the equation. Taking the inverse Laplace transformation on each side of the last equation gives

$$\lambda = f\int_0^\infty \mathrm{RIF}(t)\,dt = f\,\mathrm{MTT} \Leftrightarrow f = \frac{\lambda}{\mathrm{MTT}} \tag{8}$$

Thus, the central volume principle is correct for any shape of RIF.

Above, we have alluded to the information embedded in the RIF. The question is how we can estimate RIF and f. Clearly, we need to sample many concurrent time points of C_a and C_t in order to estimate RIF and f. But we also need a model of the RIF(t), expressed as an analytical mathematical expression, containing our physiologic "free" parameters and which can be found in an optimization procedure.

Estimation of RIF by Models

Building a model based on assumptions of the destiny of the CA in the tissue is intimately related to deriving an analytical expression for the RIF, as shown in the following.

Imagine that we have some evidence that all tracer molecules entering as a bolus (ideally as a delta function) and traveling with the same speed (plug flow) through the tissue will leave the tissue (voxel) exactly at the same time T_c. Then, we would build a simple model of RIF as RIF(t) = 1 for $0 < t < T_c$ and RIF(t) = 0 for $t > T_c$. The RIF is shown in Figure 8.4A. If we inject a short bolus with concentration $C_a(0)$ at time zero over a very short time interval Δt, then the tracer kinetic equation will look like

$$C_t(t) = C_a(t) \otimes f\,\mathrm{RIF}(t) = fC_a(0)\Delta t \quad 0 < t < T_c$$
$$C_t(t) = 0 \quad t > T_c$$

A unit step function, $U(t)$, is defined as

$$U(t) = 1; \quad t \geq 0$$
$$U(t) = 0; \quad t < 0$$

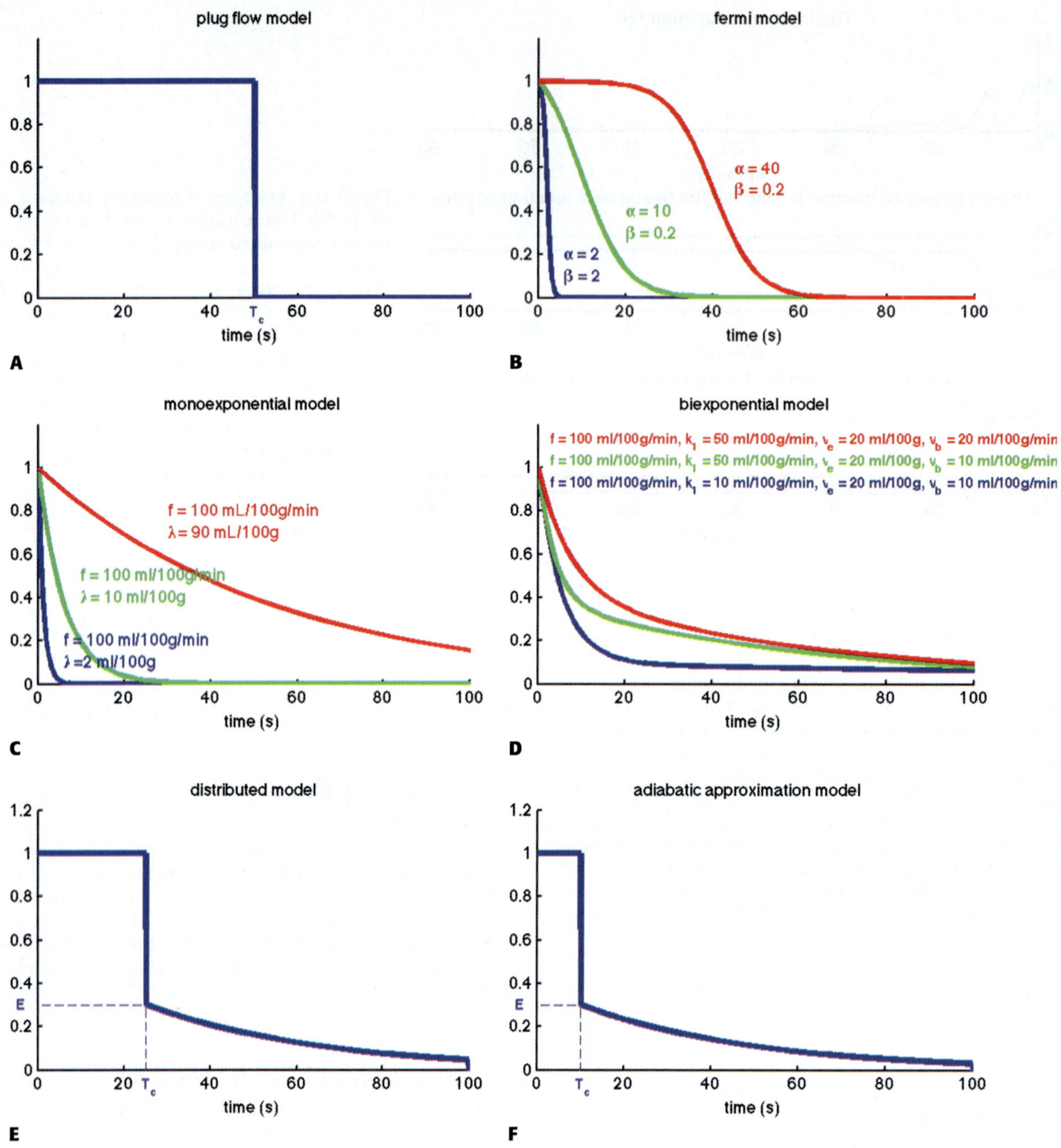

Figure 8-4. Examples of different models of the residue impulse response function. **A:** A simple model based on the assumption that all CA molecules leave the tissue simultaneously. **B:** A Fermi function, the curve is shown for three different sets of values; note the flexibility of the configuration. **C:** A monoexponential model compatible with a one-compartment model; note how the distribution volume, λ, influences the timing of the curve. **D:** A biexponential model compatible with a two-compartment model. Note how k_1 influences the slow component. **E and F:** These models take into account that a CA concentration can be a function of both time and position in a capillary. Essentially, the functions consist of a vascular phase, where a fraction of the CA moves through the tissue like a plug flow and leave the tissue simultaneously, while another fraction leaks into the extravascular space and gradually leaves the tissue afterwards.

Then, the RIF(t) can conveniently be rewritten as

$$\mathrm{RIF}(t) = U(t) - U(t - T_c)$$

A more reasonable assumption is that we have a distribution of transit times where some tracer molecules are somewhat faster than others. The Fermi function may capture this situation, with the expression

$$\mathrm{RIF}(t) = \frac{1 + e^{-\alpha\beta}}{1 + e^{(t-\alpha)\beta}} \tag{9}$$

having two adjustable parameters, where α determines the plateau (the minimal transit time) and β is related to the decay due to CA leaving the tissue. Note that if $t = 0$, RIF(0) = 1, and after the plateau, the function decays monotonously. The RIF(t) function is shown in Figure 8.4B.

A common approach is to consider the tissue as consisting of one or more compartments. Ideally, a compartment constitutes a volume fraction of the total tissue, where uniform concentration is established so fast at each time point so the concentration can be characterized as $C(t)$, that is, the compartment is well mixed, and a possible slow diffusion within a compartment is ignored. The starting point for compartment analysis is based on an extension of the Fick principle

$$\frac{dQ}{dt}=\sum_m J_{in}^m-\sum_n J_o^n \tag{10}$$

which states that the change in the amount of a CA in a given compartment is equal to the sum of all fluxes in and out of the compartment, where fluxes entering the compartment are positive and fluxes leaving the compartment are negative. As an example, we will derive the transport equation for a freely diffusible tracer. If membranes do not restrict diffusion through the tissue, the tissue (or voxel) will behave, as a one-compartment system, and the change of the amount in the tissue is according to the Fick principle[14]

$$\frac{dQ}{dt}=J_{in}-J_o \tag{11}$$

assuming either one inlet and one outlet, or if multiple inlets exist, it will sum up to J_{in} and similar for the outlet. If blood is the source of delivery of the CA, and CA is not produced or metabolized inside the tissue and also leaves by blood plasma, then we have

$$\frac{dQ(t)}{dt}=V_t\frac{dC_t(t)}{dt}=J_{in}(t)-J_o(t)=FC_a(t)-FC_o(t)$$

where V_t is the volume (or the mass) of the tissue, F is the total blood flow entering the tissue in focus (e.g., mL/min), and $C_a(t)$ is the arterial concentration and $C_o(t)$ is the concentration at the outlet. For a freely diffusible CA, it is a reasonable assumption that a fast equilibrium exists between tissue concentration and concentration at the outlet at any time point, giving $\lambda=C_t(t)/C_o(t)$, that is, the partition coefficient. Depending on the particular CA used, λ can be larger, equal, or smaller than V_t. Inserting this relationship results in a solvable first-order differential equation:

$$\frac{dC_t(t)}{dt}=\frac{F}{V_t}C_a(t)-\frac{F}{V_t}\frac{C_t(t)}{\lambda}=fC_a(t)-\frac{f}{\lambda}C_t(t)$$

With the initial conditions that $C_t(0) = 0$, the solutions is

$$C_t(t)=fC_a(t)\otimes\exp\left(-\frac{f}{\lambda}t\right)=f\int_0^t C_a(\tau)\exp\left(-\frac{f}{\lambda}(t-\tau)\right)d\tau \tag{12}$$

This equation is appropriate for labeled water or radioactive xenon. Thus, the RIF is a simple monoexponential function (see Fig. 8.4C) with two physiologic constants, the perfusion and the partition coefficient. If the time course of the tissue concentration and the arterial concentration as a function of time are measured, then these two constants can easily be estimated using standard fitting procedures. This equation is based on the pioneering work of Kety.[10]

In the MR field, we are not so lucky as to have a freely diffusible CA yet. In, for example, muscle tissue, the extraction fraction during the first pass is around 50% to 60%; in the liver, it is probably higher; and in the brain, it is close to zero. For an MR CA, which is confined to the plasma volume, the equation will be

$$\frac{dQ(t)}{dt}=V_t\frac{dC_t(t)}{dt}=J_{in}(t)-J_o(t)=F^pC_a^p(t)-F^pC_o^p(t)$$

where F^p is the blood plasma flow entering the tissue in focus (e.g., mL/min), $C_a^p(t)$ is the arterial plasma concentration, and $C_o^p(t)$ is the plasma concentration at the outlet. The conversion to full blood is given by

$$F^p=\left(1-\mathrm{Hct}_{SV}\right)F,\qquad C_a^p(t)=\frac{C_a(t)}{1-\mathrm{Hct}_{LV}} \tag{13}$$

where Hct_{SV} and Hct_{LV} are the small-vessel hematocrit and large-vessel hematocrit, respectively. The small-vessel hematocrit is used in conjunction with F because F relates to the microcirculation within the tissue, while the large-vessel hematocrit in conjunction with the input function relates to measurements in larger arteries. If we still can assume that $\lambda=C_t(t)/C_o^p(t)$, we end up with a similar equation as Eq. (12):

$$\frac{dC_t(t)}{dt}=\frac{F^p}{V_t}C_a^p(t)-\frac{F^p}{V_t}\frac{C_t(t)}{\lambda}=f^pC_a^p(t)-\frac{f^p}{\lambda}C_t(t)$$

With the initial condition that $C_t(0) = 0$, the standard solution is

$$\begin{aligned}C_t(t)&=f^p\int_0^t C_a^p(\tau)\exp\left(-\frac{f^p}{\lambda}(t-\lambda)\right)d\tau=\\ &f^pC_a^p(t)\otimes\exp\left(-\frac{f^p}{\lambda}t\right)=\\ &\frac{\left(1-\mathrm{Hct}_{SV}\right)}{\left(1-\mathrm{Hct}_{LV}\right)}fC_a(t)\otimes\exp\left(-\frac{\left(1-\mathrm{Hct}_{SV}\right)f}{\lambda}t\right)\end{aligned} \tag{14}$$

In fact, Eq. (14) has been used for brain perfusion with assumed intact BBB, and here, the MR CA behaves as an intravascular CA. Then, the partition coefficient λ is a measure of the cerebral blood volume, CBV. An example is shown in Figure 8.5. Whether one can use an intravascular CA for measurement of brain perfusion is controversial, because the results obtained are restricted by the assumption of the monoexponential RIF and may bias the results as pointed out by Lassen[15] and Weisskoff et al.,[16] and it is also uncertain which part of the vascular system is actually being measured. At least, it would be preferable to be able to model the RIF with a higher degree of freedom or without specifying an analytic model at all (see later).

In many types of tissues, the extraction fraction is neither very low nor very high. In, for example, the heart muscle tissue, the extraction fraction during the first pass is around 50% to 60%, and the models above might not be the most appropriate in this situation. A two-compartment model is a better description of the transport of the CA. Here, we let these two compartments be represented by the blood plasma in tissue, V_p, with the CA plasma concentration $C_p(t)$ in the tissue and the extravascular extracellular space in the tissue with volume V_e, with a CA concentration $C_e(t)$ (see Fig. 8.6). Note the assumption of the blood volume being represented by just one concentration regardless of the location along the capillary. Using the Fick principle and assuming first-order diffusion between compartments, the transport equations for the two compartments are

$$\begin{aligned}&V_p\frac{dC_p(t)}{dt}+\left(F+K_1\right)C_p-K_1C_e=FC_a(t),\\ &V_e\frac{dC_e(t)}{dt}-K_1C_p+K_1C_e=0\end{aligned} \tag{15}$$

Here, F and K_1 denote *plasma* perfusion and *plasma* clearance, respectively, and $C_a(t)$ is arterial plasma concentration (we omit the superscript for graphical reasons). In addition, we have the following relationships:

$$\begin{aligned}&V_eC_e=V_{tis}C_{tis}\\ &V_pC_p=\left(V_p+V_{Hct}\right)C_b\Leftrightarrow C_b=\left(1-\mathrm{Hct}_{SV}\right)C_p\\ &V_t=V_{tis}+V_p+V_{Hct}\\ &1=v_{tis}+v_p+v_{Hct}\\ &C_t=\frac{Q}{V_t}\end{aligned}$$

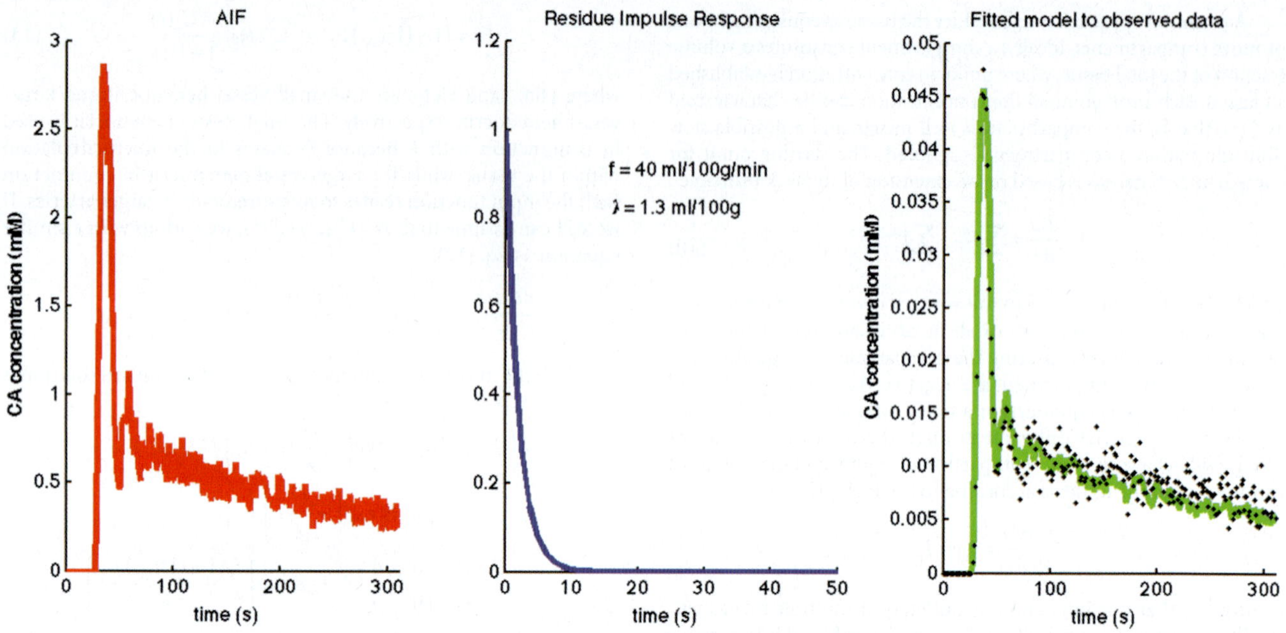

Figure 8-5. The arterial input function, AIF, is obtained from the internal carotid artery. Observed data are the tissue concentration enhancement obtained from an ROI placed in brain cortical gray matter. The green curve is a one-compartment model fitted to the data, that is, the AIF convolved with the residue impulse function of a one-compartment system. Optimum of the two free parameters, f and λ, is shown. Because the CA is nearly confined to the vascular space because of the blood–brain barrier, λ, is a measure of the cerebral blood volume in the ROI.

stating that the total tissue volume is composed of the extravascular tissue with volume, V_{tis}, the plasma volume, V_p, and the cell blood volume, V_{Hct}. It is assumed that the MR CA diffuses fast in the extravascular interstitial space. The second differential equation of Eq. (15) can be solved as done previously and gives

$$C_e(t) = \frac{K_1}{V_e} C_p(t) \otimes \exp\left(-\frac{K_1}{V_e} t\right)$$

which inserted in the first differential equation gives

$$V_p \frac{dC_p(t)}{dt} + (F + K_1)C_p - \frac{K_1^2}{V_e} C_p(t) \otimes \exp\left(-\frac{K}{V_e} t\right) = FC_a(t)$$

If we apply the Laplace transformation, then we can isolate $L\left(C_p(t)\right)$ and $L\left(C_e(t)\right)$, which we are searching for

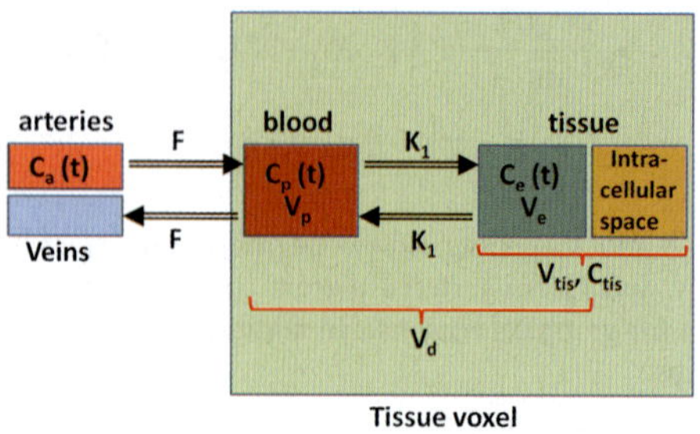

Figure 8-6. A two-compartment model. Such a model may be relevant for a moderate degree of leakiness. If k_1 is zero or very high, a one-compartment model might be more useful. Using a two-compartment model in this situation may result in so-called overfitting and less reliable results.

$$L(C_p)\left(sV_p + (F + K_1) - \frac{K_1^2}{sV_e + K_1}\right) =$$

$$FL(C_a) \Leftrightarrow L(C_p) =$$

$$\frac{s/V_p + K_1/V_pV_e}{s^2 + s(K_1/V_e + F/V_p + K_1/V_p) + FK_1/V_eV_p} FL(C_a)$$

$$L(C_e) = \frac{K_1}{sV_e + K_1} L(C_p) =$$

$$\frac{K_1}{V_eV_p} \frac{1}{s^2 + s(K_1/V_e + F/V_p + K_1/V_p) + FK_1/V_eV_p} FL(C_a)$$

Using the Laplace transformation of exponentials as

$$L(A\exp(-at) + B\exp(-bt)) = \frac{A}{s+a} + \frac{B}{s+b}$$

$$L\left(\frac{\exp(-bt) - \exp(-at)}{a-b}\right) = \frac{1}{(s+a)(s+b)}$$

we can identify

$$A = \frac{V_e\alpha - K_1}{V_eV_p(\alpha - \beta)}; \qquad B = -\frac{V_e\beta - K_1}{V_eV_p(\alpha - \beta)}$$

$$\alpha = \frac{1}{2}\left(\frac{K_1}{V_e} + \frac{F + K_1}{V_p} + \sqrt{\left(\frac{K_1}{V_e} + \frac{F + K_1}{V_p}\right)^2 - 4\frac{FK_1}{V_eV_p}}\right)$$

$$\beta = \frac{1}{2}\left(\frac{K_1}{V_e} + \frac{F + K_1}{V_p} - \sqrt{\left(\frac{K_1}{V_e} + \frac{F + K_1}{V_p}\right)^2 - 4\frac{FK_1}{V_eV_p}}\right)$$

and $C_p(t)$ and $C_e(t)$ are then

$$C_p(t) = FC_a(t) \otimes \frac{1}{V_e V_p(\alpha-\beta)}\left((V_e\alpha - K_1)\exp(-\alpha t) - (V_e\beta - K_1)\exp(-\beta t)\right)$$

$$C_e(t) = FC_a(t) \otimes \frac{1}{V_e V_p(\alpha-\beta)}\left(K_1\exp(-\beta t) - K_1\exp(-\alpha t)\right)$$

Total tissue concentration, $C_t(t)$, is then found from

$$V_t C_t(t) = V_p C_p(t) + V_e C_e(t) \Rightarrow C_t(t) = \frac{F}{V_t} C_a(t) \otimes \frac{1}{\alpha-\beta}\left(\left(\alpha - \frac{K_1}{V_e} - \frac{K_1}{V_p}\right)\exp(-\alpha t) + \left(\frac{K_1}{V_e} + \frac{K_1}{V_p} - \beta\right)\exp(-\beta t)\right) \quad (16)$$

where $f = F/V_t$, and conveniently, all other constants are normalized by V_t. Conversion to full blood reference is also straightforward. Note that the residue impulse response function is biexponential and RIF(0) = 1 (see Fig. 8.4D). The two-compartment model has four free parameters: f^p, k_1^p, v_e, and v_p. This type of model has previously been applied to a number of diseases in different organs including the brain lately.[8,17] Brix already presented a simplified version of the two-compartment model in 1991.[18] An example of using this model in a leaky brain tumor is shown in Figure 8.7.

The first tracer kinetic model, often called the Tofts model, used in conjunction with MRI, focused on estimation of BBB permeability of multiple sclerosis plaques and brain tumors[19,20]:

$$C_t(t) = k_1^p C_a^p(t) \otimes \exp\left(-\frac{k_1^p}{\lambda}t\right) = K^{\text{trans}} \frac{C_a(t)}{(1-\text{Hct}_{\text{LV}})} \otimes \exp\left(-\frac{K^{\text{trans}}}{v_e}t\right) \quad (17)$$

Note that $K^{\text{trans}}\left(= k_1^p = Ef^p\right)$ is the tissue clearance (tissue uptake transfer constant) with reference to plasma with the dimension mL plasma cleared/100 mL tissue/min (a capital letter in K^{trans} is traditional used), $C_a^p(t)$ is plasma concentration of the CA, while $C_a(t)$ is full blood concentration. The assumptions behind this model are, firstly, that the vascular volume fraction in the tissue is vanishing small and can be ignored and, secondly, that the arterial plasma concentration of the CA represents the input function to a distribution volume, which is equivalent with the extravascular extracellular space, v_e. Note that if $ps \gg f(E = 1)$, then $K^{\text{trans}} = f^p$, and we are back to Eq. (12). If $ps \ll f(E \to 0)$, $K^{\text{trans}} = ps$. Thus, the residue impulse response function in this case is $\text{RIF}(t) = \exp(-K^{\text{trans}}t/v_e)$. After the introduction of Eq. (17), it was quickly being used outside the brain, and it soon became clear that the vascular component could not be ignored and constituted a significant part of the MR signal in many types of tissue, for example, in the heart.[21] In order to ameliorate this situation, the vascular volume was included giving the following equation, often denoted as the extended Tofts model[22]:

$$C_t(t) = v_p C_a^p(t) + k_1^p C_a^p(t) \otimes \exp\left(-\frac{k_1^p}{v_e}t\right) \quad (18)$$

The specific assumption associated with this expression is that the plasma fraction in the tissue has a CA concentration equal with the arterial plasma concentration (which is measured), and the loss from the vascular space due to leakage is so small that it can be ignored; obviously, this equation implicitly suggests a very small $k_1^p \approx ps$ product. The extended Tofts model has three unknown free parameters: k_1^p, v_e, and v_p. Formally, the $\text{RIF}(t) = v_p\delta(t) + \exp(-K^{\text{trans}}t/v_e)$.

It is increasingly being recognized that Eq. (18) in some situation is inadequate to describe the CA transport in some type of tissues, or at least, the interpretation of k_1^p is somewhat ambiguous, as it is often correlated with both perfusion and permeability.[23–25] It has even been shown that a good fit of Eq. (18) to data is no guaranty of obtaining accurate results,[24] and more elaborate methods should probably be used (see below).

Equation (18) is a good starting point for deriving the famous Patlak equation.[26] If leakage is unidirectional, that is, negligible backflux, then RIF(t) = 1, and Eq. (18) becomes

$$C_t(t) = v_p C_a^p(t) + k_1^p \int_0^t C_a^p(\tau)\,d\tau$$

Again, the assumptions are a unidirectional transport, that is, an irreversible leakage, and the arterial plasma with concentration

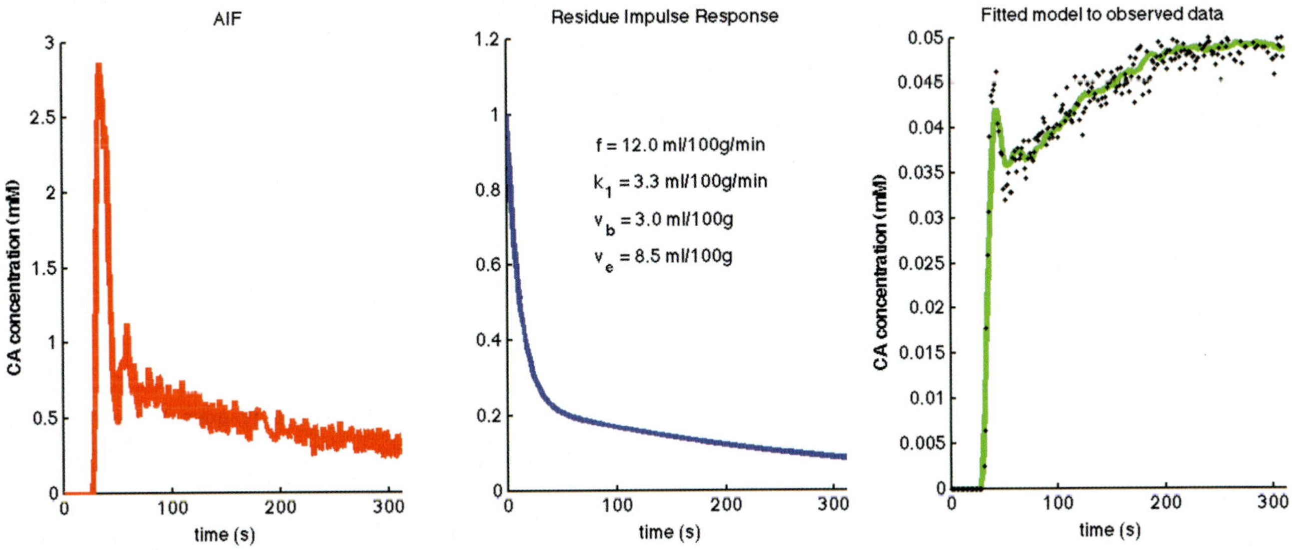

Figure 8-7. **Observed data are the tissue concentration enhancement obtained from an ROI placed in a brain tumor.** Note that data show a pronounced "vascular" peak followed by a steadier enhancement due to deficiency of the BBB. The green curve is two-compartment model fitted to the data, that is, the AIF convolved with the residue impulse function of a two-compartment system. Optimum of the four free parameters is shown.

$C_a^p(t)$ serves as a source for the leakage inside the tissue, and importantly, the CA loss from this vascular space is so small that it can be ignored. Obviously, for an inert typical MR CA agent, $k_1^p = \text{ps}$ product. Dividing both sides of the equation with the instantaneous $C_a^p(t)$ results in the Patlak equation

$$\frac{C_t(t)}{C_a^p(t)} = v_p + k_1^p \frac{\int_0^t C_a^p(\tau)\mathrm{d}\tau}{C_a^p(t)} \tag{19}$$

If one then plots the ratio $C_t(t)/C_a^p(t)$ as a function of $\int_0^t C_a^p(\tau)\mathrm{d}\tau / C_a^p(t)$, one will get at straight line with the slope k_1^p and an intercept of v_p, which are the two unknown in this equation. As pointed out by Patlak, v_p in reality includes the steady-state volume of distribution of all reversible compartments. The Patlak analysis has been used successfully in many nuclear medicine studies and seems also useful when measuring the BBB permeability in the brain when using DCE-MRI.[17,27] However, it is important to restrict its use in accordance with the assumptions. When used, one will notice an initial phase in the Patlak plot, which is related to a vascular transition, and the Patlak equation only relates to the slowly steady increase afterwards (see Fig. 8.8). In order to understand the entire curve obtained, it is more instructive to start with the two-compartment model, eliminating all terms related to the back-diffusion, which we now assume can be neglected:

$$V_p \frac{\mathrm{d}C_p(t)}{\mathrm{d}t} + (F + K_1)C_p = FC_a(t),$$
$$V_e \frac{\mathrm{d}C_e(t)}{\mathrm{d}t} - K_1 C_p = 0$$
$$V_t C_t(t) = V_e C_e(t) + V_p C_p(t)$$

Solving these coupled differential equations using the Laplace transformation as previously, and where F, K_1, and C_a relate to plasma, gives

$$C_p(t) = \frac{F}{V_p} C_a(t) \otimes \exp\left(-\frac{F+K_1}{V_p}t\right)$$
$$C_e(t) = \frac{FK_1}{V_e(F+K_1)} C_a(t) \otimes \left(1 - \exp\left(-\frac{F+K_1}{V_p}t\right)\right) \tag{20}$$
$$C_t(t) = \frac{F}{V_t} C_a(t) \otimes \left[\frac{K_1}{F+K_1} + \frac{F}{F+K_1}\exp\left(-\frac{F+K_1}{V_p}t\right)\right]$$

$f^p = F^p/V_t$ and all other constants can be normalized to V_t. Note that the RIF(0) = 1. Furthermore, if $F^p \gg K_1^p$, as will be the case for a unidirectional transport of an inert MR CA, then we get

$$C_t(t) \approx k_1^p \int_0^t C_a^p(\tau)\mathrm{d}\tau + f^p \int_0^t C_a^p(\tau) \exp\left(-\frac{f^p + k_1^p}{v_p}(t-\tau)\right)\mathrm{d}\tau \tag{21}$$

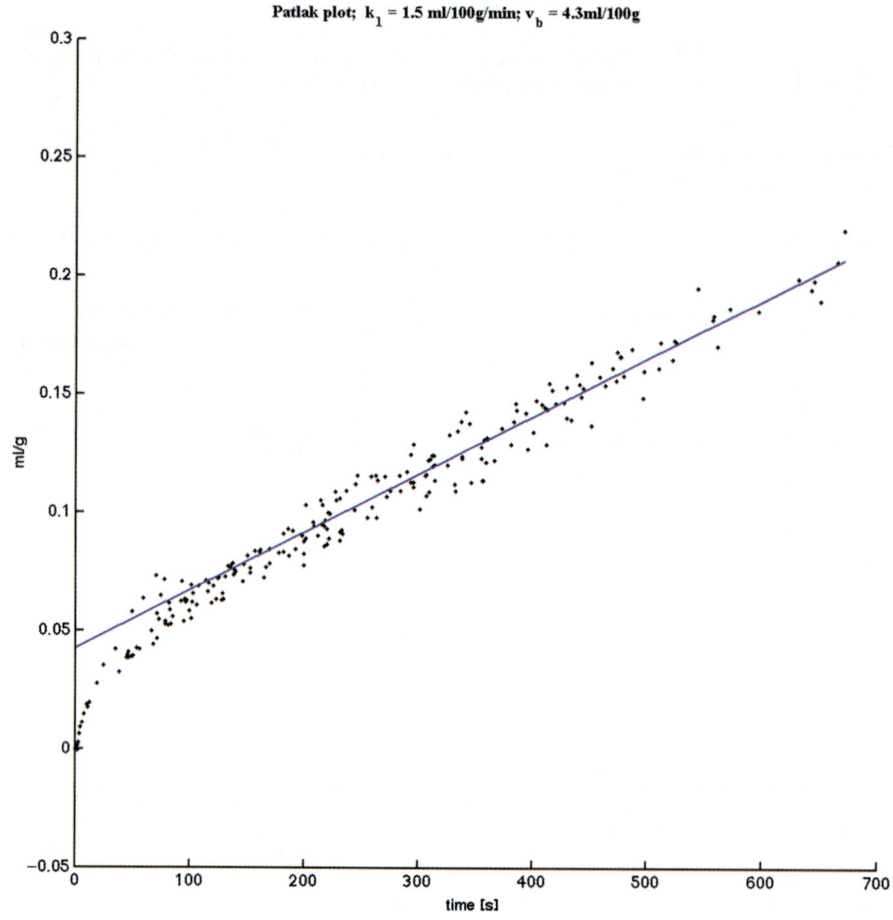

Figure 8-8. An example of a Patlak plot: $\frac{C_t(t)}{C_a^p(t)}$ as a function of $\frac{\int_0^t C_a^p(\tau)\mathrm{d}\tau}{C_a^p(t)}$. The slope of the regression line corresponds to k_1, while the intercept corresponds to the blood plasma volume v_p. Data obtained from a leaky brain tumor.

Obviously, k_1^{p} is the ps^{p} product. It is seen that the initial part in a Patlak plot is related a vascular phase, which eventually vanished leaving a term $k_1^{\mathrm{p}}\int C_{\mathrm{a}}^{\mathrm{p}}(\tau)\mathrm{d}\tau$, which is related to a steady irreversible accumulation of the CA in the extravascular extracellular tissue. Equation (20) can in fact be used as a model and fitted to data, when back-diffusion can be ignored. The model has three free parameters: f^{p}, ps^{p}, and v_{p}; however, v_{e} cannot be estimated. Finally, it is important to inspect the Patlak plot: If the straight line, corresponding to the steady increase, tends to level off for later time points, then this is an indication of a possible back-diffusion. In fact, if the uptake is followed for very long time, back-diffusion will eventually occur. In that perspective, fitting of Eq. (16) to such data seems more appropriate.

The assumption of a uniform well-mixed vascular concentration is an approximation and can potentially introduce a bias. In reality, one can imagine that the capillary concentration changes as a function of position along the capillary in addition to being a function of time.[28,29] Incorporation of time and position constitutes the so-called distributed model, signifying that concentration gradients exist within the tissue, which is in contrast to compartment models where every compartment is well mixed instantaneously and concentration is only a function of time. The starting point for this model is related to the concentration inside the capillary at location x with a total length L:

$$V_{\mathrm{p}}\frac{\partial C_{\mathrm{p}}(t,x)}{\partial t} = -FL\frac{\partial C_{\mathrm{p}}(t,x)}{\partial x} - \mathrm{PS}\big(C_{\mathrm{p}}(t,x) - C_{\mathrm{e}}(t,x)\big) + FLC_{\mathrm{a}}(t)\delta(x)$$

where we have used the same consideration as when deriving the Crone-Renkin equation. The equation for the extravascular extracellular space is given as

$$V_{\mathrm{e}}\frac{\partial C_{\mathrm{e}}(t,x)}{\partial t} = \mathrm{PS}\big(C_{\mathrm{p}}(t,x) - C_{\mathrm{e}}(t,x)\big)$$

The model assumes plug flow, meaning that every cross section at location x of the capillary have the same uniform concentration characterized by $C_{\mathrm{p}}(t,x)$ and in addition no significant extravascular diffusion along the capillary. The solution to the differential equations using the Laplace transformation results in a residue impulse response function consisting of two parts:

$$\begin{aligned}
&\mathrm{RIF}(t) = \mathrm{RIF}_1(t) + \mathrm{RIF}_2(t - T_{\mathrm{c}})\\
&\mathrm{RIF}_1(t) = U(t) - U(t - T_{\mathrm{c}})\\
&\mathrm{RIF}_2(t) =\\
&U(t)\left(1-\exp\left(-\frac{\mathrm{PS}}{F}\right)\left(1+\int_0^t \exp\left(-\frac{\mathrm{PS}}{V_{\mathrm{e}}}\tau\right)\sqrt{\frac{\mathrm{PS}^2}{V_{\mathrm{e}}F\tau}}I_1 2\sqrt{\frac{\mathrm{PS}^2}{V_{\mathrm{e}}F}\tau}\right)\mathrm{d}\tau\right)
\end{aligned} \tag{22}$$

I_1 is the modified Bessel function. Although the solution is cumbersome, the interpretation is straightforward (see Fig. 8.4E). The first part, $\mathrm{RIF}_1(t)$, until T_{c} corresponds to a fraction of the CA staying inside the vessels and moving forward as a plug flow and leaving the tissue at T_{c}. This may be called the vascular transit phase. During this phase, another fraction can leave the vascular space into the extravascular space, still contributing to the total amount in tissue. When the vascular phase ends, the RIF is dominated by a slow back-diffusion from the parenchyma corresponding to the leakage fraction, $\mathrm{RIF}_2(t)$, signifying loss of CA by perfusion. The transition is a direct measure of E, and the mean transit time of the vascular space and the extravascular space can be found as the area of the respective RIF, which correspond to $\mathrm{MTT} = v_{\mathrm{p}}/f^{\mathrm{p}}$ and $\mathrm{MTT} = v_{\mathrm{e}}/f^{\mathrm{p}}$, respectively.[30] The distributed model has not been thoroughly validated and compared to a two-compartment model, but several studies report a better fit to observed data in brain tumors,[31] in infarcted myocardium,[32] and in neuroendocrine hepatic metastases.[33] It is likely that the model is highly dependent on the assumption of plug flow, meaning no radial gradient in capillary during the initial wash-in and also a high time resolution, at the level of a second, in order to define the vascular phase with sufficient accuracy. Two variants of the distributed model exist. The first is the so-called tissue homogeneity model, where the extravascular compartment model is treated as a well-mixed compartment and therefore only a function of time.[34] However, this does not ease the solution. The second is the so-called adiabatic approximation, where the vascular phase is assumed to be much faster than the leakage process, and leakage occurs only at the venous end of the capillary.[35] This leads to a considerable simplification with a residue impulse response function as

$$\begin{aligned}
&\mathrm{RIF}(t) = 1 \quad 0 \le t < T_{\mathrm{c}}\\
&\mathrm{RIF}(t) = E\exp\left(-\frac{EF}{V_{\mathrm{e}}}(t - T_{\mathrm{c}})\right) \quad t \ge T_{\mathrm{c}}
\end{aligned} \tag{23}$$

It is evident that the initial vascular phase is similar to the original model, but the wash-out phase is substituted by an exponential function (see Fig. 8.4F). The adiabatic approximation model was implemented and validated using D_2O and MRI, and for this setup, perfusion seems to be underestimated for higher value of perfusion.[36]

In the models presented above, we have assumed a one-capillary model, that is, one typical capillary is representative for all the capillaries in a given voxel or tissue region of interest (ROI). However, multiple-pathway models have been proposed consisting of many capillaries with different flow distribution and length, and each capillary can be characterized by, for example, a distributed model.[37] The degree of clinical impact of these elaborated models is up to future research and will probably benefit from an increasing time and spatial resolution of MRI.

Estimation of RIF without a Model

So far, it is clear that estimating perfusion or permeability necessitates building a model based on some specific assumptions of how tissue is "handling" the CA used. It is also clear that any model will influence the results obtained using that model. In addition, it is difficult to prove that one model is more accurate compared to another, and even microsphere injection or radioactive water ($^{15}H_2O$) in conjunction with PET, normally considered as a gold standard, has its limitations.[38] However, if a model gives useful clinical results, then accuracy might be secondary.

In order to circumvent the problem of specifying a model, model-free or data-driven solution is increasingly being used. The starting point is based on the fact that a convolution can be written in a discrete form as a matrix equation:

$$\vec{y} = f\Delta t\,\mathbf{A}\vec{x} \tag{24}$$

Here, $\vec{y}$ is a column vector representation of C_{t}, $\mathbf{A}$ is a matrix representation of C_{a}, and $\vec{x}$ is a column vector representation of the RIF. Specifying the entries of the matrix equation, it looks like

$$\begin{bmatrix} C_{\mathrm{t}}(1)\\ C_{\mathrm{t}}(2)\\ C_{\mathrm{t}}(3)\\ \vdots\\ C_{\mathrm{t}}(N)\end{bmatrix} = f\Delta t\begin{bmatrix} C_{\mathrm{a}}(1) & 0 & 0 & \cdots & 0\\ C_{\mathrm{a}}(2) & C_{\mathrm{a}}(1) & 0 & \cdots & 0\\ C_{\mathrm{a}}(3) & C_{\mathrm{a}}(2) & C_{\mathrm{a}}(1) & \cdots & 0\\ \vdots & \vdots & \vdots & \ddots & \vdots\\ C_{\mathrm{a}}(N) & C_{\mathrm{a}}(N-1) & C_{\mathrm{a}}(N-2) & \cdots & C_{\mathrm{a}}(1)\end{bmatrix}\begin{bmatrix}\mathrm{RIF}(1)\\ \mathrm{RIF}(2)\\ \mathrm{RIF}(3)\\ \vdots\\ \mathrm{RIF}(N)\end{bmatrix} \tag{25}$$

Obviously, the equation is discretized with a total of N samples and with a time resolution of Δt. Scrutinizing this equation will disclose the nature of the convolution, however, in a discrete form. For information about matrix calculus, see Glodberg, or for a compact tutorial, see Larsson HBW: Introduction to the general linear model used in fMRI. In fact, Eq. (25) is the typical computer realization of the convolution, where the RIF may be specified by an analytical expression. For example, let $\mathrm{RIF}(i) = \exp(-f\Delta t(i-1)/\lambda)$, $i = 1,\ldots,N$; then, this can be used in an optimization procedure, where the model is specified by having a monoexponential residue impulse response function, with two free parameters, f and λ, and with N samples of C_t and C_a. The optimization problem can then be formulated as minimizing the following term:

$$\min\left\{\left\|\vec{y}^{\text{obs}} - \vec{y}^{\text{calc}}\right\|^2\right\}$$

where $\vec{y}^{\text{obs}}$ is the measured tissue concentration and A represents the measured arterial input function. Then $\vec{y}^{\text{obs}} = \vec{y}^{\text{calc}} + \vec{\varepsilon}$, with $\vec{y}^{\text{calc}} = f\Delta t\,\mathrm{A}\vec{x}$, the calculated tissue concentration using the model $f\vec{x}$. The value of f and λ, which minimized the difference between the observed and the calculated tissue concentration, that is, the error or residual $\|\vec{\varepsilon}\|$, is said to constitute the optimal solution.

However, Eq. (25) offers another solution. Under some circumstances, it is possible to isolate the RIF(i) giving a direct solution if the matrix **A** can be inverted:

$$\vec{y} = f\Delta t\,\mathrm{A}\vec{x} \Rightarrow \vec{x} = \frac{1}{f\Delta t}\mathrm{A}^{-1}\vec{y}$$

From matrix algebra, we know that a unique solution is possible if the determinant of the matrix **A** is different from zero, equivalent with all the columns of the matrix are linearly independent, that is, the matrix has the rank of N. However, this lucky situation is seldom satisfied due to noise, and perhaps interpolation (see later), and the matrix becomes what is called singular, or rank deficient. Luckily, a solution can always be found in a reduced dimensional space, using the singular value decomposition (SVD) obtaining the pseudo-inverse matrix $\mathbf{A}^{-}$:

$$\vec{y}^{\text{obs}} = f\Delta t\,\mathrm{A}\vec{x} + \vec{\varepsilon} \Rightarrow \vec{x} = \frac{1}{f\Delta t}\mathrm{A}^{-}\vec{y}^{\text{obs}} \Rightarrow \vec{y}^{\text{calc}} = \mathrm{AA}^{-}\vec{y}^{\text{obs}}$$

It can be shown that this solution also minimizes the residuals, that is, the distance between the observed tissue concentration and calculated tissue concentration. Leif Østergaard was the first to introduce this technique in the MR community focusing on perfusion measurements using exogenous CA and tracer kinetic theory.[39] For information about SVD, see Glodberg, or for a compact tutorial, see Larsson HBW: Introduction to the general linear model used in fMRI. An example of using the SVD in order to estimate perfusion in the brain is shown in Figure 8.9.

The use of the pseudoinverse comes at a price: the solution is extremely sensitive towards noise, and the unphysiologic oscillation of the RIF is a manifestation of the noise sensitivity. In order to suppress these spurious oscillations, one can select an empirical threshold below which, all eigenvalues are set to zeros, for example, the 20% lowest eigenvalues are set to zeros, at a price of underestimating the perfusion. Thus, the threshold setting is a trade-off between unwanted unphysiologic oscillations and distortions of the RIF and overfitting at one side and a blunted RIF and underestimation of perfusion f at the other side, see Figure 8.9. Another possibility is to directly incorporate our theoretical knowledge about the RIF,

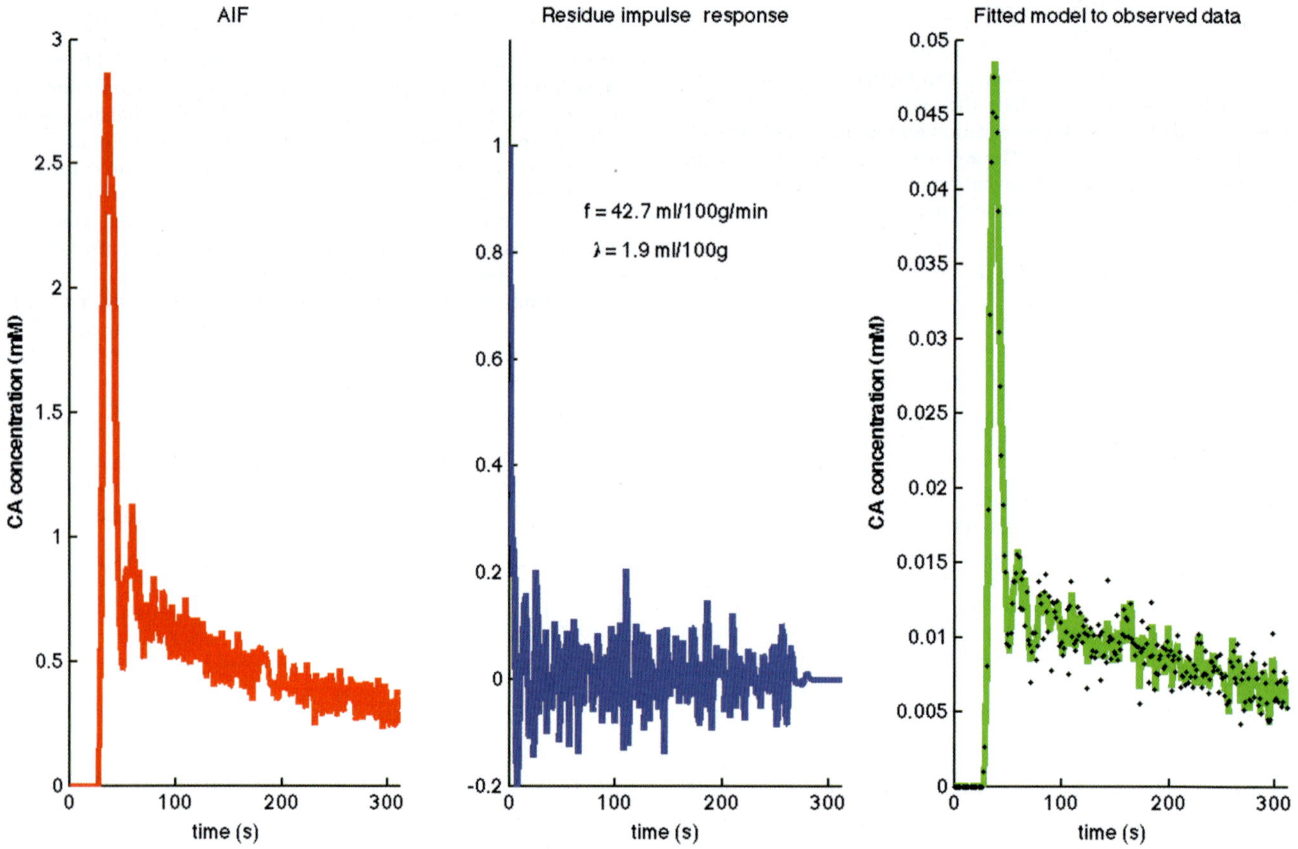

A

Figure 8-9. **Example of the use of the singular value decomposition (SVD).** AIF and observed data are the same as in Figure 8.5. **A:** SVD keeping nearly all eigenvalues, that is, no regularization, results in a noisy residue impulse response function and a tendency of overfitting of data.

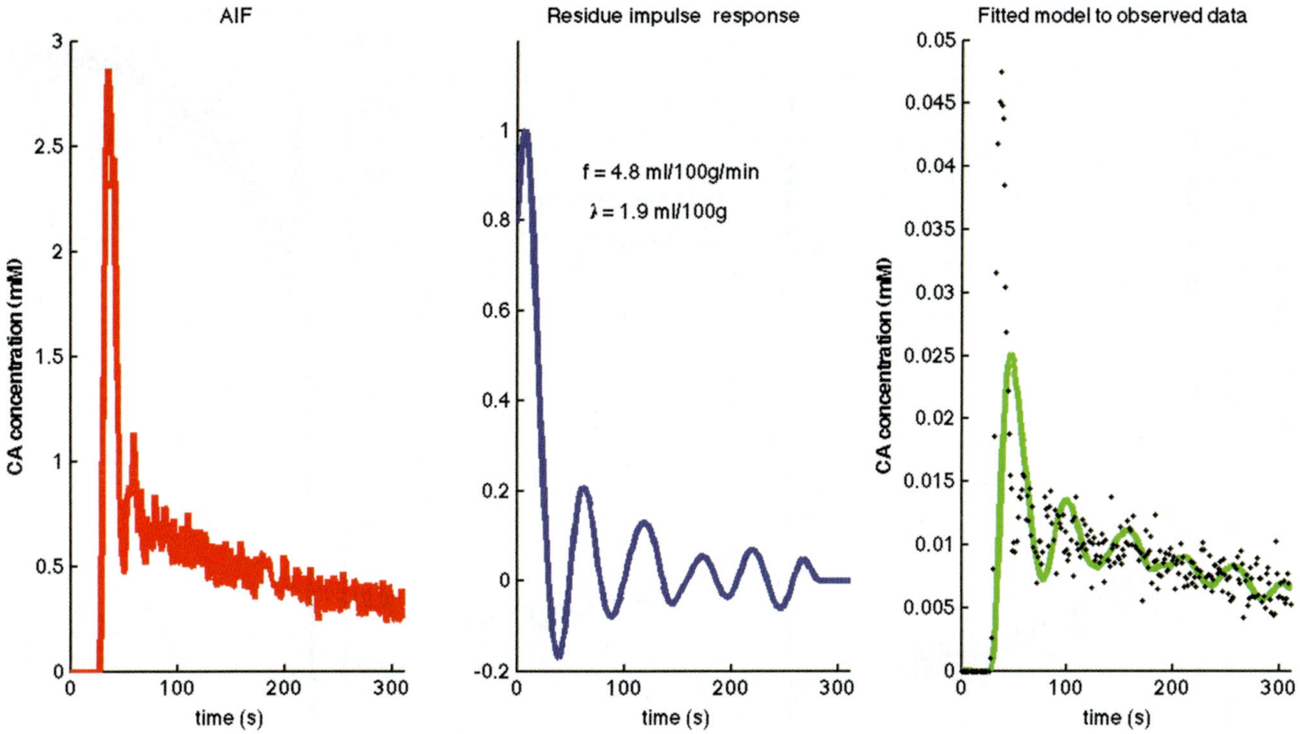

B

Figure 8-9. (*Continued*) **B:** Keeping only eigenvalues larger than 20% of the first (largest) eigenvalue results in a less noisy residue impulse response function, however, still having spurious oscillations and a considerable underestimation of brain perfusion.

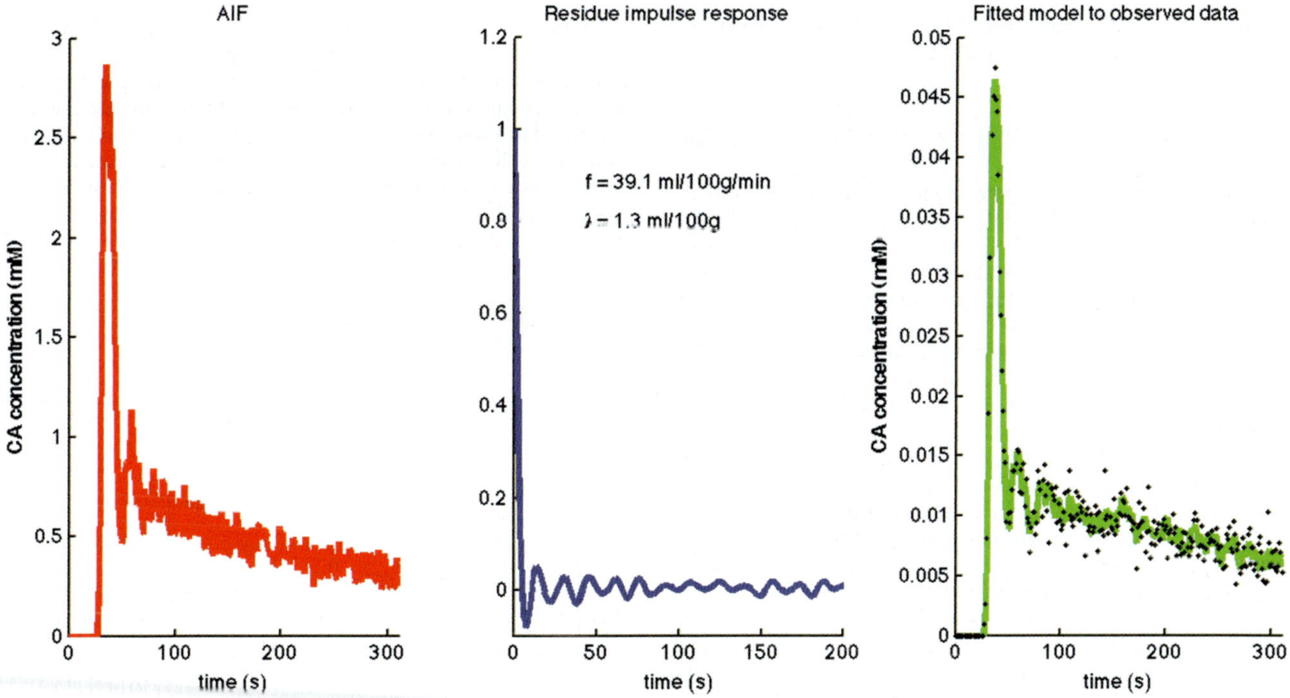

Figure 8-10. Example of the use of the generalized singular value decomposition (GSVD) with regularization using the *L*-curve method (see text). AIF and data are the same as in Figures 8.5 and 8.9. Note the reduction of the oscillations of the residue impulse response function, still fitting the data and no obvious underestimation of perfusion.

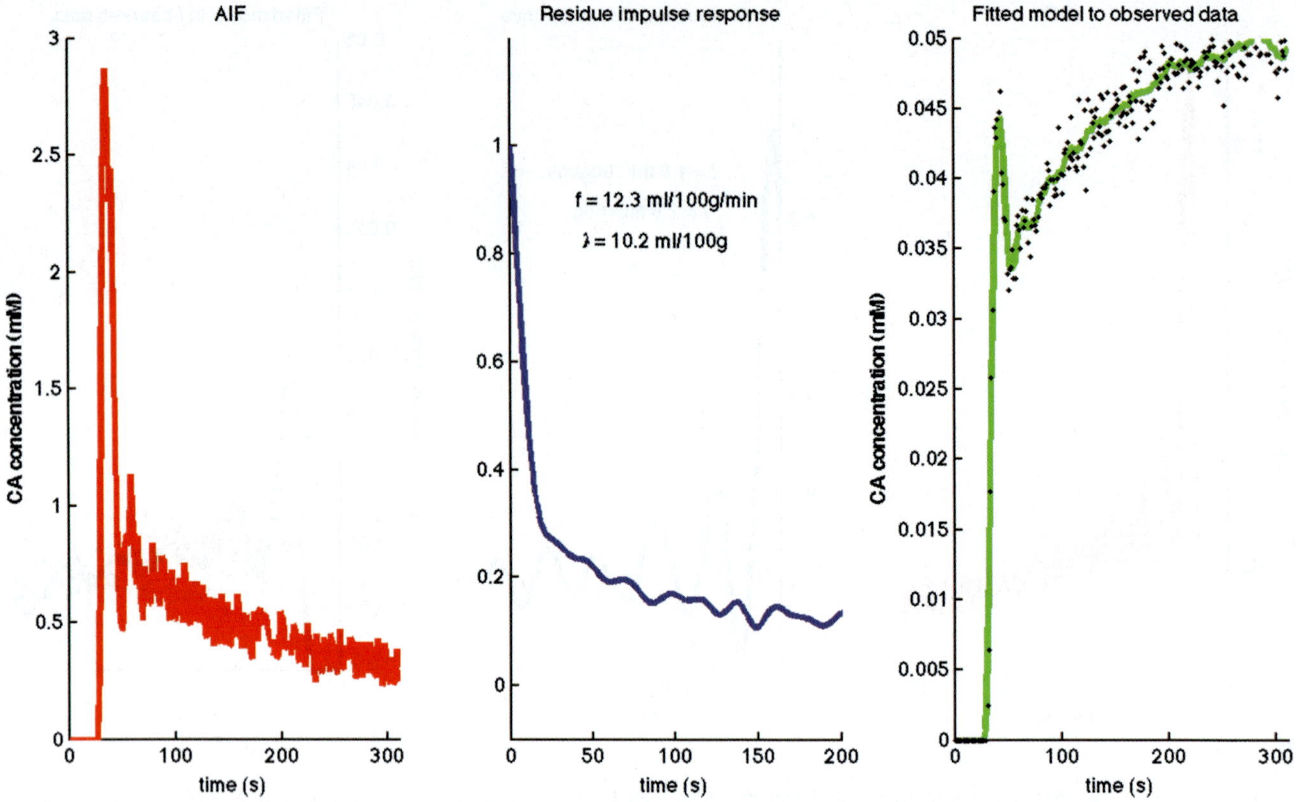

Figure 8-11. Example of the use of the generalized singular value decomposition (GSVD) with regularization using the *L*-curve method (see text). AIF and data are the same as in Figure 8.7. λ should be interpreted as the volume of distribution and corresponds approximately to the sum of v_b and v_e in Figure 8.7.

namely, that the RIF is a nonincreasing function. The "generalized singular value decomposition" (GSVD)[40,41] seeks to find the solution from the minimization of

$$\min\left\{\left\|\mathbf{A}\vec{x}-\vec{y}^{\text{obs}}\right\|^2+\lambda^2\left\|L(\vec{x})\right\|^2\right\} \tag{26}$$

where L is the first derivative operator and λ is the degree of regularization. If λ is set to zero, the solution is not regularized, and the RIF may manifest these unphysiologic oscillations. If λ is set to a very high value, the solution, that is, the RIF, will become very smooth without oscillations. The optimum value of the regularization parameter, λ, is found using the curvature of the so-called L-curve, a heuristic approach: a trade-off between obtaining a smooth RIF and match between $\mathbf{A}\vec{x}$ and $\vec{y}^{\text{obs}}$,[42] and can be implemented as an automatic procedure voxel-wise. A practical implementation is given in reference.[7] Even the GSVD with regularization, which tends to eliminate abrupt changes of the RIF, seems to underestimate perfusion in some situations (see ref.[17]). Examples of using the GSVD in order to estimate brain perfusion are shown in Figures 8.10 and 8.11. Figure 8.12 shows an example of voxel-wise calculation of CBF, creating CBF maps of the brain, and Figure 8.13 shows maps of permeability of a patient with a brain tumor.

In conclusion, it is possible to find a solution to the general tracer kinetic equation (Eq. (6)), without specifying a specific model with its associated analytical expression, but the solution is very noise sensitive, and one have to regularize the solution, by either cutting eigenvalues or incorporating a smoothing operator, with a possible impact on the shape of RIF and some underestimation of f.

Equation (25) involves sums of the form $C_a(i)\text{RIF}(j)\Delta t$, and the term represents an area of a square. If $C_a(i)$ or RIF(j) are characterized by a pronounce change from sample to sample, then this discrete calculation will overestimate or underestimate the area compared to a convolution performed by a real continuous integration. This will introduce a bias of the resulting perfusion. In order to ameliorate this problem, one can either interpolate data to a finer temporal grid, for example, by a factor of 2 to 10, or use the trapezoid rule, and Eq. (25) will be given as[28]

$$\begin{bmatrix} C_t(1) \\ C_t(2) \\ C_t(3) \\ \vdots \\ C_t(N) \end{bmatrix} = f\,\Delta t \begin{bmatrix} \frac{C_a(1)}{2} & 0 & 0 & \cdots & 0 \\ \frac{C_a(2)}{2} & \frac{C_a(1)}{2} & 0 & \cdots & 0 \\ \frac{C_a(3)}{2} & C_a(2) & \frac{C_a(1)}{2} & \cdots & 0 \\ \vdots & \vdots & \vdots & \ddots & \vdots \\ \frac{C_a(N)}{2} & C_a(N-1) & C_a(N-2) & \cdots & \frac{C_a(1)}{2} \end{bmatrix} \begin{bmatrix} \text{RIF}(1) \\ \text{RIF}(2) \\ \text{RIF}(3) \\ \vdots \\ \text{RIF}(N) \end{bmatrix} \tag{27}$$

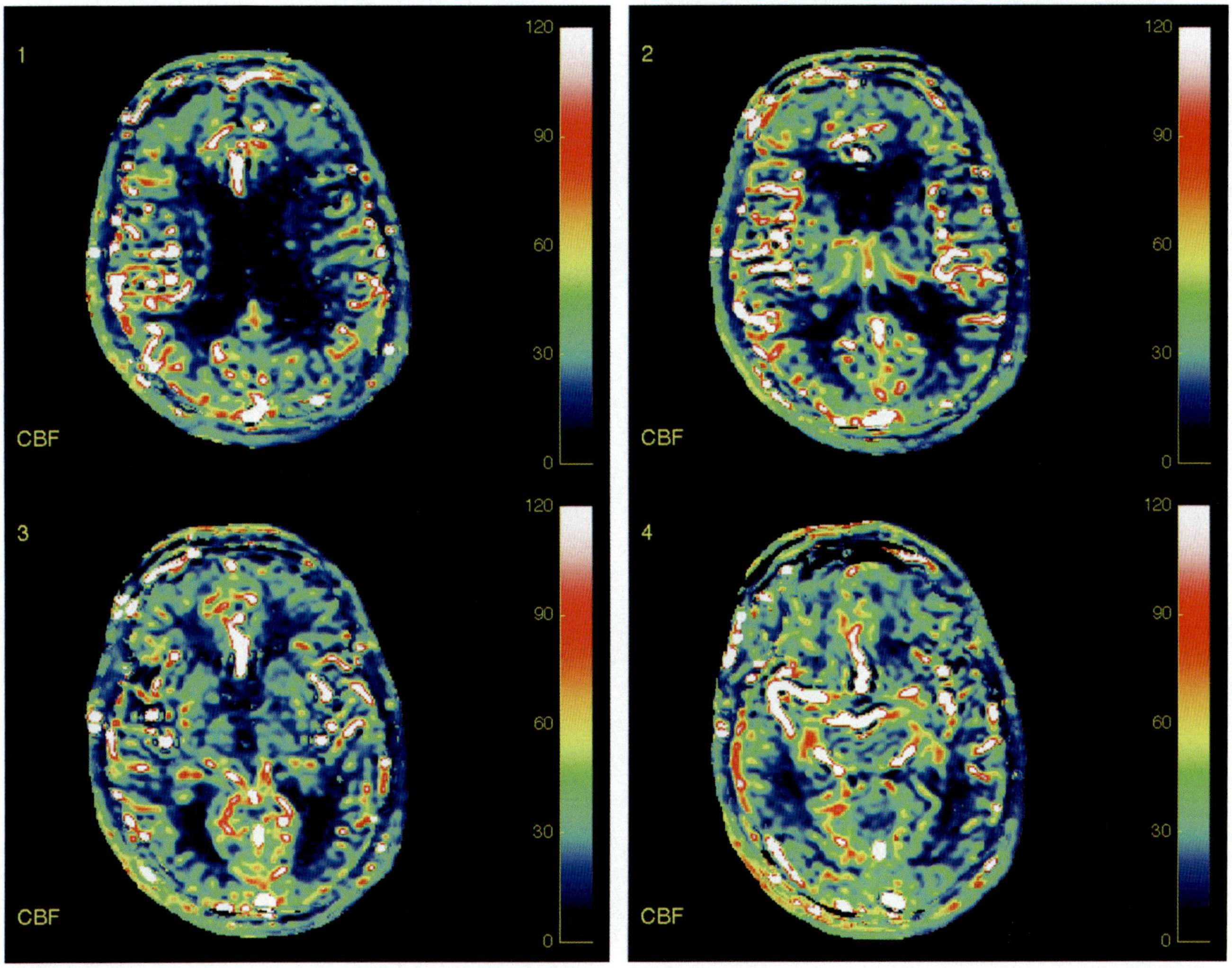

Figure 8-12. CBF maps using dynamic contrast-enhanced T_1-weighted MRI, at 3 T, using a saturation fast-field echo MR sequence, with a temporal resolution about 1 second. CBF is calculated pixelwise using the GSVD with *L*-curve regularization. Color scale is in mL/100 mL/min. The subject has a slight asymmetric perfusion pattern corresponding to cerebral media artery, with decreased perfusion corresponding to a known internal carotid stenosis at the same side.

The Arterial Input Function—Direct Measurement

The arterial input function, $C_a(t)$, represents the arterial concentration of the CA used as a function of time and is often abbreviated the AIF. It is necessary to measure or estimate the AIF if absolute physiologic measures of the tissue are wanted. The AIF can be obtained from arterially placed catheter, but it is more convenient if the AIF can be obtained from the dynamic images obtained during the bolus passage. For the heart, the left ventricle is a good location, and for the brain, the internal carotid artery (ICA) is obviously a good choice. Ideally, the AIF should be obtained from an artery as close as possible to the tissue in focus. If not, the AIF will be time shifted compared to the tissue enhancement curve, typically a couple of seconds ahead of the tissue. In all the models above, we have assumed simultaneous MR signal increase of tissue and arterial blood corresponding to the bolus arrival. If this condition is not satisfied, severe error of estimates of perfusion and transit times might be introduced. Therefore, the AIF should be shifted accordingly before applying the tracer kinetic model, or the time shift can be incorporated in the model: $C_a(t - T_{lag})$. Thus, an additional parameter enters the model and has to be fitted along with the other free parameters of the model, hopefully with an improved fit and a significant reduction of the residual error of the fit. Another problem is that the shape of the AIF will also change as the CA passes through the vascular tree before entering the tissue in focus. Typically, the AIF entering to the tissue will look like a low-pass filtered (dispersed) version of the AIF measured at a long distance from the tissue in focus. This effect is probably small in normal tissue, but might become important in ischemic tissue with possible collateral vessel formation and long traveling distance. The importance of this problem has not really been assessed and is often ignored in the MR literature, but in nuclear medicine, the problem is treated by adding a filter function like $\exp(-t/T_{smooth})$ into the convolution kernel of Eq. (6), adding an additional parameter to be fitted. It should be realized that an error of the AIF directly propagates to the final result, and if the entire AIF is underestimated with a factor of 2, then perfusion is overestimated with a factor of 2.

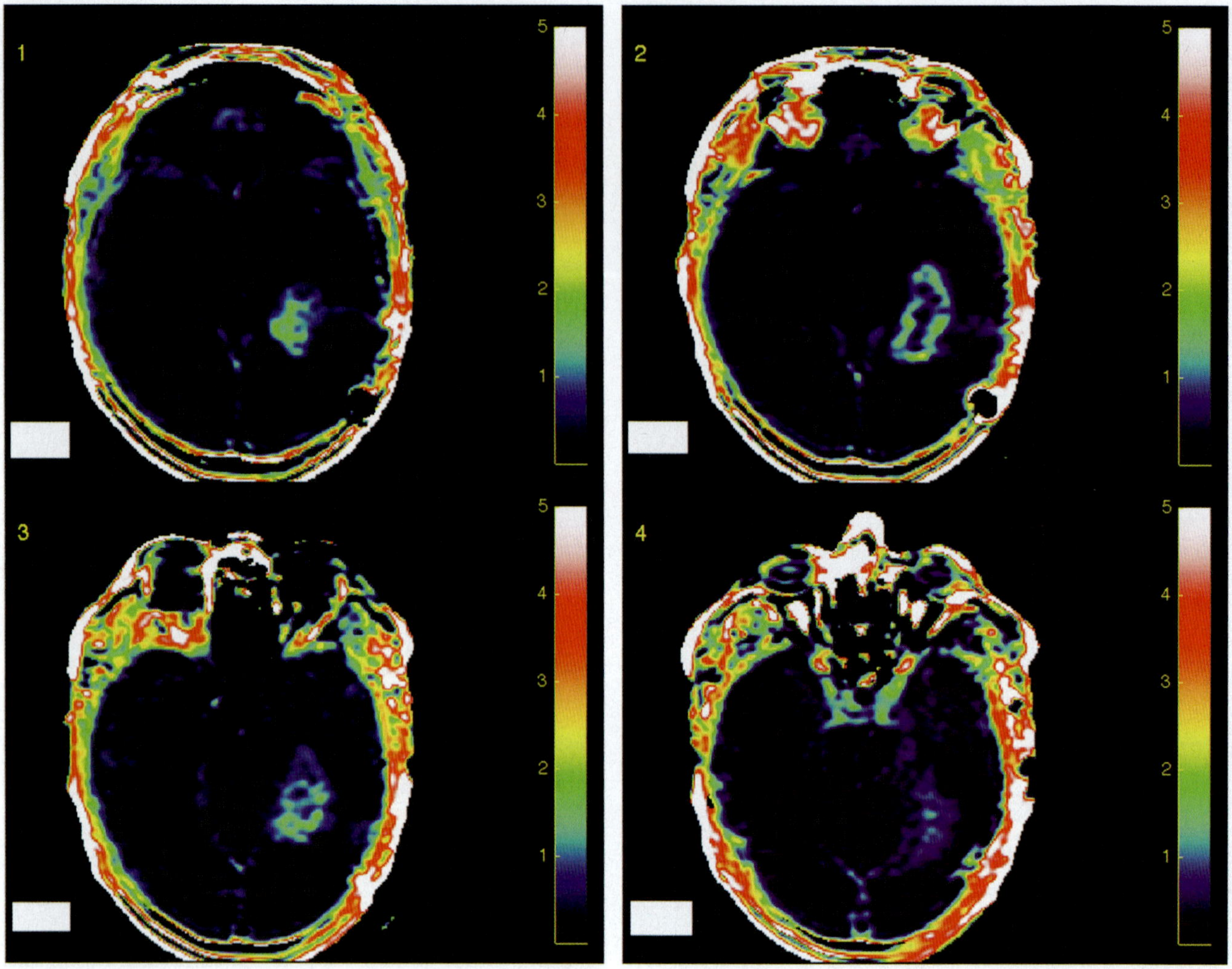

Figure 8-13. Maps of permeability (k_1) using dynamic contrast-enhanced T_1-weighted MRI, at 3 T, using a saturation fast-field echo MR sequence, with a temporal resolution about 1 s. Permeability is calculated pixelwise using the Patlak method. Color scale is in mL/100 mL/min. The patient has an enhancing brain tumor and has previously been operated.

Schmitt et al.[43] showed in a computer simulation that the perfusion and the perfusion reserve could be underestimated with 50% and 20%, respectively, with an unaccounted dispersion of the AIF. Calamante et al.[44] showed a similar dependence on a delayed and dispersed AIF on CBF calculations.

The configuration of the AIF depends on factors as injection rate, central versus peripheral injection site, resistance in the pulmonary circulation, rest, or stress conditions. The peak and duration of the AIF are found to correlate with the function of the right and left ventricle.[45] Saline infusion after the bolus injection of CA may also effect the AIF configuration.[46] The AIF is also influenced by the concentration of CA, and injection rates between 2 and 10 mL/s have shown that the peak and width of AIF are significantly lower and broader for injection rates at 2 and 3 mL/s than for rates of 5 mL/s, but no difference was observed between the rates of 5 mL/s up to 7 and 10 mL/s.[45,47] An obvious question is what is best? There is no real consensus on this matter, but a fast injection rate may probably be preferred, because of a more favorable contrast-to-noise ratio and improved RIF estimation especially in the brain because of a more clear distinction between tissue response and the AIF.

The temporal resolution used for obtaining the AIF should be high enough, in the order of seconds for the injection rate 1 to 10 mL/s; otherwise, the fine details of the AIF is missing, and especially the peak concentration and the initial slope might be inaccurate due to undersampling of the curve. Figure 8.5 shows a typical AIF obtained from an ROI placed in the ICA of a human.

The AIF is quite unique from person to person and even from trial to trial within the same subject.[48] Therefore, the AIF should be estimated for each trial; a standardized population-based general AIF is not recommendable and should be avoided.

The Arterial Input Function—Correction for a Partial Volume Effect

From the above discussion, we see that the AIF should be obtained as close as possible to the tissue in focus. This can some time be accomplished by choosing a small artery. However, as a consequence, this artery will likely suffer from a partial volume effect, which means that the voxels in the ROI will consist of a mixture of tissue and blood in the artery, thus a partial volume effect, and the arterial concentration will be underestimated. This situation is aggravated by the fact that we often want to run a dynamic MR sequence with a high time resolution, meaning that we have to sacrifice the spatial resolution, that is, reduce the matrix size. The consequence is a considerable point spread function, meaning a blurring of a small artery and additional underestimation of the arterial input function. In addition, the AIF can suffer from pulsation artifacts, probably related to an inflow effect, but is otherwise not rigorously characterized in the literature. One simple way to assess the partial volume effect is to look at a profile of the vessel as a function of the spatial resolution and note when a plateau occurs inside the vessel. In the left ventricle of the heart, this is easily obtained with conventional spatial resolution, but often, such a resolution in smaller vessels is not compatible with the timing requirement, for example, in the brain.

Sometimes, is it possible to correct for the partial volume effect. The brain has a large draining venous system, and especially, the sagittal sinus has a larger lumen compared to the brain arteries including ICA. Conservations of mass tell us that for an organ with one inlet (artery) and one outlet (vein), the AIF and the venous outflow function (VOF) should have the same area. Thus, matching the area of the AIF with the area of the VOF will mitigate, although not eliminate the partial volume effect if the vein also suffers from some degree of partial volume effect. It has been shown that this method has some value in the brain using ICA and the sagittal sinus.[49] In fact, due to the BBB, the AIF and VOF are almost identical, and therefore a scaling of the AIF and a time shift of the VOF will create a nearly perfect match of the two functions, which also signify that dispersion through the normal brain tissue is minimal (see Fig. 8.14). It should be remembered that also the basilar artery subserves blood to the brain, and the sagittal sinus blood flow constitutes about 50% of the total effluent blood from the brain.

Elimination of a possible partial volume effect from the sagittal sinus can be taken one step further, using the phase information. The following is based on the study of van Osch, originally developed for dynamic susceptibility contrast-enhanced perfusion imaging,[50] but is here adapted for DCE T_1 perfusion imaging of the brain, and further simplified, and thus easily implemented.

Using the modulus of the MR signal, the general relationship between the MR signal and concentration of a paramagnetic CA in the blood is $S(t) = f\left(M_0, \text{TR}, \text{TE}, \text{TD}, \alpha, r_1, R_1^{\text{b}}, C_{\text{mod}}(t)\right)$, where $S(t)$ is modulus MR signal, t is time, f describes the MR sequence function, M_0 is a constant related to the equilibrium magnetization, TR is the repetition time, TE is echo time, α is the flip angle of the readout pulses, r_1 is the relaxivity, and R_1^{b} is the blood longitudinal relaxation rate before arrival of the CA. Here, we illustrate the implementation using a simple fast-field MR sequence with a nonselective 90-degree prepulse preceding the first α-pulse by a time period of TD, with central phase-encoding scheme, and spoiling between lines in k-space. So for this particular sequence, the relationship is simply

$$S(t) = M_0\left(1 - e^{-\text{TD}\left(R_1^{\text{b}} + r_1 C_{\text{mod}}(t)\right)}\right) \qquad (28)$$

In practice, M_0 and R_1^{b} are measured before contrast injection, and M_0 also includes regional variation due to B_0 inhomogeneity; B_1 inhomogeneity, that is, sinus(α); and a $T_2{}^*$ decay term, which we consider minimal. Having measured R_1^{b} and M_0 before contrast injection, it is easy to find $C_{\text{mod}}(t)$, from the modulus of the MR signal.

The blood concentration can also be estimated from the phase of the MR signal.[51] Especially for a long tube placed parallel with the B_0 field containing a paramagnetic CA, the relationship between the

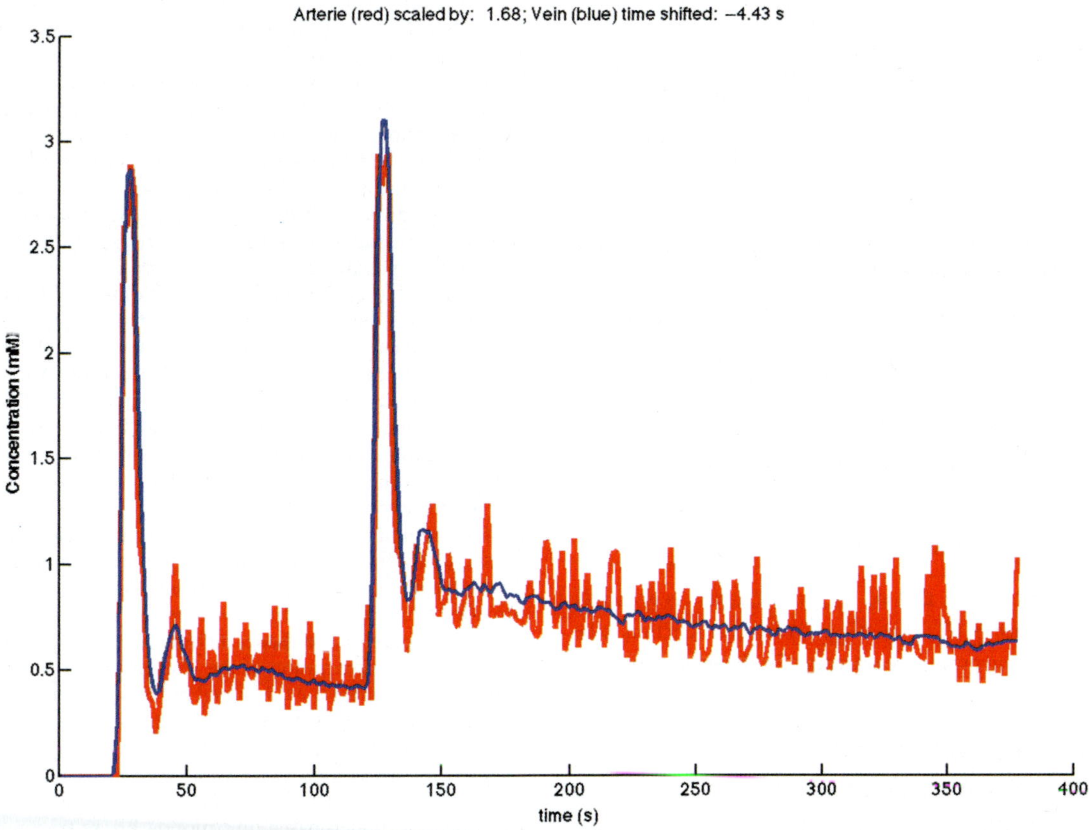

Figure 8-14. The AIF (*red*) is obtained from the internal carotid artery; the venous curve (*blue*) is obtained from the sagittal sinus. Fitting of the curves is provided by scaling the AIF, while the venous curve is time shifted back in time. In this case, two separated bolus injections, each of half dose, are administrated. Note that the AIF suffers from what is believed to be inflow effects, which are completely absent from the venous curve.

phase change as a function of time ($\Delta\Phi(t)$) and concentration as a function of time $\left(C_{\text{phase}}(t)\right)$ is

$$\Delta\Phi(t)=\frac{2}{3}\pi\,\text{TE}\gamma B_0\chi_{\text{m}}C_{\text{phase}}(t) \qquad (29)$$

where γ is the proton gyromagnetic ratio (4.258×10^7 Hz/T), B_0 is the magnitude of the main magnetic field in tesla, and χ_{m} is the molar susceptibility of the CA (3.4×10^{-7} mM^{-1}). The sagittal sinus constitutes nearly a long tube, and one can always find portions, which run parallel with the B_0 field, and in addition, transversal imaging of the brain allows such a portion to be imaged during a perfusion study. If the complex MR signal is obtained, then one can calculate the concentration from either Eqs. (28) or (29), and if no interfering factors exist, then $C_{\text{phase}}(t) = C_{\text{mod}}(t)$. As shown later, $C_{\text{phase}}(t)$ is not equal to $C_{\text{mod}}(t)$, most likely because $C_{\text{mod}}(t)$ is affected by a partial volume effect. $C_{\text{phase}}(t)$ is less susceptible to the effect of the partial volume, but suffers from poor signal to noise and is bias especially for low concentration as shown later.

In order to solve this problem, we consider an ROI placed over the sagittal sinus and having a fraction containing blood (v_{b}) and a complimentary fraction containing tissue (v_{t}), where $v_{\text{t}} + v_{\text{b}} = 1$. In addition, we assume that these two tissue fractions behave as a two-compartment system without any water exchange (see later). Therefore, the complex MR signal for this ROI is

$$S(t)=v_{\text{t}}M_0\left(1-\text{e}^{-\text{TD}R_1^{\text{t}}}\right)\text{e}^{i\Phi_{\text{t}}}+v_{\text{b}}M_0\left(1-\text{e}^{-\text{TD}\left(R_1^{\text{b}}+r_1C_{\text{mod}}(t)\right)}\right)\text{e}^{i(\Phi_{\text{b}}+\Delta\Phi(t))} \qquad (30)$$

where Φ_{b} and Φ_{t} are initial phase of the blood and tissue component in an ROI, respectively. R_1^{t} is the longitudinal relaxation rate of the tissue component.

Before arrival of the CA, we just have

$$S(0)=v_{\text{t}}M_0\left(1-\text{e}^{-\text{TD}R_1^{\text{t}}}\right)\text{e}^{i\Phi_{\text{t}}}+v_{\text{b}}M_0\left(1-\text{e}^{-\text{TD}R_1^{\text{b}}}\right)\text{e}^{i\Phi_{\text{b}}} \qquad (31)$$

$S(0)$ is an average of all baseline points before arrival of the CA. Therefore, the baseline-subtracted complex MR signal during the bolus passage is

$$\begin{aligned}&S(t)-S(0)=\\&v_{\text{b}}M_0\left(1-\text{e}^{-\text{TD}\left(R_1^{\text{b}}+r_1C_{\text{mod}}(t)\right)}\right)\text{e}^{i(\Phi_{\text{b}}+\Delta\Phi(t))}-v_{\text{b}}M_0\left(1-\text{e}^{-\text{TD}R_1^{\text{b}}}\right)\text{e}^{i\Phi_{\text{b}}}\end{aligned} \qquad (32)$$

This equation contains two unknown: v_{b} and Φ_{b}. If these were known, $C_{\text{mod}}(t)$ can be calculated from

$$\begin{aligned}\left\|S(t)-v_{\text{t}}M_0\left(1-\text{e}^{-\text{TD}R_1^{\text{t}}}\right)\text{e}^{i\Phi_{\text{t}}}\right\|&=\left\|S(t)-S(0)+v_{\text{b}}M_0\left(1-\text{e}^{-\text{TD}R_1^{\text{b}}}\right)\text{e}^{i\Phi_{\text{b}}}\right\|\\&=v_{\text{b}}M_0\left(1-\text{e}^{-\text{TD}\left(R_1^{\text{b}}+r_1C_{\text{mod}}(t)\right)}\right)\end{aligned} \qquad (33)$$

and $C_{\text{phase}}(t)$ can be calculated from

$$\begin{aligned}&\arg\left[S(t)-S(0)+v_{\text{b}}M_0\left(1-\text{e}^{-\text{TD}R_1^{\text{b}}}\right)\text{e}^{i\Phi_{\text{b}}}\right]\\&-\Phi_{\text{b}}=\\&\frac{2}{3}\pi\,\text{TE}\gamma B_0\chi_{\text{m}}C_{\text{phase}}(t)\end{aligned} \qquad (34)$$

For correct values of v_{b} and Φ_{b}, $C_{\text{phase}}(t) = C_{\text{mod}}(t)$. As v_{b} and Φ_{b} are unknown, we use $\sum\left(C_{\text{phase}}(t)-C_{\text{mod}}(t)\right)$ as a cost function to be minimized in a fitting procedure searching for the most optimal v_{b} and Φ_{b}.

The Arterial Input Function—Optimization of Dose

The T_1-weighted MR sequences typically used in DCE imaging include a prepulse, which is either an inversion or saturation pulse. The MR signal range is typically much higher for the AIF compared with the tissue MR signal increase. Because of the low tissue response, it is preferable to use a high dose of CA and an MR sequence optimized for high sensitivity, for example, long inversion time (TI). However, this may cause truncation and underestimation of the AIF due to full magnetic recovery in the blood pool. This means an artificial underestimation of the AIF and may lead to substantial errors in calculation of tissue perfusion.[52] High concentrations of gadolinium-DTPA in the blood pool may also reduce the signal due to T_2* effects,[53] and obviously, the shortest allowed echo time should be used, which will eliminate or at least minimize the T_2* effect. The use of a double-echo sequence with short echo times might rule out and correct for a possible T_2* effect. Careful optimization and validation is therefore required, ensuring that both the AIF and the tissue signal during the bolus passage are measured correctly within the dynamic range of the entire system. If this is not possible, the dual-bolus approach,[54,55] the prebolus technique,[56] or the dual-imaging sequence[52,57] through repeated measurements of the bolus passage using low and high doses of CA focusing on the AIF and the tissue response, respectively, is a possibility.

The Arterial Input Function—Indirect Measurement

Obtaining an AIF can be a challenge and is subjected to many potential errors as just explained, and sometimes, no artery is available in the field of view or close to the tissue of interest. Therefore, methods for estimating the AIF without directly measuring the AIF, so-called blind estimation of the AIF, are of considerable interest. Several methods have been suggested, but only two principal methods, the multiple reference tissue–based AIF method[58,59] and jointly estimated AIF seems of relevance. The starting point for these methods is the recognition that the equation $\vec{y}=f\Delta t A\vec{x}$ represents N linear equations, because we have N samples. Furthermore, let the entries of $\vec{x}$ be specified by an analytic model, for example, having three free parameters depending on the actual model used. In the situation where AIF is missing, we have $N + 3$ unknown, which cannot be estimated. If we obtain information from multiple tissue ROIs, including ROIs placed in pathologic tissue, preferably with a large diversity of the physiologic tissue parameters between sites, and we assume that R tissue sites are exposed to the same AIF (except for a possible difference of arrival time, which also can be incorporated), then the number of equations is RN, but the number of unknown is only $N + 3R$. Therefore, in principle, enough information is available in order to estimate the matrix $\mathbf{A}$ (the AIF with N samples). In the multiple reference tissue–based AIF method, the AIF is estimated without assuming a specific form of the AIF, and the physiologic tissue parameters from all tissue sites are estimated in conjunction with the AIF. The estimation of the AIF and the other unknown physiologic constants are based on ingenious and fast optimization procedure, minimizing the residual error of the fit. The method does not provide an absolute scale of the AIF, and consequently, the physiologic parameters are estimated only within a scale factor (except time constants as K_i/V_e). Scaling of AIF can be provided from incorporating, for example, a literature value of the interstitial space of the tissue, or from a real single measurement of the blood concentration of the CA during the late phase of the bolus passage, where the CA is well mixed in the entire blood pool, and saturation, arrival time, and temporal resolution are minor problems. The obtained blind estimated AIF can then be used to calculate the physiologic tissue parameters voxel-wise.

The jointly estimated AIF utilized a parameterized form of the AIF. Previous models based on a mono-, bi-, or triexponential AIF are not accurate enough. Instead, a superposition of 2 to 3 normalized gamma-variate functions and a Gaussian or sigmoid functions with about 10 to 15 adjustable free parameters seem to model the measured AIF encountered in vivo.[60] Thus, the total number of free parameters is considerable reduced compared with the multiple reference tissue–based AIF method and consequently alleviate the requirement of inclusion of multiple reference tissue sites, assumed to have the same AIF. However, multiple tissue enhancement curves, randomly selected within a particular tissue type, for example, within tumor tissue, is still necessary and assumed to have the same (local) AIF, in order to tune the free parameters of the AIF.[61] As with the multiple reference tissue–based AIF method, a model of the RIF is still required, and the tissue physiologic parameters are fitted simultaneously. Like the multiple reference tissue–based AIF method, the AIF and the physiologic parameters of the tissue are only determined within a scale factor, and a final scaling is still necessary.

The importance of blind estimation of the AIF resides in the fact that it provides a possibility of finding and utilizing a local AIF, incorporating a possible dispersion, and it alleviates the inherent problems mentioned above, thus obtaining a more accurate AIF for the given tissue site. It has been shown that local dispersion of the AIF can have a significant impact on the results obtained[62] and that the local AIF in normal brain tissue deviates significantly from the local AIF in an adjacent brain tumor. The danger is that using algorithms for obtaining a local AIF, which is based on only a local set of tissue enhancement curves, results in mixing characteristics of the local AIF and the tissue enhancement curves, and thus the results will be biased. However, the finding of a significant reduction of the residual error of the fit to tumor data, when using the local blind estimated AIF from tumor tissue, compared to a local blind estimated AIF from normal tissue, suggests a real improvement of accuracy.[63]

Blind estimation of the AIF necessitates a model of the RIF, and so far, only the extended Tofts model has been used in DCE T_1-weighted studies. Future research is needed for investigate blind AIF estimation in conjunction with other models. In conjunction with dynamic susceptibility-weighted perfusion imaging, it has been shown that a blind local AIF can be obtained when using independent component analysis, without the need of specifying a model for the RIF,[64] a method that also should be exploited for DCE T_1-weighted studies.

Linking Tracer Kinetic Theory and Modeling to MRI

Tracer kinetic modeling seeks to describe the biologic systems handling of the CA and works directly on CA concentration. In DCE T_1-weighted MRI, information about the CA is via the MR signal, and the signal is generally a nonlinear function of the CA concentration. This is because the MR signal is bound to the magnetization in the voxel, and the magnetization spans from $-M_0$ to $+M_0$, where M_0 is the equilibrium magnetization. The CA considered here works by enhancing the longitudinal relaxation rate R_1 ($=1/T_1$: the reciprocal of the longitudinal relaxation time T_1) of water protons preferably by binding to the paramagnetic core of the CA, so-called inner sphere relaxation. A smaller contribution comes from the so-called outer sphere relaxation, based on proximity between the paramagnetic core and the water protons.[65,66] The relaxation mechanism is governed by the large magnetic dipole moment associated with the unpaired electrons in the inner electron shells of the paramagnetic atoms through an electron–nuclear dipolar interaction. The associated large dipole creates an oscillating magnetic field with a broad frequency distribution, including frequencies at the relevant Lamor frequency, inducing relaxation. Because of a fast exchange between bound and free water, the relaxation enhancing effect is transmitted to the entire water population.[65,66] The enhanced T_1 relaxation results in an MR signal increase when using a T_1-weighted MR sequence.

It is important to realize that the effect of a CA, when using a T_2*-weighted MR sequence can provide relaxation due to the electron–nuclear dipolar interaction, but also indirectly over a much longer distance due to creation of local magnetic field inhomogeneity, a susceptibility effect, without direct contact with the paramagnetic core of the CA. The MR signal decreases during the bolus passage when using a T_2- or T_2*-weighted MR sequence, because R_2 ($=1/T_2$) and R_2* ($=1/T_2$*) increase. The most often used paramagnetic atom is gadolinium (Gd) belonging to the lanthanide series of chemical elements with the atomic number 64 (^{158}gadolinium(III) is the most abundant and stable isotope). Both theoretical and experimental studies have shown that for a homogeneous water solution of the normally used MRI CAs, a linear relationship exists between the CA concentration and the longitudinal relaxation rate:

$$\frac{1}{T_1^{CA}} = \frac{1}{T_1} + r_1 C \Leftrightarrow R_1^{CA} = R_1 + r_1 C \Leftrightarrow \Delta R_1 = r_1 C \tag{35}$$

where T_1^{CA} and T_1 are the relaxation times with and without CA, r_1 is the relaxivity defined as the change in the longitudinal relaxation rate per concentration unit of the CA (mM s)$^{-1}$, and C is the concentration of the CA. The relaxivity depends on field strength and the type of CA. Paramagnetic metals, as Gd is toxic, and toxicity is eliminated by chelation with a molecule, for example, diethylenetriamine pentaacetic acid (Gd-DTPA), which secures a fast clearance by the kidney. In general, the size and configuration of the molecule, the number of paramagnetic atoms, and water accessibility to the paramagnetic core determine the relaxivity. A pertinent question is how dependent the relaxivity is on the local biologic tissue environment. In a comprehensive study, Donahue et al. measured the relaxivity in saline, plasma, and cartilage and found a relaxivity of about 4 (mM s)$^{-1}$ for Gd-DTPA.[67] Neither changing the plasma protein concentration nor compression of the cartilage (reducing the water content) nor trypsinization of the cartilage (nearly completely removing proteoglycan and fixed charges) had significant effect on the relaxivity. At a field strength of 1 T, the relaxivity was about 20% higher compared to field strength of 4.7 and 8.5 T. Many have measured the relaxivity of Gd-DTPA in biologic tissues, for example, the relaxivity of blood plasma is 3.9 ± 0.2 (mM s)$^{-1}$[68] and 4.3 (mM s)$^{-1}$ in the myocardium at 1.5 T.[66] The relaxivity is generally assumed to be independent of the biologic microenvironment, but exceptions might occur.

The MR signal equation derived from the Bloch equation corresponding to the actual MR sequence used provides the link between the MR signal and the concentration of the CA. A relevant example is imaging using 2D fast gradient echo sequence (GRE sequence), with a nonselective 90-degree prepulse, followed by repeated slice-selective readout α-pulses (flip angle 10 to 30 degrees), each separated by a TR of a few milliseconds. The time between the prepulse and the first α-pulse is called TD. The MR signal equation becomes very simple if centric phase encoding is used, meaning that the first phase-encoding step corresponds to the center of K-space ($Ky = 0$, phase-encoding gradient is zero). TE should be as short as possible and preferably below 1 milliseconds, so T_2*-weighing can be ignored. Residual transverse magnetization should be spoiled effectively by, for example, rf and gradient spoiling before the next α-pulse. The signal equation is then

$$S = S_0 \sin(\alpha)\left(1 - \exp(-\mathrm{TD} R_1)\right) \tag{36}$$

where S is the MR signal, S_0 is the maximal MR signal, and R_1 is the relaxation rate without any CA. S_0 is a constant and proportional to proton density, receiver gain, and the local coil sensitivity. The time resolution can be as high as 0.5 seconds, depending on matrix size and number of slices. Generally, the MR signal is primarily determined by the phase-encoding step corresponding to the "zero phase-encoding step" ($Ky = 0$), because this step is the most important determinant for the overall signal strength. In contrast to nuclear medicine measurements, where sampling of radioactive counts is more uniform over the sampling interval, the level of the MR signal is determined at a distinct point in time, corresponding to traversal of the center of *K*-space. In the present context, Eq. (36) is a function of position (the voxel), time, and CA concentration. Focusing on time and concentration, the equation becomes

$$S(t)=S_0\sin(\alpha)\left(1-\exp\left(-\mathrm{TD}\left(R_1+r_1C(t)\right)\right)\right) \tag{37}$$

If we obtain measurements of $S_0 \sin(\alpha)$ (taken as one constant) and R_1 before CA injection, and assume a known value of r_1, then $S(t)$ can easily be converted to $C(t)$. $S_0 \sin(\alpha)$ and R_1 can be obtained by a regular T_1 measurement by stepping through a set of TD values and measure the corresponding signal. Note that $S_0 \sin(\alpha)$ obtained voxel-wise corrects for scanner inhomogeneity and nonuniform flip angle. The nonselective 90-degree prepulse should be as accurate as possible, for example, using an adiabatic pulse, and coverage should be large in order to label blood entering the field of view. In all perfusion imaging, it is important to obtain a reliable baseline signal before CA enters the tissue, for example, 10 to 20 samples. If we call the average baseline signal $\hat{S}(0)$, then Eq. (37) can be expressed as

$$\frac{S(t)-\hat{S}(0)}{\hat{S}(0)}=\frac{1-\exp\left(-\mathrm{TD}r_1C(t)\right)}{\exp\left(\mathrm{TD}R_1\right)-1} \tag{38}$$

If TD is short, we may use the approximation $\exp(x) \approx 1 + x$ ($x < 0.2$) and get

$$\frac{S(t)-\hat{S}(0)}{\hat{S}(0)}\approx\frac{r_1C(t)}{R_1} \tag{39}$$

This equation shows that the relative MR signal change is linearly related to the CA concentration, if the argument of the exponential function is small. For this reason, some people are using a very low dose of CA, to secure linearity. If in addition R_1 is assumed and fixed at a value, the concentration can be estimated without the initial T_1 measurement. However, assuming a fixed T_1 value has lately questioned as a valid simplification for body imaging.[69] It should also be noted that if $\hat{S}(0)$ is close to zero, the relative MR signal change may be very sensitive to noise of the baseline MR signal.

If centric phase encoding is impossible, one has to take all phase-encoding steps and the corresponding manipulation of the magnetization into account until the center of *K*-space is reached. Note that for short TR of a few milliseconds, the longitudinal magnetization evolves during traversal of *K*-space. If the center of *K*-space is reached after n phase-encoding steps, Eq. (37) becomes[70]

$$S(t)=S_0\sin(\alpha)\Bigg[\left(1-e^{\mathrm{TD}(R_1+r_1C(t))}\right)\left(\cos(\alpha)e^{-\mathrm{TR}(R_1+r_1C(t))}\right)^{n-1} +\left(1-e^{-\mathrm{TR}(R_1+r_1C(t))}\right)\frac{1-\left(\cos(\alpha)e^{-\mathrm{TR}(R_1+r_1C(t))}\right)^{n-1}}{1-\cos(\alpha)e^{-\mathrm{TR}(R_1+r_1C(t))}}\Bigg] \tag{40}$$

Retrieval of $C(t)$ can be provided by an iterative process. The flip angle should either be known or, alternatively, can be estimated together with $S_0 \sin(\alpha)$ and R_1 from the T_1 measurement voxel-wise before CA injection. Again, the 90-degree prepulse should be as accurate as possible.

If the 90-degree prepulse is not perfect, or the 90-degree prepulse is replaced by a 180-degree inversion pulse, then longitudinal magnetization survives from one frame to the next, the evolution of the magnetization from the last α-pulse of a frame to the prepulse of the next frame has to be taken into account, and the MR signal equation becomes more sophisticated.[71] When taking the history of the magnetization into account, steady-state MR signal equations are normally calculated and used, that is, the MR signal initially shows some oscillation and gradually settles at a constant steady-state value. As an example, an often used MR sequence in DCE T_1-weighted imaging is a 3D spoiled T_1-weighted gradient echo sequence. The TE is short, preferably a few milliseconds, but TR is typically around 100 milliseconds, separating each readout α-pulses. The magnetization before each α-pulse is in steady state (have the same size), in contrast to the previously mentioned fast gradient echo sequences. Such a 3D sequence provides better coverage (slice direction) and better in-plane spatial resolution, and possible better signal-to-noise ratio than do corresponding 2D sequences, sacrificing the temporal resolution, which often is no better than 2 to 3 seconds and often 5 to 10 seconds. The steady-state MR signal equation, assuming negligible T_2* contribution, corresponding to the center of *K*-space is

$$S(t)=S_0\sin(\alpha)\frac{1-e^{-\mathrm{TR}(R_1+r_1C(t))}}{1-\cos(\alpha)e^{-\mathrm{TR}(R_1+r_1C(t))}} \tag{41}$$

Again, $C(t)$ can be estimated if $S_0 \sin(\alpha)$, R_1, and the flip angle is known. $S_0 \sin(\alpha)$ and R_1 can be estimated before CA injection by varying either TR or the flip angle. A pertinent question is whether a steady-state signal equation can be used during the bolus passage where the longitudinal relaxation rate changes due to the concentration changes. According to own unpublished simulations, no major error is introduced in this situation. However, it is possible to follow the magnetization from frame to frame during the bolus passage of the CA without relying on a steady-state equation.[70]

In conclusion, there is a linear relationship between the CA concentration and change in the longitudinal relaxation rate. The MR signal can be converted to concentration by use of the relevant MR signal equation. It is important to optimize the MR sequence parameters, for example, a long TI or TD is beneficial for improving sensitivity, but in conjunction with a high dose of CA, there is a risk of getting full relaxation of the MR signal, especially with regard to the AIF, which will suffer from truncation and therefore result in a overestimation of the physiologic parameters.

Water Exchange

Biologic tissue contains several compartments, such as plasma, erythrocytes, extravascular extracellular space (interstitial space), and the intracellular space. The CA distribution is often uneven and depends on concentration, permeability of the capillary membranes, cellular membranes, and time for equilibration among other factors. In DCE T_1-weighted MRI, the effect of the CA in a compartment can affect an adjacent compartment without any CA, if a significant water exchange between the two compartments occurs. In fact, the rate of water exchange between compartments influences the overall tissue relaxation. This complicates matters but also opens for the possibility of measuring water permeability.

The water exchange can be categorized into four types: fast, intermediate, slow, and no-exchange regime.[72] The *fast*-exchange regime between compartments a and b with relaxation times T_1^{a} and T_1^{b} is characterized by

$$\frac{1}{\tau}\gg\left|\frac{1}{T_1^{\mathrm{a}}}-\frac{1}{T_1^{\mathrm{b}}}\right|=\left|R_1^{\mathrm{a}}-R_1^{\mathrm{b}}\right| \tag{42}$$

where

$$\frac{1}{\tau}=\frac{1}{\tau^{\mathrm{a}}}+\frac{1}{\tau^{\mathrm{b}}}$$

and τ^{a} and τ^{b} represent the mean lifetime of a proton in compartments a and b, respectively. This equation states that the water exchange frequency is much faster than the difference between the two compartments' intrinsic relaxation rates, that is, if each compartment's relaxation rate were measured separately. In this case, the overall relaxation rate will be[73]

$$R_1 = v^a R_1^a + v^b R_1^b \tag{43}$$

where v^a and v^b are the relative fraction of water of the two compartments ($v^a + v^b = 1$). The two compartments relax with one relaxation rate, and the relaxation process is monoexponential. Imagine that a CA is added to compartment b with concentration C. Then, still assuming fast exchange (could potentially move out of the fast-exchange regime; see later), the overall relaxation rate is

$$R_1^{CA} = v^a R_1^a + v^b\left(R_1^b + r_1 C^b\right) = v^a R_1^a + v^b R_1^b + v^b r_1 C^b = R_1 + v^b r_1 C^b$$

Now, defining an average CA concentration for both compartments as

$$\hat{C}\left(v^a + v^b\right) = \hat{C} = v^b C^b$$

results in

$$R_1^{CA} = R_1 + r_1 \hat{C} \tag{44}$$

This equation shows that even though the CA is nonuniformly distributed, the system behaves as if the CA is well mixed in both compartments, and the system relax monoexponentially, and a T_1 measurement before and after adding the CA will result in a concentration estimate corresponding to an even distribution of the CA in the two compartments. An important example is estimation of the CA concentration in arterial blood in conjunction with AIF measurement. It is generally accepted that the water exchange between plasma and the interior of the erythrocytes is very fast, with an exchange rate of 100 Hz.[74,75] Even with a plasma concentration up to 6 mM as has been observed,[6] the fast-exchange regime prevails. This means that an estimate of the CA concentration in blood, for example, in conjunction with measurement of the AIF, results in an estimation of the full blood concentration, even though the CA is confined to the plasma. The real plasma concentration can then be calculated from $C_a^p = C_a/\left(1 - \text{Hct}_{LV}\right)$ where C_a^p and C_a are arterial plasma concentration and full blood concentration, respectively. In tracer kinetic equations, it is often convenient to use the real physical concentrations and only later change concentration reference.

The no-exchange regime means no exchange of water between compartments. In this case, each compartment has its own distinct relaxation process, and the combined relaxation is multiexponential. If two compartments *a* and *b* have relaxation rate R_1^a and R_1^b, respectively, then the MR signal for a simple saturation recovery sequence with centric phase encoding becomes

$$S = S_0 v^a\left(1 - e^{-TD R_1^a}\right) + S_0 v^b\left(1 - e^{-TD R_1^b}\right) \tag{45}$$

Adding a CA to compartment b will change the relaxation rate of only that compartment, and the concentration can be measured by carefully measuring the biexponential relaxation process:

$$S^{CA} = S_0 v^a\left(1 - e^{-TD R_1^a}\right) + S_0 v^b\left(1 - e^{-TD\left(R_1^b + r_1 C^b\right)}\right) \tag{46}$$

If compartment a represents the extravascular space and b the vascular space, and we assume no exchange between these compartments, then the vascular space can be estimated from the ratio of total tissue MR signal change to the blood MR signal change before and after adding the CA[76]:

$$v^b = \frac{\Delta S}{\Delta S^b} = \frac{S^{CA} - S}{\Delta S^b} \tag{47}$$

where ΔS^b is determined from a blood sample or from an ROI with pure blood placed within the vessel. This is quite distinct from assuming a fast exchange between blood and the extravascular space. In this situation, we would have[76]

$$v^b = \frac{C_t}{C_a} = \frac{\Delta R_1^t / r_1}{\Delta R_1^a / r_1} = \frac{\Delta R_1^t}{\Delta R_1^a} \tag{48}$$

assuming the same relaxivity for blood and tissue, as is normally done. Here, we also assume a fast exchange between the interstitial space and the intracellular water in both situations.

The slow exchange regime is defined as[72]

$$\frac{1}{\tau} \ll \left|\frac{1}{T_1^a} - \frac{1}{T_1^b}\right| = \left|R_1^a - R_1^b\right| \tag{49}$$

In this situation, each compartment's relaxation rate will be modified as

$$\tilde{R}_1^a = R_1^a + \frac{1}{\tau^a}$$

$$\tilde{R}_1^b = R_1^b + \frac{1}{\tau^b}$$

where τ^a and τ^b represent the mean lifetime of a proton in compartments a and b, respectively. The intermediate water exchange regime[77] is

$$\frac{1}{\tau} \approx \left|\frac{1}{T_1^a} - \frac{1}{T_1^b}\right| = \left|R_1^a - R_1^b\right| \tag{50}$$

Hazlewood has developed a two-site exchange model, which deals with the water exchange in general.[78] The model takes into account the combined relaxation and exchange of magnetization between compartments. For two compartments a and b, the model is given by the two coupled differential equations:

$$\begin{aligned} \frac{dM^a(t)}{dt} &= \frac{M_0^a - M^a(t)}{T_1^a} - \frac{M^a(t)}{\tau^a} + \frac{M^b(t)}{\tau^b} \\ \frac{dM^b(t)}{dt} &= \frac{M_0^b - M^b(t)}{T_1^b} - \frac{M^b(t)}{\tau^b} + \frac{M^a(t)}{\tau^a} \end{aligned} \tag{51}$$

Conservation of matters implies $M_0^a/\tau^a = M_0^b/\tau^b$ and $M_0^a + M_0^b = 1$. The solution is then given by

$$\begin{aligned} M^b(t) &= P_1 e^{\Psi t} + P_2 e^{\varphi t} + M_0^b \\ M^a(t) &= P_3 e^{\Psi t} + P_4 e^{\varphi t} + M_0^a \\ \Psi &= -\frac{1}{2}\left(k_1 + \sqrt{k_1^2 - 4k_2}\right) \\ \varphi &= -\frac{1}{2}\left(k_1 - \sqrt{k_1^2 - 4k_2}\right) \\ k_1 &= \frac{1}{T_1^a} + \frac{1}{\tau^a} + \frac{1}{T_1^b} + \frac{1}{\tau^b} \\ k_2 &= \frac{1}{T_1^a T_1^b} + \frac{1}{T_1^a \tau^a} + \frac{1}{T_1^b \tau^b} \end{aligned} \tag{52}$$

The amplitude P_1 to P_4 depends on the initial conditions, and a general expression for the amplitudes can be found in reference.[70] Thus, water exchange in general results in a multiexponential relaxation process, and estimation of CA concentration is not straightforward.

Obviously, a CA confined in a compartment of a multicompartment system can become more or less invisible, unless a fast water exchange exists between all compartments, and the lack of fast exchange complicates estimation of the overall tissue concentration.

However, these problems can be ameliorated by the observation of Hazlewood that the initial slope of the MR signal relaxation curve is the same for the no-exchange and the fast-exchange regime.[78] This observation was taken up and elaborated further by Schwickert et al.[79] and Donahue et al.[76] Selecting appropriate MR imaging parameters can minimize the effect of the water exchange, so that the obtained MR signal becomes water exchange insensitive. An example is a two-compartment system, with no or slow water exchange, with the signal equation corresponding to a saturation recovery sequence:

$$S = S_0 v^{\mathrm{a}}\left(1-\mathrm{e}^{-\mathrm{TD}R_1^{\mathrm{a}}}\right)+S_0 v^{\mathrm{b}}\left(1-\mathrm{e}^{-\mathrm{TD}R_1^{\mathrm{b}}}\right)$$

If TD is set to a low value, so that the exponential argument is below 0.2, then

$$S \approx S_0\,\mathrm{TD}\left(v^{\mathrm{a}}R_1^{\mathrm{a}}+v^{\mathrm{b}}R_1^{\mathrm{b}}\right) \approx S_0\left(1-\mathrm{e}^{-\mathrm{TD}\left(v^{\mathrm{a}}R_1^{\mathrm{a}}+v^{\mathrm{b}}R_1^{\mathrm{b}}\right)}\right)$$

which is the signal one will obtain in case of a fast-exchange regime. Thus, the MR signal does not depend on details of the water exchange, and the effect is minimized for a low value of TD or TI. For a conventional GRE sequence (Eq. (41)), it is easy to show that

$$\frac{\cos\alpha}{1-\cos\alpha}\frac{\mathrm{TR}}{T_1} \ll 1 \tag{53}$$

will minimize the effect of water exchange,[76] that is, selecting a short TR and a relative high flip angle. The reason is that there is only a short time for manifestation of the evolution of the water exchange for short TR, TD, or TI, and the no-exchange model and the fast-exchange model will give the same result.

As previously mentioned, the water exchange between plasma and erythrocyte is believed to be very fast with a residence lifetime of about 10 to 15 milliseconds for a water molecule within the intracellular compartment.[80,81] The water exchange between the capillary blood space and the extravascular extracellular space has been estimated to be less than 7 Hz, corresponding a mean lifetime of 140 milliseconds.[72,76] If we assume no leakage between the vascular space and the extravascular space and a peak concentration of about 4 mM in the vascular space, and that the R_1 is roughly the same for tissue and blood before CA injection, then the difference in relaxation rates between the two compartments is about 16 Hz at the peak concentration. This should be compared with a water exchange rate of about 7 Hz. Obviously, even though we have a fast-exchange regime between compartments without any CA, we will enter an intermediate and slow water exchange regime during the bolus passage, and there is therefore a risk of underestimating the CA concentration, if we still assume a fast exchange. The largest CA segregation between the vascular space and the extravascular space is in the brain, due to the BBB, which is nearly impermeable for typical MR CA. In agreement with this, the cerebral perfusion was found to be eight times smaller for a TI = 0.9 seconds compared to TI = 20 milliseconds, but simulations showed only a 10% underestimation, if TI = 100 milliseconds. This is compatible with a water exchange rate of about 3 Hz between the vascular space and the extravascular space in human brain tissue.[70] Thus, the water exchange has a significant impact on DCE T_1-weighted MRI in the brain, and water exchange minimization methods should be employed if the aim is perfusion measurement. This is also most likely for other organs if a macrocontrast agent molecule is used. In an in vivo animal study, Bjørnerud et al.[82] studied the relaxation process in the heart using an intravascular CA and found evidence for a biexponential relaxation process with a water exchange rate between the vascular and extravascular space of 1.39 ± 0.52 Hz.

A more controversial issue is whether the interstitial water space is in fast-exchange regime with the intracellular water, for example, between the interstitial space and myocytes in the heart. Several studies have evaluated the water exchange between the interstitial space and the myocytes using isolated heart preparations. Wedeking et al.[83] found a cellular interstitial water exchange rate of 21 Hz in rat hearts and that fast exchange dominates as long as the interstitial CA concentration was below 1 mM. Donahue et al.[76] measured exchange rates of 8 to 27 Hz for the heart. Judd also studied both polylysine-Gd-DTPA and gadoteridol's effect on the water exchange regime in a heart preparation and found evidence for a slow water exchange regime for both compounds, but most pronounced for the intravascular polylysine-Gd-DTPA.[84] Vascular peak concentrations for polylysine-Gd-DTPD and gadoteridol were up to 15 and 25 mM, respectively, concentration which in our experience are far too high and never observed in humans, using conventional doses. Sobol et al.[85] showed that fast exchange existed up to an interstitial Gd-DTPA concentration of 10 mM in rat muscle. As seen, there is no general agreement about the level of cellular interstitial water exchange, and a large variation of the reported exchange rates is apparent. The exchange rate in some of these ex vivo studies could have been underestimated if carried out at a temperature of 20°C instead of 37°C, where water diffusion is higher. The concentration of CA in the interstitial space is related to the extraction fraction of the CA, and the interstitial concentration is usually lower than the plasma concentration. Own tracer kinetic modeling using a typical AIF with a peak concentration of 4 mM, a perfusion of 100 mL/100 g/min, and 50% extraction never results in a interstitial tissue concentration of more than 0.5 mM. In a further simulation study, the MR signal curves were very similar for fast, intermediate, and slow water exchange when extraction fractions were larger than 30% and for inversion times up to 800 milliseconds.[70] When extraction fraction was below 20%, the MR signal curves were clearly separated for fast and slow water exchange, when using a TI of 400 milliseconds or longer, but were similar when using a TI of 20 milliseconds. Thus, a high extraction fraction of a CA promotes conditions for a fast-exchange regime between the vascular and extravascular space, while an extraction fraction of zero, as occurs in the brain or when using macromolecular CA, tends to result in a slow water exchange condition between the vascular and extravascular space. Furthermore, it was also shown that a slow water exchange regime prevails when using an unphysiologic high arterial concentration (a factor 15), which cannot be compensated when using short inversion times (TI = 20 milliseconds). An in vivo human study showed equal myocardial perfusion values, regardless the value of TI in the interval 15 to 598 milliseconds.[86] This finding suggests that for the myocardium, the error of assuming fast water exchange both regarding the vascular and extravascular exchange and the cellular interstitial exchange are relatively small, and thus fast water exchange is likely a valid assumption in the heart. This is in contrast to the study of Landis et al.[87] In this study, the cellular interstitial water exchange was only fast up to an interstitial concentration of 0.1 mM. This suggests that it will be problematic to estimate extravascular tissue concentration in most situations, but the finding is not compatible with some of the previously mentioned results. Lately, Landis et al. study was contradicted by a study of human internal obturator muscle by Buckley et al.[88] In this study, only minimal difference was found when fitting a fast water exchange and a no-water exchange model to data, and the physiologic constants obtained were not dependent of the model of the water exchange being used. In addition, data suggested that a fast water exchange regime could be assumed for an interstitial concentration up to 0.5 mM. Finally, the study also pointed out the large uncertainty of estimated water exchange rates, making definite conclusion elusive. No doubt more elaborated models and measurements of the water exchange in various types of tissue are needed.[89] Generally, water exchange minimization methods are recommended.

Conclusion

Dynamic contrast-enhanced T_1-weighted MRI has the ability to provide important physiologic information. Compared with other methods, it is relatively simple to implement and integrate DCE-MRI in a standard MRI protocol. The advantages compared to dynamic susceptibility T_2*-weighted MRI is less susceptibility to field inhomogeneity, more reliable estimation of perfusion, and BBB permeability due to a robust relationship between concentration and longitudinal relaxation rate. Disadvantages are less coverage and a less favorable contrast to noise of tissue during the bolus passage. Implementation of fast multiband sequences will probably improve coverage, and higher field strength, for example, 7 T, might improve contrast to noise and also pave the way for direct estimation of water permeability in conjunction with estimation of other physiologic parameters.

REFERENCES

1. **Ballabh P, Braun A, Nedergaard M.** The blood-brain barrier: an overview. Structure, regulation, and clinical implications. *Neurobiol Dis* 2004;16:1–13.
2. **Erickson MA, Banks WA.** Blood-brain barrier dysfunction as a cause and consequence of Alzheimer's disease. *J Cereb Blood Flow Metab* 2013;33:1500–1513.
3. **Renkin EM.** Transport of potassium-42 from blood to tissue in isolated mammalian skeletal muscles. *Am J Physiol* 1959;197:1205–1210.
4. **Crone C.** The permeability of capillaries in various organs determined by use of the indicator diffusion method. *Acta Physiol Scand* 1963;58:292–305.
5. **Diesbourg LD, Prato FS, Wisenberg G, et al.** Quantification of myocardial blood flow and extracellular volumes using a bolus injection of Gd-DTPA: kinetic modelling in canine ischemic disease. *Magn Reson Med* 1992;23(2):239–253.
6. **Larsson HB, Stubgaard M, Søndergaard L, et al.** In vivo quantification of the unidirectional influx constant for Gd-DTPA diffusion across the myocardial capillaries with MR imaging. *J Magn Reson Imaging* 1994;4(3):433–440.
7. **Larsson HBW, Hansen AE, Berg HK, et al.** Dynamic contrast-enhanced quantitative perfusion measurement of the brain using T_1-weighted MRI at 3 T. *J Magn Reson Imaging* 2008;27:754–762.
8. **Sourbron S, Ingrisch M, Siefert A, et al.** Quantification of cerebral blood flow, cerebral blood volume, and blood–brain-barrier leakage with DCE-MRI. *Magn Reson Med* 2009;62:205–217.
9. **Kety SS, Schmidt CF.** The nitrous oxide method for the quantitative determination of cerebral blood flow in man: theory, procedures and normal values. *J Clin Invest* 1948;27(4):476–483.
10. **Kety SS.** The theory and applications of the exchange of inert gas at the lungs and tissues. *Pharmacol Rev* 1951;3(1):1–41.
11. **Meier P, Zierler KL.** On the theory of the indicator-dilution method for measurement of blood flow and volume. *J Appl Physiol* 1954;6(12):731–744.
12. **Kuschinsky W, Paulson OB.** Capillary circulation in the brain. *Cerebrovasc Brain Metab Rev* 1992;4(3):261–286.
13. **Jespersen SN, Østergaard L.** The roles of cerebral blood flow, capillary transit time heterogeneity, and oxygen tension in brain oxygenation and metabolism. *J Cereb Blood Flow Metab* 2012;32:264–277.
14. **Fick A.** Über die Messung des Blutquantums in den Herzventrikeln. Sitzungsber. *Physik Med Gesell zu Wurzburg* 1870;16:36.
15. **Lassen NA.** Cerebral transit of an intravascular tracer may allow measurement of regional blood volume but not regional blood flow. *J Cereb Blood Flow Metab* 1984;4:633–634.
16. **Weisskoff RM, Chesler D, Boxerman JL, et al.** Pitfalls in MR measurement of tissue blood flow with intravascular tracers: which mean transit time? *Magn Reson Med* 1993;29:553–559.
17. **Larsson HBW, Courivaud F, Rostrup E, et al.** Measurement of brain perfusion, blood volume, and blood-brain barrier permeability, using dynamic contrast-enhanced T1-weighted MRI at 3 tesla. *Magn Reson Med* 2009;62:1270–1281.
18. **Brix G, Semmler W, Port R, et al.** Pharmacokinetic parameters in CNS Gd-DTPA enhanced MR imaging. *J Comput Assist Tomogr* 1991; 15(4):621–628.
19. **Larsson HB, Stubgaard M, Frederiksen JL, et al.** Quantitation of blood-brain barrier defect by magnetic resonance imaging and gadolinium-DTPA in patients with multiple sclerosis and brain tumors. *Magn Reson Med* 1990;16(1):117–131.
20. **Tofts PS, Kermode AG.** Measurement of the blood–brain barrier permeability and leakage space using dynamic MR imaging. 1. Fundamental concepts. *Magn Reson Med* 1991;17(2):357–367.
21. **Larsson HBW, Fritz-Hansen T, Rostrup E, et al.** Myocardial perfusion modelling using MRI. *Magn Reson Med* 1996;35:716–726.
22. **Tofts PS, Brix G, Buckley DL, et al.** Estimating kinetic parameters from dynamic contrast-enhanced T1-weighted MRI of a diffusible tracer: standardized quantities and symbols. *J Magn Reson Imaging* 1999;10:223–232.
23. **Cramer SP, Larsson HBW.** Accurate determination of blood–brain barrier permeability using dynamic contrast enhanced T1-weighted MRI. A simulation and in vivo study on healthy subjects and MS patients. *J Cereb Blood Flow Metab* 2014;34(10):1655–1665.
24. **Sourbron PS, Buckley DL.** On the scope and interpretation of the Tofts models for DCE-MRI. *Magn Reson Med* 2011;66:735–745.
25. **Patlak CS, Blasberg RG.** Graphical evaluation of the blood-to-brain transfer constants from multiple-time uptake data. Generalizations. *J Cereb Blood Flow Metab* 1985;5:584–590.
26. **Zwick S, Brix G, Tofts PS, et al.** Simulation-based comparison of two approaches frequently used for dynamic contrast-enhanced MRI. *Eur Radiol* 2010;20:432–442.
27. **Cramer SP, Simonsen H, Frederiksen JL, et al.** Abnormal blood-brain barrier permeability in normal appearing white matter in multiple sclerosis investigated by MRI. *Neuroimage Clin* 2014;4:182–189.
28. **Sangren WC, Sheppard CW.** Mathematical derivation of the exchange of a labelled substance between a liquid flowing in a vessel and an external compartment. *Bull Math Biophys* 1953;15:387–394.
29. **Goresky CA, Ziegler WH, Bach GG.** Capillary exchange modeling. Barrier-limited and flow limited distribution. *Circ Res* 1970;27:739–764.
30. **Koh TS, Bisdas S, Koh DM, et al.** Fundamentals of tracer kinetics for dynamic contrast-enhanced MRI. *J Magn Reson Imaging* 2011;34: 1262–1276.
31. **Koh TS, Tan CKM, Cheong LHD, et al.** Cerebral perfusion mapping using a robust and efficient method for deconvolution analysis of dynamic contrast-enhanced images. *Neuroimage* 2006;32:643–653.
32. **Moran GR, Thornhill RE, Sykes J, et al.** Myocardial viability imaging using Gd-DTPA: physiological modelling of infracted myocardium, and impact on injection strategy and imaging time. *Magn Reson Med* 2002;48:791–800.
33. **Koh TS, Thng CH, Hartono S, et al.** Dynamic contrast-enhanced MRI of neuroendocrine hepatic metastases: a feasibility study using a dual-input two-compartment model. *Magn Reson Med* 2011;65:250–260.
34. **Johnson JA, Wilson TA.** A model for capillary exchange. *Am J Physiol* 1966;210(6):1299–1303.
35. **St. Lawrence KS, Lee TY.** An adiabatic approximation to the tissue homogeneity model for water exchange in the brain: I. Theoretical derivation. *J Cereb Blood Flow Metab* 1998;18(12):1365–1377.
36. **St. Lawrence KS, Lee TY.** An adiabatic approximation to the tissue homogeneity model for water exchange in the brain: II. Experimental validation. *J Cereb Blood Flow Metab* 1998;18(12):1378–1385.
37. **Bassingthwaigthe JB, Goresky CA.** Modeling in the analysis of solute and water exchange in the microvasculature. In: Renkin EM, Michel CC, Geiger SR, eds. *Handbook of physiology. Section 2. The cardiovascular system.* Bethesda, MD: American Physiological Society; 1984:549–626.
38. **Bassingthwaigthe JB, Malone MA, Moffett TC, et al.** Validity of microsphere depositions for regional myocardial flows. *Am J Physiol* 1987;253:H184–H193.
39. **Østergaard L, Weisskoff RM, Chesler DA, et al.** High resolution measurement of cerebral blood flow using intravascular tracer bolus passages. Part I: Mathematical approach and statistical analysis. *Magn Reson Med* 1996;36:715–725.
40. **Tikhonov AN, Arsenin, eds.** *Solutions of ill-posed problems.* John F, transl. editor. Washington, DC: V.H. Winston; 1977.
41. **Tiknonov AN.** Ill-posed problems in natural sciences. In: Leonov AS, ed. Proceedings of International Conference, Moscow; 1991.
42. **Hansen PC.** *Rank-deficient and ill-posed problems.* Doctoral Dissertation. UniC. Technical University of Denmark; 1996.
43. **Schmitt M, Viallon M, Thelen M, et al.** Quantification of myocardial flow and blood flow reserve in the presence of arterial dispersion: a simulation study. *Magn Reson Med* 2002;47:787–793.

44. **Calamante F, Gadian DG, Connelly A.** Delay and dispersion effects in dynamic susceptibility contrast MRI: Simulations using singular value decomposition. *Magn Reson Med* 2000;44:466–473.
45. **Elkington AG, He T, Gatehouse PD, et al.** Optimization of the arterial input function for myocardial perfusion cardiovascular magnetic resonance. *J Magn Reson Imaging* 2005;21:354–359.
46. **Boos M, Scheffler K, Haselhorst R, et al.** Arterial first pass gadolinium-CM dynamics as a function of several intravenous saline flush and Gd volumes. *J Magn Reson Imaging* 2001;13:568–576.
47. **Van Osch MJP, Vonken EPA, Wu O, et al.** Model of the human vasculature for studying the influence of contrast injection speed on cerebral perfusion MRI. *Magn Reson Med* 2003;50:614–622.
48. **Fritz-Hansen T, Rostrup E, Larsson HBW, et al.** Measurement of the arterial concentration of Gd-DTPA using MRI: a step toward quantitative perfusion imaging. *Magn Reson Med* 1996;36:225–231.
49. **Hansen A, Pedersen H, Rostrup E, et al.** Partial volume effect (PVE) on the arterial input function (AIF) in T_1-weighted perfusion imaging and limitations of the multiplicative rescaling approach. *Magn Reson Med* 2009;62:1055–1059.
50. **Van Osch MJP, Vonken EPA, Bakker CJG, et al.** Correcting partial volume artifacts of the arterial input function in quantitative cerebral perfusion MRI. *Magn Reson Med* 2001;45:477–485.
51. **Conturo TE, Barker PB, Mathews VP, et al.** MR imaging of cerebral perfusion by phase-angle reconstruction of bolus paramagnetic-induced frequency shift. *Magn Reson Med* 1992;27(2):375–390.
52. **Gatehouse PD, Elkongton AG, Ablitt NA, et al.** Accurate assessment of the arterial input function during high-dose myocardial perfusion cardiovascular magnetic resonance. *J Magn Reson Imaging* 2004;20: 39–45.
53. **Kleppestø M, Larsson C, Groote I, et al.** T_2*-correction in dynamic contrast-enhanced MRI from double-echo acquisitions. *J Magn Reson Imaging* 2014;39:1314–1319.
54. **Christian TF, Rettmann DW, Aletras AH, et al.** Absolute myocardial perfusion in canines measured by using dual-bolus first-pass MR imaging. *Radiology* 2004;232:677–684.
55. **Hsu LY, Rhoads KL, Holly JE, et al.** Quantitative myocardial perfusion analysis with a dual-bolus contrast-enhanced first-pass MRI technique in humans. *J Magn Reson Imaging* 2006;23:315–322.
56. **Köstler H, Ritter C, Lipp M, et al.** Prebolus quantitative MR heart perfusion imaging. *Magn Reson Med* 2004;52:296–299.
57. **Kim D, Axel L.** Multislice, dual-imaging sequence for increasing the dynamic range of the contrast-enhanced blood signal and CNR of myocardial enhancement at 3T. *J Magn Reson Imaging* 2006;23:81–86.
58. **Yang C, Karczmar GS, Medved M, et al.** Multiple reference tissue method for contrast agent arterial input function estimation. *Magn Reson Med* 2007;58:1266–1275.
59. **Yang C, Karczmar GS, Medved M, et al.** Reproducibility assessment of a multiple reference tissue method for quantitative dynamic contrast enhanced-MRI analysis. *Magn Reson Med* 2009;61:851–859.
60. **Fluckiger JU, Schabel MC, DiBella EVR.** Model-based blind estimation of kinetic parameters in DCE-MRI. *Magn Reson Med* 2009;62(6): 1477–1486.
61. **Schabel MC, Fluckiger JU, DiBella EVR.** A model-constrained Monte Carlo method for blind arterial input function estimation in dynamic contrast-enhanced MRI: I) simulations. *Phys Med Biol* 2010;55(16): 4783–4806.
62. **Calamante F, Willats LW, Gadian DG, et al.** Bolus delay and dispersion in perfusion MRI: implications for tissue predictor models in stroke. *Magn Reson Med* 2006;55:1180–1185.
63. **Schabel MC, DiBella EVR, Jensen RL, et al.** A model-constrained Monte Carlo method for blind arterial input function estimation in dynamic contrast-enhanced MRI: I) in vivo results. *Phys Med Biol* 2010;55(16): 4807–4823.
64. **Calamante F, Mørup M, Hansen LK.** Defining a local arterial input function for perfusion MRI using independent component analysis. *Magn Reson Med* 2004;52:789–797.
65. **Gadian DG, Payne JA, Bryant DJ, et al.** Gadolinium-DTPA as a contrast agent in MR imaging—theoretical projections and practical observations. *J Comput Assist Tomogr* 1985;9(2):242–251.
66. **Lauffer RB.** Paramagnetic metal complexes as water proton relaxation agents for NMR imaging: theory and design. *Chem Rev* 1987;87: 901–927.
67. **Donnahue KM, Burstein D, Manning WJ, et al.** Studies of Gd-DTPA relaxivity and proton exchange rates in tissue. *Magn Reson Med* 1994;32:66–76.
68. **Fintaske J, Martirosian P, Graf H, et al.** Relaxivity of Gadopentetate Dimeglumina (Magnevist), Gadobutrol (Gadovist), and Gadobenate Dimeglumine (MultiHance) in human blood plasma and 0.2, 1.5 and 3 tesla. *Invest Radiol* 2006;41:213–221.
69. **Heye T, Boll DT, Reiner C, et al.** Impact of precontrast T_{10} relaxation times on dynamic contrast-enhanced MRI pharmacokinetic parameters: T_{10} mapping versus a fixed T_{10} reference value. *J Magn Reson Imaging* 2014; 39:1136–1145.
70. **Larsson HBW, Rosenbaum S, Fritz-Hansen T.** Quantification of the effect of water exchange in dynamic contrast MRI perfusion measurements in the brain and heart. *Magn Reson Med* 2001;46:272–281.
71. **Brix G, Schad LR, Deimling M, et al.** Fast and precise T1 imaging using tomrop sequence. *Magn Reson Imaging* 1990;8:351–356.
72. **McLaughlin A, Leigh J.** Relaxation times in systems with chemical exchange: approximate solutions for the non dilute case. *J Magn Reson* 1973;9:296–304.
73. **Donahue KM, Weisskoff RM, Burstein D.** Water diffusion and exchange as they influence contrast enhancement. *J Magn Reson Imaging* 1997; 7:102–110.
74. **Colon T, Outhred R.** Water diffusion permeability of erythrocytes using an NMR technique. *Biochim Biophys Acta* 1972;288:354–361.
75. **Koenig SH, Spiller M, Brown RD, et al.** Relaxation of water protons in the intra- and extracellular regions of blood containing Gd(DTPA). *Magn Reson Med* 1986;3:791–795.
76. **Donahue KM, Weisskoff RM, Chesler DA, et al.** Improving MR quantification of regional blood volume with intravascular T1 contrast agent: accuracy, precision, and water exchange. *Magn Reson Med* 1996;36:858–867.
77. **Zimmerman JR, Brittin WE.** Nuclear magnetic resonance studies in multiple phase systems: lifetime of a water molecule in an adsorbing phase on silica gel. *J Phys Chem* 1957;61:1328–1333.
78. **Hazlewood C, Chang D, Nichols B, et al.** Nuclear magnetic resonance transverse relaxation times of water protons in skeletal muscle. *Biophys J* 1974;14:583–605.
79. **Schwickert HC, Roberts TP, Shames DM, .**Quantification of liver blood volume: comparison of ultra short TI inversion recovery echo planar imaging (ULSTAR-EPI), with dynamic 3D-gradient recalled echo imaging. *Magn Reson Med* 1995;34:845–852.
80. **Fabry ME, Eisenstadt M.** Water exchange between red cells and plasma. Measurement by nuclear magnetic relaxation. *Biophys J* 1975;15(1): 1101–1110.
81. **Bruno E, Digilio G, Cabella C, et al.** Water exchange across the erythrocyte plasma membrane studied by HR-MAS NMR spectroscopy. *Magn Reson Med* 2006;56(5):978–985.
82. **Bjørnerud A, Bjerner T, Johansson LO, et al.** Assessment of myocardial blood volume and water exchange: theoretical considerations and in vivo results. *Magn Reson Med* 2003;49:828–837.
83. **Wedeking P, Sotak CH, Telser J, et al.** Quantitative dependence of MR signal intensity on tissue concentration of Gd(HP-DO3A) in nephrectomised rat. *Magn Reson Imaging* 1992;10:97–108.
84. **Judd RM, Atalay MK, Rottman GA, et al.** Effects of myocardial water exchange on T1 enhancement during bolus administration of MR contrast agents. *Magn Reson Med* 1995;33:215–223.
85. **Sobol WT, Jackels SC, Cothran RL, et al.** NMR spin-lattice relaxation in tissues with high concentration of paramagnetic contrast media: evaluation of water exchange rates in intact rat muscle. *Med Phys* 1991; 18:243–250.
86. **Nielsen G, Fritz-Hansen T, Dirks CG, et al.** Evaluation of heart perfusion in patients with acute myocardial infarction using dynamic contrast-enhanced magnetic resonance imaging. *J Magn Reson Imaging* 2004;20:403–410.
87. **Landis CS, Li X, Telang FW, et al.** Equilibrium transcytolemmal water-exchange kinetics in skeletal muscle in vivo. *Magn Reson Med* 1999;4: 467–478.
88. **Buckley DL, Kershaw LE, Stanisz GJ.** Cellular-interstitial water exchange and its effect on the determination of contrast agent concentration in vivo: dynamic contrast-enhanced MRI of human internal obturator muscle. *Magn Reson Med* 2008;60:1011–1019.
89. **Moran GR, Prato FS.** Modeling (1H) exchange: an estimated of the error introduced in MRI by assuming the fast exchange limit in bolus tracking. *Magn Reson Med* 2004:51(4):816–827.

CHAPTER

9 Arterial Spin-Labeled MR Perfusion Imaging Techniques

Francesca B. Pizzini, MD, PhD, Marion Smits, MD, PhD,
Roman Wesolowski, PhD Eng, Michael Chapell, PhD,
Rolf Jager, MD, Henri J. M. M. Mutsaerts, MD,
and Juan Antonio Hernandez Tamames, MSc, PhD

Introduction

Arterial spin labeling (ASL) is a relatively new technique for MR perfusion assessment that is particularly useful in brain tissues. From a technical point of view, ASL-MRI is essentially a classic tracer experiment where the injected blood-borne tracer has been replaced by a procedure whereby water protons in the blood have been "labeled" on their way to the organ of interest. This labeling is achieved remotely by the application of radio-frequency (RF) waves that effect an inversion of the magnetization of the blood–water in the region where the RF is applied. This is achieved either for all blood within a region (pulsed ASL) or for blood flowing through a plane (continuous ASL), and for brain perfusion, it is usually performed in the neck. Conventional MR imaging can be used to capture this inverted blood signal once it has arrived in the organ, allowing time for it to arrive. However, the image will also contain contribution from the normal soft tissue in the image, which is much larger in magnitude than is the perfusion signal. Hence, the basic ASL experiment contains two images, one with labeling of blood–water and a second without: the subtraction of the two revealing the perfusion. The reliance on an endogenous tracer means that the ASL technique is noninvasive and, for most variants, readily available on existing hardware. However, the small signal magnitude relative to noise in the images and the relatively short "half-life" of the labeled water mean that careful and optimal acquisition and quantification are required.

The primary goal of this chapter is to provide a complete overview of ASL from the technical issues, such as acquisition and quantification, to the clinical application in the brain including neuro-oncology, neurodegeneration, psychiatry, vascular and inflammatory disease, and epilepsy. The final section is focused on common pitfalls in ASL that should be avoided in diagnosis and a procedure to assess quality. A white paper[1] regarding technical aspects of ASL has recently been published, from which technical recommendations in this chapter are drawn.

Arterial Spin Labeling Acquisition

Tissue functions strongly depend on the underlying perfusion, which is the process of supplying tissue cells with nutrients via oxygenated blood from arteries through exchange across the capillary bed; in brain, it is blood–brain barrier (BBB). The measurement of perfusion using MRI has been an active area of research for over 20 years.[2]

In general, perfusion techniques can be divided into two categories: exogenous and endogenous methods. Exogenous techniques use intravenous contrast agents such as Gd-DTPA (gadolinium diethylenetriaminepentaacetic acid). Endogenous methods use the water protons in arterial blood as the tracer (natural contrast agent). The endogenous MR method is called ASL or, rarely, arterial spin tagging. In ASL, the magnetization of water molecules of the inflowing arterial blood can be labeled by either saturation[2] or inversion pulses,[3,4] altering the magnetization of the arterial blood.[2] Labeled blood then progressively travels through the arteries and arterioles into the capillary bed where the magnetization is exchanged with that in the tissue, as water is a fast and freely diffusible tracer. ASL can be assessed either qualitatively or quantitatively. If two images are acquired, one with labeled blood and a second nonlabeled, then the difference image yields a qualitative map of perfusion. Qualitative measurements result in perfusion-weighted images that are simply a percentage difference between labeled and nonlabeled images. Quantitative measurements typically involve measuring the voxel signal intensity curve at a range of postlabeling delays and fitting to a complete perfusion model.[5,6]

ASL sequence consists of two independent parts: labeling and image acquisition. ASL labeling techniques can be classified into continuous (CASL),[7] pulsed (PASL),[8] and, recently introduced, a hybrid of both, pseudocontinuous ASL (PCASL).[9]

In continuous ASL, labeling within the tissue of interests reaches a steady state, due to long labeling time. The major advantage of this method is much higher signal-to-noise ratio (SNR) over the pulsed ASL and also simpler quantitative perfusion models. In the PASL technique, a bolus of arterial blood is labeled and passes through the tissue carrying a transient change in signal. Shorter labeling time with a greater efficiency and smaller RF power deposition are the most important advantages of this method,[10] due to which, CASL often requires additional hardware to be employed.

Labeling—Continuous ASL

CASL is the original method for ASL. Proposed in 1992,[2,3,11] this method originated from angiography.[11,12] Early techniques employed multiple saturation pulses,[2] which were then replaced by

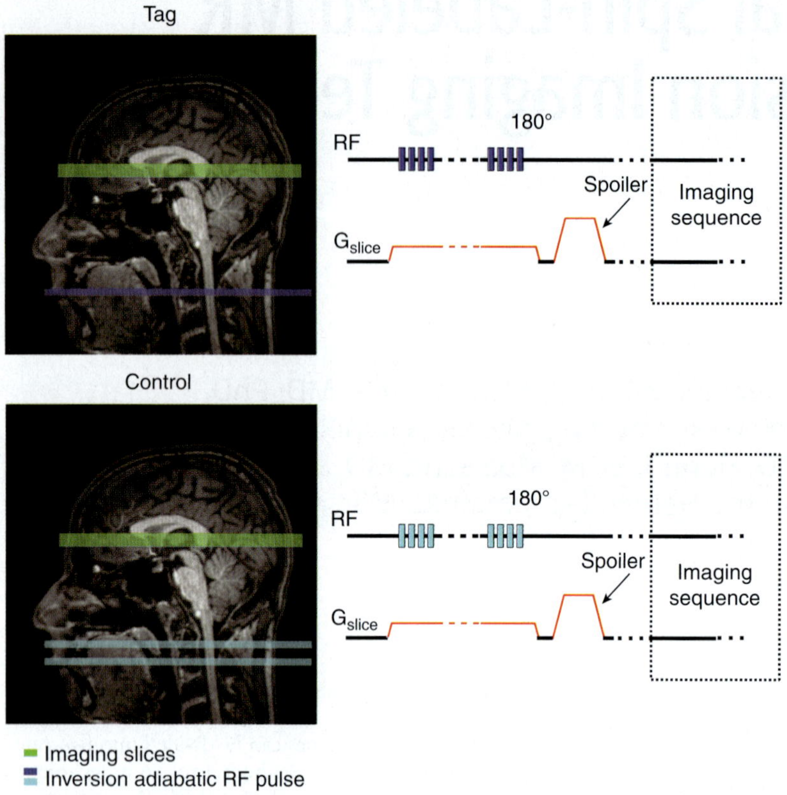

Figure 9-1. Schematic diagram of continuous ASL technique. Tag **(top)** and control **(bottom)** images are shown with the spatial inversion of tag and control (*blue* and *turquoise*, respectively) and imaging slices (*green*). Pulse sequence for tag and control shown on right.

the magnetization inversion approach.[3] CASL relies on continuous, flow-induced, adiabatic inversion with simultaneous application of magnetic field gradient in the flow direction[11] (Fig. 9.1). This adiabatic inversion pulse alone does not carry any amplitude or frequency modulation; therefore, stationary spins are not under the influence of the adiabatic inversion.[10] By implementing concurrently a magnetic field gradient G along the direction of motion, spins located at position $r_0 = \omega rf$ will be inverted. The inversion γG is usually applied for 2 to 4 seconds (labeling duration) to ensure the complete filing of vessels and exchange with inverted arterial spins to the imaging slices. The most common spatial placement of the inversion plane is in the vicinity of the circle of Willis or common carotid. Spins are inverted with efficiency α, which must be considered in the quantification process; typical efficiency values range from 80% to 98%.[3,11,13–17] The acquisition part of the sequence begins after labeling duration and additional postlabeling delay (PLD).

To estimate perfusion to produce a nonlabel image, the control plane has to be inverted twice, which results in double RF deposition—higher specific absorption rate (SAR), especially problematic in high magnetic fields of 3 T and above. In addition, CASL, with its prolonged train of RF pulses, is particularly sensitive to magnetization transfer (MT) effects resulting in saturation of the static tissue signal in imaging slices. To lower exposure to the excess of SAR, a second RF coil is needed to expand limited coverage, which is an additional, hardware-based disadvantage and difficulty in using this method.

Labeling—Pulsed ASL

Pulsed arterial spin labeling (PASL) denotes a family of sequences and spatial techniques that use a bolus to label the inflowing magnetization. This approach is far less demanding on the hardware and lowers the SAR. The bolus travels through the arteries and arterioles to the capillary bed (recovering with the T1 of blood) where the labeled magnetization is exchanged with unlabelled magnetization of the water in tissue. Once in the tissue, the labeled magnetization then experiences T1 relaxation (T1 of tissue) and eventually recovers and washes out as the fresh, unlabelled blood arrives in the imaging slice. The most commonly used PASL techniques are discussed later in this section. These techniques are described in the form they were initially introduced. Today, however, most of these sequences have variously been optimized and modified, for example, with the addition of pre- and postsaturation pulses.

Figure 9.2 represents the basic sequence for any PASL method; first, we label arterial blood, and then we perform a readout sequence of the desired slice, slices, or volume. In-plane pre- and postsaturation pulses are optional but commonly used in most of the sequences because they limit the effect of poor labeling pulse profile (180 degrees inversion). In-plane saturation becomes more of a requirement at higher fields, where the 180-degree pulses

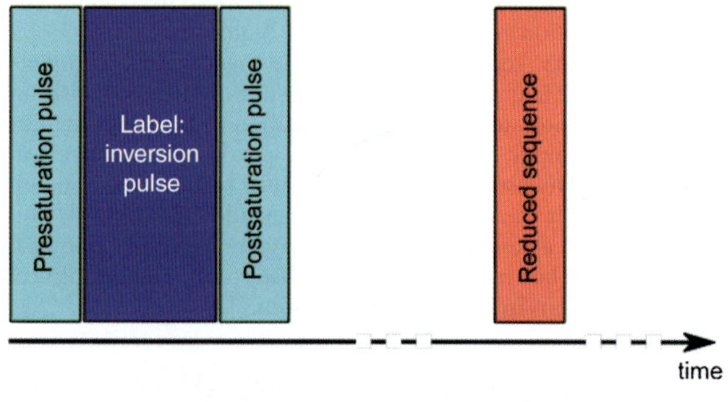

Figure 9-2. Schematic diagram of a general pulse sequence of the ASL. Pre- and postsaturation pulses play immediately before and after the label (180 degrees inversion pulse). The *red box* represents the beginning of the readout sequence.

are even more susceptible to imperfections in their profile and efficiency across the volume. Typically, the in-plane presaturation uses a WET scheme[18] and the postsaturation uses a single sinc pulse.

There is a large number of various pulsed labeling techniques reported in literature, and they all can be used in obtaining ASL images, depending on their availability. This chapter contains only a few most popular approaches.

In the STAR (signal targeting with alternating radiofrequency) technique,[4] the sequence begins with an in-plane (90-degree) saturation pulse to minimize possible perturbations in the imaging slice from the labeling inversion pulse. The RF pulse is typically followed by an additional spoiler to dephase the magnetization. After the initial saturation, a spatially selective adiabatic inversion pulse is played (Fig. 9.3). The spatial placement of the 180-degree (typically adiabatic hyperbolic secant or frequency offset corrected inversion [FOCI]) inversion[19–21] pulse differs between the tag and control images such that the tag is played below the imaging slice and the control is played above the imaging slice at an equal distance from the center of the slice. This approach avoids discrepancies in static tissue signal between tag and control as a result of the MT effects. However, this original approach would not accurately correct for MT effects away from the isocenter and in particular for multislice acquisitions. A multislice version of EPI STAR has since been developed, which applies two 180-degree pulses back-to-back to act as the control.[22] Following the tag/control inversion pulses, at a time equal to the inversion time (TI, equivalent to PLD in CASL and PCASL), a spin echo EPI or gradient echo EPI pulse sequence is typically employed to collect images.

Flow-sensitive alternating inversion recovery (FAIR)[23,24] employs a frequency-selective inversion pulse with and without an accompanying slice-selective gradient (or with a reduced one) to produce tag and control images, respectively (Fig. 9.4). Similar to STAR, the inversion is typically performed using a hyperbolic secant adiabatic pulse (bandwidth of 1 to 5 kHz); for optimal labeling, FOCI pulses are used. The ideal FAIR scheme would employ a 180-degree slab over the imaging volume to produce the tag image and over the entire coverage of the coil to produce the control image. Realistically, in the tagging part of the sequence, the selective inversion must cover more than imaging volume due to imperfect pulse profile (side lobes) and the inversion width in the control image is also spatially selective (approximately 4 times the width of the tagging part) (Fig. 9.4), allowing shorter TR (repetition time). In addition, often, a head-only coil is used for the labeling. Under such circumstances, limiting the inversion pulse width in the control sequence is vital to avoid signal drop-off due to the coil efficiency and to assure arrival of the fresh, noninverted blood at the beginning of the following tagging sequence. FAIR is resistant to MT effects with respect to the imaging slice if slices are centered at zero offset frequency. Again, the image acquisition is obtained following the TI typically using one of the fast imaging sequences.

QUIPSS II (also Q2TIPS)[25,26] is very similar to the FAIR technique, only the labeling cutoff is achieved by employing a series of spatially selective saturation pulses applied just prior to image acquisition (Fig. 9.5). The pulses are placed underneath the imaging slab providing a clear finishing edge of the inflowing labeled blood bolus.

Labeling—Pseudocontinuous ASL

More recently, a hybrid of CASL and PASL techniques, PCASL, has been developed.[9] Figure 9.6 shows a schematic representation of PCASL tag and control conditions. This method uses rapidly repeated RF pulses in place of the continuous RF and, therefore, overcomes the problems of needing two RF coils or exceeding a safe SAR and is advantageous for scanning as it provides a relatively higher SNR. After repeated application of RF pulses, the magnetization reaches a steady state. The z-component of the magnetization, M_z, in the steady-state conditions is dependent on the flip angle of

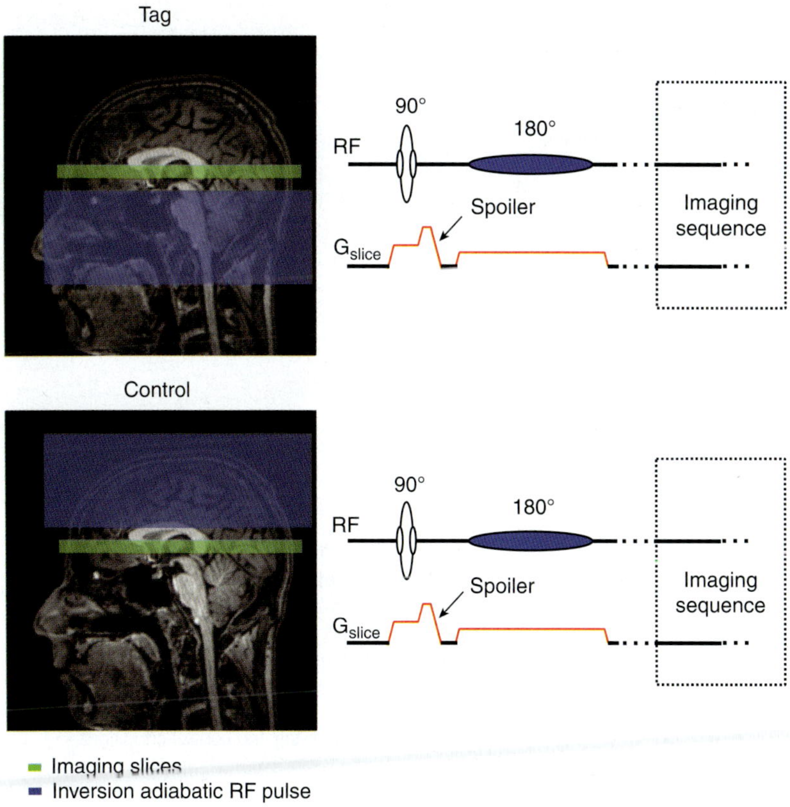

Figure 9-3. Schematic diagram of the traditional STAR labeling technique. Tag **(top)** and control **(bottom)** images are shown with the spatial inversion of both labeling conditions (*blue*) and imaging slices (*green*). Schematics of the radio frequency (RF) and slice-selective gradient of the sequence are shown. It can be seen that gradients are identical for tag and control resulting in equal eddy current effect. Here, the frequency offset is alternated tag and control conditions (*blue*).

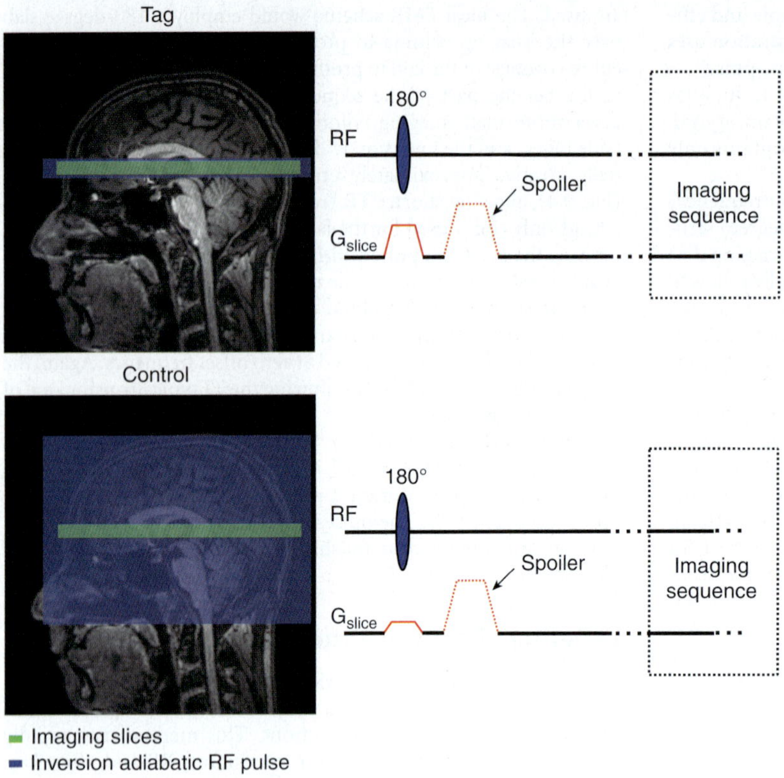

Figure 9-4. Schematic diagram of the FAIR labeling technique. Tag **(top)** and control **(bottom)** images are shown with the spatial inversion of both labels (*blue*) and imaging slices (*green*). Schematics of the RF and slice-selective gradient are shown on the right. The gradient amplitude can be seen to alternate between tag and control conditions.

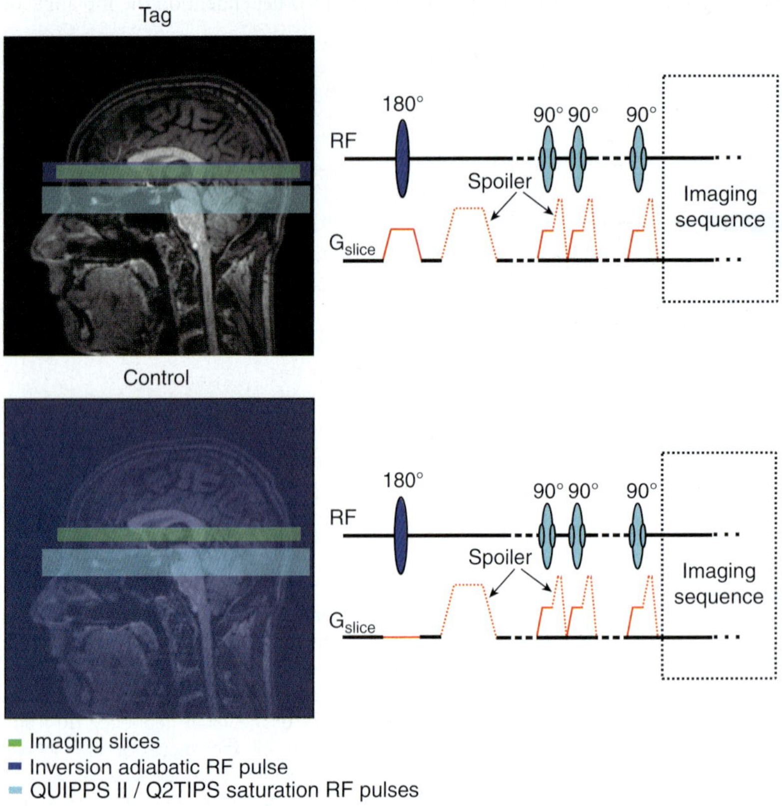

Figure 9-5. Schematic diagram of QUIPPS II (Q2TIPS) technique. Tag **(top)** and control **(bottom)** images are shown with the spatial inversion of both labels (*blue*) and imaging slices (*green*). QUIPPS II (Q2TIPS) saturation slabs are presented in turquoise. Schematics of the RF and slice-selective gradient are shown on the right. The gradient amplitude can be seen to alternate between tag and control conditions.

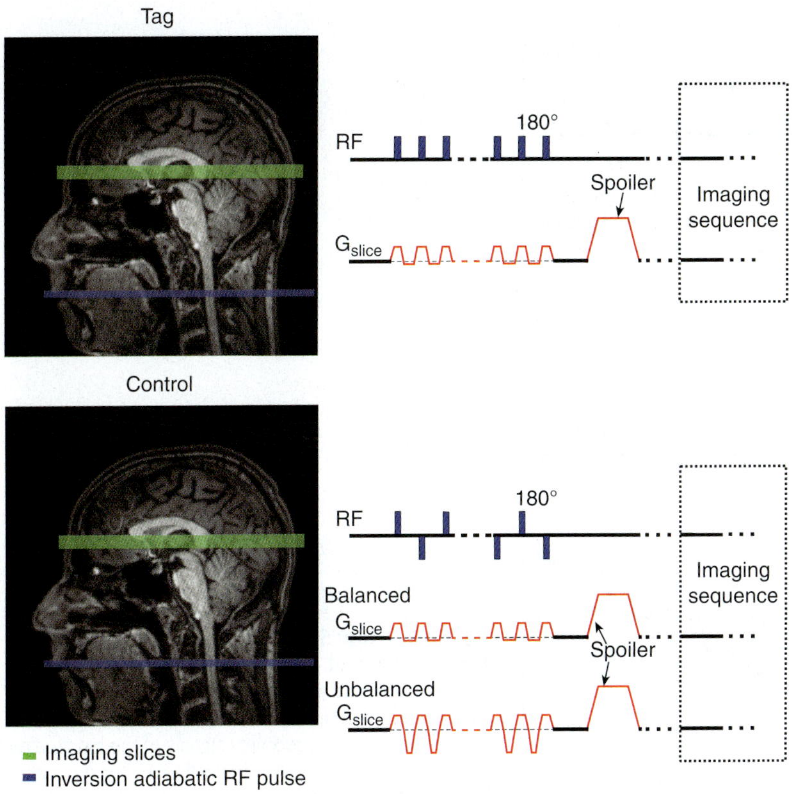

Figure 9-6. **Schematic diagram of pseudocontinuous ASL technique.** Tag **(top)** and control **(bottom)** images are shown with the spatial inversion of tag and control (*blue*) and imaging slices (*green*). Schematic representation of the RF pulses and the slice gradient of the sequence for tag and control shown on the right. Control condition indicates two variations of the sequence: balanced and unbalanced (marked in the figure).

the RF pulse, θ, and the phase shift experienced during the time between pulses, φ:

$$M_z = \frac{\pm M_0 \sin\theta \sin\frac{\varphi}{2}}{\sqrt{(1-\cos\theta)^2 + \sin^2\theta \sin^2\frac{\varphi}{2}}} \quad (1)$$

Similarly to CASL, the image acquisition sequence begins after labeling duration and PLD.

Readout

One of the most popular readout sequences used for ASL is EPI (echo planar imaging).[27] This is due to EPI being a method of rapid acquisitions, and it is essential to acquire the image before the label decays. However, alternative acquisition methods may be used, such as 3D-GRASE (gradient and spin echo).[28] The advantage of this sequence is that it acquires a 3D volume in a single shot, reducing the slice-dependent variation in perfusion signal due to differences in acquisition delays that occurs with 2D multislice methods. It also provides increased SNR compared to 2D acquisitions. However, it is generally limited to coarse in-plane resolution to reduce off-resonance effects or limited slice thickness to reduce through-slice decay and blurring. Although blurring can be reduced by introducing segmentation in z-plane, there are fewer full-volume images acquired, which makes this sequence very sensitive to motion artifacts. 3D RARE (Rapid Acquisition Relaxation Enhanced)[29] with spiral readout trajectory[30,31] has reduced sensitivity to motion artifacts due to oversampling of the center of the k-space, but can introduce in-plane blurring (resonance offset).[32]

Alternatively, more structural-based readout sequences can be used, such as TurboFLASH[33] and TrueFISP,[34,35] which have been shown to be advantageous for body ASL applications.

Background Suppression

To improve ASL image quality and reduce physiologic noise contamination, it is very common to use background suppression. Background suppression techniques[36] have been proposed to reduce the effects of physiologic noise by suppressing the static signal in ASL data prior to image acquisition. The tag and control images are acquired close to their null point ($M_z = 0$) in longitudinal (T1) recovery of magnetization by applying a nonselective inversion recovery sequence prior to the ASL acquisition.[36] Figure 9.7 shows a schematic representation of a pulse sequence employing background suppression pulses. Background suppression reduces noise from physiologic sources as well as the effects of head motion and other system instabilities of signal intensity. However, the intrinsic suppression of static signal does prevent background-suppressed ASL images being motion corrected.

Analysis and Quantification of ASL

The analysis of ASL data to produce a perfusion image is very simple, requiring only the subtraction of pairs of label and control images. Quantification goes one step further than this and seeks to provide perfusion images on an absolute perfusion scale, so that values in mL/100 g/min can be read from the images. At its most basic, the process of quantification of perfusion would entail three steps:

- Subtraction
- Kinetic model inversion
- Calibration (M_{0a} calculation)

Subtraction

As noted above, central to the principles of ASL is the subtraction of label and control images, where the "label" images contain signal from static tissue and labeled blood that has been delivered to the tissue:

$$M_{label} = M_{static} - M_{blood} \quad (2)$$

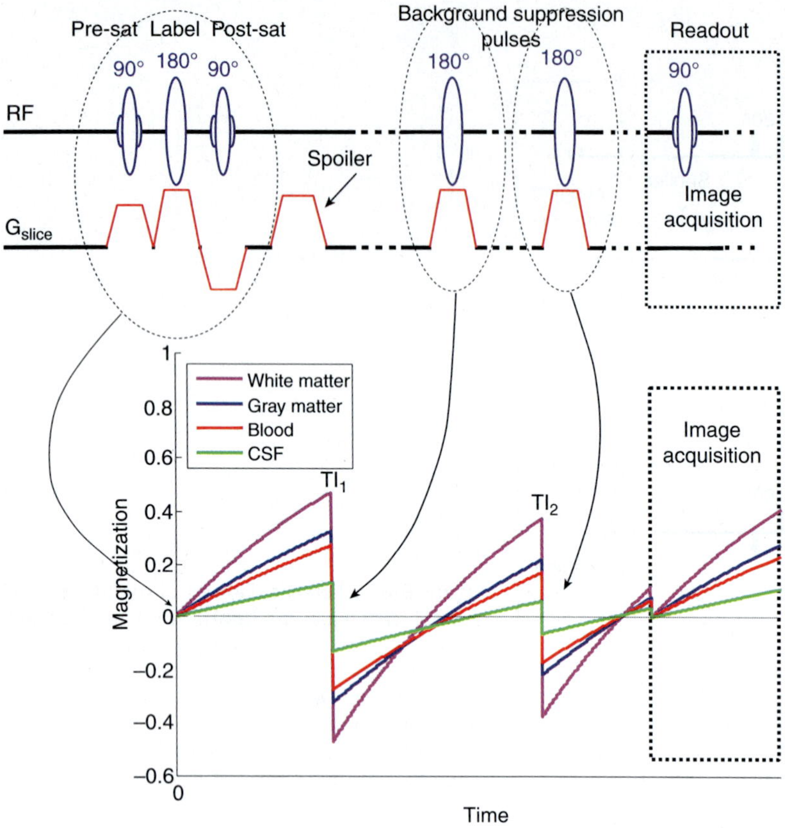

Figure 9-7. Top: Schematic of a pulse sequence with two background suppression adiabatic inversion pulses employed. For simplicity, only RF and slice-selective gradient time lines are shown. **Bottom:** Simulated normalized inversion recovery signals of the longitudinal magnetizations for various brain tissues (white matter, gray matter, blood, and CSF) with two background suppression pulses applied at times TI_1 and TI_2.

This accounts for the labeling process "inverting" the signal from the blood and assumes that (in the ideal case) this "inversion" is 100% efficient. The "control" image, in the absence of the labeling process, consists (ideally) of the same static tissue as well as unlabeled blood:

$$M_{\text{control}} = M_{\text{static}} + M_{\text{blood}} \tag{3}$$

Subtraction of these two, often referred to as tag-control subtraction, then produces:

$$\Delta M = M_{\text{control}} - M_{\text{label}} = 2 \times M_{\text{blood}} \tag{4}$$

This "difference" image is a direct measure of the delivery of blood to the tissue and thus perfusion; a brighter voxel will have had more blood delivered in any given time period (see below).

Compared to the tissue signal, the "blood" signal is small, approximately 1% to 2%. Hence, routinely multiple pairs of label and control images are acquired; these can be combined by taking the average over all the measurements.

Advanced: Motion and Artifacts

Since ASL relies on subtraction to reveal a difference signal far smaller than the static signal that is common to both label and control images, it is susceptible to motion. Any misalignment between the two images, and thus all those in the full data series, will lead to subtraction artifacts; these are often most visible around the brain periphery. Various postprocessing strategies exist for the correction of motion between image frames; from brain images, these typically rely upon rigid realignment of the images, and these equally can be applied to ASL data. However, issues can arise due to the varying contrast between label and control images, which may be interpreted by the motion correction algorithm as a motion effect that it will attempt to correct. It may be desirable to separately motion correct label and control images within the series and only as a final step seek to align them.

ASL perfusion images are also sensitive to the presence of artifacts within individual images in the series. While acquiring multiple pairs and taking the average improves robustness, an individual image with an artifact can lead to errors in the final difference image. A common solution is to manually reject individual images, or most often difference images, that upon visual inspection exhibit an artifact. This approach can also be taken with regard to motion to reject particularly corrupted images due to large subject motion at a particular time during acquisition. More automated approaches either attempt to identify these outlier images by comparison to others in the series, for example, using a correlation measure, or use a more robust method to take the average across the measurements than the mean.

Kinetic Model Inversion

Subtraction results in a relative perfusion image; the next step toward absolute quantification is to account for the relationship between measured signal and rate of delivery of the label itself. This process can be described by a kinetic model, which at its most general is given by a convolution relationship:

$$\Delta M(t) = f \times \text{AIF}(t) \otimes R(t) = f \times \int_0^t \text{AIF}(t')R(t-t')\text{d}t' \tag{5}$$

This relationship is widely employed in perfusion measurement and states that the measured signal is scaled by perfusion, f, and given by the convolution of two functions:

AIF(t)—The arterial input function, this describes the delivery of the contrast agent—here labeled blood—to the region of interest (voxel) over time.

$R(t)$—The residue function, this describes what happens to the contrast agent in the time after its arrival.

To convert from measured signal to perfusion, it is thus necessary to "invert" this equation (this inversion assumes that f does not appear in the residue function, which is not true of some more advanced ASL kinetic models—see below).

Various perfusion imaging modalities take differing approaches to the determination of AIF(t) and $R(t)$, including attempting to directly measure them from the data or derive population averages. The nature of ASL imaging means that it is typically appropriate to ascribe simple mathematical forms to both, with parameters that can be determined from the acquisition protocol.

The Arterial Input Function

ASL creates contrast by the RF inversion of blood prior to its entry to the imaging region. This ideally creates a well-defined bolus of labeled blood, and thus, signal at the labeling region takes the form of a boxcar (or "top hat") function. The duration of the boxcar is determined from the labeling scheme used: for PCASL (CASL), it is simply the labeling duration; for PASL, a spatially defined region of blood will be labeled and normally limited by the spatial extent of the labeling coil; thus, the bolus duration is unknown. For sufficiently short inflow time, it might be appropriate to ignore this parameter. However, more usually where a QUIPPS II or Q2TIPS scheme has been applied, the bolus duration will be defined by the time at which saturation is applied.

By the time the label has reached the measurement region, the label will have decayed due to T1 decay and this needs to be accounted for in the AIF shape. This is where the PASL and PCASL forms of ASL differ: for PASL, some blood is labeled more distally and thus takes longer to arrive in the imaging region; hence, it sees greater T1 decay, and the T1 decay effect is dependent upon the inflow time; for PCASL (and CASL), all blood is labeled at the same distance from the imaging region, and thus, T1 decay effects are only determined by the time of arrival: often called the bolus arrival time (BAT). It is usual in the simplest experiment to assume that this arrival time is negligible.

Finally, the magnitude of the AIF needs to be defined; this is the "concentration" of the label, which is related to the equilibrium magnetization of the arterial blood that was inverted: M_{0a}. As we have seen above, ASL takes the difference between label and control images so that the magnitude would ideally be twice M_{0a}. It is also necessary to take the efficiency of the inversion process, α, into account normally using values determined for a typical ASL experiment using the same labeling scheme (see Table **9.1**).

$$\mathrm{AIF}(t)=\begin{cases} 0 & 0<t<\Delta t \\ 2\alpha M_{0a}e^{-\frac{t}{T_1}} \quad \text{(pulsed)} & \Delta t<t<\tau+\Delta t \\ 2\alpha M_{0a}e^{-\frac{\Delta t}{T_1}} \quad \text{(continuous)} & \\ 0 & \tau+\Delta t<t \end{cases} \tag{6}$$

where Δt is the time it takes the blood to travel from the labeling region to the region of interest, BAT, and τ is the duration of the labeled bolus. Figure 9.8 illustrates these two input functions. In the simplest case, BAT is ignored, particularly if the inflow time is sufficiently long that its effect on the final measurement is small. The bolus duration is equal to the labeling duration for PCASL; for PASL, it will be determined by the size of the labeling region. However, where QUIPSS II has been used to limit the bolus duration, this parameter will be known.

TABLE 9.1 **Recommended Parameters for Quantification, Taken from Ref.[1]**

Parameter	Value
λ	0.9 mL/g
T1 at 3.0 tesla[a]	1,650 ms
T1 at 1.5 tesla[a]	1,350 ms
α for PCASL	0.85
α for PASL	0.98

[a]These are based on measured values for arterial blood.

The Residue Function

The residue function describes what happens to the label once it arrives in the measurement region—for a perfusion image, this would be the individual voxels. The simplest assumption is that labeled blood remains with the region; this is predicated on the basis that since the label is created by RF inversion of blood water protons and that water is in rapid exchange between blood and (the much larger volume of) tissue. Thus, as a first approximation, all the labeled blood water that arrives rapidly transfers into the tissue where it remains. However, at the same time, the label continues to decay with time constant T1.

$$R(t)=e^{-t/T_1} \tag{7}$$

Figure 9.8 illustrates this residue function. Any venous outflow has been ignored here since it is assumed that this will be insignificant compared to the effects of the T1 decay process. This model treats the ASL signal as having entered a single "well-mixed" compartment.[37]

Kinetic Model

The final model of the signal using the arterial input and residue functions above is shown in Figure 9.8. From this, it can be seen that perfusion simply scales the magnitude of the difference signal; thus, the "inversion" of the model is simple—as long as the effect of the other parameters can be accounted for. The early stages of the time course of the difference signal are very sensitive to BAT, hence the recommendation, for the simplest ASL acquisition, to use a long inflow time so that the signal is measured in the tail end of the curve, which is relatively insensitive to this parameter. Note also that PCASL is less sensitive to BAT than PASL and that the duration of the bolus determines both the amount of signal available and how late the measurement time needs to be to avoid sensitivity to BAT.

Inversion

These simple models can be "inverted" to give the following relationships between signal and perfusion:

PCASL:

$$f=\frac{6000\,\Delta M\,e^{\mathrm{PLD}/T_1}}{2\alpha T_1 M_{0a}\left(1-e^{-\frac{\tau}{T_1}}\right)}[\mathrm{mL/100g/min}] \tag{8}$$

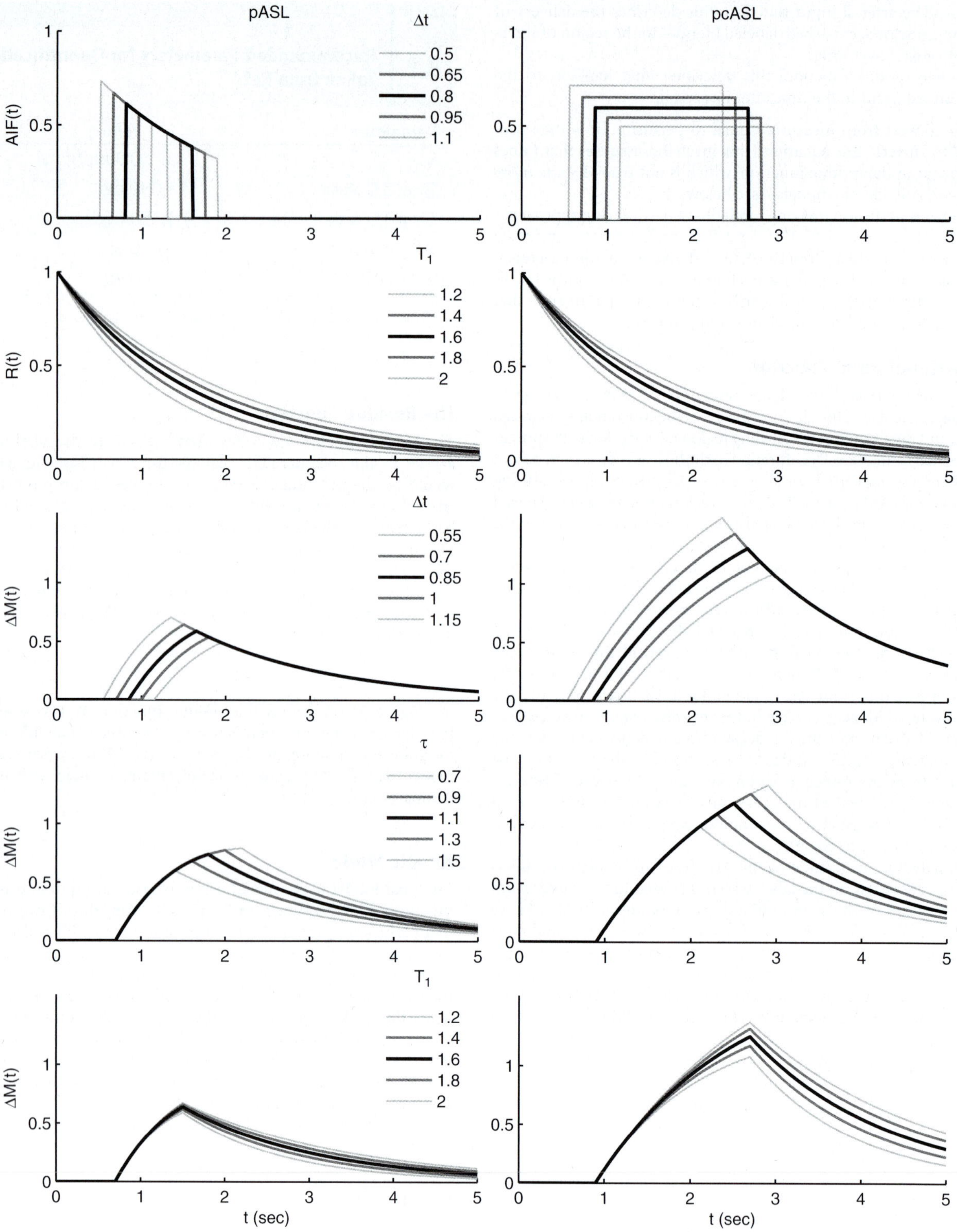

Figure 9-8. Examples of functional forms of the ASL signal for both pASL and pcASL acquisitions with variations in some of the key parameters.

PASL (with QUIPSS II):

$$f = \frac{6000\,\Delta M\,e^{TI/T_1}}{2\,\alpha\,T_1\,M_{0a}}[\mathrm{mL/100g/min}] \tag{9}$$

T1 may be chosen based on field strength from Table **9.1** based on measurements in the literature for the T1 of arterial blood. In some populations or in patients, it may be appropriate to use estimates of T1 that have been acquired in the subject using a quantitative T1 sequence. The factor of 6,000 converts the units from mL/g/s to the conventional mL/100 g/min. For an acquisition that is composed of multiple 2D slices, it will be necessary to use an appropriate PLD or TI for each slice, taking into account the time taken to acquire any previous slices.

Advanced

The simple kinetic model considered above can be extended to incorporate various other processes that affect the quantification of perfusion using ASL:

Arrival Time

Labeled blood will take some time to travel from labeling region to the region of interest, and this delay will also be different across the organ due to the length of different vascular pathways. This can be accommodated into the AIF through the inclusion of an arrival time parameter, as has been illustrated in the definition of the AIF above.[37]

Venous Outflow

A simple model for venous outflow is to assume that labeled blood leaves the voxel having reached equilibrium with the tissue at a rate determined by perfusion. This can be included within the residue function[37,38] but typically has a small effect on the shape of this function.

T1 Decay Rates

Typically, the T1 decay in tissue is shorter than in blood, and thus, separate T1 values might be defined for the AIF and residue functions.[37]

Further effects that can in theory be modeled, but are harder practically to measure and thus account for, include dispersion of the bolus of labeled blood water during transit through the vasculature[39,40] and the rate at which labeled blood water exchanges into the tissue.[41,42]

These more complex models of ASL kinetics typically require extra information to permit the computation of parameters associated with the effects they describe. For example, the inclusion of arrival time requires a measurement of bolus arrival in the voxel. This information can be obtained by sampling the ASL signal at a range of inflow times and thus sampling the kinetic signal itself. The process of model "inversion" then becomes one of model fitting—minimizing the error between the (noisy) data and the model by the judicious choice of the model parameters, most commonly performed using a sum-of-squares-error measure.

Calibration (M_{0a} Calculation)

A key parameter of the AIF that is required to quantify perfusion is the equilibrium magnetization of arterial blood that has been labeled: effectively the "concentration" the ASL tracer. Unlike the relative perfusion, this cannot be determined from the difference images. However, it is possible to calculate a surrogate measure of the equilibrium magnetization in the tissue at every voxel, M_{0t}, and relate this to the equivalent arterial blood magnetization, M_{0a}. Most commonly, a separate proton density image (with long TR) will be acquired and used to quantify M_0 of tissue—this is generally reasonable if TR > 5 seconds.[1] For shorter TR, for example, using the control image itself, a correction may be applied:

$$M'_{0t} = \frac{M_{0t}}{1 - e^{-\mathrm{TR}/T_{1,\mathrm{tissue}}}} \quad (10)$$

where $T_{1,\mathrm{tissue}}$ is the T1 of tissue—typically gray matter values would be used.

Since the proton density of tissue differs from that of arterial blood, a correction is introduced based on the partition coefficient, λ:

$$M_{0a} = \frac{M_{0t}}{\lambda} \quad (11)$$

A single whole brain partition coefficient of 0.9[1] may be assumed.

Advanced

The above approach makes a voxelwise calculation of M_{0a} that can then be applied in the quantification using the equations given above. However, noise from the proton density image will be imported into the perfusion quantification. An alternative approach is to quantify M_{0t} in a region of homogenous composition, for example, a region of white matter (WM) or CSF. An average taken across the region (to reduction corruption by noise) allows a single global value of M_{0a} to be calculated, theoretically reflecting the single value of M_{0a} for the labeled blood bolus. The region used may be defined manually or through automated segmentation of a structural image. The disadvantage of this approach is that it will not correct for variations in coil sensitivity, for example, in segmented acquisitions, and thus, a separate sensitivity image may be required or sensitivity correction applied in the acquisition.

While M_{0a} is required to quantify perfusion, a measurement of T1 might also be valuable (to account for its variation within the brain). The measurement of the two can be combined using a saturation recovery sequence. A series of measurements at different TIs permits both M_{0t} and T_{1t} to be determined from the data. In some cases, saturation recovery has been combined with the main ASL acquisition and inflow times, allowing a single acquisition to be used to collect all the required data, for example, the QUASAR sequence.[43]

Partial Volume Effects

Issues surrounding the presence within an individual voxel of multiple tissue types are present in a wide range of MR imaging methods. For perfusion imaging with ASL, the effects of partial voluming relate both to the boundary between CSF and tissue and between GM and WM. The former is more obvious because CSF will have no perfusion and thus should contribute no ASL difference signal—leading to underestimation of perfusion in voxels containing a partial volume of CSF. However, a mixture of white and gray matter is also important because the two tissue types have substantially different perfusion characteristics. The main difference is the lower perfusion in WM. It also exhibits a shorter T1 as well as a longer arterial arrival time (AAT).

The different perfusion properties substantially dictate the form of the normal ASL perfusion image, meaning that a lot of the features reflect the underlying variations in structure of the brain as shown in Figure 9.9.

It is possible using segmentation methods, applied typically to T1- or T2-weighted images, to estimate the partial volume contributions within voxels of an image. It is then possible to write down the contribution of each "tissue" type to the ASL signal:

$$M = \mathrm{PV}_{\mathrm{GM}} \times M_{\mathrm{GM}} + \mathrm{PV}_{\mathrm{WM}} \times M_{\mathrm{WM}} + \mathrm{PV}_{\mathrm{CSF}} \times M_{\mathrm{CSF}} \quad (12)$$

$$\Delta M = \mathrm{PV}_{\mathrm{GM}} \times \Delta M_{\mathrm{GM}} + \mathrm{PV}_{\mathrm{WM}} \times \Delta M_{\mathrm{WM}} \quad (13)$$

These can be used to correct for the effects of partial voluming, and a number of strategies have been proposed:

Rescaling The simplest method is to rescale the values in the subtracted image based on the estimated proportions of gray matter (GM) and WM.[44] Since the actual contribution (i.e., perfusion) of both GM and WM is unknown and we have only one measurement within the voxel, it is necessary to define one further constraint to solve the equation above for the difference image. This can be achieved by assuming the ratio of GM and WM perfusion.

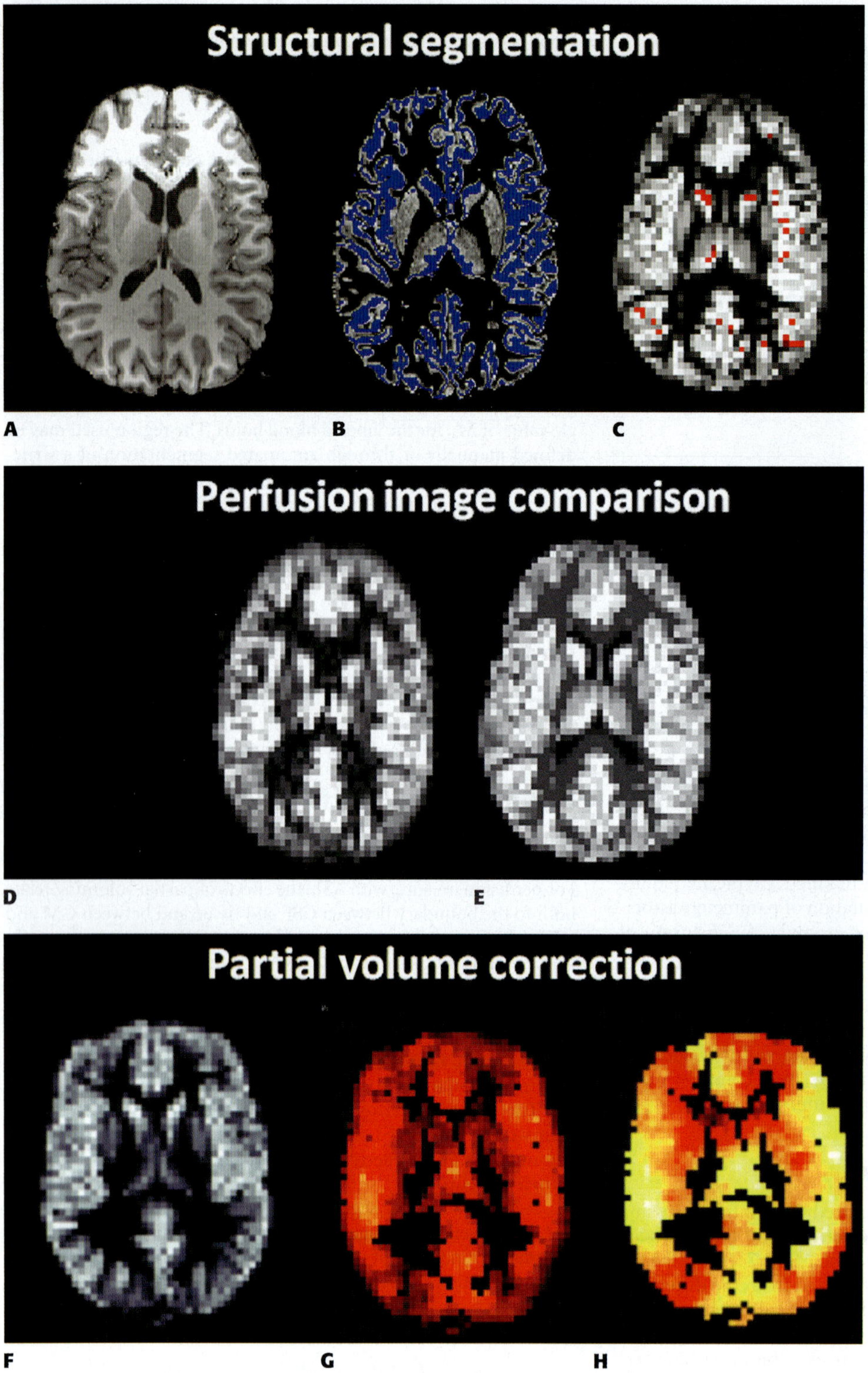

Figure 9-9. **Examples of partial volume effects in ASL and their correction.** A typical structural image **(A)** has been segmented into tissue types and GM contributions greater than 90% highlighted **(B)**. Once these partial volume estimates have been transformed into the same resolution as ASL data, very few voxels contain a high proportion (>90%) of GM **(C)**. The look of perfusion images is often highly dependent upon the underlying structure: Compare a typical ASL perfusion image **(D)** with one created using a set of partial volume estimates and spatially constant GM and WM (60 and 20 mL/100 g/min respectively) perfusion values **(E)**. Partial volume correction can be applied using a structural scan: GM partial volume estimates **(F)** (along with WM) have been used to correct the ASL perfusion image **(G)** to create a GM perfusion image **(H)**.

This in turn is the main drawback of this approach since it does not allow for variations in this ratio throughout the brain, or that a suitable value for this ratio is not well established.

Linear regression[45] takes a different approach for solving the equations above. Instead of assuming a fixed ratio between different tissue types, it assumes that perfusion varies smoothly in the brain, and thus, it is approximately reasonable to assume that GM and WM perfusion in neighboring voxels will be identical. The method proceeds by, for each voxel, choosing a neighborhood of voxels and solving a set of simultaneous equations based on the equations above across all of them to arrive at the GM and WM contributions. The size of the neighborhood needs to be chosen manually with larger sizes leading to more stable solutions. The strength of the approach is that it does not rely upon an assumed ratio, but it does introduce further smoothness into the perfusion images, which gets more substantial as the size of the neighborhood used increases.

Advanced

More advanced methods based on similar principles to the linear regression method have been proposed, including a method that attempts to adaptively determine the appropriate neighborhood for the calculations directly from the data,[46] as illustrated in Figure 9.9. Additionally, partial volume correction methods have been applied to multidelay ASL exploiting the different kinetics of GM and WM (T1 values and AAT) to increase sensitivity, thus accuracy of the perfusion estimates.[46]

An issue for partial volume correction is the accurate estimation of the partial volume values at the first place. These are normally most accurately achieved using high-resolution structural scans and preferably using a combination of T1- and T2-weighted images. However, these estimates then need to be transformed into the same resolution as that of the ASL data, requiring a good registration between the ASL and structural images. Additionally, typically, the ASL and structural images will have been acquired with different readouts leading to them having different distortions, particularly around the ventricles. Thus, while accurate PV estimates can be achieved from high-resolution images, errors will be introduced in the transformation process. Alternatives such as a segmentation of an image matching the ASL data, such as the raw control or calibration images, have been explored since these avoid transformation and distortion issues.[47] However, these are far more difficult to segment with any degree of accuracy.

Neuro-Oncologic Disease

MR perfusion imaging is extensively used in the context of neuro-oncological disease, where vascularisation and vascular proliferation are prominent features for tumour characterisation and grading. Increased vessel diameter and number of vessels in brain tumors lead to local increases in cerebral blood volume (CBV), which is usually assessed with T2-/T2*-weighted dynamic susceptibility contrast (DSC) MR imaging. DSC MR imaging is used in the clinical routine to differentiate types of brain tumors and metastases,[48–50] to grade neuroepithelial brain tumors,[51–54] and to distinguish tumor progression from treatment effects.[53,55–58]

There are now several studies that have evaluated ASL perfusion imaging in brain tumors.[59–61] ASL has several advantages over contrast agent perfusion techniques for the assessment of neuro-oncologic disease. Its noninvasiveness is often—but unjustly—dismissed in this context, because contrast agent administration is generally required in the evaluation of brain tumors, in which contrast enhancement is considered a key diagnostic feature. Contrast-enhanced perfusion imaging however requires a larger-bore intravenous cannula for, as well as a larger volume of contrast administration than conventional contrast-enhanced MR imaging. Especially in the pediatric population and in patients on or after chemotherapy, with difficult intravenous access, as well as patients with renal insufficiency, non–contrast-enhanced perfusion imaging can still be considered advantageous. A methodologic advantage is the fact that ASL is insensitive to the disturbing effects of contrast agent leakage occurring with disruption of the BBB. Extravasation of contrast agent to the extravascular compartment reduces the T2-/T2*-weighted signal due to T1 shortening and as such leads to an underestimation of CBV with T2-/T2*-weighted contrast-enhanced perfusion MR imaging techniques (Fig. 9.10). Furthermore, ASL is not sensitive to susceptibility artifacts, such as due to hemorrhage (Fig. 9.11), metallic surgical material (Fig. 9.12), or air–tissue interfaces (Fig. 9.13).

In a study comparing a multitude of perfusion techniques (T2-/T2*-weighted DSC and T1-weighted dynamic contrast-enhanced perfusion MR imaging, $H_2{}^{15}O$ positron emission tomography (PET), and pulsed ASL), Lüdemann et al.[60] demonstrated a nearly linear correlation between the various parameters assessed with these techniques. The estimated values for tumor perfusion on the other hand were significantly different between the techniques and can therefore not be compared or interchanged. Relatively small tumor perfusion ratios were obtained with $H_2{}^{15}O$ PET and T2-weighted DSC, while T1-weighted DCE perfusion MR imaging seemed to overestimate tumor perfusion. The pulsed ASL and T2*-weighted DSC yielded median estimation of tumor perfusion. Pulsed ASL, however, had the largest statistical uncertainty and failed to represent very highly perfused tumor regions.

Although it is CBV that is the most widely used parameter in the context of brain tumor perfusion imaging, cerebral blood flow (CBF) measurements with ASL seem to yield similar results.[62,63] In contrast-enhancing brain tumors, CBV measured with T2*-weighted DSC perfusion MR imaging was found to significantly correlate with CBF measured with pseudocontinuous ASL (Pearson correlation coefficient $r = 0.70$).[64] Furthermore, tumor CBF measurements with T2*-weighted DSC perfusion MR imaging correlate with those obtained with ASL,[59,65] while CBV values calculated from ASL data were found to correlate with those obtained with T2*-weighted DSC perfusion MR imaging[66] (Fig. 9.14).

Tumor Diagnosis

The differential diagnosis of certain intra-axial brain neoplasms can be challenging, but may have important—presurgical—therapeutic implications. ASL studies of brain tumor diagnosis are still relatively scarce and overall retrospective in nature. An important finding reported by Noguchi et al.[67] is that ASL measurements correlated with the relative vascular density as well as cellular proliferation in a wide variety of brain neoplasms (Fig. 9.15).

In a retrospective study comparing 19 patients with primary central nervous system lymphoma (PCNSL) to 37 patients with glioblastoma multiforme, Yamashita et al.[68] demonstrated a significantly lower absolute and relative blood flow in PCNSL. The same research group also looked at the differentiation between hemangioblastoma and metastases in the brain and found that tumor blood flow in hemangioblastoma was more than double that of most metastases.[69] A renal cell carcinoma metastasis, however, was found to have even higher blood flow than hemangioblastoma. Both these studies support the notion that ASL measurements reflect histopathological tumour characteristics.

Tumor Grading

Primary brain tumors are not only classified but also graded to predict biologic behavior and to guide therapeutic management. The World Health Organization (WHO) grading system is the most widely used and is based on the tumor's cellularity, mitosis, necrosis, pleomorphism, and vascular proliferation. Vascular proliferation is the basis of the radiologic features of high-grade tumor, namely, enhancement after contrast administration and increased tumor perfusion. Diagnostic accuracy of tumor grading based on contrast enhancement is only moderate, which is significantly improved with perfusion imaging.[51] The relative CBV (rCBV) is the most widely used parameter obtained with DSC MR imaging for brain tumor grading. The rCBV increase shows a reliable correlation with tumor grade and increased tumor vascularity.[70] CBF measured with DSC MR imaging performs less well,[71] which may be attributed to both physiologic and methodologic issues. Physiologically, it has been suggested that CBF is not consistently and homogeneously increased in areas of vascular proliferation: arteriovenous shunting, occurring particularly at the tumor margins, leads to CBF increase, but CBF may also be decreased due to the tortuosity and reduced lumen of the newly formed blood vessels.[72] Methodologically, measurement of CBF requires an arterial input function, which can be difficult to determine with DSC perfusion MR imaging. Previous studies assessing CBF with DSC perfusion MR imaging may therefore have suffered from inaccurate CBF estimation.

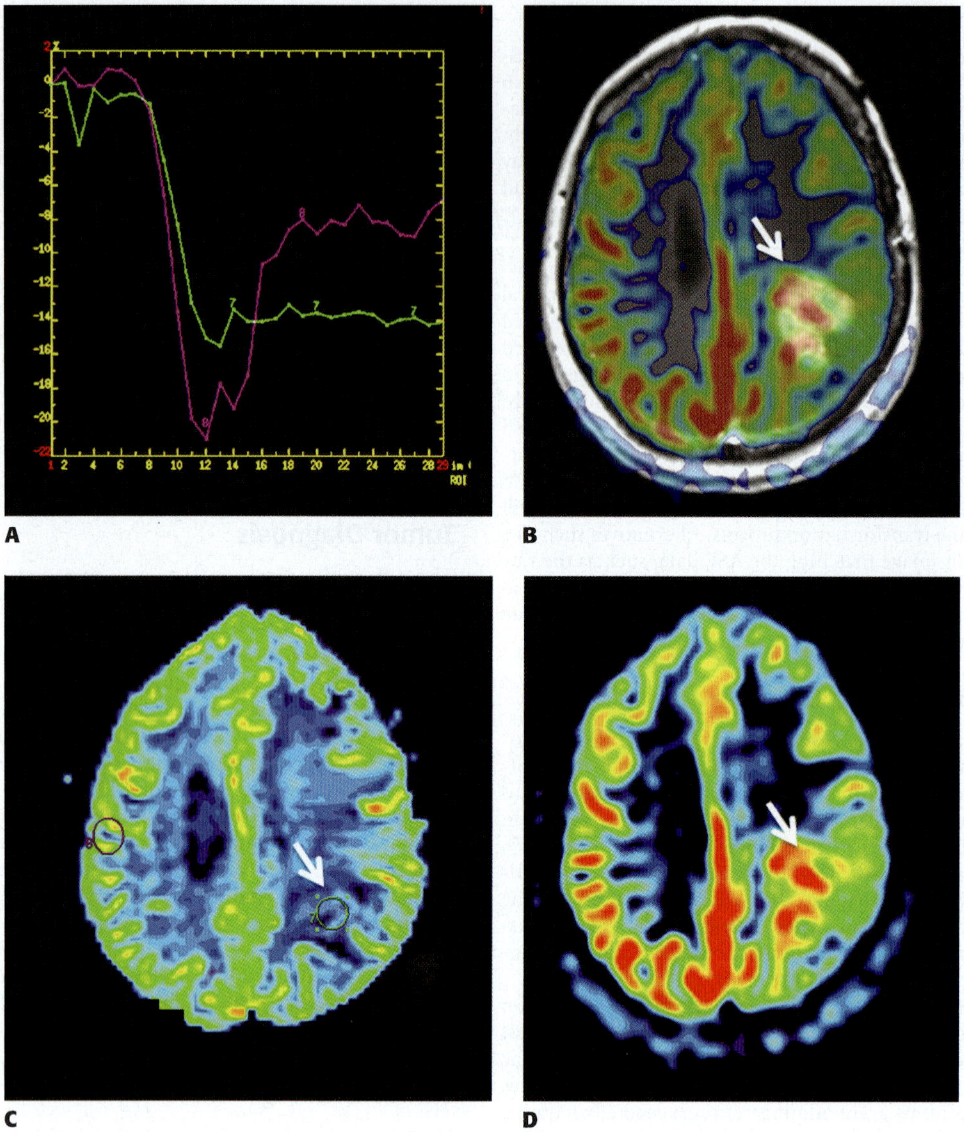

Figure 9-10. Enhancing tumor (*arrow*, **B**) with leakage of contrast resulting in an underestimation of the rCBV (**A**, *green curve*). DSC rCBV maps (*arrow*, **C**) fail to identify the high perfusion, visible on the ASL CBF maps (*arrow*, **D**). Images courtesy of Dr. Álvarez Linera, Ruber Hospital, Madrid (ES).

In studies assessing ASL for tumor grading, CBF measurements were found to distinguish high- (grades III and IV) from low (grades I and II)-grade tumors[48,59,64,73,74] and to correlate with CBV measurements assessed with DSC perfusion MR imaging.[64] Importantly, however, most studies used relative rather than absolute CBF values. Warmuth et al.[59] specifically reported that absolute tumor blood flow was less important for tumor grading than tumor blood flow relative to the mean brain perfusion. They suggest that as a "rule of thumb," mean tumor blood flow of low-grade gliomas is less than the mean CBF, while that of high-grade gliomas is greater than the mean CBF. As with DSC perfusion MR imaging, specificities for distinguishing tumor grades individually (e.g., grades III from IV) are not as high.[48]

Tumor Follow-up and Treatment Effects

Low-grade (WHO II) gliomas undergo malignant transformation, mandating a change in therapy. Timely detection of malignant transformation is thus essential. High-grade tumors as well as other intracranial neoplasms are followed up to assess treatment response and disease progression.

Malignant transformation of low- to high-grade tumors is characterized by the so-called angiogenic switch, indicating the transition of an avascular to a vascular tumor. It is this angiogenic switch that is assumed to underlie the progressive increase of maximum rCBV ratios in low-grade transforming to high-grade gliomas.[75] This finding has as yet not been reported with ASL.

One of the few studies on ASL for tumor follow-up assessed response to radiotherapy of brain metastases and demonstrated that an early change in tumor blood flow was highly predictive of treatment outcome.[76] In a case report of a patient treated with antiangiogenic treatment for recurrent glioblastoma, CBF measured with ASL indicated tumor progression well before the conventional MR imaging findings.[77]

In the follow-up of high-grade tumors, the effects of radiotherapy treatment may pose an important diagnostic challenge. Radiotherapy-induced necrosis and tumor progression cannot reliably be distinguished with conventional MR imaging, and DSC MR

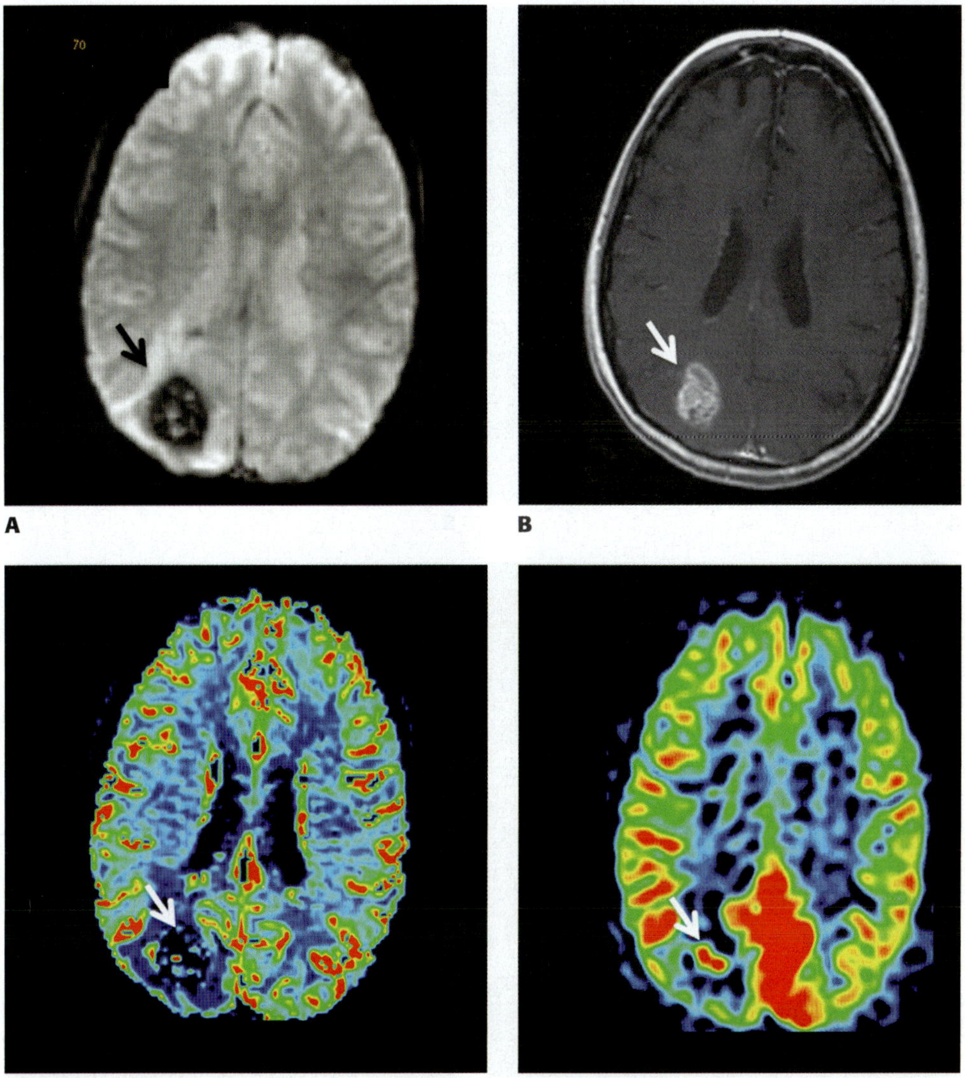

A B C D

Figure 9-11. Tumor hemorrhage as seen on the T2*-weighted image (**A**, *arrow*) and contrast-enhanced T1-weighted image (**B**, *arrow*). DSC fails to detect the area of hyperperfusion (**C**, *arrow*), which was identified with ASL (**D**, *arrow*) and confirmed as hypermetabolism on fluorodeoxyglucose positron emission tomography (not shown). Images courtesy of Dr. Álvarez Linera, Ruber Hospital, Madrid (ES).

imaging is then commonly used: necrosis is characterized by low rCBV ratios, while rCBV ratios are high in progressive tumor. In a pilot study comparing perfusion techniques, ASL was found to outperform DSC MR imaging to distinguish recurrent high-grade glioma from radiotherapy-induced necrosis with greater than 90% sensitivity.[78]

Limitations and Future Perspectives

Despite several reports indicating that ASL has similar or even better diagnostic performance compared with other MR imaging perfusion techniques, ASL has not yet made its way into the clinical routine of neuro-oncologic imaging. ASL suffers from several disadvantages compared with the widely used DSC perfusion MR imaging technique: it has much lower signal-to-noise ratio and takes longer to acquire. Also, blood flow is underestimated in regions with low blood flow and longer transit times. The advantages of ASL do not seem to sufficiently weigh against these disadvantages at present. There is, however, an increasing interest in perfusion parameters beyond CBV with the recent introduction of antiangiogenic treatment regimes. While DSC perfusion MR imaging may be used to estimate such parameters as well, quantification remains an issue, which is where ASL may find its place in neuro-oncologic imaging.

Neurodegenerative Disease

Cerebral perfusion imaging is of considerable interest for the evaluation of patients with suspected neurodegenerative disease, especially at the early stages of the underlying disease process. In several neurodegenerative diseases, changes in both brain metabolism and perfusion precede the eventually occurring structural brain changes such as atrophy, allowing for earlier and/or more accurate diagnosis of the underlying disease process.[79] Currently, the clinical assessment of such functional brain changes in the context of neurodegenerative disease is most commonly done with fluorodeoxy-D-glucose (FDG) PET. It is used as an additional diagnostic tool to diagnose dementia in the early stages and to differentiate underlying disease processes, in particular

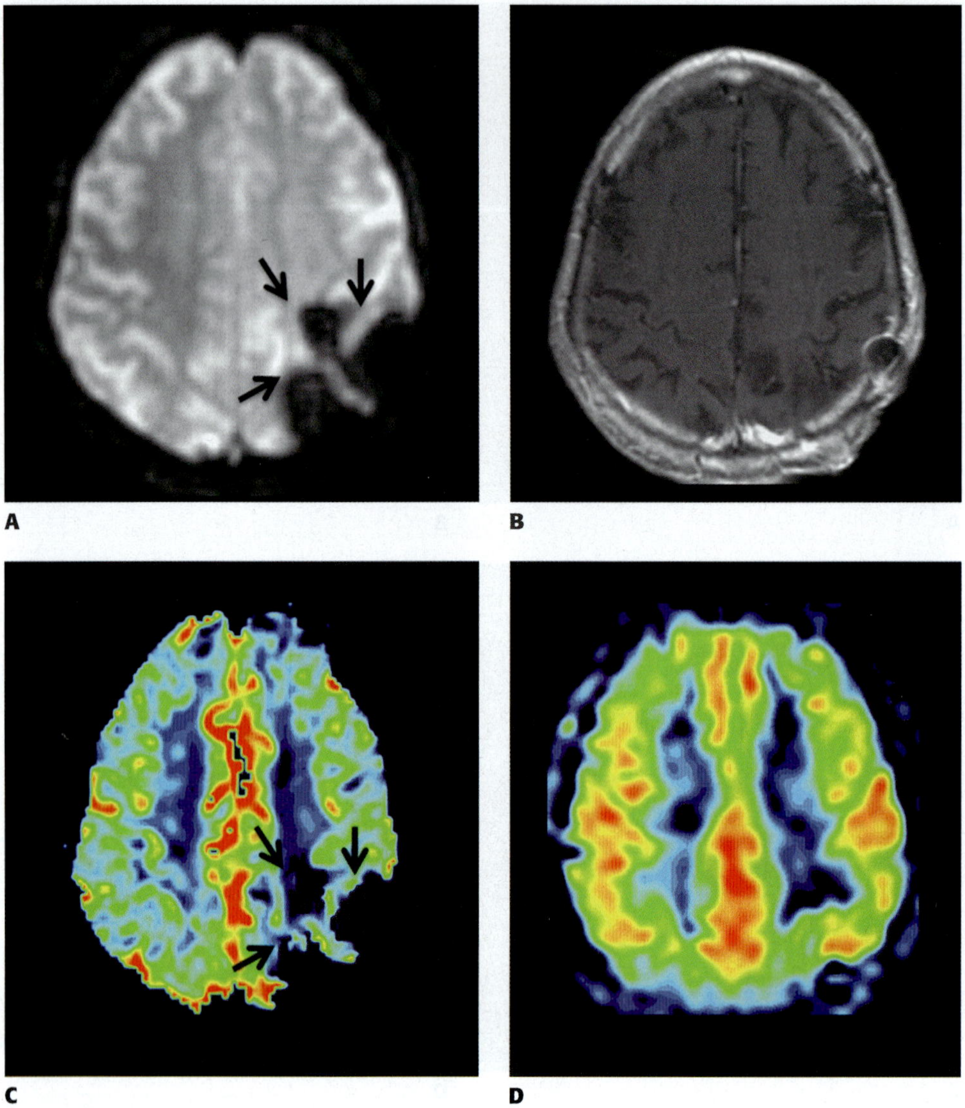

Figure 9-12. Susceptibility artifacts due to metallic surgical material, resulting in signal loss on the T2*-weighted DSC perfusion images (**A**, *arrows*) and rCBV maps (**C**, *arrows*). Artifacts are much less problematic on the T1-weighted contrast-enhanced **(B)** and ASL images **(D)**. Images courtesy of Dr. Álvarez Linera, Ruber Hospital, Madrid (ES).

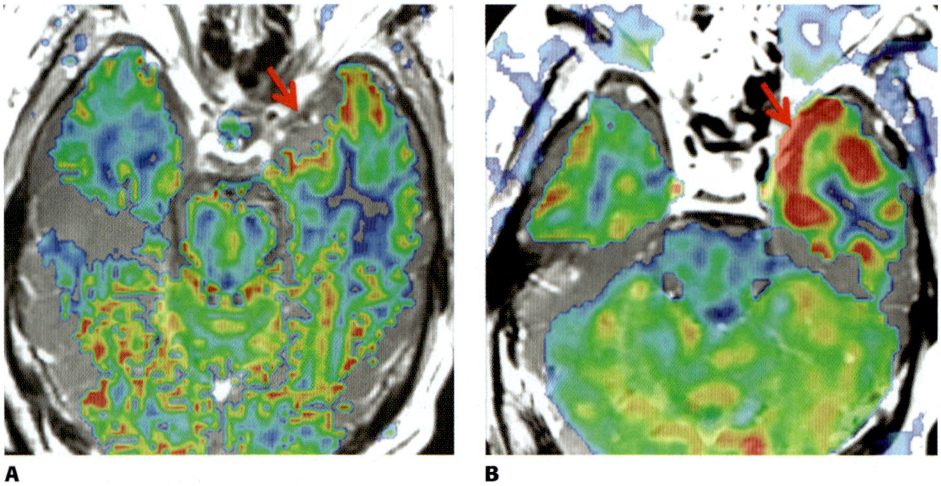

Figure 9-13. Susceptibility artifacts in the temporal pole render DSC perfusion (**A**, *arrow*) less sensitive than ASL perfusion (**B**, *arrow*) for perfusion assessment in this region. Images courtesy of Dr. Álvarez Linera, Ruber Hospital, Madrid (ES).

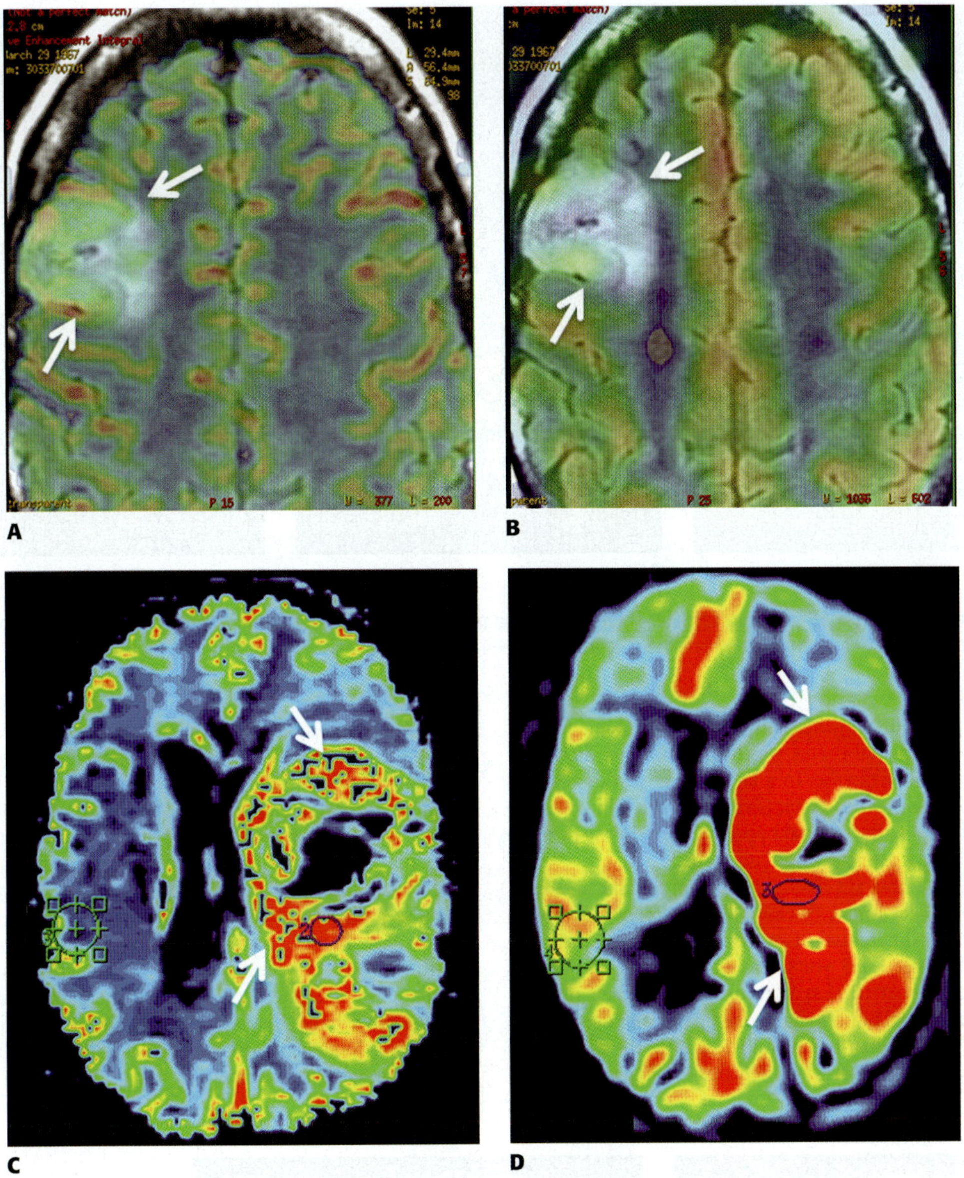

Figure 9-14. Comparison of DSC **(A, C)** and ASL **(B, D)** perfusion maps in low- **(A, B)** and high **(C, D)**-grade glioma. Both techniques indicate low perfusion in low-grade glioma (**A, B**, *arrows*) and high perfusion in high-grade glioma (**C, D**, *arrows*). Images courtesy of Dr. Álvarez Linera, Ruber Hospital, Madrid (ES).

Alzheimer disease and frontotemporal dementia. Unfortunately, due to the high cost and limited availability of FDG-PET,[80,81] functional brain imaging is not routinely used and is probably underused as a clinical diagnostic tool. ASL perfusion imaging has several advantages over FDG-PET imaging, being noninvasive and having higher temporal resolution, while it provides very similar information on functional brain changes.[82] Crucially, ASL can easily be added to the structural MRI examination that patients routinely undergo as part of their diagnostic workup. It requires only about 5 minutes additional scan time at low incremental cost[80,81] and burden to the patient. ASL provides reliable CBF measurement in both young and older subjects compared with the gold standard of $H_2{}^{15}O$ PET.[83–85] ASL also provides reliable CBF maps in neurodegenerative disease as shown in feasibility studies[86] (Fig. 9.16B).

In patients with established *Alzheimer disease*, ASL consistently showed decreased CBF in the precuneus and/or posterior cingulate cortex.[44,79,83,87–92] There are also frequent reports of decreased CBF in the lateral parietal cortices.[44,88,93] These findings of regional hypoperfusion are in concordance with those of regional hypometabolism established with FDG-PET (Fig. 9.16A). Patients with *mild cognitive impairment (MCI)*, commonly referred to as prodromal Alzheimer disease, are an important target population for disease-modifying therapy. Regions of hypoperfusion are generally those that are also found to be affected in established Alzheimer's disease, albeit to a lesser extent.[44,94,95] The most prominently affected regions are the posterior cingulate cortex, the precuneus and the inferior parietal lobe. Of note, however, is the fact that some studies additionally report regions of hyperperfusion in patients with MCI, such as in the hippocampus, amygdala and striatum.[94] Longitudinal studies following patients with MCI to conversion to Alzheimer's disease are scarce. In one study regional hypoperfusion was found to predict clinical, functional, and cognitive decline.[90] Baseline

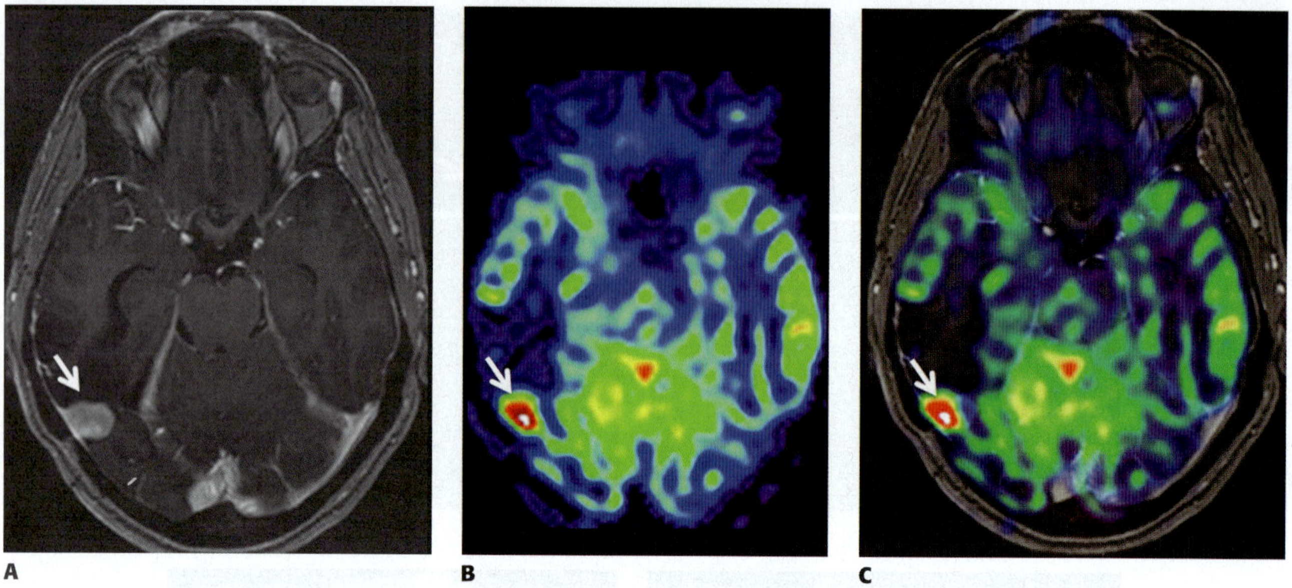

Figure 9-15. Meningioma in a 56 year old female. There is avid enhancement **(A)** of the lesion (*arrow*) with high CBF (*arrow*, **B, C**). Note the region of low perfusion anterior to the lesion, where there is posttherapeutic tissue damage.

hypoperfusion in the right precuneus, inferior parietal lobe, middle cingulum and middle frontal cortex was found to be predictive of conversion to Alzheimer's disease. In a large, cross-sectional study of both MCI and Alzheimer disease patients, a correlation with disease severity was found with regional hypoperfusion in the parietal cortex, precuneus, and posterior cingulate cortex.[95]

Much less is known as yet about the potential clinical use of ASL in other neurodegenerative diseases. *Frontotemporal dementia* is the most important differential diagnosis to Alzheimer disease in patients with early-onset (<65 years) dementia, as Alzheimer disease often presents with atypical symptoms in this patient population (Fig. 9.17). Functional brain imaging is of particular use in these patients, where diagnosis often remains unclear until the underlying disease has progressed to a stage when neuropsychological and neuroimaging findings have become distinctive. Studies of ASL in frontotemporal dementia however are still scarce. In a large study comparing 18 patients with established Alzheimer disease with 42 patients with frontotemporal dementia, hypoperfusion was found with ASL in areas similar to those that are found with FDG-PET imaging[96]: patients with Alzheimer disease had regional hypoperfusion in the precuneus and lateral parietal cortices, while patients with frontotemporal dementia had reduced CBF bilaterally in the frontal cortex and insula (Fig. 9.18). Contrasting patients with frontotemporal dementia to those with Alzheimer's disease, hyperperfusion was noted in the precuneus and posterior cingulate. Patients with Alzheimer's disease, on the other hand, displayed regional hyperperfusion in the anterior cingulate, dorsolateral prefrontal cortex and insula relative to patients with frontotemporal dementia.

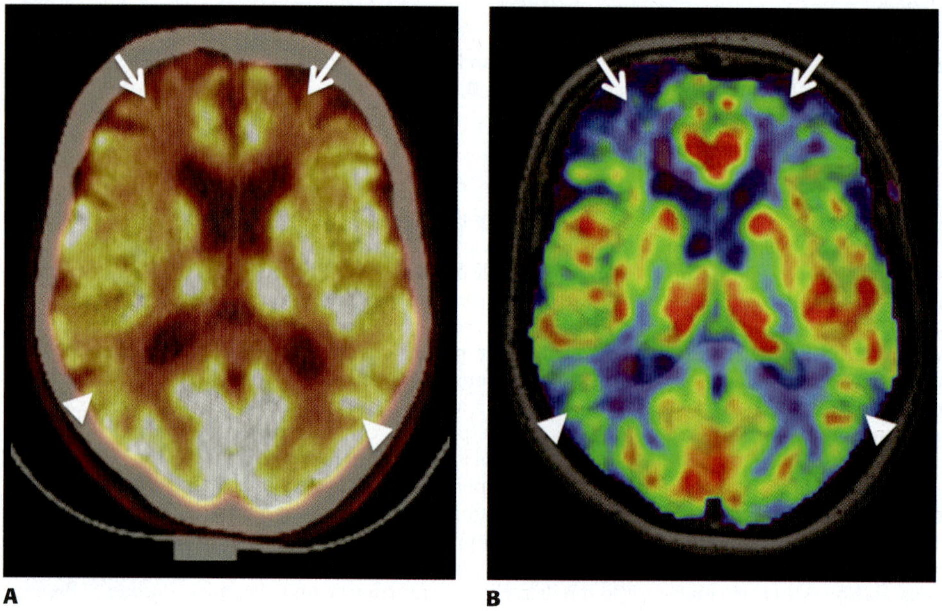

Figure 9-16. (A) FDG-PET and **(B)** ASL-CBF in the same patient show hypometabolism and hypoperfusion, respectively, in the frontal *(arrows)* and parietal *(arrowheads)* cortex bilaterally.

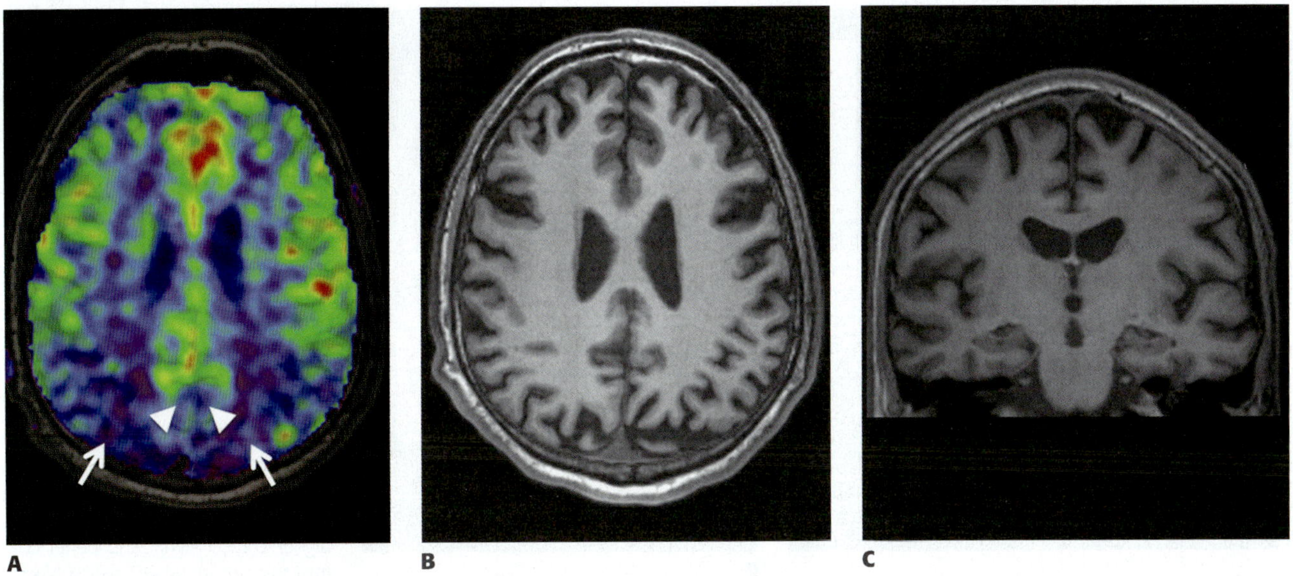

Figure 9-17. Sixty-four year old male with Alzheimer disease (AD). **(A)** Color-coded CBF map overlay on a structural T1-weighted MR image **(B)** shows pronounced regional hypoperfusion bilaterally in the parietal cortex (*arrows*) and posterior cingulate/precuneus (*arrowheads*), consistent with presenile AD. Structural imaging shows global cortical atrophy and only minimal hippocampal changes **(C)**.

The currently available literature thus provides substantial evidence towards the technical feasibility and potential advantages of using ASL for the detection and diagnosis of neurodegenerative disease. Published studies on potential use of ASL in neurodegenerative disease to date, however, are almost exclusively reporting findings at a group level, and the necessary step toward the individual patient level still needs to be made. In one study making this translation from group to individual patient level, neuroradiologists were trained to assess ASL exams qualitatively.[97] Four neuroradiologists were evaluated for their diagnostic distinction of 13 patients with Alzheimer disease from 19 healthy elderly controls. They reached an average accuracy of 70% with an interrater agreement (κ) of 0.7, which was higher than when they used the T1w structural scans to make this same distinction ($\kappa = 0.17$, accuracy = 63%).

While ASL is potentially very useful in the diagnostic workup of patients suspected of neurodegenerative disease, it has to be kept in mind that in the elderly population, ASL comes with several challenges.[98] With aging, transit times from the labeling plane to the brain tissue are prolonged due to tortuosity of the feeding brain vessels. This necessitates the use of longer labeling delay times, which results in lower perfusion contrast due to increased recovery of the ASL signal after the labeling pulse. Additionally, CBF values

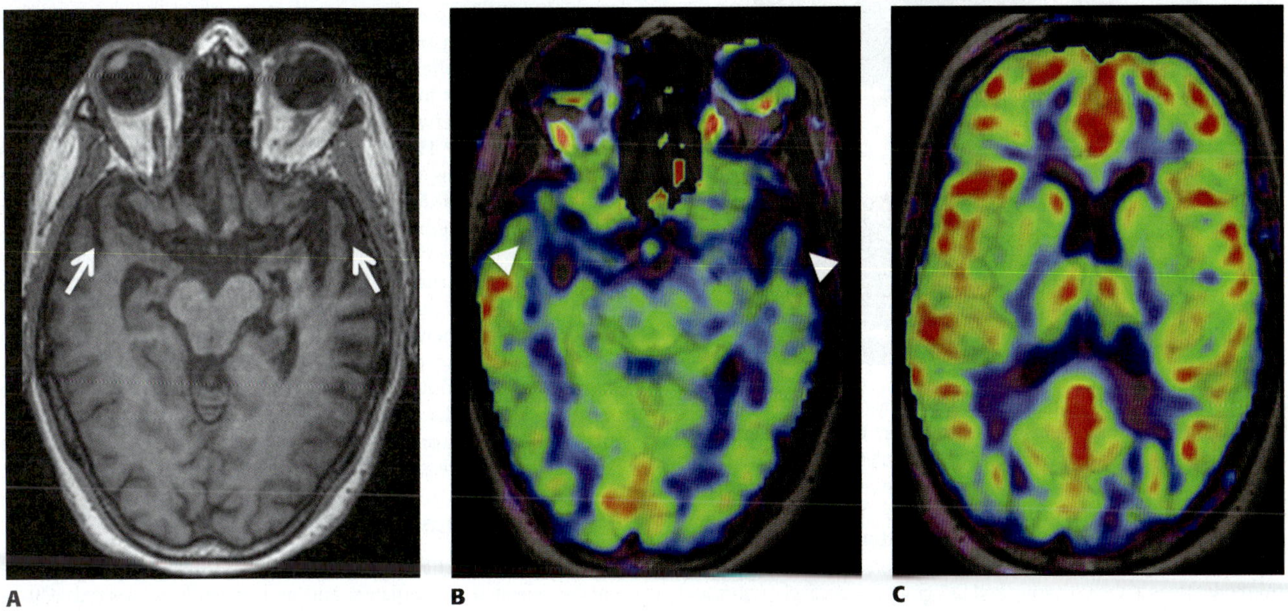

Figure 9-18. Sixty-five year old female with semantic dementia (a type of frontotemporal dementia). **(A)** Structural T1-weighted imaging shows pronounced, left more than right, temporal lobe atrophy (*arrows*). The CBF map overlay on the structural image **(B)** shows marked hypoperfusion of the temporal lobe. **(C)** Note for comparison the normal cortical perfusion in the frontal and parietal lobes.

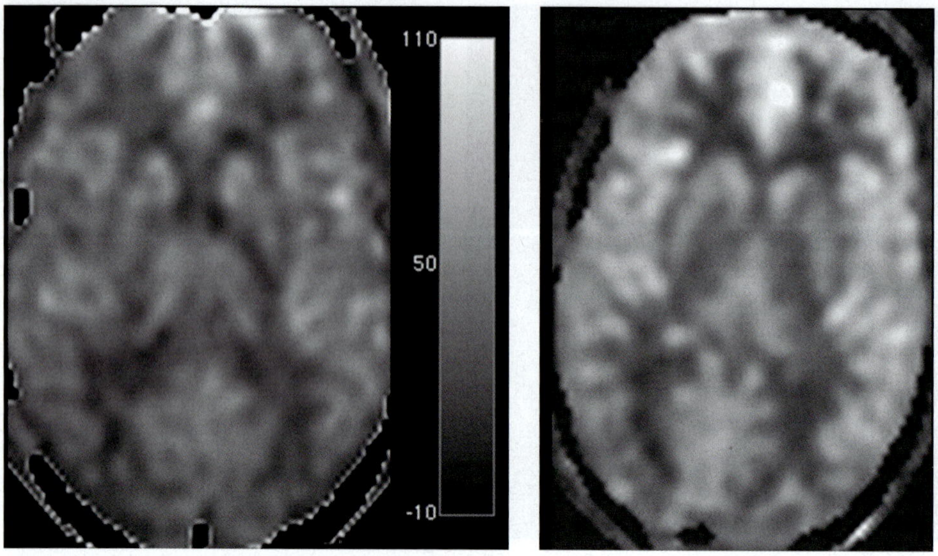

A B

Figure 9-19. ASL-CBF maps of a 64-year-old (A) and 24-year-old (B) male healthy volunteer. Note that at the same level of scaling, there is higher cortical signal and better contrast to noise in the younger subject.

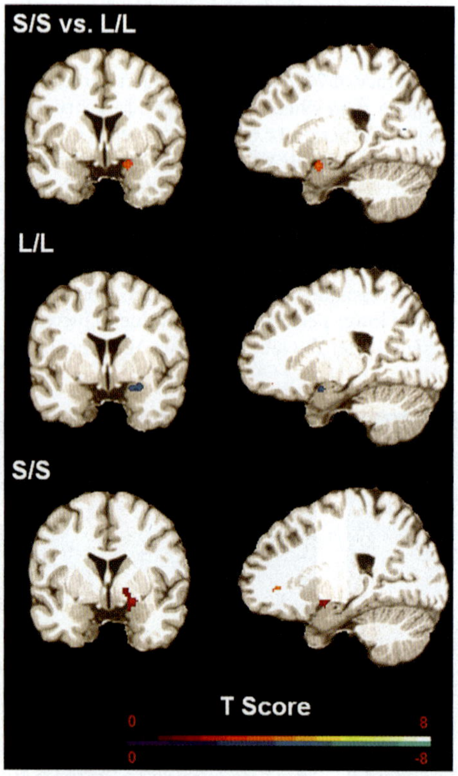

Figure 9-20. Relationships between amygdala CBF and Beck Depression Inventory scores differ between two different genetic depression risk profiles. S/S and L/L = serotonin transporter promotor short (confers depression risk) and long allele, respectively. **Top row:** interactions between the S/S and L/L groups (threshold set as small volume corrected $p < 0.05$). **Middle and bottom row:** amygdala CBF, respectively, negatively and positively correlated with Beck Depression Inventory scores in the L/L group and S/S group, respectively, (thresholds set as small volume corrected $p < 0.05$ and uncorrected $p < 0.05$, respectively). Reprinted with permission from Gillihan SJ, Rao H, Brennan L, et al. Serotonin transporter genotype modulates the association between depressive symptoms and amygdala activity among psychiatrically healthy adults. *Psychiatry Res* 2011;193(3):161–167.

are lower in the elderly, and thus, less labeled blood will be available to generate the perfusion contrast, resulting in lower SNR ASL images in this patient population (Fig. 9.19).

Psychiatric Disease

The use of ASL in clinical psychiatric studies is relatively new and steadily increasing.[99] In the field of psychiatry, perfusion imaging enables to gain knowledge of the neurobiologic and anatomical correlates of clinical psychiatry *in vivo*, which is important because its pathophysiology is unknown to a large extent.[99,100] Although some psychiatric diseases may have a vascular origin,[101] regional CBF changes measured by perfusion MRI are generally regarded to reflect changes in neuronal activity and energy demand secondary to psychiatric disease or its therapy.[102,103]

Baseline CBF Examples

Several studies have employed ASL to investigate baseline regional CBF differences in patients as compared to healthy control subjects. In patients suffering from major depressive disorders, ASL has shown that CBF is lower in the total GM and in affective, executive, and motor networks, which was correlated with the severity of depression.[104,105] Hyperperfusion, on the other hand, has been observed in regions that are considered a key component in the pathophysiology of depression, such as the subgenual anterior cingulate cortex.[106] Figure 9.20 shows a nice example where ASL was able to show subtle differences between healthy subjects with and without a genetic risk profile for depression.[107] This figure shows the correlation between amygdala CBF and a neuropsychological depression assessment score. In subjects with a genetic depression risk profile, this correlation was positive, whereas this correlation was negative in subjects without this risk profile. In borderline personality disorder, brain regions that mediate impulsivity—such as the orbitofrontal cortex—have been shown to exhibit both decreased and increased CBF as compared to controls.[108]

Challenge/Symptoms

Considering that CBF measurements with ASL are noninvasive and can be repeated immediately and as frequently as desired, ASL is highly suitable for the investigation of regional CBF changes induced by a task or pharmaceutical challenge. This is of particular interest to neurobiologically charter the psychiatric brain, since it allows to study specific psychiatric symptoms or pharmaceutical effects in isolation. In both depression and schizophrenia, regional CBF changes have

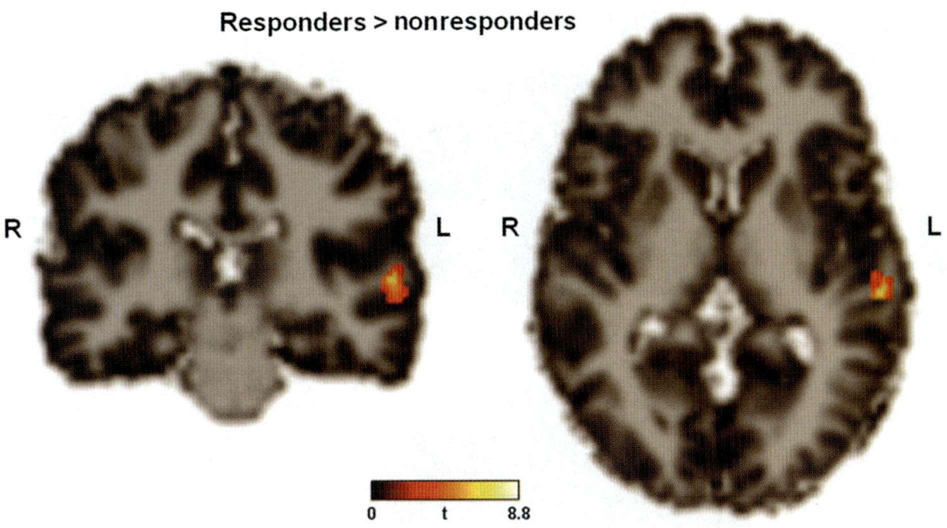

Figure 9-21. CBF reduction following heroin administration in heroin-dependent subjects. Relative hypo- (*blue*) and hyperperfusion (*red*) in heroin condition as compared to placebo condition is projected on an inflated standard brain (threshold $p < 0.05$). Hyperperfusion was not significant. (Reprinted with permission from Denier N, Schmidt A, Gerber H, et al. Association of frontal gray matter volume and cerebral perfusion in heroin addiction: a multimodal neuroimaging study. *Front Psychiatry* 2013;4:135.)

been identified as neural correlates of disturbed motor control as measured by wrist actigraphy.[109,110] In patients with schizophrenia, motor activity was correlated with CBF changes in frontal voluntary motion regions, whereas in controls, it was correlated with CBF changes in the basal ganglia motor circuit. This led the authors to the conclusion that basal ganglia motor control might be impaired in schizophrenia, with compensation from frontal regions that coordinate volitional motor behavior.[109] In elderly with an anxiety disorder, ASL demonstrated the absence of CBF changes in the prefrontal cortex during the suppression of worries, supporting the hypothesis that these emotion-regulating regions are less effective in these subjects.[111] The combination of ASL and clinical psychiatry with genetics may provide evidence for a genetic predisposition of mood disorders, as was shown by one study that reported a correlation between amygdala perfusion and task-induced symptoms of anxiety or sadness, which differed between carriers of different serotonin transporter alleles.[112] This result alludes to a future potential of ASL to aid in predicting the risk for development of psychiatric diseases in subjects that are genetically at risk for the development of these diseases.

Therapy

The abovementioned properties of ASL are not only attractive for the application of a task but also enable the study of short- or long-term metabolic changes induced by psychopharmacologic therapy in patients or healthy volunteers. This may aid in unraveling the location of therapeutic action and to monitor or even predict therapeutic efficacy. One example is the application of transcranial magnetic stimulation (TMS) in patients with schizophrenia. This 10-day therapy has shown to result in a CBF decrease in the areas of application, which correlated with the decrease of verbal auditory hallucinations.[113,114] Moreover, patients with elevated CBF in the left superior temporal gyrus were more likely to respond to 10 days of TMS as compared to patients with normal CBF values in this region (Fig. 9.21).[115] The possibility of individualized prediction of treatment effects is important for therapeutic decision making in psychiatry since it may take weeks or even months before the clinical effects of therapy become apparent.[116]

The application of a pharmaceutical challenge in healthy volunteers facilitates to isolate CBF changes induced by pharmaceuticals from preexisting CBF changes in patients. One example is the study of differences between first- and second-generation antipsychotics. In healthy volunteers, both drugs had overlapping effects on CBF in regions that are suspected to be involved in schizophrenia.[102] In some of these regions, effects were similar for both drugs, whereas in other regions, the effects were dissimilar or even opposed, providing an in vivo neurobiologic substrate for differences in clinical effects and side effects between different antipsychotics.[102] Also in attention deficit hyperactivity disorder, a similar conclusion could be drawn for the drugs methylphenidate and atomoxetine. In comparison to placebo, both drugs shared a common effect on CBF in several cortical and subcortical regions, whereas four regions remained where both drugs had had a different—or even opposed—effect on CBF.[117]

Recreational Drugs

The study of CBF changes induced by recreational drugs may not only serve to gain a better understanding on the neurobiology of psychiatric dependency and the pathophysiology of craving but also is important since recreational drugs can be potent confounders of CBF.[118] Since drug dependency is a comorbidity frequently observed in psychiatric patients, knowledge on CBF changes caused by these drugs is essential.[119] In heroin-dependent patients, heroin administration induces a CBF decrease in several frontal regions of the brain (Fig. 9.22), which is correlated with low GM volume.[120] In chronic cigarette smokers, a 12–14-hour abstinence increases CBF in several visuospatial and reward brain regions, suggesting that increased activation of these regions underlie abstinence-induced smoking craving.[121] Chronic cannabis users have lower CBF in several brain regions as compared to healthy controls, which is reversible after 4 weeks of abstinence.[122] Alcohol induces a CBF increase in frontal brain regions, which is lower in people with an increased risk of alcohol dependency, higher in men as compared to women, and can be partly compared with the effects of morphine.[123–125]

Limitations and Promising Development

Despite the many potential applications of ASL perfusion MRI in psychiatric disease, one main challenge remains. Perfusion changes due to psychiatry are often subtle and focal. These subtle changes can easily be covered by the large between-session physiologic variation of CBF on a single subject level—requiring a large sample size in order to reach statistical significance.[126] In addition, ASL inherently suffers from poor SNR, requiring low spatial and/or temporal resolution.[32] This combination of large physiologic variation and low SNR does currently not allow single-subject applications of ASL in psychiatry. For example, it may explain how two studies with similar methods—oral 20-mg citalopram challenge in young adult healthy females—can report dissimilar regional CBF changes.[82,127] Fortunately, ASL labeling and readout techniques are advancing rapidly, allowing for increasing spatial and temporal resolution. In the field of image analysis, investigators are developing analysis methods that decrease the sensitivity for physiologic variation, such as machine learning for the automatic classification of patients versus controls or therapy responders versus

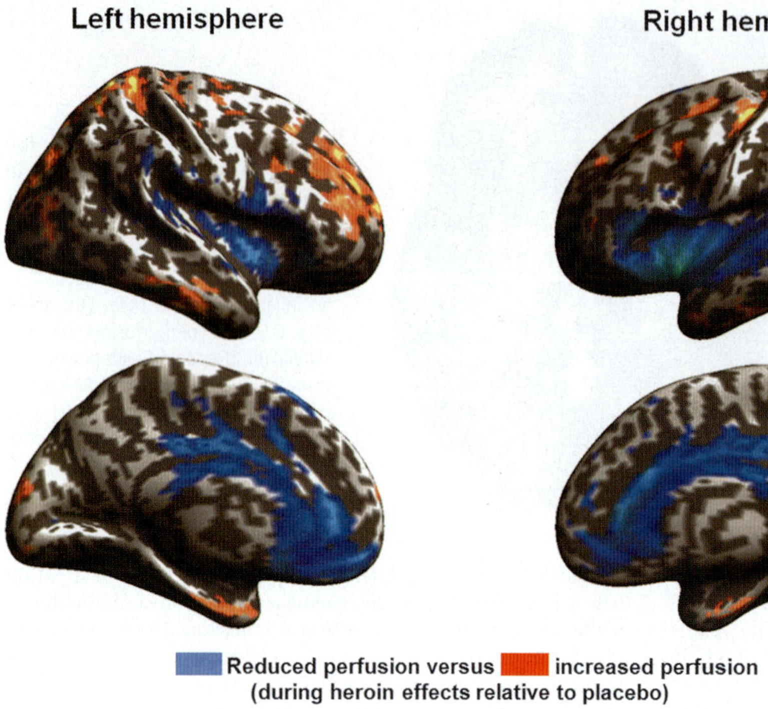

Figure 9-22. **CBF predicts responders to TMS in patients with auditory verbal hallucinations.** Shown here are the voxels that were significantly highly perfused in responders than in nonresponders prior to treatment. A single cluster of 120 voxels survived a cluster-level whole brain correction for family-wise errors in the left superior temporal gyrus (Brodmann area 22). No clusters survived in the inverse contrast (nonresponders > responders). (Reprinted with permission from Homan P, Kindler J, Federspiel A, et al. Muting the voice: a case of arterial spin labeling-monitored transcranial direct current stimulation treatment of auditory verbal hallucinations. *Am J Psychiatry* 2011;168(8):853–854.)

nonresponders.[128] The combination of the above may eventually enable the clinical use of ASL on a single-subject basis. Considering its results so far, ASL seems promising as a future tool to aid in the prediction of psychiatric disease and therapy response.

Neurovascular Disease

ASL has been used to assess cerebral perfusion in acute stroke[129,130] as well as in chronic cerebrovascular disease[131] and can be combined with an acetazolamide challenge to assess the cerebrovascular reserve (CVR).[132,133]

ASL has also been used to assess the cerebral perfusion in children.[134] In both acute and chronic conditions, neurologic symptoms not only may be related to structural brain damage but can also be caused by blood flow disturbances in brain regions that appear structurally intact on traditional MRI.[135]

Technical Aspects

The clinical usefulness of absolute perfusion measurements has been shown in a number of studies.[136–138]

One of the limitations for quantification of CBF is the random noise related to a low SNR. Higher magnetic field strength improves the SNR, and pCASL with multiple PLDs also improves the assessment of CBF in the human brain.[139] One of the main problems of ASL in studying acute or chronic cerebral and cardiovascular conditions are related to transit delay and visualization of collateral flow due to the rapid T1 decay of the label.[140,141] In the presence of delayed arterial transit, CBF quantification may be hampered but a qualitative interpretation of perfusion deficits is still possible.

In an attempt to reduce transit time sensitivity, an inversion time (IT, in pASL) or a postlabeling delay (PLD, in CASL and pCSL) approach was introduced.[142,143]

IT or PLD defines the time duration for spins to move from the labeling plane or volume to the imaged slices and is typically between 1,500 and 2,000 milliseconds. The diagnosis of ischemia on ASL is often based on reduced flow via proximal routes: blood flow via collateral routes is more difficult to detect as it takes longer, leading to increased delays between the labeling of the spins and their arrival in the imaged voxel. Choosing the appropriate labeling time for ASL is therefore critical and is often a trade-off between time and SNR, as longer delays between the labeling and the imaging result in lower SNR due to T1 signal decay of the labeled spins.[144]

Often, when the AATs are the same or longer than the PLD, labeled spins will be visualized in the arteries feeding the ischemic tissue, a finding that has been defined arterial transit artifact (ATA).[132] If a vascular suppression method is applied, the spins moving above a certain velocity (presumably vascular) are not visible on the ASL images.[145] ATA is problematic for the quantification, but can be a marker of pathology: low ASL signal, with surrounding cortical areas of high signal intensity (ATA) in the middle cerebral artery (MCA)–anterior cerebral artery (ACA) border zone, and MCA–posterior cerebral artery (PCA) border zone has been called "*border zone sign*" *and was* more sensitive than was bolus perfusion-weighted imaging (PWI) for identifying subtle perfusion anomalies.[146] ATA may represent collateral flow.[147]

Another approach is to obtain images at multiple PLDs, effectively mapping and quantifying arrival times into the tissue.[43,148,149] The approach is limited by low SNR, persistent inaccuracies in regions with severely delayed flow, and challenges with nonlinear fitting of CBF to the kinetic models.[37]

Moving to a higher field strength makes a longer delay time (as 6 seconds) more feasible because the increased T1 allows the label to persist for longer delays and improves the ability to visualize collateral blood flow.[150,151]

High and ultrahigh field ASL benefits from both an increased SNR owing to the increased spin polarity and the prolongation of the T1 of the arterial blood.[152,153]

Higher SNR and prolonged T1 will increase signal difference between label and control images, allowing more accurate CBF measurements in zones of relatively low perfusion such as the WM and arterial border zones. Furthermore, the increased SNR improves the spatial resolution, thereby reducing partial volume effects.[154]

A longer arterial T1 also increases the labeling time window, allowing better CBF detection in tissues with a long transit time such as the deep WM.[155]

Newer ASL techniques such as velocity-selective ASL (VS-ASL)[156] or flow encoding arterial spin tagging,[145] could have an advantage in cerebrovascular disease and pathologies with slow or collateral flow conditions, but their efficiency has yet to be proven.

Further implementations of ASL enable to study the normal individual variability of vascular territories and might be useful in a number of cerebrovascular conditions[157] and for the evaluation of hemodynamic effects of surgery (i.e., bypass[158] and TEA[159]).

Three different approaches have been proposed for determining the cerebral perfusion territories of individual arteries: (a) using a dedicated labeling RF coil, (b) applying selective inversion of spatially confined areas, and (c) employing multidimensional RF pulses. Methods that apply a dedicated labeling RF coil have high SNR, low RF power deposition, and unrestricted 3D coverage because of the absence of MT effects, but are mostly limited to separation of the left and right circulation, and require extra hardware, which may limit their implementation on clinical systems. Alternatively, methods that apply selective inversion of spatially confined areas have more flexibility and a higher arterial selectivity, but may suffer from excessive RF power deposition, from imprecision in delineating vascular territories, and from the presence of imaging artifacts resulting from interference between the labeling slab and the volume of interest. Two-dimensional RF labeling pulses achieve high flexibility and selectivity, but have some disadvantages such as contamination of the perfusion signal leading to poor definition of the vascular territories. Further future improvements will be important for optimizing these methods.[160]

Acute Ischemia/Stroke

One of the advantages of ASL compared to DSC is that it provides noninvasive, quantitative, and repeatable measurements of CBF with relative insensitivity to permeability. ASL, like DSC, can assess perfusion abnormalities in acute ischemic stroke,[161] and typical finding on ASL stroke studies is hypoperfusion in the regions with high DWI signal (Fig. 9.23, stroke), sometimes associated with an ATA in the periphery, which may reflect collateral flow.[129] ASL has shown good agreement with DSC in depicting large perfusion deficits.[162] It is however still subject of an on-going debate whether ASL can accurately depict the area of perfusion abnormality and identify the penumbra in acute stroke as well as DSC, because ASL tends to overestimate the perfusion deficit and penumbra, especially in patients with small infarct size.[163] Prior studies showed that ATA in patients with acute ischemic stroke correlated with improved outcomes,[164] possibly reflecting the presence of collateral flow. ATA was often present surrounding the ischemic core and tended to be associated with lack of progression to infarct and better clinical outcome.[165]

Finally, there are relatively few perfusion studies in TIA patients. A very recent study revealed that ASL performed within 24 hours of TIA onset can demonstrate perfusion abnormalities that correlate well with the clinically diagnosed TIA in patients with otherwise normal MRI studies, including diffusion-weighted imaging.[166] Earlier studies described an asymmetry index in AAT between hemispheres, which was significantly increased in the affected hemisphere of minor

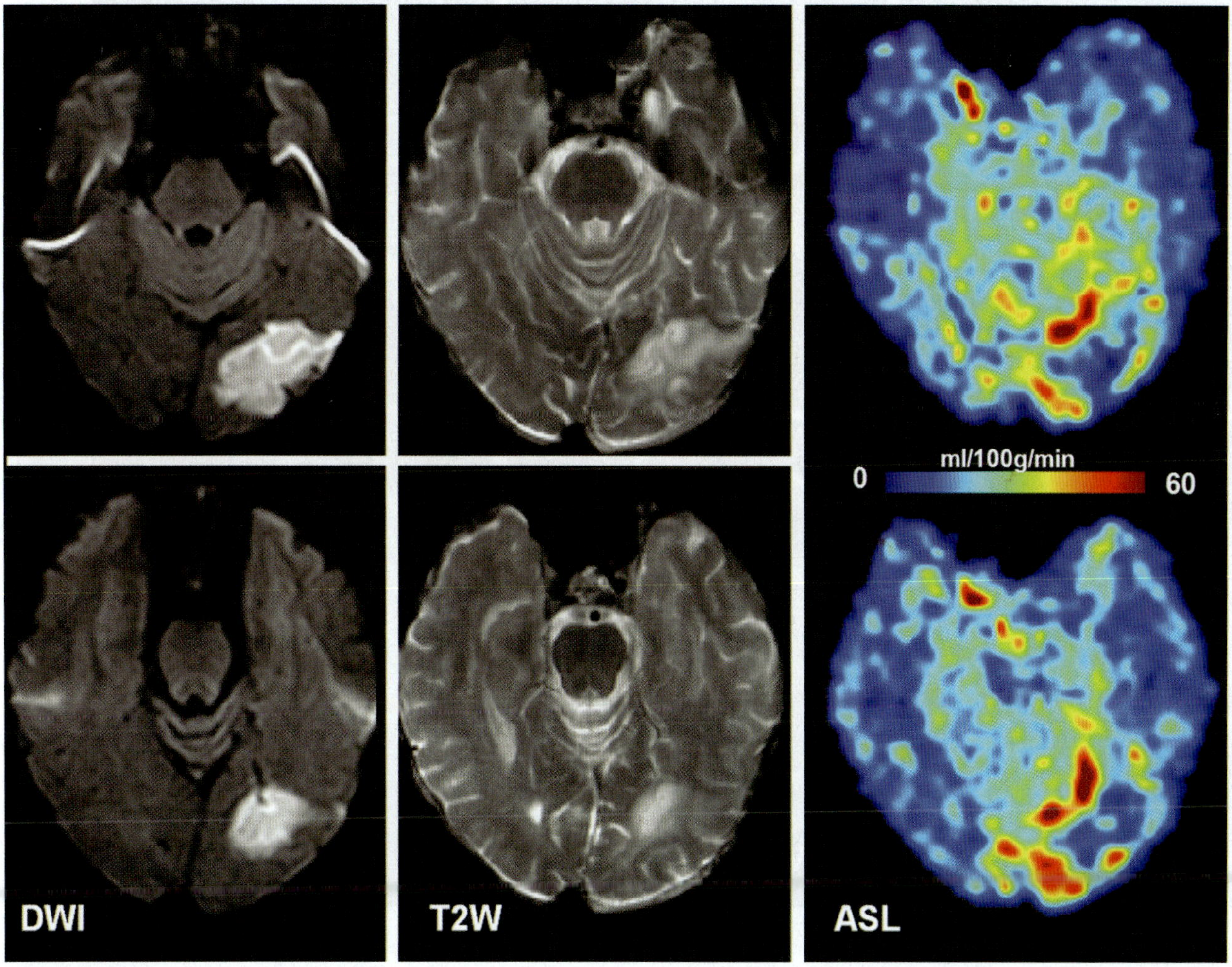

Figure 9-23. Stroke. Bright DWI and T2 lesion, in keeping with acute ischemic lesion, is seen at the left inferior occipital area. The perfusion is reduced within the lesion, but there is ATA at the periphery of the lesion, which is likely to represent collateral flow.

stroke patients[167]). In TIA patients, perfusion-related alterations on ASL (commonly, the bilateral border zone sign and/or ATA) are more frequently detected compared with PWI or intracranial MRA and are most frequently associated with the symptomatic hemisphere.[168] Almost all cases with a PWI lesion also had an ASL lesion, which exceeds the published yield of bolus PWI in this population (16%).[169]

When using ASL in acute stroke and TIA, one has to be aware of the limitations of this method as mentioned earlier on, one of the most important being a delayed transit times, which may overestimate the region of CBF abnormality in severe cases.

Other issues with ASL include the advanced age of most patients with acute stroke and the reduction of CBF associated with age: so, it has been suggested that AATs are longer in elderly patients.[170] Finally, artifacts, which are frequently due to magnetic susceptibility inhomogeneities, can also mimic an ischemic lesion.

Reduced Cerebrovascular Reserve: Chronic Cerebrovascular Disease and Brain Hypoperfusion Syndrome

Assessment of the CVR plays an important role in chronic cerebrovascular disease and brain hypoperfusion syndrome. Cerebral Venous Thrombosis (CVR) describes how far cerebral perfusion can increase from a baseline value after stimulation (often CO_2 inhalation or acetazolamide injection). Alternative stimuli are breath holding or cerebral activation by hand gripping. ASL is ideally suited for assessment of the CVT since it is quantitative and can be repeated easily. ASL has been used in conjunction with acetazolamide administration, to indentify the tissue most at risk for possible stroke.[171]

The indication for carotid artery surgery according the North American Symptomatic Carotid Endarterectomy Trial (NASCET) and European Carotid Surgery Trial (ECST) investigations takes into account only the degree of the stenosis and not the CVR. According to recent studies, the risk of cerebral infarction in these patients is considerably higher with reduced CVR.[172] Therefore, CVR can be used as an additional parameter if the indication for surgery is unclear (i.e., in asymptomatic carotid artery stenosis) and for identifying patients who might benefit from an extra- and intracranial bypass operation and high-risk patients with cerebral microangiopathy. ASL can also be used to assess treatment effects.[173]

White matter lesions (WMLs) are considered one of the hallmarks of small vessel disease but are not specific to vascular neuropathology: they could also reflect inflammatory process and gliosis and overlap other neurodegenerative processes.[98,174–176] Dysfunction of BBB is an early finding in WML of microvascular disease,[177] and it can cause vascular inflammation and demyelination.[178] At present, it is not clear whether the pattern and quantification of perfusion changes with ASL can distinguish between different types of WMLs (Fig. 9.24).

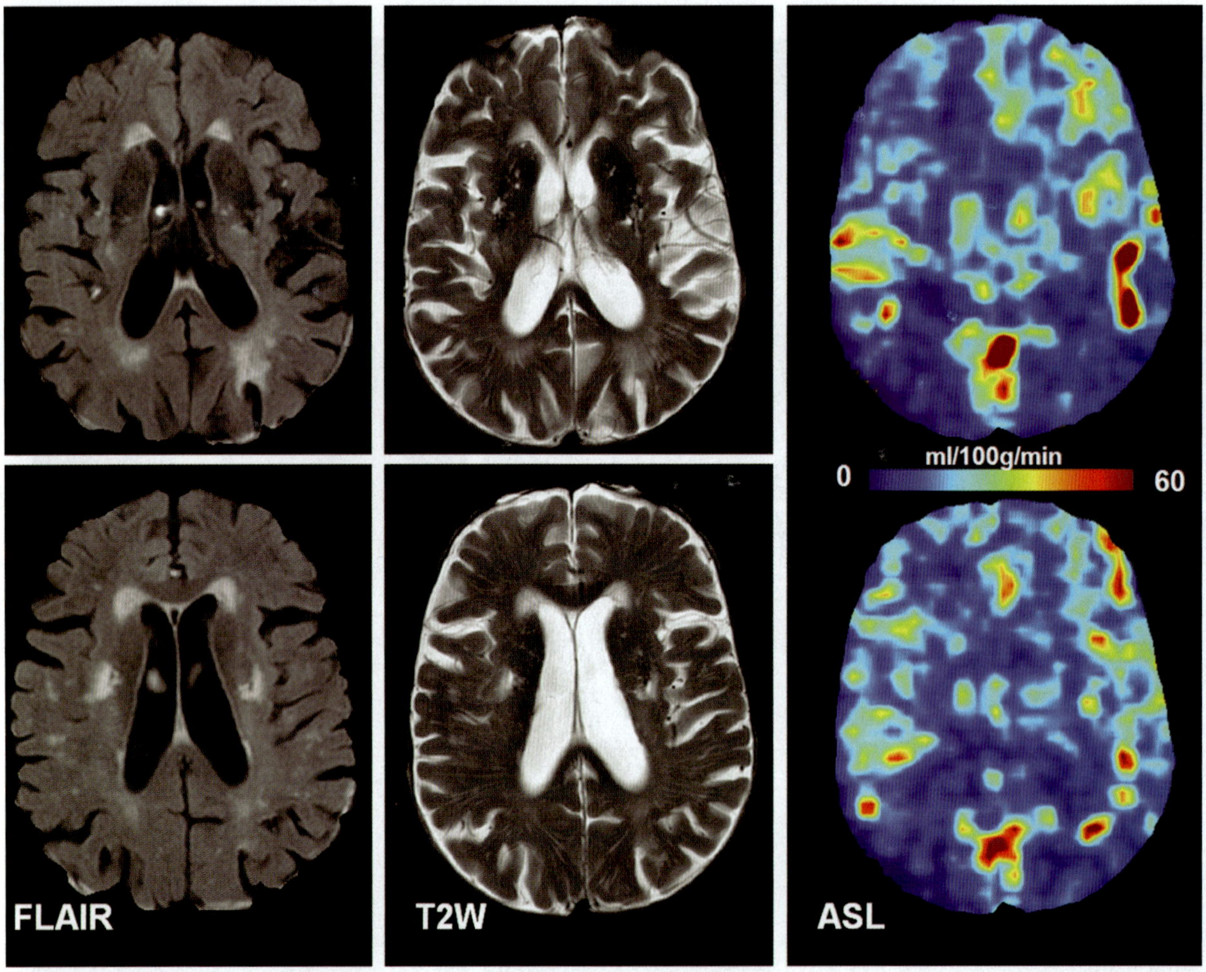

Figure 9-24. White matter disease. WM bright lesions are seen in both FLAIR and T2-weighted image **(first and second column)**, consistent with small vessel disease. CBF map **(third column)** shows low perfusion at border zone between MCA and PCA bilaterally and MCA and ACA on the right (border zone sign).

There is, however, evidence that cerebral perfusion disturbances correlate with the extent of WM disease. A study using ASL demonstrated that patients with diffuse confluent white matter hyperintensities had about 20% lower CBF measurements than patients with punctiform or beginning confluent white matter hyperintensities. A more marked reduction of CBF was found not only in the subcortical WM but also in the deep and cortical gray matter, indicating a more generalized cerebrovascular disease process.[179] A challenge in applying ASL is the relatively low sensitivity of ASL in WM, which has lower CBF and longer arterial transit time than GM, but methodologic advances (higher field strength, labeling strategies as pCASL) and optimization of sequences (high resolution and sufficient PLD)[155] improved the sensitivity of ASL and provided reproducible measures of CBF.[98]

Arteriovenous Malformation

Blood moving through an arteriovenous malformation (AVM) has an abnormally fast transit time compared to the rest of the brain, and in the region of the AVM, labeled blood no longer functions as a diffusible tracer but as an intravascular tracer. This transit time effect in AVMs has been used to generate MR angiograms, and new ASL methods with spatially nonselective labeling have been introduced, based on the acceleration of flowing spins, which are able to image brain perfusion with minimal contamination from venous signal.[180,181] ASL difference images show AVMs and draining vessels as hyperintense structures with an angiographic appearance due to high flow, while the rest of the brain may be hypoperfused due to steal phenomenon (Fig. 9.25). ASL can be used to detect AVMs, quantify the arteriovenous shunting, and evaluate CBF alteration of the adjacent and distant regions.[182,183]

Inflammation

Multiple sclerosis (MS) is by far the most frequent chronic demyelinating disease thought to be due to immune-mediated inflammation.[184] In addition to demyelination, axonal loss has emerged as a prominent neuropathologic feature, especially in chronic lesions.[185] Neurodegeneration could cause decrease in cerebral perfusion[186] and in metabolic activity. Previous studies with PET or SPECT have revealed areas of decreased perfusion in GM and WM.[187] The main findings in ASL were a reduction of perfusion in GM structure, especially deep GM thalami, compared to the healthy volunteers and an inverse correlation of cortical perfusion with the WML volume in MS, suggesting that the amount of WMLs indicates a reduced metabolic demand and

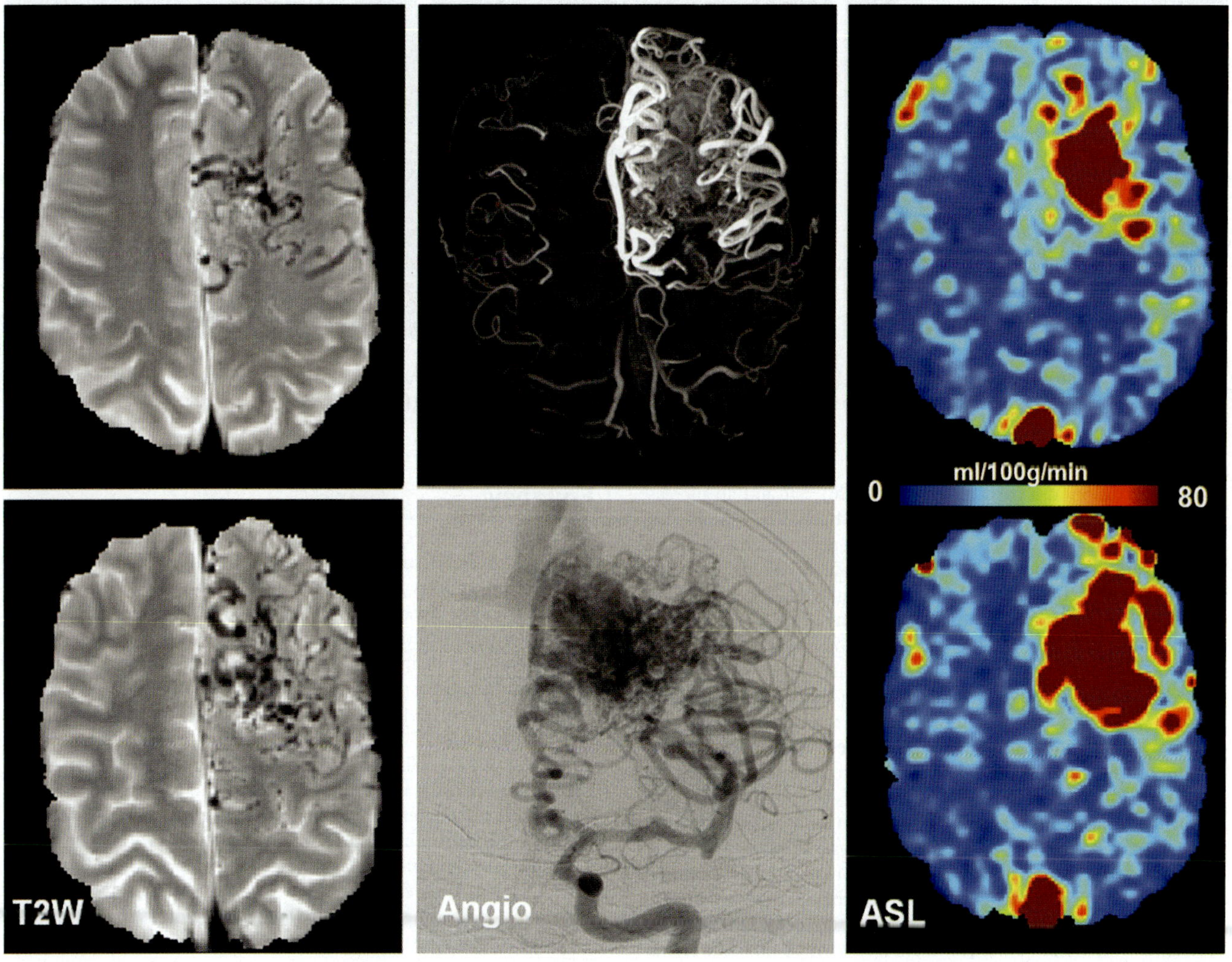

Figure 9-25. Arteriovenous malformation (AVM). T1 **(first column)**, angio (MR and DSA, **second column**), and CBF map **(third column)** show AVM with preeminent feeders from left MCA. The high flow structures of AVM and the steal phenomenon are well detected by ASL.

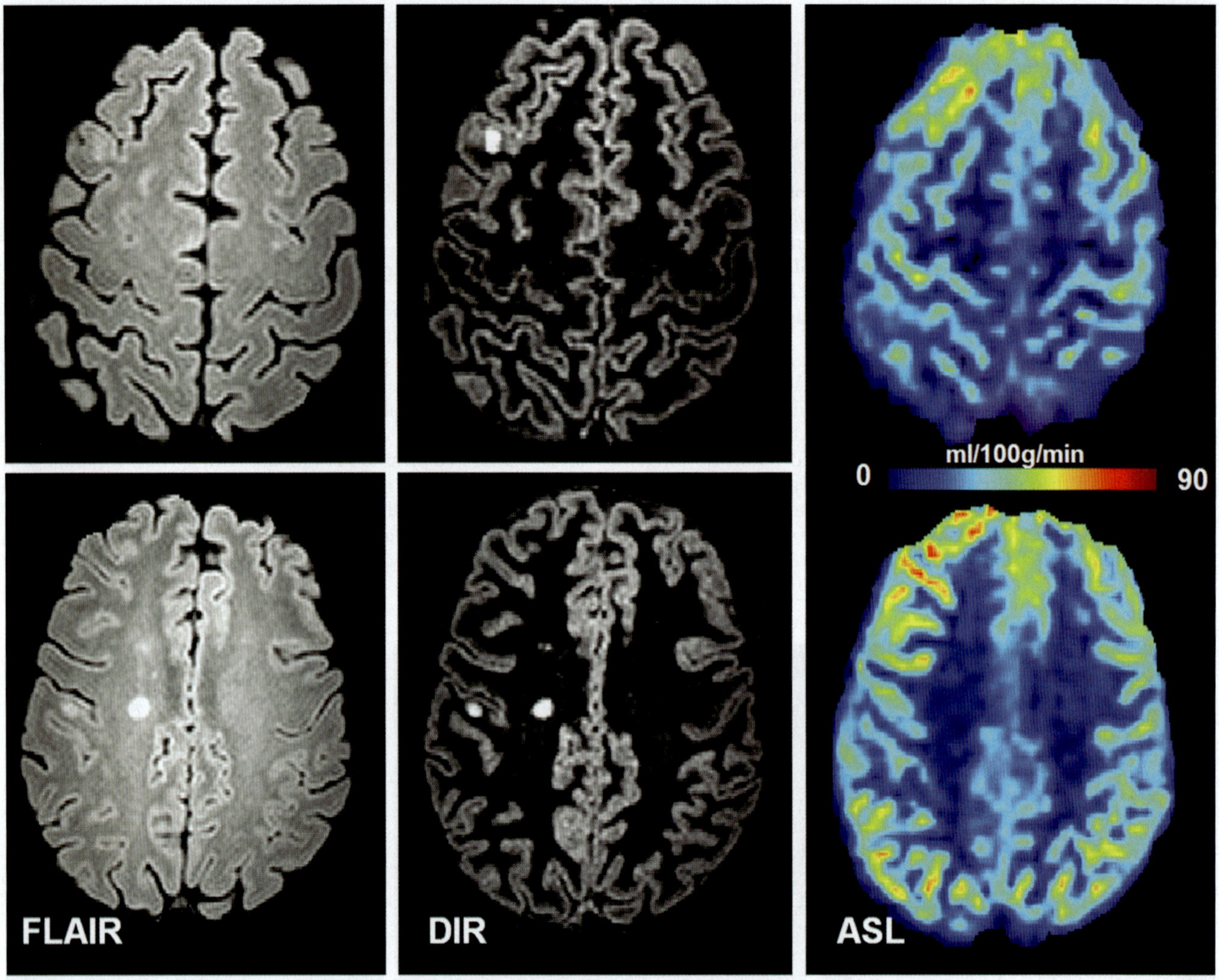

Figure 9-26. Multiple sclerosis. 3D DIR acquisition **(second column)** shows better than 3D FLAIR **(first column)** the cortical involvement of the SM lesions. All the lesions (including the one detected in deep white matter) have low CBF values **(third column)**.

reduced perfusion at a cortical level (Fig. 9.26)[188,189] and an increase in perfusion in WM.[190] Low perfusion in GM could be explained by reduction in local metabolic activity due to neurodegeneration and by redistribution of perfusion in other activated regions. Increased perfusion in WM could be due to an increase in cell number (astrocyte proliferation) and activity in normal-appearing WM,[191] or it could be due to inflammation in MS lesions. ASL is potentially more accurate than using a gadolinium bolus technique, as gadolinium is an intravascular contrast and perfusions values could be affected by BBB, which is known to occur in MS.[192] With SNR and resolution improvements, ASL may better reveal absolute perfusion alterations indicating early stage of disease progression. These perfusion changes could be linked to inflammation, which could precede cortical degeneration and correlates with future MS-related disability. In fact, meningeal inflammation in the form of ectopic lymphoid-like structures (ectopic B-cell follicle-like) has been suggested to play a prominent role in the development of extensive cortical pathology and in exacerbating disease course in MS. Substantial cortical neurodegeneration and generalized cell loss in association with meningeal inflammation and lymphoid tissue formation support the hypothesis that cytotoxic factors diffusing from the meningeal compartment contribute to GM pathology.[193,194]

Epilepsy

Different techniques could be applied to study epilepsy, including PET, SPECT, and MRI.[195–197] ASL could detect ictal and postictal alterations in the form of hemispheric asymmetries in brain perfusion dynamics,[198,199] and it could be repeated noninvasively during follow-up and/or therapy response assessment. Furthermore, ASL imaging is expected to be the best tolerated perfusion technique for pediatric examinations.[134] ASL is comparable to DSC for detecting seizure-associated perfusion changes and asymmetries.[200] For the identification of the epileptogenic zone (Fig. 9.27), ASL is comparable to PET and electroencephalography (EEG) data.[201] Experimental[202] and clinical[203] data indicate that the occurrence of repeated seizures can lead to a chronic epileptic condition and that seizure-induced vascular alterations and neuroinflammation play a key role for epileptogenic mechanisms, such as anoxic/hypoxic ischemic alterations and excitotoxic damage.[204] It becomes thus important to unravel seizure-induced vascular responses and ASL can be an elective technique to investigate such alterations.

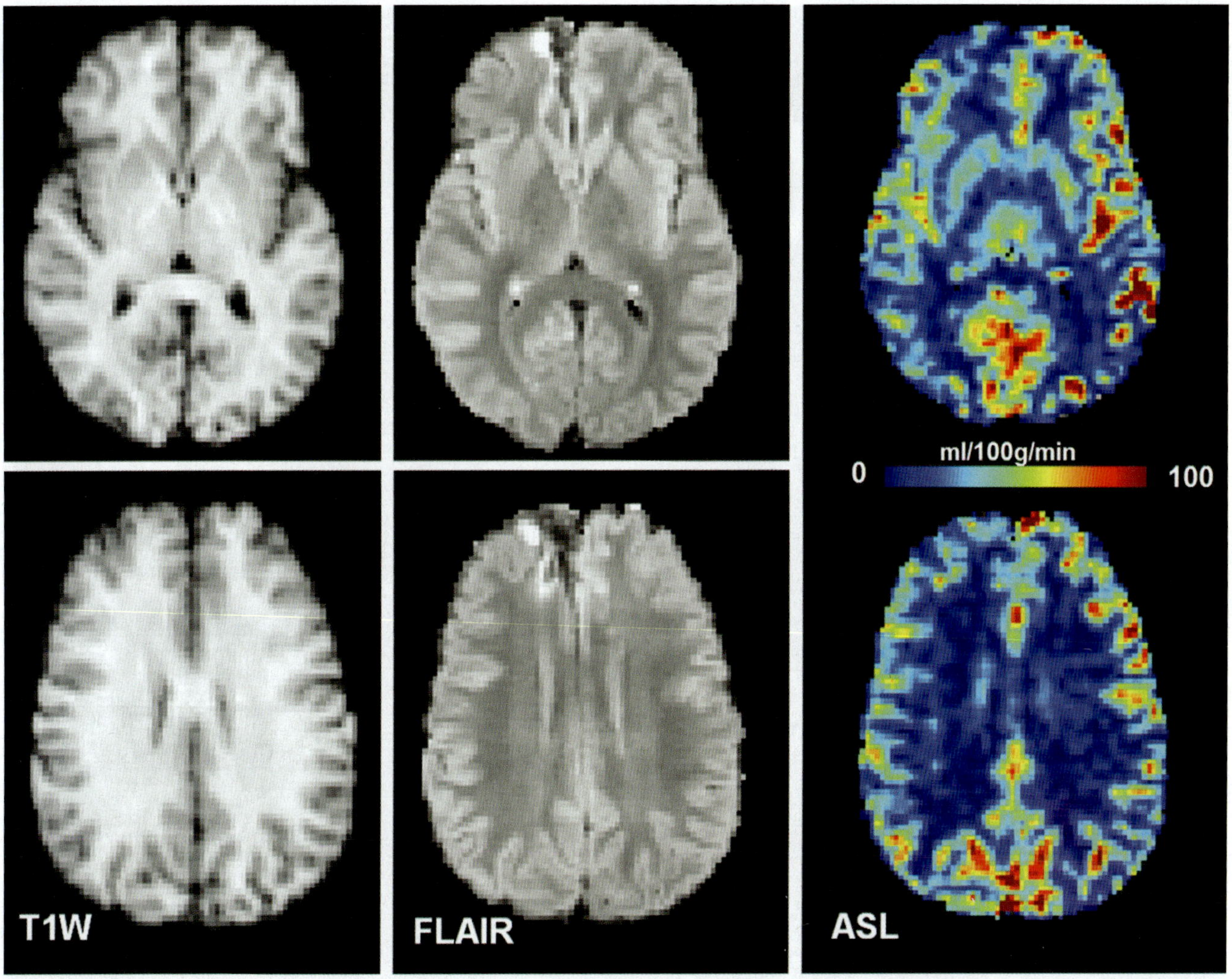

Figure 9-27. Epilepsy. Preoperative T1 MRI **(first column)** and postoperative FLAIR images **(second column)** from a patient with drug-resistant focal epilepsy involving the right frontal lobe as detected by EEG examinations. ASL acquired during interictal phase **(third column)** points out to a right frontomesial area of hypoperfusion. A good agreement between the resected area, clearly visible in the FLAIR images, and the hypoperfused region, as revealed by ASL, can be appreciated.

Quality Assurance: ASL in Practice, Artifacts and Pitfalls

Improvements and standardization of each single step of ASL method is necessary for optimizing ASL quality and permitting reproducible and comparable estimations of perfusion across different sites. As shown in previous chapters, these steps could be synthesized as follows:

1. MR and ASL acquisition mode (magnetic field, phases array coil, type of labeling, and 2D vs. 3D)
2. Data processing: preprocessing (motion correction, T1 segmentation, partial volume correction) and postprocessing (quantification model)
3. Artifact reduction

Identification and familiarity with the most common artifacts in ASL is crucial to avoid pitfalls and to interpret correctly perfusion images.

The most frequent artifacts affecting ASL flow maps could be due to motion and susceptibility, and they appear as peripheral ring, chemical shift, signal drop areas, distortion, bright spots/areas, and loss of differentiation between GM and WM (Fig. 9.28A–D).

Motion artifacts usually appear as bright rings (peripheral ring) or curvy lines, which indicate that the chemical shift was not adequately subtracted in the raw images (chemical shift–like artifact). Motion could also produce signal drop areas, bright spots/areas, and loss of differentiation between GM/WM (Fig. 9.28A).

Susceptibility artifacts (Fig. 9.28 B) are visualized as signal drop at air/bone interfaces (i.e., near the base of the skull and sinuses and nasal cavity) or as distortion if they determine changes of the boundaries of the image and/or ghosts. Some degree of signal drop and distortion could be acceptable, but excessive pneumatization of sinuses or petromastoid region could affect the quality of the images.

Signal drop areas are often due to motion or susceptibility artifacts, but they could also be due to other causes (i.e. noise, poor labeling, post processing or pathology) (Fig. 9.28 B). In particular, if a signal drop area is within the same vascular territory, it is most likely to be due to poor labeling (tortuous arteries or nearby dental work). In both cases, it will be helpful to try

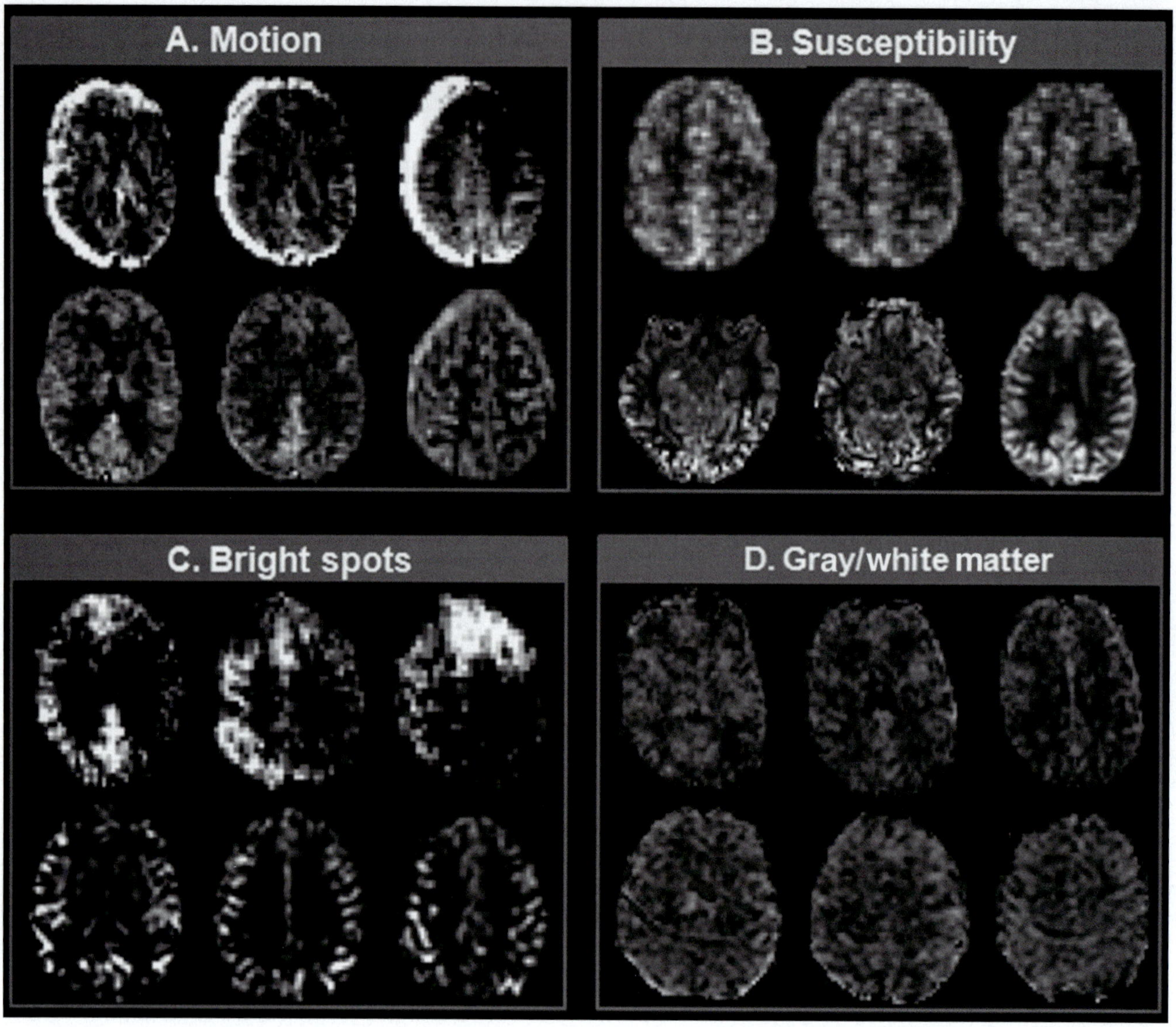

Figure 9-28. Artifacts. Motion: high-degree motion artifacts **(first row)**, low-degree artifacts **(second row)**. Susceptibility artifacts: signal drop caused by blood product deposition **(first row)**, distortion and signal drop at air/bone interfaces **(second row)**. Bright spots: high-degree artifacts **(first row)**, serpiginous regions due to a wrong PLD **(second row)**. G/W matter poor differentiation: two examples **(first and second row)** of studies acquired with wrong PLD and affected by noise and motion.

to adjust the labeling plane in order to optimize the labeling. Watershed areas are at borders of two or more major arterial territories (anterior watershed area is located between the anterior and middle cerebral arteries, posterior between the middle and posterior cerebral arteries, and deep watershed area is located between the deep and superficial perforator vessels), so they are distal territories of vascular distribution, and a drop of the signal in these areas could represent longer ATT or a low CBF: An additional scan with longer PLD could help to differentiate these possibilities.

Also, bright spots/areas and GM/WM differentiation (Fig. 9.28C,D) could be due to motion or not (e.g., poor labeling, bright areas due to residual vascular signal in vessels, baseline magnetization—M0 "shine through," coil sensitivity, noise, postprocessing), and they could appear as single artifact or in combination with others. In particular, if bright spots or serpiginous regions are seen, it could be caused by a wrong PLD: Indeed, if PLD is too low, it will generate ASL signal in larger vessels. But if PLD is appropriate for the subject, bright spots/areas could be due to a delay of the delivery of labeled blood to the tissue, as it happens when the flow is slow because of vascular alteration (collateral circuits, arteriovenous shunt). Note that if intravascular artifacts are present, whole brain CBF could be valid only if flow crushing values are not applied.

Other conditions could mimic artifacts, but should not be considered and counted as artifacts; these are (a) normal/physiologic variability: regional bright areas due to physiologic brightness/hyperperfusion in frontal, temporal, and occipital areas (default network, auditory, visual cortex activation) and pediatric hypersignal due to elevated CBF values in GM and WM (CBF has been reported to peak around 8 years of age and then gradually to decrease to normal adult levels); (b) normal acquisition variability: spin-label decay (if images are acquired from inferior to superior, there is a decreased global signal intensity in the more superior images compared with more inferior levels), intravascular spin label (despite the use of a crusher gradient to suppress intravascular spins, focal high signal intensity on ASL maps may be seen in the sylvian fissures, basal cistern regions, and dural venous sinuses), and not optimized TI; and (c) pathophysiologic changes: small vessel disease, encephalomalacia, vascular malformations, brain atrophy, neoplasm, and epilepsy.

Since now, we reviewed artifacts as results of alterations of acquisition phase (i.e., motion, susceptibility, M0 "shine through," coil sensitivity, intravascular spin label), but they could be also due to errors during pre- (i.e., motion correction, T1 segmentation, partial volume correction) and postprocessing phases (i.e., quantification model).

Thus, identification of the artifacts in ASL flow map should lead to a revision of all the previous processing phases (from the raw data to the intermediate maps, i.e., individual control–tag difference, ΔM-, M0, T1/R1, raw data), of which it is a result (Fig. 9.29). Practically, this inferential revision of ASL flow map requires the knowledge of the data processing (Which preprocessing and postprocessing were used? Was a reference value or map used to calculate T1? Was a global value or a voxel-based M0 value used?) to view and check correctly the intermediate maps used for generating the CBF and to see whether artifacts arise from them and maybe exclude them from the CBF calculation or, alternatively, correct them by applying motion correction algorithms.

This could improve the detection of subtle abnormalities or errors that occurred during pre- and postprocessing phases, resulting in a global optimization of the quality of the study.

Besides artifact identification, other pitfalls should be considered before applying ASL in clinical setting.[1]

1. Many repetitions of label control images should be acquired and averaged to enable sufficient SNR, to reduce the effects of motion, and to ensure possible data filtering. Usually, a good-quality scan, acquired with recommended parameters and modalities (see previous chapters),[205] takes approximately 4 minutes. But in clinical setting, acquisition time of applying could be essential to get feasible, so the possibility of applying fast imaging and to compensate the SNR loss with a reduced spatial resolution should be taken into account.
2. Another clinical pitfall could be due to the ability to view and interpret correctly the perfusion maps: A color scale could be very sensitive to perfusion alterations, but it could also lead to false interpretations. So, it is useful to view CBF maps critically, either in grayscale or color, with a quantitative scale bar next to the images to indicate flow values.
3. White matter's perfusion alterations are difficult to detect because of its low CBF, higher ATT, and blurring of boundaries between WM and GM in in-plane or through-plane directions.[154]

Guidelines are required for evaluating standards of quality in ASL. Considering this, it will be necessary to introduce a new scoring system that qualifies and quantifies the presence of artifacts (motion, distortion, signal drop areas, bright spots/areas, and GM/WM differentiation: artifacts scale, AS) and visibility of good quality items (anatomical landmarks as cortical gray matter, deep gray matter, i.e., basal ganglia/thalami, GM/WM differentiation: items scale, IS).

These criteria should be applied not only to CBF maps but also to intermediate maps, according to the type of processing used (usually ΔM, R1, M0), as problems in these maps can make the results unusable (Fig. 9.29).

The quality of the scan according to the presence of artifacts (AS) was assigned to a score between 0 and 3 (Table 9.2): 0, if no artifacts in all slices; 1, if artifacts visible in less than 50% of slices; 2, if artifacts in more than 50% (moderate); and 3, if artifacts in all slices (marked). The maximum total AS score achievable[15] indicates a bad quality study.

For IS, each of the 3 items (GM, basal ganglia/thalami, GM/WM differentiation) should be assessed in all slices of each map. Each item was assigned a score between 1 and 3 (Table 9.2): 0, when not visible in any slice of the maps; 1, when visible in less than 50% (just visible); 2, when visible in more than 50% and less than 90% (partially visible); and 3, when visible in more than 90% of slices (well visible).

If all GM visualization is not or just visible, it should be considered the possibility of a global failure of the labeling or that an error of acquisition or processing of T1 occurred. The higher the total IS score (max 30), the lesser the artifacts are and the better the quality of the study is. The final quality score (QS) is calculated by subtracting the total artifact's score from the items' quality score: IS – AS. QS ranges from −15 to +30.

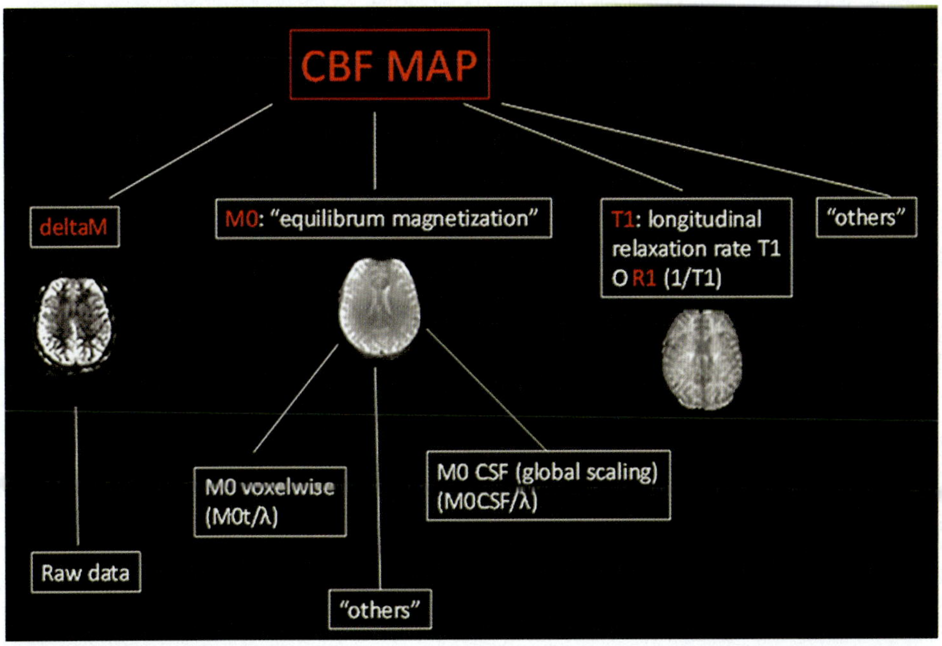

Figure 9-29. Flowchart showing a scheme of possible processing that could generate CBF map.

TABLE **9.2** **QA Scoring System**

Artifacts' Scale	Absent	Mild (<50%)	Moderate (more 50%)	Marked
Motion	0	1	2	3
Distortion	0	1	2	3
Signal drop	0	1	2	3
Artifacts affecting G/W matter differentiation	0	1	2	3
Bright spots and areas in R1	0	1	2	3
Global Quality Measurement (S/N Ratio)				
Items' Scale	*Not Visible (<10%)*	*Just Visible (more than 10%, <50%)*	*Partially Visible (more than 50%, <90%)*	*Well Visible (more than 90%)*
CBF gray matter	0	1	2	3
CBF W/G differentiation	0	1	2	3
CBF basal ganglia/thalami	0	1	2	3
ΔM gray matter	0	1	2	3
ΔM W/G differentiation	0	1	2	3
ΔM basal ganglia/thalami	0	1	2	3
R1 gray matter	0	1	2	3
R1 W/G differentiation	0	1	2	3
R1 basal ganglia/thalami	0	1	2	3
M0 basal ganglia/TH/W/G (global assessment)	0	1	2	3
Clinical Score	*Clinically Usable*	*Clinically not Usable*		

The higher the total IS (max 30), the lesser the artifacts are and the better the quality of the study is. The scoring system may reveal a threshold beyond which the clinical utility of the study (clinical score) is no longer guaranteed.

But besides CBF, other maps (as blood volume (BV) and arterial transient time (ATT) maps) could be generated by multi-TI pulsed ASL sequence (i.e., QUASAR); they visualize different anatomical landmarks: BV map assesses the visibility of the main cerebral arteries and ATT identifies the main watershed areas (anterior, posterior, and deep watershed areas). So the "basic" CBF, ΔM, R1, M0 IS proposed could be implemented and modified depending on the ASL sequence and the post-processing method allowing a more flexible IS system.

No study has so far established clear guidelines for ASL data quality assurance,[206] but recently, a scoring system for data quality has been proposed[207] specifically for QUASAR ASL in clinical trials. Nonetheless, no basic quality scale adaptable to all ASL sequences has ever been proposed. The proposed scoring system may reveal objectively a threshold beyond which the clinical utility of the study is no longer guaranteed in (Table 9.2), and it can help the researchers to accept or discard images.

One of the limitations of this tool is that it is observer dependent and there may be a challenge in differentiating artifacts from normal findings. Therefore, good training in reviewing ASL data is required to help researchers correctly interpret ASL maps. If this is done correctly, excellent interobserver agreement can be achieved. The scoring scale reported here could be used as a simple tool in clinical trials employing ASL.

Acknowledgments

COST Action BM1103: ASL Initiative in Dementia (AID).

Dr. Ilaria Boscolo Galazzo, University of Verona

Prof. Alberto Beltramello, Neuroradiology Department, University Hospital Verona.

Dr. Juan Álvarez-Linera. Neuroradiology Department. Ruber International Hospital. Madrid, Spain.

Dr. Ana Ramos. Neuroradiology Department. Doce de Octubre Hospital. Madrid, Spain.

REFERENCES

1. **Alsop DC, Detre JA, Golay X, et al.** Recommended implementation of arterial spin-labeled perfusion MRI for clinical applications: a consensus of the ISMRM perfusion study group and the European consortium for ASL in dementia. *Magn Reson Med* 2014;73(1):102–116.
2. **Detre JA, Leigh JS, Williams DS, et al.** Perfusion imaging. *Magn Reson Med* 1992;23(1):37–45.
3. **Williams DS, Detre JA, Leigh JS, et al.** Magnetic resonance imaging of perfusion using spin inversion of arterial water. *Proc Natl Acad Sci U S A* 1992;89(1):212–216.
4. **Edelman RR, Siewert B, Darby DG, et al.** Qualitative mapping of cerebral blood flow and functional localization with echo-planar MR

imaging and signal targeting with alternating radio frequency. *Radiology* 1994;192(2):513–520.

5. **Østergaard L, Sorensen AG, Kwong KK, et al.** High resolution measurement of cerebral blood flow using intravascular tracer bolus passages. Part II: Experimental comparison and preliminary results. *Magn Reson Med* 1996;36(5):726–736.
6. **Østergaard L, Weisskoff RM, Chesler DA, et al.** High resolution measurement of cerebral blood flow using intravascular tracer bolus passages. Part I: mathematical approach and statistical analysis. *Magn Reson Med* 1996;36(5):715–725.
7. **Gonzalez-At JB, Alsop DC, Detre JA.** Cerebral perfusion and arterial transit time changes during task activation determined with continuous arterial spin labeling. *Magn Reson Med* 2000;43(5):739–746.
8. **Yang Y, Engelien W, Xu S, et al.** Transit time, trailing time, and cerebral blood flow during brain activation: measurement using multislice, pulsed spin-labeling perfusion imaging. *Magn Reson Med* 2000;44(5):680–685.
9. **Wong EC.** Vessel-encoded arterial spin-labeling using pseudocontinuous tagging. *Magn Reson Med* 2007;58(6):1086–1091.
10. **Berstein MA, King KF, Zhou XJ.** *Handbook of MRI pulse sequences*: Elsevier Academic Press; 2004; MA, USA.
11. **Petersen ET, Zimine I, Ho YC, et al.** Non-invasive measurement of perfusion: a critical review of arterial spin labelling techniques. *Br J Radiol* 2006;79(944):688–701.
12. **Dixon WT, Du LN, Faul DD, et al.** Projection angiograms of blood labeled by adiabatic fast passage. *Magn Reson Med* 1986;3(3):454–462.
13. **Maccotta L, Detre JA, Alsop DC.** The efficiency of adiabatic inversion for perfusion imaging by arterial spin labeling. *NMR Biomed.* 1997;10(4–5):216–221.
14. **Utting JF, Thomas DL, Gadian DG, et al.** Velocity-driven adiabatic fast passage for arterial spin labeling: results from a computer model. *Magn Reson Med* 2003;49(2):398–401.
15. **Franke C, van Dorsten FA, Olah L, et al.** Arterial spin tagging perfusion imaging of rat brain: dependency on magnetic field strength. *Magn Reson Imaging* 2000;18(9):1109–1113.
16. **Gach HM, Dai W.** Simple model of double adiabatic inversion (DAI) efficiency. *Magn Reson Med* 2004;52(4):941–946.
17. **Trampel R, Jochimsen TH, Mildner T, et al.** Efficiency of flow-driven adiabatic spin inversion under realistic experimental conditions: a computer simulation. *Magn Reson Med* 2004;51(6):1187–1193.
18. **Wong EC, Buxton RB, Frank LR.** Implementation of quantitative perfusion imaging techniques for functional brain mapping using pulsed arterial spin labeling. *NMR Biomed* 1997;10(4–5):237–249.
19. **Ordidge RJ, Wylezinska M, Hugg JW, et al.** Frequency offset corrected inversion (FOCI) pulses for use in localized spectroscopy. *Magn Reson Med* 1996;36(4):562–566.
20. **Yongbi MN, Branch CA, Helpern JA.** Perfusion imaging using FOCI RF pulses. *Magn Reson Med* 1998;40(6):938–943.
21. **Yongbi MN, Yang Y, Frank JA, et al.** Multislice perfusion imaging in human brain using the C-FOCI inversion pulse: comparison with hyperbolic secant. *Magn Reson Med* 1999;42(6):1098–1105.
22. **Edelman RR, Chen Q.** EPISTAR MRI: multislice mapping of cerebral blood flow. *Magn Reson Med* 1998;40(6):800–805.
23. **Kwong KK, Chesler DA, Weisskoff RM, et al.** MR perfusion studies with T1-weighted echo planar imaging. *Magn Reson Med* 1995;34(6):878–887.
24. **Kim SG.** Quantification of relative cerebral blood flow change by flow-sensitive alternating inversion recovery (FAIR) technique: application to functional mapping. *Magn Reson Med* 1995;34(3):293–301.
25. **Wong EC, Buxton RB, Frank LR.** Quantitative imaging of perfusion using a single subtraction (QUIPSS and QUIPSS II). *Magn Reson Med* 1998;39(5):702–708.
26. **Luh WM, Wong EC, Bandettini PA, et al.** QUIPSS II with thin-slice TI1 periodic saturation: a method for improving accuracy of quantitative perfusion imaging using pulsed arterial spin labeling. *Magn Reson Med* 1999;41(6):1246–1254.
27. **Mansfield P.** Multi-planar image formation using NMR spin echoes. *J Phys C: Solid Phys* 1977;10:L55.
28. **Oshio K, Feinberg DA.** GRASE (Gradient- and spin-echo) imaging: a novel fast MRI technique. *Magn Reson Med* 1991;20(2):344–349.
29. **Mulkern RV, Wong ST, Winalski C, et al.** Contrast manipulation and artifact assessment of 2D and 3D RARE sequences. *Magn Reson Imaging* 1990;8(5):557–566.
30. **Duhamel G AD.** Single-shot susceptibility insensitive whole brain 3D fMRI with ASL. 12th Annual Meeting of ISMRM; 2004; 15-21 May 2004; Kyoto, Japan.
31. **Ye FQ, Frank JA, Weinberger DR, et al.** Noise reduction in 3D perfusion imaging by attenuating the static signal in arterial spin tagging (ASSIST). *Magn Reson Med* 2000;44(1):92–100.
32. **Vidorreta M, Wang Z, Rodriguez I, et al.** Comparison of 2D and 3D single-shot ASL perfusion fMRI sequences. *Neuroimage* 2012;66C:662–671.
33. **Edelman RR, Wallner B, Singer A, et al.** Segmented turboFLASH: method for breath-hold MR imaging of the liver with flexible contrast. *Radiology* 1990;177(2):515–521.
34. **Scheffler K, Heid O, Hennig J.** Magnetization preparation during the steady state: fat-saturated 3D TrueFISP. *Magn Reson Med* 2001;45(6): 1075–1080.
35. **Pereles FS, Kapoor V, Carr JC, et al.** Usefulness of segmented trueFISP cardiac pulse sequence in evaluation of congenital and acquired adult cardiac abnormalities. *AJR Am J Roentgenol* 2001;177(5):1155–1160.
36. **Garcia DM, Duhamel G, Alsop DC.** Efficiency of inversion pulses for background suppressed arterial spin labeling. *Magn Reson Med* 2005;54(2):366–372.
37. **Buxton RB, Frank LR, Wong EC, et al.** A general kinetic model for quantitative perfusion imaging with arterial spin labeling. *Magn Reson Med* 1998;40(3):383–396.
38. **Alsop DC, Detre JA.** Reduced transit-time sensitivity in noninvasive magnetic resonance imaging of human cerebral blood flow. *J Cereb Blood Flow Metab* 1996;16(6):1236–1249.
39. **Hrabe J, Lewis DP.** Two analytical solutions for a model of pulsed arterial spin labeling with randomized blood arrival times. *J Magn Reson* 2004;167(1):49–55.
40. **Chappell MA, Woolrich MW, Kazan S, et al.** Modeling dispersion in arterial spin labeling: validation using dynamic angiographic measurements. *Magn Reson Med* 2013;69(2):563–570.
41. **Parkes LM, Tofts PS.** Improved accuracy of human cerebral blood perfusion measurements using arterial spin labeling: accounting for capillary water permeability. *Magn Reson Med* 2002;48(1):27–41.
42. **St Lawrence KS, Frank JA, McLaughlin AC.** Effect of restricted water exchange on cerebral blood flow values calculated with arterial spin tagging: a theoretical investigation. *Magn Reson Med* 2000;44(3):440–449.
43. **Petersen ET, Lim T, Golay X.** Model-free arterial spin labeling quantification approach for perfusion MRI. *Magn Reson Med* 2006;55(2): 219–232.
44. **Johnson NA, Jahng G-H, Weiner MW, et al.** Pattern of cerebral hypoperfusion in Alzheimer disease and mild cognitive impairment measured with arterial spin-labeling MR imaging: initial experience. *Radiology* 2005;234(3):851–859.
45. **Asllani I, Borogovac A, Brown TR.** Regression algorithm correcting for partial volume effects in arterial spin labeling MRI. *Magn Reson Med* 2008;60(6):1362–1371.
46. **Chappell MA, Groves AR, MacIntosh BJ, et al.** Partial volume correction of multiple inversion time arterial spin labeling MRI data. *Magn Reson Med* 2011;65(4):1173–1183.
47. **Petr J, Schramm G, Hofheinz F, et al.** Partial volume correction in arterial spin labeling using a Look-Locker sequence. *Magn Reson Med* 2013;70(6):1535–1543.
48. **Weber MA, Zoubaa S, Schlieter M, et al.** Diagnostic performance of spectroscopic and perfusion MRI for distinction of brain tumors. *Neurology* 2006;66(12):1899–1906.
49. **Al-Okaili RN, Krejza J, Wang S, et al.** Advanced MR Imaging Techniques in the Diagnosis of Intraaxial Brain Tumors in Adults1. *Radiographics* 2006;26(suppl 1):S173–S189.
50. **Bulakbasi N, Kocaoglu M, Farzaliyev A, et al.** Assessment of diagnostic accuracy of perfusion MR imaging in primary and metastatic solitary malignant brain tumors. *AJNR Am J Neuroradiol* 2005;26(9): 2187–2199.
51. **Law M, Yang S, Wang H, et al.** Glioma grading: sensitivity, specificity, and predictive values of perfusion MR imaging and proton MR spectroscopic imaging compared with conventional MR imaging. *AJNR Am J Neuroradiol* 2003;24(10):1989–1998.
52. **Sugahara T, Korogi Y, Kochi M, et al.** Correlation of MR imaging-determined cerebral blood volume maps with histologic and angiographic determination of vascularity of gliomas. *AJR Am J Roentgenol* 1998;171(6):1479–1486.

53. **Lacerda S, Law M.** Magnetic resonance perfusion and permeability imaging in brain tumors. *Neuroimaging Clin N Am* 2009;19(4):527–557.
54. **Maia AC, Jr., Malheiros SM, da Rocha AJ, et al.** MR cerebral blood volume maps correlated with vascular endothelial growth factor expression and tumor grade in nonenhancing gliomas. *AJNR Am J Neuroradiol* 2005;26(4):777–783.
55. **Mitsuya K, Nakasu Y, Horiguchi S, et al.** Perfusion weighted magnetic resonance imaging to distinguish the recurrence of metastatic brain tumors from radiation necrosis after stereotactic radiosurgery. *J Neurooncol* 2010;99(1):81–88.
56. **Sugahara T, Korogi Y, Tomiguchi S, et al.** Posttherapeutic intraaxial brain tumor: the value of perfusion-sensitive contrast-enhanced MR imaging for differentiating tumor recurrence from nonneoplastic contrast-enhancing tissue. *AJNR Am J Neuroradiol* 2000;21(5): 901–909.
57. **Gasparetto EL, Pawlak MA, Patel SH, et al.** Posttreatment recurrence of malignant brain neoplasm: accuracy of relative cerebral blood volume fraction in discriminating low from high malignant histologic volume fraction. *Radiology* 2009;250(3):887–896.
58. **Barajas RF, Chang JS, Segal MR, et al.** Differentiation of recurrent glioblastoma multiforme from radiation necrosis after external beam radiation therapy with dynamic susceptibility-weighted contrast-enhanced perfusion MR imaging. *Radiology* 2009;253(2):486–496.
59. **Warmuth C, Gunther M, Zimmer C.** Quantification of blood flow in brain tumors: comparison of arterial spin labeling and dynamic susceptibility-weighted contrast-enhanced MR imaging. *Radiology* 2003;228(2):523–532.
60. **Lüdemann L, Warmuth C, Plotkin M, et al.** Brain tumor perfusion: comparison of dynamic contrast enhanced magnetic resonance imaging using T1, T2, and T2* contrast, pulsed arterial spin labeling, and H2(15) O positron emission tomography. *Eur J Radiol* 2009;70(3):465–474.
61. **Silva AC, Kim SG, Garwood M.** Imaging blood flow in brain tumors using arterial spin labeling. *Magn Reson Med* 2000;44(2):169–173.
62. **Lehmann P, Monet P, de Marco G, et al.** A comparative study of perfusion measurement in brain tumours at 3 Tesla MR: arterial spin labeling versus dynamic susceptibility contrast-enhanced MRI. *Eur Neurol* 2010;64(1):21–26.
63. **Kimura H, Takeuchi H, Koshimoto Y, et al.** Perfusion imaging of meningioma by using continuous arterial spin-labeling: comparison with dynamic susceptibility-weighted contrast-enhanced MR images and histopathologic features. *AJNR Am J Neuroradiol* 2006;27(1):85–93.
64. **Järnum H, Steffensen EG, Knutsson L, et al.** Perfusion MRI of brain tumours: a comparative study of pseudo-continuous arterial spin labelling and dynamic susceptibility contrast imaging. *Neuroradiology* 2010;52(4):307–317.
65. **Hirai T, Kitajima M, Nakamura H, et al.** Quantitative blood flow measurements in gliomas using arterial spin-labeling at 3T: intermodality agreement and inter- and intraobserver reproducibility study. *AJNR Am J Neuroradiol* 2011;32(11):2073–2079.
66. **van Westen D, Petersen ET, Wirestam R, et al.** Correlation between arterial blood volume obtained by arterial spin labelling and cerebral blood volume in intracranial tumours. *MAGMA* 2011;24(4):211–223.
67. **Noguchi T, Yoshiura T, Hiwatashi A, et al.** Perfusion imaging of brain tumors using arterial spin-labeling: correlation with histopathologic vascular density. *AJNR Am J Neuroradiol* 2008;29(4):688–693.
68. **Yamashita K, Yoshiura T, Hiwatashi A, et al.** Differentiating primary CNS lymphoma from glioblastoma multiforme: assessment using arterial spin labeling, diffusion-weighted imaging, and 18F-fluorodeoxyglucose positron emission tomography. *Neuroradiology* 2013;55(2):135–143.
69. **Yamashita K, Yoshiura T, Hiwatashi A, et al.** Arterial spin labeling of hemangioblastoma: differentiation from metastatic brain tumors based on quantitative blood flow measurement. *Neuroradiology* 2012;54(8):809–813.
70. **Law M, Yang S, Babb JS, et al.** Comparison of cerebral blood volume and vascular permeability from dynamic susceptibility contrast-enhanced perfusion MR imaging with glioma grade. *AJNR Am J Neuroradiol* 2004;25(5):746–755.
71. **Law M, Young R, Babb J, et al.** Comparing perfusion metrics obtained from a single compartment versus pharmacokinetic modeling methods using dynamic susceptibility contrast-enhanced perfusion MR imaging with glioma grade. *AJNR Am J Neuroradiol* 2006;27(9): 1975–1982.
72. **Law M.** Perfusion and MRS for brain tumor diagnosis. In: *Clinical magnetic resonance imaging*. Philadelphia, PA: Saunders; 2005:1215–1247.
73. **Wolf RL, Wang J, Wang S, et al.** Grading of CNS neoplasms using continuous arterial spin labeled perfusion MR imaging at 3 Tesla. *J Magn Reson Imaging* 2005;22(4):475–482.
74. **Kim HS, Kim SY.** A prospective study on the added value of pulsed arterial spin-labeling and apparent diffusion coefficients in the grading of gliomas. *AJNR Am J Neuroradiol* 2007;28(9):1693–1699.
75. **Danchaivijitr N, Waldman AD, Tozer DJ, et al.** Low-grade gliomas: do changes in rCBV measurements at longitudinal perfusion-weighted MR imaging predict malignant transformation? *Radiology* 2008;247(1):170–178.
76. **Weber M-A, Bock M, Plathow C, et al.** Asbestos-related pleural disease: value of dedicated magnetic resonance imaging techniques. *Invest Radiol* 2004;39(9):554–564.
77. **Fellah S, Girard N, Chinot O, et al.** Early evaluation of tumoral response to antiangiogenic therapy by arterial spin labeling perfusion magnetic resonance imaging and susceptibility weighted imaging in a patient with recurrent glioblastoma receiving bevacizumab. *J Clin Oncol* 2011;29(11):e308–e311.
78. **Ozsunar Y, Mullins ME, Kwong K, et al.** Glioma recurrence versus radiation necrosis? A pilot comparison of arterial spin-labeled, dynamic susceptibility contrast enhanced MRI, and FDG-PET imaging. *Acad Radiol* 2010;17(3):282–290.
79. **Alsop DC, Casement M, de Bazelaire C, et al.** Hippocampal hyperperfusion in Alzheimer's disease. *Neuroimage* 2008;42(4):1267–1274.
80. **McMahon PM, Araki SS, Neumann PJ, et al.** Cost-effectiveness of functional imaging tests in the diagnosis of Alzheimer disease. *Radiology* 2000;217(1):58–68.
81. **McMahon PM, Araki SS, Sandberg EA, et al.** Cost-effectiveness of PET in the diagnosis of Alzheimer disease. *Radiology* 2003;228(2):515–522.
82. **Chen Y, Wolk DA, Reddin JS, et al.** Voxel-level comparison of arterial spin-labeled perfusion MRI and FDG-PET in Alzheimer disease. *Neurology* 2011;77(22):1977–1985.
83. **Xu G, Rowley HA, Wu G, et al.** Reliability and precision of pseudo-continuous arterial spin labeling perfusion MRI on 3.0 T and comparison with 15O-water PET in elderly subjects at risk for Alzheimer's disease. *NMR Biomed* 2010;23(3):286–293.
84. **Ye FQ, Berman KF, Ellmore T, et al.** H(2)(15)O PET validation of steady-state arterial spin tagging cerebral blood flow measurements in humans. *Magn Reson Med* 2000;44(3):450–456.
85. **Donahue MJ, Lu H, Jones CK, et al.** An account of the discrepancy between MRI and PET cerebral blood flow measures. A high-field MRI investigation NMR in biomedicine. *NMR Biomed* 2006;19(8):1043–1054.
86. **Detre JA, Alsop DC.** Perfusion magnetic resonance imaging with continuous arterial spin labeling: methods and clinical applications in the central nervous system. *Eur J Radiol* 1999;30(2):115–124.
87. **Du AT, Jahng GH, Hayasaka S, et al.** Hypoperfusion in frontotemporal dementia and Alzheimer disease by arterial spin labeling MRI. *Neurology* 2006;67(7):1215–1220.
88. **Asllani I, Habeck C, Scarmeas N, et al.** Multivariate and univariate analysis of continuous arterial spin labeling perfusion MRI in Alzheimer's disease. *J Cereb Blood Flow Metab* 2008;28(4):725–736.
89. **Yoshiura T, Hiwatashi A, Yamashita K, et al.** Simultaneous measurement of arterial transit time, arterial blood volume, and cerebral blood flow using arterial spin-labeling in patients with Alzheimer disease. *AJNR Am J Neuroradiol* 2009;30(7):1388–1393.
90. **Chao LL, Buckley ST, Kornak J, et al.** ASL perfusion MRI predicts cognitive decline and conversion from MCI to dementia. *Alzheimer Dis Assoc Disord* 2010;24(1):19–27.
91. **Alsop DC, Detre JA, Grossman M.** Assessment of cerebral blood flow in Alzheimer's disease by spin-labeled magnetic resonance imaging. *Ann Neurol* 2000;47(1):93–100.
92. **Wolk DA, Detre JA.** Arterial spin labeling MRI: an emerging biomarker for Alzheimer's disease and other neurodegenerative conditions. *Curr Opin Neurol* 2012;25(4):421–428.
93. **Ances BM, Liang CL, Leontiev O, et al.** Effects of aging on cerebral blood flow, oxygen metabolism, and blood oxygenation level dependent responses to visual stimulation. *Hum Brain Mapp* 2009;30(4):1120–1132.
94. **Dai W, Lopez OL, Carmichael OT, et al.** Mild cognitive impairment and Alzheimer disease: patterns of altered cerebral blood flow at MR imaging. *Radiology* 2009;250(3):856–866.
95. **Binnewijzend MA, Kuijer JP, Benedictus MR, et al.** Cerebral blood flow measured with 3D pseudocontinuous arterial spin-labeling MR imaging in Alzheimer disease and mild cognitive impairment: a marker for disease severity. *Radiology* 2013;267(1):221–230.

96. **Hu W, Wang Z, Lee V-Y, et al.** Distinct cerebral perfusion patterns in FTLD and AD. *Neurology* 2010;75(10):881–888.
97. **Raji CA, Lee C, Lopez OL, et al.** Initial experience in using continuous arterial spin-labeled MR imaging for early detection of Alzheimer disease. *AJNR Am J Neuroradiol* 2010;31(5):847–855.
98. **Zhang Q, Stafford RB, Wang Z, et al.** Microvascular perfusion based on arterial spin labeled perfusion MRI as a measure of vascular risk in Alzheimer's disease. *J Alzheimers Dis* 2012;32(3):677–687.
99. **Theberge J.** Perfusion magnetic resonance imaging in psychiatry. *Top Magn Reson Imaging* 2008;19(2):111–130.
100. **Drevets WC.** Neuroimaging and neuropathological studies of depression: implications for the cognitive-emotional features of mood disorders. *Curr Opin Neurobiol* 2001;11(2):240–249.
101. **Beadles CF.** On the degenerative lesions of the arterial system in the insane, with remarks upon the nature of granular ependyma. *Br J Psychiatry* 1895;41(172):32–50.
102. **Handley R, Zelaya FO, Reinders A, et al.** Acute effects of single dose aripiprazole and haloperidol on resting cerebral blood flow (rCBF) in the human brain. *Hum Brain Mapp* 2013;34(2):272–282.
103. **Sadaghiani S, Scheeringa R, Lehongre K, et al.** Intrinsic connectivity networks, alpha oscillations, and tonic alertness: a simultaneous electroencephalography/functional magnetic resonance imaging study. *J Neurosci* 2010;30(30):10243–10250.
104. **Ho TC, Wu J, Shin DD, et al.** Altered cerebral perfusion in executive, affective, and motor networks during adolescent depression. *J Am Acad Child Adolesc Psychiatry* 2013;52(10):1076.e2-1091.e2.
105. **Orosz A, Jann K, Federspiel A, et al.** Reduced cerebral blood flow within the default-mode network and within total gray matter in major depression. *Brain Connect* 2012;2(6):303–310.
106. **Duhameau B, Ferre J-C, Jannin P, et al.** Chronic and treatment-resistant depression: a study using arterial spin labeling perfusion MRI at 3 Tesla. *Psychiatry Res* 2010;182(2):111–116.
107. **Gillihan SJ, Rao H, Brennan L, et al.** Serotonin transporter genotype modulates the association between depressive symptoms and amygdala activity among psychiatrically healthy adults. *Psychiatry Res* 2011;193(3):161–167.
108. **Wolf RC, Thomann PA, Sambataro F, et al.** Orbitofrontal cortex and impulsivity in borderline personality disorder: an MRI study of baseline brain perfusion. *Eur Arch Psychiatry Clin Neurosci* 2012; 262(8):677–685.
109. **Walther S, Federspiel A, Horn H, et al.** Resting state cerebral blood flow and objective motor activity reveal basal ganglia dysfunction in schizophrenia. *Psychiatry Res* 2011;192(2):117–124.
110. **Walther S, Hofle O, Federspiel A, et al.** Neural correlates of disbalanced motor control in major depression. *J Affect Disord* 2012;136(1–2):124–133.
111. **Andreescu C, Gross JJ, Lenze E, et al.** Altered cerebral blood flow patterns associated with pathologic worry in the elderly. *Depress Anxiety* 2011;28(3):202–209.
112. **Gillihan SJ, Rao H, Wang J, et al.** Serotonin transporter genotype modulates amygdala activity during mood regulation. *Soc Cogn Affect Neurosci* 2010;5(1):1–10.
113. **Homan P, Kindler J, Federspiel A, et al.** Muting the voice: a case of arterial spin labeling-monitored transcranial direct current stimulation treatment of auditory verbal hallucinations. *Am J Psychiatry* 2011; 168(8):853–854.
114. **Kindler J, Homan P, Jann K, et al.** Reduced neuronal activity in language-related regions after transcranial magnetic stimulation therapy for auditory verbal hallucinations. *Biol Psychiatry* 2013;73(6):518–524.
115. **Homan P, Kindler J, Hauf M, et al.** Cerebral blood flow identifies responders to transcranial magnetic stimulation in auditory verbal hallucinations. *Transl Psychiatry* 2012;2:e189.
116. **Ball TM, Stein MB, Ramsawh HJ, et al.** Single-subject anxiety treatment outcome prediction using functional neuroimaging. *Neuropsychopharmacology* 2014;39(5):1254–1261.
117. **Marquand AF, O'Daly OG, De Simoni S, et al.** Dissociable effects of methylphenidate, atomoxetine and placebo on regional cerebral blood flow in healthy volunteers at rest: a multi-class pattern recognition approach. *Neuroimage* 2012;60(2):1015–1024.
118. **Field AS, Laurienti PJ, Yen Y-F, et al.** Dietary caffeine consumption and withdrawal: confounding variables in quantitative cerebral perfusion studies? *Radiology* 2003;227(1):129–135.
119. **Kelly TM, Daley DC, Douaihy AB.** Treatment of substance abusing patients with comorbid psychiatric disorders. *Addict Behav* 2012;37(1): 11–24.
120. **Denier N, Schmidt A, Gerber H, et al.** Association of frontal gray matter volume and cerebral perfusion in heroin addiction: a multimodal neuroimaging study. *Front Psychiatry* 2013;4:135.
121. **Wang Z, Faith M, Patterson F, et al.** Neural substrates of abstinence-induced cigarette cravings in chronic smokers. *J Neurosci* 2007;27(51): 14035–14040.
122. **Jacobus J, Goldenberg D, Wierenga CE, et al.** Altered cerebral blood flow and neurocognitive correlates in adolescent cannabis users. *Psychopharmacology (Berl)* 2012;222(4):675–684.
123. **Khalili-Mahani N, van Osch MJ, Baerends E, et al.** Pseudocontinuous arterial spin labeling reveals dissociable effects of morphine and alcohol on regional cerebral blood flow. *J Cereb Blood Flow Metab* 2011;31(5): 1321–1333.
124. **Rickenbacher E, Greve DN, Azma S, et al.** Effects of alcohol intoxication and gender on cerebral perfusion: an arterial spin labeling study. *Alcohol* 2011;45(8):725–737.
125. **Tolentino NJ, Wierenga CE, Hall S, et al.** Alcohol effects on cerebral blood flow in subjects with low and high responses to alcohol. *Alcohol Clin Exp Res* 2011;35(6):1034–1040.
126. **Klomp A, den Hollander B, de Bruin K, et al.** The effects of ecstasy (MDMA) on brain serotonin transporters are dependent on age-of-first exposure in recreational users and animals. *PLoS One* 2012;7(10).
127. **Klomp A, Caan MWA, Denys D, et al.** Feasibility of ASL-based phMRI with a single dose of oral citalopram for repeated assessment of serotonin function. *Neuroimage* 2012;63(3):1695–1700.
128. **Hermes M, Hagemann D, Britz P, et al.** Latent state-trait structure of cerebral blood flow in a resting state. *Biol Psychol* 2009;80(2):196–202.
129. **Zaharchuk G.** Arterial spin label imaging of acute ischemic stroke and transient ischemic attack. *Neuroimaging Clin N Am* 2011;21(2):285–301.
130. **Hendrikse J, Petersen ET, Golay X.** Vascular disorders: insights from arterial spin labeling. *Neuroimaging Clin N Am* 2012;22(2): 259–269, x–xi.
131. **Detre JA, Alsop DC, Vives LR, et al.** Noninvasive MRI evaluation of cerebral blood flow in cerebrovascular disease. *Neurology* 1998;50(3):633–641.
132. **Detre JA, Samuels OB, Alsop DC, et al.** Noninvasive magnetic resonance imaging evaluation of cerebral blood flow with acetazolamide challenge in patients with cerebrovascular stenosis. *J Magn Reson Imaging* 1999;10(5):870–875.
133. **Kamano H, Yoshiura T, Hiwatashi A, et al.** Arterial spin labeling in patients with chronic cerebral artery steno-occlusive disease: correlation with (15)O-PET. *Acta Radiol* 2013;54(1):99–106.
134. **Wang J, Licht DJ.** Pediatric perfusion MR imaging using arterial spin labeling. *Neuroimaging Clin N Am* 2006;16(1):149–167, ix.
135. **Richardson JD, Baker JM, Morgan PS, et al.** Cerebral perfusion in chronic stroke: implications for lesion-symptom mapping and functional MRI. *Behav Neurol* 2011;24(2):117–122.
136. **Saida T, Masumoto T, Nakai Y, et al.** Moyamoya disease: evaluation of postoperative revascularization using multiphase selective arterial spin labeling MRI. *J Comput Assist Tomogr* 2012;36(1):143–149.
137. **van Laar PJ, van der Graaf Y, Mali WP, et al.** Effect of cerebrovascular risk factors on regional cerebral blood flow. *Radiology* 2008;246(1): 198–204.
138. **Jahng GH, Song E, Zhu XP, et al.** Human brain: reliability and reproducibility of pulsed arterial spin-labeling perfusion MR imaging. *Radiology* 2005;234(3):909–916.
139. **Jiang L, Kim M, Chodkowski B, et al.** Reliability and reproducibility of perfusion MRI in cognitively normal subjects. *Magn Reson Imaging* 2010;28(9):1283–1289.
140. **Wang DJ, Alger JR, Qiao JX, et al.** Multi-delay multi parametric arterial spin-labeled perfusion MRI in acute ischemic stroke—Comparison with dynamic susceptibility contrast enhanced perfusion imaging. *Neuroimage Clin* 2013;3:1–7.
141. **Wolf RL, Detre JA.** Clinical neuroimaging using arterial spin-labeled perfusion magnetic resonance imaging. *Neurotherapeutics* 2007;4(3):346–359.
142. **Gunther M, Bock M, Schad LR.** Arterial spin labeling in combination with a look-locker sampling strategy: inflow turbo-sampling EPI-FAIR (ITS-FAIR). *Magn Reson Med* 2001;46(5):974–984.
143. **Mildner T, Moller HE, Driesel W, et al.** Continuous arterial spin labeling at the human common carotid artery: the influence of transit times. *NMR Biomed* 2005;18(1):19–23.
144. **Alsop D, Detre J.** Reduced transit-time sensitivity in noninvasive magnetic resonance imaging of human cerebral blood flow. *JJ Cereb Blood Flow Metab* 1996;16(6):1236–1249.

145. **Wang J, Alsop DC, Song HK, et al.** Arterial transit time imaging with flow encoding arterial spin tagging (FEAST). *Magn Reson Med* 2003;50(3):599–607.
146. **Zaharchuk G, Bammer R, Straka M, et al.** Arterial spin-label imaging in patients with normal bolus perfusion-weighted MR imaging findings: pilot identification of the borderzone sign. *Radiology* 2009;252(3):797–807.
147. **Chng SM, Petersen ET, Zimine I, et al.** Territorial arterial spin labeling in the assessment of collateral circulation: comparison with digital subtraction angiography. *Stroke* 2008;39(12):3248–3254.
148. **Hendrikse J, van Osch MJ, Rutgers DR, et al.** Internal carotid artery occlusion assessed at pulsed arterial spin-labeling perfusion MR imaging at multiple delay times. *Radiology* 2004;233(3):899–904.
149. **Qiu D, Straka M, Zun Z, et al.** CBF measurements using multidelay pseudocontinuous and velocity-selective arterial spin labeling in patients with long arterial transit delays: comparison with xenon CT CBF. *J Magn Reson Imaging* 2012;36(1):110–119.
150. **Golay X, Petersen ET.** Arterial spin labeling: benefits and pitfalls of high magnetic field. *Neuroimaging Clin N Am* 2006;16(2):259–268, x.
151. **Wang J, Alsop DC, Li L, et al.** Comparison of quantitative perfusion imaging using arterial spin labeling at 1.5 and 4.0 Tesla. *Magn Reson Med* 2002;48(2):242–254.
152. **Shimada K, Nagasaka T, Shidahara M, et al.** In vivo measurement of longitudinal relaxation time of human blood by inversion-recovery fast gradient-echo MR imaging at 3T. *Magn Reson Med Sci* 2012;11(4):265–271.
153. **Dobre MC, Ugurbil K, Marjanska M.** Determination of blood longitudinal relaxation time (T1) at high magnetic field strengths. *Magn Reson Imaging* 2007;25(5):733–735.
154. **van Gelderen P, de Zwart JA, Duyn JH.** Pitfalls of MRI measurement of white matter perfusion based on arterial spin labeling. *Magn Reson Med* 2008;59(4):788–795.
155. **van Osch MJ, Teeuwisse WM, van Walderveen MA, et al.** Can arterial spin labeling detect white matter perfusion signal? *Magn Reson Med* 2009;62(1):165–173.
156. **Wong EC, Cronin M, Wu WC, et al.** Velocity-selective arterial spin labeling. *Magn Reson Med* 2006;55(6):1334–1341.
157. **van Laar PJ, van der Grond J, Hendrikse J.** Brain perfusion territory imaging: methods and clinical applications of selective arterial spin-labeling MR imaging. *Radiology* 2008;246(2):354–364.
158. **Hendrikse J, van der Zwan A, Ramos LM, et al.** Altered flow territories after extracranial-intracranial bypass surgery. *Neurosurgery* 2005;57(3):486–494; discussion 486–494.
159. **Jones CE, Wolf RL, Detre JA, et al.** Structural MRI of carotid artery atherosclerotic lesion burden and characterization of hemispheric cerebral blood flow before and after carotid endarterectomy. *NMR Biomed* 2006;19(2):198–208.
160. **Paiva FF, Tannus A, Silva AC.** Measurement of cerebral perfusion territories using arterial spin labelling. *NMR Biomed* 2007;20(7):633–642.
161. **Wang DJ, Alger JR, Qiao JX, et al.** The value of arterial spin-labeled perfusion imaging in acute ischemic stroke: comparison with dynamic susceptibility contrast-enhanced MRI. *Stroke* 2012;43(4):1018–1024.
162. **Bokkers RP, Hernandez DA, Merino JG, et al.** Whole-brain arterial spin labeling perfusion MRI in patients with acute stroke. *Stroke* 2012;43(5):1290–1294.
163. **Huang YC, Liu HL, Lee JD, et al.** Comparison of arterial spin labeling and dynamic susceptibility contrast perfusion MRI in patients with acute stroke. *PLoS One* 2013;8(7):e69085.
164. **Chalela JA, Alsop DC, Gonzalez-Atavales JB, et al.** Magnetic resonance perfusion imaging in acute ischemic stroke using continuous arterial spin labeling. *Stroke* 2000;31:680–687.
165. **Chen J, Licht DJ, Smith SE, et al.** Arterial spin labeling perfusion MRI in pediatric arterial ischemic stroke: initial experiences. *J Magn Reson Imaging* 2009;29(2):282–290.
166. **Qiao XJ, Salamon N, Wang DJ, et al.** Perfusion deficits detected by arterial spin-labeling in patients with TIA with negative diffusion and vascular imaging. *AJNR Am J Neuroradiol* 2013;34(11):2125–2130.
167. **MacIntosh BJ, Lindsay AC, Kylintireas I, et al.** Multiple inflow pulsed arterial spin-labeling reveals delays in the arterial arrival time in minor stroke and transient ischemic attack. *AJNR Am J Neuroradiol* 2010;31(10):1892–1894.
168. **Zaharchuk G, Olivot JM, Fischbein NJ, et al.** Arterial spin labeling imaging findings in transient ischemic attack patients: comparison with diffusion- and bolus perfusion-weighted imaging. *Cerebrovasc Dis* 2012;34(3):221–228.
169. **Mlynash M, Olivot JM, Tong DC, et al.** Yield of combined perfusion and diffusion MR imaging in hemispheric TIA. *Neurology* 2009;72(13):1127–1133.
170. **Campbell AM, Beaulieu C.** Pulsed arterial spin labeling parameter optimization for an elderly population. *J Magn Reson Imaging* 2006;23(3):398–403.
171. **Bokkers RP, van Osch MJ, Klijn CJ, et al.** Cerebrovascular reactivity within perfusion territories in patients with an internal carotid artery occlusion. *J Neurol Neurosurg Psychiatry* 2011;82(9):1011–1016.
172. **Stoll M, Hamann GF.** [Cerebrovascular reserve capacity]. *Der Nervenarzt* 2002;73(8):711–718.
173. **Van Laar PJ, Hendrikse J, Mali WP, et al.** Altered flow territories after carotid stenting and carotid endarterectomy. *J Vasc Surg* 2007;45(6):1155–1161.
174. **Iadecola C.** The overlap between neurodegenerative and vascular factors in the pathogenesis of dementia. *Acta Neuropathol* 2010;120(3):287–296.
175. **Gouw AA, Seewann A, van der Flier WM, et al.** Heterogeneity of small vessel disease: a systematic review of MRI and histopathology correlations. *J Neurol Neurosurg Psychiatry* 2011;82(2):126–135.
176. **Hesselink JR.** Differential diagnostic approach to MR imaging of white matter diseases. *Top Magn Reson Imaging* 2006;17(4):243–263.
177. **Farrall AJ, Wardlaw JM.** Blood-brain barrier: ageing and microvascular disease—systematic review and meta-analysis. *Neurobiol Aging* 2009;30(3):337–352.
178. **Charidimou A, Kakar P, Fox Z, et al.** Cerebral microbleeds and the risk of intracerebral haemorrhage after thrombolysis for acute ischaemic stroke: systematic review and meta-analysis. *J Neurol Neurosurg Psychiatry* 2013;84(3):277–280.
179. **Bastos-Leite AJ, Kuijer JP, Rombouts SA, et al.** Cerebral blood flow by using pulsed arterial spin-labeling in elderly subjects with white matter hyperintensities. *AJNR Am J Neuroradiol* 2008;29(7):1296–1301.
180. **Ishimori Y, Kawamura H, Monma M.** Feasibility of MR perfusion-weighted imaging by use of a time-spatial labeling inversion pulse. *Radiol Phys Technol* 2013;6(2):461–466.
181. **Schmid S, Ghariq E, Teeuwisse WM, et al.** Acceleration-selective arterial spin labeling. *Magn Reson Med* 2014;71(1):191–199.
182. **Wolf RL, Wang J, Detre JA, et al.** Arteriovenous shunt visualization in arteriovenous malformations with arterial spin-labeling MR imaging. *AJNR Am J Neuroradiol* 2008;29(4):681–687.
183. **Suazo L, Foerster B, Fermin R, et al.** Measurement of blood flow in arteriovenous malformations before and after embolization using arterial spin labeling. *Interv Neuroradiol* 2012;18:42–48.
184. **Zettl UK, Stuve O, Patejdl R.** Immune-mediated CNS diseases: a review on nosological classification and clinical features. *Autoimmun Rev* 2012;11(3):167–173.
185. **Lassmann H, Suchanek G, Ozawa K.** Histopathology and the blood-cerebrospinal fluid barrier in multiple sclerosis. *Ann Neurol* 1994;36 suppl:S42–S46.
186. **O'Brien JT.** Role of imaging techniques in the diagnosis of dementia. *Br J Radiol* 2007;80(Spec No 2):S71–S77.
187. **Lycke J, Wikkelso C, Bergh AC, et al.** Regional cerebral blood flow in multiple sclerosis measured by single photon emission tomography with technetium-99m hexamethylpropyleneamine oxime. *Eur Neurol* 1993;33(2):163–167.
188. **Ota M, Sato N, Nakata Y, et al.** Abnormalities of cerebral blood flow in multiple sclerosis: a pseudocontinuous arterial spin labeling MRI study. *Magn Reson Imaging* 2013;31(6):990–995.
189. **Amann M, Achtnichts L, Hirsch JG, et al.** 3D GRASE arterial spin labelling reveals an inverse correlation of cortical perfusion with the white matter lesion volume in MS. *Mult Scler* 2012;18(11):1570–1576.
190. **Rashid W, Parkes LM, Ingle GT, et al.** Abnormalities of cerebral perfusion in multiple sclerosis. *J Neurol Neurosurg Psychiatry* 2004;75(9):1288–1293.
191. **Allen IV, Glover G, Anderson R.** Abnormalities in the macroscopically normal white matter in cases of mild or spinal multiple sclerosis (MS). *Acta Neuropathol Suppl* 1981;7:176–178.
192. **Tofts PS, Kermode AG.** Blood brain barrier permeability in multiple sclerosis using labelled DTPA with PET, CT and MRI. *J Neurol Neurosurg Psychiatry* 1989;52(8):1019–1020.
193. **Howell OW, Reeves CA, Nicholas R, et al.** Meningeal inflammation is widespread and linked to cortical pathology in multiple sclerosis. *Brain* 2011;134(Pt 9):2755–2771.

194. **Magliozzi R, Howell OW, Reeves C, et al.** A Gradient of neuronal loss and meningeal inflammation in multiple sclerosis. *Ann Neurol* 2010;68(4):477–493.
195. **Kim S, Mountz JM.** SPECT imaging of epilepsy: an overview and comparison with F-18 FDG PET. *Int J Mol Imaging* 2011;2011:813028.
196. **Duncan JS.** Imaging in the surgical treatment of epilepsy. *Nat Rev Neurol* 2010;6(10):537–550.
197. **Connor SE, Jarosz JM.** Magnetic resonance imaging of patients with epilepsy. *Clin Radiol* 2001;56(10):787–801.
198. **Lim YM, Cho YW, Shamim S, et al.** Usefulness of pulsed arterial spin labeling MR imaging in mesial temporal lobe epilepsy. *Epilepsy Res* 2008;82(2–3):183–189.
199. **Pizzini F, Farace P, Zanoni T, et al.** Pulsed-arterial-spin-labeling perfusion 3T MRI following single seizure: a first case report study. *Epilepsy Res* 2008;81(2–3):225–227.
200. **Pizzini FB, Farace P, Manganotti P, et al.** Cerebral perfusion alterations in epileptic patients during peri-ictal and post-ictal phase: PASL vs DSC-MRI. *Magn Reson Imaging* 2013l;31(6):1001–1005.
201. **Storti SF, Boscolo Galazzo I, Del Felice A, et al.** Combining ESI, ASL and PET for quantitative assessment of drug-resistant focal epilepsy. *Neuroimage* 2013;102:49–59.
202. **Holmes GL.** Seizure-induced neuronal injury: animal data. *Neurology* 2002;59(9 suppl 5):S3–S6.
203. **Duncan JS.** Seizure-induced neuronal injury: human data. *Neurology* 2002;59(9 suppl 5):S15–S20.
204. **Choi J, Koh S.** Role of brain inflammation in epileptogenesis. *Yonsei Med J* 2008;49(1):1–18.
205. **Ferre JC, Bannier E, Raoult H, et al.** Arterial spin labeling (ASL) perfusion: techniques and clinical use. *Diagn Interv Imaging* 2013;94(12): 1211–1223.
206. **Xavier G.** How to do an ASL multi-center neuroimaging study. *Int Soc Magn Reson Med* 2010; 2010. Retrived from: http://cds.ismrm.org/protected/10MProceedings/files/1_program2.htm
207. **Fallatah SM, Gomez-Anson B, Pizzini FB, et al.** Quality control scoring for arterial spin labelling perfusion maps. *Eur Soc Magn Res Med Biol* 2013;2013:219; Toulouse, France.

CHAPTER

10 Ultrasound Perfusion Imaging: Techniques and Analytical Methods

Emilio Quaia, MD

Introduction

The ability to accurately quantify tissue perfusion—blood flow equalized for the volume or weight of the perfused tissue ($cm^3/s/cm^3$ or grams)—is essential for the assessment of the physiologic functionality and viability of a tissue. Different parameters are related to tissue perfusion including blood velocity (cm/s), the speed of red blood cells in the region analyzed, blood flow (cm^3/s), the volume of blood passing in a section of tissue per unit of time, the fractional vascular volume (cm^3), and the proportion of tissue volume occupied by blood.

Single photon emission computed tomography (SPECT), positron emission tomography (PET), multidetector computed tomography (CT), and magnetic resonance (MR) imaging all quantify tissue perfusion accurately.

PET with (15)O-water, (13)N-ammonia, (82)RbCl, or (62)Cu-ETS and imaging techniques, MR and CT, with contrast administration represent valuable tools to assess noninvasively organ perfusion. However, the utility of PET is limited because of the short half-life of most of the radiolabeled tracers.

MR advantages include absence of ionizing radiations, high spatial resolution, and use of intravascular agents (high serum albumin binding). MR limitations include the nonlinear relation between signal intensity (SI) and gadolinium concentration at high concentrations due to concomitant reduction of T_1 and T_2* (use < 0.1 mmol/kg usually 0.0125 mmol/kg), the gadolinium contrast that should be avoided when GFR is less than 30 mL/min/1.73 m^2, the difficulty of measuring the arterial input function, and limited availability for perfusion studies.

CT advantages include direct and constant linearity between renal tissue attenuation and the concentration of contrast medium. Advanced scanners are available (EBCT or MDCT) allowing a high temporal resolution. CT limitations include radiation and iodinated agents and limited use in renal failure.

Unenhanced ultrasound (US) is not useful for organ perfusion quantification, while color Doppler and power Doppler are limited by the low sensitivity to low-velocity flow in smaller vessels (<2 mm in diameter). Dynamic contrast-enhanced ultrasound (CEUS) can be used to quantify microbubble enhancement and has recently been proposed as a new imaging technique for quantifying tissue perfusion.[1] CEUS is an imaging modality that presents several advantages, including low financial cost, portability, availability, lack of restrictions in performing frequent serial examinations at short intervals, real-time assessment of mural enhancement after contrast injection, absence of radiation exposure, the use of blood pool contrast agents, and absence of usage of potentially nephrotoxic contrast agents.

Ultrasound Technology

In the last decade, the image quality in US had important improvements due to technology advancements particularly in the new array transducers with a high number of elements, in the US systems with numerous focus lines, and in the computer processing power corresponding to a powerful beamformer with higher resolution and higher dynamic range in the images. The most important technologic advances in the US field were introduced in the signal transmission process, in the signal reception process, in compounding and equalization, in color and power Doppler, and in the 3D and elastographic imaging.[2]

Signal Transmission

In the signal transmission process, the transducer arrays, formed by ceramic polymer composite elements of variable shape and thickness, and the multilayered technology led to a more accurate shaping of the US pulses in terms of frequency, amplitude, phase, and length. The development of piezoelectric crystals with a lower acoustic impedance and greater electromechanical coupling coefficients, the improvement of the physical characteristics of the absorbing backing layers, and the quarter-wave impedance matching layers represent the most significant results of the US transducer research.[2]

Increased bandwidth of transducers allows a better spatial and contrast resolution with a consequent improvement of the axial resolution due to shorter pulse length. Shorter transmission pulses used in a broadband emission generates shorter echo pulses that can be faithfully converted into electric signals. Since short pulses are attenuated to a greater extent and are characterized by less penetration than long pulses, specific techniques have been introduced by the different manufacturers to allow a more accurate shaping of the US pulse in terms of the control of the transmission frequency, amplitude, phase, and pulse length. Phase can only be determined by the comparison with a reference waveform or with another pulse. This can be achieved by using multiple beamformers allowing the direct integration of the phase information from the signal received from the adjacent lines.[2] Another way to improve penetration is by increasing the output power, even though it is limited by safety limits, or by utilizing excitation signals much more sophisticated than the single-carrier short pulses currently used in the US scanners. These signals are usually defined coded excitation and increase the signal-to-noise ratio and the frame rate. In coded-emission mode, the scanner transmits not a single pulse but a sequence of 8 to 22 short, high-frequency transmission pulses that may have different phases and are modulated in a code sequence. Comparison between transmitted pulses and received signal shapes using matched filtering (decoding) is subsequently performed with a very high sampling rate.[2] In chirp encoding, a long specially shaped pulse is transmitted with frequency and amplitude progressively varied. The matched filtering process involves comparing the echoes with a stored reference version of the transmitted chirp. When the two waveforms present identical shape but different amplitude, they are out of alignment and the output of the process is low. The filter output is a large-amplitude compressed pulse for every match between a genuine chirp echo and the reference chirp.

Electronic focusing, obtained by activating a series of elements in the array with appropriate delay, can easily be used to regulate the focal depth. The higher the number of channels involved to activate the array elements in a combined mode and with the appropriate delays, the more accurately the US beam can be focused. In the dynamic transmit focusing modality, edge crystal elements have a longer pulse excitation than center elements, making the US beam focus at two different points in the insonated field, improving lateral resolution. As the resulting wave front has the characteristics of a short excitation pulse, the axial resolution is preserved.[2] The spatial and contrast resolution of the US image had a further improvement due to matrix transducers, which allows a further reduction in the thickness of the US beam with better spatial resolution.

Signal Reception

Tissue harmonic imaging has allowed a further improvement in the signal-to-noise ratio and image quality due to the improved contrast resolution and speckle and artifact reduction even in patients with a limited explorability including obese patients. Harmonic imaging requires large transducer bandwidth and that the system is configured to receive preferentially harmonic components produced by tissues, hence at double the transmitted frequency, by a high-pass filter, and to cancel out the fundamental echo signals generated directly from the transmitted acoustic energy. Such filtering is successful in eliminating echoes from solid stationary tissues that present prevalently linear properties, even though the effect is to reduce the range of frequencies (or bandwidth) contained in the received echoes, causing a low spatial axial resolution of the resulting image. Harmonic imaging and speckle reduction techniques have improved signal-to-noise ratio and image quality also in patients who are difficult to explore by US, such as obese or large-body-habitus subjects.

Compound Imaging and Equalization

Compound imaging may be obtained by spatial (transmit compounding) or frequency compound. In spatial compound imaging, the same insonated slice is interrogated according to different insonation angles, while in frequency compound imaging, the same slice is insonated more times with different frequencies. The resulting images are managed by subtracting step by step all echoes, which appears incoherently in the different acquired images, corresponding essentially to noise. Compound imaging allows a reduction of speckles, clutter, and noise, without compromising other beneficial image characteristics such as spatial resolution, and improves contrast-to-noise ratio and better depiction of the curved surface such as the renal poles. Compounding also reduces shadowing from strongly reflecting interfaces such as organ boundaries, fascial planes, and vessel walls.

Tissue equalization is based on regional and adaptive methods to analyze, using regional speckle statistics and thermal noise identification, and applies an algorithm to perform region-by-region adjustment to lateral gain, depth gain, and overall gain.[2]

Color and Power Doppler

The color and power Doppler techniques have reached a high sensitivity for the renal parenchymal flows. In particular, the introduction of wideband Doppler technology, making use of short pulses, has led to some advantages in imaging subtle blood flows due to the improved frame rate and axial resolution. Differently from color Doppler, the sensitivity of power Doppler for the renal flows is not dependent from the angle of insonation. Moreover, power Doppler has a higher sensitivity than color Doppler for the renal parenchyma flow in particular at renal poles. The introduction of wideband color Doppler (e.g., advanced dynamic flow) has improved the sensitivity and contrast resolution for the flow signal of the renal parenchymal vessels up to the interlobular vessels, which can be imaged with a 2- to 5-MHz convex US transducer. 3D US (volume sonography), elastography, and microbubble contrast agents represent further advancements in US.

3D Imaging

3D US acquisition is obtained by using multidimensional matrix transducers with parallel processing of the signal. Digitally stored volume data can then be displayed in a multiplanar array that simultaneously shows three perpendicular planes throughout the volume: axial, sagittal, and reconstructed coronal views. The volume can be explored by scrolling through parallel planes in any of the three views and by rotating the volume to obtain an optimal view of the structure of interest.[2] Data can also be displayed as true 3D images using various rendering algorithms, including maximum-intensity projections and surface renderings.

Microbubble Contrast Agents

Microbubble contrast agents are hemodynamically inert, remain entirely intravascular, and also have the same rheology as red blood cells. Although larger microbubbles produce much greater acoustic signals, their maximum size is limited by the diameter of the capillary so that intravenously administered agents may cross the pulmonary microcirculation—which is approximately 5 μm. The limitations of a small microbubble became evident with the first commercial air-filled microbubble agent that was made by sonication of a solution of 5% human albumin. The mean microbubble size of 4.3 μm allowed it to clear the pulmonary circulation following an intravenous injection, but the air rapidly diffused out along the concentration gradient into the surrounding blood, with a resultant decrease in bubble size and backscatter signal. This inevitably meant that by the time the microbubbles had cleared the pulmonary circulation, their ability to opacify the myocardium was already substantially diminished. Therefore, the majority of studies using this agent for myocardial perfusion relied on direct intracoronary injections.

The need to improve microbubble persistence in the circulation was eventually overcome by the incorporation of high molecular weight gases with low diffusibility and solubility or by the use of gas-impermeable polymer shells into new-generation microbubbles. The gas proved to diffuse out of the microbubbles at a much slower rate, which meant that microbubbles had the ability to maintain their size and significantly increase their half-life within the circulation. The new-generation microbubbles currently approved for clinical use in the United States share a number of similarities in that they are composed of a thin shell that enclose a core of perfluorocarbon gas. A number of other microbubbles are in various phases of development and approval.

Apart from their stability, microbubble contrast agents possess a number of unique properties that distinguish them from tracers used with other noninvasive imaging technologies. The microbubbles remain entirely intravascular, unlike nuclear tracers such as thallium or ^{99m}Tc-sestamibi, which are extracted by myocytes, or radiologic contrast agents for CT or gadolinium tracers for MR imaging that diffuse into the interstitial space. Consequently, microbubble contrast agents are the ideal tracers of red blood cell kinetics and to assess organ perfusion. The microbubbles are also hemodynamically inert, so they do not affect local or systemic blood flow. By comparing the transit of microbubbles with Tc-labeled red blood cells, or by direct visualization of fluorescently labeled microbubbles and red blood cells, the in vivo myocardial kinetics and rheology of microbubbles have been shown to be very close to that of red blood cells.

Nowadays, microbubble contrast agents for ultrasound (US) (Table 10.1) have a diameter of 2 to 6 μm.[3] The microbubble shell may be stiff (e.g., denatured albumin) or flexible (phospholipids) and has a thickness of 10 to 200 nm. New-generation microbubbles are filled with a high molecular weight gas (e.g., perfluorocarbon or sulfur hexafluoride) with low solubility in the bloodstream. Microbubbles have a purely intravascular distribution even though some agents present a postvascular hepato- and/or splenospecific phase beginning 5 minutes after intravenous injection and lasting from 15 minutes up to 1 hour after injection.[3] The microbubble gas content is exhaled via the lungs 10 to 15 minutes after injection, while the components of the shell are metabolized by the liver or filtered by the kidney and eliminated by the liver. Adverse reactions in humans are rare, usually transient, and of mild intensity.[4] Hypotensive reactions have been observed after microbubble injection, and some deaths have been reported in cardiac patients.

At resonant frequency (f_o), the microbubble radial oscillation becomes efficient and exaggerated[5]; the scattering cross section of a microbubble is no longer simply dependent on microbubble size and can reach peak values a thousand times higher than values at off-resonance. The insonation power is usually expressed by the mechanical index (MI) defined as $p-/\sqrt{f}$ where $p-$ is the largest peak negative pressure and f is the center frequency of the pulse. When acoustic pressures at or near the resonant frequency are sufficiently high, nonlinear microbubble oscillation develops, producing harmonic frequencies.

Innovative US techniques, named contrast-specific modes or techniques,[6] were introduced to register selectively the harmonic signal produced by the nonlinear physical behavior of microbubbles and to distinguish microbubble signal from tissue clutter. This was determined by the impossibility of traditional color and power Doppler to manage the harmonic signals produced by microbubble insonation, since they are limited by the strong presence of artifacts including the blooming and jail bar artifacts. *Pulse inversion* is the best-known phase modulation technique. *Vascular recognition imaging* combines Doppler information with phase analysis and involves the transmission of four, alternately inverted, pulses along each imaging line. *Cadence contrast pulse sequencing* works by interrogating each imaging line a number of times with pulses with various amplitudes and phases. Both harmonic and nonlinear fundamental signals from microbubbles are represented on a grayscale or color map suppressing the linear fundamental echoes from native tissues.

Chemical Composition of Microbubble Contrast Agents

Microbubble contrast agents are now approved in most European countries and are largely employed also in Asia and Canada. The Food and Drug Administration in the United States has not yet approved microbubble contrast agents for noncardiac use. The recently introduced sulfur hexafluoride or perfluorocarbon-filled microbubbles (Table 10.1) offer both an excellent safety profile and a longer persistence in the peripheral circle than air-filled microbubbles. Microbubble contrast agents are composed by a shell of biocompatible material such as a proteins, lipids, or biopolymers. Microbubble contrast agents are injectable intravenously and can pass through the pulmonary capillary bed after a peripheral injection, since their diameter (3 to 10 μm) is below that of red blood cells.

Two principal strategies were developed to increase microbubble stability and persistence in the bloodstream: the stability in the peripheral bloodstream of the external microbubble encapsulation

TABLE 10.1 **Microbubble Contrast Agents Classified According to the Filling Gas**

Perfluorocarbon	Sulfur Hexafluoride
Definity (Lantheus Medical Imaging)	SonoVue (Bracco)
Sonazoid (GE Healthcare)	
Optison (GE Healthcare)[a]	

Note: The list includes the available microbubble contrast agents.
Imavist (Imagent; Alliance), Quantison (Quadrant), and Echogen (Sonus Pharmaceuticals) did not achieve the clinical use. Echovist and Levovist (Bayer-Schering) and Albunex (Mallinckrodt) are not presently employed. Cardiosphere (Point Biomedical) is no longer developed.
One other agent, Zhifuxian, is being developed by Chinese hospitals and is nearing clinical use.
All available agents present a phospholipid shell. SonoVue is currently approved and marketed within European countries. Definity is approved in the United States for cardiology, while Sonazoid (GE Healthcare) is licensed in Japan for liver imaging.
In perfluorocarbon-filled agents, the filling gas is perfluorobutane (e.g., Optison and Sonazoid), octafluoropropane (e.g., Definity), or perfluorohexane (e.g., Imagent).
[a]Albumin shell; likely to be rereleased to the market.

and the selection of filling gases with a low diffusion coefficient. The peripheral shell presents a thickness ranging from 10 to 200 nm and may be stiff (e.g., denatured albumin or biopolymers) or more flexible (phospholipids). Low-solubility low-diffusibility gases, such as perfluorocarbons and sulfur hexafluoride gas, are employed to improve the persistence of microbubbles in the peripheral bloodstream. The physical properties of microbubble contrast agents are closely related not only to their gas content and to the peripheral shell chemical composition but also to the frequency of the US beam, to the pulse repetition frequency and, overall, to the acoustic power employed for insonation. The different microbubble contrast agents are reported in Table 10.1.

Safety of Microbubble Contrast Agents

The safety of microbubble contrast agents is somewhat complex because not only must their safety as drugs be studied, as with other contrast agents, but additionally, the effects of sonication need to be taken into account. The safety of ultrasound contrast media is the subject of a recent report by the World Federation for Ultrasound in Medicine and Biology.[4] The adverse reactions in humans are rare, usually transient, and of mild intensity and include tissue irritation in the vicinity of the injection site, dyspnea, chest pain, hypo- or hypertension, nausea and vomiting, taste alterations, headache, vertigo, warm facial sensation, cutaneous eruptions, and asymptomatic premature ventricular contractions. However, serious allergic reactions have been observed at a very low incidence (estimated to be 1:10,000).

In 2004, the European Agency for the Evaluation of Medicinal Products (EMEA) temporarily withdrew the approval for SonoVue (Bracco, Milan, Italy) for cardiac applications due to three deaths reported in temporal relation with the application of SonoVue. All patients did not present any allergic reaction, but all of them had unstable ischemic heart disease. Nineteen cases of severe, nonfatal adverse events (0.002%) were reported, and most of the cases were considered to be allergic reactions. The EMEA committee recognized a favorable risk/benefit ratio for SonoVue when patients with acute coronary syndromes and unstable heart disease were excluded, and the committee otherwise restored the approval for cardiac indications. Even more recently, the FDA issued a black box warning for Definity in October 2007 due to postmarketing reports of deaths in four patients with significant underlying progressive cardiovascular disease that were temporally related to contrast agent use. On May 12, 2008, and June 6, 2008, revised labeling changes were again implemented for Definity and Optison, respectively, following mounting evidence of safety and unequivocally favorable risk–benefit profile in the acute setting. The present FDA documents state that Definity and Optison are not to be administered to patients in whom right-to-left bidirectional or transient right-to-left cardiac shunts and hypersensitivity to perflutren, blood products, or albumin are known or suspected. SonoVue is contraindicated in patients known to have right-to-left shunts, severe pulmonary hypertension (pulmonary artery pressure >90 mmHg), uncontrolled systemic hypertension, and in patients with adult respiratory distress syndrome. Both Definity and Optison may be used in acute coronary syndromes. SonoVue should be used with special caution in patients with recent acute coronary syndrome or clinically unstable ischaemic cardiac disease. The intra-arterial injection of ultrasound contrast agents also is contraindicated.

Experimental studies on small animals and cell preparation have shown that potential adverse bioeffects from microbubble contrast agents under a US field, including hemolysis, platelet aggregation, disruption of cell membrane, rupture of small vessels, and induction of ectopic heart beats, can be induced under extreme conditions (exteriorized heart preparation, no or minimal attenuation, low-frequency high acoustic pressures, and long pulse durations). The phenomenon of inertial cavitation—the rapid formation, growth, and collapse of a gas cavity in a fluid as a result of US exposure—is considered the cause of most of the microbubble side effects observed in animals in experimental studies, and no evidence of bioeffects from a clinically comparable US exposure and microbubble concentration has been reported in humans. These experimental findings cannot be extrapolated to the clinical setting where the attenuation of ultrasound significantly reduces patient exposure, even though these conditions could be reproduced also in the clinical setting during lithotripsy and focused ultrasound ablation.

Microbubble Persistence in the Bloodstream: Physical Factors

To act as effective contrast agents in the peripheral circulation, microbubble contrast agents have to persist in the bloodstream. Various chemical strategies have been adopted to produce stabilized gas microbubbles in the peripheral circulation, and the different compositions have an important influence upon the performance of the resulting agent.

Diffusibility of the Filling Gas

The first factor that determines the persistence of microbubbles in the peripheral circle is the diffusibility of the filling gas throughout the peripheral shell.[5] The diffusibility, expressed by the diffusion coefficient, and the solubility of the filling gas in the blood strongly affect microbubble persistence in the circle, according to the following equation:

$$T = \frac{\rho R^2}{2DC_s} \tag{1}$$

where T is the microbubble persistence in the blood, ρ is the density of the gas, R is the initial radius of the microbubble, D is the diffusion coefficient of the gas in the substance of the shell, and C_s is the saturation coefficient of exchange of gas between aqueous and gaseous phases, which is higher in gas with increased solubility in the blood.

Surface Tension

The previous equation is an effective approximation of the microbubbles persistence in the bloodstream. Anyway, the surface tension is another important mechanism responsible for the disappearance of the filling microbubble gas in a gas-saturated liquid.[5] The microbubble shell contains surface-active molecules, namely, phospholipids, which act as surfactant reducing the surface tension. The surfactant layer exerts a counterpressure against the tendency of surface tension and other forces to cause gas diffusion from a microbubble. The relation of the surface tension with microbubble dissolution is

$$\frac{dR}{dt} = D \times L \left(\frac{\frac{C_i}{C_s} - 1 - \frac{2S_T}{Rp_0}}{1 + \frac{4S_T}{3Rp_0}} \right) \left(\frac{1}{R} + \frac{1}{\sqrt{\pi D t}} \right) \tag{2}$$

where $\left(\frac{dR}{dt}\right)$ is the variation of microbubble radius (R), with time (t), which is related to microbubble disappearance from the peripheral circle; D is the diffusion coefficient of the gas; L is the Ostwald coefficient, which corresponds to the ratio of the amount of gas dissolved in the surrounding liquid and in the gas phase per unit volume; C_i/C_s is the ratio of the dissolved gas concentration to the saturation concentration; S_T is the surface tension; and p_0 is the ambient pressure. In Eq. (2), the surface tension is showed to strongly affect the dissolution of microbubbles, and the higher is the surface tension, the lower is the microbubble persistence.

Osmotic Pressure of the Filling Gas

The stability of a microbubble in the peripheral circle is related to the osmotic pressure of the filling gas, which counters the sum of the surface tension and blood arterial pressure[5]:

$$(C_G + C_A)K \times T = \frac{2S_T}{R} + p_b + p_{atm} \quad (3)$$

where C_G and C_A are concentrations of the filling gas ($_G$) and air ($_A$), K is the gas constant, T is the absolute temperature, S_T is the surface tension, R is the bubbles radius, p_b is the systemic blood pressure, and p_{atm} is the atmospheric pressure (101 kPa). The limited solubility in blood determines an elevated vapor concentration in the microbubble relative to the surrounding blood and establishes an osmotic gradient that opposes the gas diffusion out of the microbubble. After the initial size adjustment due to the effect of body temperature, the microbubbles will either swell or shrink depending on the partial pressure of the air in the bubble, followed by a period of slow diffusion of gas into the bloodstream.

Diffusion and Ostwald Coefficients

Also, diffusion and Ostwald coefficients strongly determine the rate of decrease of the bubble radius, which is a direct measure for the disappearance rate of the microbubble:

$$-\frac{d}{dt}(C_G R^3) = 3RD_G L_G C_G \quad (4)$$

$$-\frac{d}{dt}(C_A R^3) = 3RD_A L_A \left(C_A - \frac{p_{atm}}{KT}\right) \quad (5)$$

where C_G and C_A are concentrations of the filling gas ($_G$) and air ($_A$); R is the bubbles radius; D_G, D_a and L_G, L_a are diffusion and Ostwald coefficients, respectively, for the filling gas ($_G$) and the air ($_A$); p_{atm} is the atmospheric pressure (101 kPa); K is the gas constant; and T is the absolute temperature. From Eqs. (4) and (5), it can be derived that the diffusion and Ostwald coefficients determine the rate of decrease of the bubble radius, which is a direct measure for the disappearance rate of the microbubble. Thus, microbubble filled with gases having lower diffusion and/or Ostwald coefficient will persist longer in the bloodstream.

Nature of the Peripheral Capsule

The nature of the encapsulating shell is the last fundamental factor, which affects microbubble persistence in the bloodstream.[5] Of course, the more stable is the peripheral shell or the less is its solubility in the water, the longer is the microbubble persistence and the echo-enhancing effect. Galactose-covered microbubbles present a low persistence for the high solubility of the sugar in the water. New-generation microbubble-based agents present an albumin or lipid shell, which presents a low solubility in the water, further improving microbubble persistence in the bloodstream and the effect of scattering.

Physical Basis and Principles of Action of Microbubble Contrast Agents

Resonance Frequency

Encapsulation of microbubbles affects their ability to oscillate, due to the presence of viscoelastic damping effects determined by the shell, which influence the microbubble acoustic properties. To produce effective backscattering, microbubbles have to be insonated by their characteristic resonance frequency, and the exposure to US at their resonance frequency forces microbubbles to contract and expand their diameter severalfold.[5] At low acoustic power, microbubbles produce a US signal with the same frequency as the sound that excited them. By increasing the acoustic power of insonation, microbubbles exhibit nonlinear vibrations at their resonance frequency (f_0) generating signals at f_0, harmonics ($2f_0$, $3f_0$, $4f_0$, etc.), and subharmonics ($f_0/2$, $f_0/3$, etc.). At further higher acoustic power, the expansion eventually disrupts the microbubbles' shell generating a wideband harmonic signal similar to a burst.

The resonance—fundamental—frequency (f_0) is inversely related to the microbubble diameter, and it may be expressed as

$$f_0 \approx \frac{1}{2\pi R}\sqrt{\frac{3\gamma p_0}{\rho_0}} \quad (6)$$

where R is the microbubble diameter, γ is the ideal adiabatic constant of gas, p_0 is the ambient fluid pressure, and ρ_0 is the density of the surrounding medium. To derive Eq. (6), the damping caused by the surrounding medium is assumed negligible, as no effects due to bubble surface tension or thermal conductivity.

Considering the same model employed for the backscattering of an air-filled microbubble surrounded by a thin elastic shell and taking into account the increased restoring force due to shell elasticity,

$$f_0 \approx \frac{1}{2\pi R}\sqrt{\frac{3\gamma}{\rho}\left(P_0 + \frac{\pi}{3\gamma}\frac{S_e}{r}\right)} \quad (7)$$

where S_e is the shell elasticity parameter, which is defined as

$$S_e = 8\pi \frac{R_o - R_i}{1 - \nu} E \quad (8)$$

where R_i and R_o are the inner (i) and the outer (o) diameters of the microbubble (the difference $R_o - R_i$ is the thickness of the shell); ν is the Poisson ratio, which describes the ratio of transverse contraction strain to longitudinal extension strain in the direction of stretching acoustic pressure (tensile deformation is considered positive, and compressive deformation is considered negative); and E is the modulus of Young—modulus of elasticity in tension—which describes the stiffness of a microbubble.

According to Eq. (7), the higher is the shell elasticity due to encapsulation, the higher is the resonant frequency, at equivalent microbubble radius. Moreover, the lower is the shell elasticity due to encapsulation, the lower is the generation of harmonics, due to the damping provided by the shell viscosity, which produces a notable decrease in the pulsation amplitude. So, for a stiff and thick shell, the stability in the peripheral blood is higher if compared with a flexible and thin shell, but production of harmonics is lower. In practical terms, for any given US power and frequency, less acoustic signal can be expected from microbubbles with thick, stiff shells. Since microbubble with a thick and stiff shells present an increased resistance to the US acoustic power of insonation, the produced acoustical backscattering signal may be improved simply by increasing the acoustic power of insonation.

Moreover, according to Eq. (7), the ideal resonant frequency for a microbubble is inversely related to the square of its radius. The larger the microbubble radius, the lower the resonance frequency, and the resonance frequency of microbubble with a diameter of few μm is in the low MHz frequency range, which is employed in abdominal US. Specifically, the resonance frequency for phospholipid-coated microbubbles with a diameter of 1 to 5 μm is approximately 3-4MHz.

Backscattering

According to the most accepted physical model describing microbubble backscattering properties, the microbubble is considered coated by a continuous layer of incompressible solid elastic material, with a spherically symmetric motion, and surrounded by an incompressible liquid, which presents infinite extent and a constant viscosity according to the Newton law. A Newtonian fluid is a fluid in which the shear stress—the ratio of force up to the area subjected to the force—is proportional to viscosity and velocity gradient. The rheologic parameters (surface tension and viscosity) for microbubble-based agents may be calculated. The wavelength of the US field is assumed to be much larger than the microbubble diameter, and only the motion of the bubble surface is of interest. It is assumed that the vapor pressure remains constant during the compression and expansion phase and that there is no rectified diffusion during the short period of exposure to US. The gas in the bubble is assumed to be ideal and compressed and expanded according to the ideal gas law with the polytropic exponent (Γ) remaining constant during vibration.

The first parameter to be considered in the backscattering is the motion of the microbubble wall:

$$\rho R\ddot{R} + \frac{3}{2}\rho\dot{R}^2 = p_L - p_\infty \tag{9}$$

where ρ is the density of the surrounding liquid medium (=998 kg/m^3), R is the instantaneous microbubble radius, $\dot{R}$ is the first-time derivative of the radius (the velocity of the microbubble wall), $\ddot{R}$ is the second-time derivative of the radius (the acceleration of the microbubble wall), p_L is the liquid pressure at the microbubble wall, and p_∞ is the liquid pressure at infinity.

The assumption is that presence of the microbubble shell completely dominates the motion of the microbubble wall. Therefore, the microbubbles are considered to be elastic particles, which have an effective bulk modulus, K_{eff}, describing the elasticity of the shell and a friction parameter describing the viscosity of the shell.

Bulk Modulus ≈ Elasticity of the Shell

The effective bulk modulus describes the elasticity of the shell. For a spherical volume V deformed by a quasi-static pressure change, ΔP determines the volume change of the microbubble and it is uniform over the microbubble surface. The volume strain (deformation) corresponds to $-\frac{\Delta V}{V}$, where V is the initial volume and ΔV is the change in volume, while the volume stress (ΔP) corresponds to the ratio of the magnitude of the normal force to the area.[5,6] The effective bulk modulus—K_{eff}—is given by the ratio of the volume stress to the volume strain:

$$K_{eff} = -V\frac{\Delta P}{\Delta V} \tag{10}$$

Since the volume is spherical, symmetric, and defined by the radius, the volume strain can be written as

$$\frac{\Delta V}{V} = \left(\frac{R}{R_0}\right)^3 - 1 \tag{11}$$

where R_0 is the initial microbubble radius. Combining Eqs. (10) and (11) gives

$$\Delta P = -K_{eff}\left[\left(\frac{R}{R_0}\right) - 1\right] \tag{12}$$

Friction Damping ≈ Viscosity of the Shell

The friction damping parameter describes the viscosity of the shell.[5,6] Since the pressure change, ΔP, determining the volume change of the microbubble, can be split into three parts: (a) the liquid pressure at the bubble wall (p_L), (b) the damping pressure caused by friction damping of the system bubble—liquid (p_d), and (c) the hydrostatic pressure (p_0), it may be expressed as

$$\Delta P = p_L + p_d - p_0 \tag{13}$$

Substitution of Eqs. (12) and (13) into Eq. (9) and using the expanded expression for p_∞ ($p_\infty = p_0 + P_{(t)}$, where p_0 is the hydrostatic pressure and $P_{(t)}$ is the time-varying applied acoustic pressure) yield

$$\rho R\ddot{R} + \frac{3}{2}\rho\dot{R}^2 = -K_{eff}\left[\left(\frac{R}{R_0}\right)^3 - 1\right] - p_d - P_{(t)} \tag{14}$$

By equating the damping pressure, multiplied by the bubble surface, to the damping force, an expression for p_d can be derived from the equation of motion of a damped forced oscillator:

$$4\pi R^2 p_d = \beta\dot{R} \tag{15}$$

where β is the mechanical resistance, R is the instantaneous microbubble radius, and $\dot{R}$ is the first time derivative of the radius (the velocity of the microbubble wall).

The total viscous and friction damping coefficient, $\delta_{tot} = \frac{\beta}{\omega m}$, where ω is the insonating frequency of the applied acoustic field and m is the effective microbubble mass $\left(\frac{4}{3}\pi R^3\rho\right)$, the damping pressure can be written as

$$p_d = \delta_{tot}\rho\omega R\dot{R} \tag{16}$$

where $\delta_{tot} = \delta_{rad} + \delta_{vis} + \delta_{th} + \delta_{fr}$ and δ_{rad} is the damping coefficient due to reradiation; δ_{vis} is the damping coefficient due to the viscosity of the surrounding medium; δ_{th} is the damping coefficient due to heat conduction; and δ_{fr} is the damping coefficient due to internal friction or viscosity of the shell.

Including friction damping, the final expression for the Rayleigh-Plesset theory is

$$\rho R\ddot{R} + \frac{3}{2}\rho\dot{R}^2 = p_{go}\left(\frac{R_0}{R}\right)^{3\Gamma} + p_v - p_o - \frac{2S_T}{R} - \delta_{tot}\omega\rho R\dot{R} - P_{(t)} \tag{17}$$

or

$$\rho R\ddot{R} + \frac{3}{2}\rho\dot{R}^2 = -K_{eff}\left[\left(\frac{R_0}{R}\right)^3 - 1\right] - \delta_{tot}\rho\omega R\dot{R} - P_{(t)} \tag{18}$$

or

$$\rho R\ddot{R} + \frac{3}{2}\rho\dot{R}^2 = p_{go} - p_0 - \frac{2S_T}{R} - \frac{4\eta}{R}\dot{R} \tag{19}$$

or

$$\rho R\ddot{R} + \frac{3}{2}\rho\dot{R}^2 = p_{go}\left(\frac{R_0}{R}\right)^{3\Gamma} - \frac{2S_T}{R} - \frac{4\eta R}{R} - p_0 + P_{(t)}\sin\omega t \tag{20}$$

where R is the instantaneous microbubble radius; $\dot{R}$ is the first time derivative of the radius (the velocity of the microbubble wall); $\ddot{R}$ is the second time derivative of the radius (the acceleration of the microbubble wall); p_{go} is the initial internal gas pressure in the microbubble (=[$C_A + C_G$]RT, where C_A and C_G are concentrations of the filling air and gas, respectively, and T is the absolute temperature); R_0 is the initial microbubble radius; Γ is the polytropic exponent of the gas; p_v is the vapor pressure; p_o is the ambient hydrostatic pressure; S_T is the surface tension; δ_{tot} is the total damping constant;

ω is the angular frequency of the applied acoustic field; ρ is the density of the surrounding medium; $P_{(t)}$ is the time-varying applied acoustic pressure; η is the shear viscosity of liquid; ω is the driving frequency; and t is the time. These differential equations predict that the surface shell supports a strain that counters the surface tension and thereby stabilizes the microbubble against dissolution.

Scattering Cross Section—Echogenicity of Microbubbles

The scattering cross section, σ, is used as the parameter defining the acoustic behavior of the microbubble and is defined as the quotient of the acoustic power scattered in all directions per unit incident acoustic intensity.[5,6] The scattered US intensity (I_s) is a function of the incident intensity I_0, the distance between the receiving transducer and the scatterer z, and the scattering cross section of the scatterer σ according to

$$I_s = \frac{I_0 \sigma}{4\pi z^2} \tag{21}$$

The scattering cross section is directly related to the scattered acoustic power and to microbubble radius and inversely related to the applied pressure.

The general expression for the scattering cross section in the frequency domain including higher harmonics is

$$\sigma(R,\omega) = 4\pi R_0^2 \frac{\Omega^4}{(1-\Omega)^2 + (\Omega\delta)^2} \tag{22}$$

where R is the microbubble radius, R_0 is the initial microbubble radius, ω is the insonating frequency, $\Omega = \dfrac{\omega}{f_0}$ with f_0 is the resonance frequency, and δ is the damping constant.

Equation (22) may be further developed as

$$\sigma = \frac{4\pi R_0^2}{\left[\left(\frac{f_0}{f}\right)^2 - 1\right]^2} + \left(\frac{f_0}{f}\right)^4 \delta^2 \tag{23}$$

$$\sigma = \frac{4\pi}{9} k^4 R^6 \left[\left(\frac{k_s - k}{k}\right)^2 + \frac{1}{3}\left(\frac{3(\rho_s - \rho)}{2\rho_s + \rho}\right)^2\right] \tag{24}$$

where δ is the damping constant, ρ is the density respectively of the scatterer (subscript s, microbubble) and the surrounding medium (tissue or plasma), and k is the adiabatic compressibility. The k and ρ are also related to the speed of sound ($c = 1/\sqrt{\rho k}$). Consequently, the scattering cross section is strongly dependent from frequency both for free air and encapsulated microbubbles and from the difference in density between the microbubble and the surrounding medium.

At the resonant frequency, the scattering cross section of a microbubble is no longer simply dependent on their size and can reach peak values a thousand times higher compared to values at off-resonance frequencies. Since the scattering cross section is strongly dependent between the ratio between the insonating frequency and the resonant frequency (Eq. (23)), at frequency below resonance most of the scattering occurs at 180 degrees relative to the incident wave, with an angular distribution pattern depending on the scatterer shape and the contrast in the acoustic properties between the particle and the surrounding medium.

The compressibility (k value, see Eq. (24)) of air is 7.65 × 10^{-6} m^2/N, and the compressibility of water is 4.5 × 10^{-11} m^2/N, similarly to tissue and plasma, while the compressibility of a coated microbubble-based agents falls within this range (5 × 10^{-7} m^2/N in the case of Albunex). This high difference in compressibility, and so in impedance, results in a very high echogenicity, which increases the sensitivity of the US equipments to microbubble.

Scattering cross-sectional equations may be simplified to

$$\sigma = R_0^6 f_0^4 \; [\approx Z] \tag{25}$$

known as Born approximation, where R_0 is the initial microbubble radius, f_0 is the resonance frequency, and Z is the difference in acoustic impedance (ratio of acoustic pressure to sound flow) between the surrounding medium and the microbubble. Encapsulation drastically reduces the influence of resonance frequency on scattering cross section since the lower is the shell elasticity due to encapsulation, the higher is the resonant frequency. Moreover, since Eq. (22) shows that the scattering cross section is inversely related to the damping constant, the encapsulation of microbubbles with a thick and stiff shell produces a lower scattering cross section also for the viscoelastic properties of the surrounding shell.

US Beam Attenuation and Microbubble Size Distribution

The US weakening results from scattering and absorption.[5,6] The combined effect of scattering and attenuation depends on microbubbles concentration. Scattering is the prevalent phenomenon with low microbubble concentrations while the attenuation, caused by multiple scattering, dominates when the microbubble concentration increases.

$$a(f) = \int_{R_{min}}^{R_{max}} n(r)\sigma(r)\mathrm{d}r \tag{26}$$

where $a(f)$ is the US frequency-dependent attenuation coefficient expressed in nepers[Np]/length and neper is a dimensionless quantity, R_{max} and R_{min} are minimum and maximum microbubble radii, $n(r)$ is the microbubble concentration, and σ is the scattering cross section.

Equation (26) may be employed to calculate the microbubble size distribution, which is in agreement with values measured with optical methods. Microbubble-size distribution is normal shaped, and the standard deviation is larger for first-generation agents and lower for new-generation agents, which present a more uniform microbubble diameter.

Scattering to Attenuation Ratio

In a suspension of microbubbles, each microbubble has to be considered as an element, which absorbs and scatters US at the same time.[5,6] The total energy loss or attenuation for an acoustical beam traveling through a screen of microbubbles is called the extinction coefficient, $\mu_e(\omega)$, and is given by

$$\mu_e(\omega) = \mu_a(\omega) + \mu_s(\omega) \tag{27}$$

where $\mu_a(\omega)$ is the absorption coefficient and $\mu_s(\omega)$ is the scattering coefficient.

The scattering to attenuation ratio (STAR) is a measure of the acoustical effectiveness of the contrast agent. The STAR is defined as

$$\mathrm{STAR}(\omega) = \frac{\mu_s(\omega)}{\mu_e(\omega)} \tag{28}$$

and substituting Eq. (28) into Eq. (27) gives

$$\text{STAR}(\omega) = \frac{\mu_s(\omega)}{\mu_a(\omega) + \mu_s(\omega)} \tag{29}$$

where $\mu_s(\omega)$ represents the part of the energy that is scattered away omnidirectionally by the microbubbles, while $\mu_a(\omega)$ represents the part of the energy that is absorbed by the microbubbles.

Therefore, the lower the absorption of the incoming plane US wave, the higher the STAR. A maximum value of STAR = 1 is obtained when there is no absorption. However, this index is only valid for low acoustic pressures, and at high acoustic pressures, nonlinear transient effect appears.

The attenuation of the acoustical beam traveling through a screen of microbubbles can cause shadowing of underlying biologic structures and is not considered to be a useful parameter. An effective contrast agent, therefore, is defined by good scattering properties and low attenuation. For these reasons, the higher is the STAR, the more effective is the contrast agent. There is a nonlinear relation between the increase in microbubble acoustic pressure of insonation and the produced backscattering and attenuation.

Acoustic Power of Insonation

The probability for a single US pulse to destroy a microbubble increases for high acoustic power amplitudes, long US pulse lengths, and low frequencies according to the following equation:

$$E_{\text{acoustic}} = \int_0^k \left(P_0 \sin 2\pi f t\right)^2 \mathrm{d}t = K P_0^2 \frac{1}{f} \approx K(\text{MI})^2 \tag{30}$$

where E_{acoustic} is the acoustic power of insonation (W_0), P_0 is the acoustic pressure amplitude, f is the frequency, t is the time, and K is the number of cycles per burst, which determines the US pulse length.

To obtain a useful harmonic signal for imaging, the microbubbles have to be insonated at their specific fundamental frequency, defined also resonance frequency, which corresponds to the frequency range usually employed for the abdominal US examination from 3 to 3.7 MHz. The acoustic power employed to insonate the microbubbles is usually expressed by the MI, which measures the potential for mechanical damage to tissues exposed to intense US pulses.

$$\text{MI} = \frac{p-}{\sqrt{\text{f}}} \tag{31}$$

where $p-$ is the largest peak negative (rarefactional) pressure that the transmitted US pulse achieves during its travel through a medium of specified attenuation coefficient and f is the center frequency of the pulse. The peak negative acoustic pressure ($p-$) is expressed in MPascal (Pa; 1 Pa = 1 Newton/m^2), and the frequency in MHz. In clinical practice, the range for MI varies from 0.05 to 1.9. The lower the frequency of US, the greater its MI and therefore its destructive properties. Anyway, the MI is an unreliable predictor of microbubble destruction, since at the same MI value different values of acoustic powers of insonation may be measured in different US systems. The MI is actually a safety index indicating the potential for nonthermal bioeffects during insonation. Anyway, it presents the disadvantage to be poorly reproducible between the different US equipments. A more correct and reproducible manner is to express the insonation transmit power as MPa (mega Pascal), which is mentioned in the operative screen of some US equipments.

There are two quite different approaches to insonate microbubbles. One group of methods, commonly known as high transmit power insonation, use large pulse amplitudes (about 1 MPa) and produce microbubble destruction with emission of an irregular wideband harmonic signal, similar to an explosion, and named stimulated acoustic emission (SAE). At very high acoustic pressures, exaggerated microbubble oscillation leads to microbubble destruction by one of several mechanisms. Microbubble compression can increase surface tension and cause outward diffusion of the microbubble gas during each high-pressure US cycle, resulting in a gradual reduction in microbubble volume. Exaggerated radial oscillations can result in permanent defects in the microbubble shell, which results in rapid loss of gas from the microbubbles. Finally, abrupt fragmentation of microbubbles has been visualized with only a single high-energy US pulse. Harmonic power Doppler is one of the most sensitive high acoustic power techniques for perfusion imaging and offers the best signal-to-noise ratio. The threshold for destruction is variable and depends on a number of different factors such as the size, the shell material, and the filling gas of microbubble and the attenuation of the US beam power from the overlaying tissues. These methods are generally employed to insonate air-filled microbubble contrast agents with a soft shell presenting a low harmonic behavior at low transmit power insonation and are limited by the transiency of the signal, which persists only for 2 to 3 frames. Intermittent imaging at low frame rates (one image every 2 to 3 seconds) may overcome this problem by limiting the destruction of microbubbles.

The other group of methods consists in the low transmit power insonation (30 to 70 kPa). This technique reduces the microbubble destruction and the magnitude of harmonic signals produced by stationary tissues and employs the nonlinear physical behavior of microbubbles. When microbubbles are insonated at the fundamental (resonance) frequency with a low acoustic power, the microbubbles present a nonlinear physical behavior and become relatively more resistant to compression than to expansion. This leads to asymmetric or nonlinear oscillations, which contain both fundamental and harmonic frequencies multiple of the fundamental frequency. This insonation method is employed with sulfur hexafluoride or perfluorocarbon-filled microbubbles and allows a real-time scanning due to the long persistence of the signal.

Contrast-Specific Ultrasound Techniques

The different contrast-specific US techniques (Table 10.2) may be differentiated from their basic principles in pseudo-Doppler, harmonic, phase modulation, amplitude modulation, and phase and amplitude modulation techniques.[7,8]

Pseudo-Doppler Techniques

These are multipulse high transmit power techniques. Pseudo-Doppler techniques employ the SAE effect, which corresponds to the emission of a wideband signal when microbubbles are destroyed by an high transmit power insonation. These techniques are limited by the presence of motion artifacts and by the transiency of the signal. The stationary tissues and contrast information can be displayed separately or simultaneously by an electronic system that measures the Doppler power in each pixel and represents a pixel as a color pixel if the Doppler power exceeds a threshold value (priority) or as a gray-scale pixel if the Doppler power is lower according to the B-mode echo amplitude for that pixel. This Doppler threshold value is easily exceeded if microbubble contrast agents are employed resulting in the presence of artifacts as blooming (presence of Doppler signal not determined by the mean frequency shift) and the clutter (low-frequency Doppler signal produced by stationary tissues overlapping to the real Doppler signal). To limit the blooming artifact and clutter, the B-mode and Doppler power for a pixel are compared and the larger one is used to set the pixel gray level. This avoids blooming and clutter since a pixel will not display a power Doppler signal if the B-mode signal for that pixel is large, while the pixels with a strong clutter will merge relatively inconspicuously with those showing strong B-mode stationary tissue signals.

TABLE 10.2 **Contrast-Specific Ultrasound Techniques (More Extended Than Text)**

Pseudo-Doppler	Harmonic Imaging	Coded Imaging	Phase Modulation	Amplitude Modulation	Phase and Amplitude Modulation
Stimulated acoustic emission (SAE)	*Gray-scale techniques*	Coded harmonic angio	*Gray-scale techniques*	Power modulation	Cadence contrast pulse sequencing (CPS)
Cadence agent detection imaging (ADI)	Second harmonic imaging cCube Flash echo imaging Extended pure harmonic detection (ePHD) Contrast-tuned imaging (CnTI) Ultraharmonic imaging Subharmonic imaging 1.5 harmonic imaging	Chirp excitation	Pulse inversion Microflow imaging[a] Contrast tissue discriminator (CTD) Coherent contrast imaging (CCI)		Power modulation phase inversion (PMPI)
Advanced dynamic flow (ADF)	*Doppler technique* Harmonic power Doppler		*Doppler techniques:* Power pulse inversion Vascular recognition imaging (VRI) Low MI color-flow contrast		
Tissue signature imaging (TSI)					

Note: General classification of specialized contrast-specific US techniques according to the pulse transmission and signal processing.
[a]*Microflow imaging* is based on the summation of multiple consecutive frames and represents a multi-intensity projection algorithm of data obtained by a phase inversion technique. It improves the visualization of slowly perfused organs (e.g., breast) by monitoring the tracks of single microbubbles. Further discrimination of microbubbles with respect to the stationary tissues is achieved by comparing consecutive frames with each other, pixel for pixel. If the content of a pixel has not changed from one frame to the next, it is rejected, leaving, ideally, only echoes from moving microbubbles.

Harmonic Imaging Techniques

These are multipulse techniques, which employ the nonlinear physical properties of microbubbles to suppress the stationary tissue background. These techniques employ a high or low transmit power insonation. Since the second harmonic (double of the insonating frequency) has the highest amplitude among the harmonics, it is therefore the most relevant harmonic frequency for the contrast-specific US imaging even though the signal may be persistent or transient according to the employed acoustic power. Moreover, these techniques are limited by the presence of tissue harmonic components that are present at high transmit power insonation, which leads to a relative production of harmonics frequency and to the consequent poorer contrast resolution of the technique.

Gray-Scale Harmonic Imaging—Narrowband Harmonic Imaging

In harmonic mode, the system is configured to receive preferentially second harmonic echoes produced by microbubbles, hence at double the transmitted frequency, by a high-pass filter. This technique presents several limitations. Even though such filtering is successful in eliminating echoes from solid stationary tissues, which present prevalently linear properties, the effect is to reduce the range of frequencies (or bandwidth) contained in the received echoes, causing a low spatial axial resolution of the resulting image. Moreover, if the transmit pulse bandwidth (centered at the fundamental frequency f_o) and the receive bandwidth (centered at $2f_o$) overlap, then a portion of the echo from linear scattering will contaminate the harmonic receive signal, reducing the difference between microbubble agent and stationary tissue and, consequently, the contrast resolution of the technique.

Flash Echo Imaging

This technique employs intermittent high transmit power insonation to produce microbubble destruction with a progressively increasing interscan delay producing a progressive microbubble accumulation in the scanning plane. The longer is the interscan delay, the larger is the microbubble accumulation in the scanning plane with an increased echo signal produced from insonation.

Harmonic Power Doppler Imaging

This technique is known also as harmonic power Doppler imaging by high-pass signal filtering. Doppler is an effective method for separating echoes from the microbubbles moving with the blood and echoes from the tissues. With conventional color Doppler, moving scatterers in a region of interest produce a low-frequency shift (clutter signal), which has a Doppler shift frequency nearly identical to that of the moving blood. A high-pass filter allows to cancel the signal produced by tissues and to selectively register the signal produced by microbubbles.

Contrast Tuned Imaging (CnTI)

This technique employs the transmission of the specific resonance frequency of sulfur hexafluoride–filled microbubbles and the selective registration of the harmonic frequencies. This allows a significant reduction of the insonation power with reduction of the nonlinear harmonic behavior of the stationary tissues and a selective production of harmonic frequencies from microbubbles.

C-Cube

This is a harmonic intermittent high transmit power technique, which relies on the transmission of two identical US pulses down each ray line and on the comparison of returning echo signals. This enables the identification of the nonlinear harmonic response from microbubbles from the different intensities on the two echoes due to microbubble destruction by the first US pulse.

Extended Pure Harmonic Detection (ePHD)

This technique consists in the transmission of a low transmit power US pulse with a frequency equal to the resonance frequency of the microbubbles without any distortion and harmonic component. As a result, only the real harmonic signals generated by the microbubble resonance are employed for image generation. Moreover, analysis of phase-shift information is performed for an even more selective registration of the signal produced by microbubbles. The nonlinear nature of microbubble oscillation under the influence of sound pressure generates phase-shifted signals that identify the received harmonic signal as being originated by the contrast agent and not the surrounding tissue. The solution provided enables scanning with an extremely low transmit power, maintaining very high sensitivity for the harmonic microbubble signal and delivering a precise representation of contrast-perfused tissue.

Ultraharmonic Imaging

This technique employs a wideband frequency transducer. Ultraharmonics ($3f_0/2$, $5f_0/2$, $7f_0/2$,...) refer to radiofrequency signals that occur between higher harmonics ($2f_0$, $3f_0$, $4f_0$,...). Very little ultraharmonic signals arise from nonlinear propagation of US through tissue, while ultraharmonics are effectively produced by microbubbles both by high and low transmit power intonation. With ultraharmonic imaging, a combination of high and low pass filters can be used to selectively display only ultraharmonic frequencies where the signal-to-noise ratio is intrinsically greater.

Subharmonic Imaging

When microbubbles are insonated at one frequency, some return echoes with a frequency component at half the insonation frequency, as well as at the fundamental frequency and the second, third, and higher integer harmonics mentioned previously. Two causes have been identified for the subharmonic signal. One is certainly the nonlinear response of a microbubble to an incident pulse. The other is ringing (continuing oscillations) at the natural frequency of the bubble after the forced oscillation due to the incident pulse has stopped. Both effects are greater for transmitted pulses containing a larger number of cycles and for the more flexible microbubbles. The strength of the subharmonic component in the scatter spectrum of microbubbles is greater than that of the second harmonic. This, combined with the fact that nonlinear propagation of ultrasound in tissue does not generate a subharmonic component, suggests that subharmonic detection might offer an imaging method with greater contrast between microbubble and tissue echoes. Moreover, the lower frequency of the subharmonic means attenuation is less. Against these advantages must be set the fact that pulses containing more cycles generate stronger subharmonic signals, and such long pulses would not give good spatial axial resolution.

1.5 Harmonic Imaging

In this method, images are obtained using a frequency transmission band that is intermediate between the fundamental and the second harmonic components. In the 1.5 harmonic imaging techniques, a frequency band whose center frequency is higher than the fundamental by a factor of 3/2 is extracted and visualized. It includes only bubble echoes and is free of tissue echoes. This imaging technique reduces tissue echoes without generating motion artifacts such as those that are seen in the pseudo-Doppler imaging technique. Contrast between tissues and bubbles is improved by ≥20 dB compared with the second harmonic imaging technique.

Phase Modulation Techniques

Nowadays, low transmit power contrast-specific techniques are employed. The newer modalities share also a common feature—namely, the transmission of multiple pulses of US per scan line, followed by processing of the received radiofrequency signals from each line. The purpose of these techniques is to remove linear or predominantly tissue signal, from nonlinear microbubble signals to improve the contrast resolution and the signal-to-noise ratio. These techniques employ a low transmit power and allows a long persistence of the signal produced by microbubbles with the possibility of continuous and real-time scanning.

Pulse Inversion Harmonic Imaging (Pulse Inversion with Two Transmissions)

Pulse inversion harmonic imaging was developed to address two important limitations of harmonic imaging—to provide better discrimination between tissue and microbubble contrast agents and to overcome the requirement of the use of a narrowband signal for harmonic imaging with the consequently reduced spatial axial resolution. In pulse inversion, two sequential US waves that are inverted replicas of each other are transmitted into tissue, and the resulting echoes are summed. For a linear medium, the echoes from the two waves are inverted copies of each other, and the resulting sum is zero. For nonlinear media such as microbubbles, the echoes will not be inverted copies; the sum is not zero. If a high acoustic power of insonation is employed for imaging, however, tissue harmonics are not eliminated by pulse inversion and are incompletely canceled and tissue and microbubble second harmonics may still overlap.

The advantage of the pulse inversion method over the harmonic techniques is that overlap between the fundamental and second harmonic spectra does not matter, and there is no need to restrict the transmission spectrum to the lower half of the transducer frequency range. This allows short (large bandwidth) pulses to be used and hence good axial spatial resolution to be achieved. The disadvantage of the method, however, is a reduction in frame rate due to the need to interrogate each scan line twice. The tissue contrast discrimination that can be achieved by pulse inversion is limited by any tissue movement between the two transmissions. Where there is tissue movement, the positions of the tissue interfaces in the second echo sequence will not match those in the first, and the cancelation of the linear signal will not be perfect.

Microflow Imaging

This technique is based on the summation of multiple consecutive frames, and it represents a multi-intensity projection algorithm of pulse inversion data. It improves the visualization of small vessels containing few microbubbles by monitoring the tracks of single microbubbles. Further discrimination of microbubbles with respect to the stationary tissues is achieved by comparing consecutive frames with each other, pixel for pixel. If the content of a pixel has not changed from one frame to the next, it is rejected, leaving, ideally, only echoes from moving microbubbles. Moreover, in order to help the eye to recognize the line of the vessel, the signals can be made to persist on the screen.

Contrast Tissue Discriminator

Contrast tissue discriminator is a low transmit power multipulse mode based as the phase inversion mode on the pulse subtraction method using alternating phases. The echoes from tissue are canceled while highlighting those from the microbubbles are registered.

Coherent Contrast Imaging

This is a high frame rate phase modulation technique. The reduction in frame rate referred as a limitation of pulse inversion can be avoided by transmitting only one pulse per scan line, but inverting the transmitted pulse on alternate scan lines.[6] The overlap between adjacent beams means that scatterers receive pulses of alternating polarity. The sum of the two echo sequences represents an average of the two contributing lines and is therefore displayed as a synthetic line situated midway between them. Summing the echo sequences from adjacent lines therefore cancels out echoes from linear scatterers, as in the two-pulse method described in the previous section. The avoidance of a frame rate penalty comes at the expense of a slightly imperfect cancelation of the fundamental, since not all points in a pair of overlapping beams experience matching but inverted versions of the same pulse waveform.

Power Pulse Inversion (Pulse Inversion with Three Transmissions)

Power pulse inversion is a technique where a series of US pulses (≥ 3) are transmitted at a high pulse repetition interval along each line. Three interrogations of a line with alternately inverted pulses can greatly reduce the effect of tissue motion, which limits the usual pulse inversion mode. Each transmitted pulse is an inverted copy of the previous pulse. The processing amounts to forming an average of the first and third echo sequences (by adding them together and dividing by two) and adding this to the second echo sequence. If the tissue velocity is not too great, the difference in phase between echoes from the first and third pulses (less than a millisecond apart) will be small, say, less than 30 degrees or so, and the average echo sequence will then be a close approximation to one with half the phase shift, corresponding to what would have been returned if an imaginary pulse had been transmitted midway in time between these two real pulses. As for the two-pulse method, adding the average echo sequence from the two noninverted pulses to the real sequence from the second (inverted) pulse will give cancelation of linear tissue echoes but not of microbubble echoes. The use of multiple pulses reduces motion artifacts while preserving true contrast signal (noise cancels but real signals add). Doppler processing on the received echoes is performed and allows linear and nonlinear scatterers to be separated into two distinct Doppler spectra. Similar to harmonic power Doppler, the power spectrum of the returning backscatter signal is displayed. As a disadvantage, this technique determines an increased microbubble destruction due to multipulse insonation.

Vascular Recognition Imaging

A generalization of the pulse inversion method, called pulse inversion Doppler, combines the nonlinear detection performance of pulse inversion imaging with the motion discrimination capabilities of color Doppler. It is the first contrast-specific technique, which discriminates moving from stationary microbubbles. It involves transmitting four pulses, alternately inverted, along each scan line. The echoes from the first three are summed with weights (1, 2, 1) to give one fundamental-free signal, and the echoes from the last three are summed the same way to give a second fundamental-free signal. The phase difference between these two principally second harmonic signals gives a velocity estimate, and their mean magnitude gives a power estimate. Stationary bubbles are shown in green, while moving bubbles are either red or blue, depending on their flow direction. A disadvantage of using only a few transmission/receive sequences for each scan line is that the accuracy of Doppler frequency measurement is much less than in conventional color-flow imaging.

Coded Harmonic Angio

Coded harmonic angio sonography combines phase inversion harmonic imaging with a coded transmission pulse technique that boosts weak microbubble signal and suppresses tissue signals by transmitting coded pulse sequences and decoding them on receipt. Within the long pulses are frequency or phase changes that act as a code. This code is present in genuine echoes but not in noise, so by using a special "matched" filter, designed to respond strongly to the transmitted code, the signal-to-noise ratio can be also improved by this contrast-specific technique. The coded harmonic angio-coded excitation technique involves transmitting pulses in the form of several "base pulses." As echoes return, they are matched with a reference replica of the coded transmission pulse and compared, one code digit at a time. When an echo code lines up perfectly with the reference code, the electric circuit output is high. A mismatch in position of just one digit will produce only a low output.

It is possible to selectively suppress echoes with the transmission codes and hence the fundamental signal produced by the stationary tissues. Different coded transmission sequences in which one or more of the base pulses is shifted by a quarter of a cycle are employed. If second harmonic components are present in an echo, this quarter cycle shift at the fundamental frequency will become a half a cycle shift at the second harmonic frequency. Thus, the code of the second harmonic component of an echo will be modified from that transmitted, whereas the fundamental component will retain the code of the transmitted pulse. By careful choice of the transmission codes and filters, it can be arranged that the modified codes of the second harmonic component cause the second harmonic component to be selectively detected, while the unmodified codes cause the fundamental component to be canceled out.

Amplitude Modulation Techniques

Power modulation represents the paradigm of amplitude modulation contrast-specific technique. At low acoustic power insonation, the tissue signal may also be suppressed online by alternating acoustic power rather than phase. For power modulation, a train of three low-power US pulses are transmitted per image line. The pulses are transmitted at two power levels, where the first and third pulses are half-height amplitude relative to the second pulse. Since all pulses are transmitted at a low acoustic power, little nonlinear tissue backscatter is generated. Subsequently, the received echoes from the half-height transmitted pulses are scaled and subtracted from the full-height signal, which results in effective removal of tissue clutter. On the other hand, microbubbles continue to respond nonlinearly to all three pulses, resulting in residual microbubble signal even after subtraction.

Amplitude and Phase Modulation Techniques

The contrast pulse sequencing (CPS) and Power modulated Pulse Inversion (PMPI) techniques work by interrogating each scan lines a number of times with pulses having various amplitudes and phases. Three pulses are employed with a typical sequence of pulse as (½, −1, ½), which means that each line is interrogated three times, with the first and last transmitted pulses having amplitudes half that of the central pulse, which is inverted. A processor first amplifies the echo sequence from each transmission by a particular weighting factor (e.g., × 2 or ×−1) and then sums all the weighted echo sequences. It registers and represents both harmonic and nonlinear fundamental signals from microbubbles in a gray scale or color map. By suitable choice of transmission pulses and weighting factors, it is possible to isolate or suppress the linear fundamental echoes from stationary tissues. The amplitude and phase modulation contrast-specific techniques produce a high sensitivity to the microbubble nonlinear harmonic signals and an optimal suppression of the linear signal from the stationary tissues, a higher contrast enhancement homogeneity and contrast resolution than phase inversion techniques, and a strong reduction of motion artifacts and of clutter.

Artifacts after Microbubble Injection

Most microbubble-specific artifacts are found with color and power Doppler modes because the settings of US equipments become inappropriate following a strong increase of the backscattered signals and need to be recognized to avoid interpretative errors.[9]

High-Intensity Transient Signals

This artifact is determined by microbubble collapse or by aggregates of macrobubbles producing sharp spikes on the Doppler spectral tracing, heard as crackling on the audio output. These spikes are easily recognized since they cover the entire frequency spectrum. This artifact may also be detected with color and power Doppler imaging appearing as color pixels of higher intensity within the more uniform signal of the vessel.

Pseudoacceleration of the Systolic Peak Velocity

An increase in the systolic peak velocity of up to 50% can be found at peak enhancement. This artifact is probably the result of signals that were too weak to be detected before microbubble injection, and it may be almost completely canceled by reducing the Doppler gain or by employing slow infusion of microbubbles. The increase in systolic peak velocity may produce error in grading stenotic lesions of the vessels.

Blooming Artifact

In Doppler tracing only, the mean frequency shift is displayed, while the Doppler signal intensity is increased after microbubble injection since the increase in backscattering echo-signal intensity also determines the appearance of the lowest velocities that were too weak to be registered before microbubble injection. When color or power Doppler is turned on, the overload of the Doppler signal registration apparatus is determined by the strong signals and multiple rereflections between adjacent microbubbles. Such artifact can be limited by reducing the color gain and persistence and the MI or by increasing the wall filter and the pulse repetition frequency, resulting in a decreased sensitivity of the system. The slow infusion of microbubbles limits this artifact because of a decrease in the peak signal intensity. Dedicated US contrast–specific modes were introduced principally to avoid this artifact.

Jail Bar Artifact

The jail bar artifact is prevalently observed with power Doppler mode. It is determined by an error in image interpolation when the management of the backscattering signal intensity from the US system approaches the saturation. Since each frame is reconstructed from an interpolation mathematical procedure of the image view lines, the saturation of signal determines a lack of color along the interpolating view.

Transit Time Measurements with Doppler Vessel Interrogation

Tracking the transit time of a bolus of microbubbles through the organ vessels enables measurements of the physiology of organs and may derive semiquantitative parameters correlated to organ perfusion.[9] In this method, organ vessels are interrogated by spectral Doppler and the Doppler signal rise as the microbubble bolus arrives. The loudness of audio signals from spectral Doppler analysis can be used to generate time–intensity curves to follow the wash-in and wash-out of the microbubble bolus. The form of the time–intensity curves contain hemodynamic information that can be revealed using the same mathematics as has classically been applied to radionuclide tracers. The approaches relevant to microbubble time–intensity curves include bolus transit studies in which the true tissue perfusion is calculated as the ratio of the peak tissue enhancement to the area under the arterial curve. Provided the necessary arterial and tissue curves could be obtained (and this will depend on the particular anatomical arrangements on the organ or lesion), these approaches could be applied to US.[9] According to the central volume theorem, the organ perfusion is calculated as the ratio of the central (i.e., fractional vascular) volume to the mean transit time. The Mean Transit Time strictly requires transit curves from the artery and vein. Performing these transit time studies is cumbersome as it requires at least two operators and dedicated computing equipment. With the advent of perfluoro gas contrast agents and the development of contrast-specific scanning modes, the possibility of performing the scan in two dimensions became realistic.

In the kidney, it is easy to include in the spectral Doppler interrogating volume for both the artery and vein due to their adjacent position with Doppler measurement of the signal first in the artery and then in the vein. In the normal kidney, the arterial venous transit is some 4 seconds. The true mean transit time can be calculated by plotting the arterial and venous time–intensity curves, applying a gamma-variate fit to select the first pass of the contrast agent, discarding signals from recirculating contrast, and then calculating the difference between the centroids of the two curves.[9] In the breast, many studies showed that both transit time and arrival time[10,11] in cancers are shorter than in benign masses.

A similar method has been developed for the liver,[12–14] the goal here being to evaluate arteriovenous shunting in liver cirrhosis and hepatic malignancies.[15] Normally, the hepatic artery supplies some 25% of the liver's blood, but this increases in these conditions because of shunts as well as the scarring that increases resistance to portal vein flow in cirrhosis. This method developed employs spectral Doppler to assess the arrival of microbubbles in hepatic veins with the audio output of the scanner fed into a laptop computer. The arrival time is defined as a sustained increase in signal strength of 10% over base line. To this end, a hepatic vein is targeted and kept in the field of view before the microbubble injection is given with the patient breathing quietly.[9] In normal subjects, the arrival time in the hepatic vein after peripheral intravenous injection usually occurs after 30 seconds (the lower limit of normal was found to be 25 seconds). In cirrhosis, an early arrival time of the contrast bolus (<24 seconds) and a left shift of the time–intensity curve is observed because of a hepatic arterial supply and the presence of intrahepatic shunts.[12–14] This test was also shown to be accurate in assessing the severity of diffuse liver disease and in separating between mild and moderate/severe chronic hepatitis.[13,14] Hepatic vein transit time was shown to be significantly shorter with sulfur hexafluoride–filled (SonoVue, Bracco, Milan, Italy) than with air-filled microbubbles (Levovist, Schering, Berlin, Germany), even though there was more effective differentiation between moderate or severe hepatic fibrosis or cirrhosis from normal volunteers with Levovist than with SonoVue.[14]

In parallel with this, the role of the arrival time in metastatic disease of the liver has been studied.[15] It depends on an accurate measurement of the volume flow in both the hepatic artery and portal vein and has been shown to be able to detect not only overt but, importantly, also occult metastatic disease (i.e., disease not detectable at preoperative staging or at laparotomy, which becomes manifest on follow-up). The Doppler perfusion index, the ratio of hepatic arterial blood flow (the product of the time-averaged velocity and cross-sectional area of the common hepatic artery) to total liver blood flow (the sum of the product of the time-averaged velocity and cross-sectional area of the portal vein and the common hepatic artery),[16,17] though very promising, was found to be too technically demanding for general use, so simpler alternatives were sought. Tracking the arrival of a microbubble bolus in the hepatic veins seems to be a feasible alternative that is practical to perform.

Quantitative Analysis of Echo-Power

Accurate quantification of the degree of contrast enhancement requires assessment of the change in video intensity between the baseline and contrast-enhanced images. The direct visual assessment of the degree of log-compressed video intensity is the least accurate method because the background tissue signal varies widely within the US sector, because of heterogeneities of acoustic power and differences in the attenuation and absorption of US energy by tissue.

Backscatter signals from microbubbles are processed into pixels of brightness or video intensity in the US system. Several factors can affect the intensity registered by the imaging system (image brightness) including signal saturation, acoustic shadowing, nonlinear propagation of ultrasound through tissues, beam nonuniformity, stability of ultrasound probe placement, and US system settings (gain, dynamic range, focal zone position, etc.). In particular, the background signal varies widely within the acoustic window due to inhomogeneities of the acoustic power and to differences in attenuation and absorption of ultrasound energy by tissues. Respiratory motions and displacement of tissue within the US sector can be limited by asking to the patient to breathe quietly during the study.

The relationship between video intensity and microbubble concentration is linear, and it reaches a plateau as microbubble concentration increases.[18,19] The plateau phase reflects the effective microbubble concentration within the organ tissue microcirculation. After achievement of the plateau phase, microbubble concentration increases while video intensity remains constant. At even higher concentrations, the video intensity actually decreases due to attenuation of US by the microbubbles themselves. Quantitative analysis of tissue perfusion using CEUS is still limited by acoustic shadowing owing to the inadequate compensation for microbubble attenuation, and tissue attenuation correction algorithms or mathematical models estimating microbubble attenuation have been proposed.[20,21] For these reasons, it is essential to ensure that the microbubble concentration is maintained within the linear range so that video intensity remains directly proportional to microbubble concentration.

Determination of the degree of tissue contrast enhancement from microbubbles relies on accurate distinction between backscatter signals from microbubbles and the native tissue signal background. Digital image processing techniques such as image alignment, averaging, and background subtraction are essential and may be performed by specialized calculation software packages produced by the scanner manufacturers, which have access to the raw data before application of nonlinear modifications, and are able to antilog the gray-scale signals that are log compressed for video presentation.

To perform background subtraction, baseline (precontrast) and contrast-enhanced images are aligned, and all video-intensity values within a region of interest from the baseline image are digitally subtracted from the contrast-enhanced image. Further optimization of the image alignment can be obtained either manually or by using proprietary software. The tissue intensity can then be determined by placing a region of interest over the image. US systems usually perform a variety of processing operations on the echo-power signal for visualization purposes. Backscatter signals from microbubbles are processed into pixels of brightness for video presentation in the US system in order to express echo-power values that reflect instantaneous *in situ* concentration of microbubble contrast agents. The translation of echo amplitude values to a scale of display brightness or color appropriate to human visual perception is performed through a series of steps. Logarithmic compression is employed for displaying signals with a large dynamic range on US monitors that have smaller dynamic ranges. Beside logarithmic compression, other methods are employed to provide pleasing images at visual perception including the use of different postprocessing curves or color maps and signal filtering for edge enhancement.

Consequently, demodulated echo signals are typically log compressed to remap the dynamic range of meaningful ultrasound echoes at each depth (approximately 60 to 70 dB) to the range of perception for the human eye of a monitor display (approximately 30 dB). Results are then provided as compressed video images in DICOM (Digital Imaging and Communications in Medicine) JPEG (Joint Photographic Experts Group) format. DICOM JPEG files are generally considered unsuitable for echo-power estimation[18] due to a lack of publically available information on the process used to create the displayed color images (in particular, information on the log compression is not available) and also due to steps of thresholding and quantitation, in addition to the reversible logarithmic compression, during which information is lost.

Time–intensity curves may be calculated by positioning a manually defined or automatically copied ROI over a parenchymal region and by correlating the measured video intensity (VI, 0 to 255 gray-scale levels) with time in seconds. Based on the mathematics of logarithms, the mean video intensity in an ROI is

$$\text{mean VI} = \frac{1}{N} \times \sum_{j=1}^{N} 10\log_{10}\left(\frac{I_j}{I_{\text{ref}}}\right)$$

where N indicates the pixel number within the ROI, I_j is the acoustic intensity, and I_{ref} is an intensity reference level determined through equipment gain. Since video intensity data are logarithmic, to subtract tissue from microbubble contrast signal, the correct mathematical transformation is log A − log B = log A/B (A = microbubbles; B = background or baseline). Consequently, subtraction of baseline video intensity values is actually a calculation of the logarithm of a ratio between echo intensities.

The quantitation of echo-signal intensity after antilogarithmic transformation is the most accurate method and eliminates the influence of logarithmic compression, color maps, postprocessing curves, and techniques for edge enhancement on the input signal mapping for video presentation. A practical approach consists of collecting imaging-converted video data, log compressed and palletized as gray-scale or color-coded 8-bit data, in the form of DICOM files. Proper linearization needs to be applied before curve fitting and analysis, in order to reverse the effects of log compression and possibly nonlinear palette rendering. Background subtraction should therefore ideally be performed after logarithmic video intensity data have been converted to linear data using an antilog function. This task is now performed by some proprietary software packages—for example, VueBox (Bracco, Suisse SA, Geneva, Switzerland)—which apply algorithms to extract the echo power from DICOM JPEG images at the pixel level. These algorithms apply an antilog function within the linear range of the microbubble concentration versus video intensity relation. This type of software provides a more flexible integration of new sequence analysis approaches and enables analysis of contrast data acquired from a large range of imaging systems.

The lack of accessibility to machine-dependent echo signals can make it difficult to compare analyses of data from different US systems. Raw radiofrequency (RF) signal and quadrature (IQ) signal analyses are the gold standards for echo-power estimation. However, RF and IQ signals are generally not made available on machines for clinical use, primarily because of the large storage space required to handle this type of data.[18,19] Dedicated software packages—for example, CHI-Q (Contrast Harmonic Imaging Quantification software, Toshiba Medical Systems, Tochigi, Japan) or (QLab; Philips Ultrasound)—produced by scanner manufacturers are able to access the US data before the final display processing and to read proprietary information on processing stages for optimized linearization of ultrasonic data.[18]

Parametric images may be obtained after background subtraction in a pixel-by-pixel evaluation from the analysis of harmonic gray-scale imaging data through the use of dedicated software packages for the automated color-coded depiction of the different kinetic parameters.

Insonation Methods to Assess Organ Perfusion

The achievement of a steady-state microbubble concentration in the peripheral circulation is preferable in tissue perfusion studies. When microbubbles are administered as a constant infusion, the steady state is achieved after 2 to 3 minutes. This may be obtained by dedicated microbubble injectors usually equipped with a rotating syringe to avoid microbubble sedimentation, which allows a constant infusion of microbubbles in the bloodstream. At steady state, the inflow and outflow of microbubbles in any microcirculatory unit are constant, proportional to the fractional blood volume of that unit, and dependent only on the flow rate of microbubbles.

The fragility of microbubbles is a feature that can be exploited to obtain a measure of tissue perfusion. The method uses a high-power US beam to destroy the microbubbles within a slice of tissue that corresponds to the orthogonal beam profile. The destructive pulse creates a negative bolus, and "reperfusion kinetics" are used to study the way contrast flows back into the void at a rate that depends on the tissue's perfusion.

High Transmit Power Insonation

This refill phase can be assessed in two ways, both of which assume a steady state of blood microbubble concentration. In the first method, developed by Wei et al.,[22] further high transmit power frames are sent along the same path at progressively increasing intervals, and the signal strength from each is measured. The opposite approach, known as "diminution kinetics,"[23] can also be implemented, that is, observing the rate of decay of the microbubbles when exposed to a high-intensity beam, but this cannot be performed in real time so it has had limited application.

This model assumes that all microbubbles within an US field are destroyed by a single US pulse and that the thickness of the US beam is uniform. If new microbubbles enter the field at a velocity v, the distance (d) they will travel within the beam elevation as the pulsing interval (t) is prolonged is given by the equation $E = vt$; this means that as the time interval between consecutive destructive US pulses is increased, more time is allowed for microbubble replenishment, which is dependent on the velocity of microbubbles. As pulsing interval lengthens, the rise in microbubble concentration is displayed as a rise in organ parenchyma video intensity, provided that the relationship between video intensity and microbubble concentration remains linear. When the pulsing interval exceeds the time necessary to fill a distance equal to the US beam thickness, video intensity remains constant.

The refill curve has a rising exponential form described by the equation

$$I = A\left(1 - e^{-\beta t}\right)$$

where I is the signal intensity and t is the pulsing interval. Its initial exponent (β) is proportional to the speed of microbubble/blood flow into the slice, while the peak signal strength, A, is proportional to the fractional vascular volume. The product of these two is an indirect semiquantitative measure of tissue perfusion. In principle, this could be converted to true quantified perfusion if the volume perfused is known, but this is likely to prove elusive since it corresponds to the beam thickness whose shape is complex and dependent on machine settings (e.g., the focus position) and patient variables (e.g., attenuation). Actually, neither the beam thickness (which measures approximately 5 mm in thickness) nor the degree of microbubble destruction is expected to be entirely uniform. Moreover, the model predicts a sharp demarcation between the upslope and plateau phases of the time–intensity curve expressing the pulsing interval—video intensity relation. Anyway, this relationship is curvilinear. The beam's edge is also poorly defined since the energy in it tapers off towards the beam's edges. An additional practical problem is tissue movement: if the tissue being insonated moves out of the beam, the signal intensity will be increased artifactually.

Low Transmit Power Insonation

This original method is time consuming, and this makes it more difficult to keep the probe in the same place over the tissue. A faster and easier method is to switch the scanner to a very low transmit power imaging mode after the destructive burst and observe the reperfusion in real time[24,25] (Fig. 10.1). This requires a nonlinear microbubble contrast-specific mode but, as it only takes a few seconds for most tissues to replenish completely, it can be performed at the plateau of a slow bolus injection. After microbubble destruction, the system is switched to a low transmit power so that the refill rate of microbubbles returning to the imaged volume can be monitored.[1,24,25] Local tissue perfusion may be calculated by analyzing the replenishment kinetics of the volume of microbubbles after their destruction by initial high transmit power insonation. One of the main limitations of the technique is that perfusion data are acquired from a single tissue plane, a situation unlikely to accurately reflect global perfusion of the tissue or organ under consideration. The equation describing the reperfusion (Fig. 10.2) and the information that can be extracted from it are identical to the Wei method,[22] though the correspondence between the two has not been investigated systematically. However, this approach does assume that the monitoring mode does not destroy any microbubbles and that the probe needs to stay steadily over the same part of the organ. As well as its speed, the real-time reperfusion method has the advantage that in-plane tissue movement can be corrected for by deploying a speckle tracking method to follow the movement of the region of interest, for example, through the respiratory cycle, provided that the movement is confined to the scan plane (out of plane movement cannot be tracked). If three-dimensional acquisition could be achieved, complete tracking should be feasible and the reperfusion could be measured and depicted in 3D.

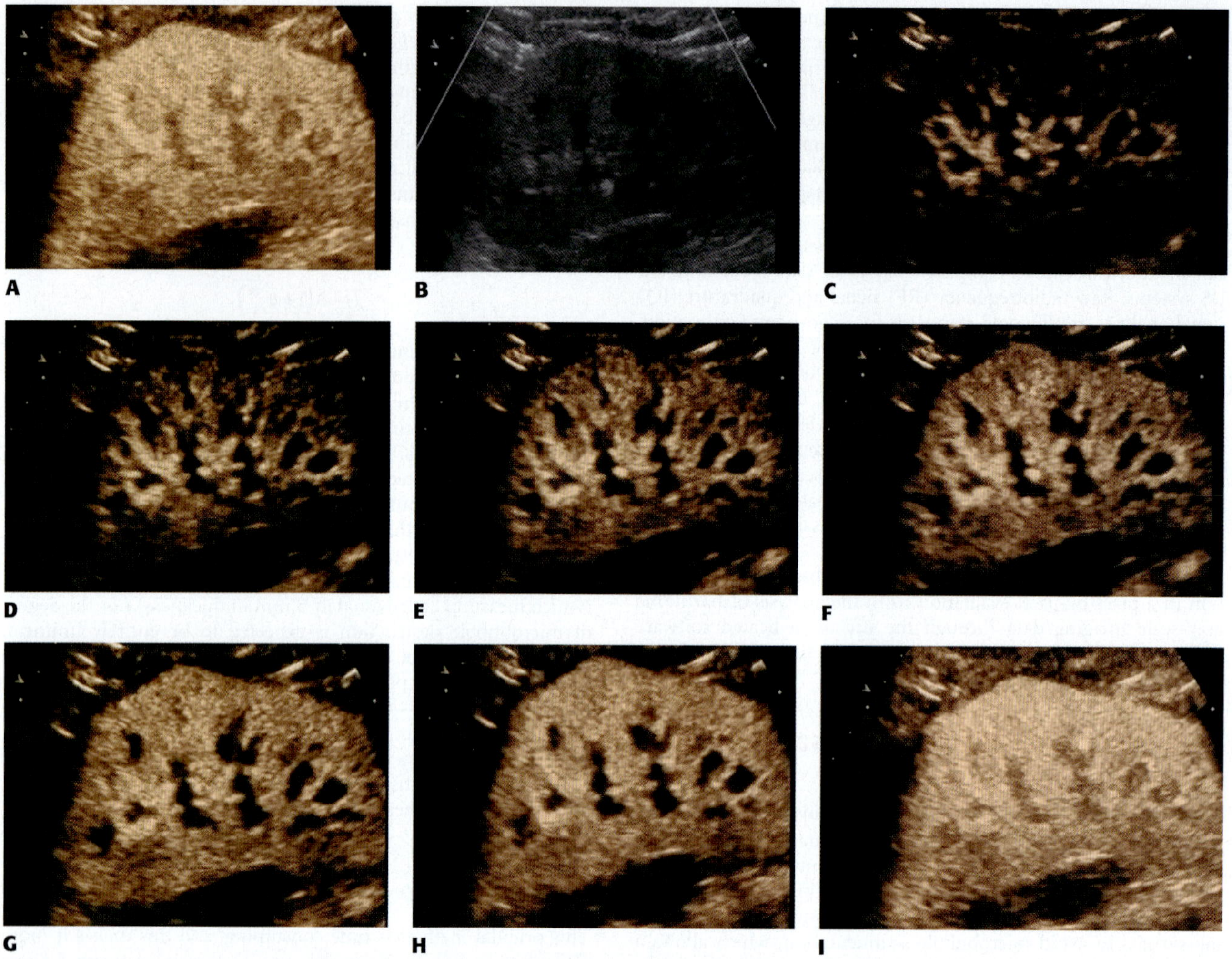

Figure 10-1. Reperfusion method for organ perfusion quantification by contrast-enhanced ultrasound. Progressive refilling of the imaged renal volume after sulfur hexafluoride–filled microbubble destruction following high transmit power insonation. After the achievement of a stationary stay of microbubble concentration in the bloodstream **(A)**, all microbubbles filling the imaged slice of the kidney are destroyed by high transmit power insonation **(B)**. Microbubbles progressively refill the renal parenchyma **(C–I)** according to a negative exponential kinetic.

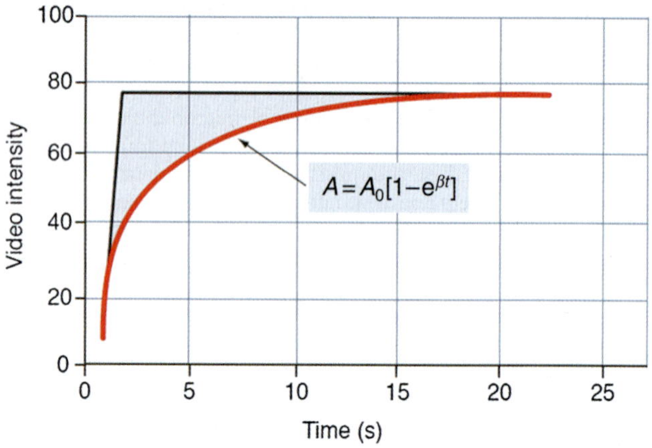

Figure 10-2. Negative exponential curve expressing the kidney reperfusion kinetic in a 25-year-old volunteer; β is the slope of the first ascending tract (approximately blood flow velocity); and *A* is the maximum amplitude of the refilling curve (approximately fractional blood volume). The distortion from the linear model (*straight line*) is due to microbubble diffusion within the vessels during the arrival time.

The analysis of the refilling process provides semiquantitative data related to tissue perfusion values. These include time-to-peak intensity, the initial slope of the refill (β ~ blood flow velocity), the maximum amplitude of the refilling curve (*A* ~ fractional blood volume), the area under the curve (approximately blood volume), and the mean transit time. The product of *A* (cm^3/g of tissue) x β ($second^{-1}$), corresponding to the area under the curve, is correlated to the amount of regional blood flow. Unfortunately, this cannot be converted to true perfusion as the volume of the perfused tissue is not known because the beam thickness and shape are complex and dependent on machine settings (e.g., the focus position) and patient variables (e.g., attenuation).

Mathematical Perfusion Models—Analytical Methods

Disruption–replenishment measurements are fitted by using a non-linear least-squares regression method, and different mathematical perfusion models have been proposed to fit the refilling kinetics after microbubble continuous infusion. All these perfusion models present several limitations including the velocity distribution within the ROI and the point spread function of the imaging system sampling the ROI.

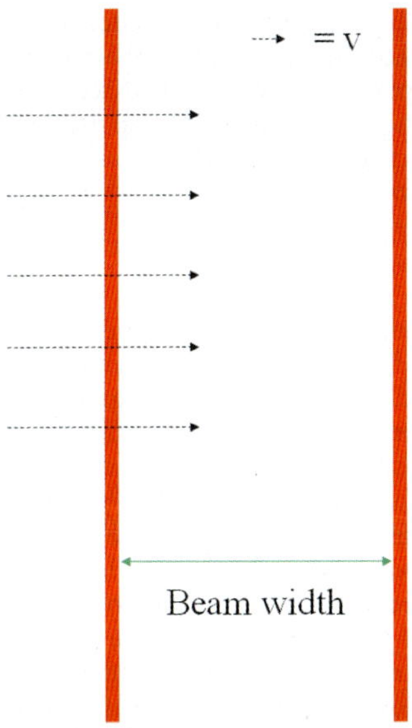

Figure 10-3. Graphical presentation of the negative exponential model. The microbubbles entering the imaged slice after microbubble destruction are assumed to have the same velocity.

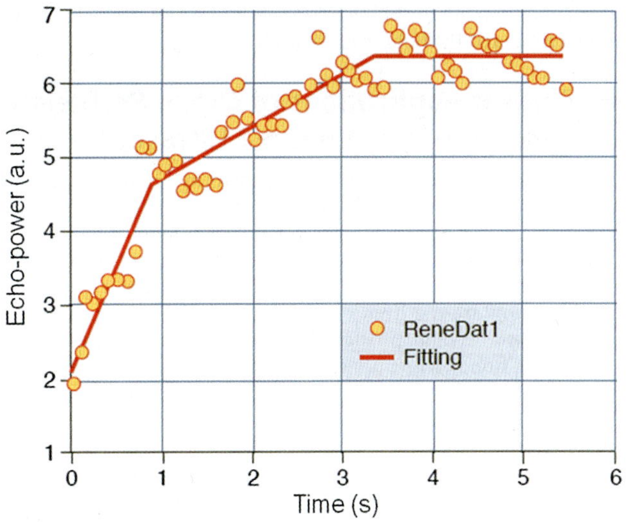

Figure 10-4. Piecewise linear function expressing the kidney reperfusion kinetic in a 25-year-old volunteer. The echo-signal intensity data set and the fittings by a piecewise linear function with three linear tracts. a.u., arbitrary unit; s, seconds.

In the first model (Fig. 10.2), the exponential behavior is a consequence of microbubble diffusion, and the refill curve has a rising exponential form described by the equation

$$\text{signal intensity} = A\left(1-e^{-\beta t}\right) \text{ expressing a negative exponential shape.}$$

Unfortunately, the exponential model (Figs. 10.2 and 10.3) does not take into account the fluid dynamics including the different blood velocity during systole and diastole and the different velocity profile of arteries and veins, and it fails to predict the experimental results if the percentage of microbubble destruction in the vessels feeding the ROI is not null.[26] Further limitations of this model include the assumption of a constant concentration of microbubbles entering the ROI immediately after the destruction pulse and the neglect of the different directions of the vessels inside the examined ROI.[26]

Lucidarme et al.[26] proposed a model described by a sigmoid function, which is based on the assumption that microbubble destruction actually occurs in the feeding vessels that reach the ROI. Quaia et al.[27] proposed a mathematical model that leads to a piecewise linear function that has the general properties of the refill curves. In this model, the vessels in the kidney can be grouped into N compartments, according to the value of the transit time of the blood within them (Figs. 10.4 and 10.5). With this assumption, we obtain a refill curve that is based on a piecewise linear function, where the transit times are the times that separate the linear tracts, the slopes are directly related to the flows, and the signal intensities at the transit times are directly related to the compartment volumes. Hence, from the fitting of the experimental data with a piecewise linear function (monotonically increasing, with slopes monotonically decreasing to zero), a description of the kidney, in terms of number of compartments, transit times, volumes, and flows, was obtained. Potdevin et al.[28,29] developed a dual model with a cross-plane and an in-plane vascularity for both the renal medullary and cortical regions, in which the whole refilling process is a weighted average of all possible elemental refill curves. Krix et al.[30] proposed a multivessel model that neglects diffusion, the microbubble movement from an area of high concentration to an area of lower concentration, and does not present exponential features, but assumes and takes into account a particular geometry of the vessels in the ROI. In all these mathematical models, the time–intensity curves frequently present a wide data dispersion during both the ascending and the second plateau phase of the curve.

Disruption–replenishment measurements may be fitted also by using a nonlinear least-squares regression method, to a lognormal perfusion model[25,31] based on the theory of indicator dilution model, which accounts for microvascular network geometry and hemodynamics, as well as the ultrasound beam sensitivity throughout the imaging plane. In this model, the infusion plateau is proportional to the fractional blood volume, while the rate of replenishment is related to the mean flow velocity.[25,31] Some commercial software employ this mathematical model by default to calculate the bolus

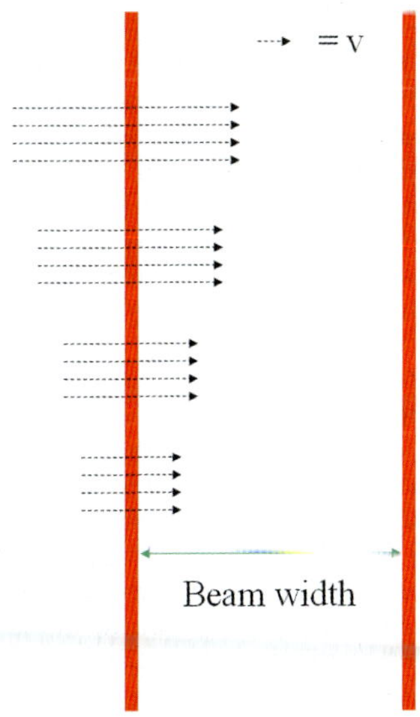

Figure 10-5. Graphical presentation of the multicompartmental model. The vectors represent the different microbubble velocity compartments entering the imaged slice after microbubble destruction.

peak enhancement, the bolus area under the curve, the bolus mean transit time, and the bolus time to peak.

Clinical Applications of Organ Perfusion Assessment by Contrast Ultrasound

In humans, CEUS has been applied to quantify brain perfusion in acute cerebral stroke.[32,33] In cardiac imaging, CEUS has an established role in left ventricle opacification and endocardial border definition to assess myocardial function and ejection fraction.[22,34] Other potential fields of application of CEUS in tissue perfusion quantification are the liver,[35] skeletal muscle,[36] free skin flaps,[37,38] joints,[39] testis,[40,41] and prostate.[42] Moreover, CEUS is capable of quantifying tumor tissue perfusion by quantifying tissue perfusion due to neoangiogenesis.[43–45]

Kidneys

CEUS quantification of tissue perfusion has been applied in the kidneys.[23,25] The renal cortex rapidly enhances from 15 to 20 seconds after microbubble injection, while the vessels of the renal medulla are progressively filled from 30 to 35 seconds and completely filled from 40 to 50 seconds after microbubble injection. This is because the renal medulla presents a lower global perfusion than the renal cortex (about 400 *vs.* 190 mL/min/100 g of renal tissue). For these reasons, it is correct to identify, after microbubbles injection, an early arterial corticomedullary phase (from 20 seconds to 40 seconds) with corticomedullary differentiation and a late corticomedullary phase (from 45 seconds up to 120 seconds) with homogeneous renal enhancement in both the renal cortex and medulla.

Microbubbles may be used as tracers for the functional assessment of the renal vascularity. Renal perfusion may be calculated by analyzing the replenishment kinetics of the volume from microbubbles after their destruction by initial high transmit power insonation.[23] The video intensity of a digital cine clip may be quantified by positioning an ROI in a region of the parenchyma and by correlating the time with the video intensity measured in a linear or logarithmic scale. The fundamental assumption is that the relation between microbubble concentration video intensity is linear up the achievement of a plateau phase. Software packages produced by the US scanner manufacturers access the raw data before application of nonlinear modifications and allow proper quantification. Different mathematical functions have been proposed to analyze the replenishment kinetic of microbubbles. The slope of the first ascending curve (approximately blood flow velocity) and the maximum amplitude of the refilling curve (approximately fractional blood volume) are calculated to quantify organ perfusion. In patients with renal artery stenosis or other vascular abnormalities, the refilling curve revealed an increased time to peak and reduced slope of the wash-in tract and maximum amplitude.

Animal models were initially employed to assess the capabilities of CEUS in the detection of renal perfusion defects,[46–49] which appear as single or multiple focal wedge-shaped areas of absent, diminished, or delayed contrast enhancement in comparison to the adjacent renal parenchyma. The identification of small renal perfusion defects in the subcapsular renal region is penalized by the limited spatial resolution of CEUS, which cannot identify renal perfusion defects smaller than 5 mm. In humans, microbubble contrast agents and contrast-specific imaging techniques improved significantly the diagnostic confidence level in identifying nonperfused renal parenchymal zones, especially in renal infarction, with a reliable depiction of renal perfusion defects.[50] Regional renal infarctions appear as single or multiple focal wedge-shaped areas of absent, diminished, or delayed contrast enhancement in comparison to the adjacent renal parenchyma after microbubble injection (Fig. 10.6). In the case of renal artery occlusion, complete filling defects appear as a nonvascularized renal parenchyma in comparison to the adjacent parenchymal organs (Fig. 10.7). This is particularly useful for renal transplants, especially as microbubbles are not nephrotoxic.

Heart

In cardiac imaging, CEUS has an established role in left ventricle opacification and endocardial border definition to assess myocardial function and ejection fraction.[51] Regarding the heart, CEUS is mainly named as contrast echocardiography in the dedicated literature. Noninvasive perfusion imaging with contrast echocardiography is now a feasible clinical tool.[32,33,52,53] Myocardial blood flow and total coronary blood volume can be quantified with myocardial contrast echocardiography.[54–56] The behavior of microbubbles in the normal circulation depends on more than just their size and deformability.[55,56] When microbubbles are administered as a constant infusion, steady state is achieved after 2 to 3 minutes, where their concentration in any blood pool (left ventricular cavity, myocardium, etc.) is constant and proportional to the blood volume fraction of that pool. The video intensity measured from the myocardium normalized to that from the left ventricular cavity provides a measure of mean blood volume fraction (since the left ventricular cavity is 100% blood).

Since microbubbles within the myocardium can be destroyed with high acoustic power insonation, they can be rapidly eliminated from the myocardium. By measuring the rate of microbubble reappearance through reperfusion technique, red blood cells velocity can be determined.[56] In experimental studies, an excellent linear relationship between absolute myocardial blood flow measured with radiolabeled microspheres and myocardial contrast echocardiography-derived microbubble velocity or myocardial blood flow was found.[30] Thus, contrast echocardiography allows quantification of myocardial blood flow velocity (β), mean blood volume (A), and myocardial blood flow ($A\beta$) in both experimental and clinical settings.

The method for quantification of myocardial blood flow with contrast echocardiography is based on an assessment of microbubble transit through the myocardial capillary bed. Myocardial vessels fill with blood when myocardial elastance is low in diastole. In systole, the high elastance compresses intramyocardial arterioles, which empty out retrogradely.[56] Likewise, intramyocardial veins are compressed during systole, which propels blood forward into the coronary sinus. Because arterioles and venules are larger than capillaries, their compression would occur earlier in systole, causing an increase in their resistance that would result in the functional isolation of capillaries.[56] Capillary pressure would thus increase concurrently with intramyocardial pressure during systole, preventing appreciable changes in capillary dimensions. Since large intramyocardial vessels do not fill anterogradely during systole, the progressive replenishment of microbubbles in the capillary bed alone is determined using intermittent high acoustic power imaging triggered in systole.[55,56]

With low acoustic power imaging, a "flash" impulse consisting of several high-power US frames can be used to destroy the microbubbles within the beam elevation, and microbubble replenishment into the microcirculation can then be followed while imaging is continued at a relatively high frame rate (>15 Hz). With real-time imaging, frames throughout the cardiac cycle are acquired after each flash impulse. In diastole, however, large intramyocardial vessels rapidly replenish with microbubbles due to their high flow velocity. Therefore, capillary replenishment is not being evaluated during diastole, and fitting a replenishment curve to sequential end-diastolic frames results in overestimation of the velocity of

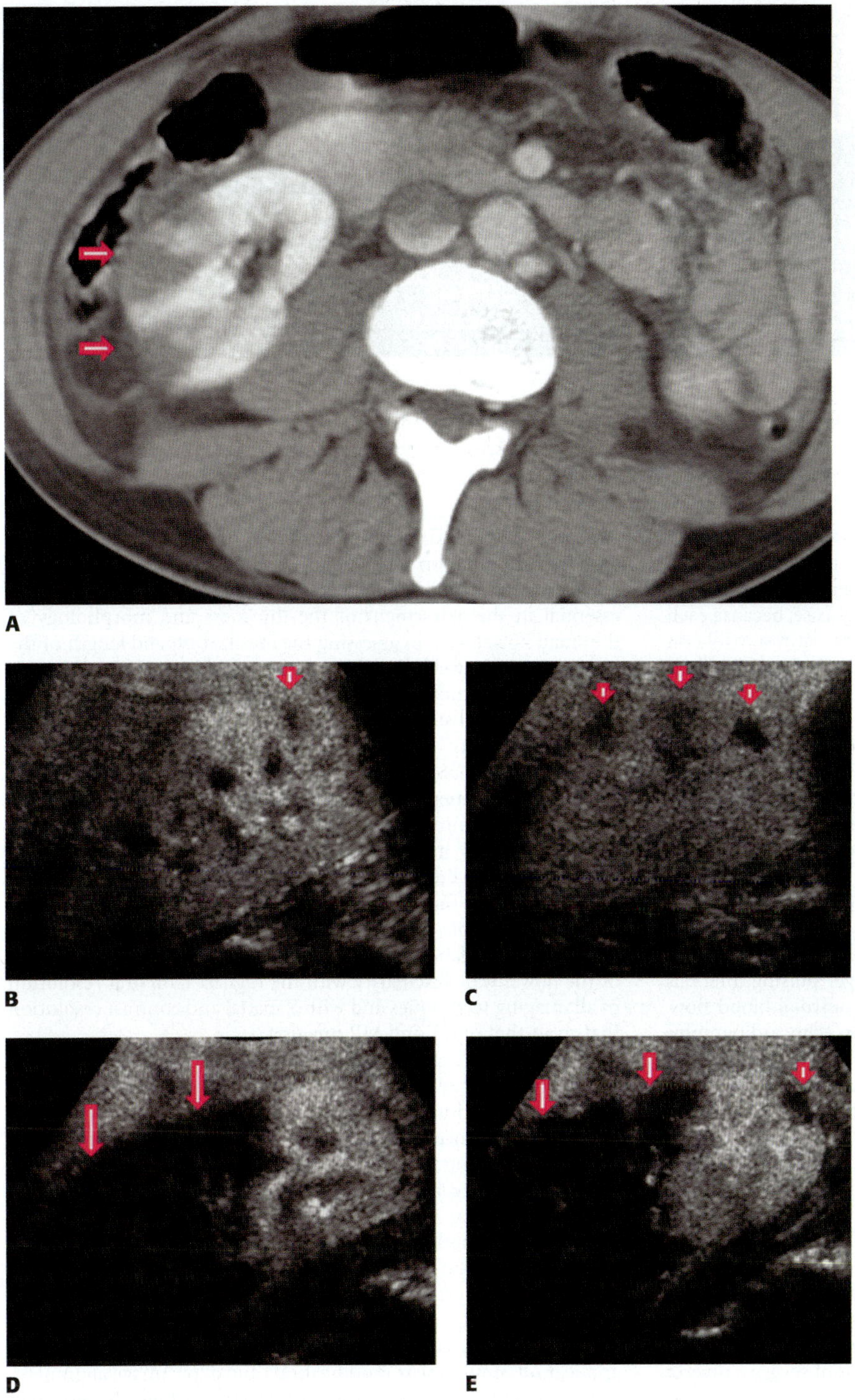

Figure 10-6. A 64-year-old patient with thrombotic aneurysm of the thoracic aorta and peripheral embolization. **A:** Contrast-enhanced CT shows renal infarctions (*arrows*) on the right kidney. **B–E:** Contrast-enhanced ultrasound scan obtained 10 days after contrast-enhanced CT: **(B and C)** the right kidney shows multiple subcapsular renal infarctions (*arrows*); **(D and E)** the left kidney shows a massive renal parenchyma infarction (*long arrows*) with the addition of a small perfusion defect on the lower renal pole (*short arrow*).

myocardial blood flow by 41%.[56] Fitting the exponential function to all frames (including diastolic and systolic) within the cardiac cycle overestimates the velocity of myocardial blood flow by 24%.[56] Myocardial blood flow derived from end-diastolic frames also correlates poorly with relative flows derived from radiolabeled microspheres ($r = 0.53$, $p = 0.04$).[56] Accurate quantification of the velocity of myocardial blood flow and of myocardial blood flow is achieved by using only end-systolic frames. The use of systolic frames also allows quantification of stenosis severity ($r = 0.94$, $p < 0.001$). Despite assessment of only end-systolic frames with both high and low acoustic power imaging techniques, differences in the quantitative parameters are still obtained using the two modalities.

During hyperemia, the normal myocardium replenishes rapidly after microbubble destruction (1 to 1.5 seconds), while in regions subserved by stenoses, the rate of filling is slower depending upon the severity of stenosis. The filling abnormalities are frequently seen to be more marked in the endocardium and, in the case of milder stenosis, may be localized only within the endocardium. It is for this reason that contrast echocardiography has been shown to be more sensitive than SPECT for the detection of coronary stenosis in patients with normal regional function and only moderate coronary artery disease.

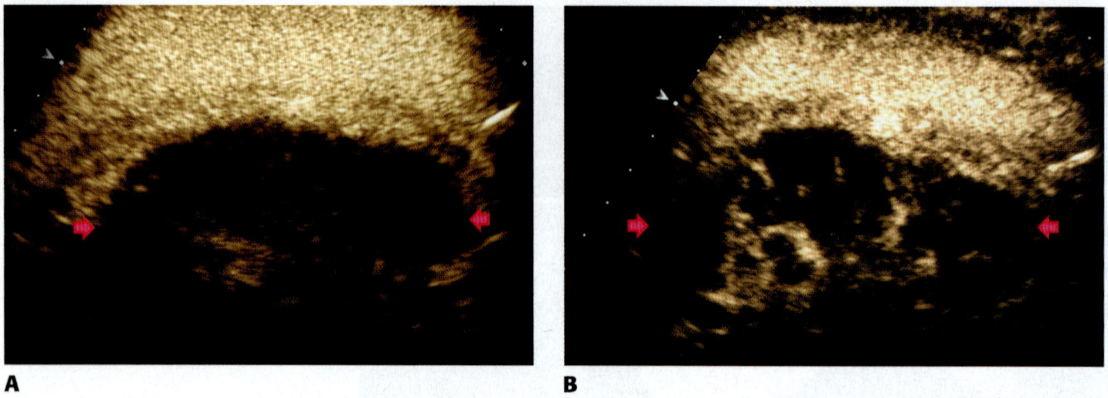

Figure 10-7. A and B: **A 75-year-old patient with abdominal aorta aneurysm treated by an endovascular stent.** The endograft closed the left renal artery. After microbubble contrast agent injection, the left kidney (*arrows*) appears avascular in comparison to the adjacent spleen.

Because of its poorer spatial resolution (cm vs. mm) compared to contrast echocardiography, SPECT cannot detect defects located only in the endocardium. Contrast echocardiography is also superior in identifying multivessel coronary artery disease, because each myocardial segment at stress is compared to itself at rest, while on SPECT, the comparison is across segments, so that left main or "balanced" multivessel coronary artery disease can be missed.

The contrast echocardiography methods to quantify regional myocardial blood flow can also be used to detect coronary stenoses in the clinical setting and can noninvasively determine the physiologic significance of stenoses in patients.[56] Since hyperemic myocardial blood flow is lower in the presence of a physiologically significant stenosis, microbubble replenishment into a bed subtended by a stenosis is slower than a normal bed and results in a relative perfusion defect at short pulsing interval. In a case of milder stenosis, only abnormalities in velocity of myocardial blood flow may be detected, while changes in myocardial blood flow may be difficult to detect, since replenishment at longer pulsing intervals may be normal due to collateral-supplied myocardial blood flow. Stenosis severity can be quantified from contrast echocardiography. By dividing hyperemic velocity of myocardial blood flow by that at rest, myocardial blood flow velocity reserve can be calculated. Myocardial blood flow velocity reserve less than 1.5 indicates the presence of greater than 70% epicardial stenosis.[55,56]

Bowel Wall

The quantitative analysis of the bowel wall contrast enhancement, with calculation of semiquantitative parameters from the time–intensity curve, related to the bowel wall flow and perfusion, in a further emerging application of CEUS. Crohn disease is an idiopathic chronic inflammatory disease of the gastrointestinal tract, which presents a relapsing nature, varying levels of severity, diverse manifestations, and unexpected complications. For these reasons, frequent imaging reevaluations are necessary in many patients with Crohn disease over the years. Barium enteroclysis, endoscopy with biopsy of the terminal ileal loop, and wireless capsule endoscopy are considered the reference standard techniques in the elective diagnosis of Crohn disease. These diagnostic methods allow the accurate evaluation of the inner bowel surface but are unable to give direct information about the transmural involvement in Crohn disease. On the other hand, CT and MR imaging present the capacity to demonstrate the transmural and extraintestinal extent of Crohn disease.

US has become an alternative imaging technique to assess the involvement of the small bowel in Crohn disease due its high contrast, spatial and temporal resolution and should be the first imaging examination in patients with suspected Crohn disease presenting with abdominal pain. Unenhanced gray-scale US is essential in the assessment of the thickness and morphology of the small bowel wall, in assessing the localization and length of the inflammatory bowel lesions or strictures, and in detecting the perivisceral complications typical of Crohn disease including abscesses, phlegmons, and fistulas even though it is less accurate to evaluate the disease activity.

Recently, CEUS has been proposed as a further imaging technique to assess patients with Crohn disease particularly in the evaluation of the inflammatory activity. The use of CEUS in patients with Crohn disease[57–59] has been recognized also by the recent nonliver guidelines of the European Federation of Societies for Ultrasound in Medicine and Biology (EFSUMB)[60] even though, presently, the use of microbubble contrast agents in the examination of the small bowel is still off-label. CEUS currently allows real-time assessment of the bowel wall vascularity with the highest temporal resolution of all imaging techniques and with a spatial and contrast resolution that rivals that of CT and MR imaging.

The addition of software packages, dedicated to the off-line analysis or directly installed in the US equipment, enables the image segmentation and the quantitative measurements of small bowel wall enhancement after microbubble contrast agent injection. When compared to visual analysis, quantitative analysis allows a more precise assessment of parietal enhancement with a lower influence of observer experience even though a significant interreader variability could be still expected. The quantitative analysis of the echo-signal intensity may eliminate the influence of logarithmic compression, color maps, postprocessing curves, and techniques for edge enhancement on the input signal for video presentation. Dedicated software packages access the raw data before application of nonlinear modifications and allow image alignment, signal averaging, and background subtraction, while the color map from the contrast-specific technique is automatically converted to a gray-scale map.

The quantitative analysis of echo-signal intensity, especially in the small bowel, should be very accurate to provide reliable and reproducible results. The first digital cine clip registered during the first-pass dynamic enhancement after microbubble contrast agent injection is transferred to a PC connected to the PACS. In each image, a manually defined polygonal ROI can be drawn encompassing the thickened bowel enhancing wall avoiding the lumen and the mesentery for the whole extension of the bowel loop included in the field of view of the US screen. However, the selection of the ROI to measure the contrast agent enhancement depends on the radiologist, which potentially may introduce some interobserver variability also in quantitative analysis. If peristalsis-related movements are evident in the scanned volume, those frames, which appear off-site to the reader, may be virtually excluded from the quantitative analysis.

Differently from the kidney and heart perfusion assessment by CEUS, routinely microbubbles are injected as a bolus (2 mL/second) to assess bowel wall perfusion. Consequently, the correct theoretical model for data fitting is the gamma variate[24] or the lognormal[25,31] perfusion models. The gamma-variate function corresponds to the following formula: $SI(t) = Ate^{-\beta t} + C$, where t is the time, e is the base of natural logarithm, $SI(t)$ is the signal intensity versus time, A is the amplitude of the curve above baseline, β is the initial slope of the ascending tract of the curve, and C is the echo-signal intensity at the baseline (the zero crossing point of the y-axis). The lognormal perfusion model, which is the most used by software packages, is based on the theory of indicator dilution model, which accounts for microvascular network geometry and hemodynamics, as well as the ultrasound beam sensitivity throughout the imaging plane. In this model, the infusion plateau is proportional to the fractional blood volume, while the rate of replenishment is related to the mean flow velocity.

Different semiquantitative kinetic parameters, corresponding to numerical values related to tissue perfusion instead to its absolute values, may be automatically calculated by the software in each patient (Fig. 10.8): (a) the percentage of maximum enhancement (corresponding to the percentage of the highest possible echo-signal intensity value before the achievement of echo-signal saturation); (b) the time-to-peak enhancement; and (c) the area under the time–intensity enhancement curve, which is related to the regional blood volume. To eliminate the influence of microbubble arrival time variability in the different patients, which is related to different physiologic parameters including the cardiac output, it is preferable to calculate the time-to-peak enhancement and the area under each time–intensity curve from the time of the initial microbubble visualization in the scanning plane during the first 20 seconds after injection. Other semiquantitative parameters, which may be calculated by dedicated software, include (but are not limited to) the difference between the baseline brightness and the value of maximum enhancement after microbubble contrast agent injection, and the slope of the first ascending tract of the time–intensity curve.

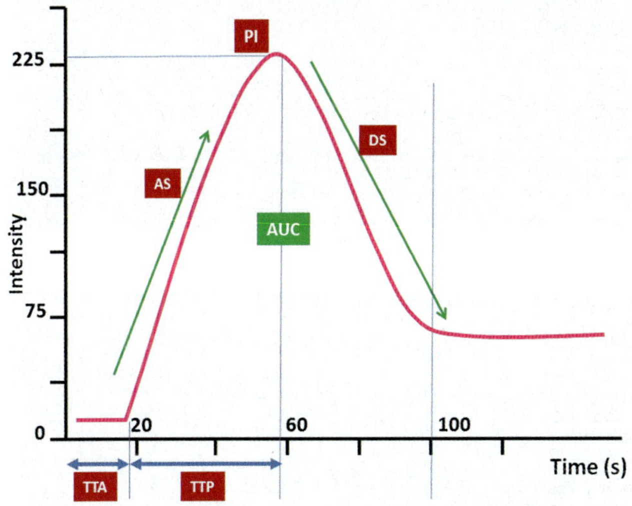

Figure 10-8. Time–intensity curve in a target region of interest showing different parameters defined for perfusion imaging. AS, ascending slope is the maximum wash-in velocity of the contrast medium in intensity/1,000 per second; DS, descending slope is the maximum wash-out velocity of the contrast medium in intensity/1,000 per second; AUC, area under the curve, which is proportional to the total volume of blood in that region; TTP, time to peak in seconds; TTA, time to arrival of microbubbles in seconds; PI, peak intensity in intensity/1,000.

Assessment of Crohn Disease Activity

Assessment of inflammatory activity is an essential component of the management of Crohn disease since in these patients the episodes of inflammation alternate with periods of remission. Therefore, the periodic assessment of Crohn disease inflammatory activity is crucial to plan a proper treatment. Several clinical indices have been proposed to assess Crohn disease activity. Most frequently, Crohn disease activity consists in the clinical response of patients by using the Crohn disease activity index (CDAI). Anyway, CDAI presents a low specificity since it is based on subjective symptoms, a low correlation with mucosal inflammation, and a poor interobserver reproducibility, while patients with inactive Crohn disease often attract high CDAI scores. Endoscopy continues to be the gold standard for lesion assessment in Crohn disease, even though patients with active Crohn disease may not accept undergoing the examination while the intubation of the distal ileum can only be completed in 80% of patients. Generally, the evaluation of Crohn disease activity should be based on the integration between clinical symptoms, physical findings, laboratory parameters, endoscopy, and imaging tests.

The different imaging modalities represent an alternative tool to assess Crohn disease activity and should provide a more objective measurement of Crohn disease activity in comparison to the CDAI score. CT and MR imaging are reliable techniques for assessing the inflammatory activity of Crohn disease, even though they present some limitations. First, both techniques require the administration of large amount of enteric contrast material or a catheter set for the nasal intubation. Second, a high-dose exposition is produced if CT is repeated during a strict follow-up schedule, as is often requested in patients with CD. Third, both CT and MR imaging require long preparation times and produce some patient discomfort due to the distension of the small bowel loops.

As a general rule, patients with active Crohn disease presents mural enhancement on the thickened bowel wall after microbubble contrast agent injection. On visual analysis, four different bowel wall enhancement patterns may be observed after microbubble contrast agent injection including (a) submucosal (with or without mucosal) enhancement sparing the muscularis propria; (b) complete transmural enhancement starting from mucosa (outward or centrifugal enhancement) and involving the entire bowel wall, which are generally related to active Crohn disease; (c) complete transmural enhancement starting from perivisceral vessels (inward or centripetal enhancement) and involving the entire bowel wall; and (d) low or absent enhancement (in comparison to the adjacent mesentery), which are generally related to quiescent Crohn disease or to mural fibrosis.[61] Unfortunately, visual analysis is penalized by the reasonable presence of interobserver variability mainly due to the rapid microbubble inflow, which does not provide a wide temporal window for a complete and unequivocal evaluation of each enhancement pattern. The careful review of the registered cine clips may allow a more reliable and reproducible assessment of the bowel wall contrast enhancement patterns.

Mural thickening correlates with inflammatory activity demonstrated by endoscopy, while the mural enhancement after microbubble contrast agent injection correlates more than mural thickening with the inflammatory activity of Crohn disease. On quantitative analysis, patients with active Crohn disease present a reduced time-to-peak enhancement and an increased percentage of maximal enhancement and area under time–intensity enhancement curve in comparison to patient with quiescent disease. The reason for this phenomenon is assumed to be an increase of blood flow and local tissue perfusion related to neoangiogenesis. According to the recent literature, CEUS presents a range of sensitivity and specificity from 80% and 60% up to 95% and 94% in distinguishing active and quiescent Crohn disease.[60–62]

Differentiation of Mural Fibrosis from Mural Inflammation

Bowel stricture may be identified in up to 50% of patients with Crohn disease. Both inflammatory and fibrotic Crohn disease may determine bowel strictures, and this represents a therapeutic challenge since Crohn disease status with active inflammation require medical treatment, while mural fibrosis indicates surgical treatment. Although CT and MR imaging present a good diagnostic accuracy (about 90%) in differentiating the bowel wall inflammation from fibrosis, CEUS currently allows real-time assessment of the bowel wall vascularity with the highest temporal resolution of all imaging techniques and with a spatial and contrast resolution that rivals that of CT and MR imaging.

Unenhanced US may detect the presence of a stricture due to bowel wall thickening in CD, and it may differentiate inflammatory stenosis based on the lack of visibility of the small bowel wall layers. Anyway, the increase in echogenicity of the mural submucosal layer is also correlated with an increase in submucosal vascularity, and inflammatory infiltration as could be verified in the surgical specimen. On the other hand, the bowel wall thickening characterized by a stratified echo pattern is mainly related to fibrosis. After microbubble injection, the percentage of maximal enhancement and the area under time–intensity curve, higher in patients with inflammatory strictures, produced the highest value of diagnostic confidence to discriminate inflammatory versus fibrotic structure.[58] Unfortunately, in most of cases, a mixture of acute inflammation and fibrosis or some areas of inflammation and different areas with fibrosis are detected in the same bowel stricture making the differential diagnosis very difficult on CEUS as in contrast-enhanced CT and MR.

Assessment of Therapeutic Outcome

Thanks to its high temporal resolution, CEUS represents a valuable additional imaging method to assess the Crohn disease activity also during the pharmacologic treatment. The long-term pharmacologic treatment of Crohn disease includes salicylates (e.g., mesalazine), immunosuppressive drugs (e.g., azathioprine), or newer immunomodulating agents (biologic therapies) such as monoclonal anti–TNF-α antibodies (infliximab). These treatments have been shown to be effective in the treatment of Crohn disease and can be monitored by clinical indices of active disease, laboratory parameters, endoscopy, or histology. Most frequently, the therapeutic outcome assessment is made by evaluating the clinical response of patients by using the CDAI, which is still considered the reference parameter for the evaluation of drug efficacy in patients with Crohn disease. Anyway, CDAI presents a low specificity since it is based on subjective symptoms, while patients with quiescent Crohn disease often attract high CDAI scores. Treatment adjustment (intensification through pharmacologic dose increments, deintensification, or the introduction of new drugs) should also be based on objective measures of Crohn disease activity and not only on patient symptoms. Imaging techniques including CT and MR enterography and CEUS may provide a more objective measurement of Crohn disease activity in comparison to the CDAI score.

Since Crohn disease presents a relapsing nature and unexpected complications, frequent imaging reevaluations are necessary during the pharmacologic treatment. CEUS could be the ideal imaging technique to monitor the Crohn disease activity during the pharmacologic treatment since it does not present any limit in performing frequent serial examinations at short intervals and does not present radiation exposure. Unfortunately, the visual assessment of bowel wall enhancement after microbubble contrast agent injection cannot differentiate responders and nonresponders among patients with Crohn disease under pharmacologic treatment. The addition of specific software for echo-signal quantitation, enabling the image segmentation and the quantitative measurements of small bowel wall enhancement after microbubble injection, allows a more precise assessment of parietal enhancement with a lower influence of observer experience even though a significant interreader variability could be still expected.

CEUS might become a crucial imaging modality for monitoring the efficacy of specific medical therapy in reducing bowel wall vascularity (Figs. 10.9 and 10.10) related to neoangiogenesis

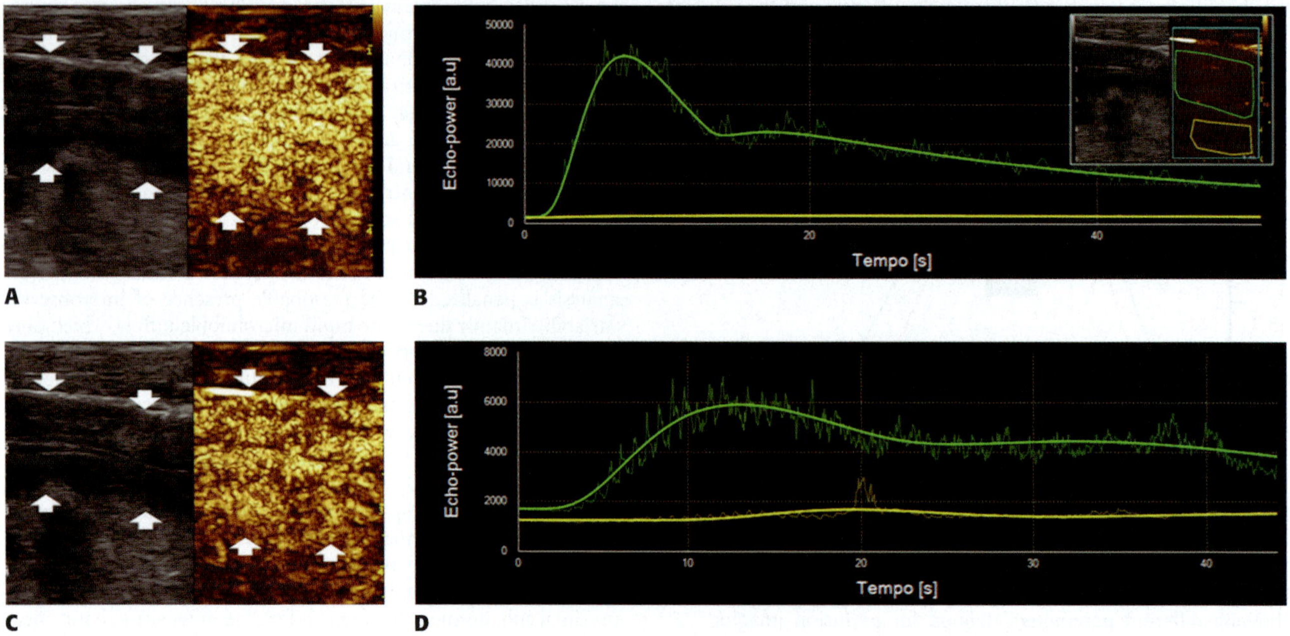

Figure 10-9. A 25-year-old male Crohn disease patient. Difference in the time–intensity curve profile before and after pharmacologic treatment. Good response to pharmacologic therapy. **A:** Contrast-enhanced ultrasound scan of the terminal ileal loop (*arrows*). **B:** The corresponding time–intensity curve obtained after echo-power quantitation by placing a region of interest over the bowel wall (*green*) and in the adjacent mesentery (*yellow*) as shown in the inlay image. **C and D:** The same patient scanned by contrast-enhanced ultrasound 6 weeks after the beginning of specific anti-inflammatory treatment (infliximab). There is a decrease intensity of the signal at visual analysis **(C)**, which is confirmed by the quantitative analysis **(D)**.

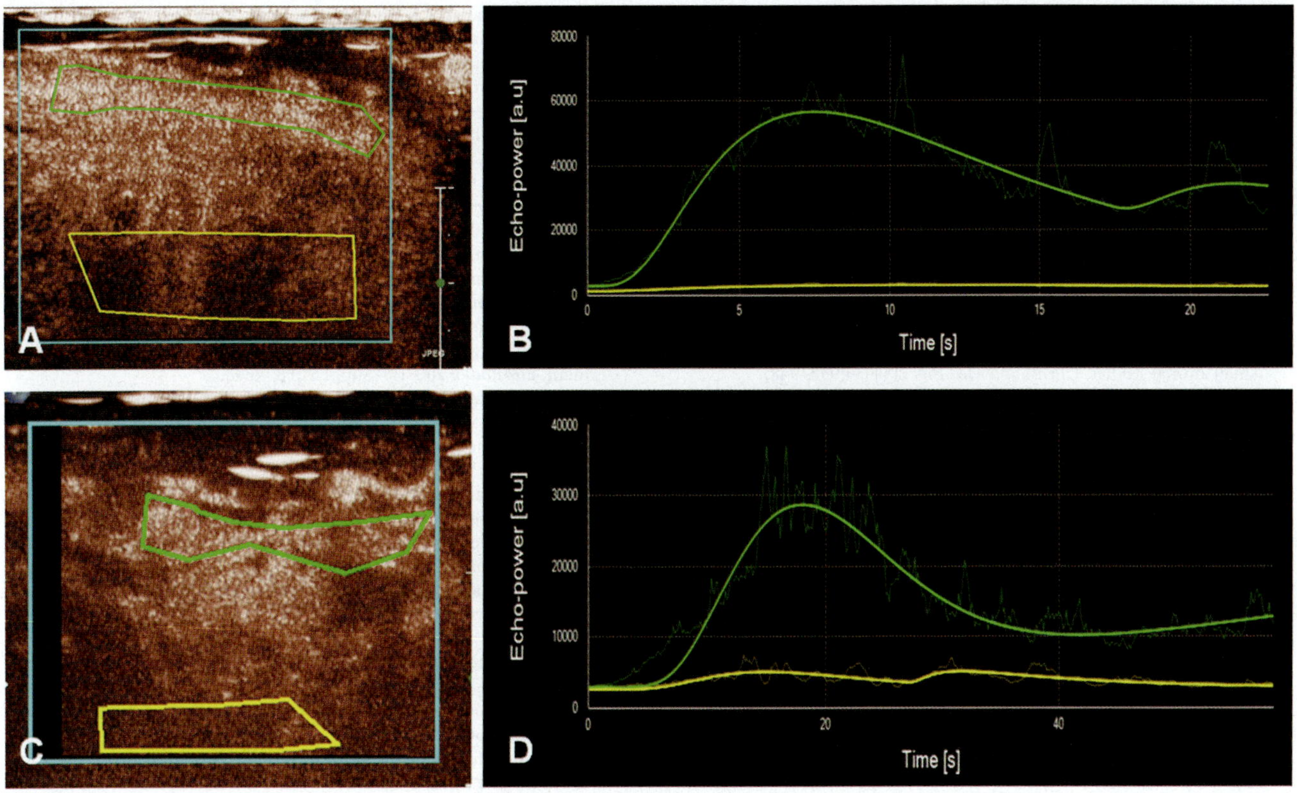

Figure 10-10. **A 45-year-old male Crohn disease patient.** Moderate response to pharmacologic therapy. Difference in the time–intensity curve profile before and after pharmacologic treatment. **A:** Contrast-enhanced ultrasound scan of the terminal ileal loop with a region of interest manually drawn over the bowel wall (*green*) and another region of interest drawn over the adjacent mesentery (*yellow*). **B:** The corresponding time–intensity curve obtained after echo-power quantitation. **C and D:** The same patient scanned by contrast-enhanced ultrasound 3 months after the beginning of specific anti-inflammatory treatment (corticosteroids and azathioprine). There is a moderate decrease intensity of the signal at visual analysis **(C)**, which is confirmed by the quantitative analysis **(D)**.

through the echo-signal quantitative analysis.[59,63] Anyway, it is preferable that the same patient is evaluated by the same radiologist using the same US equipment to avoid to introduce interreader or interequipment variability. Indeed, patients with clinically active Crohn disease and higher signal intensity after microbubble injection show a clear reduction in bowel wall thickening after steroid treatment, while patients with active Crohn disease in whom no evident echo-signal increase is detected before or after microbubble injection present a disease which is less responsive to steroid therapy and should undergo surgical resection. Moreover, patients with a clinically quiescent Crohn disease after medical treatment but with a thickened enhancing wall after microbubble contrast agent injection have an higher risk of relapse during the follow-up[61-63].

REFERENCES

1. **Quaia E.** Assessment of tissue perfusion by contrast-enhanced ultrasound. *Eur Radiol* 2011;21(3):604–615.
2. **Claudon M, Tranquart F, Evans DH, et al.** Advances in ultrasound. *Eur Radiol* 2002;12(1):7–18.
3. **Quaia E.** Microbubble ultrasound contrast agents: an update. *Eur Radiol* 2007;17(8):1995–2008.
4. **Piscaglia F, Bolondi L; Italian Society for Ultrasound in Medicine and Biology (SIUMB) Study Group on Ultrasound Contrast Agents.** The safety of Sonovue in abdominal applications: retrospective analysis of 23188 investigations. *Ultrasound Med Biol* 2006;32(9):1369–1375.
5. **Quaia E.** Physical basis and Principles of action of microbubble-based contrast agents. In: Quaia E, ed. *Contrast media in ultrasonography: basic principles and clinical applications*. Berlin/Heidelberg/New York: Springer; 2005:15–30.
6. **Frinking PJA.** *Ultrasound contrast agents: acoustic characterization and diagnostic imaging*. Rotterdam, The Netherlands: Optima Grafische Communicatie; 1999:33–37.
7. **Whittingham T.** Contrast-specific imaging techniques: technical perspective. In: Quaia E, ed. *Contrast media in ultrasonography: basic principles and clinical applications*. Berlin/Heidelberg/New York: Springer; 2005:43–70.
8. **Quaia E.** Contrast-specific ultrasound techniques. *Radiol Med* 2007; 112(4):473–490.
9. **Cosgrove DO, Eckersley RJ, Blomely MJK.** Quantitative analysis of parenchymal flow at contrast-enhanced US. In: Quaia E, ed. *Contrast media in ultrasonography: basic principles and clinical applications*. Berlin/Heidelberg/New York: Springer; 2005:383–391.
10. **Winehouse J, Douek M, Holz K, et al.** Contrast-enhanced colour Doppler ultrasonography in suspected breast cancer recurrence. *Br J Surg* 1999;86(9):1198–1201.
11. **Bäz E, Madjar H, Reuss C, et al.** The role of enhanced Doppler ultrasound in differentiation of benign vs. malignant scar lesion after breast surgery for malignancy. *Ultrasound Obstet Gynecol* 2000;15(5):377–382.
12. **Blomley MJ, Lim AK, Harvey CJ, et al.** Liver microbubble transit time compared with histology and Child-Pugh score in diffuse liver disease: a cross sectional study. *Gut* 2003;52(8):1188–1193.
13. **Lim AK, Taylor-Robinson SD, Patel N, et al.** Hepatic vein transit times using a microbubble agent can predict disease severity non-invasively in patients with hepatitis C. *Gut* 2005;54(1):128–133.
14. **Lim AK, Patel N, Eckersley RJ, et al.** Hepatic vein transit time of SonoVue: a comparative study with Levovist. *Radiology* 2006;240(1):130–135.
15. **Blomley MJ, Albrecht T, Cosgrove DO, et al.** Liver vascular transit time analyzed with dynamic hepatic venography with bolus injections of an US contrast agent: early experience in seven patients with metastases. *Radiology* 1998;209(3):862–866. Erratum in *Radiology* 1999; 209(3):862.

16. **Oppo K, Leen E, Angerson WJ, et al.** Doppler perfusion index: an interobserver and intraobserver reproducibility study. *Radiology* 1998; 208(2):453–457.
17. **Leen E, Angerson WJ, Wotherspoon H, et al.** Comparison of the Doppler perfusion index and intraoperative ultrasonography in diagnosing colorectal liver metastases. Evaluation with postoperative follow-up results. *Ann Surg* 1994;220(5):663–667.
18. **Payen T, Coron A, Lamuraglia M, et al.** Echo-power estimation from log-compressed video data in dynamic contrast-enhanced ultrasound imaging. *Ultrasound Med Biol* 2013;39(10):1826–1837.
19. **Correas JM, Burns PN, Lai X, et al.** Infusion versus bolus of an ultrasound contrast agent: in vivo dose–response measurements of BR1. *Invest Radiol* 2000;35(1):72–79.
20. **Mulè S, De Cesare A, Lucidarme O, et al.** Regularized estimation of contrast agent attenuation to improve the imaging of microbubbles in small animal studies. *Ultrasound Med Biol* 2008;34:938–948.
21. **Mari J, Hibbs K, Stride E, et al.** An approximate nonlinear model for time gain compensation of amplitude modulated images of ultrasound contrast agent perfusion. *IEEE Trans Ultrason Ferroelectr Freq Control* 2010;57:818–829.
22. **Wei K, Jayaweera AR, Firoozan S, et al.** Quantification of myocardial blood flow with ultrasound-induced destruction of microbubbles administered as a constant venous infusion. *Circulation* 1998;97(5): 473–483.
23. **Lucidarme O, Kono Y, Corbeil J, et al.** Validation of ultrasound contrast destruction imaging for flow quantification. *Ultrasound Med Biol* 2003;29:1697–1704.
24. **Cosgrove DO, Eckersley R, Blomley M, et al.** Quantification of blood flow. *Eur Radiol* 2001;11:1338–1344.
25. **Arditi M, Frinking PJ, Zhou X, et al.** A new formalism for the quantification of tissue perfusion by the destruction replenishment method in contrast ultrasound imaging. *IEEE Trans Ultrason Ferroelectr Freq Control* 2006;53:1118–1129.
26. **Lucidarme O, Franchi-Abella S, Correas JM, et al.** Blood flow quantification with contrast-enhanced US: "entrance in the section" phenomenon—phantom and rabbit study. *Radiology* 2003;228:473–479.
27. **Quaia E, Nocentini A, Torelli L.** Assessment of a new mathematical model for the computation of numerical parameters related to renal cortical blood flow and fractional blood volume by contrast-enhanced ultrasound. *Ultrasound Med Biol* 2009;35(4):616–627.
28. **Potdevin TCU, Fowlkes JB, Moskalik AP, et al.** Analysis of refill curve shape in ultrasound contrast agent studies. *Med Phys* 2004;31(3): 623–632.
29. **Potdevin TCU, Fowlkes JB, Moskalik AP, et al.** Refill model of rabbit kidney vasculature. *Ultrasound Med Biol* 2006;32:1331–1338.
30. **Krix M, Kiessling F, Farhan N, et al.** A multivessel model describing replenishment kinetics of ultrasound contrast agent for quantification of tissue perfusion. *Ultrasound Med Biol* 2003;29:1421–1430.
31. **Williams R, Hudson JM, Lloyd BA, et al.** Dynamic microbubble contrast-enhanced US to measure tumor response to targeted therapy: a proposed clinical protocol with results from renal cell carcinoma patients receiving antiangiogenic therapy. *Radiology* 2011;260:581–590.
32. **Bruce M, Averkiou M, Tiemann K, et al.** Vascular flow and perfusion imaging with ultrasound contrast agents. *Ultrasound Med Biol* 2004;30: 735–743.
33. **Seidel G, Meairs S.** Ultrasound contrast agents in ischemic stroke. *Cerebrovasc Dis* 2009;27(Suppl 2):25–39.
34. **Wei K, Ragosta M, Thorpe J, et al.** Non-invasive quantification of coronary blood flow reserve in humans using myocardial contrast echocardiography. *Circulation* 2001;103:2560–2565.
35. **Gasparini C, Bertolotto M, Crocè SL, et al.** Evaluation of liver parenchymal blood flow with contrast-enhanced US: preliminary results in healthy and cirrhotic patients. *Acad Radiol* 2003;10(8):869–876.
36. **Weber MA, Krix M, Jappe U, et al.** Pathologic skeletal muscle perfusion in patients with myositis: detection with quantitative contrast-enhanced US—initial results. *Radiology* 2005;238(2):640–649.
37. **Lindner JR, Womack L, Barrett E, et al.** Limb stress-rest perfusion imaging with contrast ultrasound for the assessment of peripheral arterial disease severity. *J Am Coll Cardiol* 2008;1:343–350.
38. **Christiansen JP, Leong-Poi H, Amiss LR, et al.** Skin perfusion assessed by contrast ultrasound predicts tissue survival in a free flap model. *Ultrasound Med Biol* 2002;28(3):315–320.
39. **Klauser A, Demharter J, De Marchi A, et al.** Contrast enhanced gray-scale sonography in assessment of joint vascularity in rheumatoid arthritis: results from the IACUS study group. *Eur Radiol* 2005;15:2404–2410.
40. **Paltiel HJ, Kalish LA, Susaeta RA, et al.** Pulse inversion US imaging of testicular ischemia: quantitative and qualitative analyses in a rabbit model. *Radiology* 2006;239:718–729.
41. **Chen L, Zhan WW, Shen ZJ, et al.** Blood perfusion of the contralateral testis evaluated with contrast-enhanced ultrasound in rabbits with unilateral testicular torsion. *Asian J Androl* 2009;11:253–260.
42. **Eckersley RJ, Sedelaar JP, Blomley MJK et al.** Quantitative microbubble enhanced transrectal ultrasound as a tool for monitoring hormonal treatment of prostate carcinoma. *Prostate* 2002;51:256–267.
43. **Krix M, Kiessling F, Vosseler S, et al.** Sensitive noninvasive monitoring of tumor perfusion during antiangiogenic therapy by intermittent bolus-contrast power Doppler sonography. *Cancer Res* 2003;63:8264–8270.
44. **Lassau N, Chami L, Benatsou B, et al.** Dynamic contrast-enhanced ultrasonography (DCE-US) with quantification of tumor perfusion: a new diagnostic tool to evaluate the early effects of antiangiogenic treatment. *Eur Radiol* 2007;17(Suppl 6):F89–F98.
45. **Lassau N, Lamuraglia M, Chami L, et al.** Gastrointestinal stromal tumors treated with imatinib: monitoring response with contrast-enhanced sonography. *AJR Am J Roentgenol* 2006;187(5):1267–1273.
46. **Wei K, Le E, Bin JP, et al.** Quantification of renal blood flow with contrast-enhanced ultrasound. *J Am Coll Cardiol* 2001;37:1135–1140.
47. **Taylor GA, Barnewolt CE, Adler BH, et al.** Renal cortical ischemia in rabbits revealed by contrast-enhanced power Doppler sonography. *AJR Am J Roentgenol* 1998;170:417–422.
48. **Taylor GA, Barnewolt CE, Claudon M, et al.** Depiction of renal perfusion defects with contrast-enhanced harmonic sonography in a porcine model. *AJR Am J Roentgenol* 1999;173:757–760.
49. **Quaia E, Siracusano S, Palumbo A, et al.** Detection of focal renal perfusion defects in rabbits after sulphur hexafluoride-filled microbubble injection at low transmission power ultrasound insonation. *Eur Radiol* 2006;16(1):166–172.
50. **Bertolotto M, Martegani A, Aiani L, et al.** Value of contrast-enhanced ultrasonography for detecting renal infarcts proven by contrast enhanced CT. A feasibility study. *Eur Radiol* 2008;18(2):376–383.
51. **Kaufmann BA, Wei K, Lindner JR.** Contrast echocardiography. *Curr Probl Cardiol* 2007;32:51–96.
52. **Wei K, Lindner J.** Contrast ultrasound in the assessment of patients presenting with suspected cardiac ischemia. *Crit Care Med* 2007;35 (5 Suppl):S280–S289.
53. **Porter TR, Xie F.** Myocardial perfusion imaging with contrast ultrasound. *JACC Cardiovasc Imaging* 2010;3(2):176–187.
54. **Jayaweera AR, Edwards N, Glasheen WP, et al.** In vivo myocardial kinetics of air-filled albumin microbubbles during myocardial contrast echocardiography. Comparison with radiolabeled red blood cells. *Circ Res* 1994;74(6):1157–1165.
55. **Lindner JR, Skyba DS, Goodman NC, et al.** Changes in myocardial blood volume with graded coronary stenosis. *Am J Physiol* 1997; 272:H567–H575.
56. **Kalvaitis S, Wei K.** Assessment of regional myocardial blood flow. In: Quaia E, ed. *Contrast media in ultrasonography*. Berlin/Heidelberg: Springer-Verlag; 2005:267–276.
57. **Quaia E.** Contrast-enhanced ultrasound of the small bowel in Crohn's disease. *Abdom Imaging* 2013;38(5):1005–1013.
58. **Quaia E, De Paoli L, Stocca T, et al.** The value of small bowel wall contrast enhancement after sulfur hexafluoride-filled microbubble injection to differentiate inflammatory from fibrotic strictures in patients with Crohn's disease. *Ultrasound Med Biol* 2012;38(8):1324–1332.
59. **Quaia E, Cabibbo B, De Paoli L, et al.** The value of time-intensity curves obtained after microbubble contrast agent injection to discriminate responders from non-responders to anti-inflammatory medication among patients with Crohn's disease. *Eur Radiol* 2013;23(6):1650–1659.
60. **Piscaglia F, Nolsøe C, Dietrich CF, et al.** (2012) The EFSUMB Guidelines and Recommendations on the Clinical Practice of Contrast Enhanced Ultrasound (CEUS): update 2011 on non-hepatic applications. *Ultraschall Med* 2012;33:33–59.
61. **Migaleddu V, Scanu AM, Quaia E, et al.** Contrast-enhanced ultrasonographic evaluation of inflammatory activity in Crohn's disease. *Gastroenterology* 2009;137(1):43–52.
62. **Ripollés T, Martínez MJ, Paredes JM, et al.** Crohn disease: correlation of findings at contrast-enhanced US with severity at endoscopy. *Radiology* 2009;253:241–248.
63. **De Franco A, Di Veronica A, Armuzzi A, et al.** Ileal Crohn disease: mural microvascularity quantified with contrast-enhanced US correlates with disease activity. *Radiology* 2012;262(2):680–688.

CHAPTER

11 Extracellular Contrast Media in Perfusion Imaging

Stacul Fulvio, MD and Henrik S. Thomsen, MD

Introduction

In all aspects of radiology (ultrasound, conventional radiography, computed tomography [CT] scanning, and magnetic resonance imaging [MRI]), medical imaging contrast-enhancing agents have been developed. They are used to enhance contrast, to characterize lesions, and to evaluate perfusion and flow-related abnormalities. They can also provide functional and morphologic information.

Classification

Iodine-Based Contrast Media

These agents are mainly used for CT and for angiography. They contain one or two triiodinated benzene rings (monomeric or dimeric agents) and may have electrical charges in their structure or not (ionic or nonionic agents) (Table 11.1). Ionic agents include one anion and one cation in each molecule.[1] These ions attract the negative and positive poles of the water molecules, and thus these agents are water soluble. Nonionic agents do not contain ions, but they are water soluble as well, thanks to their OH groups.

Therefore, we can classify iodine-based contrast media into four categories:

- Ionic monomers
- Ionic dimers
- Nonionic monomers
- Nonionic dimers

The monomers contain three atoms of iodine and the dimers contain six. Each molecule of ionic agents contains two particles in solution (one anion and one cation), while each molecule of the nonionic agent contains one particle in solution.[2] Therefore, the ratio between the number of iodine atoms and the number of particles in solution is as follows:

- Ionic monomers 1.5 (3:2)
- Ionic dimers 3 (6:2)
- Nonionic monomers 3 (3:1)
- Nonionic dimers 6 (6:1)

The ratio is closely related to the osmolality of the contrast materials because the osmolality of a solution is proportional to the sum of the concentrations of the different molecular or ionic particles contained in the solution. Indeed, the osmolality of ionic monomers is about five to seven times the osmolality of plasma (1,500 to 2,000 mOsm/kg) when considering iodine concentrations that are usually employed in CT or angiography. The osmolality of nonionic monomers and ionic dimers is two to three times the osmolality of the plasma, while nonionic dimers are iso-osmolar to plasma at any concentration (Table 11.2). Therefore, contrast media may be divided into high-osmolar agents (ionic monomers), low-osmolar agents (nonionic monomers and ionic dimers), and iso-osmolar agents (nonionic dimers).[2] It is interesting that nonionic monomers and ionic dimers are called low-osmolality agents even if their osmolality is still higher than the plasma osmolality.

The viscosity of the solution is another important parameter, although not as important as in the past, thanks to the use of modern injectors. Viscosity is affected by iodine concentration (the higher iodine concentration, the higher viscosity) and by the temperature (the higher temperature, the lower viscosity). Considering ionic monomers, their meglumine salts have a higher viscosity than sodium salts, but these agents generally have lower viscosities than nonionic monomers (Table 11.2). Additionally, the dimers usually display a higher viscosity than the monomers. Therefore, warming nonionic contrast media to body temperature to lower viscosity before their administration is advisable, particularly when nonionic dimers are used.

Iodine-based contrast media are in most cases given by bolus injection. Their pharmacokinetics is similar to those of extracellular gadolinium-based contrast media, whereas they differ regarding the protein binders used for MRI.[1] They are described according to a two-compartment model, the two compartments being the intravascular plasma space and the interstitial space. The agents do not enter cells significantly in or outside of the circulation. On injection into the circulating blood, they are simultaneously diluted in the circulating plasma volume and immediately begin to pass out of the circulation into the interstitium. At some point, varying among tissues, an "equilibrium point" is reached at which falling plasma levels and rising interstitial concentrations are transiently equal. After this point, as the contrast agents are continuously removed from blood via renal filtration, there is a reversal of movement and the contrast agents begin to come out of the interstitium and back into the plasma. Iodine-based contrast agents are excreted almost solely by the normal kidney by passive glomerular filtration with no significant active tubular involvement.

TABLE **11.1** **Structures, Types, and Names of Commercial Iodine-Based Contrast Media**

Charge/Structure	Ionic Monomers–High Osmolality			Ionic Dimer–Low Osmolality
Chemical structure	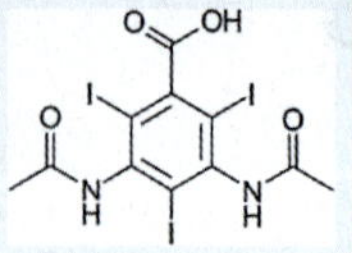	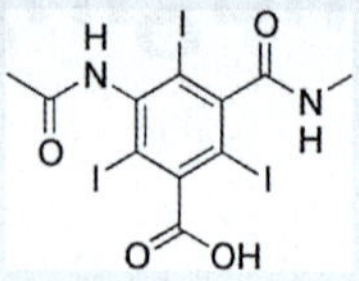	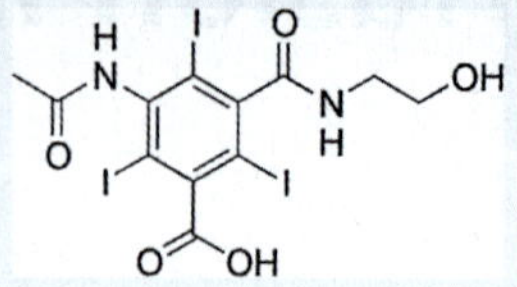	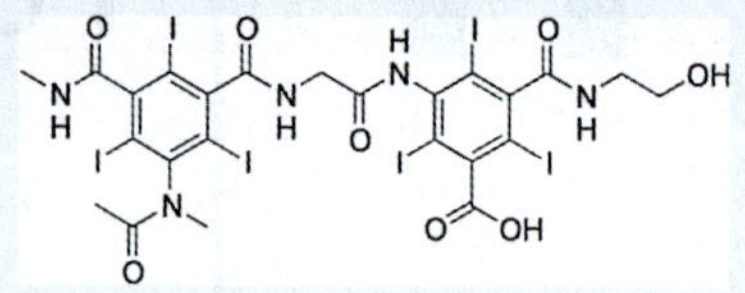
Generic name	Diatrizoic acid or diatrizoate	Iotalamic acid or iothalamate	Ioxitalamic acid or ioxitalamate	Ioxaglic acid or ioxaglate
Trade Name	Renografin, Hypaque	Conray	Telebrix	Hexabrix

Nonionic Monomers–Low Osmolality			
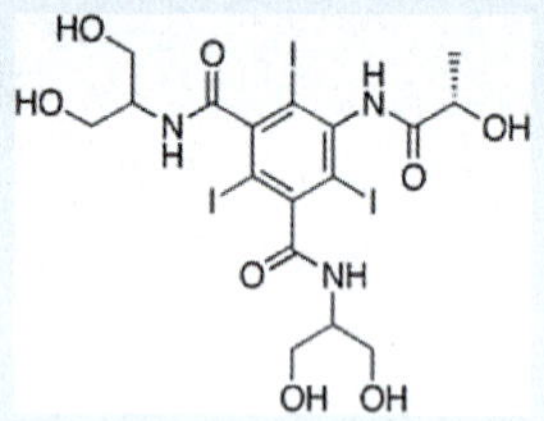	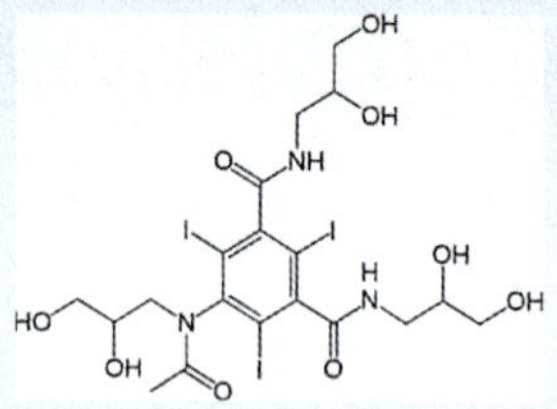	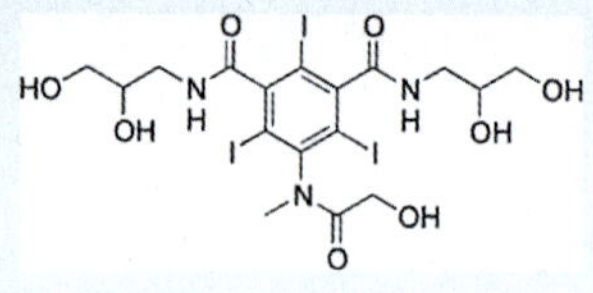	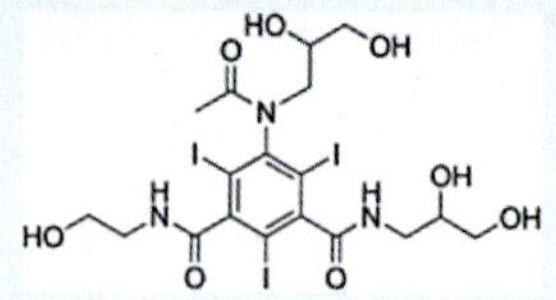
Iopamidol	Iohexol	Iomeprol	Ioxilan
IsoVue, Iopamiro, Solutrast	Omnipaque	Iomeron, Imeron	Oxilan

Nonionic Monomers–Low Osmolality		
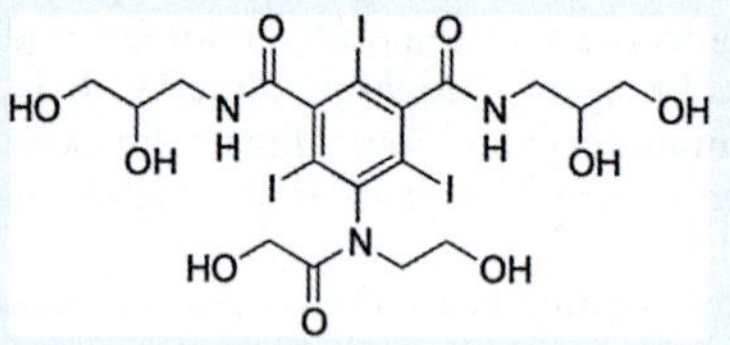	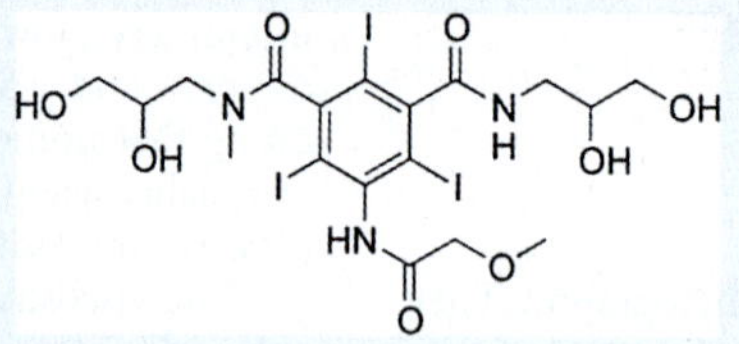	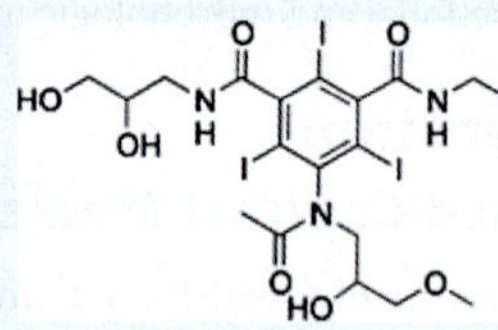
Ioversol	Iopromide	Iopentol
Optiray	Ultravist	Imagopaque

Nonionic Dimers–Isotonic Osmolality	
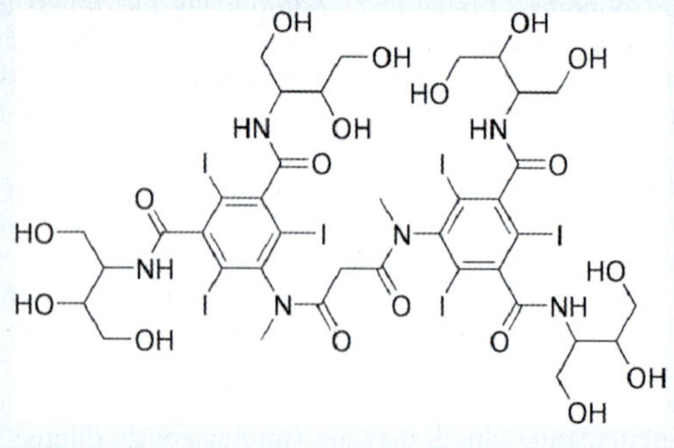	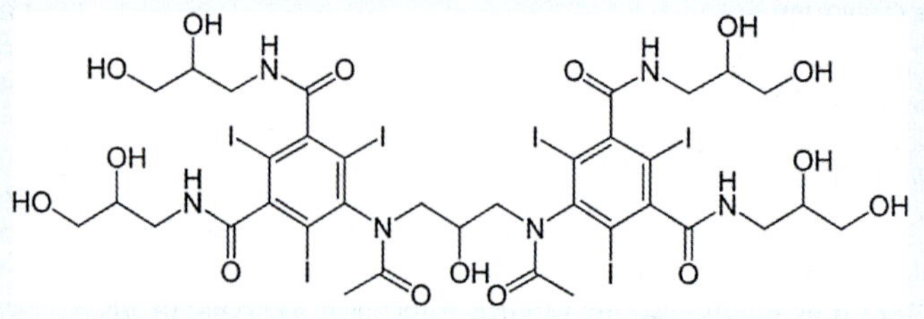
Iotrolan	Iodixanol
Isovist, Osmovist	Visipaque

All agents are distributed into extracellular space and are predominantly renally excreted. Very little, if any, protein binding exists.

Trade names are protected by copyright, and other trade names may exist.

Reprinted with permission from Thomsen HS, Dawson P, Tweedle M. MR and CT contrast agents for perfusion imaging and regulatory issues. In: Bammer R, ed. *MR & CT perfusion imaging: clinical applications and theoretical principles*. Philadelphia, PA: Lippincott Williams & Wilkins; 2015: Chapter 11.

TABLE 11.2 **Physical Data for Commercial Iodine-Based Contrast Media**

Name	Structure	Charge	Maximum[a] g-Iodine/mL	Osmolality, mOsmol/kg	Viscosity, mPa/s	Comparison, g-Iodine/mL	Osmolality, mOsmol/kg	Viscosity, mPa/s
Diatrizoate[b] Na	Monomer	Ionic	300	1,550	2.4	300	1,550	2.4
Diatrizoate NMG	Monomer	Ionic	358	1,980	9.2	282	1,500	4.0
Diatrizoate Na/NMG	Monomer	Ionic	370	2,100	8.4	292	1,420	4.0
Iothalamate	Monomer	Ionic	370	2,400	9.0	325	1,700	3.0
Ioxitalamate	Monomer	Ionic	350	2,130	7.5	300	1,500	5.2
Ioxaglate	Dimer	Ionic	320	600	7.5	320	600	7.5
Iopamidol	Monomer	Nonionic	370	796	9.4	300	616	4.7
Iohexol	Monomer	Nonionic	350	862	11.2	300	709	6.8
Iomeprol	Monomer	Nonionic	400	726	12.6	300	521	4.5
Ioxilan	Monomer	Nonionic	350	695	8.1	300	585	5.1
Ioversol	Monomer	Nonionic	350	792	9.0	300	651	5.5
Iopromide	Monomer	Nonionic	370	774	10	300	607	4.9
Iobitridol	Monomer	Nonionic	350	915	10	300	695	6
Iopentol	Monomer	Nonionic	300	683	6.5	300	683	6.5
Iotrolan	Dimer	Nonionic	320	317	11.6	300	291	8.4
Iodixanol	Dimer	Nonionic	320	290	11.8	270	290	6.3

Data at 37°C. Formulations frequently contain small quantities of excipients (e.g., Tris buffer) and can differ by geographic region. Multiple generic formulations exist for ionic monomers with slightly different data.
[a]Some ultrahigh concentrations of ionic monomers were marketed at up to 460–480 mg I/mL with osmolalities of ~3,000 and viscosities >19.
[b]Sodium, NMG (Meglumine), and mixed counterion formulations have somewhat different colligative properties. Diatrizoate, as an example, is shown in Na and NMG formulations to exemplify the expected range. NMG salts are more viscous.
Reprinted with permission from Thomsen HS, Dawson P, Tweedle M. MR and CT contrast agents for perfusion imaging and regulatory issues. In: Bammer R, ed. *MR & CT perfusion imaging: clinical applications and theoretical principles*. Philadelphia, PA: Lippincott Williams & Wilkins; 2015. Chapter 11.

Gadolinium-Based Contrast Media

MRI contrast agents can be classified according to[1]

- The metal ion
- Whether the ion is paramagnetic or superparamagnetic
- Naturally occurring ion in the body (yes or no)
- Ionicity (ionic or nonionic)
- Chelate (macrocyclic or linear)
- The capability to hold the metal ion, in particular gadolinium (low, intermediate, or high stability)
- Protein binding (yes or no)
- Distribution in the body (extracellular or organ specific)

Today, the most used agents are based on a paramagnetic metal ion (gadolinium), which does not appear naturally in the human body. The agent may be either ionic or nonionic. High-stability agents based on a macrocyclic chelate are preferred more and more. In some countries, for example, Denmark, the low-stability agents are no longer used. The most used agents are extracellular with no protein binding.

Paramagnetic contrast agents (e.g., gadolinium, manganese) are mainly positive enhancers that reduce T1 and T2 relaxation times and increase signal intensity on T1-weighted MR images.[2] Gadolinium is a paramagnetic metal ion in the lanthanide series of the periodic table. It has a high magnetic moment and a relatively slow electronic relaxation time, and it is very toxic. Manganese has similar relaxivity properties to gadolinium but, unlike gadolinium, occurs naturally in the body. It is one of the least toxic metal ions and is excreted by the hepatobiliary system.[3] Agents containing manganese are no longer commercially available in Europe and the United States.

Superparamagnetic agents (e.g., iron) are extremely effective T2 relaxation agents, which produce signal loss on T2- and T2*-weighted images. They also have a T1 effect, which is substantially less than their T2 effect.[4] However, superparamagnetic agents are no longer registered in most countries. Iron was used as the active ion in many agents. The iron agents were metabolized by the macrophages and the iron entered the body iron pool. Ferumoxytol is approved for intravenous treatment of patients with iron deficiency. Currently, it is studied whether it can be used for angiography and perfusion studies.[5] However, the MR use is off-label.

Gadolinium is a heavy metal, which in its free form is very toxic and may cause liver necrosis, hematologic changes, etc. A human being would not survive 0.1 mmol/kg free gadolinium injected into the circulation.[1] Therefore, the gadolinium ion is bound to a ligand in order to minimize its toxicity. For gadolinium-based contrast agents, the choice of chelate structure influences the compound's chemical and biologic stability and the colligative properties of its formulations, both of which in turn influence tolerance, pharmacokinetics, clinical uses, and contraindications. Two fundamental structural types are in use:

1. Linear seven-ring structures derived from diethylene triamine pentaacetate (DTPA)
2. Macrocyclic eight-ring structures derived from dodecane tetraacetic acid (DOTA).

The fundamental difference between these structural types is that the chain of nitrogen and carbon atoms constituting the backbone of the chelating agent is open on both ends in linear agents and closed into a single loop in macrocycles. The macrocyclic chelate has much better grip on the toxic gadolinium than the linear chelate.[6] The ligands may be ionic, which have a charge in solution, or nonionic. In order to reduce the osmolality, the two carboxyl groups in the ionic linear chelate have been replaced by two amide bindings, which have a weaker binding grip on the gadolinium ion than the carboxyl groups.

Gadolinium-based contrast agents may be classified in two categories: (a) nonspecific extracellular gadolinium chelates and (b) high-relaxivity agents/organ-specific agents/protein-bound agents (protein binders).[1,2] The nonspecific extracellular gadolinium chelates do not bind to proteins and are excreted by the kidney only, while the high-relaxivity agents show protein binding and are excreted to a varying extent through the bile as well as by the kidney. Nine gadolinium-based contrast agents are currently commercially available (Table 11.3).

The osmolality of the gadolinium-based contrast agents varies between 600 and 2,000 mOsmol/kg (Table 11.4). Unlike iodine-based contrast agents, high-osmolality gadolinium-based agents do not cause more acute nonrenal adverse reactions and discomfort than low-osmolality agents. This is probably because the molar amounts of gadolinium-based contrast agents used for the MR examinations are significantly less than the molar amounts of iodine-based agents used for radiography including CT.

The stability of gadolinium-based contrast agents depends on their kinetics, thermodynamics, and conditional stability (Table 11.4). Although these parameters do not directly relate to molecular structure,[1,6] the contrast agents with cyclic ligands, in which gadolinium is caged in a preorganized cavity, are more stable than those with linear ligands.

The relaxivity (r_1 and r_2) of the extracellular gadolinium-based agents is almost identical at both 1.5 and 3 T, since the change in field strength does not affect the relaxivity (Table 11.4). Protein binding increases the r_1 relaxivity of gadolinium-based agents, particularly at 1.5 T, but the relaxivity decreases more the higher the protein binding is when one moves from 1 to 3 T (Table 11.4).

The pharmacokinetics of extracellular nonspecific gadolinium-based contrast agents are similar to those of iodine-based radiographic contrast agents (two-compartment model: the two compartments being the intravascular plasma space and the interstitial space).[1] They do not enter cells significantly in or outside of the circulation. After the extracellular gadolinium-based contrast medium has been injected into the circulating blood, it is diluted in the circulating plasma volume. Straightaway, it begins to enter the interstitium, leaving the circulation, and at some point, it will reach an "equilibrium point." This point can vary from tissue to tissue. The "equilibrium point" is the point when the level of falling plasma and rising interstitial concentrations are the same. Hereafter, the extracellular contrast medium is continuously removed from the blood by means of excretion, and subsequently, the contrast medium begins to leave the interstitium and go back to the plasma, thereby revising its movement. The extracellular gadolinium-based contrast medium is excreted nearly by the normal kidney only by means of passive glomerular filtration without significant active tubular involvement.

High-relaxivity gadolinium-based contrast agents or protein binders behave similarly to the extracellular nonspecific agents immediately after intravascular injection.[7] However, because of their protein binding and biliary excretion, their pharmacokinetics differs and the liver uptake phase may be used for liver imaging. Of the available protein binders, gadobenate is used mainly as an extracellular agent, gadofosveset was specifically designed for MR angiography, and gadoxetate, which has the greatest biliary excretion, is mainly used for liver imaging. Protein binding, predominantly serum albumin binding, can produce (a) variable hepatobiliary versus renal excretion, (b) greater relaxivity where albumin is present, and (c) extended plasma half-life versus both excretion and leakage into extracellular space. All the currently available protein binders are based on the linear chelate (DTPA) and are ionic. Under similar conditions, gadobenate binds only slightly, approximately 5% to albumin; gadoxetate binds approximately 10%; and gadofosveset binds approximately 90%. These values are approximates for comparison and highly dependent on conditions of the measurement, including gadolinium concentration, which changes with time after injection, and also are complicated by binding of multiple gadolinium-based contrast agents to each albumin molecule. Gadobenate is excreted mostly into the urine at rate indistinguishable from the non–protein-binding agents, with only approximately 4% hepatobiliary excretion in man; in rats, it is much higher. The consequence of the added lipophilicity in gadoxetate is approximately 10% albumin binding along with very rapid hepatic uptake and then hepatobiliary excretion, approximately 50%, accompanied by relatively rapid renal excretion. In gadofosveset, the hepatobiliary excretion is 5%; due to the protein binding, its T½ is 18 hours or 12 times longer than that of the extracellular gadolinium-based contrast agents.

Dosage

Iodine-Based Contrast Media

This issue is addressed considering different procedures requiring administration of iodine-based agents separately.

Intravenous urography was largely replaced by CT urography, but nevertheless it is still popular in some countries. The typical recommended dose is 300 mg I/kg for an adult patient.[8] A dose of approximately 22 g of iodine is considered optimal for both low-osmolality and high-osmolality contrast media, although adjustments can be made for extremely small or large patients.[9]

Digital subtraction angiography (DSA) requires contrast administration through catheters, which are selectively placed into different vessels. Injection can be performed manually or taking benefit of power injectors. The contrast volume is related to the vessel size and tables suggesting the optimal amount and the optimal injection rate for each vessel when performing conventional angiography were available.[9] When DSA was introduced 30 years ago, its higher contrast resolution allowed for injection of lower iodine doses and thus injecting lower volumes or more diluted agents. Practical purposes usually favored the former approach.

When considering CT, dosage is a difficult issue and the type of scheduled procedure, that is, CT angiography or CT for tumor staging, should be considered. The peak of the aortic enhancement depends on the contrast concentration, on the injection rate, and, to a lesser extent, on the total contrast volume. The availability of faster scanners allowed shorter acquisition times and therefore to decrease the contrast dosage of CT angiographic studies. This is not the case when considering the hepatic enhancement, which is closely related to the iodine load delivered with the contrast injection. Therefore, faster scanners did not allow decreasing iodine dosage in an oncologic setting.

TABLE

11.3 Structures, Types, Names, and Excretion of Commercial Gadolinium-Based Contrast Media Used for MRI

Structure charge	Linear Ionic			
Renal excretion	>99%	96%	50%	95%
Protein binder	No	Yes	Yes	Yes
Hepatic excretion	<1%	4%	50%	5%
Chemical structure	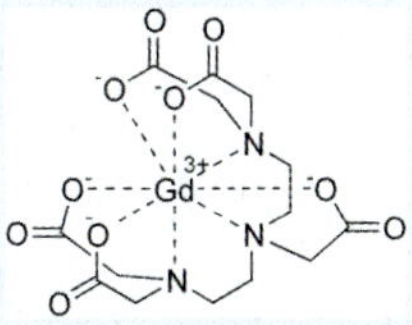	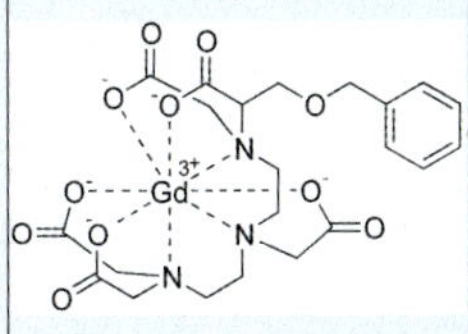	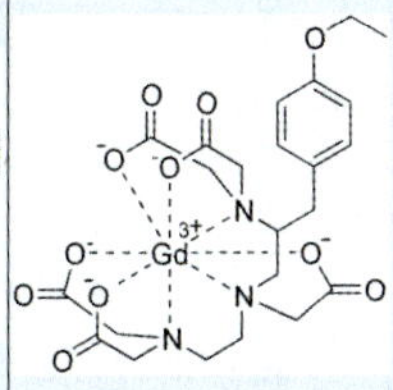	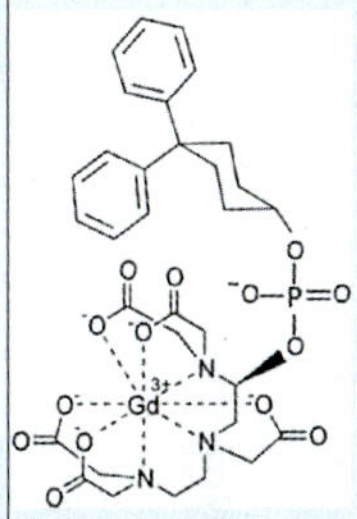
Abbreviation	$Gd(DTPA)^{2-}$	$Gd(BOPTA)^{2-}$	$Gd(DTPA\text{-}EOB)^{2-}$	MS-325
Generic name	Gadopentetate dimeglumine	Gadobenate dimeglumine	Gadoexetate disodium	Gadofosveset
Trade name	Magnevist	MultiHance	Eovist, Primovist	Ablavar

Linear nonionic		Structure of counter ion used in some contrast media
>99%	>99%	
No	No	
<1%	<1%	
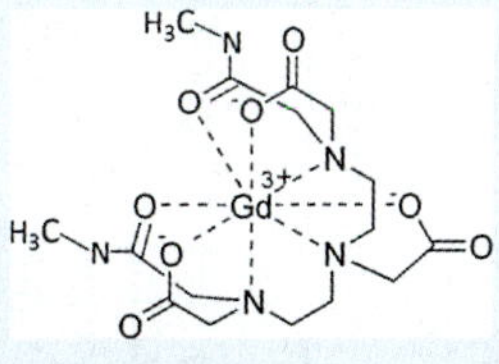	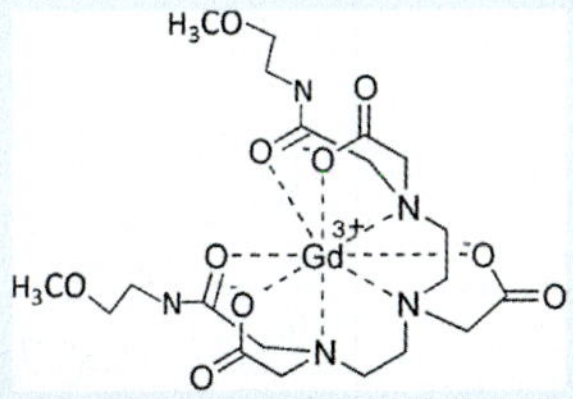	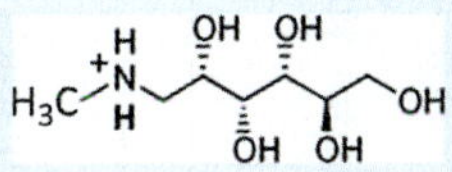
Gd(DTPA-BMA)	Gd(DTPA-BMEA)	NMG^+, $HNMG^+$
Gadodiamide	Gadoversetamide	Megluminium ion, meglumine
Omniscan	OptiMARK	

Macrocyclic ionic	Macrocyclic nonionic	Macrocyclic nonionic
>99%	>99%	>99%
No	No	No
<1%	<1%	<1%
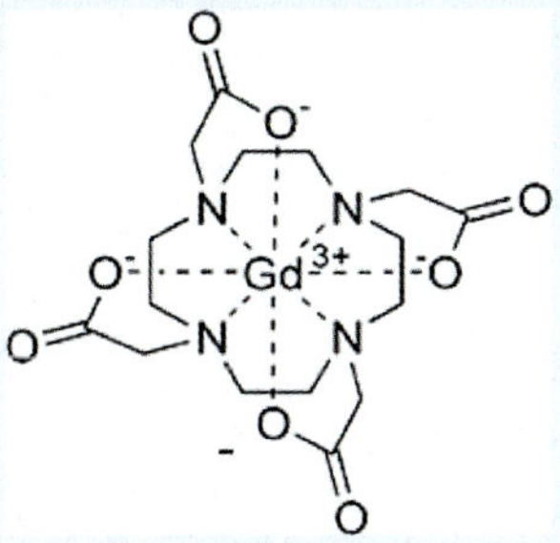	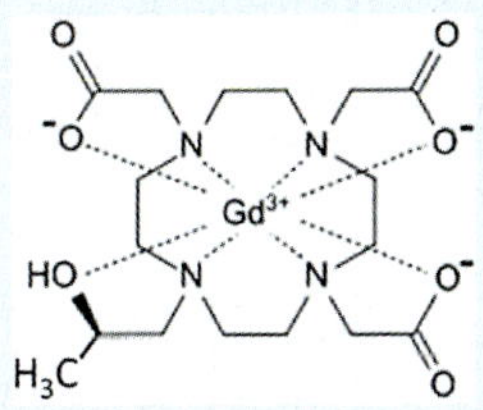	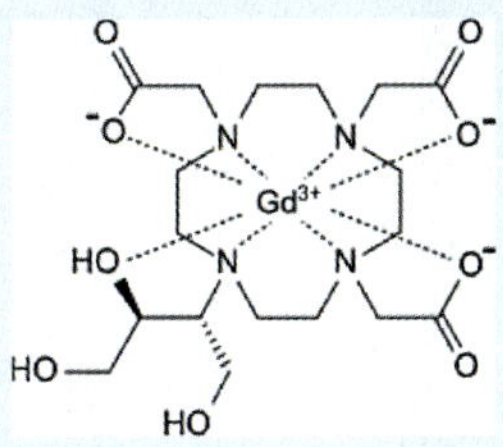
$Gd(DOTA)^-$	Gd(HP-DO3A)	Gd(BT-DO3A)
Gadoterate	Gadoteridol	Gadobutrol
Dotarem, Magnescope	ProHance	Gadovist, Gadavist

In solution, each structure also coordinates one water molecule. All agents distribute to extracellular space.
The figures shown apply to human beings. Protein binding and excretion vary with species.
Trade names are protected by copyright.
Reprinted with permission from Thomsen HS, Dawson P, Tweedle M. MR and CT contrast agents for perfusion imaging and regulatory issues. In: Bammer R, ed. *MR & CT perfusion imaging: clinical applications and theoretical principles*. Philadelphia, PA: Lippincott Williams & Wilkins; 2015. Chapter 11.

TABLE **11.4** **Physical Data for Commercial Gadolinium-Based Contrast Media for MRI at 37°C (Except Where Noted)**

Structure Type	Linear						Macrocyclic		
Charge type	Ionic				Nonionic		Ionic	Nonionic	
Trade name	Magnevist	MultiHance	Eovist Primovist	Ablavar	Omniscan	OptiMARK	Dotarem Magnescope	ProHance	Gadovist Gadavist
[Gd] in M (commercial preparations)	0.5	0.5	0.25	0.25	0.5	0.5	0.5	0.5	1.0
Osmolality, mOsm/kg	1,960	1,970	688	825	789	1,110	1,350	630	1,603
Viscosity, mPa/s	2.9	5.3	1.2	2.1	1.4	2.0	2.0	1.3	5.0
Relaxivity, Plasma									
r_1–1.5 T/mM/s	3.9–4.1	6.3–7.9	6.9	19	4.3	4.7	3.6	4.1	4.7–5.2
r_2–1.5 T/mM/s	4.6–5.3	8.7–18.9	8.7	34	5.2	5.2	4.3	5.0	6.1–7.5
r_1–3 T/mM/s	3.7–3.9	5.5–5.9	6.2	9.9	4.0	4.5	3.5	3.7	4.5–5.0
r_2–3 T/mM/s	5.2	11.0–17.5	11.0	60	5.6	5.9	4.9	5.7	6.3–7.1
Stability Constants									
Log K_{eq}, M^{-1} [a]	22.5	22.6	23.5	22.1	16.9	16.6	25.6	23.8	21.8
Log K_{eq}', pH 7[a]	18.4	18.4	18.7	18.9	14.9	15.0	19.3	17.1	15.5
$T_{1/2}$ dissociation pH 1	<5 s[a]	<s[a]	<5 s[a]	<5 s[a]	<5 s[a]	<5 s[a]	26 h	2.0 h	7.9 h
Risk of NSF[b]	High	Intermediate	Intermediate	Intermediate	High	High	Low	Low	Low

[a]25°C.

[b]According to the classification approved by the European Medicines Agency (EMA). High-risk agents are contraindicated in patients with a glomerular filtration rate (GFR) < 30 mL/min × 1.73 m² and should be used with caution in patients with a GFR between 30 and 60 mL/min × 1.73 m² (ESUR guidelines on Contrast Media version 8.1—http://www.esur.org (Jan 2014)).

Reprinted with permission from Thomsen HS, Dawson P, Tweedle M. MR and CT contrast agents for perfusion imaging and regulatory issues. In: Bammer R, ed. *MR & CT perfusion imaging: clinical applications and theoretical principles*. Philadelphia, PA: Lippincott Williams & Wilkins; 2015. Chapter 11.

When considering liver scans and the optimal contrast dosage, it should be underscored that a variety of contrast medium–related factors affect liver contrast enhancement: (a) the amount of contrast, (b) its concentration, (c) the injection rate, (d) the injection duration, and (e) the scan delay after contrast injection. Additionally, contrast enhancement depends on a number of patient-related factors including total bodyweight, lean bodyweight, and cardiac output.[10] It appears that the contrast dose should not be fixed and that an adjusted injection volume (i.e., considering patient weight) could offer better diagnostic quality and global savings.[11] The amount of administered contrast material could be adjusted after considering the total bodyweight, but individual patients may have the same weight but different tissue composition. In fact, some tissues (such as adipose tissue) are less vascular and contribute less to contrast enhancement. Thus, when considering weight alone, it could result in larger volumes than necessary being given to heavier patients with a larger amount of fat tissue. Therefore, it was suggested determining the contrast medium dose on the basis of the patient's lean bodyweight.[12] This approach appeared to reduce the patient-to-patient hepatic parenchymal and vascular enhancement variability. Kondo et al.[10] supported tailoring contrast medium dose to individual patients by using body fat percentage and recommended a dose of 750 mg I/kg of lean bodyweight to produce adequate hepatic enhancement in abdominal CT. However, it is difficult to accept using lean bodyweight as a standard index to adjust iodine load because it requires measuring body fat percentage with a body fat monitor in each patient.

Other authors[13] suggested the validity of determining the contrast medium dose based on body surface area, which is related to cardiac output without being affected by obesity, and showed that the use of body surface area is more effective than bodyweight for the aortic enhancement with less patient-to-patient variability; meanwhile, as for hepatic enhancement, the advantage was not found. Estimated body surface area can be calculated using an equation considering patient height and weight.[14]

Some authors[15] agree that these solutions may have some advantages, but they claim that it is difficult to incorporate them into the everyday working practices of a high-throughput CT department. Therefore, they suggest considering weight alone. Weight-based dosing ranging from 425 to 600 mg I/kg was suggested in the literature.[16,17] Benbow and Bull[15] designed a look-up table based on delivering approximately 450 mg I/kg to each patient that was preprogrammed into the injector pump and greatly reduced the variability of liver contrast enhancement compared to a fixed-dose approach.

When considering contrast dosage, it should be reminded that contrast-induced nephrotoxicity (CIN) is dose related. Studies evaluating the relation between CIN and dosage were produced and are considered in the renal adverse reactions section of this article.

Additionally, as to CT angiography, recent technical advances allowed contrast dose reductions using low CT voltage techniques and iterative reconstruction algorithms. CT angiography studies can be achieved with a mean photon energy of 80 kVp, which is closer to the K-absorption edge of iodine when compared to 120 kVp. As a result, a higher vascular enhancement can be acquired at a lower radiation exposure, and lower iodine dosages are therefore required. As an example, ultra–low-dose contrast studies include coronary CT angiographies rated as excellent with as low as 10 ± 4 mL of 350 mg I/mL contrast material.[18]

Gadolinium-Based Contrast Media

The currently approved extracellular gadolinium-based contrast media are delivered in vials and syringes containing 0.5 mmol/mL, whereas they are used in a dose of 0.1 mmol/kg; some of them may for special indications, for example, brain metastases, be used up to 0.3 mmol/kg (triple dose). However, the nonionic macrocyclic agent gadobutrol is delivered in a higher concentration (1 mmol/mL); the same amount of this agent in mmol per kg bodyweight is used as for the other extracellular agents.

For the protein binder gadobenate, which is mainly used as an extracellular agent, slightly lower doses may be sufficient due to its protein binding. For the other protein binders, in which a much larger part (10% to 90%) of the agent is bound mainly to albumin, the commercial vials/syringes contain only 0.25 mmol/mL or half the concentration that most extracellular agents are delivered in. The recommended dose for gadoxetate disodium is 0.1 mL/kg bodyweight.

Safety

Adverse events may involve a single organ like the kidney (e.g., contrast-induced nephrotoxicity [CIN]) and almost the whole body (e.g., nephrogenic systemic fibrosis [NSF]). The acute events are those which occur within the first 60 minutes after exposure to the agent. They may be renal or nonrenal. The events occurring after 60 minutes are divided into those which occur within 7 days after the exposure (exclusive the first 60 minutes) (late) and those which occur more than 7 days after the administration of the agent (very late). The late and very late reactions are all nonrenal.

Gadolinium-based contrast agents cause the same acute adverse events as the iodine-based contrast media. The mild reactions include nausea, mild vomiting, self-limiting urticaria, dizziness, and itching.[19] Moderate reactions are severe vomiting, marked urticaria, bronchospasm, facial edema, laryngeal edema, and vasovagal attack. Severe reactions include hypotensive shock, respiratory arrest, cardiac arrest, convulsion, and generalized anaphylactoid reaction. Moderate and severe reactions require medical treatment. Regarding the late and very late reactions, iodine- and gadolinium-based contrast agents differ.

Acute Nonrenal Adverse Reactions

Iodine-Based Contrast Media

Knowledge of acute adverse reaction mechanisms is improving, and recently, it was suggested that hypersensitivity (allergy-like) reactions that are dose independent and unpredictable can be divided into allergic and nonallergic.[19] The more severe the reaction, the more chance it is truly allergic. Moreover, raised blood tryptase levels after the reaction indicate a true allergic reaction, while raised histamine levels are less specific. A true allergy is confirmed by a positive skin test to the contrast material that triggered the reaction 1 month after the procedure.

Reaction rates when using ionic monomers were reported in the range 5% to 12%. Most of them were mild with severe reactions occurring in 0.10% to 0.15% of the cases. These figures are lower by a factor 4 when using nonionic monomers,[20] while the reduction in the rate of severe reactions appeared even higher (0.22% vs. 0.04%). A reduction in the mortality rate was not shown, probably related to the rarity of this event, which was reported in about 1 patient in 75,000 when ionic monomers were used.

Some patient categories are to be considered at increased risk for acute contrast reactions. Patients with previous acute reactions to iodine-based contrast media have an 11 times greater risk compared to patients without this history. Patients with asthma are considered to have a fivefold higher risk.[19] Additionally, patients with a history of allergy are reported to have an increased risk although lower than asthmatic patients. It should be noted that allergies to foodstuffs containing iodine and to topical iodine skin preparations are not considered to increase the risk of acute reactions to iodine-based contrast media.

Mild acute adverse reactions are the most frequent. The frequency of such reactions reported in the literature varies from 1% to 50%. The lowest figures are found in retrospective studies based on reviews of patient records.[19] With prospective studies, the frequency depends on whether adverse events were spontaneously reported or were sought by interview and on how detailed the interview was. When patients, who have had CT or MR scans, are interviewed, also those patients, who had no contrast medium, report the same mild symptoms as patients who received intravenous contrast medium. Thus, not all symptoms experienced by patients in the hour following contrast medium injection are adverse reactions to the contrast agent. Some of the symptoms may be explained by the so-called Lalli and Weber effects.[21] There is no doubt that both the Lalli and the Weber effects are seen after contrast media administration. The Weber effect is not only seen when a contrast agent is introduced but also seen when a department changes from one agent to another. Comparative studies of acute nonrenal adverse reactions to contrast media must ensure that the different agents are given under identical conditions. In retrospective studies, the Lalli and Weber effects are not controlled, so prospective randomized studies are the only way to obtain reliable data.

What to do in patients at risk for acute, moderate, or severe reactions? First of all, it should be considered if there is another radiologic procedure that can solve the patient's clinical problem without using iodine-based contrast media. If this is not the case, a different contrast agent could be used (it means that we need to be fully aware of the name of the agent that was previously used and eventually triggered a reaction). Skin tests can help in selecting another agent although the negative predictive value of the test is not very high.[22] Of course, the radiologic staff should be trained to manage an acute reaction and should have drugs and resuscitation equipment immediately available. In patients at risk, premedication with steroids eventually associated with antihistamines can be suggested. Actually, this approach is supported by a number of Scientific Societies; drugs are easy to administer and have negligible side effects, and their cost is minor. Despite use of premedication, breakthrough reactions may occur. Therefore, the radiologist should always be prepared to treat the patient. The patient should be kept for at least 30 minutes following the procedure in the radiology department.

Gadolinium-Based Contrast Media

Moderate and severe acute reactions occur in less than 0.5% of injections.[23] The prevalence is the same for all extracellular gadolinium-based contrast media. Thus, the osmolality has no influence on the prevalence in the dose (0.1 mmol/kg) used for MRI. The prevalence of mild reactions varies from 1% to 50% depending on how the study was done (lowest for retrospective studies, highest for studies with active interviews including a long list of potential adverse events). Treatment is the same for those events that are induced by iodine-based contrast media.

Records of Acute Adverse Reactions (CAVE or Warning)

It is very important that acute adverse reactions are properly noted in the patient's records, so that the necessary information is available before the next examination and appropriate precautions can be taken.[19] All reactions that require medical treatment should be recorded, but mild reactions not requiring any treatment should not be recorded, because they may not relate to the contrast medium. The only exception to this would be if a skin test has been done and shown evidence of allergic hypersensitivity. If minor symptoms, for example, dizziness or nausea, which may be due to the examination and not the contrast agent, are recorded, the patient may be denied a clinically important enhanced examination in future.

Late Adverse Reactions

Iodine-Based Contrast Media

These reactions include skin reactions (maculopapular rashes, erythema, swelling, pruritus, etc.).[24] Other symptoms are reported (e.g., headache, nausea, dizziness, fever, musculoskeletal pain, gastrointestinal disturbances), but their frequency appears to be similar in patients who did not receive contrast material, and therefore, only skin reactions are considered true late adverse reactions to contrast media. In most cases, these reactions are mild or moderate and self-limiting usually resolving within 3 to 7 days. It appears that they are hypersensitivity T-cell–mediated reactions. Their frequency is again a matter of debate as it has been reported between 0.52% and 50.8%, depending on the methodology of data collection. Probably, the frequency is about 3%, and there is evidence suggesting that it is higher following administration of nonionic dimers, both with iodixanol and with iotrolan, which was actually withdrawn from the market in 1995 because of the high incidence of late reactions in Japan. Risk factors for skin reactions include administration of nonionic dimers, previous late contrast medium reaction, and interleukin-2 treatment. Drug prophylaxis is generally not recommended, but in patients who experienced a late adverse reaction patch, delayed-reading intradermal skin testing is recommended; it can confirm the late skin reaction to contrast medium and can identify other agents showing cross-reactivity. Therefore, these tests can help in selecting another agent, avoiding both the contrast that triggered the reaction and other ones that have shown cross-reactivity.

In case a late skin reaction occurs, symptomatic treatment is advised (oral antihistamines, topic steroids, emollients).

Gadolinium-Based Contrast Media

There are no reports of late adverse reactions after exposure to gadolinium-based contrast media like there are after iodine-based contrast agents, in particular, after exposure to the dimers.

Very Late Adverse Reactions

Iodine-Based Contrast Media

Very late reactions to iodine-based contrast media include thyrotoxicosis, a rare condition that might occur in patients with untreated Graves disease or in patients with multinodular goiter and thyroid autonomy, especially old patients and patients living in areas of iodine deficiency.[25] Prophylaxis is generally not considered in these patients who require monitoring by the endocrinologist following the procedure.

It should be reminded that manifest hyperthyroidism is a definite contraindication to intravascular iodine-based contrast material administration.

Gadolinium-Based Contrast Media

In the 1980s, researchers within contrast media showed the superiority of gadolinium for MRI (highest relaxivity per ion of the tested ions, e.g., dysprosium, manganese, copper),[26] whereas researchers within biochemistry showed the toxic aspects of all the lanthanides.[27,28] It included accumulation of the lanthanides in the bone and liver, changes of the collagen in the skin, etc. Even the possibility of transmetallation in the blood was mentioned in that decade.[29]

Sadly, these observations were never combined before 2006. As a matter of fact, it took 7 years before the diagnosis of a scleromyxedema-like lesion "nephrogenic systemic fibrosis" was made and further 9 years before the link between development of nephrogenic systemic fibrosis and exposure to some linear gadolinium-based contrast media was demonstrated with certainty.[30] In the middle of the 1990s, (a) gadodiamide was approved for use in triple dose, (b) radiologists started to transfer patients with poor renal function and increased risk of contrast-induced nephropathy after iodine-based contrast media to MRI due to the much safer nonnephrotoxic MR contrast media, (c) MR angiography was introduced, (d) MR scanners with multiple steps became available for clinical use (gave the possibility of doing peripheral runoff with only one injection of contrast medium), and (e) radiologists started using gadolinium-based contrast media for radiography (e.g., CT, conventional angiography) in patients with reduced renal function in order to protect their kidneys against contrast-induced nephropathy. No agent has ever been approved for that use as well as the dose required to provide acceptable enhancement are much (approximately eight times) higher than necessary for good MR images.

In 2006, two European groups found a correlation between the occurrence of NSF and exposure to gadodiamide.[30,31] Very rapidly (within 1 to 2 years), it became very clear that unconfounded (i.e., only one agent ever used in the patient) cases were only seen after exposure to the least stable agents (gadodiamide, gadoversetamide, and to a lesser extent, gadopentetate dimeglumine), the patients all had reduced renal function or were on dialysis, and it occurred worldwide and in both young and old people.[32] The severity of the disease varies from a single small plaque on a lower extremity to nearly universal disease causing severe disability, cachexia, and death. For unknown reasons, the head is never involved, whereas the lower extremities are always involved. A patient without any lesions in the lower extremities is very likely to have another disease. The diagnosis is not easy. It requires careful inspection of the skin and a deep skin biopsy. The Yale Registry clinical and histopathologic criteria should be met.[33] The adverse reaction can start hours to several days and even years after the last exposure to the gadolinium-based contrast media. Not all patients with renal impairment develop NSF after exposure to one of the high-risk agents. Thus, there must be another as-of-yet unknown factor. It is unlikely that we will ever identify that factor. It cannot be tested in man, and many countries have switched to the more stable agents and do not see NSF anymore.

Most researchers agree that the cause of the disease is transmetallation,[29,32] a process in which the gadolinium is released from the chelate and replaced by zinc or iron. The free gadolinium thus dissociates (liberates), and it localizes in the skin, in the liver, and particularly in the bone, probably as a complex of calcium and phosphate. This may trigger circulating fibrocytes and fibrosis may develop.

After each intravenous injection of a gadolinium-based contrast medium, some very tiny amounts are left in the body,[34] particularly after the least stable agents (gadodiamide, gadoversetamide, and gadopentetate dimeglumine) are left in the body. More is left in patients with poor renal function or on dialysis than in patients with normal renal function. Whether the accumulation has any long-term effects even in patients with normal renal function is still unknown but feared by some investigators. It is currently studied in a major international investigation required by the European authorities. Therefore, it is advisable to use in all patients—independent of renal function—an agent that leaves the smallest amount of gadolinium in any patient.

Nonionic linear gadolinium-based contrast agents (gadoversetamide, gadodiamide) and ionic linear (gadopentetate dimeglumine) gadolinium-based contrast media are now contraindicated to use in patients with a glomerular filtration rate less than 30 mL/min 1.73 m^2 and should only be used with caution in patients with a glomerular filtration rate between 30 and 6 mL/min 1.73 m^2. Only single dose (0.1 mmol/kg) may be used. Before use of these unstable agents, the renal function must be tested by laboratory methods.[35,36] The unstable agents should be kept separately from the other agents, so mistakes (e.g., giving a patient on dialysis a contraindicated agent) are avoided. It can be questioned whether there is at all a need for the least stable agents.

Renal Adverse Reactions

Iodine-Based Contrast Media

Contrast-induced nephrotoxicity (CIN) is defined as a condition in which a decrease in renal function occurs within 3 days of the intravascular administration of contrast material in the absence of an alternative etiology. An increase in serum creatinine by more than 25% or 44 μmol/l (0.5 mg/dL) indicates CIN. The Contrast Media Safety Committee of the European Society of Uroradiology agreed on this definition.[37] However, the Acute Kidney Injury Network recently suggested a new approach for diagnosis and for staging severity of acute kidney injury (AKI) and considered an increase in serum creatinine by more than 26.5 μmol/L (0.3 mg/dL) as significant because it was shown that even slight changes in serum creatinine are associated with worse outcomes.[38] These criteria are probably too sensitive and will lead to an increase in the number of false-positive diagnoses.

Risk factors for CIN include patient-related and procedure-related factors. The list of patient-related risk factors indicated that preexisting renal impairment is to be considered the most important one and differentiates the risk after considering the route of contrast administration[37]: patients with eGFR less than 60 mL/min 1.73 m^2 are considered at risk before intra-arterial administration, while patients with eGFR less than 45 mL/min 1.73 m^2 are considered at risk before intravenous administration, in particular in combination with diabetic nephropathy, dehydration, congestive heart failure, low left ventricular ejection fraction, recent myocardial infarction, use of intra-aortic balloon pump, periprocedural hypotension, low hematocrit level, age over 70, and concurrent administration of nephrotoxic drugs. Known or suspected acute renal failure is considered a risk factor as well.

Actually, several publications have found the risk after intra-arterial contrast administration (particularly in the cardiology setting) to be higher than after CT. McCullough et al.[39] considering 1,826 consecutive patients referred for percutaneous coronary interventions showed a 14.5% CIN incidence and 0.7% cases requiring dialysis. On the other hand, the incidence of CIN appeared to be 5.1% in 1,075 renal insufficient patients that is in a population at higher risk, following CT.[40] In this series, no patient required dialysis, and nearly no patient had severely reduced renal function (<30 mL/min 1.73 m^2). The true reason for such difference can be debated. More unstable patients are possibly referred for angiocardiography; cholesterol embolization that might occur during angiographic procedures can mimic CIN and therefore apparently increased the rate of CIN after intra-arterial contrast administration, but the main reason is probably the lower contrast dose used in CT, which commonly ranges between 25 and 50 g I compared with reported 40 to 90 g I in intra-arterial coronary studies.[41] Additionally, roughly the same gram-iodine/GFR ratio (1:1) as a limit of relatively safe contrast media doses has preliminary been found for both intravenous CT and intra-arterial coronary procedures,[41] suggesting that the risk can be the same when equal iodine doses are injected.

Recent data questioned the risk of CIN after CT and raised the question of this risk being possibly overestimated. A review of 13 CT trials showed a similar incidence of AKI, dialysis, and death between the contrast medium group and control group[42]: only

4 of the 13 studies were prospective. A retrospective analysis involving 157,140 scans showed that the incidence of CIN was not significantly different from contrast material–independent AKI.[43] Additionally, a very recent revision of the material from the same series showed that contrast material is not a risk factor even in patients with eGFR level less than 30 mL/min 1.73 m^2.[44] Therefore, these authors claimed that iodinated contrast medium may not be the causative agent in diminished renal function after intravenous contrast administration.[43] However, another retrospective analysis involving 75,699 scans was performed by another group[45] who applied the propensity score matching method followed by Mc Donald et al. again and showed that contrast medium is a risk factor in patients with stable eGFR level less than 30 mL/min 1.73 m^2 and that there is a trend toward significance at eGFR 30 to 44 mL/min 1.73 m^2. An explanation for the different results is very likely the low number of patients with GFR below 30 mL/min 1.73 m^2 in all studies and the fact that they are retrospective. Patients with low GFR has very likely already been excluded regarding administration of iodine-based contrast media before referral. Thus, only when it is considered vital, the iodine-based contrast medium is given in patients with very low eGFR. Before 2006, the patients received gadolinium-based contrast medium. In reality, we have nearly no information about the risk of CIN in patients with GFR below 20 mL/min 1.73 m^2; they have never been included in the prospective trials, and only a few patients with GFR between 20 and 30 mL/min 1.73 m^2 have been enrolled in those studies. It is exactly the same patients who are at very increased risk of NSF after exposure to unstable gadolinium-based contrast media (see above). However, it appears difficult to accept that contrast media, which are proven to be nephrotoxic in preclinical studies and in the cardiology setting, are supposed to be entirely nonnephrotoxic in the CT setting. Nevertheless, these studies clearly show that the risk of CIN after CT has definitely been overestimated and that we should be more liberal in our policies in regard to contrast administration.[46]

Procedure-related risk factors for CIN include intra-arterial administration of contrast medium, the use of high-osmolality agents, the administration of large doses of contrast medium, and multiple contrast administrations within a few days. As to the choice of contrast material, the Contrast Media Safety Committee considered the many studies published in recent years and suggested the use of contrast media with low or iso-osmolality in patients with risk factors for CIN, without supporting any specific agent in these classes.[37] As to contrast dose, it should be reminded that CIN is related to the injected iodine dose. A safe dose does not exit, and therefore in all patients, the minimum dose necessary to solve the clinical problem should be injected.

Following evaluation of risk factors, the approach and the suggested management in patients at risk for CIN should be considered. At time of referral for elective procedures, patients with impaired renal function should be identified. Blood samples for serum creatinine can be achieved in all patients, and estimation of GFR should follow. Another possibility would be the identification of patients requiring measurement of renal function through appropriate questionnaires, thus limiting blood samples to a proportion of patients. Choice between these two possibilities relies on organization and economic evaluations.

Following identification of patients at risk, alternative imaging methods not using iodine-based contrast media should be suggested in these patients. If the procedure is to be performed, the radiologist should discuss the need to stop nephrotoxic drugs that are eventually administered to the patient with the referring physician and should schedule volume expansion, which is the main preventive measure to be applied in at-risk patients. A suitable protocol is intravenous saline, 1.0 to 1.5 mL/kg/h for at least 6 hours before and after contrast medium. An alternative protocol that became popular recently is intravenous sodium bicarbonate, 3 mL/kg/h for 1 h before contrast medium and 1 ml/kg/h for 6 hour after.[37] This approach showed no inferiority compared to volume expansion with saline and is more practical. Short (1 hour) volume expansion with sodium bicarbonate (250 mL) was recently proven noninferior to periprocedural saline hydration and can further help with outpatient management.[47]

At time of examination, at-risk patients should receive low- or iso-osmolar contrast media and the lowest dose of contrast consistent with a diagnostic result and should be injected while following the procedure, volume expansion should be continued, and eGFR should be determined 48 to 72 hours after contrast administration.

It should be underlined that no pharmacologic prophylaxis, including *N*-acetylcysteine, has yet been shown to offer consistent protection against CIN.

Gadolinium-Based Contrast Media

Decrease in renal function occurs very rarely after administration of gadolinium-based contrast media in approved doses for MRI (0.1 to 0.3 mmol/kg).[48] Experimental studies have indicated that when administered in the same molar doses as iodine-based contrast media (approximately eight times higher than used for MRI); gadolinium-based contrast media may be just as nephrotoxic if not more nephrotoxic than nonionic iodine-based contrast media. Hydration before administration of gadolinium-based contrast media for MRI in patients with moderately and severely reduced renal function is not recommended. Gadolinium-based contrast media are nowhere in the world approved for radiography including CT.

Other Adverse Reactions

Extravasation

During the injection of iodine- or gadolinium-based contrast material, the contrast medium may enter the extravascular space (extravasation). Most such injuries are minor, but in rare cases, severe injuries may include skin ulceration, soft-tissue necrosis, and compartment syndrome.[49] If it occurs, conservative treatment is preferable in most cases. One can apply ice packs, elevate the limb, as well as monitor the lesion carefully. The risk factors may be technique-related (use of a power injector, less optimal injection sites including lower limb and small distal veins, large volume of contrast medium, and high-osmolar contrast medium) and patient related (inability to communicate, fragile or damaged veins, arterial insufficiency, compromised lymphatics, and/or venous drainage and obesity). In order to decrease the risk, CT studies require nonionic iodine-based contrast media and MR procedures favor nonionic macrocyclic gadolinium-based agents. The appropriately sized plastic cannula should be placed in a suitable vein and tested with saline before use with contrast media.

Interaction

The radiologist should be fully aware of the patient's drug history. In fact, the use of a number of drugs requires special attention when iodine-based contrast media are injected.[50] Metformin can rarely induce lactic acidosis, and such risk is higher in patients with impaired renal function. That is why nephrotoxic agents such as iodine-based contrast media should be administered with caution in these patients. Metformin is not supposed to be withdrawn in patients with an eGFR of 45 mL/min/1.73 m^2 or greater if they are going to receive contrast intravenously (60 mL/min/1.73 m^2 or greater if intra-arterially).[51,52] In patients with eGFR below 30 mL/min/1.73 m^2, metformin is contraindicated. In patients with eGFR 30 to 44 mL/min/1.73 m^2 (intravenous contrast injection) or 30 to 59 mL/min/1.73 m^2 (intra-arterial injection), metformin should be withdrawn 48 hours before contrast administration and restarted 48 hours later if the renal function does not deteriorate.[51,52]

Nephrotoxic drugs (cyclosporine, cisplatin, aminoglycosides, nonsteroidal anti-inflammatory drugs, etc.) increase the risk of developing CIN in at-risk patients who are referred to contrast administration.[50] Possible withdrawal of these drugs at least 24 hours before contrast injection should be discussed with the referring physician, and benefits and harms should be balanced before making a decision.

The radiologist should be aware of the possible assumption of β-blockers by the patient because in case an adverse reaction occurs these drugs may impair the management of bronchospasm and the response to adrenaline.

Interleukin-2 treatment is a risk factor for late skin adverse reactions (see above).

With exception of a few examples, it is not known whether contrast agents interfere with the various clinical biochemical analyses.[50] The issue has never been examined systematically. In case of gadodiamide and gadoversetamide, falsely low levels of calcium (spurious hypocalcemia) have been measured by some techniques. Caution should also be exercised when using colorimetric assays for angiotensin-converting enzyme, calcium, iron, magnesium, total iron-binding capacity, and zinc in serum samples from patients who have recently received gadolinium-based contrast agents.[50] Therefore, it is recommended not to do biochemical assays within 24 hours after administration of either iodine- or gadolinium-based contrast agents and longer if the patient has renal impairment.

Pregnancy and Lactation

The knowledge is limited due to lack of studies. Our limited knowledge derives from anecdotal cases. In general, contrast media should not be used in pregnant women.[53,54] Following injection of iodine-based contrast media, the thyroid function should be checked in the neonate in the first week after delivery. This evaluation is not required following administration of gadolinium-based contrast media. Again, they should only be administered when the clinical symptoms and/or the unenhanced images are strongly indicative of a need for contrast enhancement.[53,54] Then, only the most stable agents may be used. The concern is that gadolinium crosses the placenta and is eventually in the fetus and amniotic fluid and only very slowly excreted.

For lactating women, it is different. If studies with iodine-based contrast media are performed, breastfeeding can continue normally.[53,54] As to MRI, only high-stability extracellular agents (non-protein binders) should be used. Of extracellular agents, it is only tiny amounts that are transferred via the milk to the newborn; it is considerably less than what has been approved for an examination of a child. The mother should be informed that the milk may temporarily change taste. If low-stability agents are used, the milk produced within 24 hours after administration should be thrown away.

REFERENCES

1. **Thomsen HS, Dawson P, Tweedle M.** MR and CT contrast agents for perfusion imaging and regulatory issues. In: Bammer R, ed. *MR and CT perfusion imaging: clinical applications and theoretical principles.* Philadelphia, PA: Lippincott Williams & Wilkins; 2015:Chapter 11.
2. **Thomsen HS, Bellin MF, Jakobsen JÅ, et al.** Contrast media classification and terminology. In: Thomsen HS, Webb JAW, eds. *Contrast media: safety issues and ESUR guidelines.* 3rd ed. Heidelberg, Germany: Springer Verlag; 2014:3–12.
3. **Chabanova E, Logager VB, Moller JM, et al.** Manganese based MR contrast agents: formulation and clinical applications. *Open Drug Saf J* 2011;2:29–38.
4. **Bellin MF.** Non-gadolinium-based contrast agents. In: Thomsen HS, Webb JAW, eds. *Contrast media: safety issues and ESUR guidelines.* 2nd ed. Berlin, Germany: Springer Verlag; 2009:205–211.
5. **Qju D, Zaharchuk G, Christen T, et al.** Contrast-enhanced functional blood volume imaging (CE-fBVI): enhanced sensitivity for brain activation in humans using the ultrasmall superparamagnetic iron oxide agent ferumoxytol. *Neuroimage* 2012;62:1726–1731.
6. **Morcos SK.** Gadolinium chelates and stability. In: Thomsen HS, Webb JAW, eds. *Contrast media: safety issues and ESUR guidelines.* 3rd ed. Heidelberg, Germany: Springer Verlag; 2014:175–180.
7. **Bellin MF, Leander P.** Organ-specific gadolinium-based contrast media. Gadolinium chelates and stability. In: Thomsen HS, Webb JAW, eds. *Contrast media: safety issues and ESUR Guidelines.* 3rd ed. Heidelberg, Germany: Springer Verlag; 2014:219–227.
8. **Dawson P.** Intravenous urography. In: Dawson P, Claub W, eds. *Contrast media in practice. Questions and answers.* Berlin, Germany: Springer Verlag; 1993:192–196.
9. **Older RA.** Clinical doses of contrast media. In: Thomsen HS, Muller RN, Mattrey RF. *Trends in contrast media.* Berlin, Germany: Springer Verlag;1999:75–80.
10. **Kondo H, Kanematsu M, Goshima S, et al.** Aortic and hepatic enhancement at multidetector TC: evaluation of optimal iodine dose determined by lean body weight. *Eur J Radiol* 2011;80:273–277.
11. **Arana E, Martí-Bonmatí L, Tobarra E, et al.** Cost reduction in abdominal CT by weight-adjusted dose. *Eur J Radiol* 2009;70:507–511.
12. **Ho LM, Nelson RC, DeLong DM.** Determining contrast medium dose and rate on basis of lean body weight: does this strategy improve patient-to-patient uniformity of hepatic enhancement during multi-detector row CT? *Radiology* 2007;243:431–437.
13. **Onishi H, Murakami T, Kim T, et al.** Abdominal multi-detector row CT: effectiveness of determining contrast medium dose on basis of body surface area. *Eur J Radiol* 2011;80:643–647.
14. **Kondo H, Kanematsu M, Goshima S, et al.** Body size indices to determine iodine mass with contrast-enhanced multi-detector computed tomography of the upper abdomen: does body surface area outperform total body weight or lean body weight? *Eur Radiol* 2013;23:1855–1861.
15. **Benbow M, Bull RK.** Simple weight-based contrast dosing for standardization of portal phase CT liver enhancement. *Clin Radiol* 2011; 66:940–944.
16. **Halls SB.** Methods used to develop CT scan contrast agent injection protocols. *Radiology* 1995;195:353–357.
17. **Yamashita Y, Komohara Y, Mutsumasa T, et al.** Abdominal helical CT: evaluation of optimal doses of intravenous contrast material—a prospective randomised study. *Radiology* 2000;216:718–723.
18. **Komatsu S, Kamata T, Imai A, et al.** Coronary computed tomography angiography using ultra-low-dose contrast media: radiation dose and image quality. *Int J Cardiovasc Imaging* 2013;29:1335–1340.
19. **Clement O, Webb JAW.** Acute adverse reactions to contrast media: mechanisms and prevention. Gadolinium chelates and stability. In: Thomsen HS, Webb JAW, eds. *Contrast media: safety issues and ESUR guidelines.* 3rd ed. Heidelberg, Germany: Springer Verlag; 2014:51–60.
20. **Katayama H, Yamaguchi K, Kozuka T, et al.** Adverse reactions to ionic and nonionic contrast media. *Radiology* 1990;175:621–628.
21. **Thomsen HS, Webb JAW.** The Lalli and Weber effects and the incidence of acute non-renal adverse reactions to contrast media. *Acta Radiol* 2012;53:953–954.
22. **Brockow K, Romano A, Aberer W, et al.** Skin testing in patients with hypersensitivity reactions to iodinated contrast media—a European Multicenter Study. *Allergy* 2009;64:234–241.
23. **Thomsen HS, Bongartz GM.** Acute adverse reactions to gadolinium-based contrast media. In: Thomsen HS, Webb JAW, eds. *Contrast media: safety issues and ESUR guidelines.* 3rd ed. Heidelberg, Germany: Springer Verlag; 2014:201–206.
24. **Bellin MF, Stacul F, Webb JAW, et al; On behalf of the Contrast Media Safety Committee of the European Society of Uroradiology (ESUR).** Late adverse reactions to intravascular iodine based contrast media: an update. *Eur Radiol* 2011;21:2305–2310.
25. **Van der Molen A.** Effect of iodine-based contrast media in thyroid function. In: Thomsen HS, Webb JAW, eds. *Contrast media: safety issues and ESUR guidelines.* 3rd ed. Heidelberg, Germany: Springer Verlag; 2014:157–166.
26. **Weinmann H-J, Brasch RC, Press W-R, et al.** Characteristics of gadolinium-DTPA complex: a potential NMR contrast agent. *AJR Am J Roentgenol* 1984;143:619–624.
27. **Evans CH, Drouven BJ.** The promotion of collagen polymerization by lanthanide and calcium ions. *Biochem J* 1983;213:751–758.

28. **Evans CH.** *Biochemistry of the lanthanides*. New York: Plenum Press; 1990.
29. **Tweedle MF, Gaughan GT, Hagan J, et al.** Considerations involving paramagnetic coordination compounds as useful NMR contrast agents *Int J Rad Appl Instrum B* 1988;15:31–36.
30. **Marckmann P, Skov L, Rossen K, et al.** Nephrogenic systemic fibrosis: suspected causative role of gadodiamide used for contrast-enhanced magnetic resonance imaging. *J Am Soc Nephrol* 2006;17:2359–2362.
31. **Grobner T.** Gadolinium: a specific trigger for the development of nephrogenic fibrosing dermopathy and nephrogenic systemic fibrosis? *Nephrol Dial Transplant* 2006;21:1104–1108.
32. **Thomsen HS.** Nephrogenic systemic fibrosis and gadolinium-based contrast media. In: Thomsen HS, Webb JAW, eds. *Contrast media: safety issues and ESUR guidelines*. 3rd ed. Heidelberg, Germany: Springer; 2014:207–218.
33. **Girardi M, Kay J, Elston DM.** Nephrogenic systemic fibrosis: clinicopathologic definition and workup recommendations. *J Am Acad Dermatol* 2011;65:1095–1106.
34. **White GW, Gibby WA, Tweedle MF.** Comparison of Gd (DTPA-BMA) (Omniscan) versus Gd(HP-DO3A) (ProHance) relative to gadolinium retention in human bone tissue by inductively coupled plasma mass spectroscopy. *Invest Radiol* 2006;41:272–278.
35. **European Society of Urogenital Radiology (ESUR).** Contrast media guidelines version 8.1.; 2013. Available at: http://www.esur.org
36. **Thomsen HS.** Contrast-enhanced MRI in patients with impaired renal function: recent recommendations to minimize the risk of nephrogenic systemic fibrosis. *Solut Contrast Imaging* 2010;1:1–8.
37. **Stacul F, van der Molen AJ, Reimer P, et al.** Contrast induced nephropathy: updated ESUR contrast media safety committee guidelines. *Eur Radiol* 2011;21:2527–2541.
38. **Mehta RL, Kellum JA, Shah S, et al.** Acute kidney injury network: report of an initiative to improve outcomes in acute Kidney injury. *Crit Care* 2007;11:31.
39. **McCullough PA, Wolyn R, Rocher LL, et al.** Acute renal failure after coronary intervention: incidence, risk factors, and relationship to mortality. *Am J Med* 1997;103:368–375.
40. **Katzberg RW, Lamba R.** Contrast-induced nephropathy after intravenous administration: fact or fiction? *Radiol Clin North Am* 2009; 47:789–800.
41. **Nyman U, Almén T, Jacobsson B, et al.** Are intravenous injections of contrast media really less nephrotoxic than intra-arterial injections? *Eur Radiol* 2012;22:1366–1371.
42. **McDonald JS, McDonald RJ, Comin J, et al.** Frequency of acute kidney injury following intravenous contrast medium administration: a systematic review and meta-analysis. *Radiology* 2013;267:119–128.
43. **McDonald RJ, McDonald JS, Bida JP, et al.** Intravenous contrast material-induced nephropathy: causal or coincident phenomenon? *Radiology* 2013;267:106–118.
44. **McDonald JS, McDonald RJ, Carter RE, et al.** Risk of intravenous contrast material-mediated acute kidney injury: a propensity score-matched study stratified by baseline-estimated glomerular filtration rate. *Radiology* 2014;271:65–73.
45. **Davenport MS, Khalatbari S, Cohan RH, et al.** Contrast material-induced nephrotoxicity and intravenous low-osmolality iodinated contrast material: risk stratification by using estimated glomerular filtration rate. *Radiology* 2013;268:719–728.
46. **Newhouse JH, RoyChoudhury A.** Quantitating contrast medium-induced nephropathy: controlling the controls. *Radiology* 2013;267:4–8.
47. **Kooiman J, Sijpkens YW, de Vries JP, et al.** A randomized comparison of 1-h sodium bicarbonate hydration versus standard peri-procedural saline hydration in patients with chronic kidney disease undergoing intravenous contrast-enhanced computerized tomography. *Nephrol Dial Transplant* 2014;29(5):1029–1036.
48. **Thomsen HS, Leander P.** Radiography with gadolinium-based contrast media. In: Thomsen HS, Webb JAW, eds. *Contrast media: safety issues and ESUR guidelines*. 3rd ed. Heidelberg, Germany: Springer Verlag; 2014.
49. **Jakobsen JÅ.** Contrast media extravasation injury. In: Thomsen HS, Webb JAW, eds. *Contrast media: safety issues and ESUR guidelines*. 3rd ed. Heidelberg, Germany: Springer Verlag; 2014.
50. **Morcos SK.** Contrast media and interactions with other drugs and clinical tests. In: Thomsen HS, Webb JAW, eds. *Contrast media: safety issues and ESUR guidelines*. 3rd ed. Heidelberg, Germany: Springer Verlag; 2014:125–130.
51. **Thomsen HS, Morcos SK, Almén T, et al.** Metformin and contrast media. *Radiology* 2010;256:672–673.
52. **Thomsen HS, Stacul F, Webb JAW.** Contrast medium-induced nephropathy. In: Thomsen HS, Webb JAW, eds. *Contrast media: safety issues and ESUR guidelines*. 3rd ed. Heidelberg, Germany: Springer; 2014:81–104.
53. **Webb JAW.** Pregnancy and lactation: intravascular use of contrast media. In: Thomsen HS, Webb JAW, eds. *Contrast media: safety issues and ESUR guidelines*. 3rd ed. Heidelberg, Germany: Springer; 2014:113–120.
54. **Webb JAW, Thomsen HS.** Gadolinium contrast media during pregnancy and lactation. *Acta Radiol* 2013;54:599–600.

CHAPTER

12 Brain MR Perfusion Imaging: Cerebral Ischemia

Chia-Shang Jason Liu, MD, PhD and Mircea Cristian Dobre, MD, MS

Background

Stroke is a major health care issue in the United States, affecting 6.4 million noninstitutionalized adults in 2012.[1] On average between the years of 2009 and 2010, there were 3.7 million visits to physician offices, hospital outpatient offices, and emergency departments with stroke as the primary diagnosis,[2] with the average length of stay within a hospital for the treatment of cerebrovascular disease lasting 6.1 days.[3] Stroke was the fourth leading cause of death in 2010, behind heart disease, cancer, and chronic lower respiratory disease.[4]

While stroke is still one of the leading causes of death in the United States, it has decreased in rank over the years, in part due to the increased awareness of symptoms of stroke by the health care profession as well as the public and the emphasis placed on early and rapid treatment of cerebral ischemia. The brain has little capacity to store energy, and its viability is compromised after 3 minutes of vascular occlusion. The therapeutic window is narrow, and without treatment, penumbra will progress to irreversible infarction in a few hours. Current guidelines in the treatment of stroke advocate the delivery of intravenous recombinant tissue plasminogen activator (rtPA) within 3 hours of last known well time before symptom onset, with earlier delivery of rtPA in patients with NIH Stroke Scale (NIHSS) scores of less than 20 and patients less than 75 years of age having the greatest potential for excellent outcome with treatment.[5] Even patients undergoing IV rtPA treatment up to 4.5 hours from last known well time have shown clinical benefits as compared to placebo.[6]

Current treatment guidelines rely on imaging, in particular noncontrast computed tomography (CT), to exclude the presence of intracranial hemorrhage or other causes of the patient's symptoms such as the presence of intracranial masses.[7] There is strong interest in taking into account the physiology of acute ischemia in the treatment algorithm of acute stroke, with the thought that differentiating the amount of viable brain tissue from infarcted tissue may potentially lead to better patient selection and outcomes (Fig. 12.1). This is especially important in order to decide which patients should receive intravenous or intra-arterial treatments as well as selecting patients for treatment who experience "wake up strokes," where the onset of initial stoke symptoms cannot be precisely determined and the patients therefore are technically outside of the treatment window of current treatment guidelines.

Magnetic resonance imaging (MRI) utilizing diffusion-weighted imaging (DWI) is currently the most sensitive imaging method for the detection of acute ischemia, with high sensitivity and potential for detection of stroke within hours of onset.[8–12] DWI does not, however, provide physiologic information such as cerebral blood flow (CBF), cerebral blood volume (CBV), and viability of adjacent brain parenchyma at a particular time point.

Perfusion Metrics and Technical Consideration

Dynamic contrast-enhanced (DCE) CT has been used to characterize brain physiology, with the ability to quantify perfusion parameters such as CBF, CBV, and mean transit time (MTT), parameters that are useful for the characterization of stroke as potentially useful for the prediction of the evolution of stroke.[13–15] Similarly, DCE MRI has also been used to obtain the perfusion parameters.[16,17] Details with regard to the technical considerations of CT perfusion as well as dynamic susceptibility contrast (DSC) MRI are explained in detail elsewhere in this book. With both techniques, perfusion metrics such as CBF, CBV, MTT, time to peak of the residual function (T_{max}), and delay time to peak of the residual function (DT) can be calculated (Figure 12.2). The time to peak is the time from bolus administration to peak signal intensity.

Arterial spin labeling (ASL) is an MRI technique that can also provide information with regard to brain physiology. In ASL, instead of using an intravenous contrast agent, radiofrequency energy is applied proximal to the tissue to be imaged, with the goal of flipping these spins from their normal alignment with the magnetic field.[18] This change in proton spin orientation serves as the label that is carried downstream in flowing blood. Inflow of these inverted spins creates a flow-related signal when the water is extracted from the capillary bed or, in the case of a fistula, can be seen in the venous structures. Multiple images can be acquired prior to complete decay of signal, and quantitative analysis is possible using subtraction from thin-section T1W images.[18] The short duration of labeling allows for marked sensitivity to changes in arterial transit time.[19]

While both CT and MR perfusion offer the ability to measure perfusion metrics, MR perfusion has the advantages of being an imaging technique that does not require ionizing radiation and

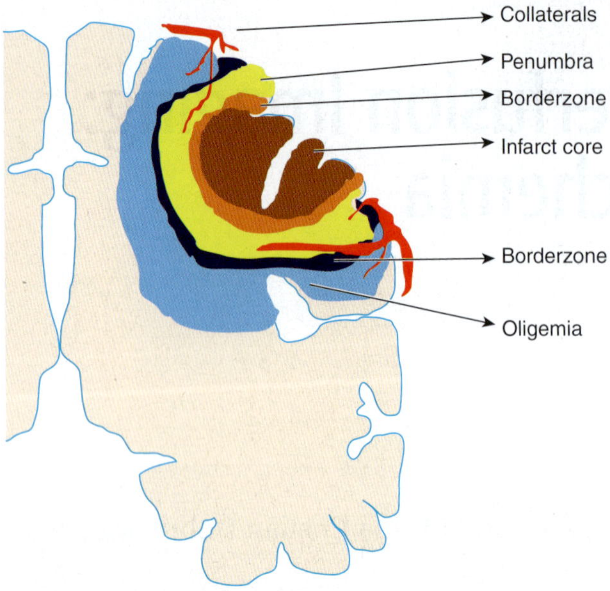

Figure 12-1. Schematic demonstration of the infarct core, penumbra, benign oligemia, and associated border zones. Dynamic changes in size over time occur depending on the status of the leptomeningeal collaterals and hemodynamic, physiologic, or metabolic factors. The infarct core is nonviable tissue. Penumbra is the ischemic but dysfunctional zone and remains viable if blood flow is restored. Benign oligemia is underperfused but functional tissue that remains viable. The threshold level for neuronal dysfunction is a CBF of approximately 20 mL/100 g/min, and benign ischemia zone is above this threshold.

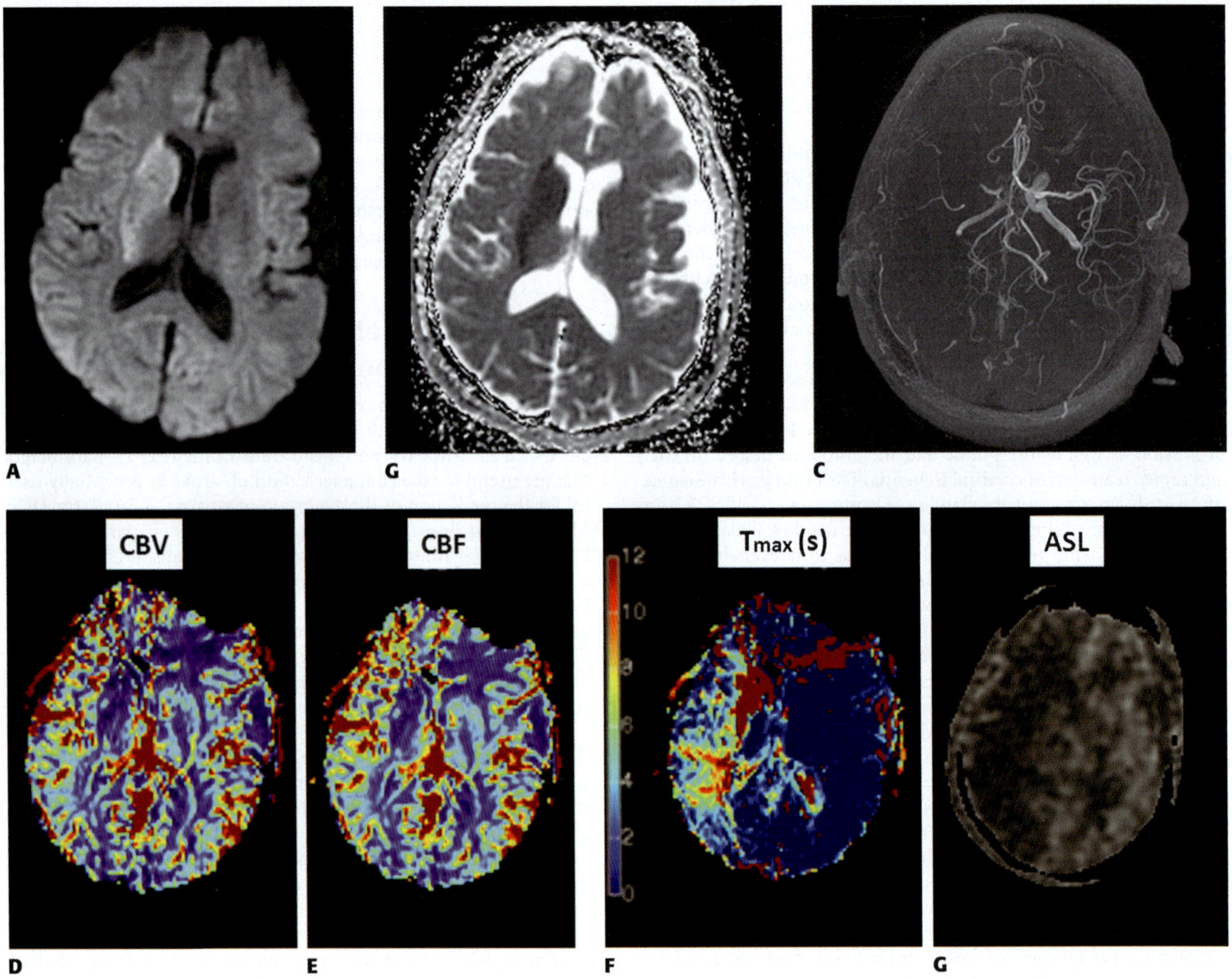

Figure 12-2. Example of contrast-enhanced MR perfusion and arterial spin labeling (ASL) in a patient with acute ischemia. Diffusion-weighted imaging **(A)** with its corresponding apparent diffusion coefficient map **(B)** in a patient demonstrates acute infarct in the right caudate head and putamen. MR angiography of the head **(C)** demonstrates an occlusion in the proximal segment of the right middle cerebral artery (MCA). Cerebral blood volume (CBV) **(D)**, cerebral blood flow (CBF) **(E)**, and T_{Max} **(F)** from contrast-enhanced MR perfusion demonstrate matched abnormality in the right caudate head and putamen, with decreased CBV and CBF as well as elevated T_{max} noted in the area of acute infarct relative to the contralateral side. The right insula and the visualized right frontal and parietal lobes, in the distribution of the more distal right MCA, demonstrate preserved CBV and CBF relative to the contralateral side, despite elevated T_{max} in the same region, compatible with penumbra. ASL **(G)** of the same region demonstrates decreased perfusion in the right MCA territory relative to the contralateral side.

therefore has decreased associated risks of radiation as compared to CT.[20] MR perfusion also has the capability for whole-brain calculation of perfusion metrics, whereas most CT perfusion studies typically only provide limited coverage of the brain, with routine CT perfusion slices centered at the level of the basal ganglia so as to maximize the interrogation of arterial territories and to minimize radiation exposure. Being an MRI technique, MR perfusion has the distinct advantage of being a part of an imaging modality that is currently the most sensitive for acute ischemia, with the evaluation incorporated with other MR sequences such as DWI as part of a stroke evaluation.[21] Despite these advantages, CT scanners are more widely available than are MRI scanners for the evaluation of stroke, especially in an emergency setting. CT perfusion metrics are also easier to quantify than are MR perfusion metrics due to the linear relationship between iodinated contrast concentration and CT attenuation, which is not the case for gadolinium contrast concentration and MR signal intensity.[7] There are also fewer contraindications for a subject to undergo a CT evaluation than an MRI evaluation, such as the presence of a pacemaker, renal failure requiring dialysis, claustrophobia, or presence of metal fragments including, among others, older ferromagnetic medical implants.

Despite their differences, MR and CT perfusion have been shown to generate similar perfusion metrics. When using a T_{max} threshold of greater than 6 seconds, there is good agreement in the predicted area of acute ischemia by MR and CT.[22] While the literature supports the use of both imaging modalities and their perfusion metrics in following stroke patients, care needs to be taken in terms of the consistent use of perfusion software, the mathematical model used for the calculation of the perfusion metrics, and the threshold used for the generation of ischemia maps.[22]

With regard to the characterization of brain perfusion in the setting of acute stroke, ASL and DSC MR perfusion demonstrate similar capabilities to characterize perfusion parameters (Fig. 12.3). A territory of decreased relative CBV or CBV with reduced diffusion identifies infarct. A territory of increased MTT or Tmax indicates slow flow through that area of the brain. Matched Tmax and relative

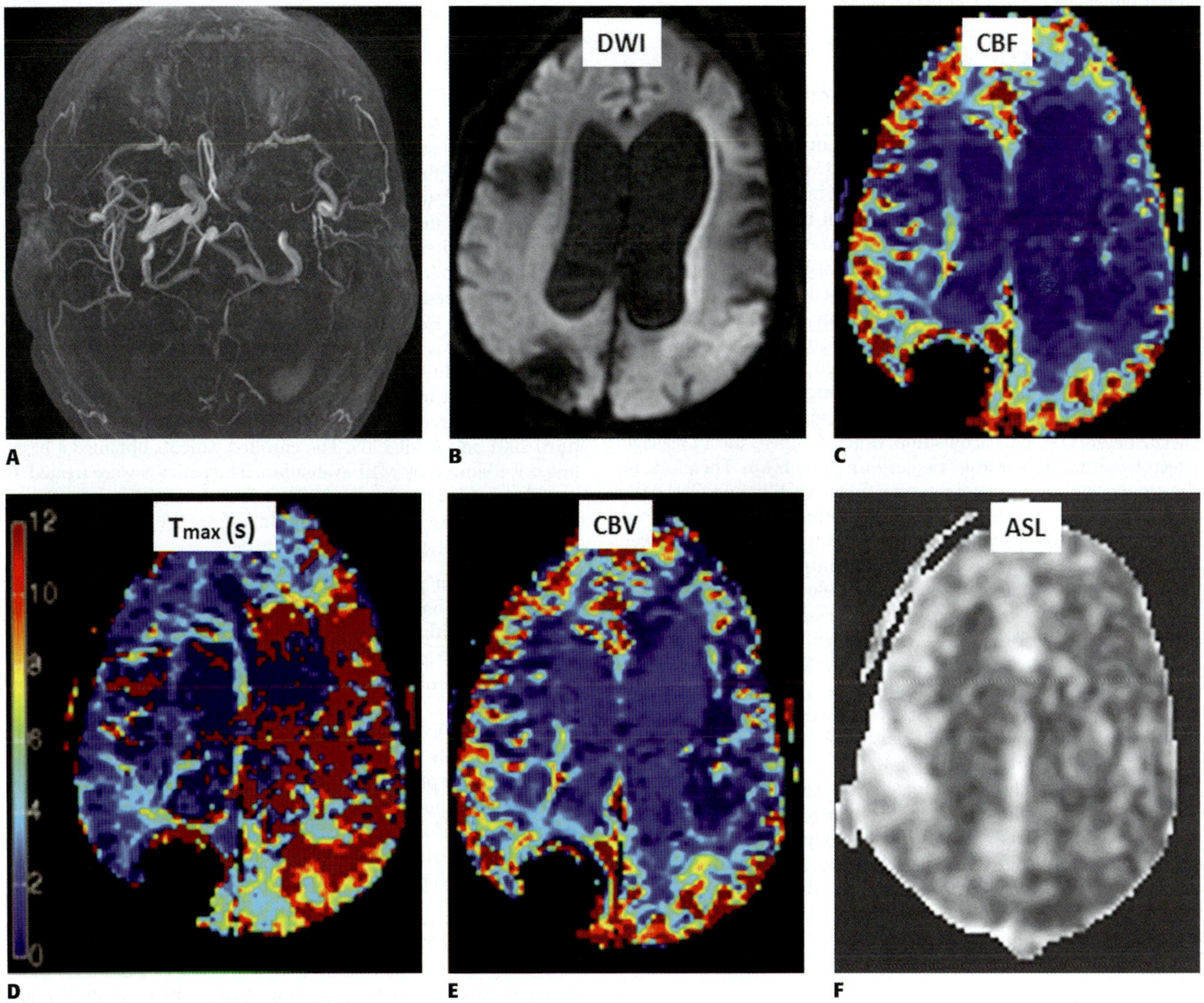

Figure 12-3. Evolution of an acute infarct as characterized with perfusion imaging. A patient with prior multifocal infarcts has an acute proximal left middle cerebral artery occlusion **(A)**. Initial diffusion-weighted imaging (DWI) **(B)** demonstrates left periventricular reduced diffusion, compatible with acute infarct, with diffusion abnormality also seen in the left parietal white matter. MR perfusion demonstrates large left middle cerebral artery distribution of decreased cerebral blood flow (CBF) **(C)** with corresponding elevated T_{max} **(D)**, involving not only the left periventricular white matter but also the left frontal and left parietal lobes. There is decreased cerebral blood volume (CBV) **(E)** within the left frontal and parietal lobes. Arterial spin labeling (ASL) **(F)** also demonstrates decreased blood flow to the left cerebral hemisphere. Subsequent DWI (not shown) demonstrated infarct progression to the left frontal and temporal lobes.

CBV (or diffusion) regions of abnormality indicate complete infarction, and a Tmax abnormality larger than the rCBV (or diffusion) defect indicates that the ischemic area is larger than the infarction, and the difference represents the penumbra or area at risk that requires intervention. ASL has shown similar ability as DSC MR perfusion in delineating regions of hypoperfusion, with similar conspicuity of the lesions using either technique.[23] Hyperemic lesions in acute ischemic stroke are more conspicuous using ASL as compared to DSC MR perfusion.[23] Other studies have shown ASL to overestimate perfusion defect volume in patients with small final infarcts.[24] In general, ASL hypoperfused area corresponds to increase in transit time on DSC. Penumbra manifests as an ASL hypoperfusion territory larger than restricted area on DWI. Abnormally hypoperfused area on ASL with a normal DWI may indicate an ischemic zone that requires further angiographic studies to assess vascular integrity. To date, however, no multicenter trials have used ASL to risk stratify patients into different treatment arms in the setting of acute stroke, perhaps in part due to the relative novelty of ASL compared to DSC MR perfusion and the lack of ability to implement the technique on conventional clinical MR scanners reliably.

MR Protocol

A comprehensive MRI protocol of brain can include DWI, ASL, DCE, and DSC sequences using 1.5 or 3 T magnets. Both DSC and DCE MR imaging methods require intravenous injection of gadolinium contrast. ASL does not need contrast, and as a matter of fact, T1 shortening effect of gadolinium contrast can destroy ASL signals. However, ASL techniques suffer low signal-to-noise ratio even at high magnetic field, and a good study may require up to 8 minutes at 1.5 T or 4 to 5 minutes at 3 T. Postcontrast perfusion sequences are otherwise faster to obtain. In the presence of a dysfunctional or "leaky" blood–brain barrier, gadolinium contrast leaks out of intravascular space. As a result of contrast extravasation, the DSC data can be compromised due to T1 shortening (increased signal), which counteracts the T2* signal shortening effect. This deleterious effect can be prevented by "preload" injection of gadolinium chelate before DSC data acquisition, which dampens the T1 leakage effects by saturating the leaky tissues with gadolinium. Therefore, in the sequence of brain imaging, some prefer DCE before DSC MR. Approximately, one-third to half of the normal weight-based dose of gadolinium (0.1 mmol/kg) is injected for DCE using a power injector at a rate of 4 to 5 mL/s for both contrast and saline chaser. This amount of contrast can serve as the preload for the subsequent DSC exam, which is obtained with the remaining dose of gadolinium. DCE is performed by a fast gradient echo sequence (3-D spoiled gradient-recalled echo [SPGR] FAST for GE or 2-D/3-D FLASH [Siemens Healthcare]), and TE is kept minimum. Typically, there are approximately 30 phases with 12 slices (6 to 8 mm) per phase. Total scan length is usually less than 4 minutes. DSC will be performed with the rest contrast at the same injection rate using a 2-D gradient echo echo-planar imaging sequence. Twelve to sixteen axial slices at 5 to 7 mm thickness are obtained for 60 phases, which usually takes less than 2 minutes (slightly longer for 3 T due to longer TR). For both DSC and DCE techniques, the contrast injection starts approximately 15 to 20 seconds after the start of MR perfusion sequence. Five to eight minutes' interval is suggested between the two injections, and in order to save time, DWI can be performed between the two perfusion sequences.

Clinical Utility of Perfusion Imaging in the Setting of Acute Stroke

Several major trials have been completed to evaluate the effectiveness of treatment options for stroke in order to improve outcome from a stroke or to extend the time limit of thrombolytic administration for the treatment of stroke. Anatomic imaging is already used as a decision criteria in the treatment of stroke (Table 12.1),[7] with studies also demonstrating clinical utility of risk stratification of stroke treatment using anatomic imaging criteria.[25] While some of the multicenter trials focus on anatomic imaging as a decision criteria for patient group selection, some of the trials have also used perfusion imaging to risk stratify the patients to the different treatment arms.

TABLE 12.1 **Imaging Findings that are Contraindications to Administration of IV tPA**

Significant head trauma or prior stroke in previous 3 mo
Symptoms/evidence of subarachnoid hemorrhage
Intracranial neoplasm, arteriovenous malformation, or aneurysm
Active internal bleeding
CT demonstrating multilobar infarction greater than one-third of cerebral hemisphere

Adapted from Jauch EC, et al. Guidelines for the early management of patients with acute ischemic stroke: a guideline for healthcare professionals from the American Heart Association/American Stroke Association. *Stroke* 2013;44:870–947.

The DWI Evaluation for Understanding Stroke Evolution (DEFUSE) trial was a multicenter, prospective trial that attempted to assess the utility of perfusion imaging in the prediction of patient outcomes following an acute stroke.[26] One thousand and twenty patients were screened, with seventy-four patients enrolled between April 2001 and April 2005. The enrolled patients obtained a baseline CT, followed by MRI evaluation. The patients were treated as quickly as possible after the MRI scan with IV tPA, no later than 6 hours from onset of stroke symptoms. From the imaging findings, patients were categorized as follows:

1. "Malignant profile"—defined as the presence of a large diffusion lesion volume (100 mL) and/or large perfusion lesion volume with long delays on the T_{max} map (>8 seconds)
2. "Mismatch profile"—defined as the presence of a perfusion lesion 10 mL or more and 120% or more of the diffusion lesion
3. "Target Mismatch profile"—defined as the presence of early reperfusion in mismatch patients who did not have the Malignant profile
4. "Small Lesion profile"—defined as the presence of diffusion and perfusion volume of less than 10 mL
5. "No Mismatch profile"—defined as the presence of perfusion volume less than 120% of the diffusion volume

From these categorizations, the DEFUSE trial demonstrated that patients with the Target Mismatch profile with early reperfusion (evidence of recanalization of the occluded vessel as well as decrease in perfusion imaging abnormality) had statistically significant difference in favorable clinical response compared to the Malignant profile as well as the Target Mismatch profile without early reperfusion, with a favorable clinical response defined as an improvement of 8 points or more in the NIHSS score between baseline and 30 days or an NIHSS score of 0 to1 at 30 days. Within the Target Mismatch profile with early reperfusion group, 60% having a modified Rankin Scale of 0 to 2 after 30 days of the stroke. For subjects with a Malignant profile, only 17% of the subjects have a modified Rankin Scale of 0 to 2 after 30 days of the stroke, and 50% of the subjects also demonstrated symptomatic intracranial hemorrhage (compared to 6.7% in the Target Mismatch profile with early reperfusion group). For subjects that have the Target Mismatch profile without early reperfusion, only 13% of the subjects have a modified Rankin Scale of 0 to 2 after 30 days of the stroke, with 6.3% of the subjects demonstrating symptomatic intracranial hemorrhage.[26]

The findings of the DEFUSE trial were extended to assess for the utility of the use of diffusion and perfusion data to identify patients who are most likely to benefit from endovascular reperfusion in the DEFUSE 2 trial.[27] DEFUSE 2 was a multicenter, prospective cohort study, in which patients treated with IV alteplase were eligible. One hundred and thirty patients were enrolled into the trial, with 28 excluded due to the lack of catheter angiography and an additional 6 excluded due to technically inadequate MR perfusion imaging. For the remaining 104 subjects, 78 have a Target Mismatch profile, and 46 of whom had evidence of early reperfusion. The subjects that had a Target Mismatch profile with early reperfusion had a statistically significant difference in having a favorable clinical response, defined as an improvement in the NIHSS score of 8 points or more or a score of 0 to 1 at 30 days, as compared to subjects with a Target Mismatch profile without early reperfusion. These subjects also had statistically significant smaller median lesion growth volume ($p = 0.005$) and had more subjects demonstrating a modified Rankin Scale of 0 to 2 after 30 days of the stroke as compared to the Target Mismatch profile without early reperfusion group (57% vs. 31%, respectively. $p = 0.04$). For subjects without a Target Mismatch profile, there were no statistically significant differences in outcome with or without early reperfusion.[27]

Extending the effective time to treatment for stroke is of tremendous clinical interest, and perfusion imaging has been used to see if subjects with certain perfusion characteristics would benefit from thrombolytic therapy beyond the 3-hour time period from the initial onset of symptoms. The Echoplanar Imaging Thrombolytic Evaluation Trial (EPITHET) ascertained whether or not rtPA given 3 to 6 hours after stroke onset promoted reperfusion and attenuated infarct growth in patients with MR perfusion and DWI mismatch, with a mismatch defined as a ratio of greater than 1.2 when comparing lesion volume on perfusion imaging to that of DWI as well as a perfusion lesion volume of great than 10 mL as compared to lesion volume by DWI.[28] It was a prospective, randomized, double-blind, placebo-controlled, phase II trial. One hundred and one subjects were enrolled in the study, with 37 subjects receiving rtPA included in the mismatch analysis and 43 subjects receiving placebo included in the mismatch analysis. Results of the study demonstrated that under the study conditions, treatment with rtPA was significantly associated with increased reperfusion but was not significantly associated with reducing infarct growth. There was also no statistically significant difference in clinical outcome between those receiving rtPA beyond the 3-hour window to those receiving placebo as measured by the number of subjects with a modified Rankin Scale score of 0 to 2 after 90 days. The subjects that demonstrated reperfusion, defined as greater than 90% reduction between baseline and day 3 perfusion lesion volumes, compared to those that did not demonstrate reperfusion, did demonstrate a statistically significant decrease in infarct size as well as resulting in a statistically significant number of subjects with good neurologic and functional outcome after 90 days.[28]

A reanalysis of the EPITHET data in 2011 reached different conclusions with regard to the efficacy of thrombolytic treatment.[29] In the reanalysis, the ischemic volume was redefined as the portions of the brain that demonstrated perfusion abnormality and excluded regions within the perfusion abnormality that also demonstrated diffusion abnormality (coregistered mismatch volume), rather than defining the ischemic volume as the volume of the brain demonstrating perfusion abnormality after removing the volume of brain also demonstrating diffusion abnormality that included the contiguous volume of brain demonstrating diffusion abnormality that is not within the perfusion abnormality (volumetric mismatch volume). With the repeat analysis and the new definition of infarct volume, the authors of the study demonstrated that while the calculated baseline mismatch volume did not significantly change between the coregistration method and the volumetric method, there was statistically significant decrease in the median relative as well as absolute growth of the infarct volume in subjects undergoing rtPA treatment compared to those receiving placebo ($P = 0.01$ and 0.03, respectively), differing from the original conclusions of EPITHET. Even with the repeat analysis, no statistically significant difference in clinical outcome is seen between the group receiving rtPA and those receiving placebo, however, as assessed by the number of subjects with an NIHSS at day 90 of 0 or 1 or improvement greater than or equal to 8 from baseline and number of subjects with a modified Rankin Scale of 0 to 2 after 90 days.[29]

Another trial that assessed the efficacy of extending the treatment of acute stroke beyond 3 hours was the desmoteplase in Acute Ischemic Stroke (DIAS-2) trial.[30] DIAS-2 was a prospective, randomized, double-blind, placebo-controlled study, in which advanced MR or CT was used for intravenous fibrinolysis triage in the 3- to 9-hour time window. In the trial, inclusion criteria required presence of penumbra defined as at least 20% of the tissue with perfusion disturbance as compared to the core of the infarct, measured by MR or CT.[30] Thirty patients were screened, of which 166 failed screening criteria and therefore were not used for analysis. The remainder of the subjects were separated into those that received 90 μg/kg of desmoteplase, 125 μg/kg of desmoteplase, or placebo, with 57, 66, and 63 subjects participating, respectively. The different treatment arms did not demonstrate any significant differences among the treatment groups both in terms of improvement in NIHSS score or modified Rankin Scale score of 0 to 2 at 90 days after treatment. There was also no significant increase in survival between groups receiving desmoteplase at 90 days compared to the placebo group. With regard to image processing, an interesting finding of the DIAS-2 trial was that there were profound differences in mismatch volumes between MRI and CT, with inconsistencies between MRI and CT data on the change in core lesion volume at day 30.[30]

The Mechanical Retrieval and Recanalization of Stroke Clots Using Embolectomy (MR RESCUE) trial was a phase 2b, randomized, controlled, open-label (blinded outcome), multicenter trial where patients with large vessel, anterior circulation ischemic stroke were randomly assigned within 8 hours after onset of symptoms to undergo mechanical embolectomy or standard medical care.[31] Patients who had received IV tPA without evidence of successful recanalization were eligible for the trial if imaging demonstrated a persistent target occlusion. One hundred and twenty-seven patients were selected into the trial, with 64 assigned to receive embolectomy and 54 assigned to receive standard medical care (9 patients were excluded due to technical factors). The different treatment groups were further subcategorized into those who had a favorable penumbral pattern, defined as having an infarct core of 90 mL or less as well as having the proportion of predicted infarct tissue within the at-risk region of 70% or less, versus a nonpenumbral pattern. The trial demonstrated that final infarct volume were less in the patients demonstrating a penumbral pattern of infarct versus a nonpenumbral pattern, with those demonstrating a penumbral pattern having a lower modified Rankin Scale after 90 days compared with those with a nonpenumbral pattern (3.6; 95% CI, 3.3 to 4.0 vs. 4.2; 95% CI, 3.8 to 4.7; $p = 0.047$)). Patients who demonstrated evidence of reperfusion, defined as a reduction of more than

90% in the volume of the perfusion lesion from baseline with T_{max} > 6 seconds, also had a smaller final infarct growth as well as better clinical outcome as evidenced by lower modified Rankin Scale after 90 days. The trial, however, did not demonstrate any benefits of embolectomy, with patients with a penumbral pattern receiving standard medical care actually having a statistically significant final infarct size that is slightly smaller than patients with a penumbral pattern who received embolectomy. A possible explanation for the lack of efficacy of embolectomy may be the relatively low success rate of revascularization in the embolectomy group, which may in part be due to the first-generation embolectomy devices that were used in the trial.[31]

While the major stroke trials to date have not demonstrated clinical utility of perfusion imaging to select for patients who would benefit from the extension of the window of treatment of thrombolytic therapy or endovascular therapy, data continue to support that evidence of reperfusion of brain affected by acute stroke result in improved clinical outcome. A study of 114 patients using CT and CT perfusion demonstrated that patients who demonstrated reperfusion by imaging had statistically significant decrease in follow-up infarct volume, with reperfusion, not recanalization, being a significant predictor of good clinical outcome as defined as a modified Rankin Score of less than or equal to 2 after 90 days.[32] Ongoing clinical trials to investigate the clinical efficacy of extending the window of intravenous and intra-arterial thrombolytic therapy (EXTEND, EXTEND-IA) continue to use perfusion imaging as a selection criteria for enrolment in order to maximize study effects.[33,34]

Pitfalls of Perfusion Imaging

Despite the theoretical advantage of predicting patient outcome by assessing the viability of brain tissue, perfusion imaging has not lived up to its promise thus far. As noted in the DIAS-2 trial, one possible explanation is that there is considerable variability in the estimation of core lesion size and penumbra. An analysis of the mismatch volumes (penumbra) calculated from MR perfusion data demonstrated that, depending on the algorithm used to generate the perfusion maps based on different estimations of time to peak and T_{max}, there is a mean difference of up to 40 mL for the calculated mismatch volume, with up to 100-mL difference in mismatch lesion volume on an individual basis.[35] The findings echo another published result, where the authors demonstrate that depending on the deconvolution technique used to calculate CT perfusion metrics, there is considerable variability in penumbra and infarct prediction.[36] Due to the variability that can occur during perfusion calculations, some institutions have relied more on DWI rather than perfusion in predicting patient outcome from an acute stroke and to guide management of the patients.[21]

Standardization of perfusion processing would be a method of overcoming the variability of perfusion calculations. An automated algorithm has been used to reanalyze the DEFUSE and EPITHET data and has demonstrated success in categorizing patients with Target Mismatch and Malignant profiles.[37] The consistent use of automated perfusion software as well as standardization of thresholds of perfusion parameters may lead to more consistent estimations of infarct and penumbra and aid in the analysis of large clinical trials.

Conclusion

MR perfusion has been used in the clinical setting in order to estimate the viability of brain tissue in the setting of acute stroke. While the technique thus far has not led to an alteration of clinical management of stroke based on time from onset of symptoms nor has it demonstrated utility in selecting for patients who would better benefit from endovascular therapy, the technique has demonstrated that in patients who have demonstrable reperfusion of brain tissue, those patients will have better neurologic as well as functional outcomes. As the processing of the perfusion data becomes more standardized, the ongoing multicenter trials may prove the utility of MR perfusion and alter the current treatment of acute stroke.

REFERENCES

1. **Blackwell DL, Lucas JW, Clarke TC**. Summary health statistics for U.S. adults: National Health Interview Survey, 2012. National Center for Health Statistics. *Vital Health Stat* 2014;10(260)1–161.
2. Selected patient and provider characteristics for ambulatory care visits to physician offices and hospital outpatient and emergency departments: United States, 2009–2010.
3. National Hospital Discharge Survey: 2010 table, Average length of stay and days of care—Number and rate of discharges by first-listed diagnostic categories.
4. Deaths: final data for 2010. *Natl Vital Stat Rep* 2013;61(4):1–117.
5. **NINDS t-PA Stroke Study Group**. Generalized efficacy of t-PA for acute stroke. Subgroup analysis of the NINDS t-PA Stroke Trial. *Stroke* 1997;28:2119–2125.
6. **Hacke W, et al.** Thrombolysis with Alteplase 3 to 4.5 hours after acute ischemic stroke. *N Engl J Med* 2008;359(13):1317–1329.
7. **Jauch EC, et al.** Guidelines for the early management of patients with acute ischemic stroke: a guideline for healthcare professionals from the American Heart Association/American Stroke Association. *Stroke* 2013;44:870–947.
8. **Marks MP, et al.** Acute and chronic stroke: navigated spin-echo diffusion weighted MR imaging. *Radiology* 1996;199:403–408.
9. **Sorensen AG, et al.** Hyperacute stroke: evaluation with combined multisection diffusion-weighted and hemodynamically weighted echo-planar MR imaging. *Radiology* 1996;199:391–401.
10. **Warach S, et al.** Clinical outcome in ischemic stroke predicted by early diffusion-weighted and perfusion magnetic resonance imaging: a preliminary analysis. *J Cereb Blood Flow Metab* 1996;16:53–59.
11. **Warach S, et al.** Acute human stroke studied by whole brain echo planar diffusion-weighted magnetic resonance imaging. *Ann Neurol* 1995;37:231–241.
12. **Singer MB, et al.** Diffusion-weighted MRI in acute subcortical infarction. *Stroke* 1998;29:133–136.
13. **Axel L**. Cerebral blood flow determination by rapid-sequence computed tomography: theoretical analysis. *Radiology* 1980;137:679–686.
14. **Lev MH, et al.** Utility of perfusion-weighted CT imaging in acute middle cerebral artery stroke treated with intra-arterial thrombolysis: prediction of final infarct volume and clinical outcome. *Stroke* 2001;32(9):2021–2028.
15. **Wintermark M, et al.** Dynamic Perfusion CT: optimizing the temporal resolution and contrast volume for calculation of perfusion CT parameters in stroke patients. *AJNR Am J Neuroradiol* 2004;25:720–729.
16. **Schellinger PD, et al.** Stroke magnetic resonance imaging within 6 hours after onset of hyperacute cerebral ischemia. *Ann Neurol* 2001;49(4):460–469.
17. **Schramm P, et al.** Comparison of perfusion computed tomography and computed tomography angiography source images with perfusion-weighted imaging and diffusion-weighted imaging in patients with acute stroke of less than 6 hours' duration. *Stroke* 2004;35(7):1652–1658.
18. **Deibler AR, et al.** Arterial spin-labeling in routine clinical practice, part 1: technique and artifacts. *AJNR Am J Neuroradiol* 2008;29(7):1228–1234.
19. **Detre JA, et al.** Applications of arterial spin labeled MRI in the brain. *J Magn Reson Imaging* 2012;35(5):1026–1037.
20. **Sodickson A, et al.** Recurrent CT. Cumulative radiation exposure, and associated radiation-induced cancer risks from CT of Adults. *Radiology.* 2009;251(1):175–184.
21. **Gonzales RG, et al.** The Massachusetts General Hospital acute stroke imaging algorithm: an experience and evidence based approach. *J Neurointerv Surg* 2013;5:i7–i12.
22. **Lin L, et al.** Comparison of computed tomographic and magnetic resonance perfusion measurements in acute ischemic stroke: back-to-back quantitative analysis. *Stroke* 2014;45:1727–1732.
23. **Wang DJ, et al.** The value of arterial spin-labeled perfusion imaging in acute ischemic *stroke*: comparison with dynamic susceptibility contrast-enhanced MRI. *Stroke* 2012;43:1018–1024.

24. **Huang YC, et al.** Comparison of arterial spin labeling and dynamic susceptibility contrast perfusion MRI in patients with acute stroke. *PLoS One* 2013;8:e69085.
25. **Pexman JH, et al.** Use of the Alberta Stroke Program Early CT Score (ASPECTS) for assessing CT scans in patients with acute stroke. *AJNR Am J Neuroradiol* 2001;22(8):1534–1542.
26. **Albers GW, et al.** Magnetic resonance imaging profiles predict clinical response to early reperfusion: the Diffusion and Perfusion Imaging Evaluation for Understanding Stroke Evolution (DEFUSE) Study. *Ann Neurol* 2006;60:508–517.
27. **Lansberg MG, et al.** MRI profile and response to endovascular reperfusion after stroke (DEFUSE 2): a prospective cohort study. *Lancet Neurol* 2012;11:860–867.
28. **Davis SM, et al.** Effects of alteplase beyond 3 hours after stroke in The Echoplanar Imaging Thrombolytic Evaluation Trial (EPITHET): a placebo-controlled randomised trial. *Lancet Neurol* 2008;7:299–309.
29. **Nagakane Y, et al.** EPITHET: positive result after reanalysis using baseline diffusion-weighted imaging/perfusion-weighted imaging co-registration. *Stroke* 2011;42:59–64.
30. **Hacke W, et al.** Intravenous desmoteplase in patients with acute ischaemic stroke selected by MRI perfusion–diffusion weighted imaging or perfusion CT (DIAS-2): a prospective, randomised, double-blind, placebo-controlled study. *Lancet Neurol* 2009;8:141–150.
31. **Kidwell CS, et al.** A trial of imaging selection and endovascular treatment for ischemic stroke. *N Engl J Med* 2013;368:914–923.
32. **Eilaghi A, et al.** Reperfusion is a stronger predictor of good clinical outcome than recanalization in ischemic stroke. *Radiology* 2013;269:240–248.
33. **Ma H, et al.** A multicentre, randomized, double-blinded, placebo-controlled Phase III study to investigate EXtending the Time for Thrombolysis in Emergency Neurological Deficits (EXTEND). *Int J Stroke* 2011;7:74–80.
34. **Campbell BCV, et al.** A multicenter, randomized, controlled study to investigate EXtending the time for Thrombolysis in Emergency Neurological Deficits with Intra-Arterial therapy (EXTEND-IA). *Int J Stroke* 2013;9:126–132.
35. **Forkert ND, et al.** Comparison of 10 TTP and Tmax Estimation Techniques for MR perfusion-diffusion mismatch quantification in acute stroke. *AJNR Am J Neuroradiol* 2013;34:1697–1703.
36. **Bivard A, et al.** Perfusion CT in Acute Stroke: a comprehensive analysis of infarct and penumbra. *Radiology* 2013;267:543–550.
37. **Lansberg MG, et al.** RAPID automated patient selection for reperfusion therapy: a pooled analysis of the Echoplanar Imaging Thrombolytic Evaluation Trial (EPITHET) and the Diffusion and Perfusion Imaging Evaluation for Understanding Stroke Evolution (DEFUSE) Study. *Stroke* 2011;42:1608–1614.

CHAPTER

13 Brain CT Perfusion Imaging: Cerebral Ischemia

Christopher D. d'Esterre, BMSc, PhD, Mohammed Almekhlafi, MD, Bijoy K. Menon, MD, and Mayank Goyal, MD, FRCPC

Introduction

Stroke is caused by variable disturbances in blood flow to intracranial structures due to lack of blood supply (ischemia) or leakage of blood from vessels (hemorrhage). Accordingly, these cerebrovascular accidents have distinct etiologies: the former caused by thromboembolism or systemic hypoperfusion leading to local or global cerebral ischemia, respectively, and the latter caused by a rupture of weakened vascular walls within or around brain tissue. In the past 40 years, the use of medical imaging to distinguish stroke subtypes has become a mainstay at almost all medical institutions, revolutionizing acute diagnosis and treatment, as well as improving prediction of long-term patient outcome. For both clinical and experimental stroke, details of the anatomical structure and function of the brain are currently possible with multimodal imaging. Computed tomography (CT), magnetic resonance imaging (MRI), and positron emission tomography (PET) have helped guide acute stroke triage and advanced our knowledge of pathophysiologic mechanisms guiding stroke treatment strategies. However, PET imaging in acute stroke remains limited to research studies in academic centers due to its cost and logistical/technical complexities. PET tracers and scanners will continue to evolve, but it is unlikely that PET will see widespread clinical use for acute stroke patients in the near future. MRI is more readily available in the setting of acute stroke and does not require a radioactive substance to be injected. Further, most sequences, unlike CT, are able to cover both supra- and infratentorial brain regions, allowing a more robust diagnostic imaging window and increased prognostic sensitivity. In terms of patient throughput, individuals who are claustrophobic or have metal implants and pacemakers are excluded from MRI. Further, MRI scanners have limited availability, primarily accessible at large city hospitals or academic centers. CT imaging is a diagnostic tool that is widely available, relatively inexpensive compared to its acute stroke counterpart, MRI, noninvasive, and fast. The acute CT imaging stroke series generally consists of a noncontrast CT (NCCT), followed by multiphase CT angiography (mCTA), for patients with stroke symptoms; however, critical information about the underlying pathophysiology may be overlooked. In a few added minutes, further assessment of cerebral hemodynamics with CT perfusion (CTP) can give insight into early ischemic changes (EICs), tissue states, and blood–brain barrier (BBB) disturbances, unseen on NCCT/CTA. Moreover, due to optimized scanning protocols, the added radiation dose is minimized.

Herein, we discuss CTP data acquisition, mathematical models, limitations and diagnostic caveats, and the potential of CTP to improve acute stroke management related to cerebral ischemia.

CT Perfusion Acquisition

CTP imaging depends on the speed of multidetector row (from 16 to 320 rows) scanners to follow the entry and exit of radiographic dye through an imaging volume or "slab of tissue." For each CTP study, 35 to 45 mL of a nonionic iodinated contrast agent, at a concentration of 300 to 370 mg iodine/mL, is power injected into an arm vein (typically the cephalic vein); injection rates can vary from 4 to 6 mL/s, followed by a saline flush of 20 to 40 mL at identical rates. The faster the injection rate, the "tighter" the contrast bolus, which results in a sharper, narrower, and higher peak in the time–attenuation curve (TAC). However, these fast injection features require an image acquisition of one image approximately every 2.5 seconds to characterize the peak of the arterial curve accurately, which is essential for the accurate calculation of CTP hemodynamic parameters. Imaging is performed at a constant milliampere-second (100 to 200 mAs) and a kilovoltage (kV) of 80; this kV setting generates photons with mean energy close to the k-edge of iodine, maximizing the photoelectric effect, and subsequent contrast visibility. Axial shuttle (step and shoot) mode is used to cover 8-cm section of the brain including the intracranial ICA at 5-mm slice thickness. Data acquisition generally starts 4 to 6 seconds after injection and before the contrast reaches the tissue of interest to measure the baseline of the TAC, which is subtracted off the entire curve as the first postprocessing step. For perfusion studies without the need to investigate BBB integrity, an acquisition time interval of 70 to 90 seconds is recommended.[1] If measurement of BBB permeability is also required along with perfusion measurements, a two-phase acquisition is more appropriate, in which the first phase lasting 45 to 50 seconds at a rapid imaging rate of one image every 1 to 3 seconds is followed by a slower second phase of one image every 10 to 15 seconds for another 2 minutes.[2]

CTP Raw Data Processing

Depending on the clinical symptoms, the imaged volume is selected at the level of the basal ganglia, which includes posterior, anterior, and middle cerebral arteries. CTP describes hemodynamics within the entire vasculature including large arteries, arterioles, capillary beds, venules, and veins. As an intravascular contrast bolus passes through a mass of brain tissue, the signal intensity of each voxel within a CT image will change over time. The intensity of the CT image, expressed in Hounsfield units (HU), is linearly proportional to the efficiency with which ionization radiation, in the form of x-rays, is attenuated. With current CTP software, processing of these hemodynamic functional maps is practically automated. The operator needs only to select an arterial input function (AIF) and a venous output function (VOF). The AIF is selected from within a large artery (usually the basilar or internal carotid artery), preferably at a location along the artery where it is orthogonal to the scan plane to limit partial volume averaging (PVA)—this "dilution" effect will become apparent when comparing the peak enhancement (increase of attenuation above baseline) of arteries of different sizes. The VOF is selected from a large vein, usually the superior sagittal sinus, to minimize the effect of PVA on its accurate measurement. As such, the underestimation of the AIF from PVA can be corrected by normalizing the area of the AIF with that of the VOF.[3]

Perfusion Parameters

For each pixel, its TAC is used to quantify several perfusion parameters: cerebral blood flow (CBF), the volume rate of blood moving though the mass of tissue (mL/min/100 g); cerebral blood volume (CBV), the total volume of moving blood in the mass of tissue (mL/100 g); the time to peak (TTP) of the pixel TAC corrected for the dispersion in the artery TAC (T_0) or the time to maximum of the tissue residue function; and a new parameter, which is discussed in detail in later sections, the permeability surface area product (PS) of the BBB (mL/min/100 g) (Fig. 13.1). Calculation of these parameters is described below. Another perfusion parameter useful for acute ischemic evaluation is the TTP (T_{max}) of the impulse residue function (IRF). This is different from the TTP of the tissue TAC. The latter is confounded by the TTP of the AIF and therefore reflects not only the local hemodynamics of the tissue but also that of the central (systemic) circulation. The T_{max} of the IRF is the summation of the delay between the arrival times of contrast at the artery and tissue region as well as mean transit time (MTT) of the local vasculature. The delay reflects the adequacy of collateral circulation to the region, while MTT is inversely related to the perfusion pressure in the local vasculature.[4] Unlike the calculation of absolute CBF or CBV, the calculation of T_{max} is independent of the calibration between the AIF and tissue TAC; as such, it is increasingly being used in perfusion-weighted DCE-MR for the determination of the tissue at risk in stroke.[5,6] However, calculation of T_{max} requires deconvolution of the tissue TAC, which is more complex than determining the TTP of the tissue TAC. It has been shown recently by comparison with PET that T_{max} maps did not perform better than the more easy-to-obtain nondeconvolved TTP maps in identifying ischemic penumbra.[7] Moreover, the T_{max} definition can be different between vendors due to IRF assumptions and modeling, especially between MRP and CTP modalities.[8]

CTP Mathematical Models

Deconvolution- and non–deconvolution-based models are used to calculate perfusion parameters. Although physiologically more appropriate, deconvolution models involve complex algorithms and require more time for the calculation, whereas the simplicity of nondeconvolution models stems from their simplified assumptions about hemodynamics in the brain that may not hold true in general.

Deconvolution Approach

Deconvolution methods correct for the inability to deliver a contrast bolus directly into the supplying artery of a tissue of interest—the bolus introduced at a peripheral vein undergoes "delay" and "dispersion" prior to its arrival at the artery to become the AIF or the TAC of the artery. Deconvolution corrects for this by calculating an IRF, which depends on the concept of convolution, and simulates the tissue TAC, which would be obtained under the ideal injection condition. For brain imaging, the governing convolution equation for the tissue TAC is as follows:

$$Q(t) = C_a(t) \otimes [CBF \cdot R(t)] \quad (1)$$

where $\otimes$ is the convolution operator; $C_a(t)$ and $Q(t)$ are the artery and the tissue TAC, respectively; and CBF·$R(t)$ is the CBF-scaled IRF.[9] The height and area of the flow-scaled IRF are CBF and CBV, respectively, and MTT is the ratio of CBV to CBF as required

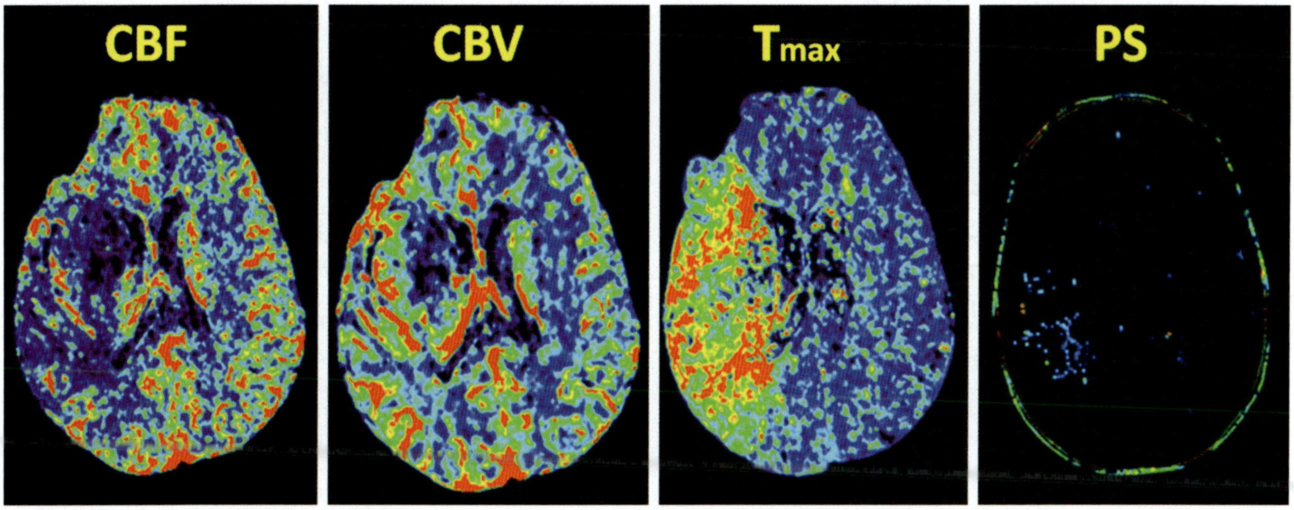

Figure 13-1. Sample cerebral blood flow (CBF), cerebral blood volume (CBV), time-to-peak of tissue-residue-function (T_{max}), and PS CTP functional maps for the patient with ischemic stroke. Color-coded functional maps of CBF, CBV, T_{max}, and permeability surface area product (PS) calculated using CT perfusion software (GE Healthcare). CBF is expressed in units of mL/100 g/min, CBV in mL/100 g, T_{max} in seconds, and PS in mL/100 g/min.

by the central volume principle.[10] In a CTP study, the arterial and tissue TAC, $C_a(t)$ and $Q(t)$, are measured, the problem concerns the deconvolution of $Q(t)$ to calculate CBF·$R(t)$. Convolution of the AIF with flow-scaled IRF gives a unique (unambiguous) tissue TAC because it is the summation of different versions of the known CBF·IRF with each version being the original CBF·IRF shifted in time and scaled with the AIF.[8] On the other hand, deconvolution estimates the unknown CBF $R(t)$, such that its convolution with the arterial TAC would approximate (fit) the tissue TAC as closely as possible. Therefore, deconvolution solutions are ambiguous, as there are many CBF·$R(t)$s, which after convolution with $C_a(t)$ are able to give equally good fits to the tissue TAC. Furthermore, many of these CBF $R(t)$s can have shapes that are not consistent with the physiologic behavior of an IRF, for instance, oscillating between positive and negative values, due to noise in either the arterial or tissue TAC.[11] These effects can be mitigated with noise suppression in the deconvolution algorithm to obtain a physiologically more plausible IRF as shown in Figure 13.2, from which more accurate perfusion parameters can be estimated as discussed above.[12]

Another hemodynamic parameter, new to stroke imaging, is the permeability surface area product (PS). PS is the product of permeability and the total surface area of perfused capillary endothelium within an unit mass of tissue and is the total diffusional flux across all perfused capillaries.[13] Currently available CTP software uses either compartmental or the Johnson-Wilson (J-W) model to describe the distribution of contrast in brain tissue.[13–15] Compartmental models can only measure PS and CBV, not CBF, because contrast distribution in the brain is determined only by diffusion when PS is much smaller than CBF.[13] The Patlak approach simplifies the compartmental model further by assuming the absence of contrast agent backflux from the interstitial to the intravascular space (IVS).[16] Under the Patlak assumption, the normalized tissue concentration is linearly related to the normalized time, with the slope and intercept of the linear regression line being equal to PS and CBV, respectively.[16] However, the assumption of no backflux of contrast from the interstitial to IVS in the Patlak model is physiologically not possible for a leaky BBB.[2] In theory, use of the Patlak model can lead to an underestimation of PS.[2] The J-W model does not invoke the Patlak assumption of no tracer backflux, and unlike compartmental models, it allows CBF to be estimated together with CBV and PS.[13] The J-W model divides the brain into two principal spaces: the IVS and the extravascular space (EVS), separated by a capillary endothelium of variable PS, therefore applicable to both permeable and impermeable BBBs. Assumptions for the J-W model include bidirectional diffusion of contrast agent between the EVS and IVS and an axial contrast concentration gradient in the capillaries, and contrast concentration is assumed to have a homogeneous spatial distribution within EVS.[17,18] The adiabatic approximation to the J-W model assumes that the contrast concentration in the EVS is changing slowly relative to the rate of change of concentration in the IVS.[18] Under this approximation, the IRF $R(t)$ can be represented simply as

$$R(t)=\begin{cases}1.0 & 0\le t<T_c\\ E\cdot e^{-\left(\frac{F\cdot E}{V_c}\right)\cdot(t-T_c)} & t>T_c\end{cases}\qquad(2)$$

where T_c is the MTT of blood through the brain and F is CBF, so that CBV is $F\cdot T_c$ according to the central volume principle.[3] E is the contrast extraction fraction, and V_c is the contrast agent distribution volume in the EVS. E relates to the PS of the BBB by the following relationship:

$$E=1-e^{-\frac{PS}{F}}\qquad(3)$$

If $C_a(t)$ is the AIF to the brain, then the measured brain tissue curve $Q(t)$ can be calculated as the convolution of $C_a(t)$ and $R(t)$:

$$Q(t)=C_a(t)\otimes\left[F\cdot R(t-T_0)\right]\qquad(4)$$

where $\otimes$ is the convolution operator, and T_0 is the appearance time of contrast agent in the brain relative to that in the input artery. Equation (4) is valid under the assumption that brain blood flow is constant and $Q(t)$ is linear with respect to $C_a(t)$. With $Q(t)$ and $C_a(t)$ having been measured in a CTP study, CT Perfusion 4D (GE Healthcare, Waukesha, WI) estimates the parameters CBF, CBV, T_c, PS, and T_0 of each voxel by iteratively changing their values until an optimum fit to $Q(t)$ is achieved by means of Eqs. (2)–(4).

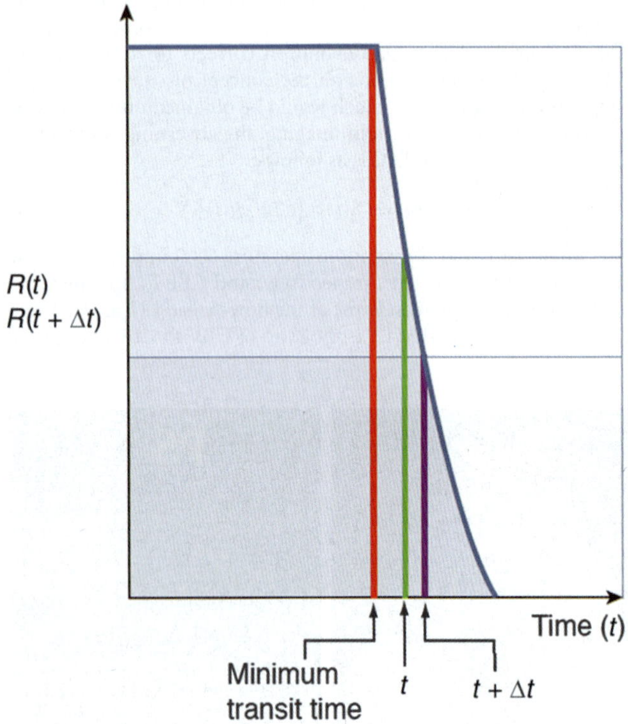

Figure 13-2. The IRF can be viewed as the fraction of contrast medium that remains in the tissue as time evolves following a bolus injection into the arterial input. Beyond the minimum transit time (the duration of the plateau), the difference of $R(t + \Delta t)$ and $R(t)$ is the fraction of contrast medium that has a transit time of t. This difference is the height of the strip with a transit time of t. Further, the area of each of the horizontal strips is the product of the transit time and the fraction of contrast medium having that transit time. It follows that the area of all the horizontal strips, that is, the area under the curve (AUC) of $R(t)$, is the MTT. Alternatively, as the Central Volume Principle states that the product of CBF and MTT is CBV, the AUC of CBF·$R(t)$ is the CBV.

Nondeconvolution Approach

Similar to the deconvolution models, nondeconvolution (model independent) approaches are based on the Fick principle of conservation of mass.[19] The maximal slope method calculates CBF as the ratio of the maximum initial slope of the tissue TAC to the peak height of the arterial TAC.[3,19] Although conceptually simple, the assumption of having no venous outflow at the time of maximum initial slope is rarely true; therefore, a global CBF underestimation is possible with this method. However, when compared to deconvolution methods, the maximum slope model provides similar functional map quality and quantitative values for acute infarct delineation, guiding thrombolysis treatment.[20]

Acquisition and Processing Caveats and Concerns

Spatial Coverage and Patient Motion

The volume of brain tissue that can be imaged in one CTP acquisition is limited in the craniocaudal direction (*z*-axis for all scanners) by the number of detector rows in a CT scanner to between 4 and 16 cm with current models of scanners. Coverage in this direction can be doubled (to include two adjacent sections of the brain) using shuttle mode or two separate boluses.[21,22] The shuttle technique can have two variations, step and shoot (axial shuttle) or continuous table translation (helical shuttle) between the two sections. Axial shuttle mode generally has less motion artifact than helical shuttle mode as images are acquired with the patient table (brain) stationary during the former. Also, the image interval of all slices in axial shuttle mode is uniform (2 to 3 seconds), while the helical shuttle mode is nonuniform for the cranial and caudal slices—the image intervals for slices in the centre of the two-section volume will be roughly uniform at 2 to 3 seconds, and those for the more cranial and caudal slices of that volume can vary from 1–2 to 4–5 seconds. The two injections technique requires double the dosage of iodinated contrast increasing the risk of affecting kidney function. However, a recent multicenter study has shown that the incidence of contrast-induced nephrotoxicity was low approximately 2.6% among at-risk patients undergoing contrast-enhanced CT scans in a "real-world" clinical setting, where guideline-recommended strategies for contrast induced nephrotoxicity prevention may not be consistently followed.[23]

Patient-related motion is a major source of image artifact in an acute stroke CTP study. During acquisition, the patient's head is normally held with a plastic head holder mounted to the scanner table to minimize the head movement. The holder can reduce but not completely eliminate head movement in some cases. Figure 13.3 shows how the arterial and tissue TACs can be affected by movement in the *x*–*y* plane, despite the use of such a head holder. Temporal registration and/or removal of images can correct for *x*–*y* plane patient motion. With *z*-axis motion, removal of images is more difficult than *x*–*y* motion as slice locations change during the cine acquisition.

Ionizing Radiation

Although a 60- to 70-second imaging protocol is sufficient for a perfusion-only study, acquisitions of 90- to 180-second durations have been advocated for combined perfusion and BBB permeability studies.[2,24–26] To minimize radiation exposure from the lengthened scan time required for blood–brain permeability measurement, temporal sampling is decreased to one image every 10 to 15 seconds after the first phase as has been discussed above in section (1).[25] The total effective dose from a multimodal CT stroke study, for a 64-row detector CT, is approximately 7 mSv—this is double the average annual background radiation.[27] Radiation dose reduction strategies, such as the adaptive statistical iterative reconstruction, can maintain image quality while reducing effective dose by greater than 25%.[28] Also, radiation dose could be reduced by two-thirds, without compromising the accuracy of the CTP functional maps, by increasing the sampling interval from 1 to 3 seconds in the first phase of a CTP study.[21]

Delay and Dispersion of the AIF

As described in section (1), an AIF measured from a large artery is required in the deconvolution of the tissue TAC to calculate tissue perfusion. Because of time causality, deconvolution formulated as the inversion of a system of linear equations using singular value decomposition (SVD) works properly only if the tissue TAC lags behind the AIF in time, that is, the contrast arrival time of the tissue TAC is later than that of the AIF (positive delay). If there is negative delay between the AIF and tissue TAC, standard deconvolution formulation with SVD will overestimate CBF and underestimate MTT.[29] The problem with perfusion studies of stroke patients is that both positive and negative delays between the chosen AIF and tissue TAC could occur in the same study. If the AIF is measured from an artery downstream from an occlusion, TAC of normal brain will lead the ipsilateral AIF in time (negative delay) while the TAC of ischemic brain may have the same or delayed contrast arrival time as that of the ipsilateral AIF (positive delay). In this situation, it is important to formulate the deconvolution as inversion of a block-circulant matrix with the SVD technique. It has been shown using simulations that block-circulant deconvolution with SVD produces CBF estimates that are independent of whether the delays between the AIF and tissue TACs are positive or negative.[30]

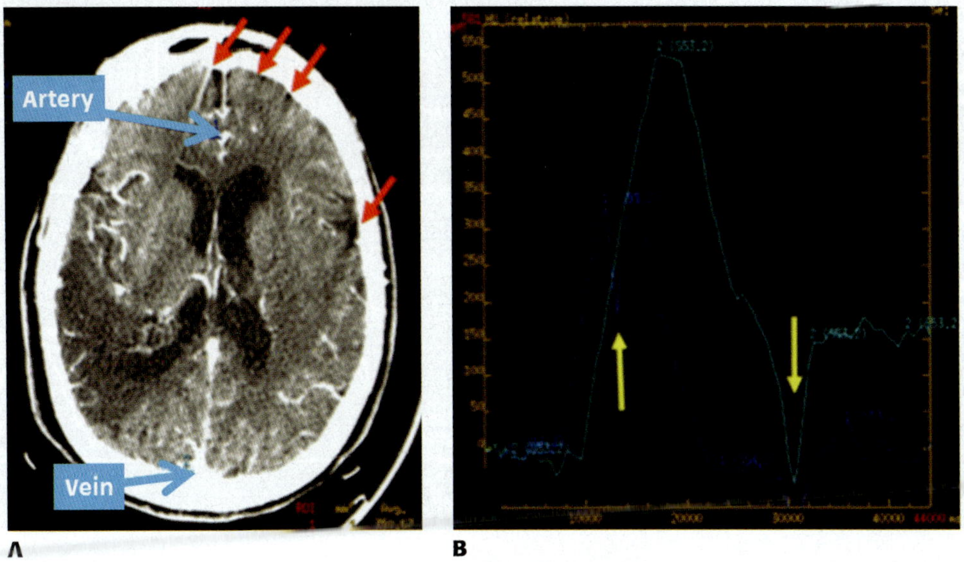

Figure 13-3. A: Movement of the patient's head during acquisition caused significant artifacts (*red arrows*) in the DCE CT images. **B:** The arterial and venous TACs were significantly affected and exhibited large fluctuations (*yellow arrows*).

Besides using block-circulant deconvolution with SVD to minimize the effects of the negative delays between the ipsilateral AIF and tissue TACs, choosing an AIF from an artery in the contralateral (unaffected) hemisphere could avoid the presence of negative delays. However, the blood supply to an ischemic region is mainly via collateral circulation such that besides delay in arrival times, the AIFs measured in ipsilateral arteries are also dispersed with respect to the AIFs measured in contralateral arteries. The use of a nondispersed contralateral AIF rather than the true dispersed ipsilateral AIF to deconvolve the tissue TAC will underestimate the true blood flow.[31] It has been proposed that dispersed ipsilateral AIF can be measured by independent component analysis (ICA) of the ischemic region.[31] ICA is a data-driven technique, which is based on analyzing the time behavior of all TACs in a region and trying to decompose the TACs into linear combinations of a few dominant temporal patterns (independent components). In a perfusion study, a few of the independent components that are similar in their temporal behavior to that expected of AIF in locations that are mostly in arteries are summed together to produce the local AIF. The disadvantages of using ICA to define the local AIF are as follows: first, the choice of which independent components to retain to represent the AIF is arbitrary; second, the spatial mask used to select locations (presumably arteries) from which the chosen independent components are summed to generate the local AIF is also arbitrary. As such, the ICA algorithm for the generation of local AIF has to be validated; so far, no validation studies have been reported.

Given the above considerations on the effects of delay and dispersion of the AIF on the estimation of perfusion parameters, it is recommended that the AIF can be chosen from the contralateral (normal) hemisphere as several studies have demonstrated that ipsilateral or contralateral placement of the AIF does not affect calculation of CBF and block-circulant or other delay-insensitive deconvolution algorithms should be used.[32,33]

CTP Data Truncation

For CTP perfusion studies with an acquisition interval limited to 45 to 50 seconds, the TAC of an ischemic region can be truncated, that is, data acquisition terminates before the TAC reaches the washout phase. As CBV is related to the area of the TAC, truncation leads to underestimation of the area and hence CBV of the ischemic region.[22] In previous work, the ability of the acute CTP-derived CBV lesion (i.e., CBV close to zero) to predict nonviable ischemic tissue has been demonstrated.[34–36] Most recently, CBV evolution was examined in 13 patients within gray and white matter destined to infarct, as defined by NCCT at 7 days postadmission, as well as overestimation of the infarct core, as defined by the CBV abnormality at admission.[37] CBV reversibility out to 7 days postadmission was observed in four patients; however, this reversal was more common in patients with an incomplete washout (truncation) of the tissue TAC at admission and/or 24 hours poststroke ictus (Fig. 13.4). It is important to note that complete wash-in and washout of the AIF and VOF does not mean the ischemic tissue TAC is free of truncation. The area and the ratio of area to

A

B

C

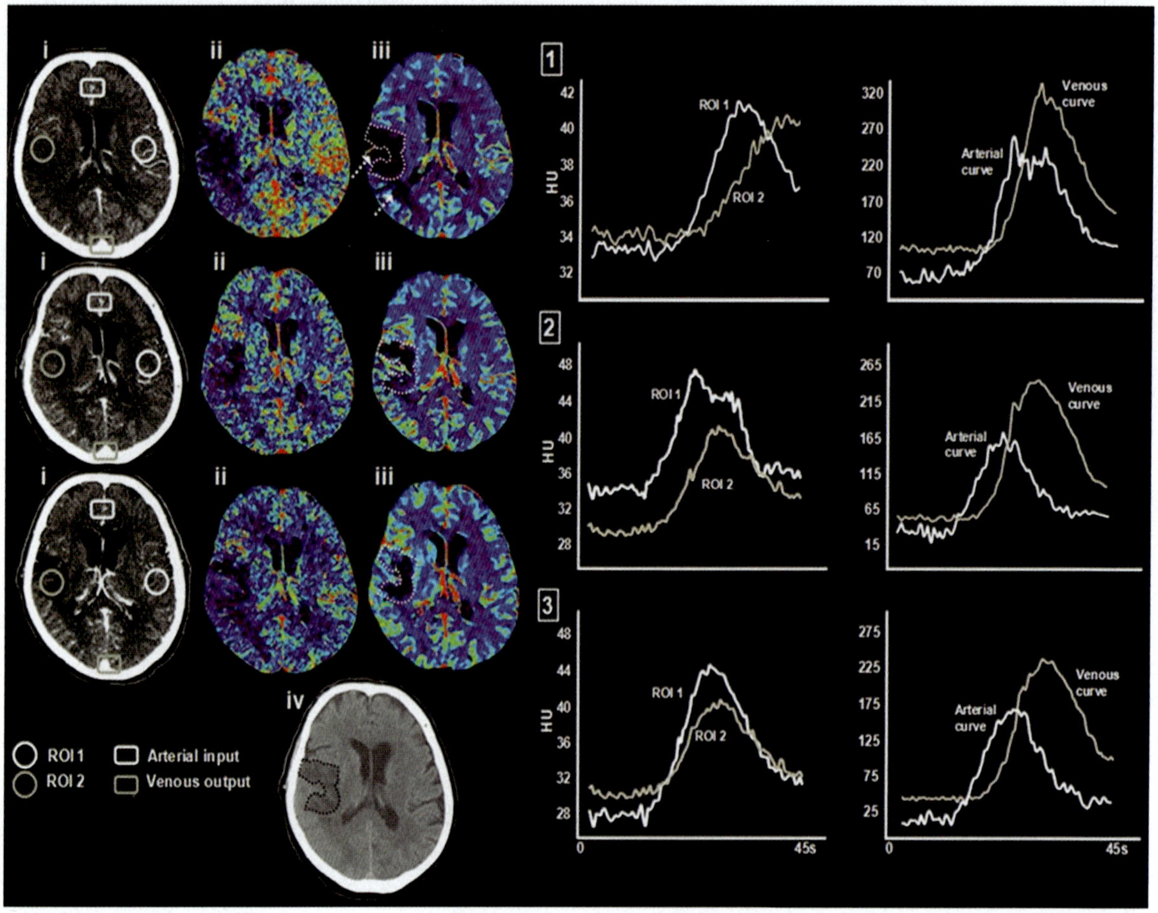

Figure 13-4. CTP-derived contrast-enhanced image, CBF (scale 0 to 150 mL/min/100 g) and CBV (scale 0 to 8 mL/100 g) functional maps (*i–iii*) at admission, 24 hours, and 7 days poststroke onset (A to C). NCCT from 7 days poststroke shows outlined infarct region (*iv*). Corresponding time–density curves (Hounsfield units versus time) were taken at each time point. Confluent areas outside of superimposed infarct ROI showing CBV lesion overestimation (*dashed arrows*); at this time, TDC_i truncation is apparent. CBV_i reversibility is observed at 24 hours and 7 days, compared to admission, for this patient.

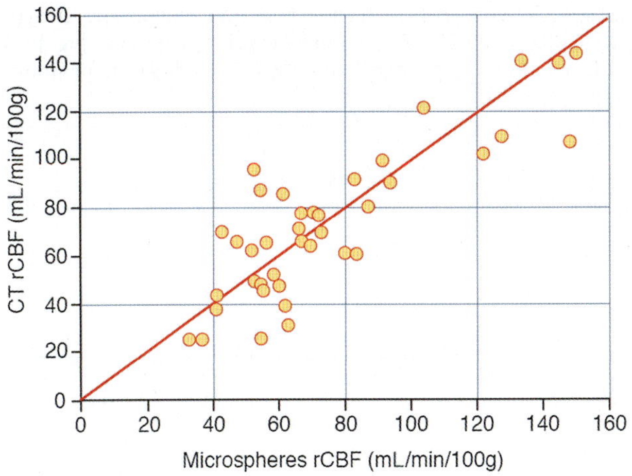

Figure 13-5. Dynamic CT measurement plotted against microsphere measurement of rCBF (mL/min/100 g). $r = 0.837$, $p < 0.001$, slope of the regression line was close to unity (0.97 ± 0.03).

height of the flow-scaled IRF represent CBV and MTT, respectively. Therefore, the truncation artifact will underestimate both parameters. On the contrary, CBF is related to the front slope of the tissue TAC (or equivalently the height of the flow-scaled IRF) and therefore is minimally affected by the truncation artifact. Campbell et al.[38] and Kamalian et al.[39] both demonstrated the ability of absolute and relative (to contralateral hemisphere) CBF values to better approximate diffusion-weighted imaging (DWI) infarct core, compared to CBV and MTT parameters. In the study by Campbell et al., the CTP data were acquired out to 45 seconds, as such, truncation may have affected the calculation of both CBV and MTT, while the study by Kamalian et al. used an appropriate two-phase acquisition (0.5-second sampling for 40 seconds, a 2-second pause, and eight more images every 3 seconds).

Preclinical Validation

Fluorescent microspheres have been used for the past 30 years for validating regional CBF (rCBF) measurement methods.[40] Cenic et al.[12] validated CTP-derived rCBF measurements, using this ex vivo microsphere technique. Specifically, closely spaced (<1 minute apart) measurements of the deconvolution-based dynamic CTP-rCBF and microsphere-based rCBF were determined in a healthy rabbit model.[12] A strong correlation was found between the dynamic CTP-rCBF and the fluorescent microsphere rCBF measurements (Fig. 13.5). The mean rCBF obtained from dynamic CTP and microsphere techniques for $n = 39$ measurements was 73.3 ± 31.5 mL/min/100 g and 74.3 ± 31.6 mL/min/100 g, respectively. This correlation compares well with the findings from others who have validated their dynamic CT and stable xenon–CT techniques with microsphere measurements.[41,42] CBV has yet to be validated in the brain.

CTP Applications in Ischemic Stroke

The Use of CT Perfusion to Define Acute Tissue States in Acute Ischemic Stroke

The understanding of the ischemic cascade brought forth distinct definitions of tissue status during hyperacute cerebral ischemia. Within the most hypoperfused territory, called the ischemic or infarct core, neurons are irreversibly damaged, even upon reperfusion, and are no longer viable.[43] Across species, the threshold for irreversible neuronal death has been identified as a CBF value of approximately 8 to 10 mL/min/100 g.[44–48] The infarct core, consisting of apoptotic/necrotic tissue, is surrounded by a variably sized tissue region with blood flow above the threshold to induce immediate infarction—the ischemic penumbra. The original definition of this tissue state is based on the absence of electroencephalography signals and sensory evoked potentials with maintenance of membrane pump function and ionic gradients retained at near-normal levels.[49,50] Due to this electrical silence, clinical symptoms relating to the affected tissue region are apparent; therefore, it is impossible to discern the amount of viable penumbral tissue based on clinical symptoms alone. The survival of penumbral tissue on the border zone of infarction is largely dependent on leptomeningeal collateral supply, as well the severity of periinfarct depolarization.[51] If blood flow is not restored promptly, the viable ischemic penumbra invariably progresses to infarction; however, with reperfusion in a timely manner, this tissue will fully recover, along with clinical function. This time-critical viability of the ischemic penumbra introduced the "time is brain" paradigm.[52] Depending on the technique for measuring CBF, the upper threshold for electrical silence and neuronal dysfunction occurs at a CBF of 22 to 25 mL/min/100 g.[47] The duration of ischemia will determine tissue fate below this threshold.[53] A third tissue state is described as having a CBF above the upper threshold for neuronal dysfunction, but lower than normal CBF values, called benign oligemia. Regardless of the duration of ischemia, this tissue does not progress to infarction and maintains normal cellular function, in spite of appreciated hypoperfusion and absence of reperfusion.[54]

Perfusion Parameters Selection and Shortcomings in Ischemic Stroke

In practical terms, perfusion imaging merely represents a snapshot of the tissue status. Therefore, distinguishing penumbra from infarct core and benign oligemia by using perfusion parameters and thresholds poses several limitations. First, these perfusion threshold levels are time dependent. We do not know the factors that determine the rate of transformation of tissue with a CBF of less than 10 mL/min/100 g, which may survive for 30 minutes but probably not for 3 hours. Perfusion threshold levels that separate core from penumbra could therefore depend on when tissue was imaged after ischemia onset. Second, perfusion measurements do not reflect metabolic activity of brain tissue. Dead, dying, or doomed tissue may have normal flow. Perfusion thresholds for infarction may be different in various regions of the brain. The dynamic nature of the penumbra is reflected in variable infarct growth rates over time. The transformation of penumbra into core is dependent on many complex and interrelated factors, including leptomeningeal collateral supply, mean arterial blood pressure, glycemic level, ischemic tissue susceptibility to necrosis, and periinfarct depolarization. These same factors lead to variable growth of penumbra into regions of oligemia and result in clinical worsening. In addition, in vitro studies hint at the possibility of selective neuronal death in the penumbra and protein dysfunction in the region with benign oligemia.[29] The use of blood flow threshold levels to define irreversibility and salvageability of brain tissue and to predict infarct growth rates is affected conceptually by these physiologic issues. Recent reports suggest that a CBF threshold is optimal to separate infarct from penumbra, prior to reperfusion efforts.[38,39,55] It has been shown in animal stroke studies that the threshold for pannecrosis is between 0.17 and 0.24 mL/min/g with persistent occlusion.[53] This threshold decreases to 0.12 mL/min/g when ischemia is limited to a few hours.[47] However, the threshold of infarction (pannecrosis) for ischemia lasting less than an hour, which is becoming more relevant in the era of rapid revascularization, is unknown. A recent study by d'Esterre et al. (submitted to AJNR 2013) determined individual gray and white matter threshold values to differentiate infarct core from penumbra. The goal of the study was to determine which CTP hemodynamic parameter (delay-insensitive deconvolution software, CT Perfusion 4D, GE Healthcare) best differentiated between regions of ischemic tissue that recovered upon recanalization (penumbra and oligemia) and regions of ischemic tissue that infarcted, as confirmed on 5- to

7-day NCCT. Logistic regression was applied to patients who recanalized by 24 hours postonset. In gray matter, the regression model using the CBF parameter resulted in the highest sensitivity (95.2%, 20/21) and specificity (95.2%, 20/21) for infarction, with an overall accuracy of 95.2% (40/42) of tissue states classified correctly (Fig. 13.6), while in white matter, the regression model using the CBF·CBV product resulted in the highest sensitivity (93.8%, 15/16) and specificity (87.5%, 14/16) for infarction, with an overall accuracy of 90.6% (29/32) of tissue states classified correctly (Fig. 13.7). A threshold of T_{max} greater than 6 seconds to delineate penumbra

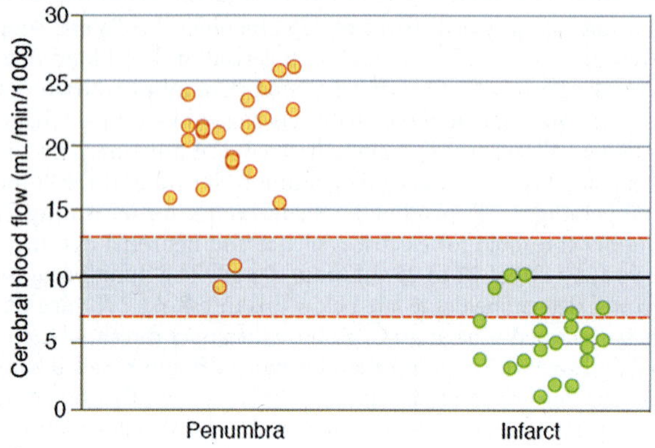

A

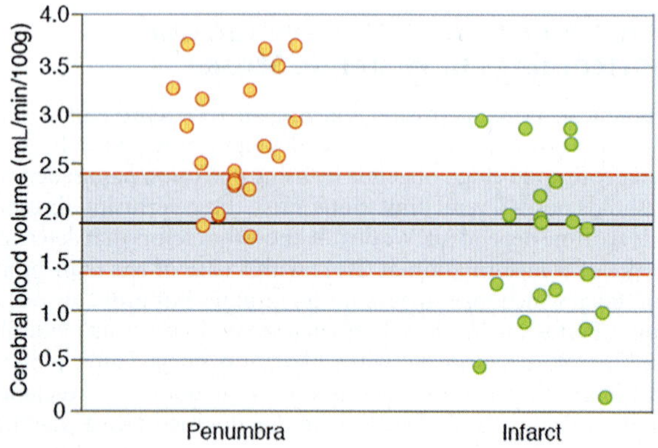

B

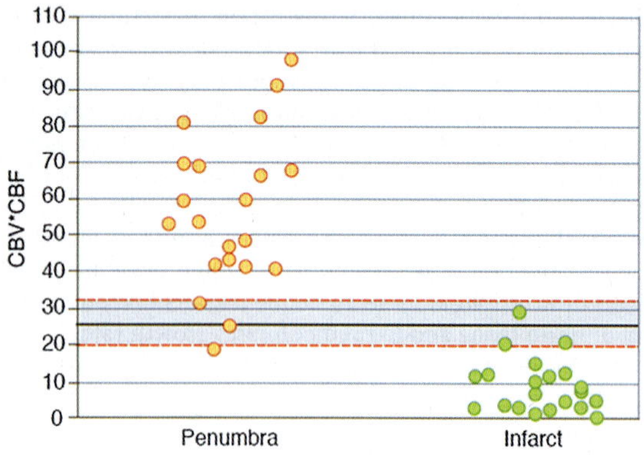

C

Figure 13-6. Thresholds for infarction for *gray matter* cerebral blood flow (CBF), cerebral blood volume (CBV), and CBF–CBV. Gray matter values for all infarct (n = 21) and penumbra (n = 21) regions of interest with the *solid line* representing the optimal threshold to separate infarct from penumbra, the *upper and lower dashed lines* represent the 5% and 95% probability for infarction, derived from univariate logistic regression with **(A)** CBF, **(B)** CBV, and **(C)** CBF–CBV product as predictor. CBF provided the best classification of penumbra and infarct regions with a sensitivity of 95.2% (20/21 regions) and specificity of 95.2% (20/21 regions), and overall accuracy of 95.2% (40/42 regions).

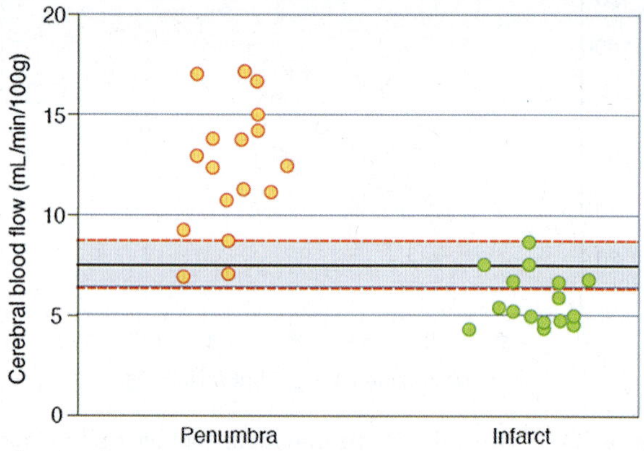

A

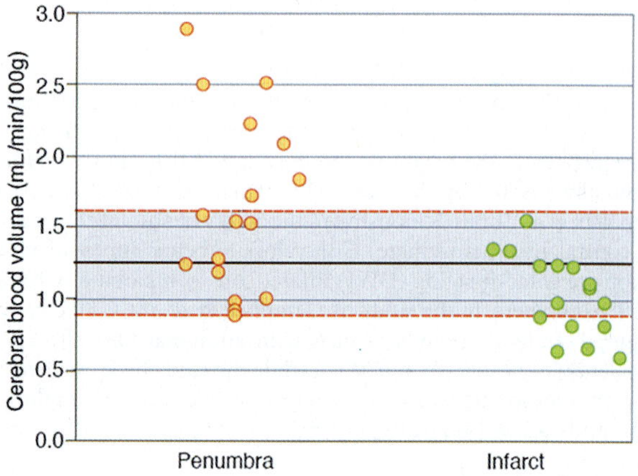

B

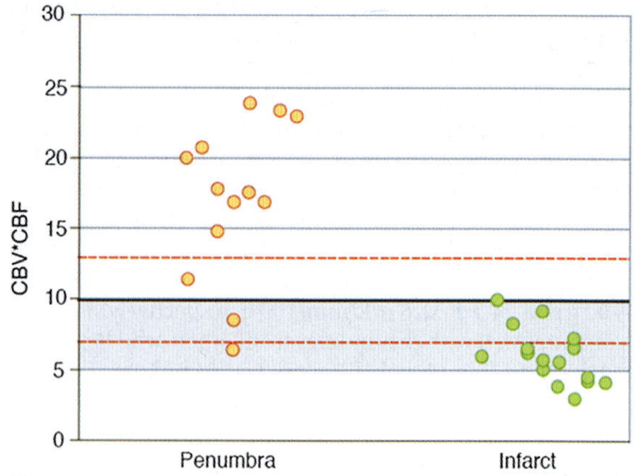

C

Figure 13-7. Thresholds for infarction for *white matter* cerebral blood flow (CBF), cerebral blood volume (CBV), and CBF–CBV. White matter values for all infarct (n = 16) and penumbra (n = 16) regions of interest with the *solid line* representing the optimal threshold to separate infarct from penumbra, the *upper and lower dashed lines* represent the 5% and 95% probability for infarction, derived from univariate logistic regression with **(A)** CBF, **(B)** CBV, and **(C)** CBF–CBV product as predictor. The CBF–CBV parameter provided the best classification of penumbra and infarct regions with a sensitivity of 93.7% (15/16 regions), specificity of 87.5% (14/16 regions), and overall accuracy of 90.6% (29/32 regions).

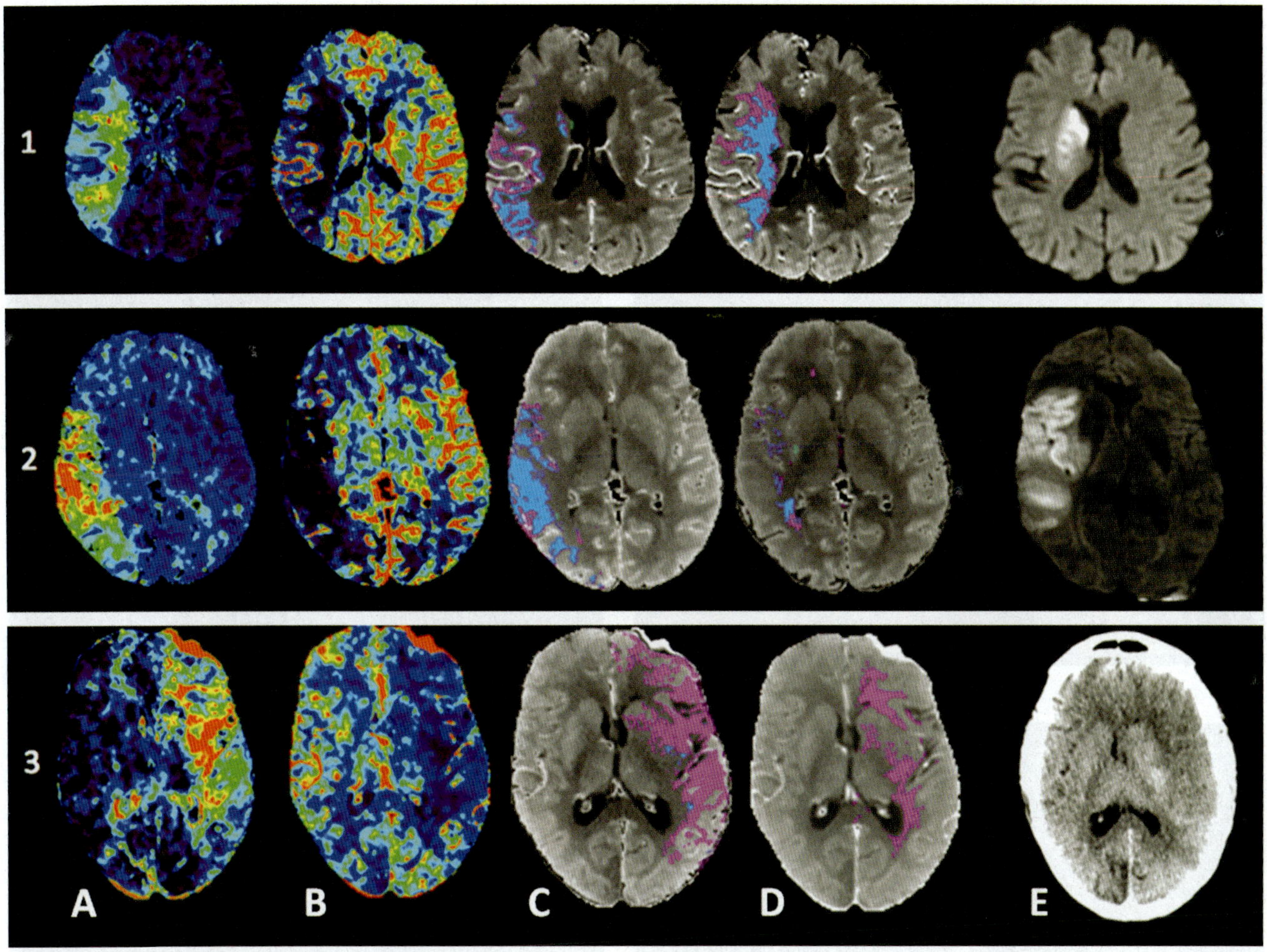

Figure 13-8. **CTP imaging taken between 2 and 3 hours of symptom onset for three patients (1 to 3) with proximal occlusions of the anterior circulation.** CTP T_{max} and CBF maps are depicted in **(A)** and **(B)**. Tissue with a T_{max} greater than 6-second (penumbra) is superimposed onto the CTP-average maps in pink for both gray and white matter (**C** and **D**, respectively). CBF less than 10 mL/min/100 g and less than 7 mL/·min/100 g, for gray and white, respectively (infarction), are flooded in blue on the CTP-average maps (**C** and **D**, respectively). **E:** depicts the follow-up MR diffusion/NCCT imaging taken at approximately 24 hours. For patient 1 (M1, TICI 3, recanalization 90 minutes from CT), the infarct core overestimates the final infarct volume. For patient 2 (M1, TICI 2b, recanalization 139 minutes from CT), the infarct core slightly underestimates the final infarct volume. For patient 3 (M2, TICI 2b, recanalization 192 minutes from CT), T_{max} penumbra prediction matches the final infarct volume.

from benign oligemia has been established using MR perfusion and CTP modalities.[55–57] However, a major methodologic downfall of this and many other CTP threshold derivation studies is that the thresholds are commonly derived from suboptimal imaging data sets where recanalization is not known until 24 hours post-CTP, and degree of reperfusion is unknown.[58,59] Therefore, infarct core delineation based on current CTP thresholds for acute tissue status may not be valid (Fig. 13.8).

The assortment of perfusion (CTP and MRP) postprocessing algorithms, and consequent lack of standardized perfusion thresholds, has limited the use of absolute perfusion values in the emergency clinical setting—standardization issues will be discussed in a later section. However, *qualitative* assessment of CTP functional maps may offer additional information to CTA/NCCT alone. A drastic reduction in CBV is thought to discriminate between viable and nonviable tissue states at the time of CTP imaging.[36,47] The rationale is that a drop in cerebral perfusion pressure in severely hypoperfused tissue leads to cerebrovascular autoregulatory failure followed by a supposedly permanent, focal decrease in CBV.[60] Conversely, an acute increase in CBV was proposed to have a protective effect on perfusion-compromised, yet viable tissue; the so-called "penumbral hypothesis."[59,61] However, in 30 acute ischemic stroke (AIS) patients, Butcher et al.[62] showed that rCBV (relative to contralateral side) increased within areas of focal swelling (isodense areas on acute NCCT) due to compensatory vasodilation and speculated shunting of the cerebral microvasculature. Furthermore, all acute NCCT-hypoattenuated regions were always associated with a decrease in rCBV.[62] In a porcine model of endothelin-1–induced ischemia, our research has been shown that a CBF/CBV mismatch (decreased CBF, increased CBV) was present within brain regions having a DWI hyperintensity for 60% of subjects. Within the true infarct core (defined using the gold standard histology), a complete CBF/CBV mismatch (hypervolemia without a CBV defect), partial mismatch (hypervolemia with a CBV defect), and absent mismatch (no hypervolemia) were observed in 3/10 (30%), 3/10 (30%), and 4/10 (40%) of animals, respectively. Figure 13.9 depicts contemporaneous CTP and MR diffusion imaging, and histology defined infarction for four subjects.

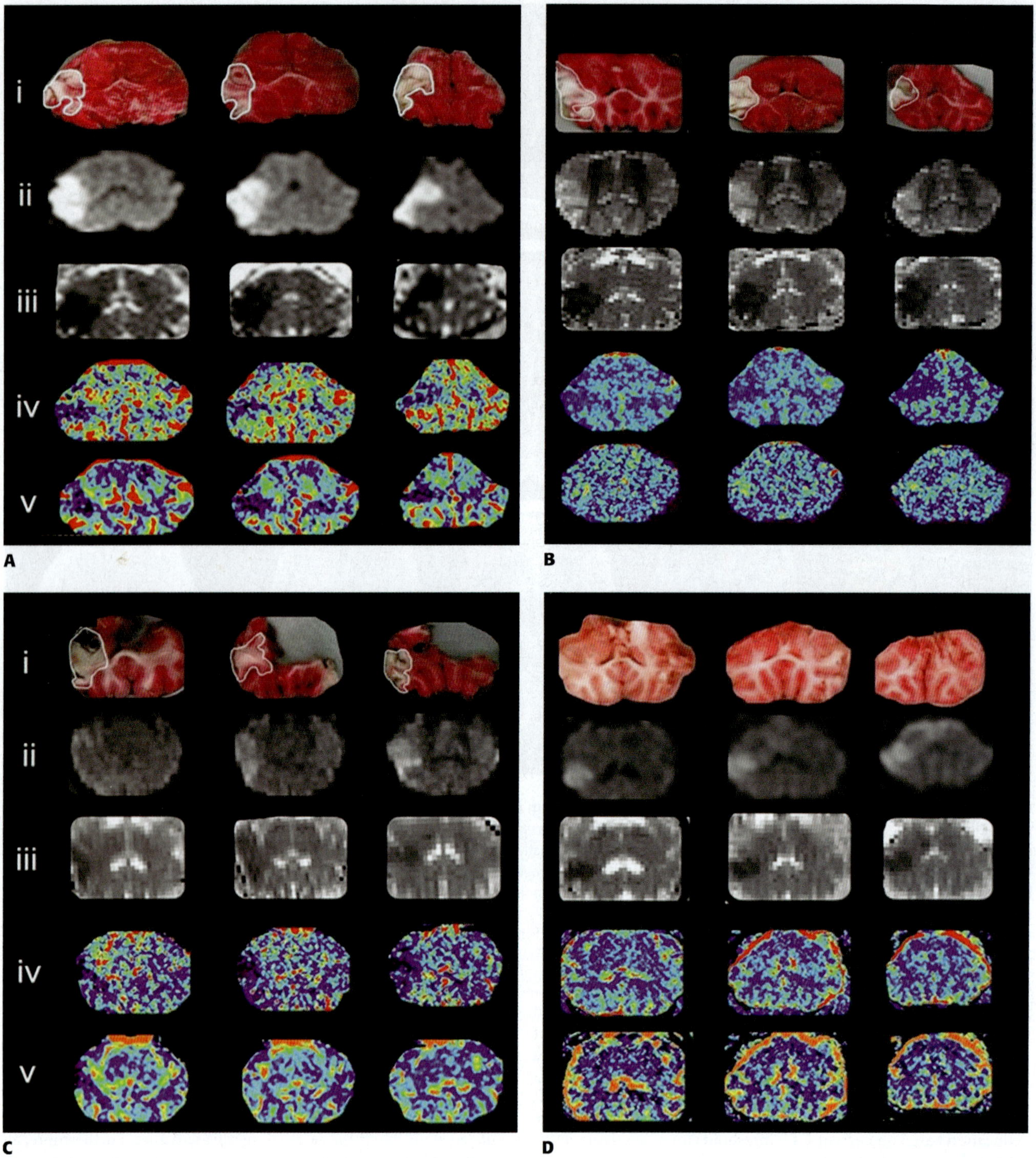

Figure 13-9. Examples of matched CT and MRI and TTC-stained brain sections. Coronal sections of (*i*) TTC-stained excised brain section with infarct outlined in white, (*ii*) MR-DWI, (*iii*) MR-ADC, (*iv*) CTP-CBF, and (*v*) CTP-CBV. Colored CBF and CBV maps display 0 to 100 mL/min/100 g and 0 to 8 mL/100 g, respectively. **(A)** Animal no. 3 shows matched CBF/CBV defect in infarct volume in all imaging modalities; **(B)** animal no. 4 shows a complete CBF/CBV mismatch in the corresponding TTC- and MR-defined infarct volumes; **(C)** animal no. 6 shows a partial CBF/CBV mismatch, which corresponds to TTC- and MR-defined infarct volumes; **(D)** animal no. 10 shows MR-defined DWI and ADC infarct volumes without corresponding TTC- and CTP-defined infarction.

Assessment of CTP maps using ASPECTS has also been explored by several investigators.[63–65] There was consensus that, compared to NCCT-ASPECTS, CBV-ASPECTS was a better predictor of clinical outcome at 24 hours and could be considered an early predictor of fatal stroke.[63–66] Moreover, one study suggested that CTP-ASPECTS was able to identify the amount of potentially salvageable ischemic tissue.[63]

Extending the Time Window for Stroke Treatment Strategies

Intravenous Tissue Plasminogen Activator

The identification of reversibly damaged tissue during the acute stroke setting has led to several early treatment strategies aimed to slow the progression of compromised tissue toward infarction. Early restoration of blood flow using thrombolytic therapy is an effective way to reverse ischemic stroke. Thrombolytic agents (mainly fibrinolytic enzymes) activate the endogenous protein plasminogen to breakdown fibrin, the structural scaffold of most blood clots. However, the negative pleiotropic effects of these agents may increase the probability of hemorrhage through the degradation of important clotting factors, and disruption of the BBB.[67] Nonetheless, evidence from the National Institute of Neurological Disorders and Stroke tissue plasminogen activator (tPA) study showed that intravenous (IV) tPA administered within the first 3 hours after stroke could significantly improve average neurologic outcome in a large cohort of patients; this result was sufficient for the Food and Drug Administration of the United States to approve tPA in 1996.[68] Patients treated with IV tPA up to 3 hours postictus were 30% more likely to have minimal or no disability compared to those receiving placebo. However, this strict time constraint has limited the use of tPA to less than 7% of AIS patients, as the risk of hemorrhagic transformation (HT) outweighed the clinical benefit beyond the 3-hour treatment window.[69,70] Several important studies have investigated the use of tPA beyond the 3-hour treatment window, namely the 2008 European Cooperative Acute Stroke Study (ECASS) III, followed by a similar study in 2009 examining a broad range of subgroups of patients, both comparing groups given alteplase or placebo 3 hours postictus[71]; observational studies investigating the Safe Implementation of Treatments in Stroke through an Internet-based audit of the International Stroke Thrombolysis Registry; and the Canadian Alteplase for Stroke Effectiveness Study, both comparing patients receiving alteplase before and after the 3 hour window.[71–74] Consensus was that IV-tPA has proven benefits if administered up to 4.5 hours from stroke onset. Only recently, the IV- tPA therapeutic window was extended to 4.5 hours from stroke onset.[2,75] Nonetheless, the ECASS III study did report a significant difference in intracranial hemorrhage for patients given alteplase, yet mortality did not differ between the treated and the placebo group.[73] The Simplified Management of Acute Stroke Using Revised Treatment (SMART) criteria study is ongoing, including all stroke patients for thrombolysis in a time window up to 4.5 hours, with hemorrhage being the only exclusion criterion.[76]

Endovascular Therapy

Intra-arterial (IA) delivery of tPA to the site of occlusion (as opposed to a systemic IV delivery) has also been shown to be beneficial.[77] The rationale for endovascular treatment is the low revascularization rates and poor outcomes with intravenous tPA in proximal occlusions. An advantage of IA-tPA treatment is the reduced systemic exposure, which allows for a higher concentration of tPA at the site of occlusion. Early studies showed that IA-tPA may be beneficial up to 6 hours after stroke onset, resulting in increased recanalization rates and no increase in mortality, compared with controls.[78] Combining IV and IA-tPA has also been tested, with moderate improvement in clinical outcome.[78] Endovascular therapy gained momentum after the introduction of thrombectomy devices that increased the rate of successful reperfusion in comparison to IA tPA alone. The first-generation devices including the Mechanical Embolus Removal in Cerebral Ischemia (MERCI) device and Penumbra clot retrieval device have been replaced by the more efficient stentrievers, fully retrievable stents that proved superior to the MERCI device in randomized trials.[79–82] A patient with moderate-to-severe stroke symptoms with a small core identified at CT and large vessel occlusion identified at CTA is most likely to benefit from endovascular treatment.[83] However, endovascular therapy is yet to be proven to improve the 90-day functional outcome of ischemic stroke patients when compared to IV tPA in a randomized control trial.[84,85]

Secondary Hemorrhage Risk Prediction

The risk of hemorrhage secondary to ischemic stroke often precludes treatment with thrombolysis, as it occurs in 2.2% to 44.0% of AIS patients and is the single most important risk factor to consider in deciding whether thrombolytic therapy should be given.[68,75,86,87] AIS-related hemorrhage is divided into parenchymal hemorrhage (PH) and hemorrhagic infarction (HI), the former increasing mortality risk by 10-fold.[88] While more severe hemorrhage is undoubtedly associated with worse outcome, there is controversy whether less severe forms of hemorrhage are clinically important.[5,88–91] Some investigators believe non-PH HT may represent a clinically irrelevant epiphenomenon, with different pathogenesis.[92] If this is the case, the ability to predict PH, the symptomatic hemorrhage subtype, at the acute stroke phase is critical to guide early treatment. Several groups have explored the use of biomarkers, as well as CT and MRI in an attempt to predict secondary hemorrhage; however, low sensitivity and specificity have limited their use in acute triage.[93–99] A positive correlation exists between the size of the hyperacute parenchymal hypoattenuation on CT (defined as tissue that is nonviable, even if reperfusion occurs), and incidence of HT, and subsequent clinical deterioration.[86] Aviv et al.[2] recently determined whether CTP-derived BBB permeability surface area product (PS) at admission differed between patients with ($n = 23$) and without ($n = 18$) subsequent hemorrhage. Figure 13.10 depicts a patient with HI-2 and a patient with PH-1, according the ECASS III criteria.[73] The mean PS for the HT group was 0.49 mL/min/100 g, which was significantly higher than that for the non-HT group, 0.09 mL/min/100 g. The optimal PS cutoff to predict HT during the acute stroke phase was 0.23 mL/min/100 g, which had a 77% sensitivity and 94% specificity. Unfortunately, higher PS values were not correlated with the more severe types of hemorrhage, PH 1 and 2. In a similar study examining acute BBB permeability in 32 patients with AIS, Hom et al.[25] were able to predict symptomatic HT and malignant edema (using a predefined lower threshold of 5 mL/100 g/min) with 100% sensitivity and 79% specificity. However, only 3 patients developed symptomatic HT, a diagnosis that has since been refuted.[100] There is a need for a multicenter study to examine the use of the PS parameter during AIS triage. Yassi et al.[101] showed that a T_{max} greater than 14-second volumes of greater than 5 mL allowed prediction of PH with sensitivity of 79% and specificity of 68%.

Ischemic Stroke Diagnostic Caveats

For patients with many cerebrovascular risk factors, chronic microvascular ischemia is common. Most notably, chronic hypoperfusion generally occurs within white matter and may be encountered during an acute stroke CTP investigation.[102,103] An experienced radiologist should distinguish these lesions from an acute ischemic stroke, as they do not incorporate cortical gray matter, or follow the normal vascular/neuronal tracts.

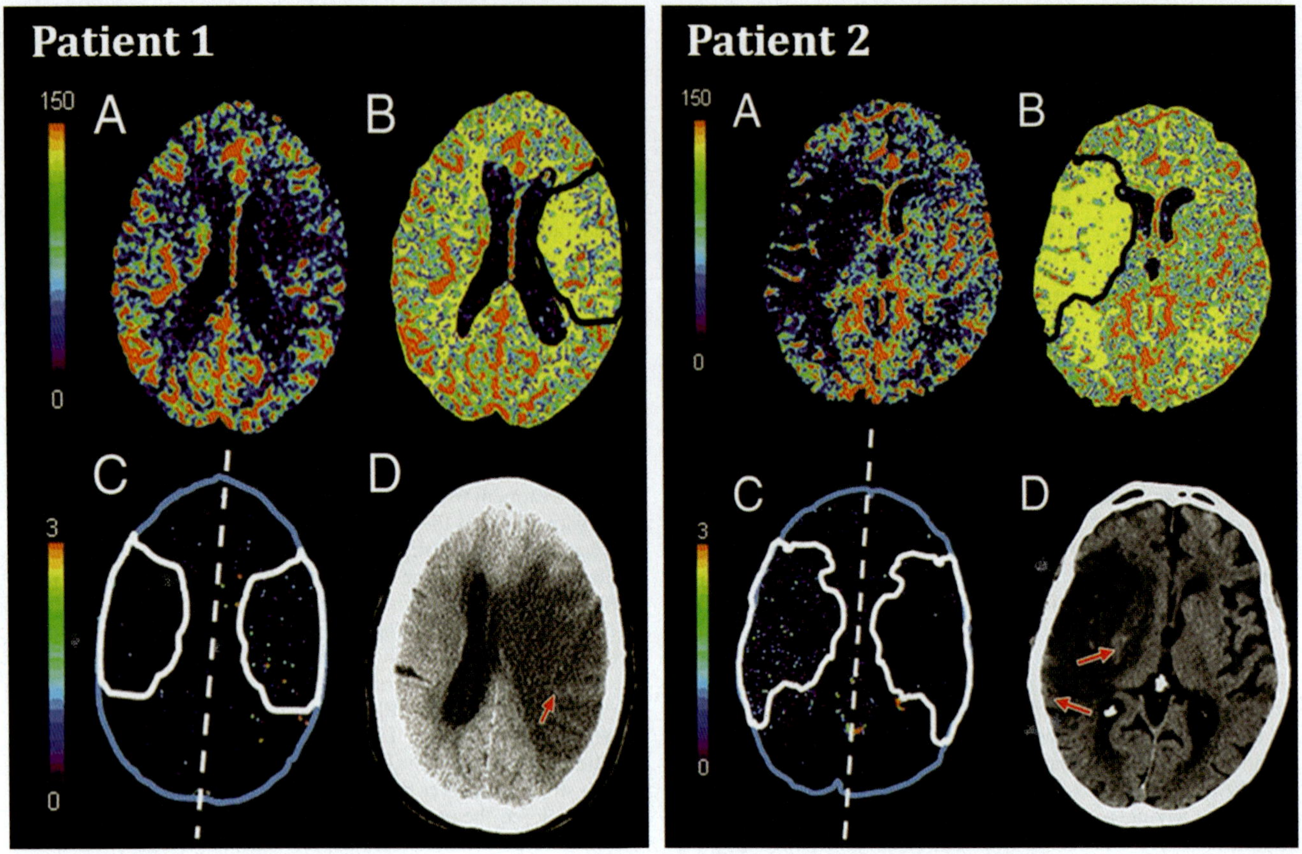

Figure 13-10. Patient 1 with small leakage in ischemic region. **A:** Admission CTP-derived CBF map of 5-mm-thick brain section displayed with color scale from 0 (*dark blue*) to 150 (*red*) mL/min/100 g. **B:** Corresponding CBF map shows ischemic ROI outlined with help of a *yellow overlay* of pixels with CBF of less than 25 mL/min/100 g. **C:** PS map corresponding to **(A)** shows superimposed ischemic ROI and mirrored ROI in contralateral hemisphere. **D:** Corresponding delayed NCCT scan of the same section shows infarct and HI (*arrow*). Patient 2 with ischemic region lesion that is larger than that in patient 1. **A:** Admission CTP-derived CBF map of 5-mm-thick brain section displayed with color scale from 0 (*dark blue*) to 150 (*red*) mL/min/100 g. **B:** Corresponding CBF map shows ischemic ROI outlined with help of a *yellow overlay* of pixels with CBF of less than 25 mL/min/100 g. **C:** PS map corresponding to **(A)** shows superimposed ischemic ROI and mirrored ROI in contralateral hemisphere. **D:** Corresponding delayed NCCT scan of same section shows infarct and PH (*arrows*).

The highly symptomatic but small infarcts occurring in the deep gray and central white matter can also cause problems when attempting to diagnose AIS. These lesions may be missed as the resolution of CTP is relatively low. With that said, it is important to use both the CTP functional maps along with the NCCT/CTA, clinical history, and symptoms to decide on triage—areas of acute infarction may be directly beside an old infarct and thus difficult to discern, even for the most experienced radiologist.

Intra- and extracranial carotid stenosis can mimic an acute ischemic stroke, as the hemisphere supplied by these vessels becomes significantly hypoperfused. Thus, it is important to examine the CTA, along with the CTP, to determine the vascular occlusion status. Along the same lines, seizures can cause hyperperfusion in one hemisphere, creating hypoperfusion within the normal contralateral hemisphere, mimicking an acute stroke.

Decision Making in Ischemic Stroke: Balancing Time versus Imaging Information

As described above, within the 0- to 4.5-hour time window, there is level 1 evidence for the use of intravenous tPA.[104] The main goals of imaging during this time window are to locate the site of occlusion; exclude the presence of intracranial hemorrhage, an absolute contraindication for IV-tPA; and assess the presence and extent of EICs. Currently, the NCCT acquisition is the most common imaging modality used to make tPA administration decisions for patients with ischemic stroke. Contraindications for tPA on NCCT are (a) ICH and (b) any region of hypointensity, which likely reflects nonviable tissue, greater than one-third of the middle cerebral artery (MCA) territory.[105,106] Notwithstanding general acceptance of the above criteria, interobserver agreement for the criterion of one-third MCA territory involvement is rather poor.[105] A systematic scoring system, The Alberta Stroke Program Early CT Score (ASPECTS), is a 10-point rating system for assessing the extent of EICs on NCCT.[107] It is easy to implement and provides valuable information for predicting patient outcome after thrombolysis. However, ASPECTS has moderate interrater reliability even among experts.[108–111] Reliability is less in early presenters (within 90 minutes from stroke symptom onset)[112] and is affected by patient motion and in the aged.[107]

CTA is a reliable, safe, quick, and widely available tool to determine the presence of an arterial occlusion. CTA is used in acute stroke decision making for two purposes (1) to determine the presence of occlusion and (2) to determine the presence of salvageable brain via collateral scoring. The latter is done by assessing extent of pial arterial filling in presumed ischemic territory in comparison to normal brain. Presence of moderate to good pial arterial filling in symptomatic brain can be considered as a surrogate for the presence of salvageable tissue. Image acquisition and interpretation is rapid (<5 minutes), potentially saving many minutes when compared to techniques like MRI and CTP. This technique has whole brain coverage and good temporal resolution, does not need additional resources or additional CT contrast compared to conventional CTA, and is minimally affected by patient motion. A recent development in the field of arterial vascular imaging is the introduction of mCTA (patent pending), which generates multiple time-resolved images of backfilling arteries beyond a blocked artery filled by collaterals. This may improve the certainty of patient selection for endovascular therapy.

The validity of perfusion imaging to determine acute tissue viability, leading to individualized treatment strategies, has yet to be proven clinically. Perfusion is used by many centers for patient selection, for thrombolysis, and/or for endovascular intervention, and clinical trials such as DEFUSE-2 and EPITHET have shown that this strategy of delineating infarct core and penumbra can be used to select patients for IV-tPA treatment beyond 3 hours of stroke symptom onset.[113,114] In a more recent study, an infarct core on CTP-CBV maps not exceeding one-third of the MCA territory and tissue at risk as defined by MTT–CBV mismatch greater than 20% was used as criteria to treat with tPA beyond the 4.5-hour window. Rates of symptomatic HT (2.9% in the <4.5-hour group vs. 2.3% in the >4.5-hour group) and good long-term outcome (64.5% vs. 60.5%, respectively; $p = 0.620$) were similar between groups.[115] Clearly, there is a need for larger randomized controlled trials based on an optimized CTP paradigm. However, the failure of the DIAS-II trail, in which CT and MR penumbral imaging (mismatch hypothesis) was used as selection criteria, to demonstrate the superiority of desmoteplase treatment (given between 3 and 9 hours) over placebo groups cast doubt on the utility of perfusion imaging for patient selection for hyperacute stroke therapies.[116] This patient selection paradigm was also not shown to improve outcomes after endovascular therapy.[85] In addition to the many reasons mentioned for the lack of substantial treatment effect of these trials, the lack of a treatment endovascular arm resulting in faster reperfusion may also be a reason. Faster reperfusion is imperative—good clinical outcome following angiographically successful reperfusion is significantly time dependent.[117] Prolyse in Acute Cerebral Thromboembolism II supports the use of endovascular therapy for proximal occlusions beyond 4.5 hours.[118] Post hoc analysis of data from Prolyse in Acute Cerebral Thromboembolism II and Echo-planar Imaging Thrombolytic Evaluation Trial shows treatment effects with small cores identified by using either nonenhanced CT or DWI.[6,118] In the absence of compelling evidence for the use of IV tPA with or without perfusion imaging in this time window and the need for identifying a proximal occlusion before initiating endovascular therapy, the use of nonenhanced CT and CTA preferably or DWI and MR angiography and the small-core–occlusion imaging paradigm could be faster and more clinically relevant.

There seems to be a misconception that perfusion imaging in real time only takes a few minutes. This may be true for image acquisition time but not for time from entry into the imaging suite to making a treatment decision. For CTP, this time includes setting up the imaging unit and injector, acquiring and transferring images, postprocessing, and finally interpreting the data. For MR perfusion, other additional steps are required: making sure the patient is MR safe, patient positioning, motion, claustrophobia, and obtaining localizing images. These steps may extend the total imaging time by 30 minutes. Therefore, perfusion imaging–based paradigms may not be practical in a real-world scenario unless ongoing efforts at reducing image postprocessing time succeed.

CTP Standardization

A significant drawback of using CTP thresholds is the intervendor CTP algorithm variability. A similar conclusion is evident when applying perfusion MR thresholds to CTP data and vice versa. This lack of standardization has been recently highlighted by Bivard et al.[119] Since absolute CTP values depend on the details of the processing (or deconvolution) algorithm, using relative thresholds have been proposed as an alternative. Schaefer et al.[35] had success with defining infarction using normalized (to contralateral hemisphere) CTP-CBF values, and Bivard et al.[120] showed that a CBF less than 50% of contralateral values best defined the acute ischemic core using whole brain CTP. Nonetheless, white matter disease, age-related changes, and previous infarcts can compromise this technique.

Variability in the CTP image analysis (after functional map processing) can also contribute to the lack of CTP standardization, even when using the same CTP vendor. First, follow-up recanalization status (confirmed with imaging) is rarely known at the time of true recanalization. Moreover, final infarct volumes can be defined anywhere between 6 hours and 7 days, during which infarct expansion occurs at various rates. Second, many studies use either "region-of-interest" analysis or voxel-based analysis to define perfusion thresholds. Further, the contribution of large vessels (CBF > 100 mL/min/100 g or CBV > 8 mL/100 g) is sometimes removed from analysis, focusing only on parenchymal perfusion.[2,58,59] Third, when implementing brain perfusion thresholds, it is important to separate gray and white matter. In resting gray matter, average CBF values are approximately 50 to 60 mL/min/100 g, whereas white matter values are closer to 20 to 25 mL/min/100 g. This substantial discrepancy in flow values is mainly because white matter synapses consume ≤0.5% of the energy of gray matter synapses.[121] It follows that white matter may be more tolerant to ischemia than is gray matter, as there is a greater relative decrease in CBF from normal in gray matter than in white matter.[122] Further, since gray matter has a greater metabolic demand for maintenance of cell structure integrity, it can be expected that the damage would occur earlier and be more severe than white matter for a given CBF. Thresholds originating from human studies frequently use regions with combined gray and white matter, which could lead to under/overestimation of infarcted tissue in follow-up prospective studies.

The Calgary Approach

We adopt a pragmatic approach based on Bayesian principles, as described in the author's recent editorial.[123] Briefly, we aim to get by with the bare minimum information that is relevant to decision making and to put the rest of the information accrued to scientific use later. In the acute stroke setting, the decision to pursue thrombectomy (vs. IV tPA or no treatment) is an evolving decision with some factors pushing us toward intervening and some arguing against. We have found that analysis of basic imaging consisting of NCCT and CTA allows for a rapid and clear decision in most cases. Use of an algorithm shortening the explicit analysis not only reduces the implicit bias but also helps establish the level of confidence in available information and the need for further tests ("no further test threshold"). In our center, advanced imaging and research studies are performed in parallel with routine investigations and treatment, interfering minimally with efficiency of clinical decision making and care. This process helps us to recognize the importance of additional information while never being biased by an "information heuristic."

Clinical stroke severity at presentation provides a general estimate of dysfunctional brain tissue, while tissue defined as nonsalvageable core can be discerned on a good quality NCCT. On its own, this paradigm may help identify the patients at risk of harm from thrombolytic treatment. Further information can be

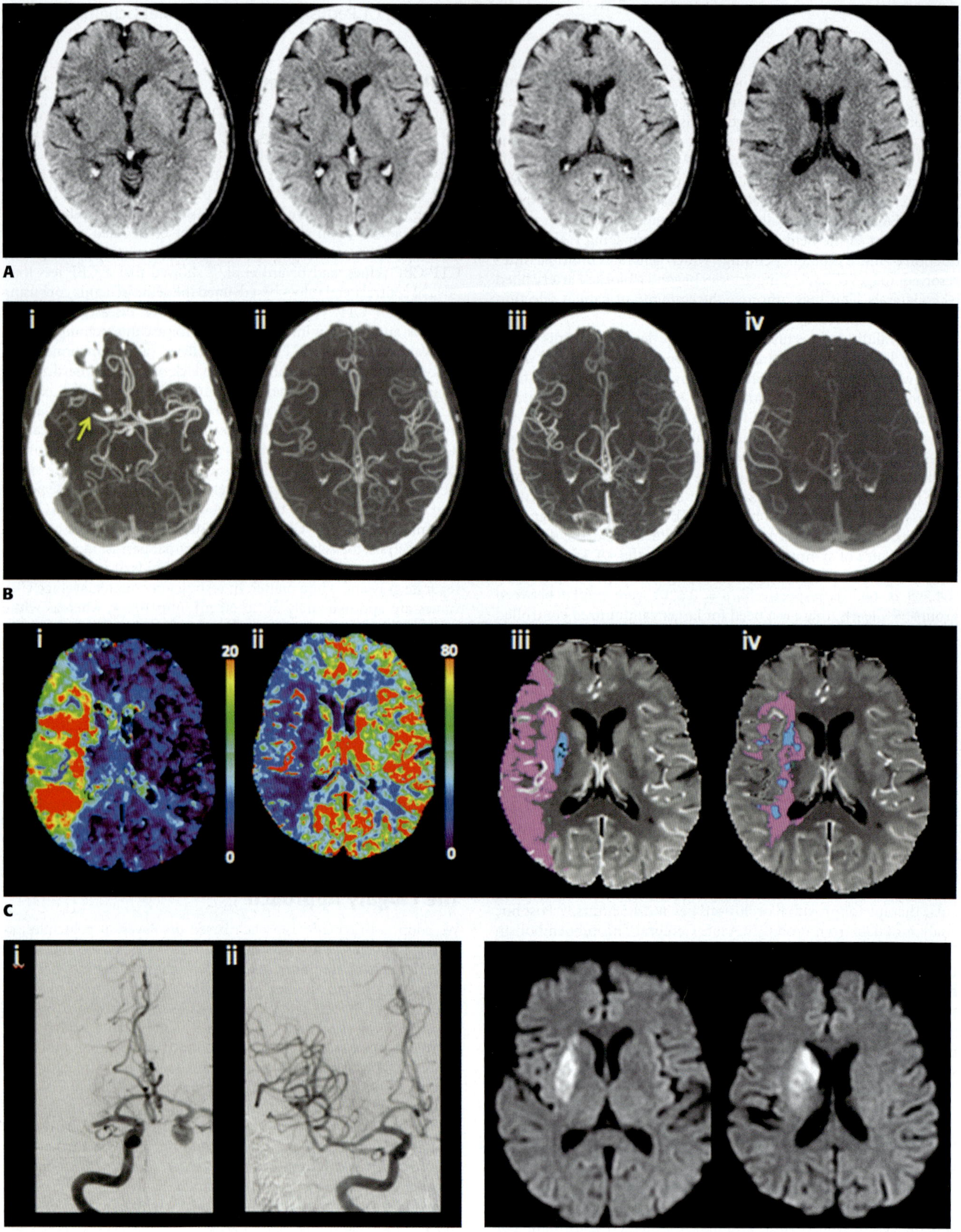

Figure 13-11. Multimodal CT imaging at 1 hour 28 minutes post–symptom onset for patient with NIHSS score of 18. ASPECTS of 8 is observed on the NCCT **(A)**. A proximal right M1 occlusion is shown **(B-*i*)**. mCTA (three phases) maximum intensity projection images are shown in **B**-*ii*, *iii*, and *iv*. An mCTA score of 4 is indicative of intermediate collaterals, salvageable tissue, and positive treatment response. CTP, T_{max}, and CBF maps are depicted in **C**-*i* and *ii*, respectively. Tissue with a T_{max} greater than 6 seconds is superimposed onto the CTP average maps in *pink* for both gray and white matter (**C**-*iii* and *iv*, respectively). CBF less than 10 mL/min/100 g and less than 7 mL/min/100 g, for gray and white, respectively, are flooded in *blue* on the CTP average maps (**C**-*iii* and *iv*). A small core and large penumbra is indicative of a positive treatment response. **D**-*i* shows the pretreatment angiogram. IV + IA tPA was administered, and TICI 3 reperfusion was achieved in 62 minutes post CT imaging **(D-*ii*)**. MR diffusion imaging at 24 hours postadmission imaging shows the final infarct as hyperintense **(E)**.

gained by examining the state of collateral circulation on mCTA. The collateral score can more accurately predict which patients will benefit from thrombolysis or endovascular intervention and confirms what is seen on NCCT. The small-core–proximal occlusion paradigm with clinical imaging mismatch is a very good surrogate for information that can be obtained by the penumbra–core mismatch paradigm using perfusion imaging and takes much less imaging time especially when further correlated with collateral imaging on mCTA (Fig. 13.11). Although no one disputes the value of the concept of penumbra and mismatch in acute ischemic stroke treatment, current perfusion techniques lack robust evidence validating their use in reliably identifying the penumbra. In addition, perfusion is affected by nonstandardized nomenclature, conceptual issues, and measurement errors have also limited more widespread use of CTP. Therefore, routine use of perfusion imaging in clinical practice could be premature when seen in the context of other imaging paradigms currently available.

REFERENCES

1. **Wintermark M, Albers GW, Alexandrov AV, et al.** Acute stroke imaging research roadmap. *AJNR Am J Neuroradiol* 2008;29(5):e23–e30.
2. **Aviv RI, d'Esterre CD, Murphy BD, et al.** Hemorrhagic transformation of ischemic stroke: prediction with CT perfusion. *Radiology* 2009;250(3):867–877.
3. **Lee TY.** Functional CT: physiological models. *Trends Biotechnol* 2002;20(8 suppl).
4. **Murphy MJ, Tichauer KM, Sun L, et al.** Mean transit time as an index of cerebral perfusion pressure in experimental systemic hypotension. *Physiol Meas* 2011;32(4):395–405.
5. **Albers GW, Thijs VN, Wechsler L, et al.** Magnetic resonance imaging profiles predict clinical response to early reperfusion: the diffusion and perfusion imaging evaluation for understanding stroke evolution (DEFUSE) study. *Ann Neurol* 2006;60(5):508–517.
6. **Davis SM, Donnan GA, Parsons MW, et al.** Effects of alteplase beyond 3 h after stroke in the Echoplanar Imaging Thrombolytic Evaluation Trial (EPITHET): a placebo-controlled randomised trial. *Lancet Neurol* 2008;7(4):299–309.
7. **Zaro-Weber O, Moeller-Hartmann W, Heiss WD, et al.** Maps of time to maximum and time to peak for mismatch definition in clinical stroke studies validated with positron emission tomography. *Stroke* 2010;41(12):2817–2821.
8. **Forkert ND, Kaesemann P, Treszl A, et al.** Comparison of 10 TTP and Tmax estimation techniques for MR perfusion-diffusion mismatch quantification in acute stroke. *AJNR Am J Neuroradiol* 2013;34(9):1697–1703.
9. **Konstas AA, Goldmakher GV, Lee TY, et al.** Theoretic basis and technical implementations of CT perfusion in acute ischemic stroke, part 2: technical implementations. *AJNR Am J Neuroradiol* 2009;30(5):885–892.
10. **Nabavi DG, Cenic A, Henderson S, et al.** Perfusion mapping using computed tomography allows accurate prediction of cerebral infarction in experimental brain ischemia. *Stroke* 2001;32(1):175–183.
11. **Gamel J, Rousseau WF, Katholi CR, et al.** Pitfalls in digital computation of the impulse response of vascular beds from indicator-dilution curves. *Circ Res* 1973;32(4):516–523.
12. **Cenic A, Nabavi DG, Craen RA, et al.** Dynamic CT measurement of cerebral blood flow: a validation study. *AJNR Am J Neuroradiol* 1999;20(1):63–73.
13. **Lee TY, Purdie TG, Stewart E.** CT imaging of angiogenesis. *Q J Nucl Med* 2003;47(3):171–187.
14. **Groothuis DR, Vriesendorp FJ, Kupfer B, et al.** Quantitative measurements of capillary transport in human brain tumors by computed tomography. *Ann Neurol* 1991;30(4):581–588.
15. **Yeung WT, Lee TY, Del Maestro RF, et al.** In vivo CT measurement of blood-brain transfer constant of iopamidol in human brain tumors. *J Neurooncol* 1992;14(2):177–187.
16. **Patlak CS, Blasberg RG.** Graphical evaluation of blood-to-brain transfer constants from multiple-time uptake data. *J Cereb Blood Flow Metab* 1985;5(4):584–590.
17. **St Lawrence KS, Lee TY.** An adiabatic approximation to the tissue homogeneity model for water exchange in the brain: I. Theoretical derivation. *J Cereb Blood Flow Metab* 1998;18(12):1365–1377.
18. **St Lawrence KS, Lee TY.** An adiabatic approximation to the tissue homogeneity model for water exchange in the brain: II. Experimental validation. *J Cereb Blood Flow Metab* 1998;18(12):1378–1385.
19. **Miles KA, Griffiths MR.** Perfusion CT: a worthwhile enhancement? *Br J Radiol* 2003;76(904):220–231.
20. **Abels B, Klotz E, Tomandl BF, et al.** Perfusion CT in acute ischemic stroke: a qualitative and quantitative comparison of deconvolution and maximum slope approach. *AJNR Am J Neuroradiol* 2010;31(9):1690–1698.
21. **Wintermark M, Smith WS, Ko NU, et al.** Dynamic perfusion CT: optimizing the temporal resolution and contrast volume for calculation of perfusion CT parameters in stroke patients. *AJNR Am J Neuroradiol* 2004;25(5):720–729.
22. **Wintermark M, Reichhart M, Thiran JP, et al.** Prognostic accuracy of cerebral blood flow measurement by perfusion computed tomography, at the time of emergency room admission, in acute stroke patients. *Ann Neurol* 2002;51(4):417–432.
23. **Lencioni R, Fattori R, Morana G, et al.** Contrast-induced nephropathy in patients undergoing computed tomography (CONNECT)—a clinical problem in daily practice? A multicenter observational study. *Acta Radiol* 2010;51(7):741–750.
24. **d'Esterre CD, Chia TL, Jairath A, et al.** Early rate of contrast extravasation in patients with intracerebral hemorrhage. *AJNR Am J Neuroradiol* 2011;32(10):1879–1884.
25. **Hom J, Dankbaar JW, Soares BP, et al.** Blood-brain barrier permeability assessed by perfusion CT predicts symptomatic hemorrhagic transformation and malignant edema in acute ischemic stroke. *AJNR Am J Neuroradiol* 2011;32(1):41–48.
26. **Wintermark M, Albers GW, Alexandrov AV, et al.** Acute stroke imaging research roadmap. *Stroke* 2008;39(5):1621–1628.
27. **Frey GD, Rumboldt Z.** Radiation effects from perfusion CT. *Radiology* 2005;234(2):638; author reply 638.
28. **Rapalino O, Kamalian S, Payabvash S, et al.** Cranial CT with adaptive statistical iterative reconstruction: improved image quality with concomitant radiation dose reduction. *AJNR Am J Neuroradiol* 2012;33(4):609–615.
29. **Wu O, Ostergaard L, Koroshetz WJ, et al.** Effects of tracer arrival time on flow estimates in MR perfusion-weighted imaging. *Magn Reson Med* 2003;50(4):856–864.
30. **Wu O, Ostergaard L, Weisskoff RM, et al.** Tracer arrival timing-insensitive technique for estimating flow in MR perfusion-weighted imaging using singular value decomposition with a block-circulant deconvolution matrix. *Magn Reson Med* 2003;50(1):164–174.
31. **Willats L, Connelly A, Calamante F.** Minimising the effects of bolus dispersion in bolus-tracking MRI. *NMR Biomed* 2008;21(10):1126–1137.
32. **Sanelli PC, Lev MH, Eastwood JD, et al.** The effect of varying user-selected input parameters on quantitative values in CT perfusion maps. *Acad Radiol* 2004;11(10):1085–1092.
33. **Ferreira RM, Lev MH, Goldmakher GV, et al.** Arterial input function placement for accurate CT perfusion map construction in acute stroke. *AJR Am J Roentgenol* 2010;194(5):1330–1336.
34. **Schaefer PW, Mui K, Kamalian S, et al.** Avoiding "pseudo-reversibility" of CT-CBV infarct core lesions in acute stroke patients after thrombolytic therapy. The need for algorithmically "delay-corrected" CT perfusion map postprocessing software. *Stroke* 2009;40(8):2875–2878.
35. **Schaefer PW, Roccatagliata L, Ledezma C, et al.** First-pass quantitative CT perfusion identifies thresholds for salvageable penumbra in acute stroke patients treated with intra-arterial therapy. *AJNR Am J Neuroradiol* 2006;27(1):20–25.
36. **Wintermark M, Flanders AE, Velthuis B, et al.** Perfusion-CT assessment of infarct core and penumbra: receiver operating characteristic curve analysis in 130 patients suspected of acute hemispheric stroke. *Stroke* 2006;37(4):979–985.
37. **d'Esterre CD, Aviv RI, Lee TY.** The evolution of the cerebral blood volume abnormality in patients with ischemic stroke: a CT perfusion study. *Acta Radiol* 2012;53(4):461–467.
38. **Campbell BC, Christensen S, Levi CR, et al.** Cerebral blood flow is the optimal CT perfusion parameter for assessing infarct core. *Stroke* 2011;42(12):3435–3440.
39. **Kamalian S, Kamalian S, Maas MB, et al.** CT cerebral blood flow maps optimally correlate with admission diffusion-weighted imaging

in acute stroke but thresholds vary by postprocessing platform. *Stroke* 2011;42(7):1923–1928.
40. **Heymann MA, Payne BD, Hoffman JI, et al.** Blood flow measurements with radionuclide-labeled particles. *Prog Cardiovasc Dis* 1977;20(1):55–79.
41. **Gobbel GT, Cann CE, Iwamoto HS, et al.** Measurement of regional cerebral blood flow in the dog using ultrafast computed tomography. Experimental validation. *Stroke* 1991;22(6):772–779.
42. **DeWitt DS, Fatouros PP, Wist AO, et al.** Stable xenon versus radiolabeled microsphere cerebral blood flow measurements in baboons. *Stroke* 1989;20(12):1716–1723.
43. **Fisher M.** The ischemic penumbra: a new opportunity for neuroprotection. *Cerebrovasc Dis* 2006;21(suppl 2):64–70.
44. **Sun Z, Zhang X, Zhang Y, et al.** Estimation of the ischemic penumbra based on CT perfusion a pilot study. *Acad Radiol* 2010;17(12): 1535–1542.
45. **He ZK, Xu YK, Qiu WJ, et al.** [CT perfusion study of acute local cerebral infarction in rhesus monkeys]. *Nan Fang Yi Ke Da Xue Xue Bao* 2007;27(5):720–724.
46. **Arakawa S, Wright PM, Koga M, et al.** Ischemic thresholds for gray and white matter: a diffusion and perfusion magnetic resonance study. *Stroke* 2006;37(5):1211–1216.
47. **Hossmann KA.** Viability thresholds and the penumbra of focal ischemia. *Ann Neurol* 1994;36(4):557–565.
48. **Rohl L, Ostergaard L, Simonsen CZ, et al.** Viability thresholds of ischemic penumbra of hyperacute stroke defined by perfusion-weighted MRI and apparent diffusion coefficient. *Stroke* 2001;32(5):1140–1146.
49. **Symon L.** The relationship between CBF, evoked potentials and the clinical features in cerebral ischaemia. *Acta Neurol Scand Suppl* 1980;78:175–190.
50. **Hossmann KA, Heiss WD, Bewermeyer H, et al.** EEG frequency analysis in the course of acute ischemic stroke. *Neurosurg Rev* 1980;3(1):31–36.
51. **Forster A, Szabo K, Hennerici MG.** Pathophysiological concepts of stroke in hemodynamic risk zones—do hypoperfusion and embolism interact? *Nat Clin Pract Neurol* 2008;4(4):216–225.
52. **Saver JL.** Time is brain—quantified. *Stroke* 2006;37(1):263–266.
53. **Jones TH, Morawetz RB, Crowell RM, et al.** Thresholds of focal cerebral ischemia in awake monkeys. *J Neurosurg* 1981;54(6):773–782.
54. **Kamalian S, Kamalian S, Konstas AA, et al.** CT perfusion mean transit time maps optimally distinguish benign oligemia from true "at-risk" ischemic penumbra, but thresholds vary by postprocessing technique. *AJNR Am J Neuroradiol* 2012;33(3):545–549.
55. **Bivard A, Spratt N, Levi C, et al.** Perfusion computer tomography: imaging and clinical validation in acute ischaemic stroke. *Brain* 2011;134(Pt 11):3408–3416.
56. **Bivard A, Levi C, Spratt N, et al.** Perfusion CT in acute stroke: a comprehensive analysis of infarct and penumbra. *Radiology* 2012;267(2):543–550.
57. **Eilaghi A, d'Esterre CD, Lee TY, et al.** Toward patient-tailored perfusion thresholds for prediction of stroke outcome. *AJNR Am J Neuroradiol* 2013;35(3):472–477.
58. **Murphy BD, Fox AJ, Lee DH, et al.** White matter thresholds for ischemic penumbra and infarct core in patients with acute stroke: CT perfusion study. *Radiology* 2008;247(3):818–825.
59. **Murphy BD, Fox AJ, Lee DH, et al.** Identification of penumbra and infarct in acute ischemic stroke using computed tomography perfusion-derived blood flow and blood volume measurements. *Stroke* 2006;37(7):1771–1777.
60. **Zaharchuk G, Mandeville JB, Bogdanov AA, Jr.** et al. Cerebrovascular dynamics of autoregulation and hypoperfusion. An MRI study of CBF and changes in total and microvascular cerebral blood volume during hemorrhagic hypotension. *Stroke* 1999;30(10):2197–2204; discussion 2204–2195.
61. **Hatazawa J, Shimosegawa E, Toyoshima H, et al.** Cerebral blood volume in acute brain infarction: a combined study with dynamic susceptibility contrast MRI and 99mTc-HMPAO-SPECT. *Stroke* 1999;30(4):800–806.
62. **Butcher KS, Lee SB, Parsons MW, et al.** Differential prognosis of isolated cortical swelling and hypoattenuation on CT in acute stroke. *Stroke* 2007;38(3):941–947.
63. **Sillanpaa N, Saarinen JT, Rusanen H, et al.** CT perfusion ASPECTS in the evaluation of acute ischemic stroke: thrombolytic therapy perspective. *Cerebrovasc Dis* 2011;1:6–16.
64. **Aviv RI, Mandelcorn J, Chakraborty S, et al.** Alberta Stroke Program Early CT Scoring of CT perfusion in early stroke visualization and assessment. *AJNR Am J Neuroradiol* 2007;28(10):1975–1980.
65. **Kim JT, Park MS, Choi KH, et al.** The CBV-ASPECT Score as a predictor of fatal stroke in a hyperacute state. *Eur Neurol* 2010;63(6): 357–363.
66. **Lin K, Rapalino O, Law M, et al.** Accuracy of the Alberta Stroke Program Early CT Score during the first 3 hours of middle cerebral artery stroke: comparison of noncontrast CT, CT angiography source images, and CT perfusion. *AJNR Am J Neuroradiol* 2008;29(5):931–936.
67. **Kaur J, Zhao Z, Klein GM, et al.** The neurotoxicity of tissue plasminogen activator? *J Cereb Blood Flow Metab* 2004;24(9):945–963.
68. **Tissue plasminogen activator for acute ischemic stroke.** The National Institute of Neurological Disorders and Stroke rt-PA Stroke Study Group. *N Engl J Med* 1995;333(24):1581–1587.
69. **Schumacher HC, Bateman BT, Boden-Albala B, et al.** Use of thrombolysis in acute ischemic stroke: analysis of the Nationwide Inpatient Sample 1999 to 2004. *Ann Emerg Med* 2007;50(2):99–107.
70. **Fang MC, Cutler DM, Rosen AB.** Trends in thrombolytic use for ischemic stroke in the United States. *J Hosp Med* 2010;5(7):406–409.
71. **Bluhmki E, Chamorro A, Davalos A, et al.** Stroke treatment with alteplase given 3.0-4.5 h after onset of acute ischaemic stroke (ECASS III): additional outcomes and subgroup analysis of a randomised controlled trial. *Lancet Neurol* 2009;8(12):1095–1102.
72. **Wahlgren N, Ahmed N, Davalos A, et al.** Thrombolysis with alteplase 3-4.5 h after acute ischaemic stroke (SITS-ISTR): an observational study. *Lancet* 2008;372(9646):1303–1309.
73. **Hacke W, Kaste M, Bluhmki E, et al.** Thrombolysis with alteplase 3 to 4.5 hours after acute ischemic stroke. *N Engl J Med* 2008;359(13): 1317–1329.
74. **Shobha N, Buchan AM, Hill MD.** Thrombolysis at 3–4.5 hours after acute ischemic stroke onset—evidence from the Canadian Alteplase for Stroke Effectiveness Study (CASES) registry. *Cerebrovasc Dis* 2011;31(3):223–228.
75. **Hacke W, Kaste M, Fieschi C, et al.** Intravenous thrombolysis with recombinant tissue plasminogen activator for acute hemispheric stroke. The European Cooperative Acute Stroke Study (ECASS). *JAMA* 1995;274(13):1017–1025.
76. **Tong D.** Are all IV thrombolysis exclusion criteria necessary? Being SMART about evidence-based medicine. *Neurology* 2011;76(21):1780–1781.
77. **Mathews MS, Sharma J, Snyder KV, et al.** Safety, effectiveness, and practicality of endovascular therapy within the first 3 hours of acute ischemic stroke onset. *Neurosurgery* 2009;65(5):860–865; discussion 865.
78. **Lee M, Hong KS, Saver JL.** Efficacy of intra-arterial fibrinolysis for acute ischemic stroke: meta-analysis of randomized controlled trials. *Stroke* 2010;41(5):932–937.
79. **Nogueira RG, Lutsep HL, Gupta R, et al.** Trevo versus Merci retrievers for thrombectomy revascularisation of large vessel occlusions in acute ischaemic stroke (TREVO 2): a randomised trial. *Lancet* 2012;380(9849): 1231–1240.
80. **Saver JL, Jahan R, Levy EI, et al.** Solitaire flow restoration device versus the Merci Retriever in patients with acute ischaemic stroke (SWIFT): a randomised, parallel-group, non-inferiority trial. *Lancet* 2012;380(9849): 1241–1249.
81. **Gobin YP, Starkman S, Duckwiler GR, et al.** MERCI 1: a phase 1 study of Mechanical Embolus Removal in Cerebral Ischemia. *Stroke* 2004;35(12):2848–2854.
82. **Tenser MS, Amar AP, Mack WJ.** Mechanical thrombectomy for acute ischemic stroke using the MERCI retriever and penumbra aspiration systems. *World Neurosurg* 2011;76(6 suppl):S16–S23.
83. **Goyal M.** Poor clinical outcome despite successful arterial recanalization. What went wrong? How can we do better? *Neuroradiology* 2010;52(5):341–343.
84. **Broderick JP, Palesch YY, Demchuk AM, et al.** Endovascular therapy after intravenous t-PA versus t-PA alone for stroke. *N Engl J Med* 2013;368(10):893–903.
85. **Kidwell CS, Jahan R, Gornbein J, et al.** A trial of imaging selection and endovascular treatment for ischemic stroke. *N Engl J Med* 2013;368(10):914–923.
86. **Larrue V, von Kummer RR, Muller A, et al.** Risk factors for severe hemorrhagic transformation in ischemic stroke patients treated with recombinant tissue plasminogen activator: a secondary analysis of the European-Australasian Acute Stroke Study (ECASS II). *Stroke* 2001;32(2):438–441.

87. **Hacke W, Albers G, Al-Rawi Y, et al.** The Desmoteplase in Acute Ischemic Stroke Trial (DIAS): a phase II MRI-based 9-hour window acute stroke thrombolysis trial with intravenous desmoteplase. *Stroke* 2005;36(1):66–73.
88. **Berger C, Fiorelli M, Steiner T, et al.** Hemorrhagic transformation of ischemic brain tissue: asymptomatic or symptomatic? *Stroke* 2001;32(6):1330–1335.
89. **Molina CA, Alvarez-Sabin J, Montaner J, et al.** Thrombolysis-related hemorrhagic infarction: a marker of early reperfusion, reduced infarct size, and improved outcome in patients with proximal middle cerebral artery occlusion. *Stroke* 2002;33(6):1551–1556.
90. **Hacke W, Donnan G, Fieschi C, et al.** Association of outcome with early stroke treatment: pooled analysis of ATLANTIS, ECASS, and NINDS rt-PA stroke trials. *Lancet* 2004;363(9411):768–774.
91. **Dzialowski I, Pexman JH, Barber PA, et al.** Asymptomatic hemorrhage after thrombolysis may not be benign: prognosis by hemorrhage type in the Canadian alteplase for stroke effectiveness study registry. *Stroke* 2007;38(1):75–79.
92. **Thomalla G, Sobesky J, Kohrmann M, et al.** Two tales: hemorrhagic transformation but not parenchymal hemorrhage after thrombolysis is related to severity and duration of ischemia: MRI study of acute stroke patients treated with intravenous tissue plasminogen activator within 6 hours. *Stroke* 2007;38(2):313–318.
93. **Montaner J, Molina CA, Monasterio J, et al.** Matrix metalloproteinase-9 pretreatment level predicts intracranial hemorrhagic complications after thrombolysis in human stroke. *Circulation* 2003;107(4):598–603.
94. **Demchuk AM, Morgenstern LB, Krieger DW, et al.** Serum glucose level and diabetes predict tissue plasminogen activator-related intracerebral hemorrhage in acute ischemic stroke. *Stroke* 1999;30(1):34–39.
95. **Montaner J.** Stroke biomarkers: can they help us to guide stroke thrombolysis? *Drug News Perspect* 2006;19(9):523–532.
96. **Selim M, Fink JN, Kumar S, et al.** Predictors of hemorrhagic transformation after intravenous recombinant tissue plasminogen activator: prognostic value of the initial apparent diffusion coefficient and diffusion-weighted lesion volume. *Stroke* 2002;33(8):2047–2052.
97. **Knauer C, Knauer K, Muller S, et al.** A biochemical marker panel in MRI-proven hyperacute ischemic stroke—a prospective study. *BMC Neurol* 2012;12(1):14.
98. **Kawano H, Hirano T, Nakajima M, et al.** Modified ASPECTS for DWI including deep white matter lesions predicts subsequent intracranial hemorrhage. *J Neurol* 2012;259(10):2045–2052.
99. **Dankbaar JW, Hom J, Schneider T, et al.** Dynamic perfusion CT assessment of the blood-brain barrier permeability: first pass versus delayed acquisition. *AJNR Am J Neuroradiol* 2008;29(9):1671–1676.
100. **Lin K.** Predicting transformation to type 2 parenchymal hematoma in acute ischemic stroke by CT permeability imaging. *AJNR Am J Neuroradiol* 2011;32(6):E124; author reply E125.
101. **Yassi N, Parsons MW, Christensen S, et al.** Prediction of poststroke hemorrhagic transformation using computed tomography perfusion. *Stroke* 2013;44(11):3039–3043.
102. **Sachdev P, Chen X, Wen W.** White matter hyperintensities in mid-adult life. *Curr Opin Psychiatry* 2008;21(3):268–274.
103. **Murray AD, Staff RT, Shenkin SD, et al.** Brain white matter hyperintensities: relative importance of vascular risk factors in nondemented elderly people. *Radiology* 2005;237(1):251–257.
104. **Adams HP, Jr., del Zoppo G, Alberts MJ, et al.** Guidelines for the early management of adults with ischemic stroke: a guideline from the American Heart Association/American Stroke Association Stroke Council, Clinical Cardiology Council, Cardiovascular Radiology and Intervention Council, and the Atherosclerotic Peripheral Vascular Disease and Quality of Care Outcomes in Research Interdisciplinary Working Groups: the American Academy of Neurology affirms the value of this guideline as an educational tool for neurologists. *Stroke* 2007;38(5):1655–1711.
105. **Kalafut MA, Schriger DL, Saver JL, et al.** Detection of early CT signs of >1/3 middle cerebral artery infarctions: interrater reliability and sensitivity of CT interpretation by physicians involved in acute stroke care *Stroke* 2000;31(7):1667–1671.
106. **Pexman JH, Barber PA, Hill MD, et al.** Use of the Alberta Stroke Program Early CT Score (ASPECTS) for assessing CT scans in patients with acute stroke. *AJNR Am J Neuroradiol* 2001;22(8):1534–1542.
107. **Barber PA, Demchuk AM, Zhang J, et al.** Validity and reliability of a quantitative computed tomography score in predicting outcome of hyperacute stroke before thrombolytic therapy. ASPECTS Study Group. Alberta Stroke Programme Early CT Score. *Lancet* 2000;355(9216):1670–1674.
108. **Gupta AC, Schaefer PW, Chaudhry ZA, et al.** Interobserver reliability of baseline noncontrast CT Alberta Stroke Program Early CT Score for intra-arterial stroke treatment selection. *AJNR Am J Neuroradiol* 2012;33(6):1046–1049.
109. **Wardlaw JM, Mielke O.** Early signs of brain infarction at CT: observer reliability and outcome after thrombolytic treatment—systematic review. *Radiology* 2005;235(2):444–453.
110. **Patel SC, Levine SR, Tilley BC, et al.** Lack of clinical significance of early ischemic changes on computed tomography in acute stroke. *JAMA* 2001;286(22):2830–2838.
111. **Coutts SB, Hill MD, Demchuk AM, et al.** ASPECTS reading requires training and experience. *Stroke* 2003;34(10):e179; author reply e179.
112. **Bal S, Bhatia R, Menon BK, et al.** Time dependence of reliability of noncontrast computed tomography in comparison to computed tomography angiography source image in acute ischemic stroke. *Int J Stroke* 2012;10(1):55–60.
113. **Nagakane Y, Christensen S, Brekenfeld C, et al.** EPITHET: positive result after reanalysis using baseline diffusion-weighted imaging/perfusion-weighted imaging co-registration. *Stroke* 2011;42(1):59–64.
114. **Lansberg MG, Straka M, Kemp S, et al.** MRI profile and response to endovascular reperfusion after stroke (DEFUSE 2): a prospective cohort study. *Lancet Neurol* 2012;11(10):860–867.
115. **Garcia-Bermejo P, Calleja AI, Perez-Fernandez S, et al.** Perfusion computed tomography-guided intravenous thrombolysis for acute ischemic stroke beyond 4.5 hours: a case-control study. *Cerebrovasc Dis* 2012;34(1):31–37.
116. **Hacke W, Furlan AJ, Al-Rawi Y, et al.** Intravenous desmoteplase in patients with acute ischaemic stroke selected by MRI perfusion-diffusion weighted imaging or perfusion CT (DIAS-2): a prospective, randomised, double-blind, placebo-controlled study. *Lancet Neurol* 2009;8(2):141–150.
117. **Khatri P, Abruzzo T, Yeatts SD, et al.** Good clinical outcome after ischemic stroke with successful revascularization is time-dependent. *Neurology* 2009;73(13):1066–1072.
118. **Furlan A, Higashida R, Wechsler L, et al.** Intra-arterial prourokinase for acute ischemic stroke. The PROACT II study: a randomized controlled trial. Prolyse in Acute Cerebral Thromboembolism. *JAMA* 1999;282(21):2003–2011.
119. **Bivard A, Levi C, Spratt N, et al.** Perfusion CT in acute stroke: a comprehensive analysis of infarct and penumbra. *Radiology* 2013;267(2):543–550.
120. **Bivard A, Levi C, Krishnamurthy V, et al.** Defining acute ischemic stroke tissue pathophysiology with whole brain CT perfusion. *J Neuroradiol* 2014.
121. **Harris JJ, Attwell D.** The energetics of CNS white matter. *J Neurosci* 2012;32(1):356–371.
122. **Bristow MS, Simon JE, Brown RA, et al.** MR perfusion and diffusion in acute ischemic stroke: human gray and white matter have different thresholds for infarction. *J Cereb Blood Flow Metab* 2005;25(10):1280–1287.
123. **Goyal M, Fargen KM, Menon BK.** Acute stroke, Bayes' theorem and the art and science of emergency decision-making. *J Neurointerv Surg* 2013;6(4):256–259.

CHAPTER

14 Clinical Applications of ASL Brain Perfusion Imaging

Ervin L. Lowther, MD, Christopher T. Whitlow, MD, PhD, and Joseph A. Maldjian, MD

Introduction

Arterial spin labeling (ASL) is an established, noninvasive perfusion imaging technique that allows quantitative assessment of blood flow without the use of ionizing radiation or contrast material. This increasingly available and powerful tool has a myriad of clinical applications in cerebral perfusion imaging, including cerebrovascular disease, epilepsy, and neuro-oncology.

Background

Cerebral perfusion or cerebral blood flow (CBF) refers to the amount of blood supplied to the capillaries and interstitial spaces of the brain. Cerebral perfusion is closely linked to brain function via autoregulation by local tissue metabolites to maintain a constant supply of oxygen and nutrients to the brain.[1] CBF was first measured by Kety and Schmidt in 1945 using inhaled nitrous oxide (N_2O) as an exogenous tracer since it freely diffuses between the vascular compartment and the tissue.[2] By measuring the cerebrovascular arteriovenous gradient and quantifying the fraction of N_2O extracted by the tissue, CBF was derived using the Fick principle and expressed in units of mL/100 g of tissue/minute.[2,3]

Since that time, less invasive techniques to determine CBF have been developed, which include single photon emission computed tomography (SPECT), dynamic susceptibility contrast-enhanced MRI (DSC-MRI), and dynamic contrast-enhanced MRI (DCE-MRI). Though differing in their methodologies, each technique relies on an exogenously administered tracer to determine CBF.

CT and nuclear medicine–based perfusion techniques expose the patient to ionizing radiation, limiting their use in certain patient populations and utility for serial examinations. Currently employed CT perfusion techniques are qualitative, and the common hemodynamic parameters measured in clinical practice are relative cerebral blood volume (CBV), mean transit time (MTT), and relative CBF. Nuclear medicine–based perfusion techniques can provide both quantitative and qualitative information on cerebral perfusion, but the PET tracers currently employed for perfusion imaging have a very short half-life, on the order of seconds to minutes, and require an on-site cyclotron or generator.[4]

Bolus contrast CT and MRI perfusion techniques are typically qualitative and rely on bolus tracking after administration of an exogenous endovascular tracer, iodine- and gadolinium-based contrast materials, respectively, to estimate CBF. The reliance of these techniques on administered contrast limits their use in certain patient populations, particularly patients with acute or chronic renal failure. It is well recognized that the use of gadolinium-based contrast material in patients with renal failure can cause nephrogenic systemic fibrosis, a devastating, progressive multisystem disease that has limited treatment options and no known cure.[5,6] The ability of ASL to use magnetically labeled water protons as an endogenous tracer obviates these concerns and allows the acquisition of cerebral perfusion data even in the setting of dialysis-dependent renal failure.

ASL perfusion imaging can be performed with clinical imaging times less than 5 minutes and without the use of ionizing radiation or contrast material, making it ideal for use in routine clinical practice as a supplement to standard anatomic imaging. The relatively short acquisition time allows it to be added to an MR stroke protocol without significantly delaying treatment. If noncontrast MR angiography is also performed, a comprehensive evaluation of the cerebral vasculature can be achieved in a single setting without the need for the administration of contrast material.

The quantitative nature of ASL allows recognition of global hypoperfusion and hyperperfusion states that are not readily apparent with relative perfusion techniques. Moreover, the ability of ASL to reliably measure absolute perfusion permits serial imaging before and after an intervention such as endarterectomy and thrombolysis.[7] Vessel selective ASL perfusion techniques allow mapping of the individual vascular territories in the brain, quantification of overall perfusion to each territory, and measurement of the contribution of each feeding artery to the territory.[8,9]

Principles of ASL Perfusion Imaging

Most ASL cerebral perfusion imaging techniques utilize radiofrequency (RF) pulses to magnetically label (tag) water protons in blood vessels outside of the brain. After allowing a period of time for the labeled blood to reach the microscopic vasculature and interstitial spaces of the brain known as the postlabeling delay (PLD), the signal from the labeled blood in the brain is measured and used to determine CBF (Fig. 14.1). The parenchyma is imaged in both the labeled and control (i.e., unlabeled) states, and the labeled images are subtracted from the control images to remove

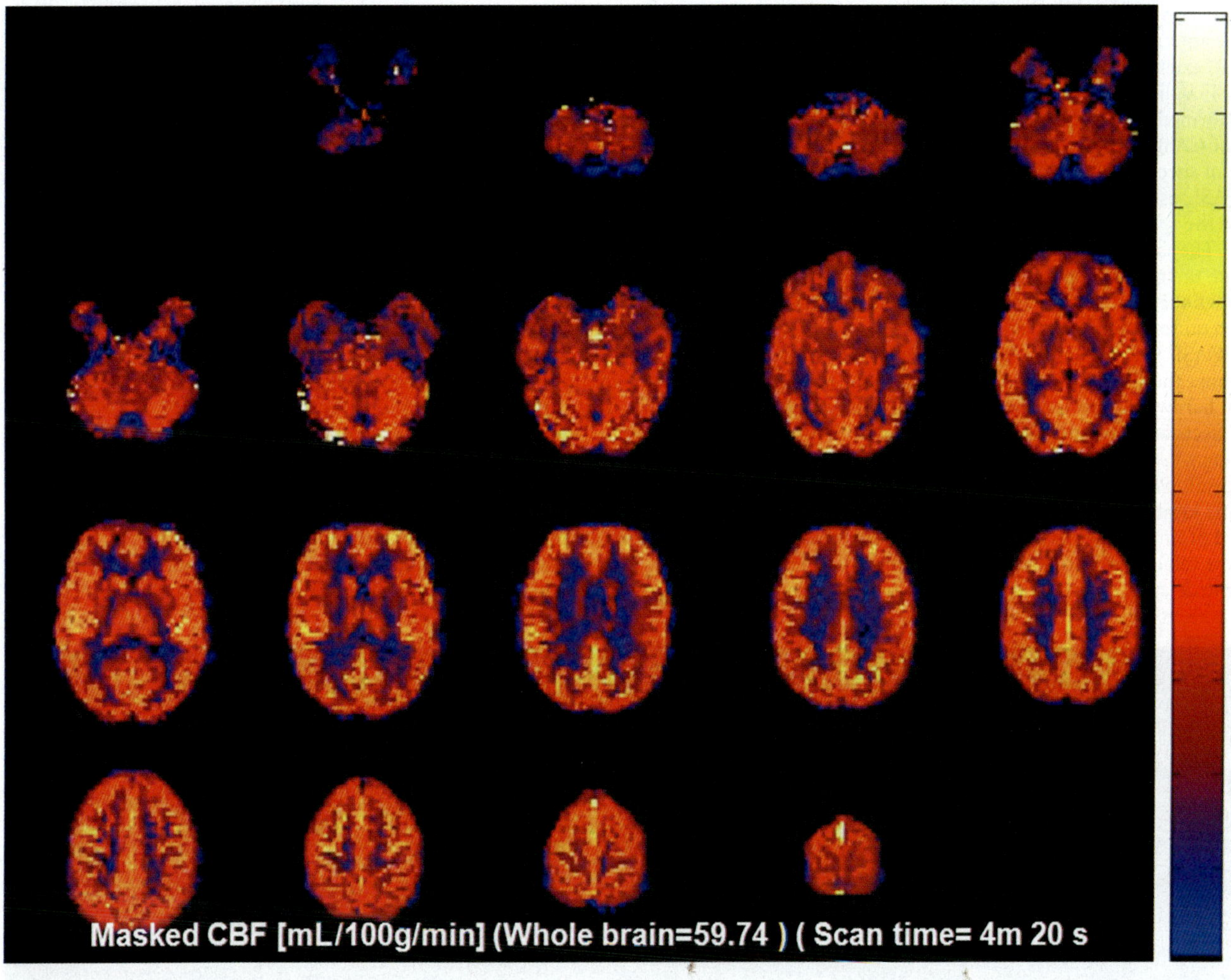

Figure 14-1. Normal ASL cerebral blood flow (CBF) maps. Sequential CBF maps through the cerebellum and cerebrum in a healthy 21-year-old female. The scale to the right of the images is set to mL/100 g/min.

the static background tissue signal and isolate the signal that came from the labeled inflowing blood. The measured signal is influenced by the intrinsic T1 properties of the blood and tissue, flow rate, transit time for blood from the tagging to the imaging region, tagging efficiency, magnetic field strength, and tissue magnetization interactions known as magnetization transfer (MT) effects.[7,10,11] Variations in transit time are one of the largest potential sources of error in quantification of CBF, and sensitivity to transit time variation is a major consideration and recurring theme in clinical ASL imaging.[7,12] Transit time prolongation is a nonspecific finding that results from any process that increases the amount of time it takes for the tag to reach the tissues. The formula utilized to calculate CBF is complex, and a number of assumptions and corrections must be taken into consideration.[10] Detailed examination of the calculation of CBF is beyond the scope of this chapter.

The signal-to-noise ratio (SNR) of ASL perfusion imaging is inherently low. The magnetic tag decays with the longitudinal relaxation of T1, usually on the order of 1 to 2 seconds for water in blood or tissue, and there is a finite time required for the transit of labeled blood from the tagging to the imaging region. As a result, only small amounts of labeled water accumulate in the tissue, and the signal from the inflowing blood is only a small fraction (1% to 2%) of the overall tissue signal at the time of imaging. To overcome this limitation, multiple acquisitions are averaged to generate the CBF maps. Background suppression with a series of appropriately timed inversion pulses can markedly increase the ASL effect and the sensitivity of ASL for detecting dynamic changes in CBF.[7]

Increased SNR can also be achieved with the use of higher magnetic field strengths.[10] Additionally, higher magnetic field strengths have the added benefit of lengthening T1 relaxation times and allowing more tag signal to accumulate in the tissues, but this comes at the cost of increased energy deposition in the tissues and susceptibility to artifacts.[13]

ASL images are acquired in two distinct and independent phases, a preparation component and an acquisition component. The independent nature of the components allows optimization of each to best suit the specific imaging application. The various preparation methods primarily differ in the way that inflowing blood is magnetically labeled. Currently employed methods include continuous ASL (CASL), pulsed ASL (PASL), pseudocontinuous ASL (PCASL), and velocity-selective ASL (VS-ASL).[14]

CASL was the first implementation of ASL, and it uses long and continuous RF pulses (1 to 2 seconds) to continuously invert the spins of inflowing blood as it passes through the tagging plane. The high labeling efficiency and SNR that results from the continuous tagging is offset by the need for continuous RF transmitting hardware that is not commonly available on commercial clinical scanners and the deposition of large amounts of RF energy into the patient. The Food and Drug Administration (FDA) sets guidelines for the amount of RF power that can be deposited in tissues during an MRI examination, also known as specific absorption rate (SAR). These FDA limits can be exceeded with CASL techniques, especially if performed at high field strengths. The widespread implementation of CASL in clinical imaging has been limited by the requirement of specific hardware and high SAR.

PASL uses relatively short RF pulses (2 to 5 milliseconds) to invert the spins in a defined slab of tissue outside of the imaging plane. The short RF pulses result in significantly decreased SAR and obviate the need for specialized hardware.[15] PCASL was developed to match the high labeling efficiency of CASL to the reduced hardware requirements and lower SAR of PASL.

PCASL uses a combination of RF pulses and gradient fields to mimic the CASL inversion method without the need for additional hardware. This technique reduces RF power deposition and MT effects and provides a good balance between SNR and tagging efficiency.[16]

CASL, PASL, and PCASL techniques label inflowing blood at a specific location and acquire images in the tissue of interest after a period of time known as the PLD. VS-ASL labels blood based solely on flow velocity and not location, eliminating the effect of the transit time delay in quantifying CBF. To do so, a velocity-selective RF pulse is used to label blood in the imaging plane traveling above a cutoff velocity (Vc). Data are only acquired from spins that decelerate through the Vc during the PLD. As a result, VS-ASL is inherently insensitive to transit time delays but suffers from lower SNR and difficulty in choosing appropriate velocity cutoff values.

Most ASL acquisition methods rely on fast MRI sequences, such as spiral or echo-planar imaging (EPI), that have a high SNR.[12] Single-shot and three-dimensional (3-D) volumetric sequences have been employed with success in ASL perfusion imaging.[17] In addition to providing improved SNR, the 3-D volumetric sequences allow the acquisition of data from the whole brain as a single slab of tissue. Single-shot techniques have been developed that use background suppression to mask the signal obtained from static signal, thereby eliminating the need for a control image.[18] However, these improvements come at the cost of more complex signal quantification during postprocessing.[7,19]

Vessel-selective ASL perfusion techniques have been developed that allow labeling of the individual arteries supplying the brain, quantitative assessment of the contribution of each individual vessel to cerebral perfusion, and accurate delineation of individual vascular territories[20,21] (Fig. 14.2).

One of the most important factors in the appearance of the perfusion image obtained is the presence or absence of bipolar "crusher"

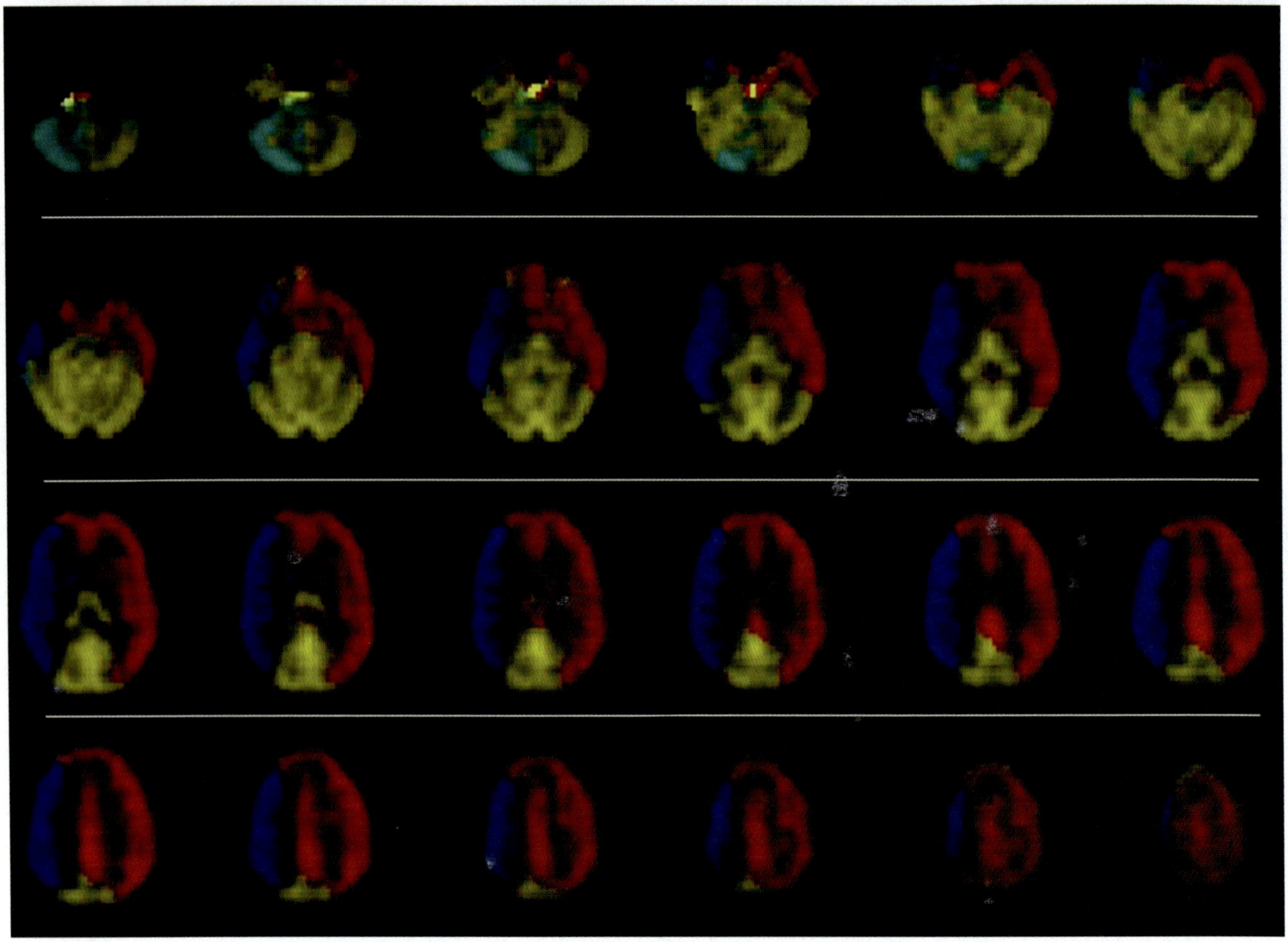

Figure 14-2. **Vascular territory imaging.** Sequential vessel-selective ASL perfusion maps through the cerebrum and cerebellum with colors corresponding to the source artery (*blue*, right internal carotid artery; *red*, left internal carotid artery; yellow, left vertebral artery; *light green*, right vertebral artery). Note that the left internal carotid supplies the anterior cerebral artery territory bilaterally due to a hypoplastic right A1 segment and that the left vertebral artery supplies nearly the entire posterior circulation due to a diminutive right vertebral artery that primarily terminates as a posterior inferior cerebellar artery branch. (Image courtesy of Youngkyoo Jung, PhD)

gradients during the acquisition component. Ideally, imaging would be performed once the entire volume of tagged signal has reached the interstitial spaces of the brain. In practice, some of the tagged signal remains in the blood vessels at the time of imaging. Crusher gradients are used to remove residual tagged signal in the large vessels before imaging that would otherwise elevate perfusion values in CBF quantification. However, removal of any signal from the relatively small amount of signal obtained with ASL can lower the quality of the perfusion image.[15,16] When using crusher gradients, the chosen length of the PLD has a significant effect on the appearance of the CBF perfusion map and can be a source of error when calculating CBF. Although choosing a shorter PLD permits a shorter acquisition time, it can underestimate the CBF because there is less time for the tracer to reach the tissues, especially in regions with slow flow, and more signal remains in the large vessels. When the intravascular signal is crushed, the resulting image overestimates perfusion defects and shows watershed territories as having decreased perfusion (Fig. 14.3). Choosing a longer PLD allows more time for the tag to reach the tissues, resulting in a more accurate global assessment of CBF and homogeneous perfusion image. However, a longer PLD increases acquisition time and lowers the SNR of the images due to decay of the tag with the longitudinal relaxation of T1.

Artifacts

Familiarity with the commonly encountered artifacts is of paramount importance when interpreting ASL images. As with any MR imaging method, patient motion is the most common source of artifacts encountered in clinical practice. Patient movement between acquisition of the control and labeled images results in a characteristic ring artifact of peripheral high signal intensity on the perfusion map. Filters have been developed to automatically detect and discard the compromised subtraction pairs that result from patient motion.[22]

As a consequence of the use of EPI and similar fast acquisition techniques, ASL perfusion imaging is vulnerable to inhomogeneities in the local magnetic field that result from calcifications, hemorrhage, metal hardware, and air–soft tissue interfaces. The susceptibility artifacts manifest as an artificially dark area on perfusion images that can mimic decreased or absent perfusion (Fig. 14.4). This is of particular importance when ASL perfusion imaging is employed in the postoperative evaluation of tumors. The presence of blood products in or along the margins of the resection cavity can produce artifacts that potentially mask a small focus of increased perfusion. ASL perfusion imaging is,

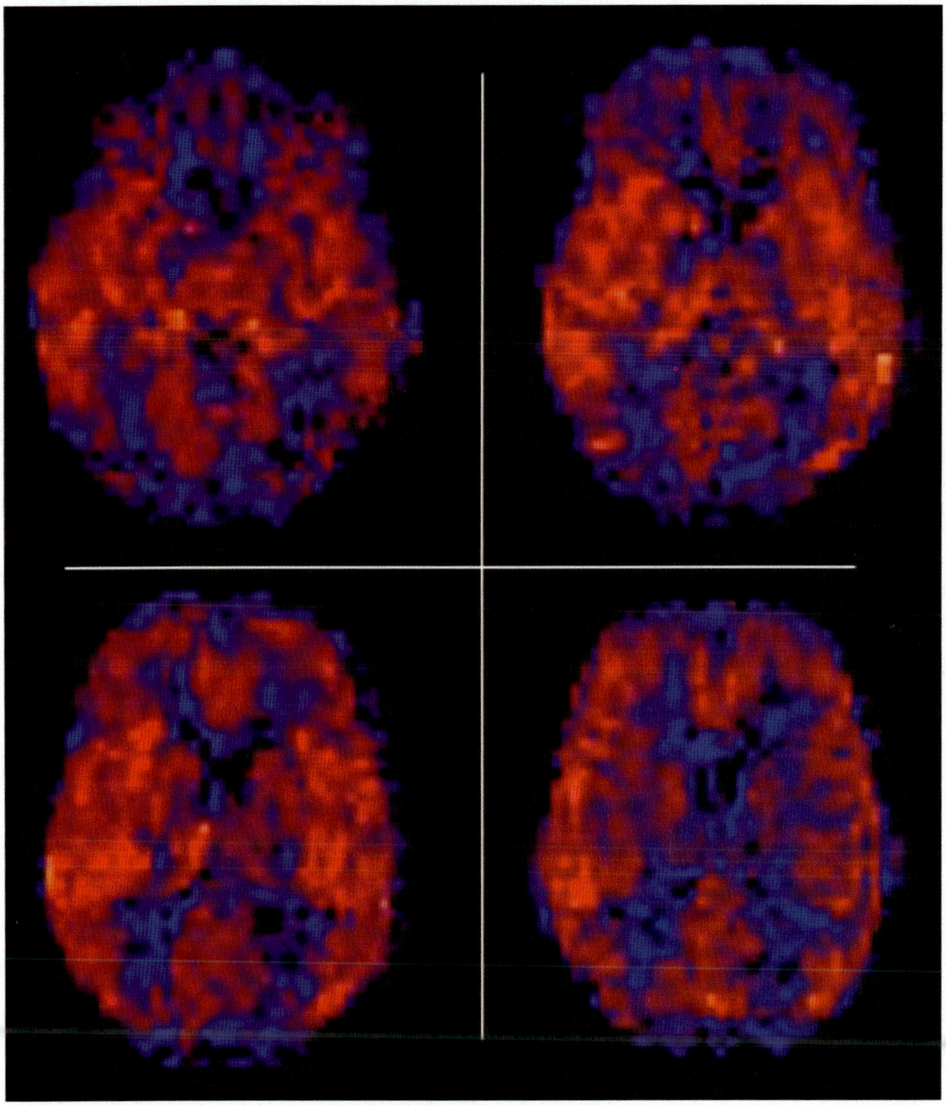

Figure 14-3. ASL CBF maps in an 82-year-old patient demonstrate apparent hypoperfusion of the anterior and posterior watershed territories due to relatively slow (prolonged) transit times and the use of crusher gradients. Mean CBF was 38.50 mL/100 g/min.

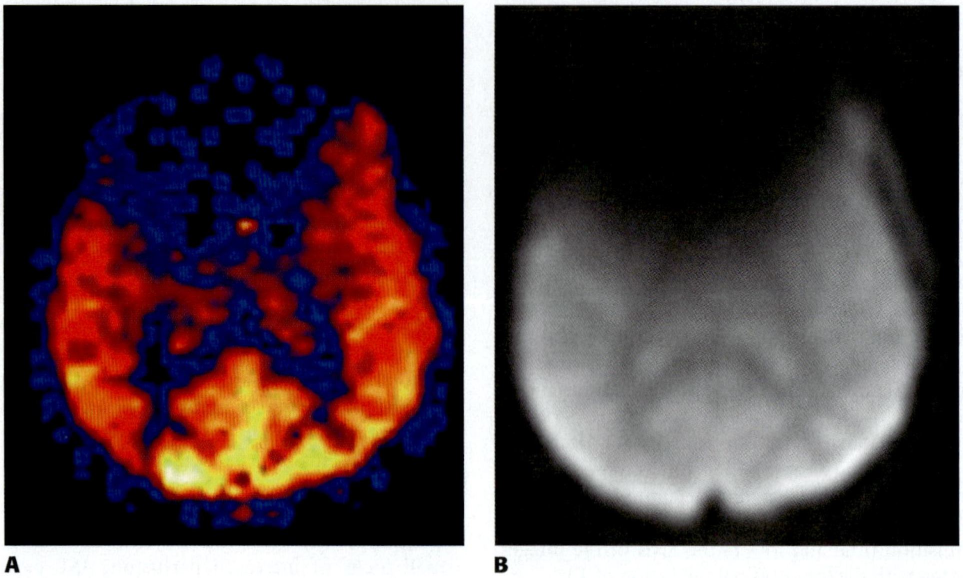

Figure 14-4. Perfusion defect on ASL due to susceptibility artifact. PASL CBF map **(A)** demonstrates a large area of apparent hypoperfusion that correlates with susceptibility artifact due to orthodontic hardware on the baseline magnetization echo-planar image **(B)**.

however, less vulnerable to susceptibility artifact than are DSC-MRI perfusion techniques that rely on T2* effects to generate perfusion maps.[23]

Gadolinium-based contrast materials result in shortening of T1 relaxation times in both labeled and control tissues.[24,25] ASL images are already signal poor, and this T1 shortening further decreases the measureable signal difference between both the labeled and control states. The result is almost no usable signal to generate the perfusion image. Therefore, it is mandatory to perform ASL imaging before gadolinium administration.[13]

Clinical Applications

Normal Findings

Marked age-dependent variability in cerebral perfusion is the norm in ASL perfusion imaging.[26,27] CBF begins at a low level in the perinatal period and plateaus in preadolescence (ages 4 to 11 years) with an average cortical CBF of approximately 100 mL/100 g/min. After the preadolescent peak, CBF values gradually decline to adult levels of approximately 75 mL/100 g/min. After age 30, there is a slow decline in CBF toward a minimum of 50 mL/100 g/min. Of note, the use of crusher gradients in elderly patients can cause the watershed territories to appear hypoperfused because of the relatively prolonged transit times in these regions (Fig. 14.3). Lengthening of the PLD can compensate for the relative transit time delay observed in these regions.[28,29] Routine ASL perfusion images show little perfusion to the cerebral white matter due to the relatively poor perfusion of the white matter with respect to the gray matter.[30] It is possible to determine CBF of the white matter, but this requires special protocols with up to 150 image pair acquisitions and averages to acquire enough signal to generate the perfusion maps of the white matter.[31] Occasionally, increased signal intensity may be seen in the occipital lobes that corresponds with physiologic hyperperfusion due to activation of the visual cortex during the examination[16] (Fig. 14.5). A similar pattern has been described in the frontal lobes in young and middle-aged patients.

Acute and Chronic Ischemia

Perfusion imaging is frequently utilized in the evaluation of cerebrovascular disease.[16,32] Whether ischemia is caused by atheromatous thrombosis, embolic disease, vasospasm, or vasculitis, the underlying cause of the ischemic infarction is decreased cerebral perfusion. As such, ASL MR perfusion imaging is well suited for the evaluation of cerebral ischemia. Identification of tissue with decreased cerebral perfusion is critical, as it is a predictor of future ischemia.[33]

The goals of imaging in acute stroke are twofold. First, establish the presence, size, and location of an infarct. Second, document the existence and quantify the extent of penumbra surrounding the infarct. Penumbra, or tissue at risk for infarction, is the ischemic tissue surrounding an infarct that remains viable due to blood flow from collateral pathways[34,35] (Fig. 14.6). Salvaging penumbra before it can go on to infarction is the primary goal of acute ischemic stroke care.

The perfusion–diffusion mismatch concept is widely used in imaging of acute stroke.[33,36] Diffusion and ASL perfusion maps are compared for mismatch, and the region of hypoperfusion in excess of the area of restricted diffusion is considered to be penumbra (Figs. 14.6 and 14.7). Qualitative visual interpretation is usually sufficient to diagnose penumbra, but cutoff values for the diagnosis of penumbra have been published.[35] It would be convenient if the distinction between infarct and penumbra could be made with ASL perfusion imaging alone, and it has been established that cerebral infarction rapidly occurs with cortical perfusion below 10 mL/100 g/min.[34,37–39] However, the diminution of ASL signal encountered with low flow states makes it difficult to accurately resolve small differences in perfusion, especially when CBF drops below 15 to 20 mL/100 g/min. This limit in resolution is near the threshold for distinguishing infarct from penumbra.[16] Therefore, the diagnosis of acute ischemia is best made with diffusion imaging. Recall that the ASL signal is dependent on transit times, so hypoperfusion may be a reflection of delayed transit to the tissue, such as can be seen with high-grade arterial stenosis or carotid occlusion, rather than true reduced CBF. In this setting, the ASL maps are more akin to MTT maps[7,40] (Fig. 14.7).

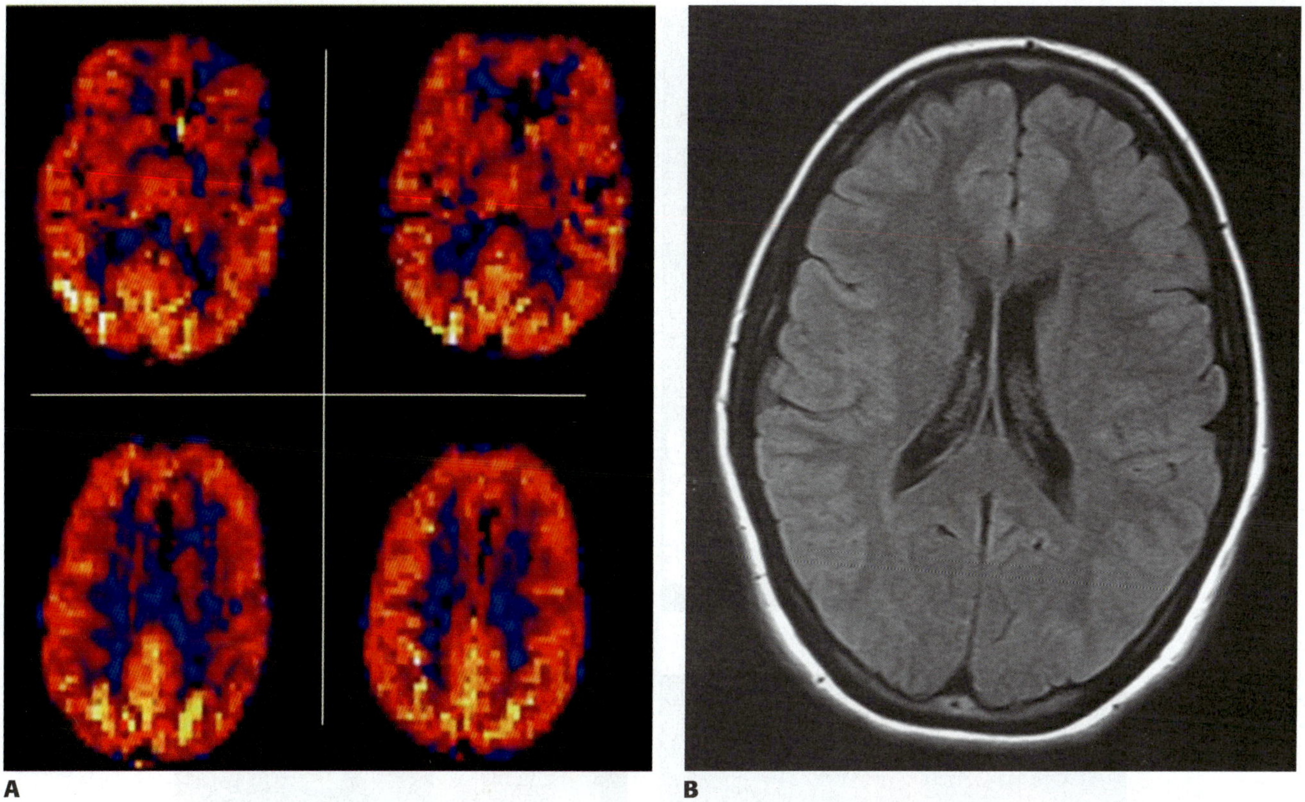

Figure 14-5. Physiologic regional hyperperfusion. A: ASL CBF maps show increased perfusion to the occipital lobes bilaterally without corresponding abnormality on the axial T2/FLAIR image **(B)**.

Studies have shown that the ASL and DSC-MRI perfusion techniques yield highly comparable perfusion values in normal cerebral tissue.[41] MRI bolus gadolinium contrast perfusion techniques, such as DSC-MRI, can be used to generate relative perfusion maps, and MTT, CBV, and CBF are the common parameters utilized in clinical practice. A completed infarct demonstrates prolonged MTT, decreased CBV, and decreased CBF; whereas penumbra demonstrates prolonged MTT and normal to increased CBV. Currently, routine ASL perfusion imaging measures CBF. It is possible to measure CBV and MTT with ASL imaging, but these parameters are difficult to quantify.[42,43]

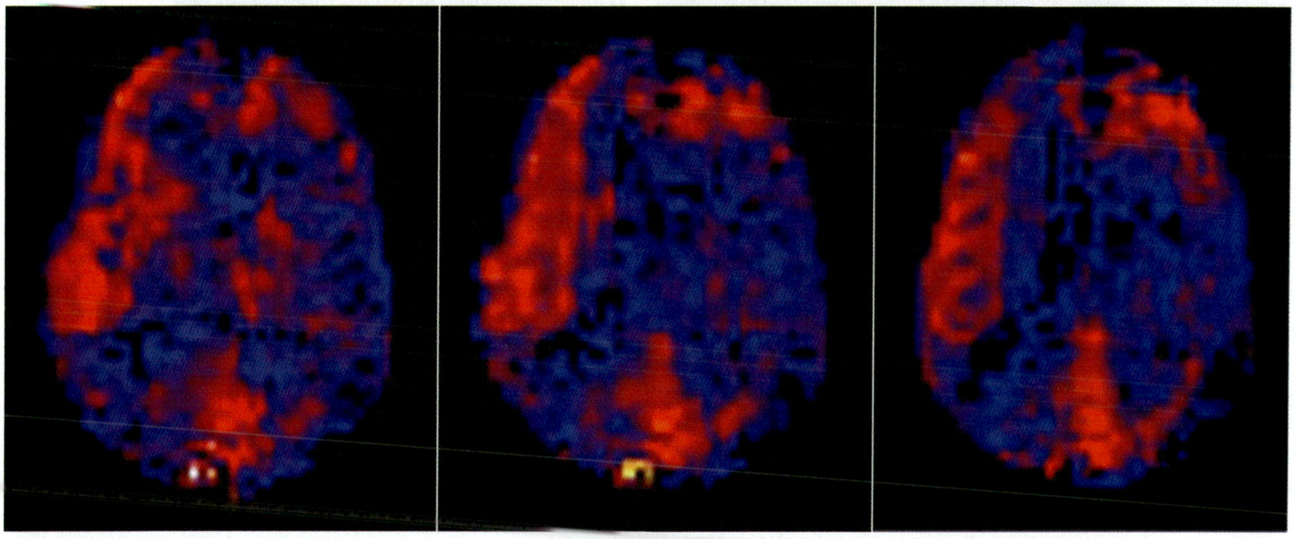

Figure 14-6. Left middle cerebral artery territory hypoperfusion in an elderly patient with reported left internal carotid artery stenosis undergoing evaluation for a transient ischemic attack. ASL CBF maps demonstrate hypoperfusion of the left middle cerebral artery (MCA) territory. The patient was asymptomatic at the time of the examination. Note the relative hypoperfusion of the right anterior and posterior watershed territories.

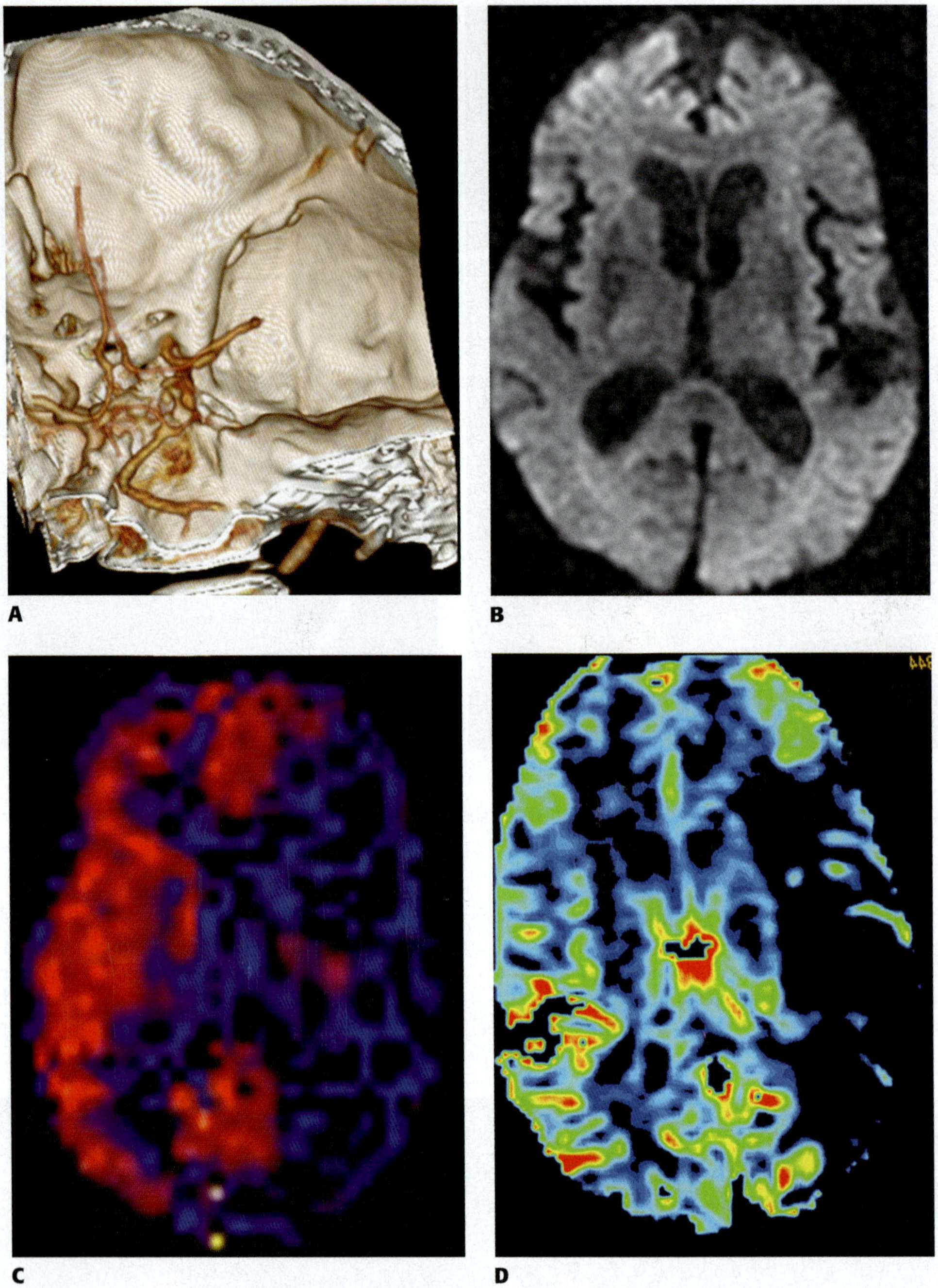

Figure 14-7. **Left MCA occlusion with penumbra but no evidence of infarct. A:** Volume-rendered oblique CT angiography (CTA) shows cutoff of the distal M1 segment of the left middle cerebral artery (MCA). **B:** Diffusion-weighted image (DWI) obtained shortly after the CTA demonstrates no evidence of hyperintense signal to suggest an infarct. The ASL CBF map **(C)** and DSC-MRI negative enhancement integral map **(D)** show decreased perfusion and prolonged transit time throughout the left MCA territory, respectively. The lack of infarct by DWI and decreased left MCA territory perfusion is consistent with territory at risk for ischemia (penumbra). Note the similar extent and distribution of prolonged transit time on DSC-MRI and hypoperfusion on ASL. In the setting of transit time delays encountered in vascular stenosis or occlusion, ASL images most closely resemble MTT, rather than CBF.

Cerebral perfusion patterns encountered in cerebral infarction primarily differ based on whether crusher gradients are used to suppress the intravascular signal and highlight the need to understand institution-specific spin labeling protocols before interpreting clinical images.[44] Slow intravascular flow in the region of infarction causes a delay in transit time of tagged blood to the tissues. As a result, a large amount of the tagged blood remains in the large vessels at the time the crusher gradients are applied. Suppression of the intravascular signal by the crusher gradients before it can reach the tissue results in an apparent perfusion defect in the region of transit time delay that correlates closely with the MTT map that would be obtained with qualitative perfusion methods[16] (Fig. 14.8). A second pattern would emerge if the same patient were to be imaged without the use of crusher gradients to suppress the intravascular signal.

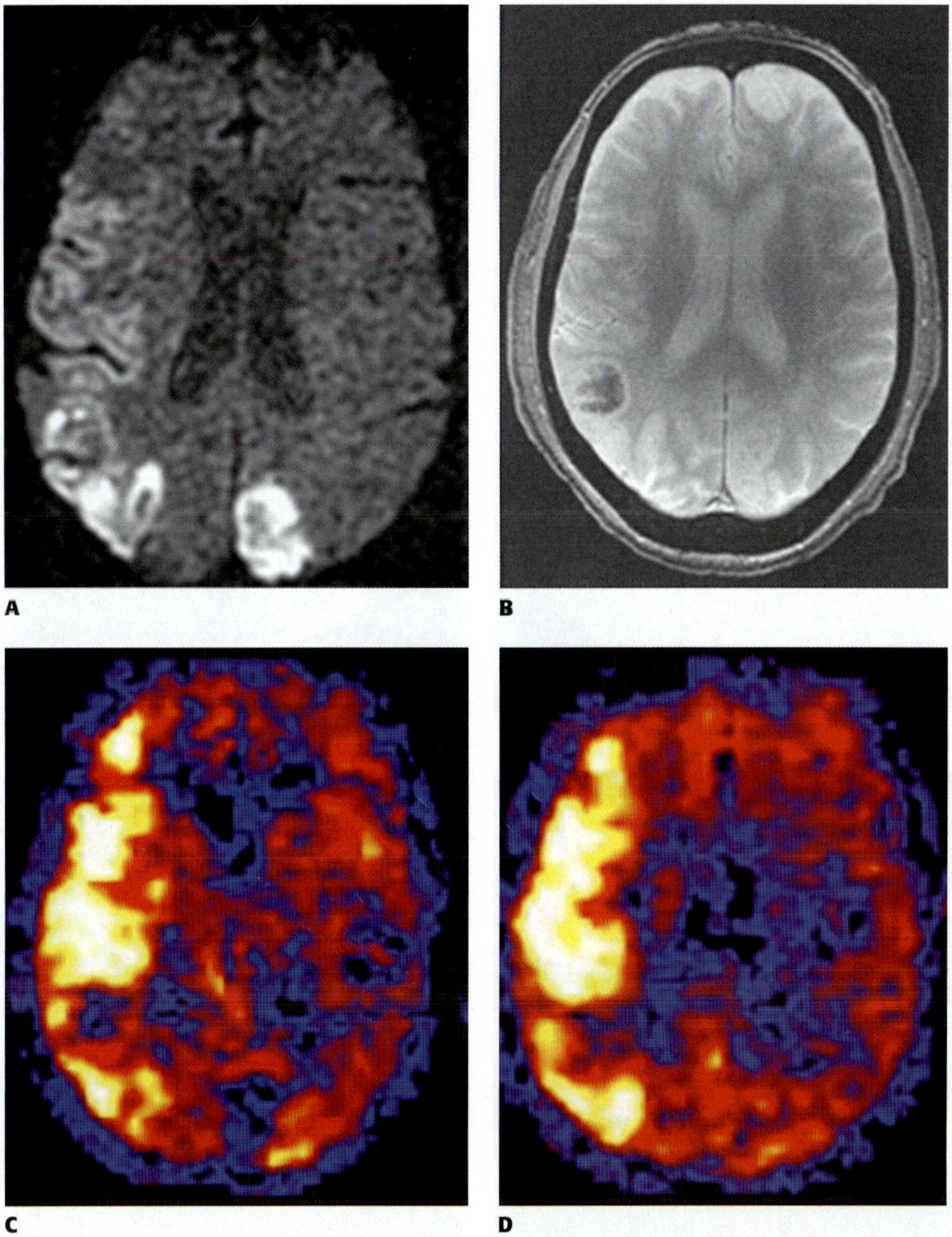

Figure 14-8. Multifocal embolic infarcts with luxury perfusion and susceptibility artifact from hemorrhagic conversion of an infarct. **A:** The diffusion-weighted image demonstrates hyperintense diffusion signal representing acute infarcts in the occipital lobes bilaterally and slightly hyperintense signal representing a subacute infarct in the right temporal and parietal lobes. **B:** The gradient image shows susceptibility artifact in the right parietal lobe due to hemorrhagic conversion of the infarct. **C:** The ASL CBF map demonstrates hyperperfusion of the subacute infarct in the right parietal and temporal lobes representing luxury perfusion. **C, D:** Demonstrate apparent hypoperfusion corresponding to the areas of hemorrhage due to susceptibility artifact. Note the hypoperfusion of the acute infarct in the left occipital lobe.

The slow moving blood in the region of the infarct would manifest as serpiginous high signal intensity along the course of the blood vessels.[45]

Counterintuitive though it may be, the third pattern seen in cerebral ischemia is hyperperfusion. Restoration of blood flow by autolysis of thrombus, administration of thrombolytic drugs, or mechanical thrombolysis/embolectomy can cause localized vasodilation due to dysfunction in the autoregulation of cerebral vascular resistance.[46] Conventional MRI imaging obtained in this setting demonstrates the familiar pattern of intravascular contrast enhancement.[47] ASL perfusion imaging demonstrates hyperperfusion to the area of infarction, a phenomenon known as luxury perfusion[46,48] (Fig. 14.8). Global hyperperfusion seen in the setting of hypoxic–ischemic encephalopathy represents an extreme form of this hyperperfusion[49] (Fig. 14.9).

The differential diagnosis of global hyperperfusion with ASL perfusion imaging includes robust perfusion in a normal young patient, hypercapnia, global hypoxic–ischemic encephalopathy, and, rarely, reper fusion syndrome following carotid endarterectomy. Hypercapnia is a potent stimulator of cerebral vasodilation, so much so that even small

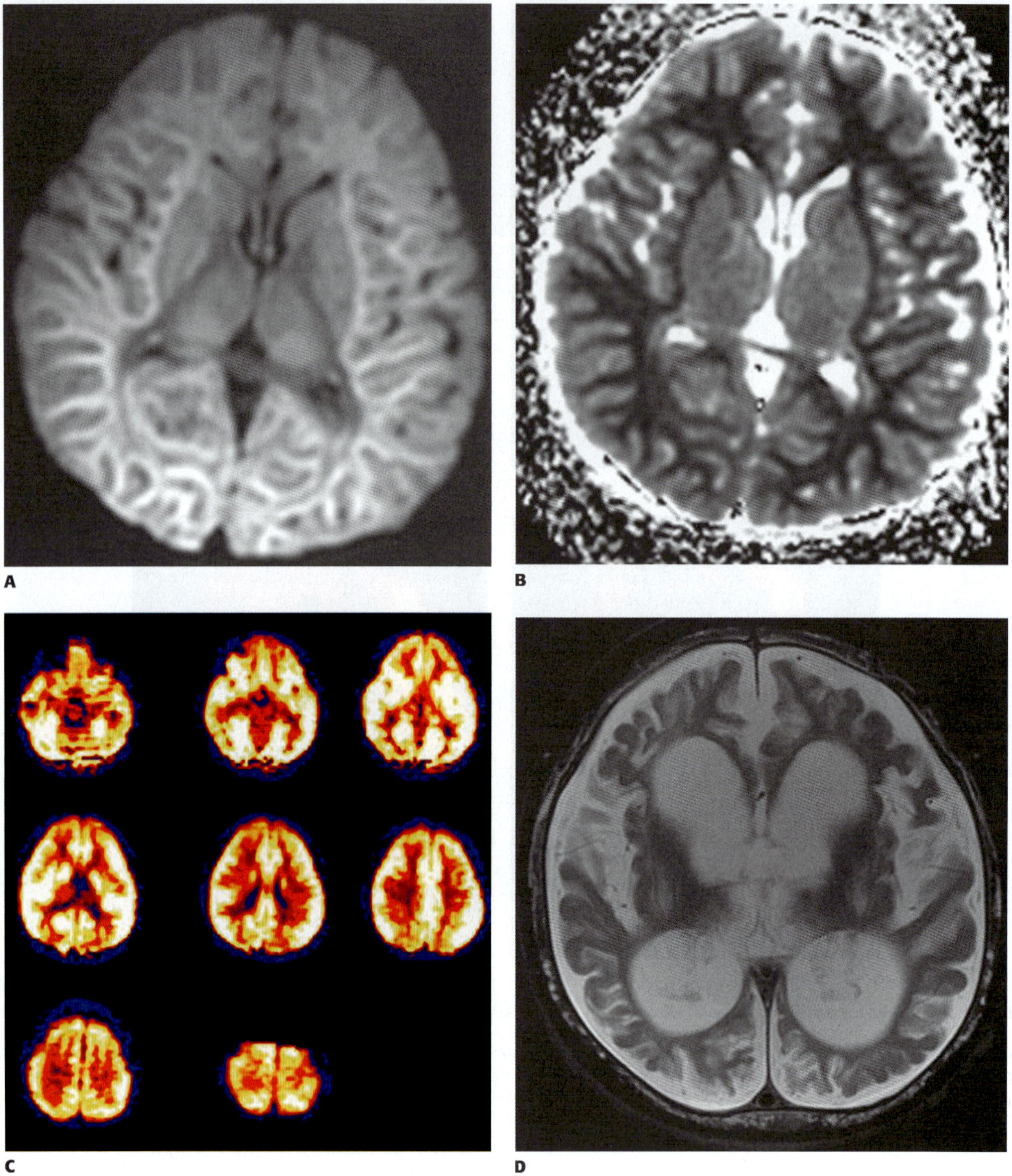

Figure 14-9. **Anoxic brain injury.** Axial diffusion-weighted image **(A)** with ADC map **(B)** shows confluent restricted diffusion throughout the bilateral periventricular and subcortical white matter with a lesser degree of involvement of the dorsal thalami. ASL CBF map **(C)** shows marked global hyperperfusion. Mean CBF of the gray matter was 174.54 mL/100 g/min. Axial T2-weighted image **(D)** obtained 2 years after the hypoxic–ischemic event demonstrates profound atrophy of the cerebral hemispheres and deep gray nuclei.

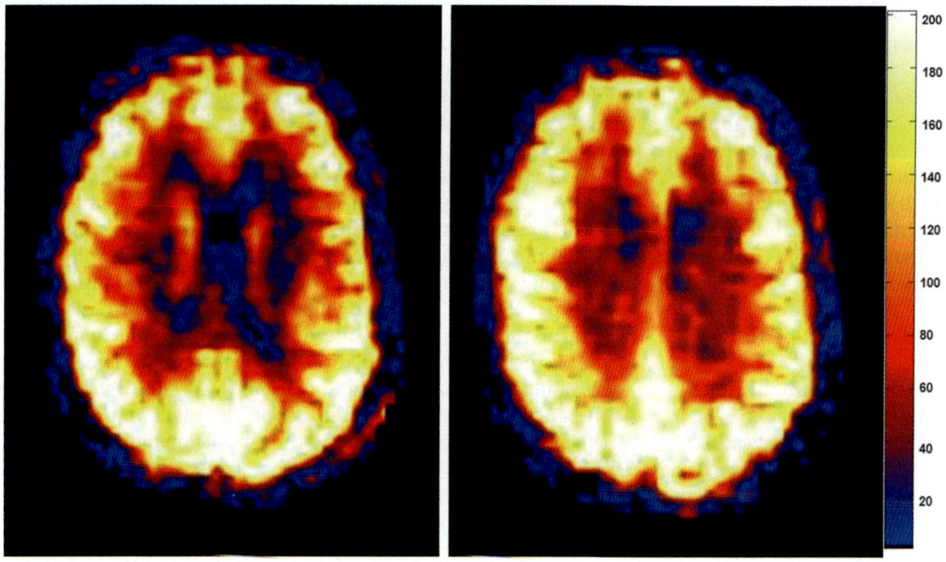

Figure 14-10. **Hypercapnia.** ASL CBF maps demonstrate marked, symmetric bihemispheric hyperperfusion. Conventional MRI images were normal (not shown). The PCO_2 measurement on arterial blood gas performed before the MRI was 72.5 mm Hg (normal range 35 to 45 mm Hg). Mean CBF of the gray matter was 158.9 mL/100 g/min.

increases in the partial pressure of CO_2 can cause substantial changes on perfusion imaging[50] (Fig. 14.10). Improvement of CBF following carotid endarterectomy can cause ipsilateral or bilateral hemispheric hyperperfusion.[51,52] Studies have shown that the degree of hyperemia is inversely related to the baseline CBF; that is, increases in CBF after carotid endarterectomy revascularization were greater when the preoperative CBF was lower.[51]

Vascular Malformations

Cerebral vascular malformations, in particular arteriovenous malformations (AVMs), are associated with significant morbidity and potential for neurologic disability due to the risk of hemorrhage, as the low resistance in the AVM causes very high flow through the malformed vessels that can be 10 times greater than normal brain parenchyma. An unruptured AVM carries a 2% to 3% risk of hemorrhage per year, 1% risk of death per year, and 10% mortality with the first hemorrhage. Moreover, the mortality rate associated with a second hemorrhage is roughly 13% and up to 20% for subsequent hemorrhages.[53] The flow diversion that occurs through large AVMs can result in hypotension in the adjacent tissues as a steal phenomenon, which may be associated with neurologic deficits in the absence of hemorrhage.

AVMs are treated by embolization, surgery, radiosurgery, or sometimes by a combination of methods in planned stages. Delineation of the anatomy and vascular supply of an AVM is readily achieved with digital subtraction, CT, and MR angiography. Assessment of the magnitude of vascular steal from or degree of hypoperfusion within the tissues surrounding an AVM is also important for treatment planning and monitoring response to therapy.[54–56]

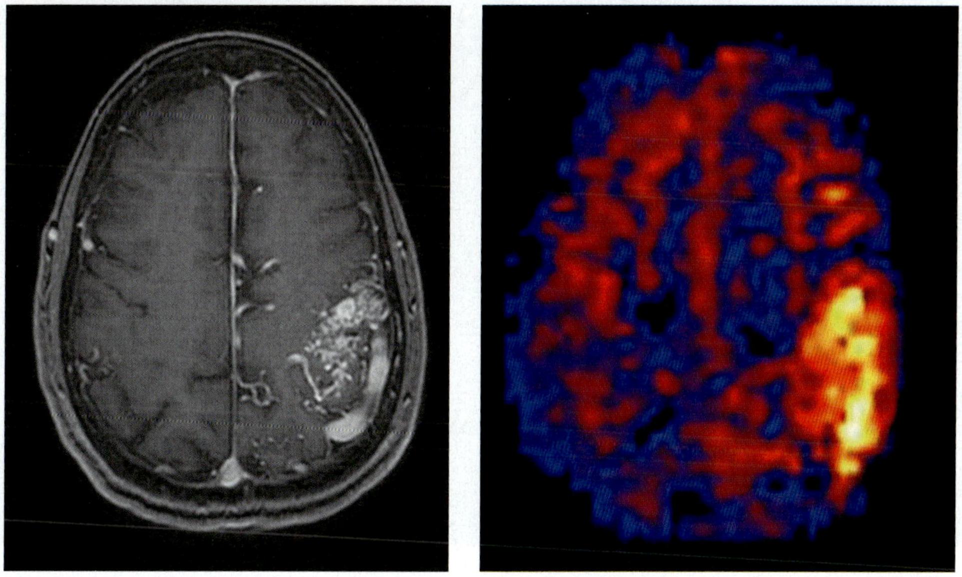

A B

Figure 14-11. **Arteriovenous malformation.** Axial postcontrast T1-weighted image **(A)** demonstrates a large arteriovenous malformation in the left posterior frontal and parietal lobes with large draining vein over the left parietal lobe. ASL CBF map **(B)** shows corresponding hyperperfusion of the malformation.

Angiographic techniques are unable to provide quantitative assessment of these parameters, but ASL perfusion techniques have been used successfully.[57–59]

Crusher gradients can significantly influence the appearance of vascular malformations on ASL perfusion images. The shunting of labeled blood through the nidus of an AVM without an intervening capillary bed usually results in hyperintense signal in the nidus and draining veins (Fig. 14.11). If large crusher gradients are applied when imaging an AVM, the signal in the draining veins can be eliminated, whereas ASL images obtained without the use of crusher gradients demonstrate intense signal in the draining veins.[16] Embolic material used in the treatment of AVMs and hemorrhage can result in regions of apparent decreased or absent perfusion of an AVM due to susceptibility artifacts.

ASL signal is not usually seen in the venous system due to the decay of the tag when passing through the capillary bed. Le et al.[60] found that the presence of venous ASL signal on nonvascular-suppressed PCASL imaging suggested the presence of a direct arteriovenous connection and facilitated the detection of small vascular malformations.

Posterior Reversible Encephalopathy Syndrome

Posterior reversible encephalopathy syndrome (PRES) is a cerebrovascular disorder that can present with a variety of nonspecific symptoms including headache, nausea and vomiting, altered level of consciousness, visual abnormalities, seizures, and/or focal neurologic deficits. The conditions associated with PRES are many and include hypertension, preeclampsia and eclampsia, acute renal failure, sepsis and shock, autoimmune conditions, and ingestion of neurotoxic or immunosuppressive drugs such as cyclosporine and tacrolimus.

There is no consensus regarding the pathogenesis of PRES.[61,62] However, PRES is probably related to vascular endothelial dysfunction under the influence of numerous diseases and drugs/toxins with subsequent loss of cerebral autoregulation and failure to maintain compartmentalization of fluid within the intravascular space.[63] PRES is typified by bilateral and symmetric vasogenic edema of the subcortical white matter of the parenchyma supplied by the posterior circulation, especially the parietooccipital lobes, and, as the name implies, is usually reversible (Fig. 14.12). If the underlying cause of PRES is not identified and addressed, it can progress to overt infarction. Atypical imaging findings of PRES such as involvement of the deep gray nuclei, frontotemporal lobes, hemorrhage, and contrast enhancement can also be seen.[64] Perfusion imaging with PRES demonstrates both hypoperfusion and hyperperfusion, depending on the duration and severity of the illness.[63] PRES tends to demonstrate hyperperfusion when imaged in the acute phase and hypoperfusion when imaged in the subacute phase[16] (Fig. 14.12). Nonetheless, the reproducible nature of ASL perfusion imaging makes it an ideal method for evaluation of PRES, as it allows serial imaging to be performed to monitor the response to therapy.

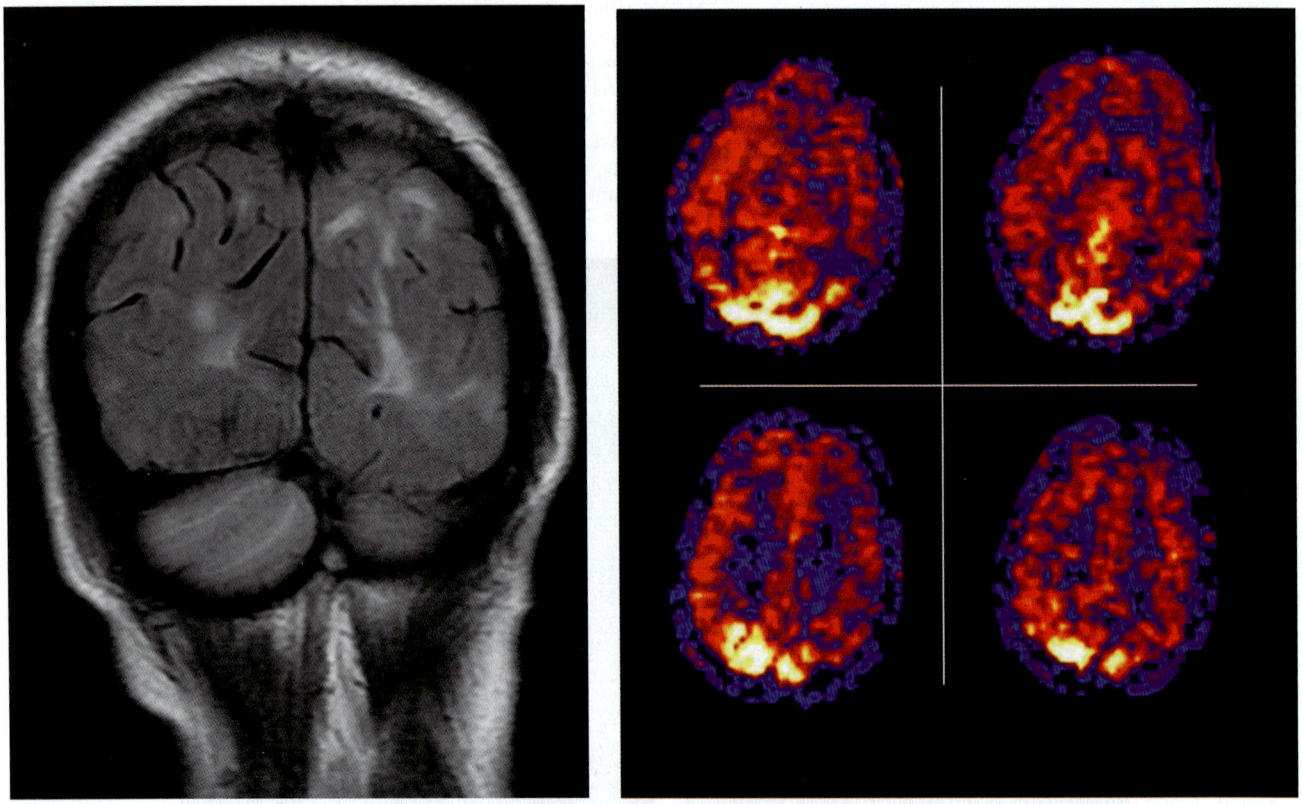

A B

Figure 14-12. Posterior reversible encephalopathy syndrome (PRES). **A:** T2/FLAIR coronal image demonstrates hyperintense signal in the subcortical white matter of the bilateral occipital lobes and right cerebellar hemisphere. The involvement of the subcortical white matter is characteristic of PRES. **B:** ASL CBF maps show relatively symmetric hyperperfusion of the occipital lobes bilaterally. The patient had a systolic blood pressure greater than 220 mm Hg at the time of presentation.

Migraine

Migraines are a neurovascular disorder characterized by recurrent unilateral headaches that can be accompanied by phonophobia, photophobia, nausea, and vomiting.[65] The precise pathogenesis of a migraine is still an ardently debated topic.[66,67] The vascular theory of migraine pathogenesis postulates that the aura is associated with arteriolar vasoconstriction and the subsequent headache is associated with vasodilation and hyperperfusion. A second theory hypothesizes that a wave of neuronal depression, known as cortical spreading depression, contiguously extends over the affected cortex and results in the symptoms. The alterations in perfusion are thought to be the response of the cerebrovascular autoregulatory mechanisms to the neuronal depression.[68] Regardless of the exact pathogenic mechanism, alterations in cerebral perfusion during the aura and headache phases of a migraine have been reported[69–71] (Fig. 14.13).

Patients may be imaged in the aura phase of a migraine because the presenting symptoms can mimic cerebral infarction. Images obtained during the aura phase demonstrate regional hypoperfusion in the cortex corresponding to the aura symptoms. However, regional hyperperfusion may be seen in the affected cortex if

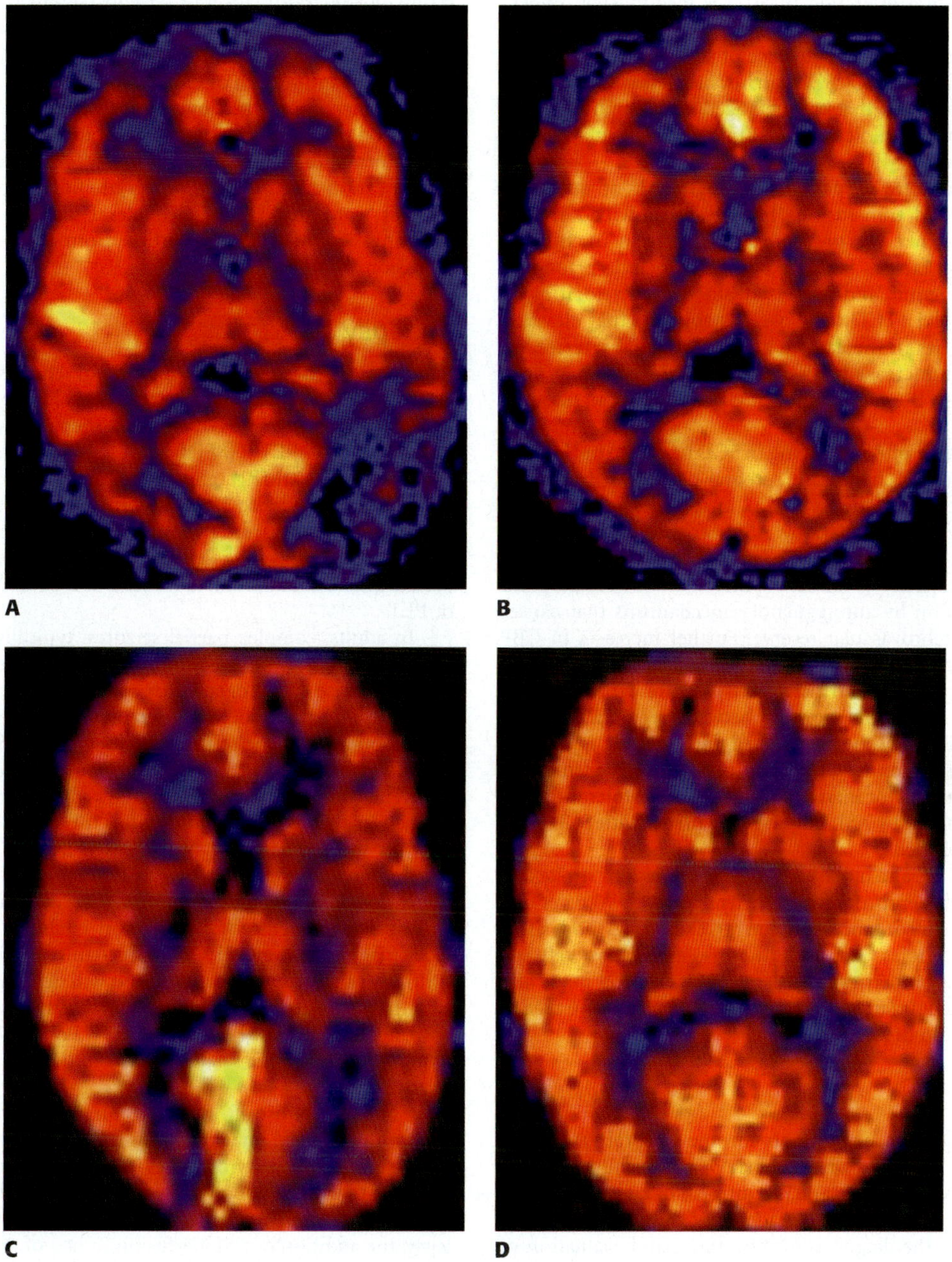

Figure 14-13. Migraine headaches on ASL. **A:** ASL CBF map on the top left shows decreased perfusion of the left occipital lobe with normal appearance of the brain on conventional sequences (not shown). The patient presented with headache and weakness and was imaged due to concerns for an infarct. Given the findings on imaging, the patient was treated for a migraine and discharged. **B:** The follow-up ASL CBF shows normal perfusion. **C:** ASL map from a different patient shows increased perfusion to the right parasagittal occipital lobe. This patient had a history of migraines but was imaged due to worsening headaches. **D:** Follow-up ASL image shows normalization of perfusion.

images are obtained during the headache phase.[71] It is imperative to correlate the perfusion images with conventional MRI sequences because these changes can also be seen with seizure, infarction, and meningitis.[71]

Sickle Cell Disease

Sickle cell disease (SCD) is a hereditary hemoglobinopathy that is characterized by chronic hemolytic anemia and vascular occlusion. SCD has a variety of manifestations in the brain including silent infarcts, areas of high signal intensity seen on MRI without focal neurologic deficits, and overt clinical stroke.[72] Though the pathophysiology of cerebral infarction in SCD is incompletely understood, it is a well-recognized and important complication of SCD.[73] In fact, SCD is the most frequent cause of stroke in children, and changes in the brain caused by SCD can be observed at a very young age.[74] Wang et al.[75] found that children aged 7 to 48 months with SCD and no history of clinical stroke can have silent infarcts and large vessel stenoses by MRI.

Identification of SCD patients at high risk of stroke is imperative, as blood transfusions have been shown to reduce the risk of a first stroke and prevent recurrent stroke in children with SCD.[76,77] Risk factors for stroke in SCD include prior history of infarct, anemia, and increased blood flow velocities by transcranial Doppler (TCD). It is well established that elevated blood flow velocities in the carotid and intracranial arteries are associated with an increased risk of stroke, and TCD imaging is widely employed in the surveillance of CBF velocities in patients with SCD.[78]

Although the role of ASL imaging in SCD has yet to be defined, the acute and chronic changes in cerebral perfusion that result from SCD have been described with ASL imaging. Hyperperfusion observed in patients with SCD by ASL perfusion imaging is a response to and a risk factor for cerebral hypoxia due to reduced oxygen-carrying capacity of the blood. Increased CBF results from adaptive vasodilation by autoregulatory mechanisms that causes a reduction in cerebrovascular reserve. Further increases in CBF demand or decreases in oxygen delivery as a result of worsening anemia or a drop in cerebral perfusion pressure can cause distal infarction. An inverse relationship between regional CBF and intelligence quotient has been reported in SCD.[79] It is feasible that direct quantification of CBF could play a role in identifying patients who are at risk for infarction, and reference tolerance limits of CBF determined by ASL in low-risk patients with SCD have recently been published.[80]

Silent infarcts are also a marker for increased risk of stroke and are associated with neurocognitive deficits. However, Wang et al.[81] found a lack of concordance between TCD findings and silent infarcts on MRI. Studies have also found no association between the hemispheric asymmetries in CBF on ASL perfusion maps and the presence of silent infarcts. This continues to be an active area of research in perfusion imaging.

Moyamoya

Moyamoya disease is an uncommon chronic cerebral vasculopathy characterized by progressive stenosis of the terminal portion of the internal carotid arteries and recruitment of collateral vessels to compensate for the lack of antegrade flow.[82] Angiographic techniques are used in the diagnosis of moyamoya and evaluation of collateral vessel formation. Criteria for the diagnosis of moyamoya disease by angiography have been established and include stenosis or occlusion of the terminal portions of the internal carotid artery or proximal segments of the anterior or middle cerebral arteries, abnormal collateral vessels in the vascular territories supplied by the stenotic or occluded vessels, and bilateral findings.[83] Moyamoya syndrome is the term applied when the above imaging findings coexist with other conditions that could potentially explain the vasculopathy such as neurofibromatosis type 1, trisomy 21, and SCD.

Serial imaging is often employed to monitor disease progression and identify individuals who would potentially benefit from surgical revascularization. However, the severity of cerebrovascular stenosis on angiography does not necessarily predict the hemodynamic status of the tissue, and angiography cannot provide a quantitative assessment of CBF.[84] ASL perfusion imaging has been utilized in the evaluation of moyamoya with some success, but the sensitivity of conventional ASL imaging to transit time delays results in underestimation of CBF in regions supplied by the stenotic vessels[85,86] (Fig. 14.14). The use of a moderately long PLD can overcome the limitations imposed by the transit time delays and allow the quantification of CBF.

Visualization of the slow intravascular flow can help with the evaluation of Moyamoya by demonstrating the extent of collateral vessel formation. Moreover, the use of vessel selective ASL techniques can distinguish slow antegrade flow through a high-grade stenosis from that through collateral pathways and even allow quantification of the contribution from each vessel to regional perfusion.[87,88]

Epilepsy

Patients presenting with a history of epilepsy often undergo extensive testing, including electroencephalography (EEG), magnetoencephalography (MEG), electrocorticography (ECoG), 18fluorodeoxyglucose PET (18FDG PET), SPECT, conventional MRI, functional MRI (fMRI), and/or intracarotid sodium amobarbital procedure (ISAP), also known as the Wada test. A large body of literature exists regarding the use of nuclear medicine perfusion imaging techniques in the evaluation of epilepsy, and the standard pre-surgical evaluation includes ictal SPECT and interictal SPECT or PET.

In adults, complex partial seizures, typically arising from the temporal lobe, are the most common cause of medically intractable seizures. These epileptogenic foci demonstrate decreased metabolic rate and blood flow between seizures and increased metabolism and blood flow during seizure activity (Fig. 14.15).

SPECT imaging is well suited to the ictal evaluation of seizure foci. The most commonly employed radiotracers have a first-pass extraction that is proportionate to CBF and do not redistribute once in the brain. These properties allow the radiotracer to be administered at the onset of seizure activity and imaged shortly thereafter.[4] The 110-minute half-life of ^{18}FDG limits the utility of PET in ictal imaging. ASL perfusion is also of limited utility in ictal imaging. However, it is well recognized that ASL images fortuitously obtained in the ictal period will demonstrate hyperperfusion that correlates with the hypermetabolism/hyperperfusion seen with nuclear medicine techniques.[89–91] Pollock et al.[90] found that hyperperfusion of the seizure focus can be seen up to 1 hour after seizure onset.

The real promise of ASL perfusion in the evaluation of epilepsy rests with interictal imaging. It has been shown that ASL perfusion can detect interictal asymmetries in mesial temporal lobe perfusion in patients with temporal lobe epilepsy[92] (Fig. 14.15). As conventional MRI is often performed in the evaluation of patients with epilepsy, the addition of ASL perfusion in lieu of an interictal nuclear medicine examination could spare the patient time, cost, and ionizing radiation dose. Despite the fact that ASL perfusion imaging is not a first-line technique employed in ictal and interictal imaging, seizure-related perfusion abnormalities are not uncommonly encountered in clinical practice and should be recognized to avoid potential misdiagnosis.

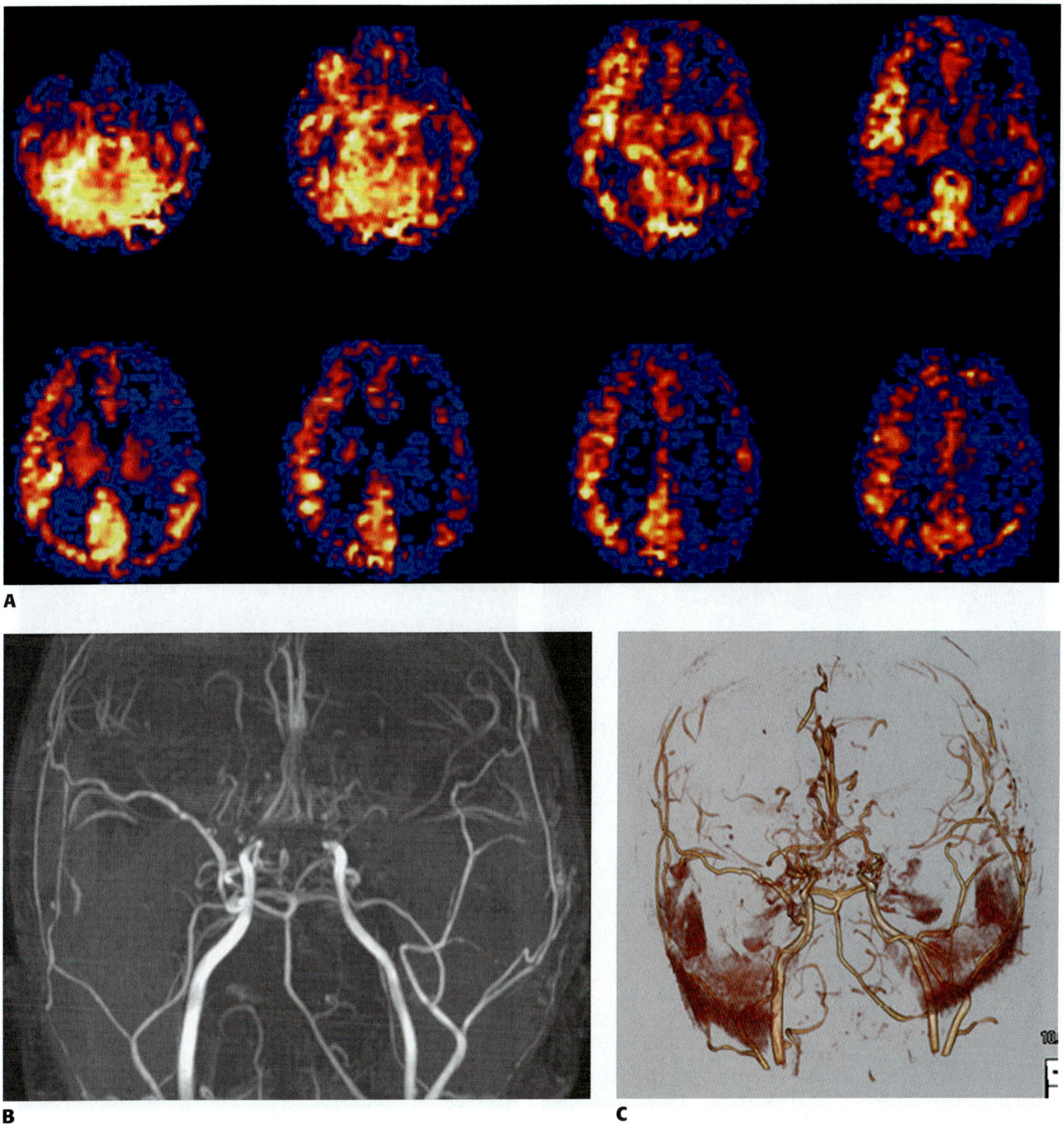

Figure 14-14. Moyamoya disease. **A:** ASL CBF images show hypoperfusion in the territories of the middle and anterior cerebral arteries bilaterally, left more so than right. Coronal MIP **(B)** and 3-D MR angiographic **(C)** images show marked narrowing of the bilateral supraclinoid carotid arteries with attenuation flow in the M1 segment of both the middle cerebral arteries and the A1 and A2 segments of both anterior cerebral arteries. Note the persistent right trigeminal artery from which the right middle meningeal artery arises. The right trigeminal artery supplies a large portion of the posterior circulation, as the right vertebral artery terminates in a posterior inferior cerebellar artery branch.

Neuro-Oncologic Applications

ASL perfusion imaging has a role in the initial diagnosis and grading of a lesion, guidance of stereotactic biopsy, and surveillance of a lesion after treatment.[16,44,48,93] MR perfusion imaging performed in the evaluation of intracranial neoplasms has traditionally utilized DSC-MRI techniques, and several studies have demonstrated a strong intermodality correlation between ASL and DSC-MRI perfusion values, CBF and relative CBV, respectively, in both normal tissues and intracranial neoplasms.[23,94–96] ASL perfusion may allow a more accurate assessment of perfusion in glioblastomas, as it is theoretically less influenced by breakdown of the blood–brain barrier (BBB) and relatively less vulnerable to susceptibility effects than is DSC-MRI due to the reliance of DSC-MRI on T2* effects.[95]

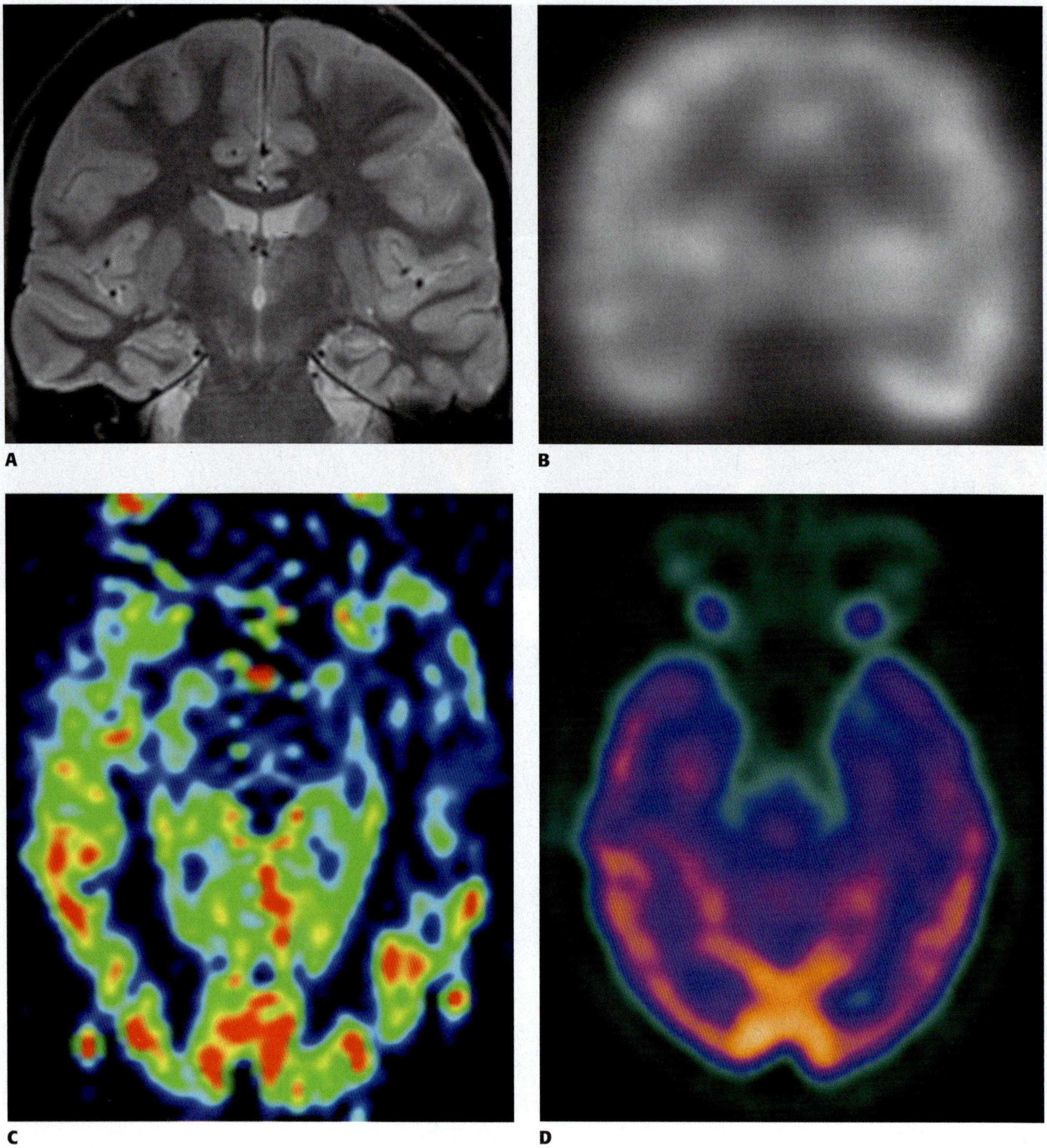

Figure 14-15. Mesial temporal sclerosis. **A:** T2-weighted coronal oblique image shows a small left hippocampus with indistinctness of the internal architecture and faintly increased T2 signal consistent with mesial temporal sclerosis. **B:** Ictal SPECT image shows increased activity in the left temporal lobe representing the seizure focus. **C:** ASL CBF map shows hypoperfusion of the left temporal lobe. **D:** Interictal PET image shows decreased activity in the left temporal lobe that is similar to the area of hypoperfusion on ASL.

It bears mentioning that intraparenchymal enhancement following the administration of gadolinium-based contrast material does not necessarily reflect regional perfusion. Intraparenchymal contrast enhancement simply represents breakdown of the BBB. While it is true that enhancement of a lesion is associated with higher-grade tumors and is a useful feature to consider when predicting the grade of a tumor on MRI, it does not necessarily reflect areas of neoangiogenesis. Tumors with a high degree of neovascularization can demonstrate hyperperfusion without associated enhancement[97] (Fig. 14.16). Thus, the enhancing portions of a lesion are not necessarily the most malignant portions of the tumor. This fact becomes important to consider when planning stereotactic biopsy in order to avoid potential sampling error and misdiagnosis of tumor grade.

Hyperperfusion of intracranial lesions has a high positive predictive value for the diagnosis of a neoplasm, but not all hyperperfused lesions are neoplasms.[97,98] Figure 14.17 shows characteristic

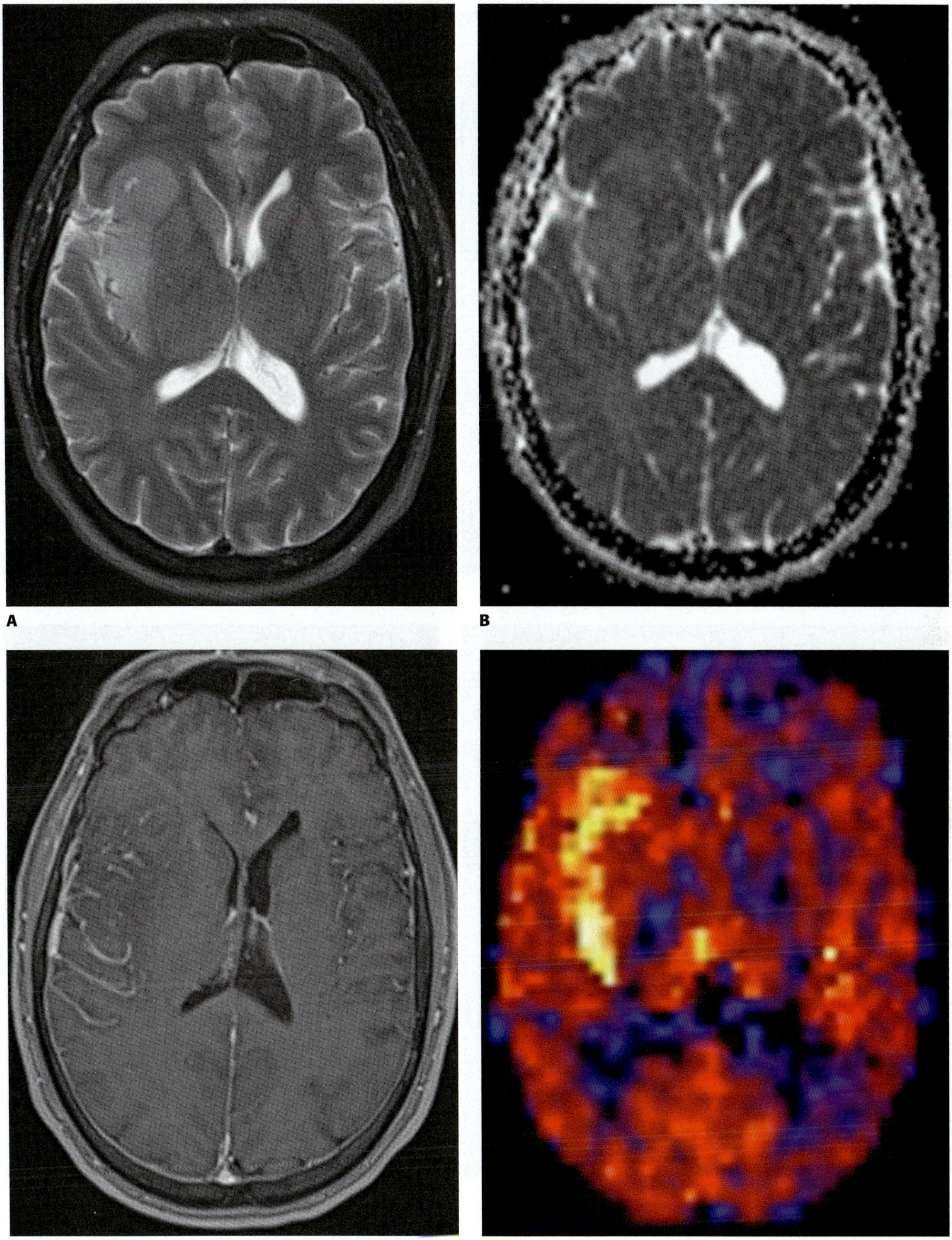

Figure 14-16. Hyperperfusion of a high-grade neoplasm without contrast enhancement. **A:** Infiltrative mass in the right insula demonstrates hyperintense signal on the T2-weighted image. There is no evidence of low signal intensity on the ADC map **(B)** or appreciable enhancement on the T1-weighted postcontrast image **(C)**. However, the ASL CBF map **(D)** shows hyperperfusion of the mass, and subsequent biopsy revealed glioblastoma (WHO grade IV).

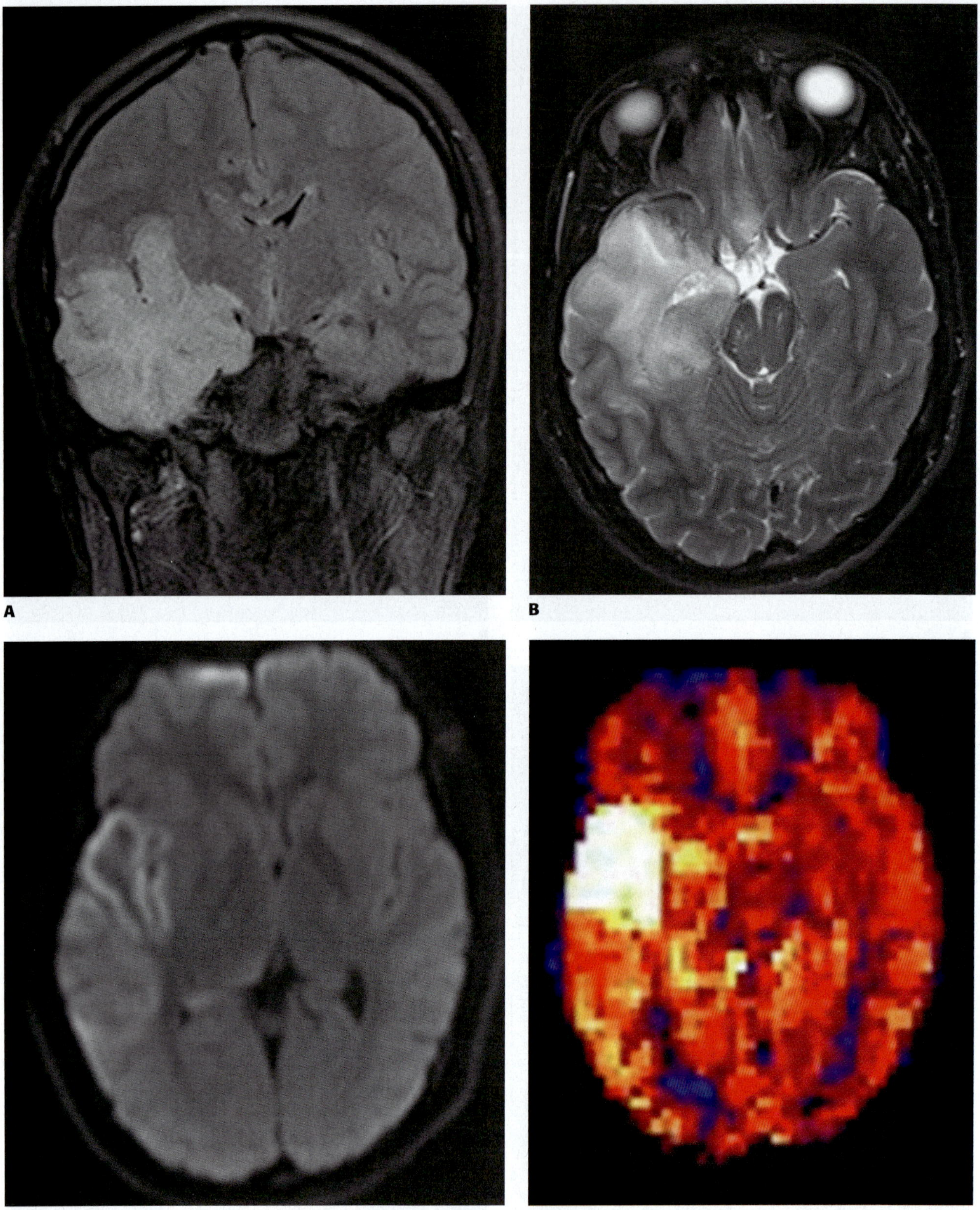

A B C D

Figure 14-17. Herpes encephalitis. Coronal T2/FLAIR image **(A)** and T2-weighted axial fat-saturated images **(B)** show hyperintense signal in the right temporal lobe, hippocampus, and insula representing edema that results in local mass effect and uncal medialization with mass effect on the cerebral peduncle. **C:** Axial diffusion-weighted image shows cortical restricted diffusion (ADC not shown) in the right anterior lobe and insula. **D:** ASL CBF map **(bottom right)** demonstrates marked hyperperfusion in the areas of edema.

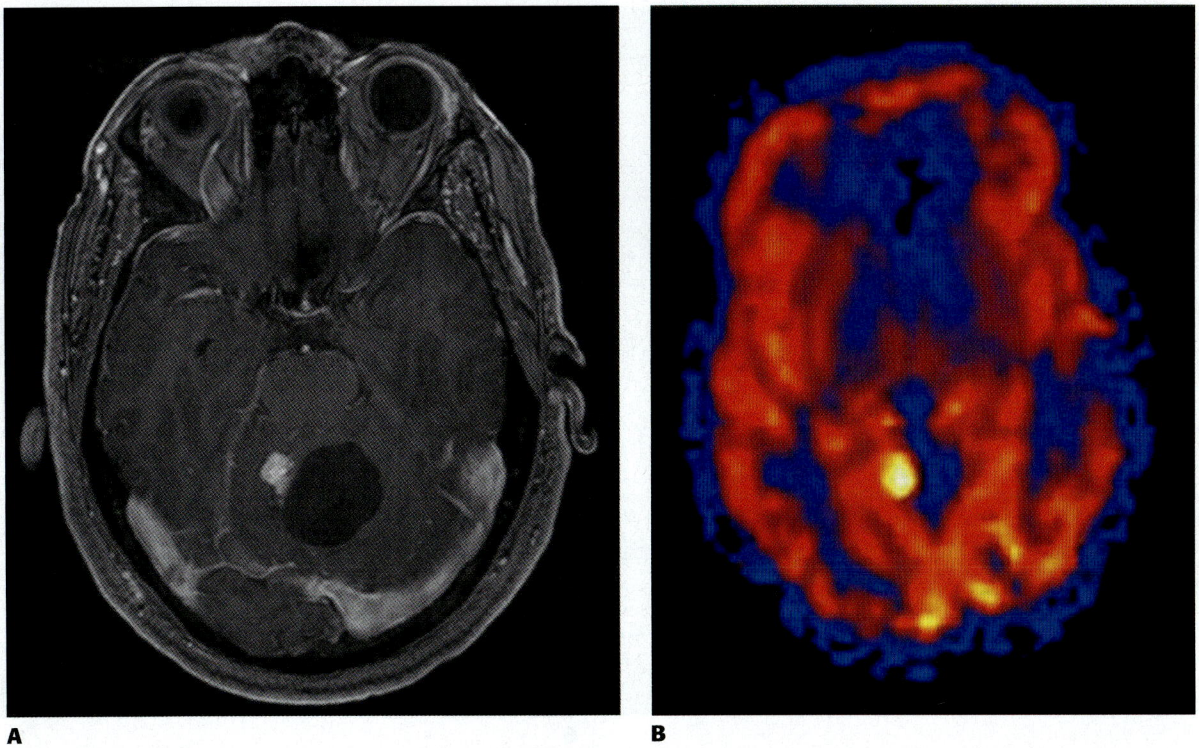

Figure 14-18. Hemangioblastoma. **A:** Axial postcontrast T1-weighted image shows a cystic mass in the cerebellum with an avidly enhancing mural nodule that was proven to represent a hemangioblastoma after surgical resection. **B:** ASL CBF map demonstrates hypoperfusion of the cyst and marked hyperperfusion of the enhancing mural nodule.

abnormal signal in the right temporal lobe with marked hyperperfusion in a patient with herpes encephalitis. Moreover, not all hyperperfused neoplasms are high grade. Meningiomas are a WHO grade I neoplasm characterized by hypervascularity that manifests as intense enhancement following contrast administration and hyperperfusion on ASL imaging. Likewise, the mural nodule classically associated with a hemangioblastoma in the posterior fossa, a WHO grade I tumor, is usually intensely enhancing and markedly hyperperfused by ASL imaging[16] (Fig. 14.18). However, assessment of tumor vascularity is particularly useful in the initial evaluation of glial tumors. Neovascularity is an important histopathologic feature used in the grading of gliomas, and it is well established that a direct relationship exists between tumor vascularity, perfusion, and histologic grade of glial tumors[93–96,99–101]. The direct correlation between histopathologic vascular density and degree of perfusion on ASL imaging in glial tumors allows ASL perfusion imaging to accurately predict the grade of glial tumors [96,102]. Furthermore, changes in tumor blood flow by ASL perfusion imaging after stereotactic radiosurgery were predictive of overall treatment outcome.[103] That is, decreased blood flow after treatment predicted tumor response, whereas increased blood flow predicted tumor progression.

It is imperative to correlate with conventional anatomic images to identify the presence of hemorrhage, calcification, and adjacent metallic hardware that could confound the interpretation of the perfusion images by creating artifactual perfusion defects and masking hyperperfusion of an adjacent neoplasm. An added caveat is that high-grade neoplasms frequently demonstrate heterogeneous perfusion due to the presence of necrosis. As such, these high-grade neoplasms may demonstrate decreased perfusion in areas of necrosis with surrounding hyperperfusion in nonnecrotic portions of the lesion[16] (Fig. 14.19).

Pseudoprogression

Glioblastomas, the most common glial neoplasms in adults, are a malignant WHO grade IV neoplasm typically treated by a combination of surgical debulking and concurrent chemoradiotherapy.[104] Surveillance imaging is routinely performed 12 weeks following the completion of initial treatment to ascertain the response of the lesion to treatment and assess for disease progression, which would alter the course of the remaining therapy.[105] Reliable differentiation between posttreatment changes and tumor progression with conventional MR imaging is challenging, as they can have a similar appearance.[105–109] It is well documented that treated lesions can demonstrate an increase in size and degree of contrast enhancement following treatment that are unrelated to actual tumor progression and stabilize or resolve on subsequent imaging without additional treatment, a phenomenon termed pseudoprogression.[106] These treatment effects are often asymptomatic and occur in up to 20% to 30% of patients treated with the chemotherapeutic agent temozolomide (Temodar), the first-line agent employed in the treatment of glioblastomas.[109,110] The exact pathophysiologic process that results in pseudoprogression has yet to be elucidated, but it likely represents an exaggerated response to chemoradiotherapy-related tumor and endothelial cell killing. Pseudoprogression may potentially lead to a change in effective therapy or unnecessary surgery to definitively differentiate true progression from pseudoprogression. The Response Assessment in Neuro-Oncology Working Group published an updated set of standardized response criteria for high-grade gliomas to address the limitations of the previously employed McDonald criteria, which equated an increase in the contrast-enhancing portions of a lesion to disease progression and mandated a change in therapy.[109]

As with treatment naïve glioblastomas, tumor recurrences demonstrate vascular proliferation, as evidenced by increased

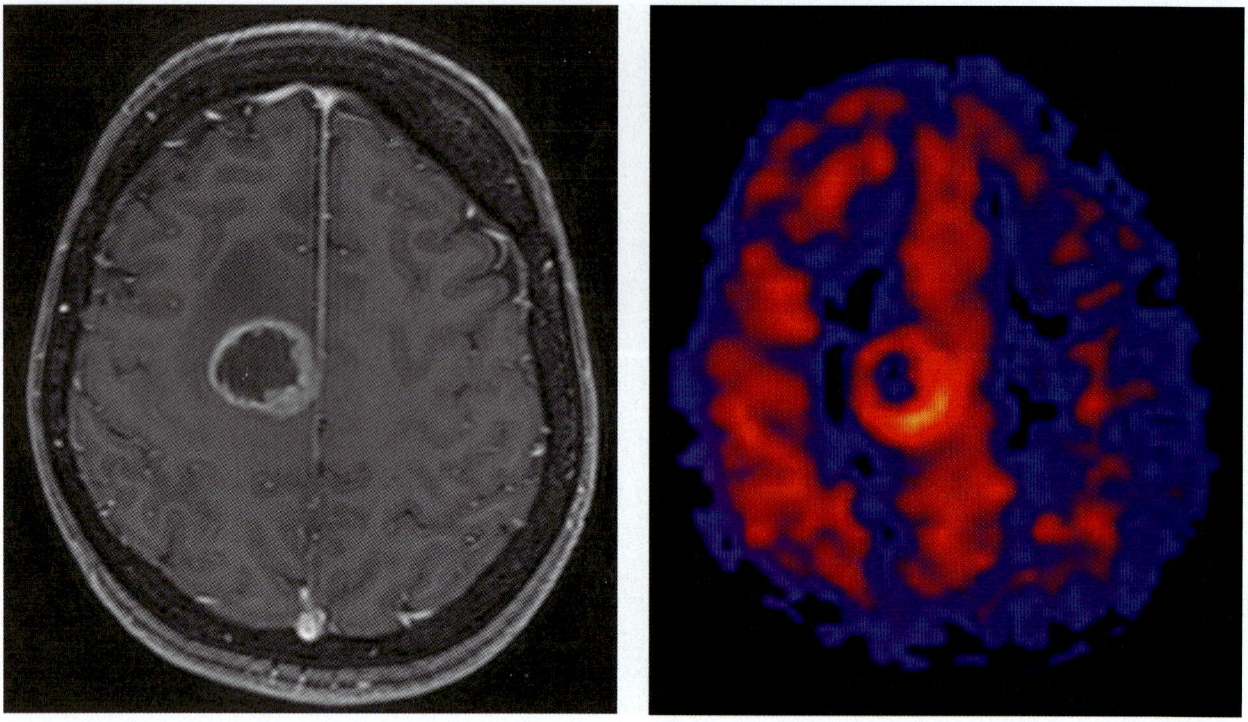

A B

Figure 14-19. Glioblastoma. **A:** Axial postcontrast T1-weighted image with an ovoid, peripherally enhancing mass in the right posterior parasagittal frontal lobe with central necrosis and surrounding edema. **B:** ASL CBF map demonstrates hyperperfusion corresponding to the enhancing tumor and hypoperfusion matching the central necrosis.

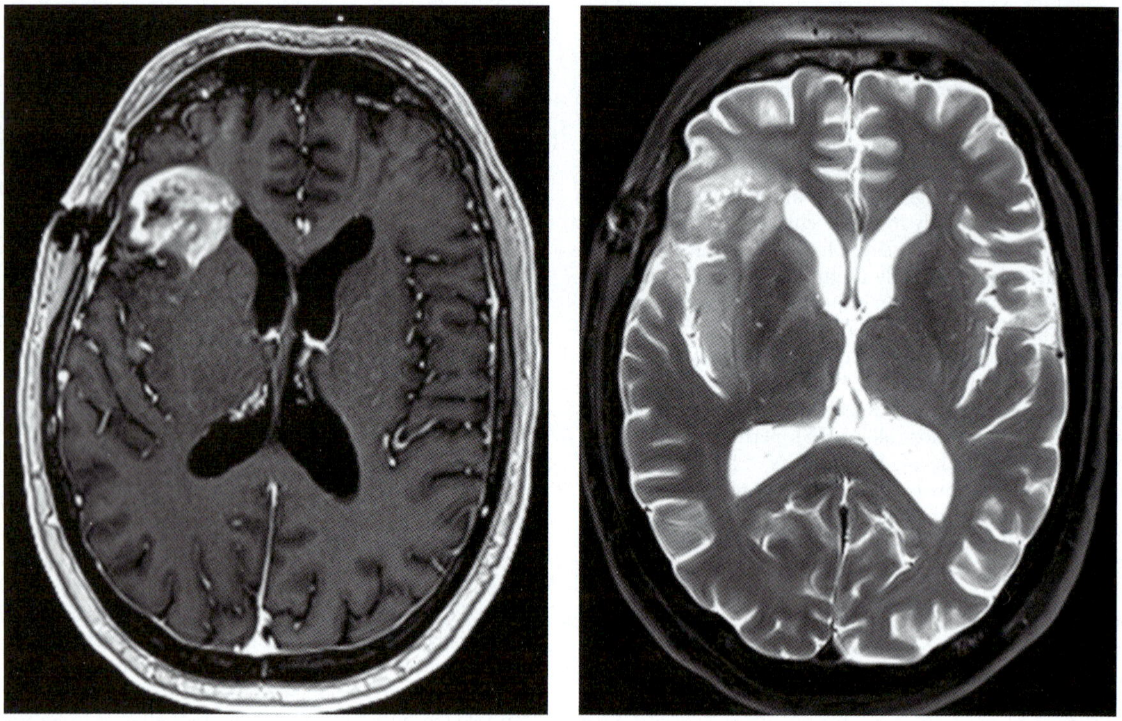

A B

Figure 14-20. Pseudoprogression in a glioblastoma. This examination was obtained 12 weeks following surgical debulking and completion of concurrent chemoradiotherapy with temozolomide. **A:** T1-weighted postcontrast image shows an avidly enhancing mass lesion in the right frontal lobe resection cavity. Note the postsurgical changes in the overlying calvarium and soft tissues. **B:** The T2-weighted image shows heterogeneous T2 signal in the area of enhancement with surrounding edema and local mass effect.

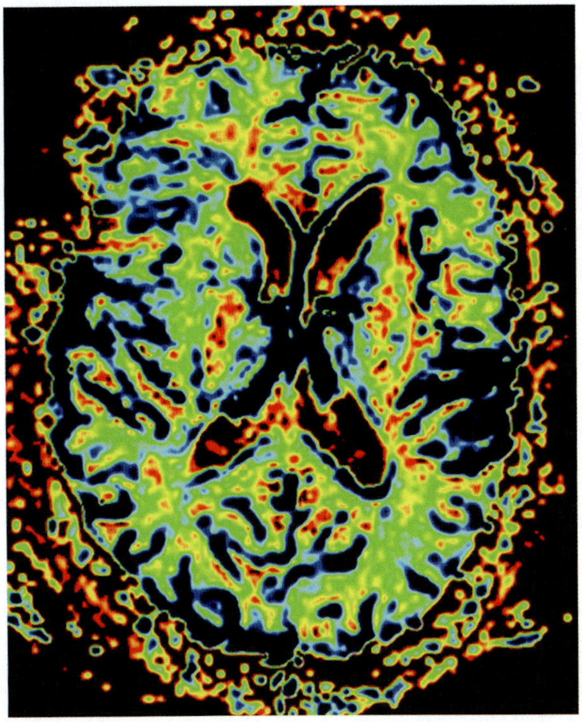

C

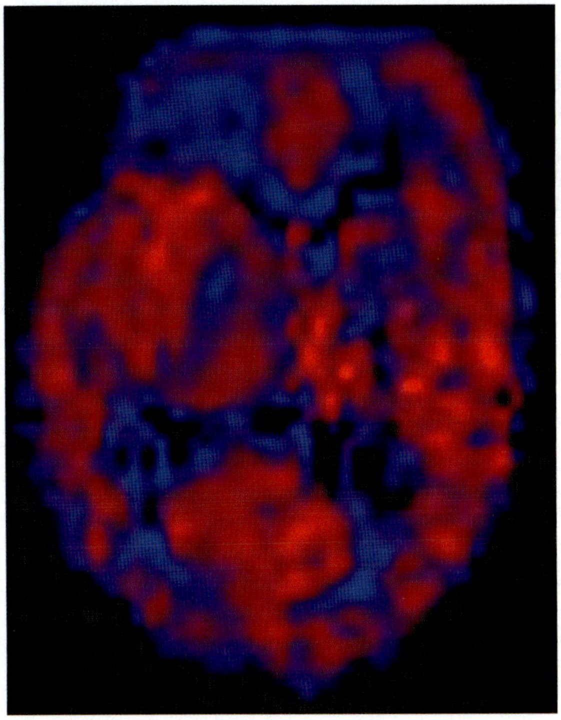

D

Figure 14-20. (*Continued*) **C:** The DSC-MRI rCBV map shows some heterogeneous signal in the resection cavity. **D:** The ASL CBF map reveals that there is minimal perfusion to the area of enhancement. Subsequent stereotactic biopsy revealed pseudoprogression.

vascular density on histopathologic analysis. However, pseudoprogression is characterized by vascular dilation and extensive fibrinoid necrosis within the treatment bed as well as endothelial injury within normal surrounding vasculature. Tumor progression therefore may manifest as increased blood flow on perfusion imaging, and pseudoprogression may manifest as decreased or absent perfusion with respect to normal brain (Fig. 14.20). However, perfusion analysis is only one facet of the evaluation of treated lesions and does not correlate with disease progression/response at all times. The interpretation of MR perfusion imaging in glioblastomas after treatment is confounded by susceptibility artifacts that result from the presence of intralesional hemorrhage or hemosiderin. Although ASL perfusion techniques are vulnerable to susceptibility artifacts, they are less so than is DSC-MRI. Nonetheless, these two perfusion techniques may have a complementary relationship, as Choi et al.[106] found that the combination of ASL and DSC-MRI improved the diagnostic accuracy in differentiating pseudoprogression from early tumor recurrence. The use of MRI perfusion techniques, including ASL and DSC-MRI, to differentiate treatment-related changes from pseudoprogression remains an active area of research.

Conclusions

ASL perfusion imaging has wide-ranging clinical applications in the field of neuroradiology and supplements conventional anatomic sequences with physiologic information. Understanding the basic technical aspects and methods of implementation of the technique are essential for the correct interpretation of the ASL images. The reproducibility and quantitative nature of the technique will continue to drive new developments and increase widespread clinical implementation of ASL perfusion imaging.

REFERENCES

1. **van Beek AH, Claassen JA, Rikkert MG, et al.** Cerebral autoregulation: an overview of current concepts and methodology with special focus on the elderly. *J Cereb Blood Flow Metab* 2008;28(6):1071–1085.
2. **Kety SS, Schmidt CF.** The determination of cerebral blood flow in man by the use of nitrous oxide in low concentrations. *Am J Physiol—Legacy Content* 1945;143(1):53–66.
3. **Kety SS, Schmidt CF.** The nitrous oxide method for the quantitative determination of cerebral blood flow in man: theory, procedure and normal values. *J Clin Invest* 1948;27(4):476–483.
4. **Mettler FA, Guiberteau MJ.** *Essentials of nuclear medicine imaging.* 5th ed. Philadelphia, PA: Saunders/Elsevier; 2006.
5. **Grobner T.** Gadolinium—a specific trigger for the development of nephrogenic fibrosing dermopathy and nephrogenic systemic fibrosis. *Nephrol Dial Transplant* 2006;21(4):1104–1108.
6. **Swaminathan S, Horn TD, Pellowski D, et al.** Nephrogenic systemic fibrosis, gadolinium, and iron mobilization. *N Engl J Med* 2007;357(7): 720–722.
7. **Wolf RL, Detre JA.** Clinical neuroimaging using arterial spin-labeled perfusion magnetic resonance imaging. *Neurotherapeutics* 2007;4(3): 346–359.
8. **Hendrikse J, van der Grond J, Lu H, et al.** Flow territory mapping of the cerebral arteries with regional perfusion MRI. *Stroke* 2004;35(4): 882–887.
9. **Hendrikse J, Petersen ET, Cheze A, et al.** Relation between cerebral perfusion territories and location of cerebral infarcts. *Stroke* 2009;40(5):1617–1622.
10. **Golay X, Hendrikse J, Lim TC.** Perfusion imaging using arterial spin labeling. *Top Magn Reson Imaging* 2004;15(1):10–27.
11. **Maldjian JA, Laurienti PJ, Burdette JH, et al.** Clinical implementation of spin-tag perfusion magnetic resonance imaging. *J Comput Assist Tomogr* 2008;32(3):403–406.
12. **Petersen ET, Zimine I, Ho Y-CL, et al.** Non-invasive measurement of perfusion: a critical review of arterial spin labelling techniques. *Br J Radiol* 2006;79(944):688–701.

13. **Deibler AR, Pollock JM, Kraft RA, et al.** Arterial spin-labeling in routine clinical practice, Part 1: technique and artifacts. *AJNR Am J Neuroradiol* 2008;29(7):1228–1234.
14. **McGehee BE, Pollock JM, Maldjian JA.** Brain perfusion imaging: how does it work and what should I use? *J Magn Reson Imaging* 2012;36(6):1257–1272.
15. **Petcharunpaisan S, Ramalho J, Castillo M.** Arterial spin labeling in neuroimaging. *World J Radiol* 2010;2(10):384–398.
16. **Pollock JM, Tan H, Kraft RA, et al.** Arterial spin-labeled MR perfusion imaging: clinical applications. *Magn Reson Imaging Clin N Am* 2009;17(2):315–338.
17. **Detre JA, Rao H, Wang DJ, et al.** Applications of arterial spin labeled MRI in the brain. *J Magn Reson Imaging* 2012;35(5):1026–1037.
18. **Fernandez-Seara MA, Wang Z, Wang J, et al.** Continuous arterial spin labeling perfusion measurements using single shot 3D GRASE at 3 T. *Magn Reson Med* 2005;54(5):1241–1247.
19. **Hernandez-Garcia L, Lee GR, Vazquez AL, et al.** Quantification of perfusion fMRI using a numerical model of arterial spin labeling that accounts for dynamic transit time effects. *Magn Reson Med* 2005;54(4):955–964.
20. **Paiva FF, Tannus A, Silva AC.** Measurement of cerebral perfusion territories using arterial spin labelling. *NMR Biomed* 2007;20(7):633–642.
21. **Okell TW, Chappell MA, Kelly ME, et al.** Cerebral blood flow quantification using vessel-encoded arterial spin labeling. *J Cereb Blood Flow Metab* 2013;33(11):1716–1724.
22. **Tan H, Maldjian JA, Pollock JM, et al.** A fast, effective filtering method for improving clinical pulsed arterial spin labeling MRI. *J Magn Reson Imaging* 2009;29(5):1134–1139.
23. **Jarnum H, Steffensen EG, Knutsson L, et al.** Perfusion MRI of brain tumours: a comparative study of pseudo-continuous arterial spin labelling and dynamic susceptibility contrast imaging. *Neuroradiology* 2010;52(4):307–317.
24. **Weinmann HJ, Brasch RC, Press WR, et al.** Characteristics of gadolinium-DTPA complex: a potential NMR contrast agent. *AJR Am J Roentgenol* 1984;142(3):619–624.
25. **Wolf GL, Fobben ES.** The tissue proton T1 and T2 response to gadolinium DTPA injection in rabbits. A potential renal contrast agent for NMR imaging. *Invest Radiol* 1984;19(4):324–328.
26. **De Vis JB, Petersen ET, de Vries LS, et al.** Regional changes in brain perfusion during brain maturation measured non-invasively with arterial spin labeling MRI in neonates. *Eur J Radiol* 2013;82(3):538–543.
27. **Biagi L, Abbruzzese A, Bianchi MC, et al.** Age dependence of cerebral perfusion assessed by magnetic resonance continuous arterial spin labeling. *J Magn Reson Imaging* 2007;25(4):696–702.
28. **Ferre JC, Bannier E, Raoult H, et al.** Arterial spin labeling (ASL) perfusion: techniques and clinical use. *Diagn Interv Imaging* 2013;94(12):1211–1223.
29. **Campbell AM, Beaulieu C.** Pulsed arterial spin labeling parameter optimization for an elderly population. *J Magn Reson Imaging* 2006;23(3):398–403.
30. **Roberts DA, Detre JA, Bolinger L, et al.** Quantitative magnetic resonance imaging of human brain perfusion at 1.5 T using steady-state inversion of arterial water. *Proc Natl Acad Sci U S A* 1994;91(1):33–37.
31. **van Osch MJ, Teeuwisse WM, van Walderveen MA, et al.** Can arterial spin labeling detect white matter perfusion signal? *Magn Reson Med* 2009;62(1):165–173.
32. **Watts JM, Whitlow CT, Maldjian JA.** Clinical applications of arterial spin labeling. *NMR Biomed* 2013;26(8):892–900.
33. **Chalela JA, Alsop DC, Gonzalez-Atavales JB, et al.** Magnetic resonance perfusion imaging in acute ischemic stroke using continuous arterial spin labeling. *Stroke* 2000;31(3):680–687.
34. **Astrup J, Siesjo BK, Symon L.** Thresholds in cerebral ischemia—the ischemic penumbra. *Stroke* 1981;12(6):723–725.
35. **Schlaug G, Benfield A, Baird AE, et al.** The ischemic penumbra: operationally defined by diffusion and perfusion MRI. *Neurology* 1999;53(7):1528–1537.
36. **Harris AD, Coutts SB, Frayne R.** Diffusion and perfusion MR imaging of acute ischemic stroke. *Magn Reson Imaging Clin N Am* 2009;17(2):291–313.
37. **Baron JC.** Perfusion thresholds in human cerebral ischemia: historical perspective and therapeutic implications. *Cerebrovasc Dis* 2001;11 (Suppl 1):2–8.
38. **Botteri M, Bandera E, Minelli C, et al.** Cerebral blood flow thresholds for cerebral ischemia in traumatic brain injury. A systematic review. *Crit Care Med* 2008;36(11):3089–3092.
39. **Morawetz RB, Crowell RH, DeGirolami U, et al.** Regional cerebral blood flow thresholds during cerebral ischemia. *Fed Proc* 1979;38(11):2493–2494.
40. **Wolf RL, Alsop DC, McGarvey ML, et al.** Susceptibility contrast and arterial spin labeled perfusion MRI in cerebrovascular disease. *J Neuroimaging* 2003;13(1):17–27.
41. **Weber MA, Gunther M, Lichy MP, et al.** Comparison of arterial spin-labeling techniques and dynamic susceptibility-weighted contrast-enhanced MRI in perfusion imaging of normal brain tissue. *Invest Radiol* 2003;38(11):712–718.
42. **Wang J, Alsop DC, Song HK, et al.** Arterial transit time imaging with flow encoding arterial spin tagging (FEAST). *Magn Reson Med* 2003;50(3):599–607.
43. **Meng Y, Wang P, Kim SG.** Simultaneous measurement of cerebral blood flow and transit time with turbo dynamic arterial spin labeling (Turbo-DASL): application to functional studies. *Magn Reson Med* 2012;68(3):762–771.
44. **Deibler AR, Pollock JM, Kraft RA, et al.** Arterial spin-labeling in routine clinical practice, Part 2: hypoperfusion patterns. *AJNR Am J Neuroradiol* 2008;29(7):1235–1241.
45. **Zaharchuk G.** Arterial spin label imaging of acute ischemic stroke and transient ischemic attack. *Neuroimaging Clin N Am* 2011;21(2):285–301, x.
46. **Lassen NA.** On the regulation of cerebral blood flow in diseases of the brain with special regard to the "Luxury Perfusion Syndrome" of brain tissue, i.e. a syndrome characterized by relative hyperemia or absolute hyperemia of the brain tissue. *Prog Brain Res* 1968;30:121–124.
47. **Elster AD, Moody DM.** Early cerebral infarction: gadopentetate dimeglumine enhancement. *Radiology* 1990;177(3):627–632.
48. **Deibler AR, Pollock JM, Kraft RA, et al.** Arterial spin-labeling in routine clinical practice, Part 3: Hyperperfusion patterns. *AJNR Am J Neuroradiol* 2008;29(8):1428–1435.
49. **Pollock JM, Whitlow CT, Deibler AR, et al.** Anoxic injury-associated cerebral hyperperfusion identified with arterial spin-labeled MR imaging. *AJNR Am J Neuroradiol* 2008;29(7):1302–1307.
50. **Pollock JM, Deibler AR, Whitlow CT, et al.** Hypercapnia-induced cerebral hyperperfusion: an underrecognized clinical entity. *AJNR Am J Neuroradiol* 2009;30(2):378–385.
51. **Ances BM, McGarvey ML, Abrahams JM, et al.** Continuous arterial spin labeled perfusion magnetic resonance imaging in patients before and after carotid endarterectomy. *J Neuroimaging* 2004;14(2):133–138.
52. **Wagner WH, Cossman DV, Farber A, et al.** Hyperperfusion syndrome after carotid endarterectomy. *Ann Vasc Surg* 2005;19(4):479–486.
53. **Wilkins RH.** Natural history of intracranial vascular malformations: a review. *Neurosurgery* 1985;16(3):421–430.
54. **Kader A, Young WL, Pile-Spellman J, et al.** The influence of hemodynamic and anatomic factors on hemorrhage from cerebral arteriovenous malformations. *Neurosurgery* 1994;34(5):801–807; discussion 807–808.
55. **Suazo L, Foerster B, Fermin R, et al.** Measurement of blood flow in arteriovenous malformations before and after embolization using arterial spin labeling. *Interv Neuroradiol* 2012;18(1):42–48.
56. **Pollock JM, Whitlow CT, Simonds J, et al.** Response of arteriovenous malformations to gamma knife therapy evaluated with pulsed arterial spin-labeling MRI perfusion. *AJR Am J Roentgenol* 2011;196(1):15–22.
57. **Noguchi T, Irie H, Takase Y, et al.** Hemodynamic studies of intracranial dural arteriovenous fistulas using arterial spin-labeling MR imaging. *Interv Neuroradiol* 2010;16(4):409–419.
58. **Ludemann L, Jedrzejewski G, Heidenreich J, et al.** Perfusion imaging of cerebral arteriovenous malformations: a study comparing quantitative continuous arterial spin labeling and dynamic contrast-enhanced magnetic resonance imaging at 3 T. *Magn Reson Imaging* 2011;29(9):1157–1164.
59. **Krainik A, Villien M, Tropres I, et al.** Functional imaging of cerebral perfusion. *Diagn Interv Imaging* 2013;94(12):1259–1278.
60. **Le TT, Fischbein NJ, Andre JB, et al.** Identification of venous signal on arterial spin labeling improves diagnosis of dural arteriovenous fistulas and small arteriovenous malformations. *AJNR Am J Neuroradiol* 2012;33(1):61–68.
61. **Bartynski WS, Boardman JF.** Catheter angiography, MR angiography, and MR perfusion in posterior reversible encephalopathy syndrome. *AJNR Am J Neuroradiol* 2008;29(3):447–455.

62. **Brubaker LM, Smith JK, Lee YZ, et al.** Hemodynamic and permeability changes in posterior reversible encephalopathy syndrome measured by dynamic susceptibility perfusion-weighted MR imaging. *AJNR Am J Neuroradiol* 2005;26(4):825–830.
63. **Feske SK.** Posterior reversible encephalopathy syndrome: a review. *Semin Neurol* 2011;31(2):202–215.
64. **Yoon SD, Cho BM, Oh SM, et al.** Clinical and radiological spectrum of posterior reversible encephalopathy syndrome. *J Cerebrovas Endovasc Neurosurg* 2013;15(3):206–213.
65. **Edvinsson L, Villalon CM, MaassenVanDenBrink A.** Basic mechanisms of migraine and its acute treatment. *Pharmacol Ther* 2012;136(3):319–333.
66. **D'Andrea G, D'Arrigo A, Dalle Carbonare M, et al.** Pathogenesis of migraine: role of neuromodulators. *Headache* 2012;52(7):1155–1163.
67. **Goadsby PJ.** Migraine pathophysiology. *Headache* 2005;45 (Suppl 1): S14–S24.
68. **Lauritzen M.** Cortical spreading depression in migraine. *Cephalalgia* 2001;21(7):757–760.
69. **Friberg L, Olesen J, Lassen NA, et al.** Cerebral oxygen extraction, oxygen consumption, and regional cerebral blood flow during the aura phase of migraine. *Stroke* 1994;25(5):974–979.
70. **Jacob A, Mahavish K, Bowden A, et al.** Imaging abnormalities in sporadic hemiplegic migraine on conventional MRI, diffusion and perfusion MRI and MRS. *Cephalalgia* 2006;26(8):1004–1009.
71. **Pollock JM, Deibler AR, Burdette JH, et al.** Migraine associated cerebral hyperperfusion with arterial spin-labeled MR imaging. *AJNR Am J Neuroradiol* 2008;29(8):1494–1497.
72. **Helton KJ, Paydar A, Glass J, et al.** Arterial spin-labeled perfusion combined with segmentation techniques to evaluate cerebral blood flow in white and gray matter of children with sickle cell anemia. *Pediatr Blood Cancer* 2009;52(1):85–91.
73. **van den Tweel XW, Nederveen AJ, Majoie CB, et al.** Cerebral blood flow measurement in children with sickle cell disease using continuous arterial spin labeling at 3.0-Tesla MRI. *Stroke* 2009;40(3):795–800.
74. **Gevers S, Nederveen AJ, Fijnvandraat K, et al.** Arterial spin labeling measurement of cerebral perfusion in children with sickle cell disease. *J Magn Reson Imaging* 2012;35(4):779–787.
75. **Wang WC, Langston JW, Steen RG, et al.** Abnormalities of the central nervous system in very young children with sickle cell anemia. *J Pediatr* 1998;132(6):994–998.
76. **Adams R, McKie V, Nichols F, et al.** The use of transcranial ultrasonography to predict stroke in sickle cell disease. *N Engl J Med* 1992;326(9):605–610.
77. **Adams RJ, McKie VC, Hsu L, et al.** Prevention of a first stroke by transfusions in children with sickle cell anemia and abnormal results on transcranial Doppler ultrasonography. *N Engl J Med* 1998;339(1):5–11.
78. **Ohene-Frempong K, Weiner SJ, Sleeper LA, et al.** Cerebrovascular accidents in sickle cell disease: rates and risk factors. *Blood* 1998;91(1):288–294.
79. **Pegelow CH, Macklin EA, Moser FG, et al.** Longitudinal changes in brain magnetic resonance imaging findings in children with sickle cell disease. *Blood* 2002;99(8):3014–3018.
80. **Arkuszewski M, Krejza J, Chen R, et al.** Sickle cell anemia: reference values of cerebral blood flow determined by continuous arterial spin labeling MRI. *Neuroradiol J* 2013;26(2):191–200.
81. **Wang WC, Gallagher DM, Pegelow CH, et al.** Multicenter comparison of magnetic resonance imaging and transcranial Doppler ultrasonography in the evaluation of the central nervous system in children with sickle cell disease. *J Pediatr Hematol Oncol* 2000;22(4):335–339.
82. **Currie S, Raghavan A, Batty R, et al.** Childhood moyamoya disease and moyamoya syndrome: a pictorial review. *Pediatr Neurol* 2011;44(6): 401–413.
83. **Scott RM, Smith ER.** Moyamoya disease and moyamoya syndrome. *N Engl J Med* 2009;360(12):1226–1237.
84. **Calamante F, Ganesan V, Kirkham FJ, et al.** MR perfusion imaging in Moyamoya Syndrome: potential implications for clinical evaluation of occlusive cerebrovascular disease. *Stroke* 2001;32(12):2810–2816.
85. **Noguchi T, Kawashima M, Irie H, et al.** Arterial spin-labeling MR imaging in moyamoya disease compared with SPECT imaging. *Eur J Radiol* 2011;80(3):e557–e562.
86. **Yun TJ, Sohn CH, Han MH, et al.** Effect of delayed transit time on arterial spin labeling: correlation with dynamic susceptibility contrast perfusion magnetic resonance in moyamoya disease. *Invest Radiol* 2013;48(11): 795–802.
87. **Okell TW, Chappell MA, Schulz UG, et al.** A kinetic model for vessel-encoded dynamic angiography with arterial spin labeling. *Magn Reson Med* 2012;68(3):969–979.
88. **Zaharchuk G, Do HM, Marks MP, et al.** Arterial spin-labeling MRI can identify the presence and intensity of collateral perfusion in patients with moyamoya disease. *Stroke* 2011;42(9):2485–2491.
89. **Pizzini F, Farace P, Zanoni T, et al.** Pulsed-arterial-spin-labeling perfusion 3T MRI following single seizure: a first case report study. *Epilepsy Res* 2008;81(2–3):225–227.
90. **Pollock JM, Deibler AR, West TG, et al.** Arterial spin-labeled magnetic resonance imaging in hyperperfused seizure focus: a case report. *J Comput Assist Tomogr* 2008;32(2):291–292.
91. **Wu RH, Bruening R, Noachtar S, et al.** MR measurement of regional relative cerebral blood volume in epilepsy. *J Magn Reson Imaging* 1999;9(3):435–440.
92. **Wolf RL, Alsop DC, Levy-Reis I, et al.** Detection of mesial temporal lobe hypoperfusion in patients with temporal lobe epilepsy by use of arterial spin labeled perfusion MR imaging. *AJNR Am J Neuroradiol* 2001;22(7):1334–1341.
93. **Tourdias T, Rodrigo S, Oppenheim C, et al.** Pulsed arterial spin labeling applications in brain tumors: practical review. *J Neuroradiol* 2008;35(2):79–89.
94. **Lehmann P, Monet P, de Marco G, et al.** A comparative study of perfusion measurement in brain tumours at 3 Tesla MR: arterial spin labeling versus dynamic susceptibility contrast-enhanced MRI. *Eur Neurol* 2010;64(1):21–26.
95. **Warmuth C, Gunther M, Zimmer C.** Quantification of blood flow in brain tumors: comparison of arterial spin labeling and dynamic susceptibility-weighted contrast-enhanced MR imaging. *Radiology* 2003;228(2):523–532.
96. **Canale S, Rodrigo S, Tourdias T, et al.** Grading of adults primitive glial neoplasms using arterial spin-labeled perfusion MR imaging. *J Neuroradiol* 2011;38(4):207–213.
97. **Noguchi T, Yoshiura T, Hiwatashi A, et al.** Perfusion imaging of brain tumors using arterial spin-labeling: correlation with histopathologic vascular density. *AJNR Am J Neuroradiol* 2008;29(4):688–693.
98. **Louis DN, Ohgaki H, Wiestler OD, et al.** The 2007 WHO classification of tumours of the central nervous system. *Acta Neuropathol* 2007;114(2):97–109.
99. **Hakyemez B, Erdogan C, Ercan I, et al.** High-grade and low-grade gliomas: differentiation by using perfusion MR imaging. *Clin Radiol* 2005;60(4):493–502.
100. **Law M, Young RJ, Babb JS, et al.** Gliomas: predicting time to progression or survival with cerebral blood volume measurements at dynamic susceptibility-weighted contrast-enhanced perfusion MR imaging. *Radiology* 2008;247(2):490–498.
101. **Wolf RL, Wang J, Wang S, et al.** Grading of CNS neoplasms using continuous arterial spin labeled perfusion MR imaging at 3 Tesla. *J Magn Reson Imaging* 2005;22(4):475–482.
102. **Yoo RE, Choi SH, Cho HR, et al.** Tumor blood flow from arterial spin labeling perfusion MRI: a key parameter in distinguishing high-grade gliomas from primary cerebral lymphomas, and in predicting genetic biomarkers in high-grade gliomas. *J Magn Reson Imaging* 2013;38(4):852–860.
103. **Weber MA, Thilmann C, Lichy MP, et al.** Assessment of irradiated brain metastases by means of arterial spin-labeling and dynamic susceptibility-weighted contrast-enhanced perfusion MRI: initial results. *Invest Radiol* 2004;39(5):277–287.
104. **Clarke JL, Chang SM.** Neuroimaging: diagnosis and response assessment in glioblastoma. *Cancer J* 2012;18(1):26–31.
105. **Chang JH, Kim CY, Choi BS, et al.** Pseudoprogression and pseudo-response in the management of high grade glioma: optimal decision timing according to the response assessment of the neuro-oncology working group. *J Korean Neurosurg Soc* 2014;55(1):5–11.
106. **Choi YJ, Kim HS, Jahng GH, et al.** Pseudoprogression in patients with glioblastoma: added value of arterial spin labeling to dynamic susceptibility contrast perfusion MR imaging. *Acta Radiologica* 2013;54(4):448–454.
107. **Lutz K, Radbruch A, Wiestler B, et al.** Neuroradiological response criteria for high-grade gliomas. *Clin Neuroradiol* 2011;21(4):199–205.
108. **Quant EC, Wen PY.** Response assessment in neuro-oncology. *Curr Oncol Rep* 2011;13(1):50–56.
109. **Wen PY, Macdonald DR, Reardon DA, et al.** Updated response assessment criteria for high-grade gliomas: response assessment in neuro-oncology working group. *J Clin Oncol* 2010;28(11):1963–1972.
110. **Brandsma D, Stalpers L, Taal W, et al.** Clinical features, mechanisms, and management of pseudoprogression in malignant gliomas. *Lancet Oncol* 2008;9(5):453–461.

CHAPTER

15 Perfusion Imaging in Brain Masses

Sotirios Bisdas, MD, PhD, MSc, Vasileios K. Katsaros, MD, PhD, Henryk Barthel, MD, PhD, and Nikolas Papanikolaou, PhD

Introduction

The goal of tumor imaging is to provide a detailed portrait of a mass by combining comprehensive morphologic information with pathophysiologic and metabolic indices. Three-dimensional, multislice computed tomography (CT) and in an exquisite way the magnetic resonance imaging (MRI) are likely to continue as the mainstay for providing morphologic information on the presence and extent of tumor, tumor volume, and anatomic relationships. Following the current trends in tumor imaging, morphologic CT and MRI continue to evolve in this context with the advent of high-resolution imaging as well as new techniques, like susceptibility weighted imaging (SWI). However, the fundamental requirement for detailed information about cardinal tumor biologic processes including angiogenesis, hypoxia, apoptosis, cellular membrane integrity, necrosis, and other malignancy-specific processes is still unanswered. Based on the characterization of these parameters, clinicians will be able to make more precise management decisions in a noninvasive manner, thereby fine-tuning cancer therapy whether it is with targeted drugs, surgery, or radiotherapy.

Therefore, the nexus between neurooncology and neuroimaging grows continually stronger. Established as well as novel ones seek imaging methodologies, currently being evolving and improved, seek to identify brain neoplasms at the limits of their detectability and label them cancers, providing indices for their in which all of the metabolic, proteomic, and genomic information needed to make management decisions.

Angiogenesis, the sprouting of new capillaries from existing blood vessels, and vasculogenesis, the de novo generation of blood vessels, are the two primary methods of vascular expansion by which nutrient supply to tissues by blood is adjusted to meet the physiologic needs or the increased needs in case of malignant tumors. The tissue vascularity may be assessed indirectly, nonetheless quantitatively and noninvasively in situ by perfusion imaging. Several imaging techniques are able to assess brain masses with respect to their angiogenic status, the clinically relevant of which are reviewed in this chapter. MRI techniques with or without contrast media are the most popular, whereas positron emission tomography (PET) and CT perfusion imaging in brain tumors are less widespread in the regular clinical setting.

MRI and PET Techniques for Perfusion Imaging

Improvements in magnetic resonance technology and sequence design have produced a series of fast and ultrafast image acquisition techniques, which allow the collection of sequential sets of morphologic data. Variations in microvascular structure and pathophysiology give rise to temporospatial variations in enhancement patterns, which can provide valuable information on tumor characteristics. MRI techniques, based on paramagnetic contrast agents, such as gadolinium, are usually used in the brain to determine blood volume, but the evaluation of perfusion in terms of blood flow remains difficult,[1] partly due to extravascular gadolinium leakage in patients with compromised blood–brain barrier (BBB). Besides low molecular weight (<1,000 Da) gadolinium contrast agents commonly used in clinical MRI, ultrasmall superparamagnetic iron oxide nanoparticles may act as a blood pool agent on postinjection MR sequences, with no significant leakage in areas of compromised BBB, and thus possess the potential to overcome inherent challenges of conventional perfusion imaging. The technique is currently under research and beyond the scope of this chapter.[2] On the other hand, arterial spin labeling (ASL)[3] and intravoxel incoherent motion (IVIM) analysis of diffusion-weighted imaging (DWI),[4] which do not use any external tracers, but exploit the T_1 relaxation effects of the water molecules in arterial blood as well as the natural sensitivity of the MR signal to spin motion, are promising surrogate markers for tumor perfusion. Further diffusible tracers that can be monitored with MRI include fluorinated halocarbons,[5] deuterated water (^2H_2O),[6] and ^{17}O-water.[7]

PET as a noninvasive molecular imaging tool offers, by employing appropriate tracers, the possibility to visualize and quantify blood flow in brain tumors. In principle, different PET tracers are available to measure brain tumor and brain blood flow. Similarly to MRI, these tracers are divided into nondiffusible and diffusible ones. For nondiffusible PET tracers, blood flow is calculated for these tracers on the basis of the indicator dilution theory.[8] Diffusible tracers, on the other hand, exchange from the arterial vascularity to the parenchyma, allowing for direct measurement of blood flow as originally described by Kety.[9] Taken together, PET imaging represents the gold standard to visualize and quantify brain tumor blood flow in vivo. Despite advantageous characteristics of the diffusible tracers, like the [^{15}O]H_2O, for monitoring blood flow changes over time in sequential scans, PET imaging remains a technologic and infrastructural challenge, preventing it from gaining a wider acceptance in a clinical routine setting. With the recent emergence of fully integrated MR-PET systems, it is now possible for the first time to cross-evaluate novel MR concepts to obtain blood flow information for brain tumors against this gold standard.[10]

Perfusion MRI with Exogenous Tracer

There are two generic approaches for the acquisition of gadolinium-enhanced perfusion MRI data. Relaxivity-based methods use T_1-weighted acquisitions, generally called as dynamic contrast-enhanced MRI (DCE-MRI), while susceptibility-based techniques use T_2 or more commonly T_2*-based acquisitions during the bolus passage of gadolinium and are called dynamic susceptibility contrast-enhanced MRI (DSC-MRI). Both methods have specific advantages and disadvantages as reviewed below.

Dynamic Susceptibility Contrast-Enhanced MRI

Susceptibility contrast agents (gadolinium compounds) act by changing the local magnetic environment around the contrast molecule. This effect extends some significant distance, which may be in the order of several millimeters depending on the sensitivity of the image acquisition sequence used, affecting water molecules lying outside the blood vessels. This effect makes DSC-MRI sensitive to small amounts of contrast distributed through the capillary bed, whereas contrast molecules concentrated in single large vessels present some amplification effect but only around the vessel periphery. DSC-MRI acquisition techniques need a reasonable trade-off between heavy T_2* weighting, which demands a long echo time (TE), and sufficient temporal resolution and spatial coverage. At the present time, the most common approach to this problem has been the use of echo-planar image (EPI) acquisitions with sequential single slice aiming at a temporal resolution of 2 seconds or below, repeated continuously for 45 to 60 seconds. Among EPI sequences, most first-pass DSC data are acquired using gradient-echo (GRE) EPI, while spin-echo (SE) EPI is still popular at some institutions. Despite the slightly higher contrast requirements for SE-EPI, this sequence is attractive because of its contrast sensitivity to 1- to 2-μm neovessels and its lower sensitivity to the susceptibility artifacts in the vicinity of bone–brain–air interfaces.[11] GRE-EPI methods are more sensitive to macrovessels and require half the dose of gadolinium compared to SE.[12] Remarkably, simultaneous acquisitions of both SE and GRE may be used for vessel size determination.[13]

Modeling and Postprocessing of DSC-MRI

Raw perfusion data should undergo several postprocessing steps in order to improve image quality and be prepared for further analysis. Postprocessing comprises several steps including motion correction, spatial and temporal smoothing, lesion segmentation, coregistration with anatomical data, generation of parametric maps, leakage correction, vessel exclusion, and normalization to contralateral unaffected tissue. The initial raw data are used to draw signal intensity over time curves that needs to be transformed to tracer concentration over time curves, in order to calculate useful parameters like blood volume, blood flow, and mean transit time. Signal intensities are transformed into concentration (T_2* or T_2 rate changes, ΔR_2^* or ΔR_2, respectively) that it is linearly related to the T_2* rate changes based on the following formula:

$$\Delta R_2 = -\frac{\ln(S_t / S_0)}{\mathrm{TE}} \tag{1}$$

where S_0 is the average prebolus signal intensity and S_t is the SI at time t (Fig. 15.1). Two main approaches are utilized in order to calculate perfusion-related parameters: either modeling of the signal intensity curve using a gamma variant function to reduce the second-pass effects of the contrast agent or deconvolution with the arterial input function (AIF). Curve fitting may result in smoother parametric maps in the setting of noisy raw data and will also reduce the effect of contrast agent recirculation. The drawback of fitting the first-pass data is that the data may not fit the model function well—in particular in areas of abnormal perfusion.

Various hemodynamic-related parameters can be quantified to assess tissue vascularity. The most robust parameter that can be extracted reliably from first-pass techniques is relative cerebral blood volume (rCBV), which is obtained from the integral of the data time series during the first pass of the contrast agent: [13,14]

$$\mathrm{rCBV} = \int_{t_0}^{t_e} \Delta R_2(t)\,\mathrm{d}t \tag{2}$$

where t_0 is the time of first arrival of contrast and t_e is the time at which ΔR_2 returns to baseline values. The mean transit time (MTT) is then estimated from the width of the curve at half the maximum height [full width at half maximum (FWHM)]. Subsequently, rCBF (relative cerebral blood flow) can be as rCBV/MTT calculated. Notably, rCBV and rCBF measurements are relative and not absolute, and therefore, normalization to an internal reference is important for comparative studies. Usually, the internal reference is the contralateral unaffected white matter.

Contrast Agent Leakage Correction

Theoretically, the semiquantification of perfusion properties in the equation for ΔR_2^* is valid under the assumption that contrast agent remains intravascular or in cases of disruption of the BBB; the T_1 enhancement does not significantly affect signal intensity. However, this does not hold true in cases of gadolinium leaky brain tumors, where in regions of contrast agent leakage, the dynamic curve will go below zero after R_2 conversion since the SI is increasing above the baseline level due to T_1-related enhancement (Fig. 15.1). Thus, an unavoidable underestimation of CBV takes place by diminishing the magnitude of DSC signal loss in regions where T_1 effect is overwhelming. Initially, using of small flip angles (though this results in decreased SNR, which can be partially compensated by increasing contrast agent dose) and long repetition times may partially solve this problem. Secondly, the effects of extravasation and T_1-weighted leakage can be minimized with the application of a preloading dose of contrast agent,[15] baseline subtraction techniques,[16] or by using multiecho methods,[13,17,18] though the dual-echo technique is technically challenging for most machines, and reducing the sampling time inevitably restricts the number of samples and therefore the slices that can be obtained. Furthermore, automatic removal of vessels from perfusion maps that have been based on GRE-EPI sequences may help to reduce false-positive diagnosis for increased neoangiogenesis. The method is based on a cluster analysis of the estimated perfusion-related parameters to separate vascular (both arteries and veins) from nonvascular structures.[19] Whole-lesion histogram analysis is also feasible as a more comprehensive method of quantification and information extraction comparing to traditional two-dimensional region-of-interest (ROI) generation on a single slice (Figs. 15.2 and 15.3).[20] Apparently, histogram analysis does not suffer from bias, introduced by the person drawing the ROI; however, it requires the availability of a robust and accurate segmentation algorithm. In addition, the final outcome of a 2D ROI-based measurement method is a single number that is suffering from averaging effects especially when heterogeneous lesions are studied.[21]

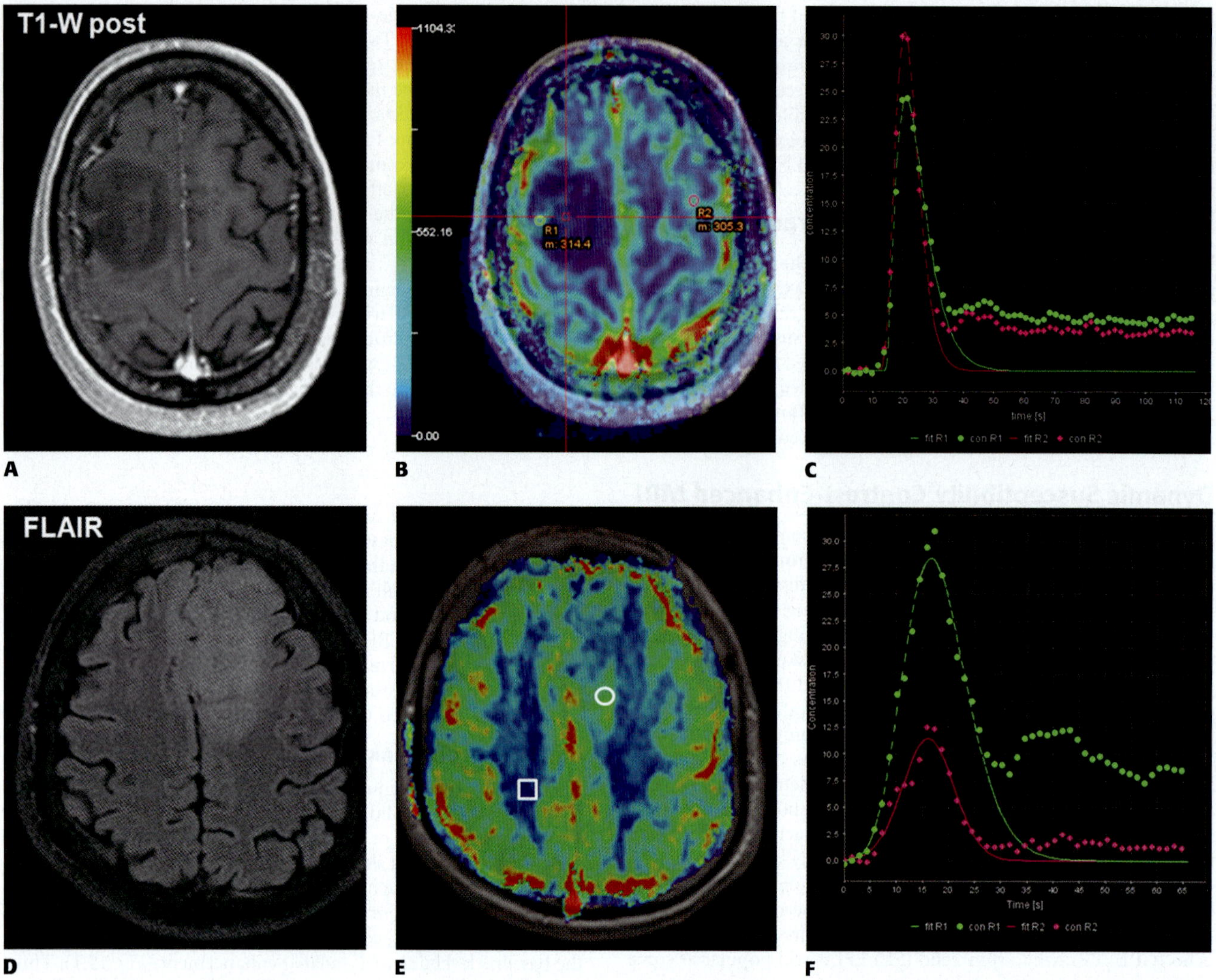

Figure 15-1. A–C: WHO grade 2 glioma. **A:** Morphologic MR imaging of an intracranial mass on the right frontal lobe showing no pathologic gadolinium enhancement. **B:** The generated rCBV map shows no significantly elevated blood volume values. **C:** The ROI analysis of the presumable tumor "hot spot" (R1) to the contralateral corresponding brain structure (R2) reveals lower peak concentration without any extravasation effects in the tracer concentration time curves (fitted and raw data are presented). **D–F:** WHO grade III tumor. **D:** FLAIR-weighted morphologic imaging of an intracranial mass on the left frontal lobe. **E:** The corrected for leakage rCBV map shows a pronounced hypervascularity adjacent to the midline (circular tumor ROI and rectangular white matter ROI). **F:** The ROI analysis (tumor ROI in green and white matter ROI in purple) demonstrates early wash-in, higher concentration peak, and prolonged washout phase since the signal intensity is increasing above the baseline level due to T_1-related effects. The tumor sampling showed a WHO grade III tumor.

Critical Appraisal of DSC-MRI

Another important and probably under recognized issue involves the dispersion and delay between the measured AIF and the true inflow to the voxel. Ideally, AIF should be measured in each imaged voxel to eliminate the effects of delay and dispersion of the contrast agent from the injection site. This discrepancy can cause either over- or underestimation of rCBF, depending on the delay between the AIF and the tissue.[22] Block circulant SVD technique may be theoretically immune to differences in bolus arrival time but still cannot account for dispersion,[23] whereas iterative blind deconvolution offers also an alternative solution.[24] Nevertheless, there are indices that the use of a different software application determines different results, even if the algorithms seem to be the same; notably, the introduction of AIF in the data postprocessing determines a higher estimates variability that can make interhospital and intrahospital examinations not completely comparable.[25]

DSC-MRI was first used to study the microcirculation of the brain and has been in a limited way validated in terms of rCBV estimates against histopathology in brain tumors[26] and in terms of rCBF against PET measurements in stroke patients.[27,28] Concerning the clinical relevance of CBF and CBV as surrogates of tumor vasculature, it is noteworthy that any immature tumor blood vessels with very slim lumina may not carry any blood flow at all and obviously underestimate tumor aggressiveness as calculated,[29,30] whereas mature microvessels often do have enlarged lumina, hence higher CBV, that may come along with low CBF.[29] Last but not least, CBF might be decreased in high-grade tumors due to the accompanying interstitial hypertension, whereas in cases of dominant tracer extravasation, the DSC data should be appropriately modeled in order to extract correct and not permeability-biased blood flow measurements. The strong susceptibility effect in the vicinity of tumors due to profound tracer extravasation makes generally

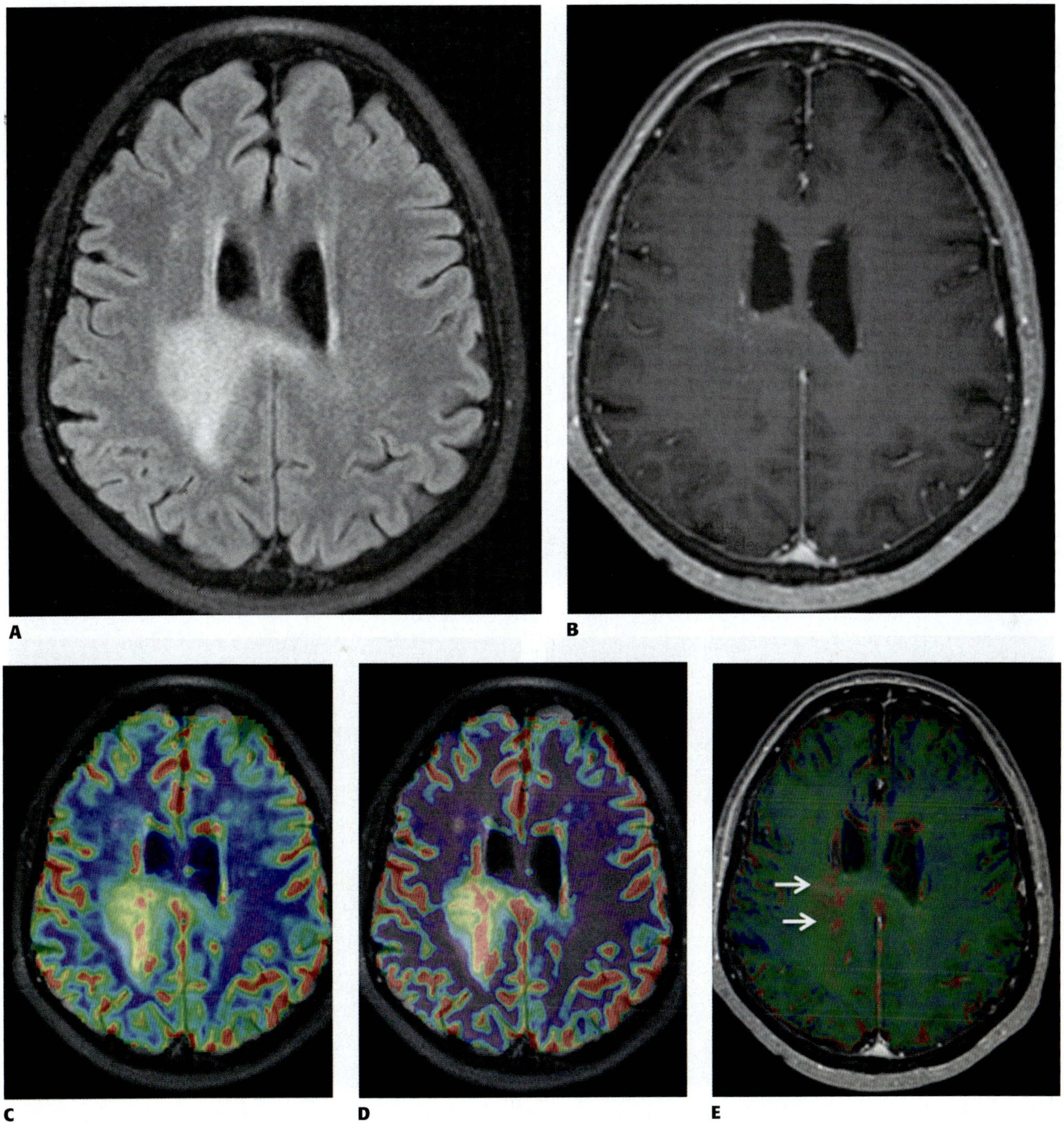

Figure 15-2. (A) FLAIR and **(B)** T1W postcontrast MRI of a right-sided cerebral mass crossing the midline demonstrates subtle enhancement suggestive of WHO grades II–III tumor. The DSC-MRI–derived rCBF map **(C)** shows elevated perfusion in the tumor resembling the one in the brain cortex, and in the leakage-corrected rCBV map **(D)**, the tumor vascularity is also pronounced. **(E)** The map of K2 leakage coefficient, which is related to permeability, demonstrates clearly foci of disruption of the blood–brain barrier (*arrows*). The histologic analysis showed a WHO grade IV tumor.

DSC-MRI not suitable for permeability measurements, although there is scarce evidence that K^{trans} may be correlated with the one obtained by DCE-MRI[31] as well as may possess diagnostic value together with CBV for glioma grading.[32] Other researchers have utilized microvascular leakage (referred to as K_2 leakage coefficient, which is related to PS and K^{trans})[15,33,34] (Figs. 15.2 and 15.3), enabling discrimination between glioblastomas (GBMs) and metastases, as well as glioma grading was facilitated.[35,36] In any case, it is clear that the flow-dependent, first-pass permeability measurement obtained by DSC-MRI has not the same pathophysiologic background like the one estimated by DCE-MRI in steady state, as permeability or K^{trans} estimation using DSC-MRI is confounded by competing T_1, T_2, and T_2* relaxation effects and the dependency of these interactions on pulse sequence parameters and the underlying physical

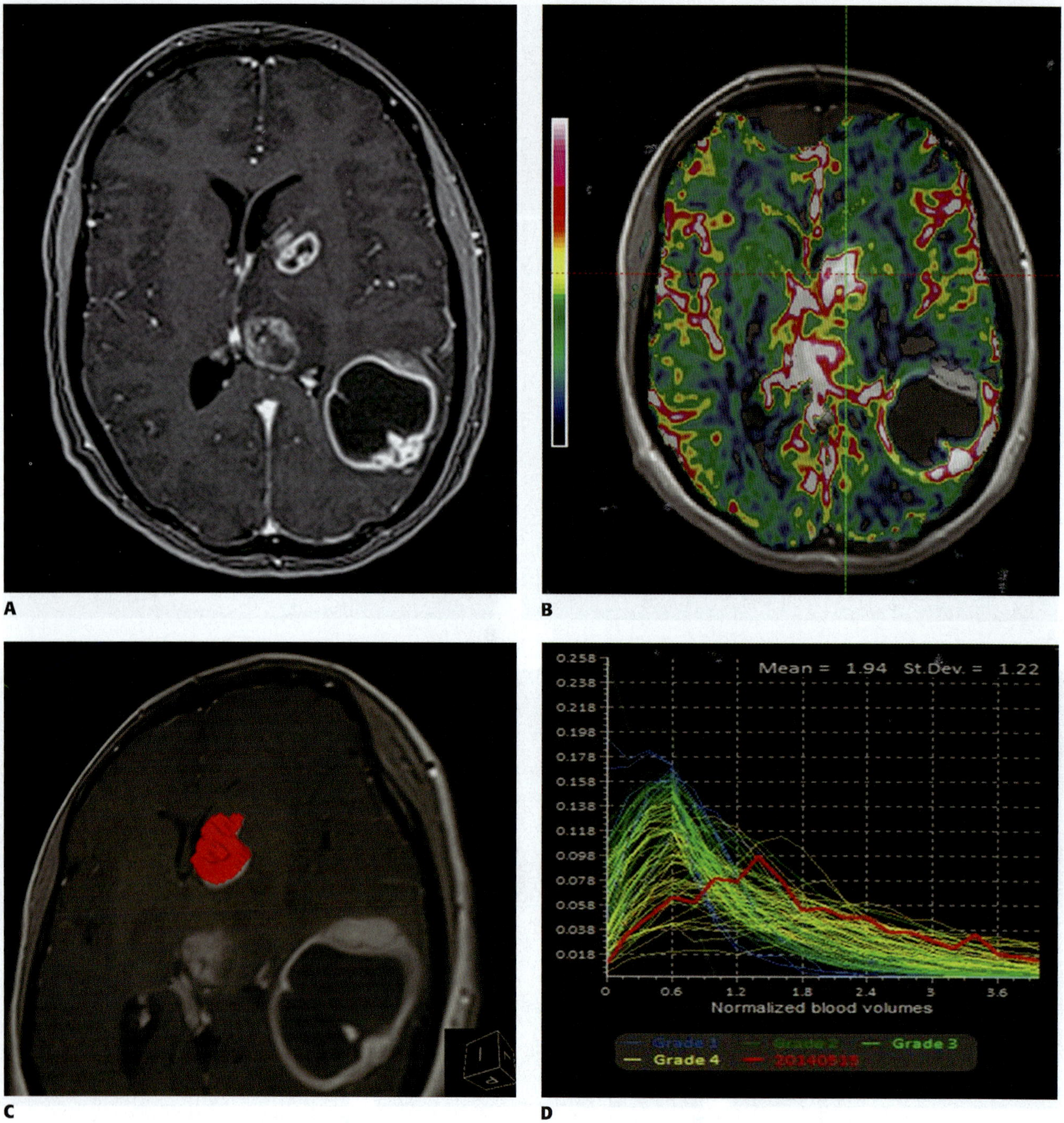

Figure 15-3. **(A)** **Typical MR appearance of a multifocal glioblastoma in the left hemisphere (postgadolinium T_1-weighted MR imaging) with increased neoangiogenesis as depicted in the leakage-corrected rCBV map** **(B)**. **C:** After 3D tumor segmentation based on postgadolinium T_1-weighted images, whole-tumor histograms of normalized blood volume (nBV) are generated. **D:** Further histogram normalization was done by normalizing the area under the histogram to unity. Significant vascular heterogeneity is reflected on the whole tumor normalized histogram as a wide, low-amplitude histogram containing various nBV values (low, moderate, and high).

and physiologic properties of the tissue. Thus, the findings have to be meticulously appreciated in therapy monitoring studies as it has been shown to overestimate K^{trans} and underestimate plasma volume.[37] The correlations to PET measurements show that DSC-MRI tends to overestimate absolute CBF and underestimate MTT of the contrast agent bolus through the tissue of interest, but the relative distribution of the perfusion variables was remarkably similar between DSC-MRI and PET, at least in the group analysis. Thus, cross-calibration of DSC-MRI with PET may be useful; when rescaling procedures are employed, it may be more important to develop deconvolution algorithms that produce CBF estimates with accuracies that vary little with MTT than to produce algorithms that provide inherently more accurate CBF estimates, but whose relative accuracy varies significantly with MTT.[38]

Clinical Applications of DSC-MRI

Pretherapeutic Tumor Imaging Workup

While contrast-enhanced T_1-weighted imaging depicts tumor regions with a disrupted BBB, DSC-MRI can quantify variations in rCBV and accurately map the alterations in tumor angiogenesis serving theoretically as a more robust and accurate grading method than histopathology, which is subject to sampling bias (Fig. 15.1). The rough estimate of permeability derived from the shape of the time–intensity curve (TIC) can provide important clues to the nature of the lesion. Microvessels within tumors of extra-axial and nonglial origin—meningioma, choroid plexus papilloma, metastases, lymphoma, and so forth—do not form a BBB, so a very large fraction of the bolus leaks into the extravascular space during the first pass,[39,40] while low rCBV favors the diagnosis of metastasis or lymphoma (the latter especially when correlation with DWI demonstrates high cellularity). Because glioma microvessels form a BBB that is impaired but not absent, the TIC returns significantly toward baseline in these tumors, although not as much as in normal brain. The difference between these patterns can contribute significantly to the discrimination of tumor types in cases of peripherally located enhancing tumors when the differential diagnosis includes meningioma and peripheral GBM and in periventricular enhancing lesions when the differential diagnosis includes choroid plexus papillocarcinoma and GBM. Low-grade gliomas exhibit significantly lower rCBV when compared with higher-grade gliomas with little or no elevation compared to the contralateral normal-appearing brain.[41] Finally, if a circumscribed cortical or subcortical lesion has imaging features otherwise suggestive of low-grade glioma but has rCBV maps that demonstrate prominent elevated blood volume equal or greater than cortical gray matter, then the diagnosis of oligodendroglioma should be suspected because the characteristic "chicken-wire" neocapillary architecture found in oligodendroglioma produces a high rCBV regardless of tumor grade.[42] "False-positive" DSC-MRI findings indicating high-grade brain neoplasm are also noted in pilocytic astrocytomas (in this common pediatric tumor, the vascular hyperplasia is not associated with angiogenic features) and in hemangioblastomas.[43] Nevertheless, in known or suspected astrocytoma, the strong correlation between the maximum rCBV measured in a tumor and the histologic tumor grade has been extensively documented.[41,44,45] As noted earlier, the presence of tumor with rCBV similar to or greater than cortex should strongly suggest the presence of WHO grade III–IV tumor (Fig. 15.2). Despite the limitations of low spatial resolution, artifacts, and quantification issues, using DSC-MRI, maximum rCBV has been demonstrated to be very helpful in preoperative planning to ensure biopsy, resection, or ablation of the highest-grade portion of a heterogeneous tumor.[46,47]

Tumor Surveillance

The longitudinal DSC-MRI in untreated lesions has also recently received attention as the significant increases in rCBV up to 12 months before contrast enhancement appearance on T_1-weighted images may predict the malignant transformation of low-grade astrocytomas and thus the survival rates.[48] Concerning progression-free survival (PFS) prediction, rCBV remains a robust predictor rCBV for short-term and 2-year PFS in patients with gliomas (without oligodendroglial components), independent of pathologic findings.[49–51] After treatment, it has been shown that low rCBV in combination with high apparent diffusion coefficient (ADC) from DWI is typical of delayed radiation necrosis.[52,53] Significant amount of clinical experience using rCBV to detect tumor recurrence (including also stereotactically irradiated metastatic disease) has been promising[54–57] for establishing DSC-MRI for the differentiation between posttherapeutic changes and tumor relapse. However, there is considerable rCBV heterogeneity and certain overlap between recurrent lesions and posttherapeutic changes since the coexistence of viable tumor tissue with therapy-induced vascular changes (mostly dilatation and breakdown of BBB), and fibrinoid tissue necrosis limits the specificity of the method, and it is frequently necessary to take into account MR spectroscopy, DWI, and PET findings in the clinical routine.[55,58,59] DSC-MRI may also serve as surveillance tool with obvious prognostic role in patients undergoing concomitant chemoradiation of high-grade astrocytic tumors,[60,61] whereas the technique is especially interesting in the era of antiangiogenic therapy, as rCBV has been demonstrated to correlate with expression of angiogenic factors[44] and to be sensitive to antineoangiogenic therapy effects.[62] Correlation with steroid dosing during interpretation may be needed, although to date, technically rigorous reports looking at this subject have reached different conclusions as to whether high-dose steroid administration acutely reduces neovessel rCBV in addition to its undisputed effect on permeability.[63,64] This controversy will not be trivial to resolve definitively because alteration in permeability has a significant effect on the calculation of rCBV.

Differentiation between Nonneoplastic and Neoplastic Focal Lesions

Differentiating between infectious as well as tumefactive multiple sclerosis lesions and neoplastic focal brain lesions that are detected by conventional structural MRI may be a challenge in routine practice, and DSC-MRI may be employed as a complementary noninvasive tool, providing lower rCBV values in the infectious lesions than in tumors with a satisfactory accuracy of 95%.[65–68]

Dynamic Contrast-Enhanced MRI

DCE-MRI approaches are based on T_1 shortening produced by the injection of a contrast agent (commonly based on gadolinium chelates). T_1-based changes are primarily a result of contrast material diffusion into the extravascular–extracellular space (EES); thus, DCE-MRI is primarily focused on quantification of vascular permeability (Fig. 15.4). The amount of signal enhancement observed on DCE-MRI is dependent on a number of physiologic (tissue perfusion, capillary surface area, permeability to contrast agent, and volume of the EES) and physical factors (precontrast T_1 relaxation rate of the tissue, contrast agent dose, rate of intracellular–extracellular water exchange, imaging sequence parameters used, and measurement gain and scaling factors). Dynamic imaging is typically performed during an interval of approximately 5 to 10 minutes rather than during the first pass of the bolus. The most common sequence for DCE-MRI is a fast, 3D, T_1-weighted GRE sequence (saturation recovery/inversion recovery snapshot sequence) with short TE (usually <1.5 milliseconds) and TR (usually <7 milliseconds) and flip angle between 15 degrees and 30 degrees as far as constrained by hardware limitations and spatial coverage requirements. The careful choice of the flip angle according to the expected gadolinium concentration in tumor tissue is mandatory since the flip angle is decisive for the intrinsic variability in the tissue measurements and the AIF estimation.[69] In addition, the actual T_1 values of the tissues at baseline (before contrast material infusion) are required for most analysis algorithms in order to perform the pharmacokinetic analysis.[70,71] This calculation can be performed by using a series of T_1-weighted images obtained at different flip angles or by an inversion recovery SE-based method, which serves as the reference method.[72] Moreover, the need for fast sampling of the arterial and tissue concentration curves necessitates a temporal resolution of 5 seconds or less.[73]

Modeling and Postprocessing of DCE-MRI

Signal enhancement seen on DCE-MRI can be assessed in two ways: by the analysis of TIC (semiquantitative) and/or by quantifying tissue T_1 relaxivity (R_1) or contrast agent concentration change

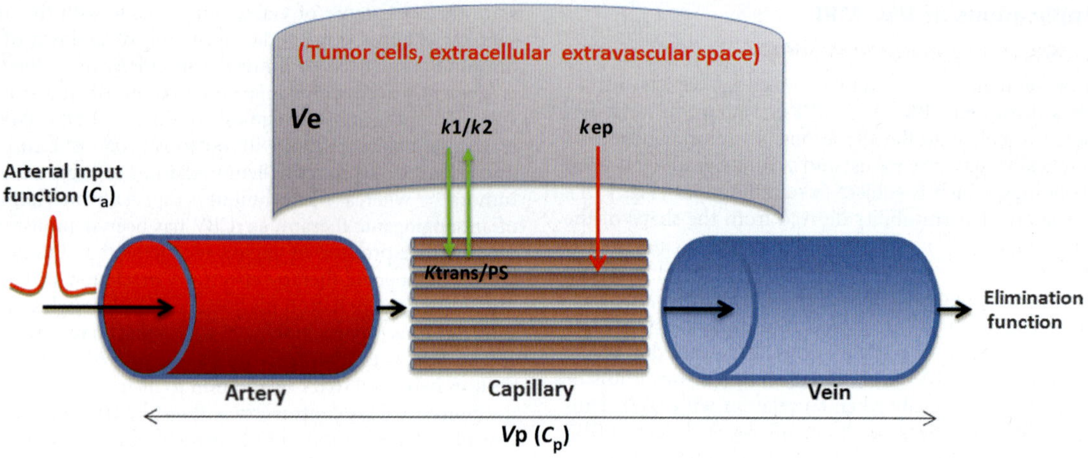

Figure 15-4. Schematic of the major compartments and the derived parameters for permeability studies using DCE-MRI. The plasma volume (v_p) refers to the total vascular bed, including the feeding arteries, the draining veins, and the capillary bed, and is characterized by the tracer concentration (C_p), and for reasons of simplicity, "constrained" tracer kinetic model derivations (see original Tofts model) are supposed to be small to negligible compared to the "well-mixed" interstitial space. In the compartmental modeling, the tracer extravasation due to capillary permeability (characterized by the permeability surface area product, PS) is described by the isodirectional flux of the contrast agent characterized by the rate constant K^{trans}. In more elaborated models (the so-called exchange models), the different concentration gradients between capillary bed and interstitium may be further exploited by the introduction of the k_1 and k_2 constant rates that describe the efflux and influx rates of the tracer, respectively. The constant rate of tracer backflux from the extracellular–extravascular matrix into the vascular bed is also called k_{ep}, and its diagnostic value in clinical brain tumor studies has to be further investigated. Almost all DCE-MRI generate estimations of interstitial volume (v_e), whose, however, estimation demands long acquisition times. An important prerequisite for accurate estimation of C_p is the accurate measurement of arterial input function (AIF) in large arteries proximal to the tissue of interest (optimally at the inlet to the tissue) in order to minimize any dispersion and delay effects.

using pharmacokinetic modeling techniques. Semiquantitative parameters describe signal intensity changes using a number of descriptors. These parameters include curve shape classification done visually, onset time (a number of definitions exist), gradient of the upslope of enhancement curves, maximum signal intensity, and washout gradient (combinations of these can also be found in the literature). The uptake integral or initial area under the signal intensity (IAUC) or gadolinium contrast medium concentration (IAUGC) curve has been also studied.[60] IAUGC is a relatively robust and simple technique, which characterizes all enhancing regions without the problems associated with model fitting failures in pharmacokinetic models. However, IAUGC does not have a simple relationship to the physiology parameters of interest (perfusion, permeability, and leakage space) and thus offers no biologic specificity.[74]

On the other hand, the conventional approach to quantify perfusion from DCE data relies upon three key assumptions: (a) that contrast concentration is predictably related to signal change; (b) that the integrated contrast concentration is predictably related to the blood volume in the measurement space; and (c) that the shape of the contrast concentration distribution curve is governed by the MTT of contrast through the measurement space.[75] Quantitative techniques use pharmacokinetic modeling applied to changes in tissue contrast agent concentration or R_1. In general, it is not recommended that pharmacokinetic modeling be done on signal intensity data. The simplest pharmacokinetic model, such as that described by Tofts and Kermode according to the following equation

$$\frac{dC_t(t)}{dt} = K^{trans}\left(C_p(t) - \frac{C_t(t)}{v_e}\right) \tag{3}$$

calculates the size of the extravascular extracellular space (v_e) and the bulk transfer coefficient (K^{trans}), a constant, which describes the relationship between the AIF and the contrast concentration changes occurring in the tissue.[71] C_p and C_t denote the plasma and tissue contrast agent concentrations, respectively. Again, following Tofts and Kermode,[71] v_e is defined as $v_e = K^{trans}/k_{ep}$. k_{ep} is the volume rate constant for exchange between tissue and central compartments. Measurements of K^{trans} will reflect changes (also significantly correlated with) in blood flow (F), blood volume, endothelial permeability, and surface area (PS), and these individual effects cannot be distinguished.[76,77] When PS $\gg F$, which is the case in GBMs, K^{trans} will primarily reflect blood flow, which is the limiting factor in this setting. On contrary, when PS $\ll F$, then K^{trans} will mainly reflect permeability. Under mixed flow- and permeability-limited conditions, K^{trans} will reflect $E{\cdot}F$, where E denotes the initial (first-pass) extraction fraction[1] (Fig. 15.5).

One major assumption in the generalized kinetic (GK) model of Tofts is that the tissue vascular fraction (v_p) is small and can be ignored (which may be the case in diffusible tracers where the distribution volume is large compared to intravascular space); however, this is not necessarily the case in tumors and in nondiffusible tracers, thus may give rise to significant errors in voxels that contain large vascular spaces (Figs. 15.6 and 15.7). The extended GK (or extended Tofts) model attempts to account for a vascular plasma space, and we again study its derivation as proposed by Tofts and Kermode.[71]

$$v_e \frac{dC_e(t)}{dt} = K^{trans}C_p(t) - K^{trans}C_e(t) \tag{4}$$

where C_e denotes the contrast agent concentration in EES. Thus, the contrast agent concentration in each voxel can be described by

$$C_t(t) = v_pC_p(t) + v_eC_e(t) \tag{5}$$

An interesting "extension" of the extended GK model would be to consider the situation of a negligible backflux rate ($k_{ep} \approx 0$) while influx (K^{trans}) remains substantial.[78] This situation is often assumed possible during the initial time period following tracer injection

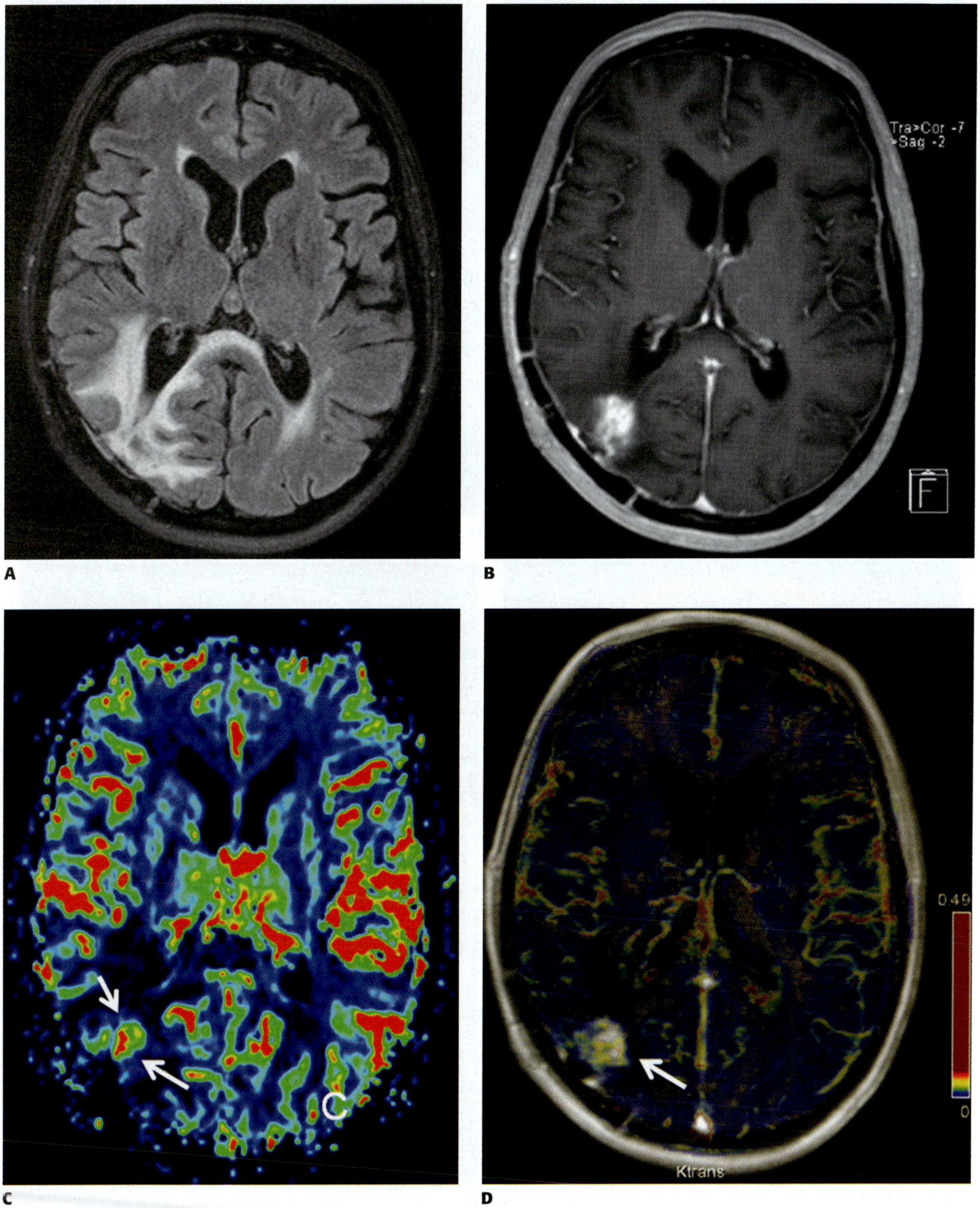

Figure 15-5. FLAIR **(A)** and postcontrast T_1-weighted **(B)** MR imaging of a patient after surgical resection and adjuvant radiotherapy of a metastasis in the right parietooccipital region shows increased enhancement and significant surrounding edema. Leakage-corrected rCBV map **(C)** demonstrates clearly the elevated blood volume in the suspected region (*arrows*), and at the same time, increased K^{trans} (*arrow*) **(D)** supports the diagnosis of recurrent tumor, which was histopathologically verified.

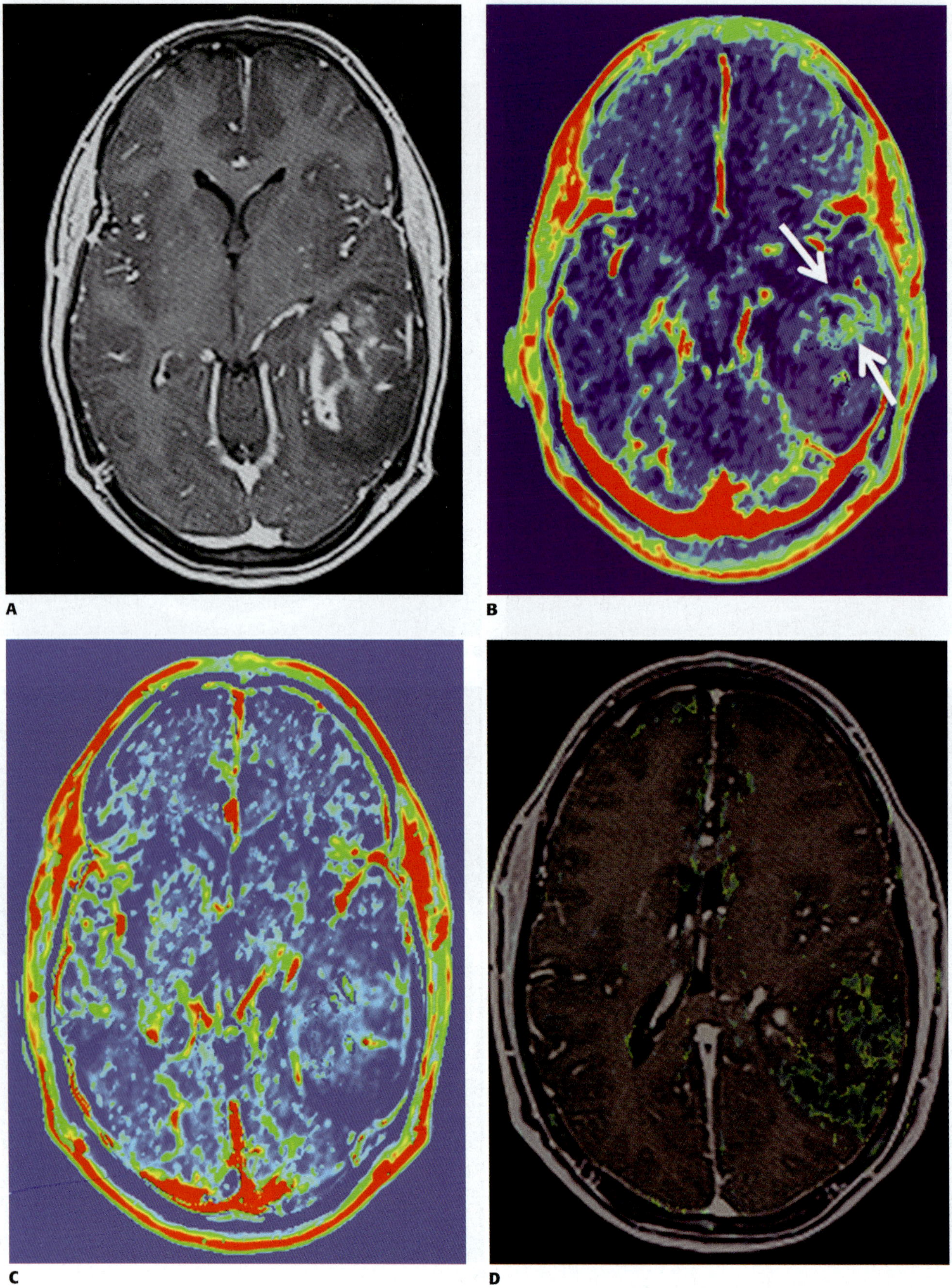

Figure 15-6. A: **Postgadolinium T_1-weighted MR imaging demonstrates a glioblastoma on the left temporal lobe with necrotic, unenhanced, and blood–brain barrier disrupted areas. B:** The DCE-MRI–derived v_p map indicates the highly vascularized tumor part (*arrows*), which represents only the minor portion of the whole tumor. Furthermore, the F map **(C)** indicates the low perfusion (in terms of quantified blood flow) in the whole tumor (including the area with relatively high vascularization), whereas the E map (superimposed on the anatomical image) **(D)** depicts the increased extravasation of the tracer in the well-vascularized tumor regions as well as in the remaining part of the tumor, where presumably the immature, leaky vasculature resides. In cases of low F and high E (which reflects the vessels permeability), K^{trans} primarily reflects blood flow in the Tofts-Kermode model as this is the main limiting factor of the contrast agent flux.

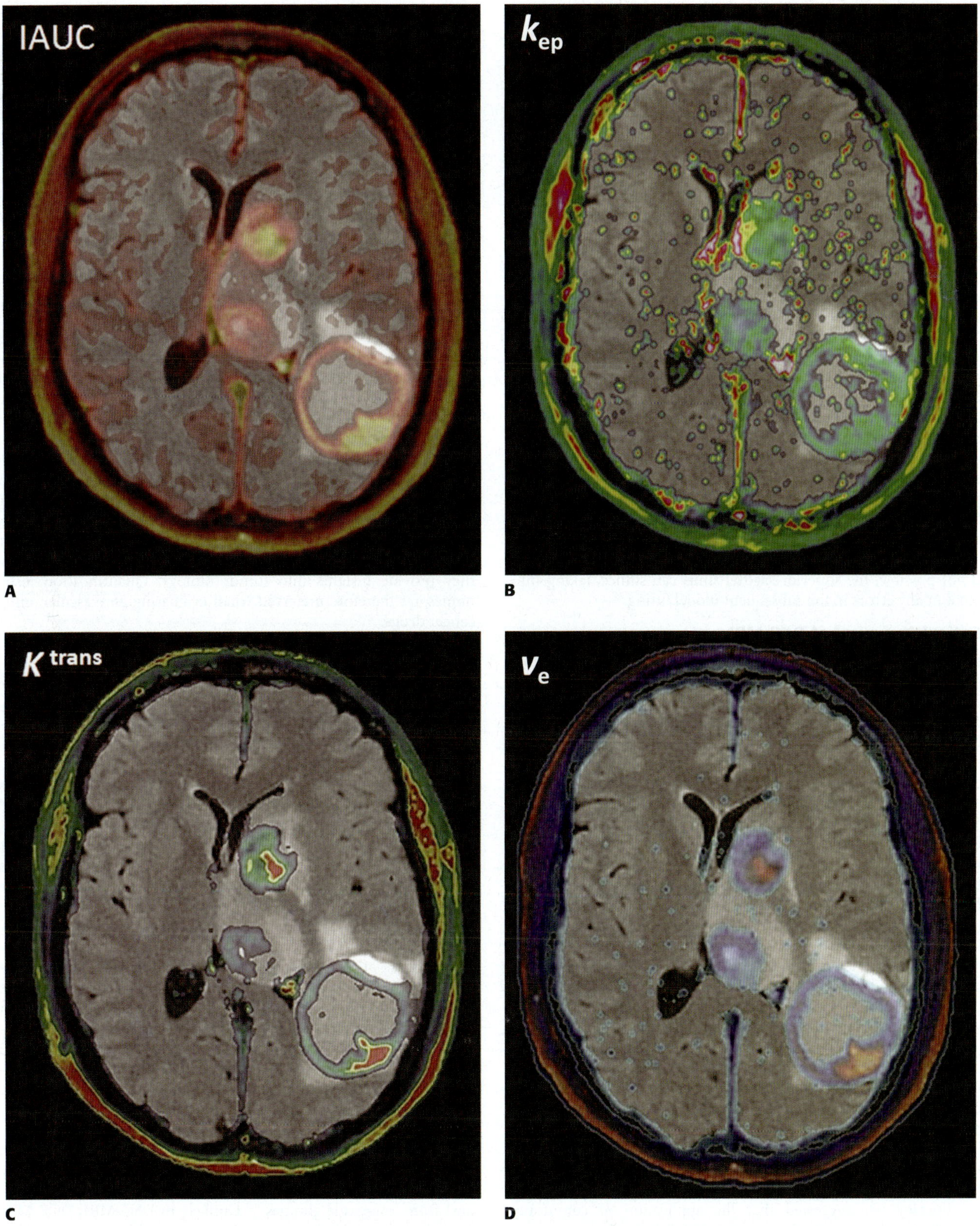

Figure 15-7. DCE-MRI–derived parameter maps including IAUC **(A)**, k_{ep} **(B)**, K^{trans} **(C)**, and v_e **(D)** are shown in a patient with multifocal glioblastoma. Though the tumor shows significant vascularization (especially in the foci in the basal ganglia), the leaky vessels (as depicted in K^{trans}) are limited to smaller regions, which has to be considered in the surveillance of any antiangiogenic therapy. The leaky vessels in the newly formed tumor parts are often associated with high disorganization of the cellular matrix, which is further reflected in higher v_e values. IAUC, initial area under the signal intensity.

whereby the tissue system functions like an accumulative pool. With $k_{ep} \approx 0$, the extended GK model may be further simplified into the Patlak plot.[1]

Measuring $C_p(t)$ (often called the AIF) directly using DCE-MRI requires measurement sequences, which yield signal intensity outputs that scale linearly over a large range of tissue and plasma concentrations. $C_p(t)$ has to be sampled in an artery at sufficient temporal resolution to accurately characterize the rapid change in tracer concentration following a bolus injection (ideally <2 seconds), which is currently impractical within the constraints of useful spatial image resolution.[79] Further confounding factors are inflow artifacts and motion. Several approaches have been utilized for obtaining or estimating $C_p(t)$. The most common method of obtaining $C_p(t)$ is to use a general input function derived from real measurement of plasma concentration done in volunteers.[80] An alternative method is to use a reference tissue with known physiologic parameters from which an estimate of $C_p(t)$ can be derived.[81] The advantages of the reference tissue approach are that the temporal sampling can be relaxed; as the rate of change in tracer concentration in the reference tissue is not as rapid as in plasma, the size of the reference tissue sample can be large, which improves the SNR of the C_t(t) obtained and averages motion effects. The disadvantages are that clinical treatments may affect blood flow in reference tissues and the implicit assumption that the reference tissue derived C_p(t) is relevant to the tissues of interest (i.e., the tumor).[79] Ideally, the AIF should be estimated in the center of the acquisition volumes to reduce end-section effects and in a large vessel with the least partial volume averaging (e.g., carotid artery); however, if this is not possible, the superior sagittal sinus can suffice, taking into account any errors in the subsequent model fitting.[82]

Critical Appraisal of DCE-MRI

For DCE-MRI, it is recognized that high resolution and short imaging time are the competing examination strategies on current equipment and software. Dynamic contrast enhancement patterns can be affected by a wide range of physiologic factors, which include vessel density, blood flow, endothelial permeability, and the size of the EES in which contrast is distributed. Additionally, system properties, including T_2* dephasing, vascular leakage or the lack thereof, T_1 shortening, water exchange, R_2^* relaxivity changes, dispersion caused by flow, and artifacts in acquiring an input function, influence the signal response.[83] Specifically, in DCE-MRI, contrast agent is detected indirectly via its effect of increasing R_1 relaxation rate in the surrounding water molecules. A tissue voxel typically consists of four water-containing compartments, two cellular compartments (red blood cells (RBC) and parenchyma cells) and two extracellular compartments (intravascular plasma and EES). It is generally accepted that water exchange between RBC and blood plasma is extremely rapid due to high water permeability of the RBC membrane, and therefore plasma and RBC can be considered a single water compartment with a single T_1 ignoring the rate of exchange of water protons between the intra- and extracellular spaces in blood. It has been shown that substantial errors can occur when ignoring the effects of water exchange.[84] However, the importance of vascular–interstitial and interstitial–cellular water exchange in the analysis of DCE-MRI data is still a topic of debate since there is evidence that clinically relevant DCE-MRI might be exchange insensitive with little or no influence from interstitial–cellular water exchange.[85,86]

Buckley has suggested that the application of commonly accepted models and their respective model-based assumptions to DCE-MRI data leads to systematic overestimation of K^{trans} in tumors.[37] Thus, it is difficult to be certain about how accurately the model-based kinetic parameter estimates compare with the physiologic parameters that they purport to measure, though some studies have shown broad correlations between microvascular density, stromal cellularity, tissue oxygenation and proliferation, and DCE-MRI parameters.[87–90] In general, DCE-MRI kinetic models are usually linear compartmental models, which can be broadly classified as lumped parameter or distributed parameter (DP) models.[1] Compartments are used to describe the physical distribution spaces of the tracer in the tissue and are assumed to be well mixed, such that tracer concentration is only a function of time, but not space. Thus, conventional compartmental models are also called lumped parameter models. On the other hand, a DP model attempts to account for tracer concentration gradient within the compartments, such that concentration can be a function of both time and space. For description, equations, and diagrams of DP models and their variations, the reader is referred to illustrative literature reviews.[1,91] Preferably, DCE-MRI should be preceded by a theoretical description of the model system and an experiment designed to generate a system response that will allow model parameters to be estimated. Data-driven model selection is also dictated by the generation of clinically important inferences based on stable parametric estimates. These may well vary from tissue to tissue and from pathology to pathology. For instance, when K^{trans} values are relatively low and flow and vascular volume are relatively high, DP models will be selected in brain tumors.[91,92]

A practical question often asked is whether it is necessary to quantify imaging data since semiquantitative analyses seem to work well in the clinic. However, semiquantitative methods are not interchangeable between centers and are limitedly reproducible. Quantification techniques aim to minimize errors that can result from the use of different equipment and imaging protocols, while they provide insights into tumor biology. Quantification techniques are therefore preferred when evaluating antivascular, anticancer drugs.[74,93]

Clinical Applications of DCE-MRI

Pretherapeutic Tumor Imaging Workup

The use of DCE-MRI in the characterization of primary tumors of the central nervous system is somewhat limited but shows encouraging result in this direction[94,95] (Figs. 15.6 and 15.7). The correlation of increased permeability with higher tumor grade has been demonstrated to be a robust biomarker for tumor grading.[94] DCE-MRI estimates of tumor physiology depict in a limited fashion the tumor histologic features as tumor typing by DCE-MRI is spatial resolution dependent.[96] Reports that permeability measures are slightly less predictive of tumor grade than rCBV[32] come are not surprising as, in addition to neoangiogenesis, there are a large number of physiologic processes that may increase capillary permeability: local inflammatory response to the tumor, tumor ischemia, release of toxic metabolites, response to corticosteroids, use of chemotherapeutic agents, and radiation injury, to name a few. Several studies showed a strong independent relationship between both rCBV and K^{trans} and histologic grade in gliomas with satisfactory discriminative power in distinguishing between low- (grade II) and high-grade (grade IV) tumors,[31,97,98] though there is a certain overlap between tumors of grades II and III. An interesting approach utilizes a subcompartmentalization of EES into permeability and leaky space, and using local AIF results in improved discrimination between high- and low-grade gliomas.[99] Beyond K^{trans}, a recent study has shown that v_e may be of comparable efficiency in differentiating high-grade gliomas (they showed higher v_e values) from low-grade gliomas.[100] Unlikely to DSC-MRI, DCE-MRI is not broadly utilized for guiding stereotactic biopsy though there is initial evidence that colocalization of DCE-MRI abnormalities and proliferation indexes may exist.[101] A recent study indicates also the potential for K^{trans} to serve as surrogate marker for nuclear density and tumor infiltration borders, thus guiding therapeutic interventions.[102]

Tumor Surveillance

DCE-MRI is also able to monitor the effects of antivascular and anticancer drugs.[103–105] It is noteworthy that enhancement on DCE-MRI can be affected by most types of successful treatments. This reflects on the fact that tumor cell kill ultimately results in apoptosis of proliferating endothelial cells and vascular shutdown. Measuring absolute K^{trans} values in patients undergoing treatment can help predict tumor recurrence or progression, as any progressive increase of K^{trans} could indirectly suggest worsening angiogenesis and, hence, more malignant or aggressive tumor in a previously stable or treated primary tumor site (Fig. 15.8). Furthermore, DCE-MRI may be used as a predictor tool for progression-free and overall survival rates though the literature is limited because accurate measurement of tumor vascular leakiness is technically more challenging than measuring tumor blood volume (Fig. 15.9). Microvascular leakage is correlated with poor prognosis irrespective of the morphologic or histopathologic features,[106,107] a finding akin to the DSC-MRI studies.[49] Contrary to these findings, Mills et al. reported that patients with higher K^{trans} showed better survival.[108]

Treatment of high-grade gliomas with concurrent chemoradiation induces acute and late changes in normal brain and tumors, which often have unspecific findings, are indistinguishable from true tumor relapse, and pose significant diagnostic dilemmas (Fig. 15.10). Theoretically, vascular permeability due to tumor angiogenesis and increased vascular density estimates may differentiate radiation necrosis from recurrent tumor, with radiation necrosis showing low blood volume and K^{trans}, as it consists primarily of hyalinized vasculopathy and coagulative necrosis, which leads to areas of hypoperfusion and reduced vascular density.[55,109] However, radiation necrosis represents a heterogeneous process with features resembling inflammation, and immature vessels may grow into previously necrotic areas, and viable tumor cells may still be found in the areas with decreased blood volume. Furthermore, a significant portion of patients undergoing adjuvant or concurrent chemoradiation may show increased size of the enhancing lesion and/or edema. Such findings, which can be misinterpreted as progression of the tumor, are often attributed to pseudoprogression.[110] Pseudoprogression is a complex phenomenon consisted of treatment-induced necrosis, postoperative infarcts, and increased vascular permeability due to tapering of steroid dose. DSC-MRI–derived rCBV may differentiate pseudoprogression from early tumor progression,[111,112] but DCE-MRI (at least in semiquantitative indices) is also a promising method that can overcome the DSC-MRI limitations, particularly in previously treated patients due to the presence of hemorrhage, calcification, and surgical clips.[113]

Combined T_1- and T_2-Weighted MR Approaches

Approaches using both T_1 and T_2 or $T_2{}^*$ weighting have been developed as a method of minimizing the confounding effects of vascular leakage in regions of an interrupted BBB. The separation of T_1- and $T_2{}^*$-induced signal changes using dual-echo pulse sequences has been shown to be a potential method to simultaneously estimate blood flow, blood volume (from the $T_2{}^*$ time series), and parameters related to the extravasation kinetics (from the T_1 time series) in human brain tumors.[114–116] Recently, another study demonstrated that a dual-echo DSC-MRI experiment, when combined with a precontrast T_1 map, enables the reliable determination of the K^{trans} and v_e parameters typically acquired in a quantitative DCE-MRI study.

Perfusion MRI with Endogenous Tracer

Arterial Spin Labeling

ASL is a totally noninvasive, perfusion-weighted MRI method that calculates cerebral perfusion maps (in terms of blood flow) without the need of intravenous contrast agent administration and, instead, uses arterial blood water as an endogenous diffusible tracer by inverting the magnetization of the blood using radiofrequency (RF) pulses (Fig. 15.11). After a delay to allow for labeled blood to flow into the brain tissue, labeled images are acquired that contain signal from both labeled water and static tissue water.[117] The inflow of the label brings negative magnetization, which mixes with the static tissue positive magnetization and results in a small decrease in signal intensity of approximately 1% to 2%. Control images without prior labeling of arterial spins are also separately acquired, and the signal difference between control and labeled images provides a measure of labeled blood from arteries delivered to the tissue by perfusion. In the last decades, a plethora of labeling schemes, readout options, and models to quantify perfusion, or blood flow, in the brain has been proposed. Many implementation choices of ASL are influenced by the fact that the lifetime of the tracer, which is governed by the longitudinal relaxation time of blood (1,300 to 1,750 milliseconds at clinical field strengths),[118] is similar to the transport time from the labeling position to the tissue (known as the arterial transit time [ATT]). The fundamental trade-off is that a short delay does not allow for complete delivery of the labeled blood water to the tissue, whereas a long delay results in strong T_1 decay and therefore reduced signal-to-noise ratio (SNR). Clinically available and extensively utilized ASL labeling approaches can be grouped into two types: continuous and pseudocontinuous ASL (CASL and

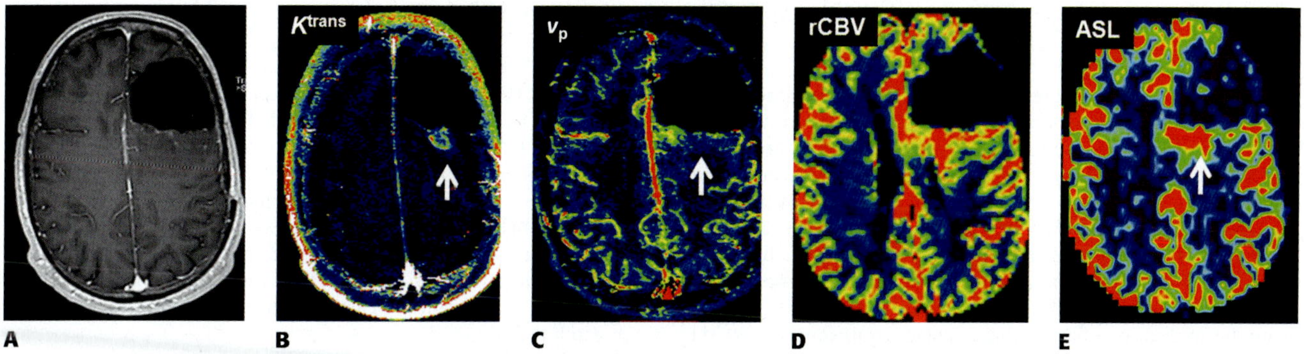

Figure 15-8. A: Morphologic MR imaging of newly appearing gadolinium enhancement on the posterior border of the tumor resection cavity. **B** and **C:** DCE-MRI–derived parameters indicate neoangiogenesis (*arrow* in K^{trans} map) with leaky vasculature as well as development of mature tumor vascular bed (*arrow* in v_p map) at different tumor sites. Interestingly, the DSC-MRI–derived leakage-corrected map **(D)**, which suffers from inferior spatial resolution, provides evidence of tumor angiogenesis over the complete resection margin, whereas the ASL map **(E)** shows clearly the pathologically high perfusion on the tumor site with nondisrupted vasculature (*arrow*).

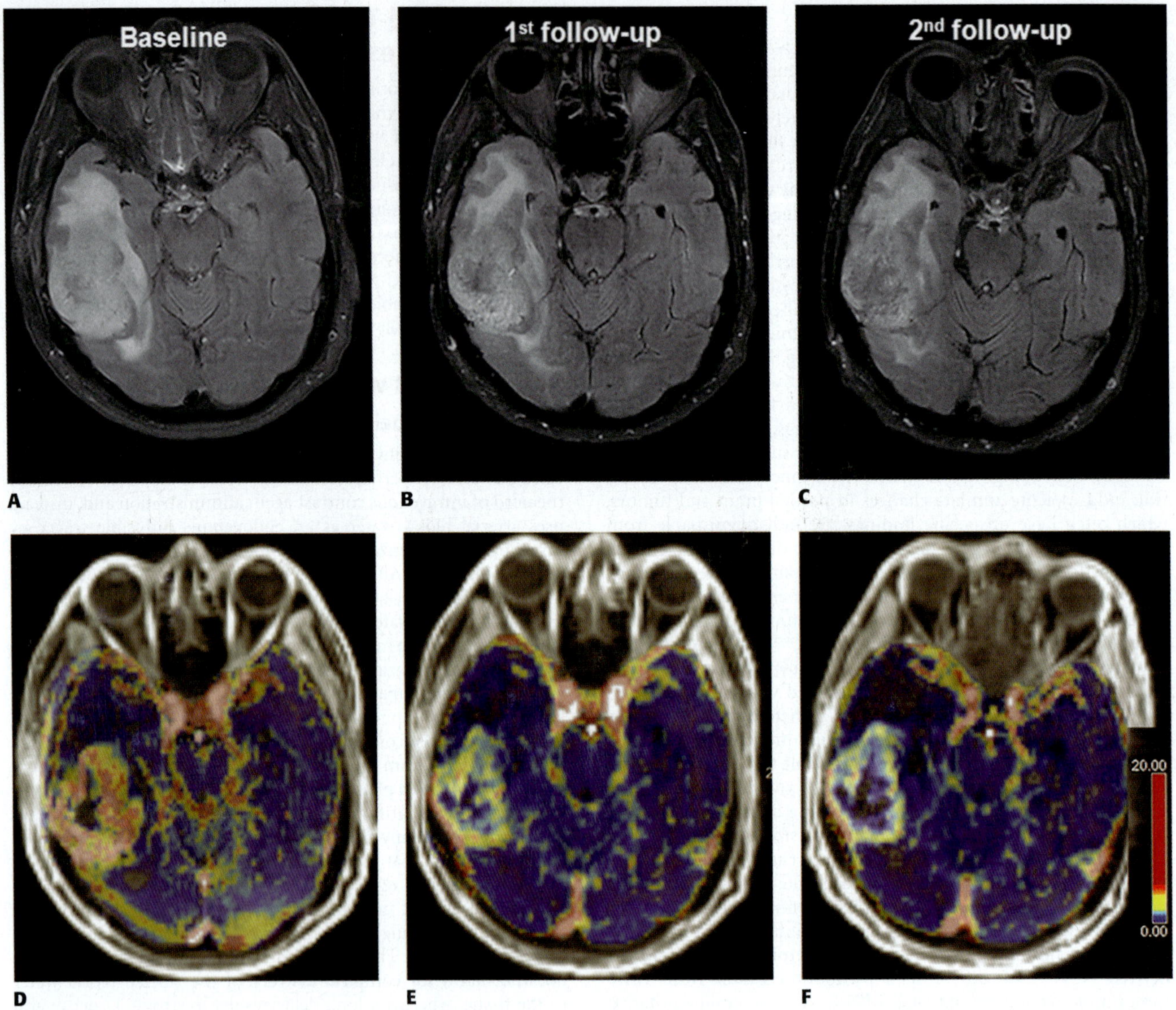

Figure 15-9. Serial morphologic MR imaging (FLAIR) before (A) and after (B and C) initiation of concurrent chemoradiation in a patient with glioblastoma on the right temporal lobe. The mid- **(B)** and end-treatment **(C)** anatomical scans show intrinsic therapy-related structural changes (usually hemorrhages and necrosis) without obvious reduction in the tumor size. DCE-MRI–generated K^{trans} estimates in the therapy course **(D–F)** demonstrate a significant (>50%) reduction of the tumor perfusion/neoangiogenesis. Thus, intratreatment DCE-MRI may be used to classify the responders and potentially serve as prognostic tool. (Courtesy: Dr. Katarina Surlan-Popovic, Ljubljana, Slovenia).

PCASL, respectively) where constant RF pulse and gradient are applied over the labeling period[119,120] (in PCASL, the continuous RF and gradient pulses are divided into shorter lengths) and pulsed ASL (PASL) where an RF pulse inverts a slab of tissue (usually 15 to 20 cm thick), including arteries, proximal to the area of interest.[121] The time between the end of this pulse train and image acquisition is referred to as the postlabeling delay (PLD). For PASL, the timing of the labeling pulse is characterized by a single time point, since the labeling pulse is nearly instantaneous (tens of ms). The time from the application of this pulse to image acquisition is referred to as the inversion time (TI). Because PLD refers to the time at which the end of the labeled bolus leaves the labeling plane in PCASL, the analogous time in PASL is the time at which the end of the labeled bolus passes through the distal end of the labeling slab. In PASL, this time is generally unknown, as the temporal width of the labeled bolus in PASL is not controlled. With the QUIPSS-II (Quantitative Imaging of Perfusion Using a Single Subtraction Method II) modification,[122] the bolus width is controlled and is referred to as TI_1. In general, CASL has higher SNR than PASL but is more hardware and specific absorption rate (SAR) intensive. Both forms of continuous ASL constitute long label scenarios, but PCASL provides superior labeling efficiency and is recommended for clinical imaging. Another method, the velocity-selective ASL, labels spins on the basis of velocity rather than location and, as such, is theoretically insensitive to differences in arterial arrival times but is currently a research technique.[123]

Modeling and Postprocessing of ASL MRI

For the most attractive feature of ASL, namely, to quantify perfusion without the need of intravenous contrast agent administration, a relatively basic model is proposed. The major assumptions of this model are that the entire labeled bolus is delivered to the target

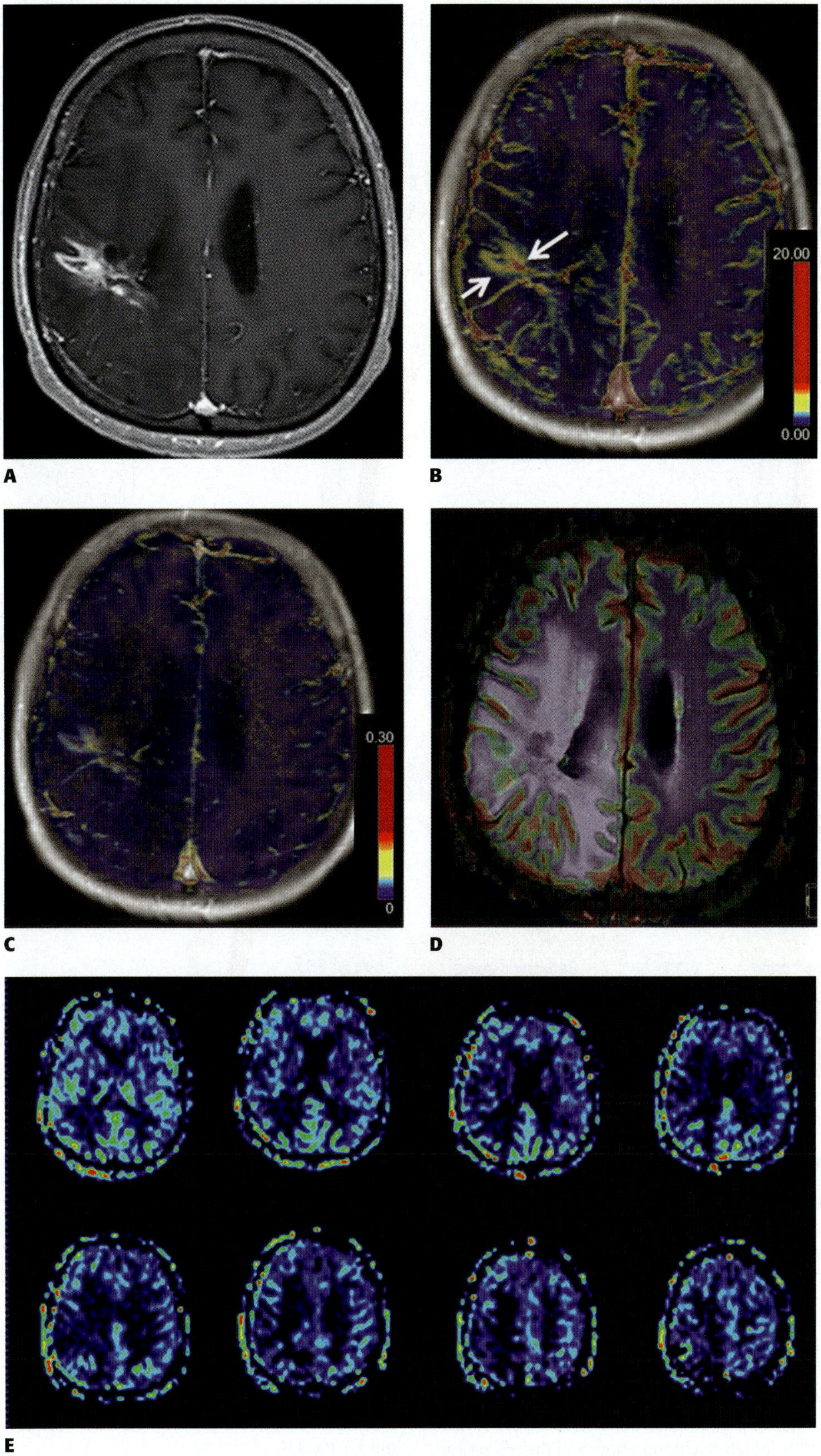

Figure 15-10. **Combined approach using three different perfusion techniques to address the diagnostic dilemma, tumor relapse versus treatment-related changes.** Postgadolinium T_1-weighted image shows avid enhancement and significant amount of surrounding edema in a patient after stereotactic radiation therapy of bronchial carcinoma metastasis on the right parietal lobe **(A)**. Hyperperfusion is evident on the DCE-MRI–derived IAUC map (*arrows*) that is akin to blood volume maps; however, IAUC estimates are difficult to be straightforwardly interpreted **(B)**. K^{trans} estimates in this region show only subtle alterations without strong evidence of tumor neoangiogenesis **(C)**. The DSC-MRI–derived leakage-corrected rCBV map (overlaid on the FLAIR image) **(D)** demonstrates no pathologically elevated blood volume, and the ASL technique **(E)** shows also no elevated perfusion in terms of blood flow in the suspected area. Subsequently performed surgery with multiple biopsies from the gadolinium enhancing tumor showed extensive radiation necrosis and treatment-induced tissue changes.

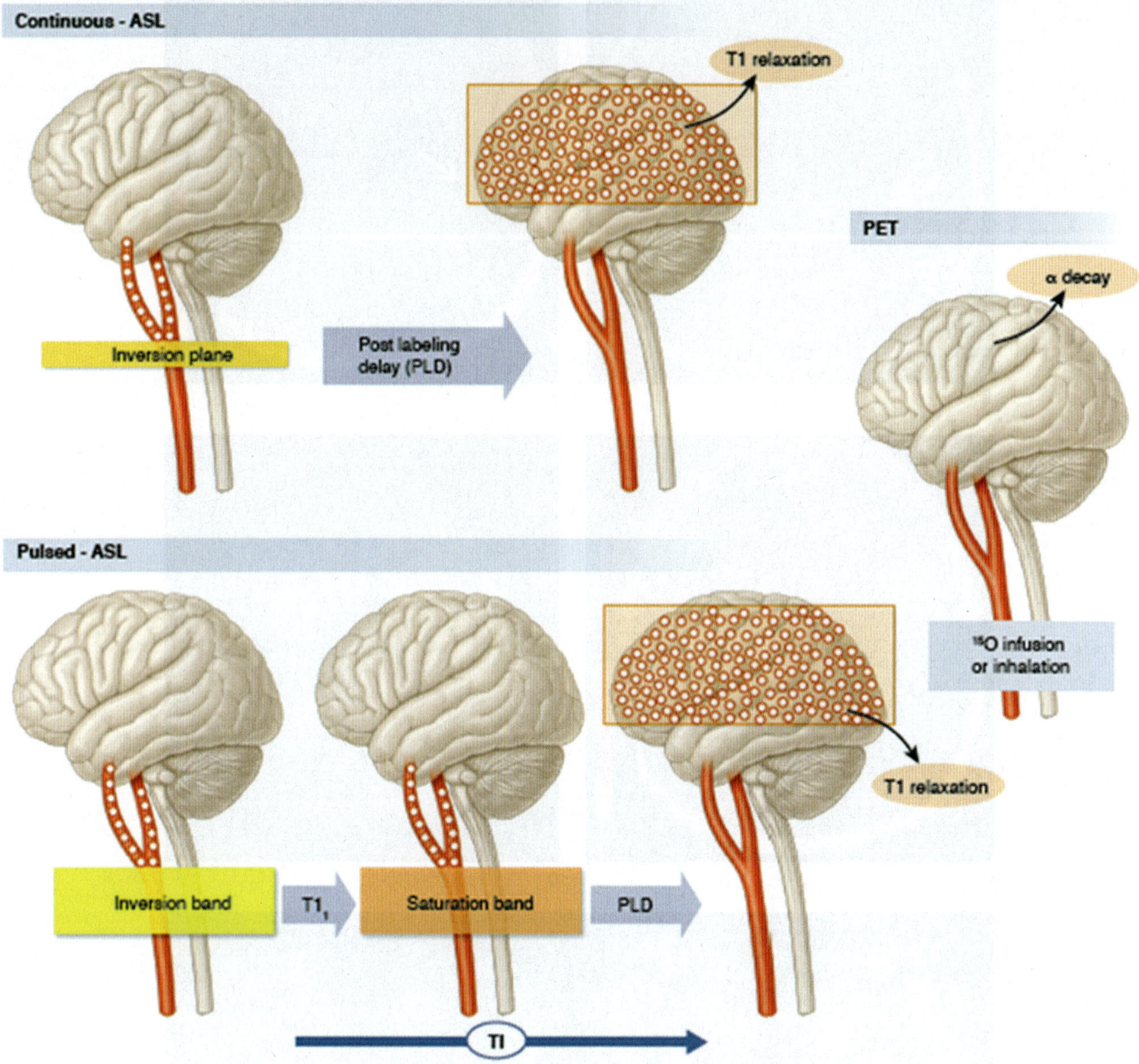

Figure 15-11. Illustration of arterial spin labeling (ASL), including the general principles of continuous and pulsed ASL, comparing to ^{15}O-PET as both methods provide absolute quantification of tissue perfusion. In ASL, endogenous arterial blood water is magnetically labeled and the magnetic label decays with T_1 (T_1 relaxation) instead of radioactive decay (α) after exogenous administration of ^{15}O. In continuous ASL (CASL) **(upper row)**, the arterial spins are continuously labeled as they flow through the labeling or inversion plane for a certain duration of time (labeling time). The PLD refers to the time between labeling and imaging and is used to allow labeled arterial water to reach the microcirculation and reduce the contributions of arterial signals (seen often as hyperperfused spots) to the perfusion image. In pulsed ASL (PASL) **(lower row)**, a slab of tissue, including arterial blood, is labeled. A single pulse simultaneously inverts the entire labeled bolus, and this bolus decays with time constant T_1 for the entire time between the inversion pulse and image acquisition. The general drawback of PASL of creating a labeled bolus with unknown and relatively short temporal width has been overcome by the QUIPSS-II modification (see text), where a slab-selective saturation pulse (matching the labeling slab) is used to remove the tail end of the labeled bolus, which has now a width of $T1_1$. Thus, the PLD in CASL is analogous to the quantity TI-$T1_1$ in PASL. Recommended imaging parameters; 3 T field strength, segmented 3D readout acquisition, spatial resolution of 3- to 4-mm in-plane and 4- to 6-mm through-plane, scan time ≅ 5 minutes.

tissue, there is no outflow of labeled blood water, and the relaxation of the labeled spins is governed by blood T_1.[124] Under these assumptions, CBF (in mL/100 g/min) in each voxel can be calculated for PCASL using[125]

$$\mathrm{CBF} = \frac{6{,}000 \cdot \lambda \cdot \left(\mathrm{SI}_{\mathrm{control}} - \mathrm{SI}_{\mathrm{label}}\right) \cdot e^{PLD/T_{1,\mathrm{blood}}}}{2 \cdot \alpha \cdot T_{1,\mathrm{blood}} \cdot \mathrm{SI}_{\mathrm{PD}} \cdot \left(1 - e^{-\tau/T_{1,\mathrm{blood}}}\right)} \tag{6}$$

and for PASL[122]

$$\mathrm{CBF} = \frac{6{,}000 \cdot \lambda \cdot \left(\mathrm{SI}_{\mathrm{control}} - \mathrm{SI}_{\mathrm{label}}\right) \cdot e^{\mathrm{TI}/T_{1,\mathrm{blood}}}}{2 \cdot \alpha \cdot \mathrm{TI}_1 \cdot \mathrm{SI}_{\mathrm{PD}}} \tag{7}$$

where λ is the blood–brain partition coefficient in mL/g; $\mathrm{SI}_{\mathrm{control}}$ and $\mathrm{SI}_{\mathrm{label}}$ are the time-averaged signal intensities in the control and label images, respectively; $T_{1,\mathrm{blood}}$ is the longitudinal relaxation time of blood in seconds; α is the labeling efficiency; SI_{PD} is the signal intensity of a proton density–weighted image; and τ is the label duration. PLD, TI, and TI_1 are as defined above. To scale the signal intensities of the subtracted ASL images to absolute CBF units, the signal intensity of fully relaxed blood spins is needed. Usually, a separately acquired proton density (PD) image (represented by SI_{PD} in the above equations) is used to obtain this scaling factor on a voxel-by-voxel basis. The factor of 6,000 converts the units from mL/(g s) to mL/100 g/min, which is customary in the physiologic literature.

Critical Appraisal of ASL

Field strength of 3 T is recommended when available, though satisfactory results can be obtained at 1.5 T. The advantage of increased field strength is higher SNR, which results from a combination of higher intrinsic SNR and longer T_1 of blood. The lower SNR at 1.5 T can be compensated for by a combination of decreased spatial resolution and/or increased scan time. The use of multichannel receive head coils with eight or more channels is advised for ASL and enables parallel acquisition, which however can come at a cost in SNR, and as ASL is significantly SNR limited, parallel acceleration should be used judiciously. Because ASL is a subtractive technique, it is sensitive to motion, and segmented 3D acquisition methods incur additional motion sensitivity. Therefore, patient motion should be minimized as much as possible. Motion sensitivity can also be partially mitigated by the use of background suppression. Another important feature in the ASL sequences is the suppression of signal from larger arteries at the time of imaging through the use of vascular crushing gradients. Besides the apparent advantage of vascular crushing gradients in removing any physiologic arterial signal that obscures tissue pathologies (e.g., tumors), they may remove also important clinical information, such as the presence of delayed flow and arteriovenous shunting. The effective TE will be prolonged when using vascular crushing, thereby introducing T_2 (or T_2*) contrast into the ASL image and a reduction in SNR. This should be taken into account in the calculation of CBF.[124,126] For single PLD imaging, the PLD is chosen so that it will be longer than ATT for the majority of cases. When this condition is true, the effects of vascular crushing gradients on the ASL image will be minimal. Therefore, the implementation of vascular crushing gradients should be a user-controlled option, as they will likely be useful under some circumstances, but not others.[124]

CBF quantification errors can occur due to delays in ATT. ATTs are regionally dependent and difficult to measure accurately, but may be on the order of the label T_1; thus, CBF underestimations can occur. It should be understood that areas of low ASL signal may reflect some combination of low CBF and unusually long ATT, and not specifically low CBF. Acquisition of different ASL images at different inflow times enables direct estimation of both ATT and CBF; however, this approach is usually time consuming and the results may be confusing during the early inflow times, whereas the imaging is noisy and challenging to fit in a robust fashion.[18] Further information needed for precise quantification of brain tissue perfusion includes water exchange rates and times between blood and tissue, tissue T_1 values, and tissue segmentation. The latter is important for quantification of the white matter perfusion, which is hallmarked by low SNR and prolonged ATT, especially in elderly patients or subjects with cerebrovascular disease. Furthermore, the white matter ASL signal can easily be overwhelmed by gray matter signal due to blurring in either in-plane or through-plane directions.[127] The sensitivity for detection of white matter perfusion deficits should therefore be considered to be too small for general clinical use and therefore should be cautiously used as reference region for rCBF ASL measurements.

Clinical Applications of ASL

By eliminating the need for exogenous tracer, ASL provides an advantageous solution for performing serial scans to track tumor growth and/or drug response, though the lack of permeability indices may be viewed as drawback of the method. Besides, it is applicable in children as well as patients with renal failure or high risk of nephrogenic systemic fibrosis (NSF). Previous studies have shown that DSC-MRI and ASL yield comparable perfusion values in normal brain tissue[128,129] and may correlate with vascular density[130] and DSC-MRI–derived blood volume metrics, but discrepancies may also be observed in a considerable percentage of brain tumors.[131–135] Tumor blood flow estimated by ASL shows a positive correlation with tumor grade and aggressiveness for intra-axial neoplasms,[136] whereas oligodendrogliomas create difficulties akin to the ones observed in DSC-MRI[137] (Fig. 15.12). Weak correlation was also observed between DCE-derived blood flow and pseudocontinuous ASL measurements in human gliomas, whereas there was no correlation in normal gray and white matter regions.[138] Interestingly, ATT showed a negative correlation between tumor grade, more profoundly in GBMs but was not significantly different compared to the contralateral white matter.[136] ASL-derived tumor blood flow and ATT could reliably discriminate GBMs from metastases or lymphomas.[136] Concerning extra-axial tumors, CASL-derived blood flow measurements in meningiomas showed significant correlation with microvessel area and higher blood flow values in angiomatous meningiomas compared to the fibrous subtypes.[139] The interchangeability of blood flow values between the two modalities is limited,[129,131] and this may be partly attributed to the different underlying principles as well as to acquisition parameters, for example, the use of vascular crusher gradients in ASL. It is still not clear in ASL imaging whether relative measures of blood flow may also be useful like the absolute ones.[136,137] In that case, the choice of the reference tissue is of major importance and any shortcomings of the ASL, for example, in estimating white matter perfusion, should be considered. An interesting extension of ASL technique is the estimation of arterial blood volume[140]; hereby, a weak correlation with DSC-MRI–derived rCBV parameters was observed.[141]

In the posttreatment setting, ASL methodology has been applied to evaluate metastases before and after radiation, demonstrating that a decrease of tumor blood flow to gray matter ratio was predictive for treatment response.[142] On contrary, there is scarce evidence in the application of ASL for differentiation between treatment-related necrosis and recurrence but the initial experience is encouraging.[55] For this clinical situation, it seems more appropriate to use absolute ASL quantification in order to overcome shortcomings related to the therapeutic effect to reference tissues. Finally, ASL-based blood flow quantification may also be used as a noninvasive marker to prognosticate the progression-free survival, independently on histopathologic tumor grading, as preliminary evidence shows in patients with gliomas.

Intravoxel Incoherent Motion (IVIM) Analysis of DWI Data

In 1988, Le Bihan et al.[143] defined IVIM as the microscopic translational motions that occur in each image voxel during an MR acquisition. In biologic tissues, these motions include molecular diffusion of water and microcirculation of blood in the capillary network. Microcirculation of the blood in capillary network (perfusion) can also be considered as an incoherent motion since the capillary organization can be seen at the voxel size as random. These two phenomena account for the biexponential decay of the signal observed on DWI when different diffusion *b*-values are applied. The IVIM modeling allows the extraction of two diffusion coefficients, one related to molecular diffusion restriction, D (also known as D_{slow}), and another related to the tissue perfusion called D^* (also known as D_{fast}), and finally the vascular volume fraction f. The contribution from larger (feeding or draining) vessels, in which blood velocity is higher, is more or less spoiled by the presence of the magnetic-pulsed gradients. Standard single-shot (ss) diffusion-weighted SE-EPI with adequate number of averages (i.e., 3 to 4)

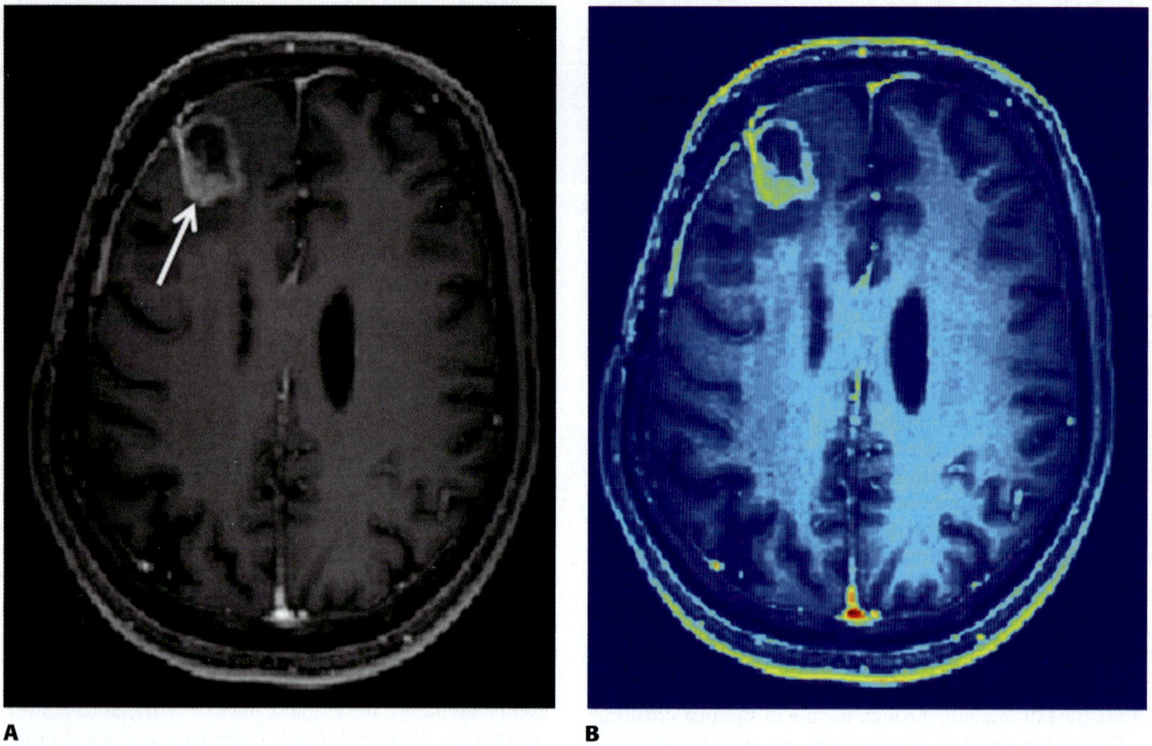

Figure 15-12. A: Contrast-enhanced T_1-weighted MR imaging demonstrates a partially necrotic mass with marked vascularization (*arrow*) on the right frontal lobe. **B:** ASL measurement (overlaid on the anatomic image) with blood flow quantification showed that the perfusion in the hypervascularized rim reached 160 mL/min/100 g tissue.

and multiple optimally distributed b-values (i.e., 10 values under 200 s/mm^2 and 5 values over 200 s/mm^2) ranging from 0 s/mm^2 to a maximum of 1,500 s/mm^2 is needed to model the biexponential decay of the MR signal with increasing b-value.

Postprocessing of IVIM DWI Data

On the processing side, an image-based correction of eddy current–induced distortions is recommended. Using the IVIM algorithm, described by the biexponential equation below, D_{slow}, D_{fast} and f maps can be generated, where D_{slow} and D_{fast} are the diffusion parameter related with molecular diffusion and with the incoherent microcirculation, respectively; S is the mean signal intensity ($S(0)$ before the application of diffusion gradients); and f is the perfusion fraction:

$$S = (1-f)\exp(-b * D_{slow}) + f * \exp(-b * (D_{slow} + D_{fast}))S(0) \quad (8)$$

The user may fit the data using three different approaches: (i) full biexponential fit, (ii) initial estimation of D_{slow} using a reduced set of b-values larger than a predetermined value and then using the resulting D_{slow} as a fix parameter to fit the missing parameters,[144] and (iii) fix D_{fast} with a given value and use it in the biexponential model to fit the missing values.[145] However, the quality of D_{fast} maps is theoretically highly dependent on the acquisition protocol and ROI. If the image quality is not sufficient, the D_{fast} map may have information that cannot be interpreted.

Clinical Applications and Critical Appraisal of IVIM Analysis

In recent years, there has been a renewed interest in IVIM on brain tumors[4,146,147] because of the improved MR hardware, which allows short-time acquisitions with multiple b-values and sufficient SNR. The initial results show the applicability of IVIM for the staging of gliomas as well as in the differentiation recurrent gliomas from treatment effects (Fig. 15.13). The immediately reraised question is whether the IVIM-based f may be surrogate markers to the established DCE- and DSC-based ones for the tumor imaging. The potential of IVIM to characterize tumors was underscored by Cho et al. in a complex flow phantom, which was constructed to mimic certain characteristics of the tumor microenvironment such as tortuous microvasculature, heterogeneous vascular permeability, and interstitial fluid pressure buildup.[148] Unlike conventional DWI measurements, which show satisfactory robustness as well as reproducibility and repeatability metrics, the D_{fast} and f maps seem to suffer from inherent noise, which is accentuated by the selected range of low b-values and the fitting process.[149] Cerebrospinal fluid (CSF) partial volume contamination is also a confounding error source for D_{fast} and f maps,[150] which due to its rapid decay with increasing b-value leads to an overestimation of f. Thus, f maps may have to rectify the irritating constant linear flow of CSF by inversion or flow-compensated gradient pulses.[151,152] This is possible but not always feasible or meaningful, since CSF suppression in the areas with rapid flow is usually incomplete, the normal brain parenchyma signal is also considerably attenuated, the slice thickness has to be suitably increased, and cardiac gating may be necessary. Not surprisingly, inversion recovery DWI with broad bandwidth inversion pulse may lead to reduced f values even in sites remote to CSF spaces. At an initial stage, IVIM will probably act as complementary and not "stand-alone" modality for tumor imaging, given the remarkable efficiency of other functional and physiologic MRI modalities. The compartmental water exchange in the DWI experiments is not adequately captured due to the short evolution time (≈100 milliseconds) compared to the dynamic contrast-enhanced MRI, which tracks the intra- and extravascular

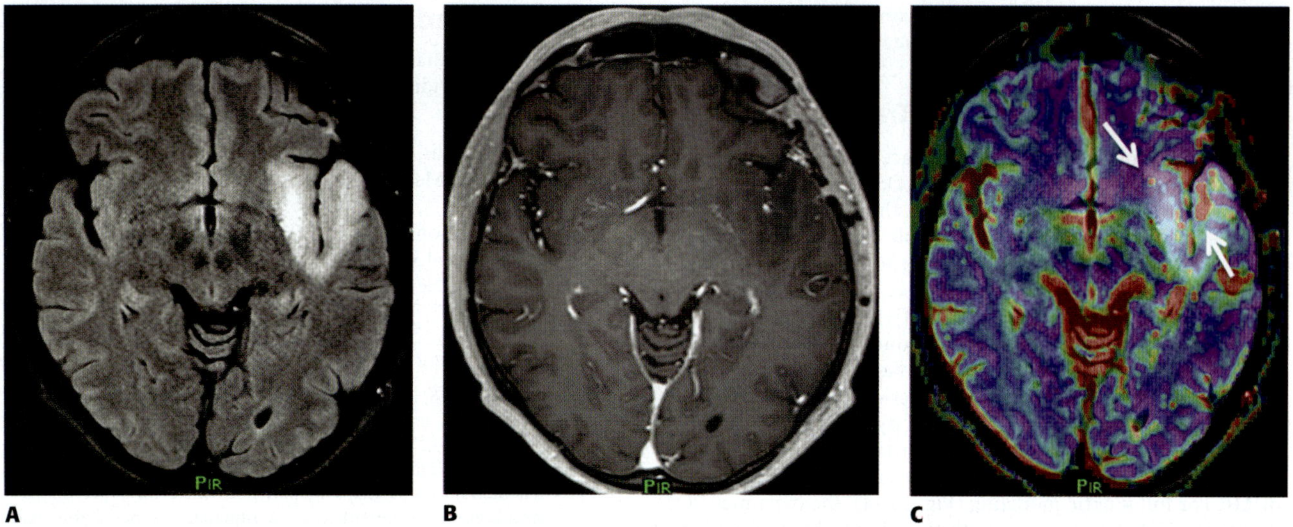

Figure 15-13. FLAIR **(A)** and postcontrast T_1-weighted **(B)** MR imaging of a patient with a glioma on the left temporal lobe cannot reliably stage the tumor. **C:** IVIM-derived *f* map overlaid on the FLAIR scan shows areas with increased *f* values (*arrows*) indicative of WHO grade 3 tumor, which was subsequently histologically proven. Note, however, the confounding effect of CSF-filled sulci, which hamper the diagnostic value of the *f* maps in the juxtacortical regions.

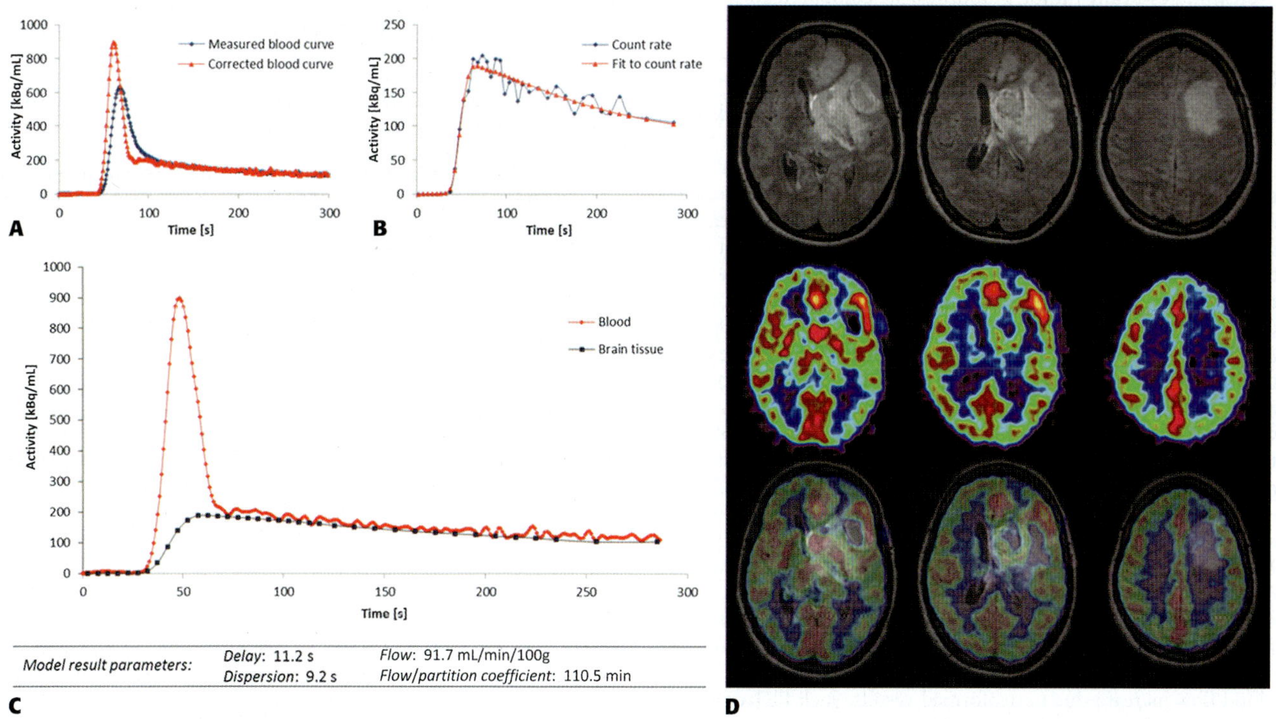

Figure 15-14. Example of full kinetic modeling of $[^{15}O]H_2O$ PET data to quantify blood flow **(A–C)** and clinical example with combined MR-PET imaging in a patient with glioblastoma **(D)**. **(A)** Arterial input function, **(B)** tissue response in a cortical brain region, and **(C)** resulting curves after correction for tracer arrival times and bolus dispersion. **Bottom**: Input and output parameters of the model. (Figure reproduced from Zeisig, et al. Cerebral blood flow measurement with oxygen-15 water positron emission tomography. In: Dierckx R, Otte A, de Vries E, et al., eds. *PET and SPECT of neurobiological systems*. 2014:103–124 with permission of Springer, Berlin/Heidelberg). In **(D)**, the heterogeneity of blood flow in the tumor micro-environment is remarkable varying from regions (attributed to edema) with very low blood flow to avidly perfused tumor parts close to the midline. (Courtesy: Dr. Geoffrey Warnock, Zurich, Switzerland).

as well as the exchange dynamics of the contrast agent over longer time acquisitions and also delivers permeability indices.

PET Imaging with Diffusible Tracers

The most popular PET diffusible tracers are [^{15}O]H_2O and [^{11}C]butanol. As compared to [^{15}O]H_2O, [^{11}C]butanol has the advantage of being permeable through the blood–brain barrier to 100%, making this tracer in principle the perfect candidate. However, [^{11}C]butanol is not used in routine practice because of its complex radiochemical synthesis.[153] Different methods to produce ^{15}O and to synthesize [^{15}O]H_2O are available. The latter is realized by either in-target or out-of-target production approaches. The classical approach to image brain blood flow by [^{15}O]H_2O PET consists of a bolus injection of 0.5 to 1 GBq of the tracer, followed by 2- to 5-minute dynamic image acquisition. In parallel, to achieve fully quantitative blood flow readouts, dynamic arterial blood sampling is required to establish an AIF. For full kinetic modeling (Fig. 15.14), the dynamic [^{15}O]H_2O brain PET data together with the AIF are used to describe the tracer kinetics via a single-tissue compartment model. As previously noted, one limitation of [^{15}O]H_2O for absolute quantification of blood flow needs to be considered: only about 90% of the tracer freely exchanges between intravascular space and tissue, with even lower rates at higher flow rates, resulting in a slightly underestimation of blood flow especially in high-flow regions.[154,155] With regard to blood flow measurement in brain tumors by means of [^{15}O]H_2O PET, a recent intraindividual comparison with perfusion CT revealed that the CT technique overestimates brain tumor blood flow as compared to the PET measures.[156]

Clinical Applications of PET Imaging

The most attractive advantage that PET CBF imaging holds over ASL is the length of the half-life of the injected radioactive tracer (2.1 minutes for [^{15}O]H_2O), which considerably exceeds the effective half-life of blood water proton label (T_1 = 1 to 2 seconds, depending on field strength) used in ASL. This allows for PET CBF measurements to be acquired at times of completed label accumulation in the tissue, whereas ASL may be hampered by residual arterial label contributing to the perfusion signal. Consequently, white matter CBF can likely be more accurately estimated by PET than by ASL. A side-by-side comparison of PET blood flow with ASL measurements demonstrated that at arterial transit time greater than 1,500 milliseconds, regional PASL-based CBF values were comparable with PET-based measurements (with similar spatial resolutions). However, at very high resolution as well as when PCASL was used, gray matter CBF values were found to increase by 10% to 20%, a consequence attributed to reduction in partial volume effects with cerebrospinal fluid and white matter.[157,158] Thus, in the era of hybrid MR-PET imaging, any disparities between PET and ASL will be examined in detail pointing toward a true measure of brain perfusion. Some other brain tumor blood flow PET studies combined [^{15}O]H_2O imaging with information with other PET readouts, like oxygen metabolism from ^{15}O inhalation,[159,160] demonstrating tumor blood flow increase due to neoformed vessels. Such PET data may provide useful information about the progression of brain tumors but has found no routine application so far. In a dual PET tracer trial, Bruehlmeier et al. employed [^{15}O]H_2O together with [^{18}F] fluoromisonidazole to study blood flow and hypoxia in various brain tumors.[161] Interestingly, it was shown that these parameters might be independent from each other. Presumably, such multitracer brain tumor imaging approaches might in future improve intensity-modulated radiotherapy or other targeted treatment approaches.

Acknowledgments

We would like to thank the following medical imaging software companies for providing us perfusion MR imaging postprocessing packages:

BrainMagix, Imagylis, Belgium (Fig. 15.1)
Olea Sphere, Olea Medical, France (Figs. 15.2B–D, 15.6, 15.7, and 15.13)
Syngo MR Perfusion, ASL and Tissue4D, Siemens Healthcare, Germany (Figs. 15.5, 15.9, and 26.10)
Tumor EX, Nordic NeuroLabs, Bergen, Norway (Fig. 15.3B–D)

REFERENCES

1. **Koh TS, Bisdas S, Koh DM, et al.** Fundamentals of tracer kinetics for dynamic contrast-enhanced MRI. *J Magn Reson Imaging* 2011;34(6):1262–1276.
2. **Varallyay CG, Nesbit E, Fu R, et al.** High-resolution steady-state cerebral blood volume maps in patients with central nervous system neoplasms using ferumoxytol, a superparamagnetic iron oxide nanoparticle. *J Cereb Blood Flow Metab* 2013;33(5):780–786.
3. **Hirai T, Kitajima M, Nakamura H, et al.** Quantitative blood flow measurements in gliomas using arterial spin-labeling at 3 T: intermodality agreement and inter- and intraobserver reproducibility study. *AJNR Am J Neuroradiol* 2011;32(11):2073–2079.
4. **Bisdas S, Koh TS, Roder C, et al.** Intravoxel incoherent motion diffusion-weighted MR imaging of gliomas: feasibility of the method and initial results. *Neuroradiology* 2013;55(10):1189–1196.
5. **Eleff SM, Schnall MD, Ligetti L, et al.** Concurrent measurements of cerebral blood flow, sodium, lactate, and high-energy phosphate metabolism using 19F, 23Na, 1H, and 31P nuclear magnetic resonance spectroscopy. *Magn Reson Med* 1988;7(4):412–424.
6. **Ackerman JJ, Ewy CS, Kim SG, et al.** Deuterium magnetic resonance in vivo: the measurement of blood flow and tissue perfusion. *Ann N Y Acad Sci* 1987;508:89–98.
7. **Pekar J, Ligeti L, Ruttner Z, et al.** In vivo measurement of cerebral oxygen consumption and blood flow using 17O magnetic resonance imaging. *Magn Reson Med* 1991;21(2):313–319.
8. **Meier P, Zierler KL.** On the theory of the indicator-dilution method for measurement of blood flow and volume. *J Appl Physiol* 1954;6(12):731–744.
9. **Kety SS.** The theory and applications of the exchange of inert gas at the lungs and tissues. *Pharmacol Rev* 1951;3(1):1–41.
10. **Bailey DL, Barthel H, Beuthin-Baumann B, et al.** Combined PET/MR: where are we now? Summary report of the second international workshop on PET/MR imaging April 8–12, 2013, Tubingen, Germany. *Mol Imaging Biol* 2014;16(3):295–310.
11. **Sugahara T, Korogi Y, Kochi M, et al.** Perfusion-sensitive MR imaging of gliomas: comparison between gradient-echo and spin-echo echo-planar imaging techniques. *AJNR Am J Neuroradiol* 2001;22(7):1306–1315.
12. **Simonsen CZ, Ostergaard L, Smith DF, et al.** Comparison of gradient- and spin-echo imaging: CBF, CBV, and MTT measurements by bolus tracking. *J Magn Reson Imaging* 2000;12(3):411–416.
13. **Donahue KM, Krouwer HG, Rand SD, et al.** Utility of simultaneously acquired gradient-echo and spin-echo cerebral blood volume and morphology maps in brain tumor patients. *Magn Reson Med* 2000;43(6):845–853.
14. **Ostergaard L, Sorensen AG, Kwong KK, et al.** High resolution measurement of cerebral blood flow using intravascular tracer bolus passages. Part II: experimental comparison and preliminary results. *Magn Reson Med* 1996;36(5):726–736.
15. **Boxerman JL, Schmainda KM, Weisskoff RM.** Relative cerebral blood volume maps corrected for contrast agent extravasation significantly correlate with glioma tumor grade, whereas uncorrected maps do not. *AJNR Am J Neuroradiol* 2006;27(4):859–867.
16. **Hu LS, Baxter LC, Pinnaduwage DS, et al.** Optimized preload leakage-correction methods to improve the diagnostic accuracy of dynamic susceptibility-weighted contrast-enhanced perfusion MR imaging in posttreatment gliomas. *AJNR Am J Neuroradiol* 2010;31(1):40–48.
17. **Miyati T, Banno T, Mase M, et al.** Dual dynamic contrast-enhanced MR imaging. *J Magn Reson Imaging* 1997;7(1):230–235.

18. **Zaharchuk G.** Theoretical basis of hemodynamic MR imaging techniques to measure cerebral blood volume, cerebral blood flow, and permeability. *AJNR Am J Neuroradiol* 2007;28(10):1850–1858.
19. **Emblem KE, Due-Tonnessen P, Hald JK, et al.** Automatic vessel removal in gliomas from dynamic susceptibility contrast imaging. *Magn Reson Med* 2009;61(5):1210–1217.
20. **Emblem KE, Scheie D, Due-Tonnessen P, et al.** Histogram analysis of MR imaging-derived cerebral blood volume maps: combined glioma grading and identification of low-grade oligodendroglial subtypes. *AJNR Am J Neuroradiol* 2008;29(9):1664–1670.
21. **Emblem KE, Nedregaard B, Nome T, et al.** Glioma grading by using histogram analysis of blood volume heterogeneity from MR-derived cerebral blood volume maps. *Radiology* 2008;247(3):808–817.
22. **Calamante F, Gadian DG, Connelly A.** Delay and dispersion effects in dynamic susceptibility contrast MRI: simulations using singular value decomposition. *Magn Reson Med* 2000;44(3):466–473.
23. **Wu O, Ostergaard L, Weisskoff RM, et al.** Tracer arrival timing-insensitive technique for estimating flow in MR perfusion-weighted imaging using singular value decomposition with a block-circulant deconvolution matrix. *Magn Reson Med* 2003;50(1):164–174.
24. **Gruner R, Taxt T.** Iterative blind deconvolution in magnetic resonance brain perfusion imaging. *Magn Reson Med* 2006;55(4):805–815.
25. **Orsingher L, Piccinini S, Crisi G.** Differences in dynamic susceptibility contrast MR perfusion maps generated by different methods implemented in commercial software. *J Comput Assist Tomogr* 2014;38(5):647–654.
26. **Cha S, Johnson G, Wadghiri YZ, et al.** Dynamic, contrast-enhanced perfusion MRI in mouse gliomas: correlation with histopathology. *Magn Reson Med* 2003;49(5):848–855.
27. **Zaro-Weber O, Moeller-Hartmann W, Heiss WD, et al.** The performance of MRI-based cerebral blood flow measurements in acute and subacute stroke compared with 15O-water positron emission tomography: identification of penumbral flow. *Stroke* 2009;40(7):2413–2421.
28. **Takasawa M, Jones PS, Guadagno JV, et al.** How reliable is perfusion MR in acute stroke? Validation and determination of the penumbra threshold against quantitative PET. *Stroke* 2008;39(3):870–877.
29. **Miyagami M, Katayama Y.** Angiogenesis of glioma: evaluation of ultrastructural characteristics of microvessels and tubular bodies (Weibel-Palade) in endothelial cells and immunohistochemical findings with VEGF and p53 protein. *Med Mol Morphol* 2005;38(1):36–42.
30. **Petersen ET, Zimine I, Ho YC, et al.** Non-invasive measurement of perfusion: a critical review of arterial spin labelling techniques. *Br J Radiol* 2006;79(944):688–701.
31. **Cha S, Yang L, Johnson G, et al.** Comparison of microvascular permeability measurements, K(trans), determined with conventional steady-state T_1-weighted and first-pass T_2*-weighted MR imaging methods in gliomas and meningiomas. *AJNR Am J Neuroradiol* 2006;27(2):409–417.
32. **Law M, Young R, Babb J, et al.** Comparing perfusion metrics obtained from a single compartment versus pharmacokinetic modeling methods using dynamic susceptibility contrast-enhanced perfusion MR imaging with glioma grade. *AJNR Am J Neuroradiol* 2006;27(9):1975–1982.
33. **Johnson G, Wetzel SG, Cha S, et al.** Measuring blood volume and vascular transfer constant from dynamic, T(2)*-weighted contrast-enhanced MRI. *Magn Reson Med* 2004;51(5):961–968.
34. **Liu HL, Wu YY, Yang WS, et al.** Is Weisskoff model valid for the correction of contrast agent extravasation with combined T_1 and T_2* effects in dynamic susceptibility contrast MRI? *Med Phys* 2011;38(2):802–809.
35. **Server A, Graff BA, Orheim TE, et al.** Measurements of diagnostic examination performance and correlation analysis using microvascular leakage, cerebral blood volume, and blood flow derived from 3 T dynamic susceptibility-weighted contrast-enhanced perfusion MR imaging in glial tumor grading. *Neuroradiology* 2011;53(6):435–447.
36. **Server A, Orheim TE, Graff BA, et al.** Diagnostic examination performance by using microvascular leakage, cerebral blood volume, and blood flow derived from 3-T dynamic susceptibility-weighted contrast-enhanced perfusion MR imaging in the differentiation of glioblastoma multiforme and brain metastasis. *Neuroradiology* 2011;53(5):319–330.
37. **Buckley DL.** Uncertainty in the analysis of tracer kinetics using dynamic contrast-enhanced T_1-weighted MRI. *Magn Reson Med* 2002;47(3):601–606.
38. **Chen JJ, Frayne R, Smith MR.** Reassessing the clinical efficacy of two MR quantitative DSC PWI CBF algorithms following cross-calibration with PET images. *Phys Med Biol* 2005;50(6):1251–1263.
39. **Hartmann M, Heiland S, Harting I, et al.** Distinguishing of primary cerebral lymphoma from high-grade glioma with perfusion-weighted magnetic resonance imaging. *Neurosci Lett* 2003;338(2):119–122.
40. **Yang S, Law M, Zagzag D, et al.** Dynamic contrast-enhanced perfusion MR imaging measurements of endothelial permeability: differentiation between atypical and typical meningiomas. *AJNR Am J Neuroradiol* 2003;24(8):1554–1559.
41. **Knopp EA, Cha S, Johnson G, et al.** Glial neoplasms: dynamic contrast-enhanced T_2*-weighted MR imaging. *Radiology* 1999;211(3):791–798.
42. **Saito T, Yamasaki F, Kajiwara Y, et al.** Role of perfusion-weighted imaging at 3 T in the histopathological differentiation between astrocytic and oligodendroglial tumors. *Eur J Radiol* 2012;81(8):1863–1869.
43. **Kumar VA, Knopp EA, Zagzag D.** Magnetic resonance dynamic susceptibility-weighted contrast-enhanced perfusion imaging in the diagnosis of posterior fossa hemangioblastomas and pilocytic astrocytomas: initial results. *J Comput Assist Tomogr* 2010;34(6):825–829.
44. **Maia AC Jr, Malheiros SM, da Rocha AJ, et al.** MR cerebral blood volume maps correlated with vascular endothelial growth factor expression and tumor grade in nonenhancing gliomas. *AJNR Am J Neuroradiol* 2005;26(4):777–783.
45. **Shin JH, Lee HK, Kwun BD, et al.** Using relative cerebral blood flow and volume to evaluate the histopathologic grade of cerebral gliomas: preliminary results. *AJR Am J Roentgenol* 2002;179(3):783–789.
46. **Lupo JM, Cha S, Chang SM, et al.** Dynamic susceptibility-weighted perfusion imaging of high-grade gliomas: characterization of spatial heterogeneity. *AJNR Am J Neuroradiol* 2005;26(6):1446–1454.
47. **Maia AC Jr, Malheiros SM, da Rocha AJ, et al.** Stereotactic biopsy guidance in adults with supratentorial nonenhancing gliomas: role of perfusion-weighted magnetic resonance imaging. *J Neurosurg* 2004;101(6):970–976.
48. **Danchaivijitr N, Waldman AD, Tozer DJ, et al.** Low-grade gliomas: do changes in rCBV measurements at longitudinal perfusion-weighted MR imaging predict malignant transformation? *Radiology* 2008;247(1):170–178.
49. **Bisdas S, Kirkpatrick M, Giglio P, et al.** Cerebral blood volume measurements by perfusion-weighted MR imaging in gliomas: ready for prime time in predicting short-term outcome and recurrent disease? *AJNR Am J Neuroradiol* 2009;30(4):681–688.
50. **Spampinato MV, Schiarelli C, Cianfoni A, et al.** Correlation between cerebral blood volume measurements by perfusion-weighted magnetic resonance imaging and two-year progression-free survival in gliomas. *Neuroradiol J* 2013;26(4):385–395.
51. **Voglein J, Tuttenberg J, Weimer M, et al.** Treatment monitoring in gliomas: comparison of dynamic susceptibility-weighted contrast-enhanced and spectroscopic MRI techniques for identifying treatment failure. *Invest Radiol* 2011;46(6):390–400.
52. **Tsui EY, Chan JH, Ramsey RG, et al.** Late temporal lobe necrosis in patients with nasopharyngeal carcinoma: evaluation with combined multi-section diffusion weighted and perfusion weighted MR imaging. *Eur J Radiol* 2001;39(3):133–138.
53. **Provenzale JM, Mukundan S, Barboriak DP.** Diffusion-weighted and perfusion MR imaging for brain tumor characterization and assessment of treatment response. *Radiology* 2006;239(3):632–649.
54. **Sugahara T, Korogi Y, Tomiguchi S, et al.** Posttherapeutic intraaxial brain tumor: the value of perfusion-sensitive contrast-enhanced MR imaging for differentiating tumor recurrence from nonneoplastic contrast-enhancing tissue. *AJNR Am J Neuroradiol* 2000;21(5):901–909.
55. **Seeger A, Braun C, Skardelly M, et al.** Comparison of three different MR perfusion techniques and MR spectroscopy for multiparametric assessment in distinguishing recurrent high-grade gliomas from stable disease. *Acad Radiol* 2013;20(12):1557–1565.
56. **Barajas RF Jr, Chang JS, Segal MR, et al.** Differentiation of recurrent glioblastoma multiforme from radiation necrosis after external beam radiation therapy with dynamic susceptibility-weighted contrast-enhanced perfusion MR imaging. *Radiology* 2009;253(2):486–496.
57. **Fatterpekar GM, Galheigo D, Narayana A, et al.** Treatment-related change versus tumor recurrence in high-grade gliomas: a diagnostic conundrum—use of dynamic susceptibility contrast enhanced (DSC) perfusion MRI. *AJR Am J Roentgenol* 2012;198(1):19–26.
58. **Fink JR, Carr RB, Matsusue E, et al.** Comparison of 3 Tesla proton MR spectroscopy, MR perfusion and MR diffusion for distinguishing glioma recurrence from posttreatment effects. *J Magn Reson Imaging* 2012;35(1):56–63.

59. **Hatzoglou V, Ulaner GA, Zhang Z, et al.** Comparison of the effectiveness of MRI perfusion and fluorine-18 FDG PET-CT for differentiating radiation injury from viable brain tumor: a preliminary retrospective analysis with pathologic correlation in all patients. *Clin Imaging* 2013;37(3):451–457.
60. **Mangla R, Singh G, Ziegelitz D, et al.** Changes in relative cerebral blood volume 1 month after radiation-temozolomide therapy can help predict overall survival in patients with glioblastoma. *Radiology* 2010;256(2):575–584.
61. **Baek HJ, Kim HS, Kim N, et al.** Percent change of perfusion skewness and kurtosis: a potential imaging biomarker for early treatment response in patients with newly diagnosed glioblastomas. *Radiology* 2012;264(3):834–843.
62. **LaViolette PS, Cohen AD, Prah MA, et al.** Vascular change measured with independent component analysis of dynamic susceptibility contrast MRI predicts bevacizumab response in high-grade glioma. *Neuro Oncol* 2013;15(4):442–450.
63. **Ostergaard L, Hochberg FH, Rabinov JD, et al.** Early changes measured by magnetic resonance imaging in cerebral blood flow, blood volume, and blood–brain barrier permeability following dexamethasone treatment in patients with brain tumors. *J Neurosurg* 1999;90(2):300–305.
64. **Wilkinson ID, Jellineck DA, Levy D, et al.** Dexamethasone and enhancing solitary cerebral mass lesions: alterations in perfusion and blood-tumor barrier kinetics shown by magnetic resonance imaging. *Neurosurgery* 2006;58(4):640–646; discussion 6.
65. **Hakyemez B, Erdogan C, Bolca N, et al.** Evaluation of different cerebral mass lesions by perfusion-weighted MR imaging. *J Magn Reson Imaging* 2006;24(4):817–824.
66. **Floriano VH, Torres US, Spotti AR, et al.** The role of dynamic susceptibility contrast-enhanced perfusion MR imaging in differentiating between infectious and neoplastic focal brain lesions: results from a cohort of 100 consecutive patients. *PLoS One* 2013;8(12):e81509.
67. **Liu X, Kolar B, Tian W, et al.** MR perfusion-weighted imaging may help in differentiating between nonenhancing gliomas and nonneoplastic lesions in the cervicomedullary junction. *J Magn Reson Imaging* 2011;34(1):196–202.
68. **Cha S, Pierce S, Knopp EA, et al.** Dynamic contrast-enhanced T_2*-weighted MR imaging of tumefactive demyelinating lesions. *AJNR Am J Neuroradiol* 2001;22(6):1109–1116.
69. **Schabel MC, Morrell GR.** Uncertainty in T(1) mapping using the variable flip angle method with two flip angles. *Phys Med Biol* 2009;54(1):N1–N8.
70. **Evelhoch JL.** Key factors in the acquisition of contrast kinetic data for oncology. *J Magn Reson Imaging* 1999;10(3):254–259.
71. **Tofts PS, Kermode AG.** Measurement of the blood–brain barrier permeability and leakage space using dynamic MR imaging. 1. Fundamental concepts. *Magn Reson Med* 1991;17(2):357–367.
72. **Wang D, Shi L, Wang YX, et al.** Concatenated and parallel optimization for the estimation of T_1 map in FLASH MRI with multiple flip angles. *Magn Reson Med* 2010;63(5):1431–1436.
73. **Schabel MC, Parker DL.** Uncertainty and bias in contrast concentration measurements using spoiled gradient echo pulse sequences. *Phys Med Biol* 2008;53(9):2345–2373.
74. **Leach MO, Brindle KM, Evelhoch JL, et al.** Assessment of antiangiogenic and antivascular therapeutics using MRI: recommendations for appropriate methodology for clinical trials. *Br J Radiol* 2003;76(Spec No 1):S87–S91.
75. **Jackson A, O'Connor J, Thompson G, et al.** Magnetic resonance perfusion imaging in neuro-oncology. *Cancer Imaging* 2008;8:186–199.
76. **Gerstner ER, Sorensen AG, Jain RK, et al.** Advances in neuroimaging techniques for the evaluation of tumor growth, vascular permeability, and angiogenesis in gliomas. *Curr Opin Neurol* 2008;21(6):728–735.
77. **Zwick S, Brix G, Tofts PS, et al.** Simulation-based comparison of two approaches frequently used for dynamic contrast-enhanced MRI. *Eur Radiol* 2010;20(2):432–442.
78. **Lee TY, Purdie TG, Stewart E.** CT imaging of angiogenesis. *Q J Nucl Med* 2003;47(3):171–187.
79. **Padhani A, Choyke PL.** *New techniques in oncologic imaging.* New York: Taylor & Francis; 2006.
80. **Weinmann HJ, Laniado M, Mutzel W.** Pharmacokinetics of GdDTPA/dimeglumine after intravenous injection into healthy volunteers. *Physiol Chem Phys Med NMR* 1984;16(2):167–172.
81. **Yang C, Karczmar GS, Medved M, et al.** Estimating the arterial input function using two reference tissues in dynamic contrast-enhanced MRI studies: fundamental concepts and simulations. *Magn Reson Med* 2004;52(5):1110–1117.
82. **Yuan J, Chow SK, Zhang Q, et al.** The use of dynamic tracer concentration in veins for quantitative DCE-MRI kinetic analysis in head and neck. *PLoS One* 2013;8(3):e59885.
83. **Ewing JR, Bagher-Ebadian H.** Model selection in measures of vascular parameters using dynamic contrast-enhanced MRI: experimental and clinical applications. *NMR Biomed* 2013;26(8):1028–1041.
84. **Landis CS, Li X, Telang FW, et al.** Determination of the MRI contrast agent concentration time course in vivo following bolus injection: effect of equilibrium transcytolemmal water exchange. *Magn Reson Med* 2000;44(4):563–574.
85. **Larsson HB, Rosenbaum S, Fritz-Hansen T.** Quantification of the effect of water exchange in dynamic contrast MRI perfusion measurements in the brain and heart. *Magn Reson Med* 2001;46(2):272–281.
86. **Buckley DL, Kershaw LE, Stanisz GJ.** Cellular-interstitial water exchange and its effect on the determination of contrast agent concentration in vivo: dynamic contrast-enhanced MRI of human internal obturator muscle. *Magn Reson Med* 2008;60(5):1011–1019.
87. **Su MY, Cheung YC, Fruehauf JP, et al.** Correlation of dynamic contrast enhancement MRI parameters with microvessel density and VEGF for assessment of angiogenesis in breast cancer. *J Magn Reson Imaging* 2003;18(4):467–477.
88. **Kiessling F, Krix M, Heilmann M, et al.** Comparing dynamic parameters of tumor vascularization in nude mice revealed by magnetic resonance imaging and contrast-enhanced intermittent power Doppler sonography. *Invest Radiol* 2003;38(8):516–524.
89. **Cooper RA, Carrington BM, Loncaster JA, et al.** Tumour oxygenation levels correlate with dynamic contrast-enhanced magnetic resonance imaging parameters in carcinoma of the cervix. *Radiother Oncol* 2000;57(1):53–59.
90. **Matsubayashi R, Matsuo Y, Edakuni G, et al.** Breast masses with peripheral rim enhancement on dynamic contrast-enhanced MR images: correlation of MR findings with histologic features and expression of growth factors. *Radiology* 2000;217(3):841–848.
91. **Sourbron SP, Buckley DL.** Classic models for dynamic contrast-enhanced MRI. *NMR Biomed* 2013;26(8):1004–1027.
92. **Paudyal R, Poptani H, Cai K, et al.** Impact of transvascular and cellular-interstitial water exchange on dynamic contrast-enhanced magnetic resonance imaging estimates of blood to tissue transfer constant and blood plasma volume. *J Magn Reson Imaging* 2013;37(2):435–444.
93. **Leach MO, Morgan B, Tofts PS, et al.** Imaging vascular function for early stage clinical trials using dynamic contrast-enhanced magnetic resonance imaging. *Eur Radiol* 2012;22(7):1451–1464.
94. **Roberts HC, Roberts TP, Ley S, et al.** Quantitative estimation of microvascular permeability in human brain tumors: correlation of dynamic Gd-DTPA-enhanced MR imaging with histopathologic grading. *Acad Radiol* 2002;9(suppl 1):S151–S155.
95. **Ludemann L, Hamm B, Zimmer C.** Pharmacokinetic analysis of glioma compartments with dynamic Gd-DTPA-enhanced magnetic resonance imaging. *Magn Reson Imaging* 2000;18(10):1201–1214.
96. **Aref M, Chaudhari AR, Bailey KL, et al.** Comparison of tumor histology to dynamic contrast enhanced magnetic resonance imaging-based physiological estimates. *Magn Reson Imaging* 2008;26(9):1279–1293.
97. **Patankar TF, Haroon HA, Mills SJ, et al.** Is volume transfer coefficient (K(trans)) related to histologic grade in human gliomas? *AJNR Am J Neuroradiol* 2005;26(10):2455–2465.
98. **Zhang N, Zhang L, Qiu B, et al.** Correlation of volume transfer coefficient Ktrans with histopathologic grades of gliomas. *J Magn Reson Imaging* 2012;36(2):355–363.
99. **Sahoo P, Rathore RK, Awasthi R, et al.** Subcompartmentalization of extracellular extravascular space (EES) into permeability and leaky space with local arterial input function (AIF) results in improved discrimination between high- and low-grade glioma using dynamic contrast-enhanced (DCE) MRI. *J Magn Reson Imaging* 2013;38(3):677–688.
100. **Choi HS, Kim AH, Ahn SS, et al.** Glioma grading capability: comparisons among parameters from dynamic contrast-enhanced MRI and ADC value on DWI. *Korean J Radiol* 2013;14(3):487–492.
101. **Weber MA, Henze M, Tuttenberg J, et al.** Biopsy targeting gliomas: do functional imaging techniques identify similar target areas? *Invest Radiol* 2010;45(12):755–768.

102. **Durst CR, Raghavan P, Shaffrey ME, et al.** Multimodal MR imaging model to predict tumor infiltration in patients with gliomas. *Neuroradiology* 2014;56(2):107–115.
103. **Hoff BA, Bhojani MS, Rudge J, et al.** DCE and DW-MRI monitoring of vascular disruption following VEGF-Trap treatment of a rat glioma model. *NMR Biomed* 2012;25(7):935–942.
104. **Ali MM, Janic B, Babajani-Feremi A, et al.** Changes in vascular permeability and expression of different angiogenic factors following anti-angiogenic treatment in rat glioma. *PLoS One* 2010;5(1):e8727.
105. **Sorensen AG, Batchelor TT, Zhang WT, et al.** A "vascular normalization index" as potential mechanistic biomarker to predict survival after a single dose of cediranib in recurrent glioblastoma patients. *Cancer Res* 2009;69(13):5296–5300.
106. **Cao Y, Nagesh V, Hamstra D, et al.** The extent and severity of vascular leakage as evidence of tumor aggressiveness in high-grade gliomas. *Cancer Res* 2006;66(17):8912–8917.
107. **Dhermain F, Saliou G, Parker F, et al.** Microvascular leakage and contrast enhancement as prognostic factors for recurrence in unfavorable low-grade gliomas. *J Neurooncol* 2010;97(1):81–88.
108. **Mills SJ, Patankar TA, Haroon HA, et al.** Do cerebral blood volume and contrast transfer coefficient predict prognosis in human glioma? *AJNR Am J Neuroradiol* 2006;27(4):853–858.
109. **Bisdas S, Naegele T, Ritz R, et al.** Distinguishing recurrent high-grade gliomas from radiation injury: a pilot study using dynamic contrast-enhanced MR imaging. *Acad Radiol* 2011;18(5):575–583.
110. **Wen PY, Macdonald DR, Reardon DA, et al.** Updated response assessment criteria for high-grade gliomas: response assessment in neuro-oncology working group. *J Clin Oncol* 2010;28(11):1963–1972.
111. **Kong DS, Kim ST, Kim EH, et al.** Diagnostic dilemma of pseudoprogression in the treatment of newly diagnosed glioblastomas: the role of assessing relative cerebral blood flow volume and oxygen-6-methylguanine-DNA methyltransferase promoter methylation status. *AJNR Am J Neuroradiol* 2011;32(2):382–387.
112. **Tsien C, Galban CJ, Chenevert TL, et al.** Parametric response map as an imaging biomarker to distinguish progression from pseudoprogression in high-grade glioma. *J Clin Oncol* 2010;28(13):2293–2299.
113. **Narang J, Jain R, Arbab AS, et al.** Differentiating treatment-induced necrosis from recurrent/progressive brain tumor using nonmodel-based semiquantitative indices derived from dynamic contrast-enhanced T_1-weighted MR perfusion. *Neuro Oncol* 2011;13(9):1037–1046.
114. **Vonken EP, van Osch MJ, Bakker CJ, et al.** Simultaneous quantitative cerebral perfusion and Gd-DTPA extravasation measurement with dual-echo dynamic susceptibility contrast MRI. *Magn Reson Med* 2000;43(6):820–827.
115. **Barbier EL, den Boer JA, Peters AR, et al.** A model of the dual effect of gadopentetate dimeglumine on dynamic brain MR images. *J Magn Reson Imaging* 1999;10(3):242–253.
116. **Zhu XP, Li KL, Kamaly-Asl ID, et al.** Quantification of endothelial permeability, leakage space, and blood volume in brain tumors using combined T_1 and T_2* contrast-enhanced dynamic MR imaging. *J Magn Reson Imaging* 2000;11(6):575–585.
117. **Alsop DC, Detre JA.** Reduced transit-time sensitivity in noninvasive magnetic resonance imaging of human cerebral blood flow. *J Cereb Blood Flow Metab* 1996;16(6):1236–1249.
118. **Zhang X, Petersen ET, Ghariq E, et al.** In vivo blood T(1) measurements at 1.5 T, 3 T, and 7 T. *Magn Reson Med* 2013;70(4):1082–1086.
119. **Dai W, Garcia D, de Bazelaire C, et al.** Continuous flow-driven inversion for arterial spin labeling using pulsed radio frequency and gradient fields. *Magn Reson Med* 2008;60(6):1488–1497.
120. **Williams DS, Detre JA, Leigh JS, et al.** Magnetic resonance imaging of perfusion using spin inversion of arterial water. *Proc Natl Acad Sci U S A* 1992;89(1):212–216.
121. **Wong EC, Buxton RB, Frank LR.** A theoretical and experimental comparison of continuous and pulsed arterial spin labeling techniques for quantitative perfusion imaging. *Magn Reson Med* 1998;40(3): 348–355.
122. **Wong EC, Buxton RB, Frank LR.** Quantitative imaging of perfusion using a single subtraction (QUIPSS and QUIPSS II). *Magn Reson Med* 1998;39(5):702–708.
123. **Wong EC, Cronin M, Wu WC, et al.** Velocity-selective arterial spin labeling. *Magn Reson Med* 2006;55(6):1334–1341.
124. **Alsop DC, Detre JA, Golay X, et al.** Recommended implementation of arterial spin-labeled perfusion MRI for clinical applications: a consensus of the ISMRM perfusion study group and the European consortium for ASL in dementia. *Magn Reson Med* 2014. [Epub ahead of print, DOI: 10.1002/mrm.25197]
125. **Buxton RB, Frank LR, Wong EC, et al.** A general kinetic model for quantitative perfusion imaging with arterial spin labeling. *Magn Reson Med* 1998;40(3):383–396.
126. **Wang J, Alsop DC, Song HK, et al.** Arterial transit time imaging with flow encoding arterial spin tagging (FEAST). *Magn Reson Med* 2003;50(3):599–607.
127. **van Gelderen P, de Zwart JA, Duyn JH.** Pitfalls of MRI measurement of white matter perfusion based on arterial spin labeling. *Magn Reson Med* 2008;59(4):788–795.
128. **Weber MA, Gunther M, Lichy MP, et al.** Comparison of arterial spin-labeling techniques and dynamic susceptibility-weighted contrast-enhanced MRI in perfusion imaging of normal brain tissue. *Invest Radiol* 2003;38(11):712–718.
129. **Wong AM, Yan FX, Liu HL.** Comparison of three-dimensional pseudo-continuous arterial spin labeling perfusion imaging with gradient-echo and spin-echo dynamic susceptibility contrast MRI. *J Magn Reson Imaging* 2014;39(2):427–433.
130. **Noguchi T, Yoshiura T, Hiwatashi A, et al.** Perfusion imaging of brain tumors using arterial spin-labeling: correlation with histopathologic vascular density. *AJNR Am J Neuroradiol* 2008;29(4):688–693.
131. **Jarnum H, Steffensen EG, Knutsson L, et al.** Perfusion MRI of brain tumours: a comparative study of pseudo-continuous arterial spin labelling and dynamic susceptibility contrast imaging. *Neuroradiology* 2010;52(4):307–317.
132. **Lehmann P, Monet P, de Marco G, et al.** A comparative study of perfusion measurement in brain tumours at 3 Tesla MR: arterial spin labeling versus dynamic susceptibility contrast-enhanced MRI. *Eur Neurol* 2010;64(1):21–26.
133. **Warmuth C, Gunther M, Zimmer C.** Quantification of blood flow in brain tumors: comparison of arterial spin labeling and dynamic susceptibility-weighted contrast-enhanced MR imaging. *Radiology* 2003;228(2):523–532.
134. **White CM, Pope WB, Zaw T, et al.** Regional and voxel-wise comparisons of blood flow measurements between dynamic susceptibility contrast magnetic resonance imaging (DSC-MRI) and arterial spin labeling (ASL) in brain tumors. *J Neuroimaging* 2014;24(1):23–30.
135. **Ludemann L, Warmuth C, Plotkin M, et al.** Brain tumor perfusion: comparison of dynamic contrast enhanced magnetic resonance imaging using T_1, T_2, and T_2* contrast, pulsed arterial spin labeling, and H_2(15)O positron emission tomography. *Eur J Radiol* 2009;70(3):465–474.
136. **Weber MA, Zoubaa S, Schlieter M, et al.** Diagnostic performance of spectroscopic and perfusion MRI for distinction of brain tumors. *Neurology* 2006;66(12):1899–1906.
137. **Wolf RL, Wang J, Wang S, et al.** Grading of CNS neoplasms using continuous arterial spin labeled perfusion MR imaging at 3 Tesla. *J Magn Reson Imaging* 2005;22(4):475–482.
138. **Roy B, Awasthi R, Bindal A, et al.** Comparative evaluation of 3-dimensional pseudocontinuous arterial spin labeling with dynamic contrast-enhanced perfusion magnetic resonance imaging in grading of human glioma. *J Comput Assist Tomogr* 2013;37(3):321–326.
139. **Kimura H, Takeuchi H, Koshimoto Y, et al.** Perfusion imaging of meningioma by using continuous arterial spin-labeling: comparison with dynamic susceptibility-weighted contrast-enhanced MR images and histopathologic features. *AJNR Am J Neuroradiol* 2006;27(1):85–93.
140. **van Westen D, Petersen ET, Wirestam R, et al.** Correlation between arterial blood volume obtained by arterial spin labelling and cerebral blood volume in intracranial tumours. *MAGMA* 2011;24(4): 211–223.
141. **Furtner J, Bender B, Braun C, et al.** Prognostic value of blood flow measurements using arterial spin labeling in gliomas. *PLoS One* 2014;9(6):e99616.
142. **Weber MA, Thilmann C, Lichy MP, et al.** Assessment of irradiated brain metastases by means of arterial spin-labeling and dynamic susceptibility-weighted contrast-enhanced perfusion MRI: initial results. *Invest Radiol* 2004;39(5):277–287.
143. **Le Bihan D, Breton E, Lallemand D, et al.** Separation of diffusion and perfusion in intravoxel incoherent motion MR imaging. *Radiology* 1988;168(2):497–505.

144. **Luciani A, Vignaud A, Cavet M, et al.** Liver cirrhosis: intravoxel incoherent motion MR imaging—pilot study. *Radiology* 2008;249(3):891–899.
145. **Lemke A, Laun FB, Klauss M, et al.** Differentiation of pancreas carcinoma from healthy pancreatic tissue using multiple *b*-values: comparison of apparent diffusion coefficient and intravoxel incoherent motion derived parameters. *Invest Radiol* 2009;44(12):769–775.
146. **Federau C, Meuli R, O'Brien K, et al.** Perfusion measurement in brain gliomas with intravoxel incoherent motion MRI. *AJNR Am J Neuroradiol* 2013;35(2):256–262.
147. **Kim HS, Suh CH, Kim N, et al.** Histogram analysis of intravoxel incoherent motion for differentiating recurrent tumor from treatment effect in patients with glioblastoma: initial clinical experience. *AJNR Am J Neuroradiol* 2013;35(3):490–497.
148. **Cho GY, Kim S, Jensen JH, et al.** A versatile flow phantom for intravoxel incoherent motion MRI. *Magn Reson Med* 2012;67(6):1710–1720.
149. **Patel J, Sigmund EE, Rusinek H, et al.** Diagnosis of cirrhosis with intravoxel incoherent motion diffusion MRI and dynamic contrast-enhanced MRI alone and in combination: preliminary experience. *J Magn Reson Imaging* 2010;31(3):589–600.
150. **Bisdas S.** Are we ready to image the incoherent molecular motion in our minds? *Neuroradiology* 2013;55(5):537–540.
151. **Falconer JC, Narayana PA.** Cerebrospinal fluid-suppressed high-resolution diffusion imaging of human brain. *Magn Reson Med* 1997;37(1):119–123.
152. **Le Bihan D, Breton E, Lallemand D, et al.** MR imaging of intravoxel incoherent motions: application to diffusion and perfusion in neurologic disorders. *Radiology* 1986;161(2):401–407.
153. **Herscovitch P, Raichle ME, Kilbourn MR, et al.** Positron emission tomographic measurement of cerebral blood flow and permeability-surface area product of water using [15O]water and [11C]butanol. *J Cereb Blood Flow Metab* 1987;7(5):527–542.
154. **Eichling JO, Raichle ME, Grubb RL Jr, et al.** Evidence of the limitations of water as a freely diffusible tracer in brain of the rhesus monkey. *Circ Res* 1974;35(3):358–364.
155. **Bolwig TG, Lassen NA.** The diffusion permeability to water of the rat blood–brain barrier. *Acta Physiol Scand* 1975;93(3):415–422.
156. **Gruner JM, Paamand R, Kosteljanetz M, et al.** Brain perfusion CT compared with (1)(5)O-H(2)O PET in patients with primary brain tumours. *Eur J Nucl Med Mol Imaging* 2012;39(11):1691–1701.
157. **Donahue MJ, Lu H, Jones CK, et al.** An account of the discrepancy between MRI and PET cerebral blood flow measures. A high-field MRI investigation. *NMR Biomed* 2006;19(8):1043–1054.
158. **Zhang K, Herzog H, Mauler J, et al.** Comparison of cerebral blood flow acquired by simultaneous [O]water positron emission tomography and arterial spin labeling magnetic resonance imaging. *J Cereb Blood Flow Metab* 2014;34(8):1373–1380.
159. **Leenders KL.** PET: blood flow and oxygen consumption in brain tumors. *J Neurooncol* 1994;22(3):269–273.
160. **Hino A, Imahori Y, Tenjin H, et al.** Metabolic and hemodynamic aspects of peritumoral low-density areas in human brain tumor. *Neurosurgery* 1990;26(4):615–621.
161. **Bruehlmeier M, Roelcke U, Schubiger PA, et al.** Assessment of hypoxia and perfusion in human brain tumors using PET with 18F-fluoromisonidazole and $^{15}O\text{-}H_2O$. *J Nucl Med* 2004;45(11):1851–1859.

CHAPTER

16

Perfusion MR Imaging in Cognitive and Developmental Brain Disorders and Neuropsychiatry

Kay Jann, PhD, Danny J. J. Wang, PhD, MSCE, and John A. Detre, MD

Introduction to Perfusion Imaging Using Arterial Spin Labeling

A Short Summary of ASL Techniques

Since its advent early 1990s, arterial spin labeling (ASL) has evolved into a family of techniques for noninvasive MRI measurement of perfusion including pulsed, continuous, and more recently pseudocontinuous versions.[1] In all cases, arterial blood water is magnetically labeled by RF pulses and allowed to flow into the imaging volume, during which time there is a T1 decay of the label. Subtraction of labeled images from control images yields a perfusion-weighted difference image, and absolute cerebral blood flow (CBF) quantification is generally achieved through single- or two-compartment tracer kinetic modeling by primarily taking into account the T1 relaxation of the label.[2] Among various ASL techniques, pseudocontinuous ASL (pCASL) has recently emerged as the technique of choice for brain perfusion studies as it merges the advantages of pulsed ASL, including hardware compatibility with current MRI scanners, and the higher tagging efficiency of continuous ASL, which includes a longer tagging bolus and thus higher signal to noise ratio (SNR).[3,4] Alternative spin labeling strategies such as velocity-selective ASL have been introduced,[5] but thus far have not been applied widely in clinical studies.

The main limitations of ASL that hamper its widespread applications include relatively low SNR given the small fraction of arterial blood (approximately 1%), as well as arterial transit effects whereby labeled spins fail to reach brain tissue by the time of image acquisition. ASL methods derive a dual benefit from high magnetic field strengths.[6] In addition to increased sensitivity at high field, T1 also increases, allowing more label to accumulate in brain tissue as well as increased postlabeling delay times to minimize arterial transit effects. ASL methods also benefit from parallel imaging and array receiver coils.[7] The use of background suppression (BS) of static tissue signals can also greatly improve the temporal stability[8,9] of ASL MRI data, resulting in shorter scan times. Since optimal suppression of static signals occurs at a single timepoint, BS ASL is most compatible with 3D acquisitions such as GRASE (a hybrid of gradient and spin echo) or fast spin echo with a stack-of-spirals readout. As a result, whole-brain perfusion images can be achieved within just a few minutes, with reduced susceptibility artifacts compared to conventional ASL sequences using gradient-recalled echo planar imaging (EPI) or spiral scans. One potential shortcoming of 3D ASL acquisitions, however, is the spatial blurring due to modulations of k-space signals by the T2 relaxation curve, especially along the z-direction. With single-shot acquisitions, the full-width-at-half-maximum of the point spread function is on the order of 1.3 to 1.5 pixels along the slice direction.[10] Therefore, trade-offs have to be made between achieving adequate temporal and spatial resolutions using single- or multishot 3D acquisitions. The recent ASL white paper[11] recommended "pseudocontinuous labeling, background suppression, and a segmented 3D readout without vascular crushing gradients" as preferred implementation of ASL for clinical applications.

Quantitative Resting CBF Using ASL

Methodologically, ASL is similar to ^{15}O-water PET. Nevertheless, the arterial input function (AIF) can be explicitly defined by the duration and amplitude of the labeling RF pulses in ASL, whereas in general, an arterial line has to be inserted to sample AIF in PET studies. This factor greatly facilitates the absolute quantification of CBF using ASL. ASL MRI measurements of CBF have been shown to correlate closely with PET CBF both at rest[12] and with task activation.[13] A small study conducted in six elderly subjects has evaluated the accuracy of pCASL with 3D BS SPIRAL readout by comparison with $H_2{}^{15}O$ PET-CBF scans.[14] The cross-modality perfusion imaging comparison yielded very good global and regional agreement in global gray matter ($r = 0.742, p < 0.091$) and the posterior cingulate cortex (PCC) ($r = 0.789, p < 0.057$). A recent study[15] compared two pCASL sequences, using 2D gradient-echo EPI and 3D GRASE as the readout, respectively, versus the gold standard of $H_2{}^{15}O$ PET in 8 elderly subjects. When compared to PET, EPI and GRASE pCASL showed a comparably high degree of spatial correlation across brain pixels (pCASL EPI $r = 0.53$, $SD = 0.06$, $p < 0.001$; pCASL GRASE $r = 0.51$, SD= 0.08, $p < 0.001$). Another recent study investigated the accuracy and precision of pCASL during baseline and hypercapnia by head-to-head comparison with $H_2{}^{15}O$ PET in 16 healthy volunteers.[16] In general, intra- and intersession repeatabilities were comparable for both modalities during both conditions. Importantly, cerebrovascular reactivity (CVR) as measured by pCASL in combination with a hypercapnia challenge was proven to be in quantitative agreement with similar CVR measurements by $^{15}O\text{-}H_2O$.

With the advent of MR-PET scanners, it is now feasible to conduct concurrent ASL/PET scanning. A recent concurrent PET/MRI study[17] demonstrated an excellent agreement (r = 0.70) between ^{15}O-water PET and pCASL although a quadratic rather than linear function was used for fitting the relationship of two CBF measurements. Part of the discrepancy at the high range of CBF values may be attributed to the relatively short postlabeling delay of 1 second employed for pCASL scans (resulting in focal intravascular intensities). Taken together, recent studies comparing pCASL and PET CBF scans suggest an overall high correlation between the two modalities, paving the way for quantitative usage of pCASL MRI in both clinical and research settings.

Comparison of ASL CBF and PET CMRglc

Both regional cerebral perfusion and metabolism are closely coupled to neural activity and are important surrogate markers of brain function. FDG-PET remains the standard method for measuring the cerebral metabolic rate of glucose (CMRglc). There has been growing interest in comparing ASL CBF with FDG-PET measurement of CMRglc. Newberg and colleagues performed concurrent ASL measurements and 18F-FDG uptake during a visual stimulation task to show the correlation between CBF and CMRglc. The correlation was high within the middle ranges of perfusion and metabolism but dropped off at higher perfusion rates. ASL was more sensitive in showing changes in the visual cortex driven by the stimuli, but PET showed relatively higher signal in the basal ganglia.[18] Discrepancies between ASL and PET in cortical versus deep gray matter may be attributable, in part, to attenuation correction procedures required for PET but not for MRI.

In a recent study,[19] we compared resting state cerebral perfusion using pCASL and cerebral glucose metabolism using 18F-FDG PET in 20 normal volunteers. In whole-brain analysis, greater regional metabolism relative to perfusion was observed in the caudate, medial prefrontal, and temporal lobes, whereas perfusion was relatively higher in the hippocampus and cerebellum. In a region-of-interest analysis, the overall mean correlation between perfusion and metabolism across voxels was r = 0.60 with regional variability. Cross-voxel correlations between perfusion and metabolism in mean ASL and PET images of all 20 subjects were the highest in the striatum (caudate: r = 0.81; putamen: r = 0.86) and lowest in medial temporal structures (amygdala: r = 0.31; hippocampus: r = −0.05). Figure 16.1 shows the mean PET CMRglc and ASL CBF maps of the 20 normal subjects. While an overall high correlation was observed between the two modalities, there was also regional variability.

Concepts of Resting Brain Function

As described above, ASL provides a noninvasive approach for measuring regional brain function that yields comparable results to standard PET and SPECT measurements. Due to its quantitative nature, ASL offers an ideal tool to assess the brain's resting state both globally and regionally. Baseline brain function, representing "trait" or "state" effects, is a fundamental aspect of brain function as 70% to 80% of the metabolic demand is consumed for maintaining this baseline state,[20] while task-induced deviations from this state commonly assessed in fMRI investigations consume a much smaller fraction of the brain's energy. Moreover, the level of baseline perfusion has been shown to modulate the degree of task-induced signal changes.[21–23] Hence, to better understand interindividual differences and specifically impairments in cognitive functioning in disease, it is crucial to understand the basic metabolic activity of the brain, and understanding the brain's baseline organization has thus become a major research focus in the past decade.

To this end, efforts to identify regional alterations in baseline metabolism related to clinical syndromes have also been paralleled by attempts to understand the brain as an interconnected system rather than individual brain areas that serve specific functions. This emerging trend in clinical neuroscience and psychiatry has been driven by the concept that cognitive functions of the brain can be thought of as implemented in complex networks optimized both for segregated and distributed information processing. Modern brain imaging methods such as positron emission tomography (PET) and functional magnetic resonance imaging (fMRI) have revealed a variety of distinct functionally connected networks (FCNs, functional connectivity [FC] defined as coherent signal

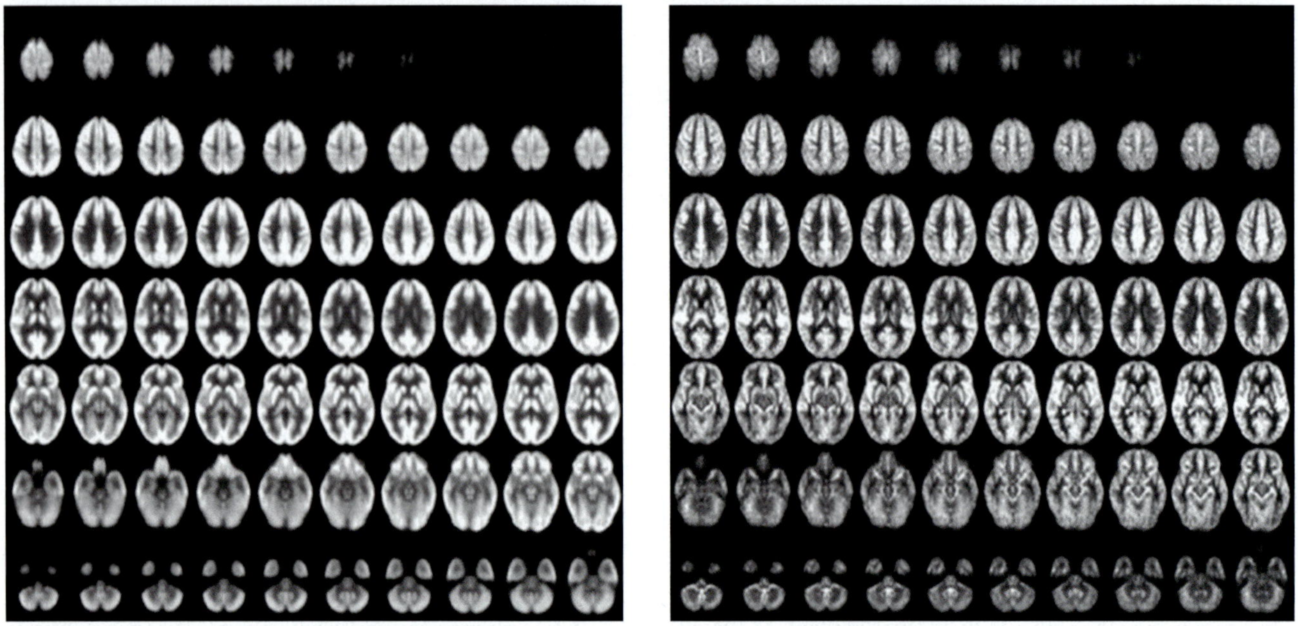

A B

Figure 16-1. Mean CMRGlc (PET) (**A**) and mean CBF (ASL) (**B**) from 20 normal subjects. CBF images are normalized to a standard MNI152 T1 template while CMRGlc images to an MNI PET template and are presented in sequential slices from vertex to skull base.

intensity fluctuations) underlying human cognition and perception. FCNs representing motor, auditory, and visual systems as well as higher cognitive functions like attention and working memory have been repeatedly described.[24–28] A major and intensely studied FCN is the so-called default mode network (DMN), initially identified in PET data as areas that exhibited consistently greater metabolic activity at baseline and less metabolic activity during task execution.[29] Although historically the first reports of FCNs have been based on PET perfusion, oxygen, and glucose metabolism data sets, functional network analysis is currently almost exclusively performed using fMRI blood oxygenation level–dependent (BOLD) signal data where networks are identified by their correlated low-frequency signals.[30] However, such BOLD connectivity measures are also highly susceptible to motion effects,[31] and since the BOLD signal relies on changes in the ratio of blood oxygenation between two distinct neuronal states and is modulated by multiple physiologic factors such as cerebral blood flow (CBF), cerebral blood volume (CBV), and cerebral metabolic rate of oxygen ($CMRO_2$),[32,33] quantitative (i.e., absolute) measures of network activity remain challenging. As outlined in the section above, recent methodologic advances in ASL yield reproducible, absolute, and quantitative values of CBF comparable to the results obtained with $H_2{}^{15}O$ PET.[34] It allows for repeated acquisitions since no exposure to radioactivity is required, and it provides a temporal resolution on the order of a few seconds. Furthermore, temporal correlations used to identify brain networks tend to occur over long timescales for which ASL provides significant signal stability advantages over BOLD fMRI.[35] Accordingly, there is strong interest in the use of ASL MRI as a means of quantifying network activity in the brain.

To date, however, only a handful of studies have demonstrated the feasibility to identify ASL-FCNs[36–39] mainly due to the relatively low sensitivity and temporal resolution of ASL scans. In a recent study, we systematically investigated similarity of ASL and BOLD networks as well as their reliability across time and scanners,[27] by taking advantage of the improved sensitivity of pCASL with 3D BS GRASE. ASL and BOLD produced spatially highly similar FCNs as displayed in Figure 16.2. The test–retest reliability of these FCNs indicated by intraclass correlation coefficients (ICC) yielded to be excellent in BOLD (average ICC across networks: 0.905 ± 0.033 between sessions; 0.885 ± 0.052 between scanners) while lower but still adequate in CBF networks ($0.545 \pm 0.048/0.575 \pm 0.059$). Nevertheless, ASL provided highly reproducible network-specific CBF measures (ICC = 0.956 ± 0.010 between sessions; 0.939 ± 0.026 between scanners). The question remains of how

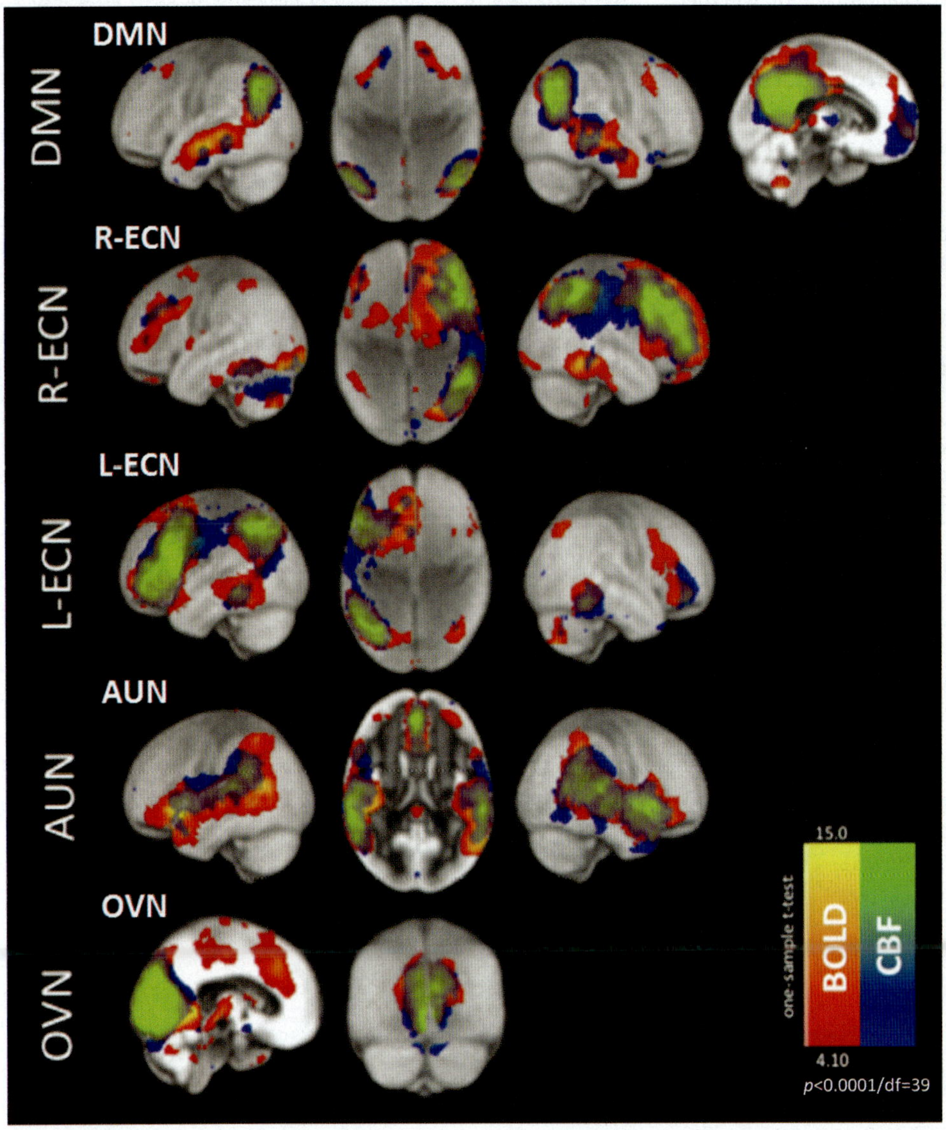

Figure 16-2. Illustration of the similarity of the spatial pattern of BOLD (*red-yellow*) and CBF (*blue-green*) based functionally connected networks overlaid on a 3D rendered brain. Modality-specific group networks were computed as one-sample *t*-test across the specific single-subject maps. Default mode network (DMN), left and right executive control networks (L/R-ECNs), occipital visual network (OVN), and auditory network (AUN).

these networks' baseline metabolic activity and the integrity of their functional organization are intercorrelated and whether they could provide estimates of the energy costs of maintaining their function.[40,41]

ASL in Developmental and Neuropsychiatric Disorders

Although recent advantages in perfusion-based fMRI using ASL allow reliable and repetitive quantitative CBF measurements during both baseline and task activation, this noninvasive, emerging technique is also starting to be applied in developmental and clinical neuroscience. In the following section, we provide an overview of the recent research findings along with their implications for the future of ASL perfusion imaging in neuropsychiatric research. We first focus on developmental changes in CBF, since a wide variety of psychiatric disorders are considered to be developmental disorders that emerge during brain maturation—a critical phase that could lead to cognitive, emotional, and other deficits and clinical symptomatology. Thereafter, we overview some of the most common developmental and psychiatric syndromes based on their prevalence, recapitulate the observed symptoms, and describe their underlying neurophysiologic alterations as identified by perfusion neuroimaging. The next section will then highlight the unique capabilities of ASL for monitoring treatment effects along with its use for personalized treatment selection based on the likelihood of the individual's response to one treatment or another.

Normal CBF Development

Significant progress has been made in the computational morphometric analysis of structural MRI. Two major neurodevelopmental trends have been revealed by brain structural analyses, including a continuous increase in the volume of white matter (WM) with age that has been attributed to myelination and improved connectivity between brain regions[42,43] and an inverted U-shaped function for age-related variations in gray matter (GM), thought to be the result of "pruning" of excitatory synaptic connections.[43–45] Several longitudinal imaging studies[44,45] reported a sequential maturation from lower-order sensorimotor to higher-order association cortices. Pediatric ASL studies demonstrated an age-related increase of CBF from neonates to toddlers, followed by tapering of CBF from childhood to adulthood.[46–49] This developmental trajectory of CBF is generally consistent with existing literature based on nuclear medicine approaches.[50,51] A recent study looking at regional CBF with adjustment of variations in GM density (GMD) showed that the relationship between GMD-adjusted CBF and age can be characterized by an inverted U-shape followed by a U-shaped trajectory in most brain regions throughout childhood and adolescence.[52,53]

In order to reliably apply ASL for tracking developmental trajectory of CBF, the accuracy and longitudinal repeatability of ASL perfusion MRI needs to be established in children. In a recent study, we performed pCASL perfusion MRI in 22 healthy children aged 7 to 17 years using repeated scans 2 to 4 weeks apart.[54] By taking into account developmental changes of key physiologic parameters (e.g., blood T1), the accuracy of pCASL against the reference standard of phase-contrast (PC) MRI measured by ICC was 0.65. CBF measurements using pCASL demonstrated a good level of longitudinal repeatability (ICC = 0.65, within-subject coefficient of variance/wsCV = 14%). This study laid a solid foundation for quantitative CBF mapping in typically developing populations as well as children with neurodevelopmental disorders.

Recently, we performed a joint analysis of perfusion and structural MR data in 82 children (40 boys and 42 girls) aged 7 to 17 years old.[55] For structural MR images, we applied a cortical reconstruction algorithm that provides accurate and efficient reconstruction of cortical surfaces and automatically parcellated them into 24 gyral regions based on the LPBA40 atlas. To correct for GM volumes due to partial volume effects, CBF values in each region of interest (ROI) were normalized by the corresponding surface area, which accounts for the extent of folding in each ROI. At each gyral region, we then applied multiple regression analysis using the GM area–adjusted CBF with respect to age and gender. After the correction for multiple comparisons with the control of false discovery rate, widespread sex differences were detected throughout the cortex on both hemispheres as shown in Figure 16.3. The results show that there is typically an inverted U-shape of the GM area–adjusted CBF measures across the brain regions, which is consistent with prior studies demonstrating synaptic pruning during brain development. In regions with significant sex differences, the results show that there is a delay of the CBF time course in boys (vs. girls) during the earlier stages of brain development. With brain maturation, the

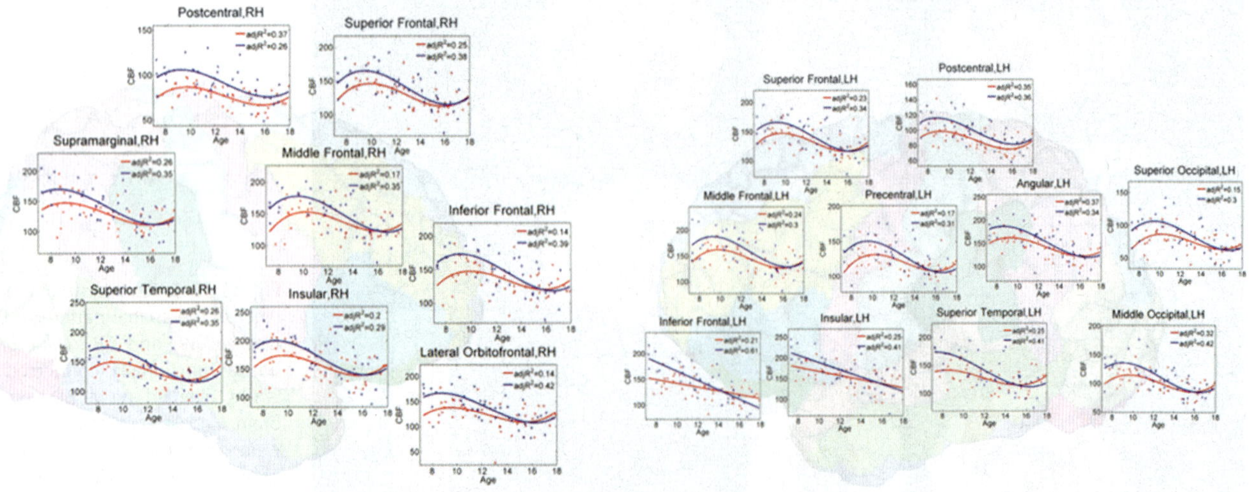

A B

Figure 16-3. Results of sex differences of GM area–adjusted CBF in brain development. The time courses of CBF obtained from regression analysis in each ROI with significant sex difference are overlaid onto parcellated cortical surfaces (boy: *blue*; girl: *red*). **A** and **B:** Lateral views of the right and left hemisphere.

CBF of boys and girls eventually converges to similar levels. These results demonstrate that GM area–adjusted CBF measure is a highly sensitive measure that allows the identification of the trajectory and sex differences in typical brain development.

Neuropsychiatry

Mood Disorders

The most common mood disorder is depression, which is a leading cause of disability affecting 7% to 18% of the population at least once in their life, with an estimated total of 350 million people of all ages suffering from depression worldwide (source WHO). Women are at a higher risk of developing depressive symptoms than are men. There are at least two subtypes of depression that can be distinguished based on the episodes of depressed states. Unipolar depression is characterized by depressed mood, loss of interest and enjoyment, and reduced energy leading to diminished activity and, in more severe cases, anxiety symptoms, disturbed sleep and appetite, and often also feelings of guilt or low self-esteem. In the most severe cases, suicidal ideation occurs. The second subtype is bipolar mood disorder, which typically consists of both manic and depressive episodes separated by periods of normal mood. Manic episodes involve elevated or irritable mood, overactivity, pressured speech, inflated self-esteem, and a decreased need for sleep. Depressed episodes are similar between unipolar and bipolar depression, which poses a major challenge for differential diagnosis, since treatment strategies differ. Therefore, additional markers of each disease are needed. Functional neuroimaging may provide such disease markers. However, to date, very little work in bipolar disorder or other subtypes of mood disorders has been carried out. Therefore, this subsection will focus on findings in unipolar depression.

ASL perfusion studies have delineated the involvement of frontolimbic–cingulate–striatal networks in states of depression, which is consistent with earlier PET and SPECT research. While frontal areas mainly support executive functions, error monitoring, and regulation of emotion, the limbic–striatal network is associated with affect, emotion, and stress. More specifically, dorsolateral prefrontal cortex (dlPFC) and anterior cingulate cortex (ACC) show reduced CBF in depression, whereas the amygdalae, the subgenual ACC (sACC), the posterior cingulate cortex (PCC), and the basal ganglia show hyperperfusion.[56–59] Moreover, Lui et al.[59] found that patients responding to medical treatment show increased CBF in the limbic network while nonresponders present with frontal hypoperfusion only. Antidepressant medication administered in healthy controls during ASL reduced CBF in serotonergic pathways, that is, the limbic–striatal network including amygdala, insula, and orbitofrontal cortex,[60] areas where only responders exhibit increased CBF but not nonresponders.[59] This is in agreement with the findings of Järnum,[61] who reported perpetual hyperperfusion in frontal lobes and ACC in nonremitting depression. Weiduschat et al.[62] further reported that baseline dlPFC perfusion could predict response to repetitive transcranial magnetic stimulation (rTMS) although they did not see an increase of CBF after treatment in this area. These preliminary findings demonstrate the potential use of ASL to characterize behavioral or pharmacologic states and to predict or monitor patients' response to standard medical or alternative treatments. Ultimately, such approaches may be used for treatment selection in individual patients. ASL has also been used to investigate genetic polymorphisms of the serotonin receptor in healthy subjects as it plays a critical role in mood disorders,[63] demonstrating genotype-associated alterations of baseline perfusion in the amygdala and ventromedial prefrontal cortex (PFC), areas critical in emotion regulation.

We recently performed an FC analysis of ASL data to assess perfusion differences in the DMN in major depression.[64] This network is involved in self-referential processes and has repeatedly been shown to show alterations in its integrity in depression using BOLD fMRI[65,66] and is thought to be involved in rumination.[67] Furthermore, the DMN comprises nodes that have altered perfusion (in depression), including the ACC and the PCC as described above. We found reduced perfusion in the DMN in depressed patients compared to healthy controls, which, however, vanished after correcting for global CBF differences. Nevertheless, PCC perfusion showed an inverse relation with depression severity. Moreover nonresponders showed reduced DMN perfusion as compared to responders, which might indicate that antidepressant treatment does not act on this specific network, in line with the findings discussed above (Fig. 16.4).

Schizophrenia

Schizophrenia is a severe mental disorder with a prevalence of 7 per 1,000 and approximately 24 million people affected worldwide. First episodes usually occur in adolescence or early adulthood, and men have a 1.4 to 2 times higher lifetime risk of developing schizophrenia as compared to women. This neuropsychiatric disorder is characterized by profound disruptions in thinking, affecting language, perception, and the sense of self. It often includes psychotic experiences, such as auditory or visual hallucinations or delusions. Symptoms are conceptually divided into positive and negative symptoms. Positive symptoms include hallucinations, delusions, thought disorder, and movement disorder. Negative symptoms present as

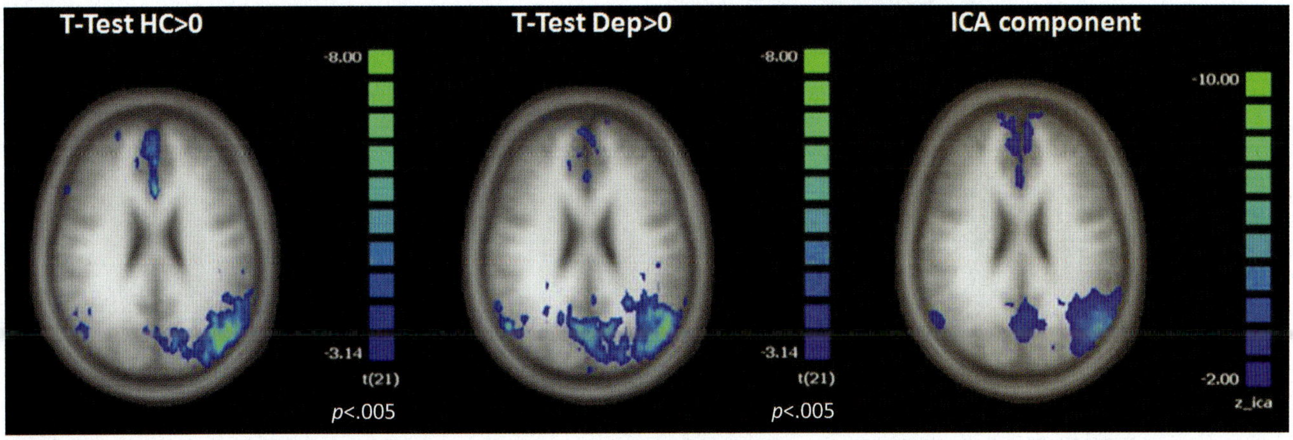

Figure 16-4. **Default mode network based on ASL cerebral blood flow in patients with depression and control subjects.** (Adapted from Orosz A, et al. Reduced cerebral blood flow within the default-mode network and within total gray matter in major depression. *Brain Connect* 2012;2(6):303–310.)

flattening of affect, lack of pleasure, lack of ability to begin and sustain activities, and impoverishment of speech. All these symptoms can lead to moderate-to-severe cognitive impairments in attention focus, executive functions, and working memory. Based on these wide variety of symptoms, schizophrenia can be seen as an ensemble of disorders, that is, schizophrenia spectrum disorders. Roughly, these symptoms can be assigned to three domains: speech, motor behavior, and affect. This wide variety of symptoms and affected functional systems might explain the great variability of findings in perfusion imaging of schizophrenia. Hence, investigation of well-characterized subsamples of patients with schizophrenia within one domain might help to better understand the diverse mechanisms underlying this disorder.

The most prominent functional neuroimaging finding in this spectrum of disorders is reduced CBF in frontal lobe, which led to the concept of hypofrontality.[68–70] Besides, frontal hypoperfusion that is related to negative symptoms and impaired cognitive functioning, several brain areas in sensory and motor areas have been identified with increased baseline CBF in association to positive symptoms.[71–73] A few groups have also investigated specific symptoms of schizophrenia such as auditory hallucinations, formal thought disorders (FTDs), and motor retardation. Walther and colleagues.[74] showed that motor activity in healthy controls was correlated with perfusion in key modules of the basal ganglia–cortical motor circuits, which was absent in patients with schizophrenia, suggesting impaired normal motor control. Instead, patients displayed correlations in the rostral cingulate motor area that is involved in motivational aspects of volitional motor activity. Horn et al. aimed at investigating the neural correlates of FTD in schizophrenia. They revealed a hyperactive left hemispheric language network, with increased CBF in frontal pars opercularis and superior temporal gyrus correlating with individual symptom severity.[75] These findings were complemented by overlapping structural changes and aberrant network patterns in an FC analysis of the same cohort.[76] Accordingly, a hyperactive, structurally altered, and disconnected language network could provide a state marker for FTD. Moreover, his findings suggest a pathophysiologically relevant association between structure, baseline metabolism, and functional integrity. The same group further published a series of papers on auditory verbal hallucinations (AVH) in schizophrenia. Consistent with the view that positive symptoms are associated with increased activity manifested by hyperperfusion, they reported increased CBF in the primary auditory cortex and sensorimotor language areas.[77,78] Moreover, they used perfusion values in the superior temporal gyrus to identify responders to transcranial magnetic stimulation (TMS) treatment[77] (Fig. 16.5) and showed that CBF in several language-specific areas could be restored to normal after TMS intervention but not in a placebo group.[79] The degree of CBF normalization was also predictive of the amount of symptom improvement.

Processes leading to a misattribution of thoughts have been hypothesized to be involved in the generation of AVH, and the DMN has been postulated as a critical player in this process. Aberrant DMN integrity could lead to self-monitoring deficits such as AVH.[80] We therefore investigated the static and dynamic characteristics of the DMN in patients with schizophrenia.[81] Besides confirming frontal hypoperfusion, significant differences in dynamic fluctuations of the posterior DMN node were found to be associated with positive and negative symptom scale (PANSS) scores. In a second study, we confirmed the association of DMN in correlation to PANSS positive severity scores (conference abstract[82]). Moreover, we demonstrated a partial correlation between DMN spatial alterations and DMN perfusion controlling for global CBF. Together, these findings support the hypothesis that DMN hyperactivity and connectivity could facilitate the advent of hallucinations.

Anxiety Disorders

While fear is a natural reaction to stress, some people experience excessive anxiety and irrational fear. Such disruptive anxiety is often triggered by traumatic experiences, as seen in posttraumatic stress disorder. Other forms of anxiety disorders include general anxiety

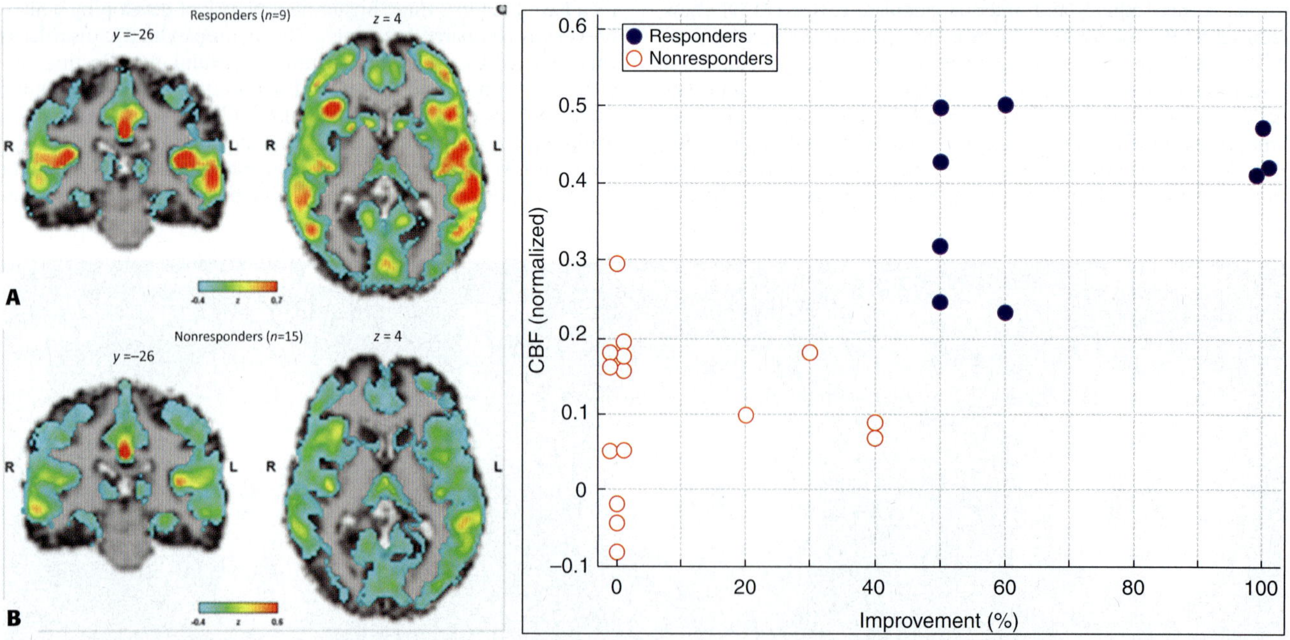

Figure 16-5. Left: Pretreatment average CBF maps for patients responding **(A)** to rTMS treatment as compared to nonresponders **(B)** (maps are z-transformed). **Right:** Scatter plot of symptom improvement (hallucinations) versus pretreatment CBF in the left STG revealing a clear discrimination between responders and nonresponders. (From Homan P, et al. Cerebral blood flow identifies responders to transcranial magnetic stimulation in auditory verbal hallucinations. *Transl Psychiatry* 2012;2:e189.)

disorder, social anxiety disorder, and specific forms of phobia (most commonly are animal phobias: snakes, spiders, and mice).

The amygdala and hippocampus are known to play significant roles in most anxiety disorders. While the amygdala is the main area that evaluates and responds to fear and stressful situations, the hippocampus is involved in memory formations of these events. More recently, top-down cognitive control over the limbic and paralimbic networks has become the focus of anxiety research. The ACC and the insula are thought to inhibit amygdala responses to fear and stress conditions.

Increased activity or overreactivity of the limbic fear network in anxiety disorders has been a common finding in PET and SPECT studies as well as task-based BOLD fMRI, while the control network (ACC) was found to exhibit reduced activity suggesting loss of inhibitory control over the fear network. However, neuroimaging studies suggest a distinction between anxiety disorders including intense fear (panic disorder or specific phobias) and those characterized by worrying and rumination (general and social anxiety). While the former show hypoactivity of the PFC and consequentially disinhibition of the amygdala, the latter shows a hyperactive PFC.[83] These dissociable patterns of brain function might be used to develop new treatment methods but requires further validation.

Perfusion findings support this view of different phenotypes. In a group of patients with general anxiety disorder, it was shown that during worry induction, ACC was hyperactive, while during a worry suppression task, these subjects fail to activate the prefrontal cortex, including the ACC, as compared to a control group.[84] Increased baseline activity in these areas in the patient cohort suggests an altered top-down regulation of anxiety.

In one preliminary study, we demonstrated that cognitive–behavioral therapy can efficiently reduce rCBF in the dorsolateral prefrontal cortex in spider phobic patients.[85] This finding is consistent with current PET/SPECT[86] results and illustrates the potential of ASL for monitoring treatment responses.

However, caution is advised when investigating anxiety inside the MRI scanner environment as the confined space and loud noise of MRI might present stressful situations not only for participants with anxiety disorders but also in other populations and even healthy control subjects. Anxiety and stress can also lead to increased hyperventilation and tachycardia, both of which can alter global CBF estimates.[87] A recent review article[88] addressed this question and found that trait anxiety, as present in anxiety disorders, as well as changes in state anxiety have large effects on global CBF that can confound interpretation of regional changes specifically in group comparisons. Including additional parameters such as heart rate variability, respiration rate, and partial CO_2 can be used to estimate the contribution of state anxiety to global CBF and thus minimize the risk of masking potential real findings.

Substances with Potential for Abuse or Dependence

There are a wide variety of substances (drugs) with potential for dependence or abuse. Common classes of drugs of abuse include sedative hypnotics (e.g., alcohol), opioids (heroin, opium, morphine), stimulants (cocaine, (met-)amphetamine, nicotine, caffeine), as well as hallucinogens (e.g., LSD, THC). Many drugs mimic the chemical structure of endogenous neurotransmitters leading to altered communication within neural networks. Other drugs can amplify network activity by causing increased neurotransmitter release at synapses or prevent neurotransmitter recycling. Of course, many therapeutic medications also exploit these mechanisms.

Several aspects of substance abuse can be investigated with neuroimaging, including acute versus steady-state effects of drugs as well as chronic effects of substance abuse on brain function, including drug craving and abstinence. Thus, a complex image of brain function in substance dependence disorders is found in the literature, and here, we provide a general overview of findings using ASL while its potential in future research in this field is discussed in the section on pharmacologic ASL.

Some of the most commonly used psychostimulants in the general population are caffeine and nicotine. Caffeine is an adenosine receptor antagonist and can also enhance sensitivity of GABAergic synapses.[89,90] Moreover, it is a vasoconstrictor and can also have global effects on perfusion. A caffeine-induced global CBF reduction in the range of 20% is consistently observed.[91–94] Moreover, caffeine use differs in the population, and Field et al.[91] observed reduced CBF in both low and high caffeine users after oral administration of caffeine as compared to placebo, while high users but not low users have increased CBF even under placebo. They hypothesized that this could be either a withdrawal effect or a brain adaptive modulation of the vasculatory system to the chronic administration of the vasoconstrictive agent caffeine. As a vasoconstrictor, caffeine can also affect the concentration of deoxyhemoglobin and thus can alter the BOLD signal response.[95–97] Haller et al.[93] demonstrated increased BOLD activation after caffeine in a working memory task as well as strengthened FC in its associated network. Hence, caffeine consumption habits could be a confounding factor in BOLD investigations and have to be considered carefully.

Nicotine craving involves the reward circuitry including the nucleus accumbens, prefrontal cortex, amygdala, as well as areas involved in associative learning and memory, that is, the hippocampus.[98] Nicotinic receptors in the ventral tegmental area are of particular interest owing to its high density of these receptors and widespread frontal projections. Reduced CBF values in frontal and cingulate areas have further been found to correlate negatively with number of cigarettes consumed.[99,100] In addition, a high comorbidity between smoking and alcohol abuse exists, and in case of alcohol dependence, the effects of nicotine have to be taken into account when investigating the physiologic alterations of alcohol.

Alcohol is a vasodilatory agent that can increase CBF through modulation of GABA-A receptors as well as affecting dopaminergic, serotonergic, and opiate neurotransmitter systems.[101] Acute intoxication in healthy subjects was found to result in increased perfusion of bilateral frontal areas[102–105] (Fig. 16.6) while chronic effects comprise reduced CBF in frontal areas[99,100] even in early adulthood, and these effects persist after months of abstinence.[106]

The reversibility of alterations due to continued substance use is of interest, and longitudinal studies take advantage of the repeatability of ASL MRI to assess whether altered CBF can be reversed.[100] This study found a normalization of perfusion in nonsmoking alcoholics, whereas no improvement was seen in the smoking group, confirming an earlier SPECT study.[107] They conclude that smoking adversely affected recovery in alcohol-dependent subjects. In general, findings from caffeine, nicotine, and alcohol resulting from ASL are fairly consistent with PET and SPECT studies.

Opioids such as heroin and morphine act directly on the brain's opioid receptors, and perfusion alterations are observed in areas of the brain involved in emotional regulation and impulse control (extended limbic network): insula, anterior cingulate cortex, and medial prefrontal cortex.[108] While steady-state effects of heroin use showed a reduction in CBF in those areas, acute effects conversely showed CBF increases. In a follow-up study, gray matter volume changes were also assessed, as such effect can be a confounding factor in CBF analysis due to partial volume effects,[109] and positive correlations between CBF and gray matter volume in frontal and midline structures (ACC) were observed. CBF increases in ACC, operculum, and brainstem were observed after morphine administration.[102]

THC (tetrahydrocannabinol) increased perfusion in ACC, frontal cortex, and insula.[110] Moreover, perfusion levels correlated with subjective ratings of feeling "high." The affected areas might explain the behavioral effects, as they are involved in emotional and cognitive control as well as interoceptive awareness.

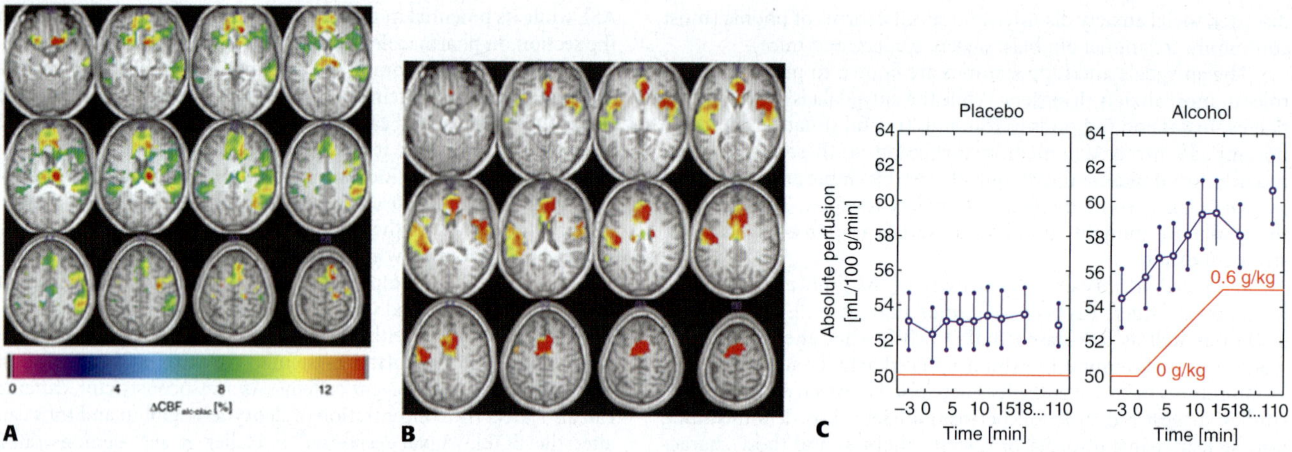

Figure 16-6. A: **Group average maps showing relative CBF increase caused by alcohol compared to placebo baseline perfusion. B:** Relative CBF increase 110 minutes after alcohol infusion still shows elevated perfusion in frontal, temporal, and insular areas. **C:** Average global absolute CBF over time for placebo and alcohol condition. *Red line* is breath alcohol concentration. (Adapted from Marxen M, et al. Acute effects of alcohol on brain perfusion monitored with arterial spin labeling magnetic resonance imaging in young adults. *J Cereb Blood Flow Metab* 2014;34(3):472–479.)

As a general rule, most recreational drugs showed acute increase of CBF in distributed networks, while chronic abuse led to decreased perfusion. This hypoperfusion has been considered as neural correlate of cognitive impairments seen in addicted subjects.

Neurodevelopmental Disorders

Attention Deficit and Hyperactivity Disorder

Attention deficit hyperactivity disorder (ADHD) is one of the most common childhood disorders and can continue through adolescence and adulthood. ADHD affects 9.0% of American children aged 13 to 18 years and continues into adulthood in about 30% to 60% of the cases (about 4.1% American adults aged 18 years and older). ADHD has a lifetime prevalence of about 9%, and boys are three to four times more at risk than are girls. The average age of onset of this disorder is at age 7. Symptoms of ADHD include difficulty staying focused and paying attention (inattention), difficulty controlling behavior (impulsivity), and hyperactivity. Although it is normal for all children to be inattentive, hyperactive, or impulsive, the severity with which these three domains are affected distinguishes three subtypes of this disorder: predominantly hyperactive–impulsive, predominantly inattentive, and combined hyperactive–impulsive and inattentive (most common type).

ADHD is thought to involve cortical and subcortical catecholamine pathways (dopamine and noradrenaline). The most consistent findings point toward an altered function of frontal and parietal lobes, striatum, and caudate nucleus, areas that are known to be involved in regulating attention and impulsivity

Only one study to date has investigated ADHD directly using ASL MRI,[111] reporting increased CBF in the caudate and inferior frontal regions in adults with ADHD after 1 week off of medication. While the affected areas are the same as reported in nuclear imaging (PET/SPECT), their findings of increased CBF, however, are in the opposite direction. The authors hypothesize that this could represent a long-term brain adaptation or an effect of chronic treatment with stimulant medication. Another interesting finding of this study was that the CBF alteration in the caudate nucleus was normalized after medical treatment using methylphenidate, whereas the inferior frontal gyrus remained hyperperfused after treatment, suggesting a regionally specific effect of methylphenidate on brain function and again illustrating the potential of ASL MRI for studying treatment responses. Additional evidence for regionally distributed effects of medication used in ADHD treatment was found in healthy volunteers[112] in whom stimulant (methylphenidate) and nonstimulant (atomoxetine) drugs elicited regionally and directionally (increase or decrease) differentiable effects on brain perfusion. While both drugs had overlapping effects in medial prefrontal cortex (CBF increase), dissociable effects for the two drugs were found in the caudate (in line with the findings in[111]), midbrain, and thalamus. The differential effects are likely linked to receptor distributions involved in the mode of action of the different drug compounds and might be useful in predicting the effects of medication in individual subjects.

Autism Spectrum Disorders

Autistic spectrum disorder (ASD) represents a continuum of developmental cognitive and neurobehavioral disorders associated with deficits in social communication and interaction. Symptoms can be recognized in early development during the first 2 years of life; however, clinical diagnosis can only be established by the age of 3. Diagnostic criteria for autism include persistent deficits in social interaction and language as well as repetitive behavioral patterns. The prevalence of ASD varies considerably with case ascertainment, ranging from 45 to 110 per 10,000 people in the United States. ASD is about five times more common in boys than in girls.

The underlying neurophysiologic changes in ASD are still not well understood. PET and SPECT studies report increased global metabolism while frontal lobe and temporal lobe, specifically the superior temporal sulcus, show hypoperfusion.[113,114] More recent findings suggest that due to neurodevelopmental deficits in neuronal growth and pruning, a wide variety of brain networks including limbic areas, insulae, and cerebral midline areas, namely the PCC are affected leading to long-range underconnectivity and local hyperconnectivity.[115]

Preliminary findings using ASL in ASD have been presented in conference abstracts by our group.[116,117] These studies investigated children with ASD in comparison to matched control participants. Besides baseline CBF, we also assessed FC to address the question whether alterations in CBF can be associated with changes in network configuration. This approach represents a first attempt to integrate both characteristics of the resting brain into a combined view of ASD pathophysiology and has to be interpreted with caution. In both analyses, we targeted the DMN, which has been associated with self-referential cognitive processes, interoception, and theory of mind.[118,119] ASL-based FC analysis revealed highly similar DMNs

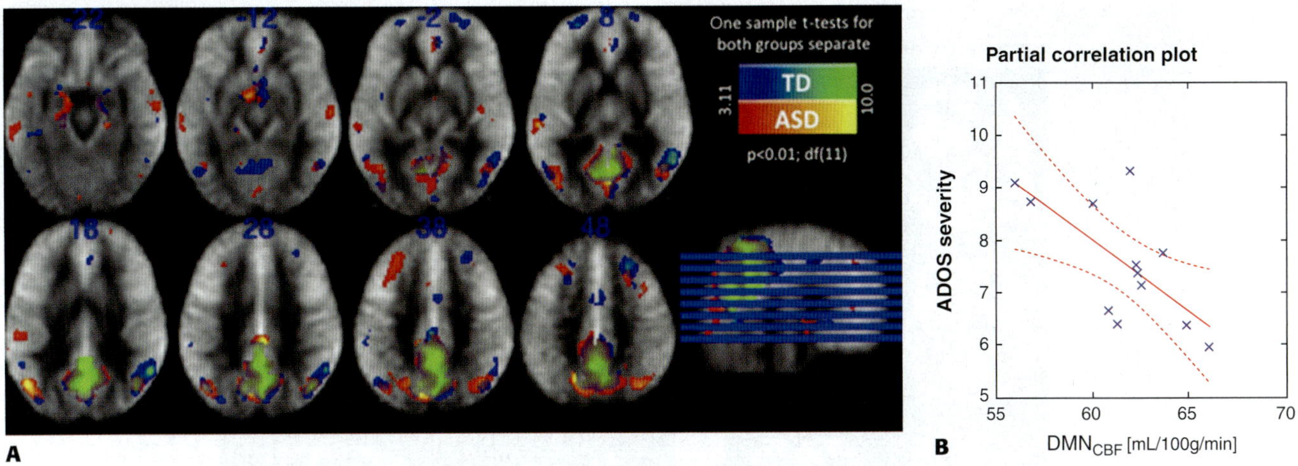

Figure 16-7. A: CBF-based default mode networks for ASD and controls overlaid on mean perfusion maps. **B:** Partial correlation between DMN, CBF, and ADOS severity score controlled for global CBF and brain volume.

in ASD and control participants. Perfusion in the DMN showed negative correlations with regional FC in areas of the posterior and anterior DMN in both groups.[116] While children with ASD demonstrated significantly reduced connectivity in posteromedial dorsal precuneus,[117] DMN perfusion showed a significant negative correlation ($r = -0.69$; $p = 0.03$) with Autism Diagnostic Observation Schedule (ADOS) severity scores.[116] These findings suggest a relation between perfusion and network connectivity within the DMN of children with ASD that highlights a disconnected but hyperactive PCC associated with symptom severity (Fig. 16.7).

To summarize the results of ASL as a biomarker of neuropsychiatric disorders, ASL perfusion imaging provides a unique opportunity to noninvasively monitor brain function in both acute and chronic states, though observed CBF changes must be considered in the context of underlying structural changes and any potential direct vasoactive effect. At this time, only a limited body of research using ASL-based perfusion imaging in clinical populations is available. Nevertheless, we believe that in the near future, this promising technique will become more widely applied in multimodal MRI studies and will yield quantitative biomarkers of brain function reflecting state and trait effects. Moreover, since ASL can easily been used repeatedly, it is optimal for longitudinal studies during development, treatment response, and course of disease. The specific application of ASL in treatment monitoring will be briefly discussed in the following section.

ASL as a Tool for Monitoring Interventions

"ASL in Developmental and Neuropsychiatric Disorders" section described preliminary findings using ASL as an imaging biomarker for an array of developmental and psychiatric diseases. Study designs implementing repeated ASL acquisitions can also be used to monitor treatment effects of psychotherapy or pharmacologic interventions. Such treatment "state" effects can interact with underlying phenotypic "trait" effects in brain disorders or with developmental changes. Additionally, studies contrasting patients who respond to treatment with patients who do not respond provide the potential to identify subsets of patients with distinct physiologic bases classified into the same disease spectrum based on symptom classification. Finally, novel methods, beyond standard pharmacologic treatment, which allow modulating brain activity (Transcranial Magnetic Stimulation [TMS], transcranial Direct Current Stimulation [tDCS]), can be employed to selectively target disease-related areas, elaborate their role in the disturbed brain networks, and facilitate novel treatment options for patients not responding to conventional treatment.

Monitoring Medication Effects with ASL

Imaging methods are increasingly used to monitor treatment effects and the mode of action of pharmacologic compounds. While PET provides unrivaled specificity for target receptor binding, the cost and challenges of developing radioligands, the need for radioactive substance injection, and low temporal resolution are major drawbacks. MR-based techniques provide noninvasive alternatives to PET and have been widely applied in pharmacologic MRI (phMRI) studies.[120,121] The most widely applied MRI contrast is BOLD due to its availability, simplicity, and high spatial and temporal resolution. However, BOLD is an indirect measure of neuronal activity and is modulated by several physiologic parameters such as CBF, CBV, and $CMRO_2$, which complicates the interpretation of drug action. Furthermore, BOLD only provides relative measures and lacks an absolute baseline, a characteristic of brain function especially important in phMRI. Accordingly, most BOLD phMRI studies measure drug effects indirectly based on alterations in task activation or focus on intravenously administered drugs whose actions occur on a short timescale. In contrast, ASL provides absolute values of CBF at rest or during task activation with high reproducibility over minutes, hours to days, and weeks.[122,123] Moreover, novel ASL implementations are resistant to magnetic field inhomogeneities (susceptibility) effects,[124] thus improving measurement of orbitofrontal and limbic areas such as the amygdala, which are associated in a variety of psychiatric disorders. These qualities make ASL a promising tool for investigation of treatment effects and monitoring of drug action over longer periods of time. ASL phMRI has this far mainly been used in proof-of-concept studies to demonstrate the effects on brain function using standard psychiatric drugs in healthy volunteers. For example, Chen et al.[60] found citalopram-induced CBF reductions in areas of the limbic network, detectable after a single oral dose of the drug. However, ASL MRI has also been applied to experimental therapies.[125]

Besides detecting increases or decreases in perfusion, repeated ASL scans after drug intake can yield its pharmacodynamics, an important factor in drug development of novel therapies[126] (Fig. 16.8). Moreover, ASL has proven its ability to provide differential effects of drugs with presumed distinct modes of action.[112,127] First- and second-generation antipsychotic drugs are different in

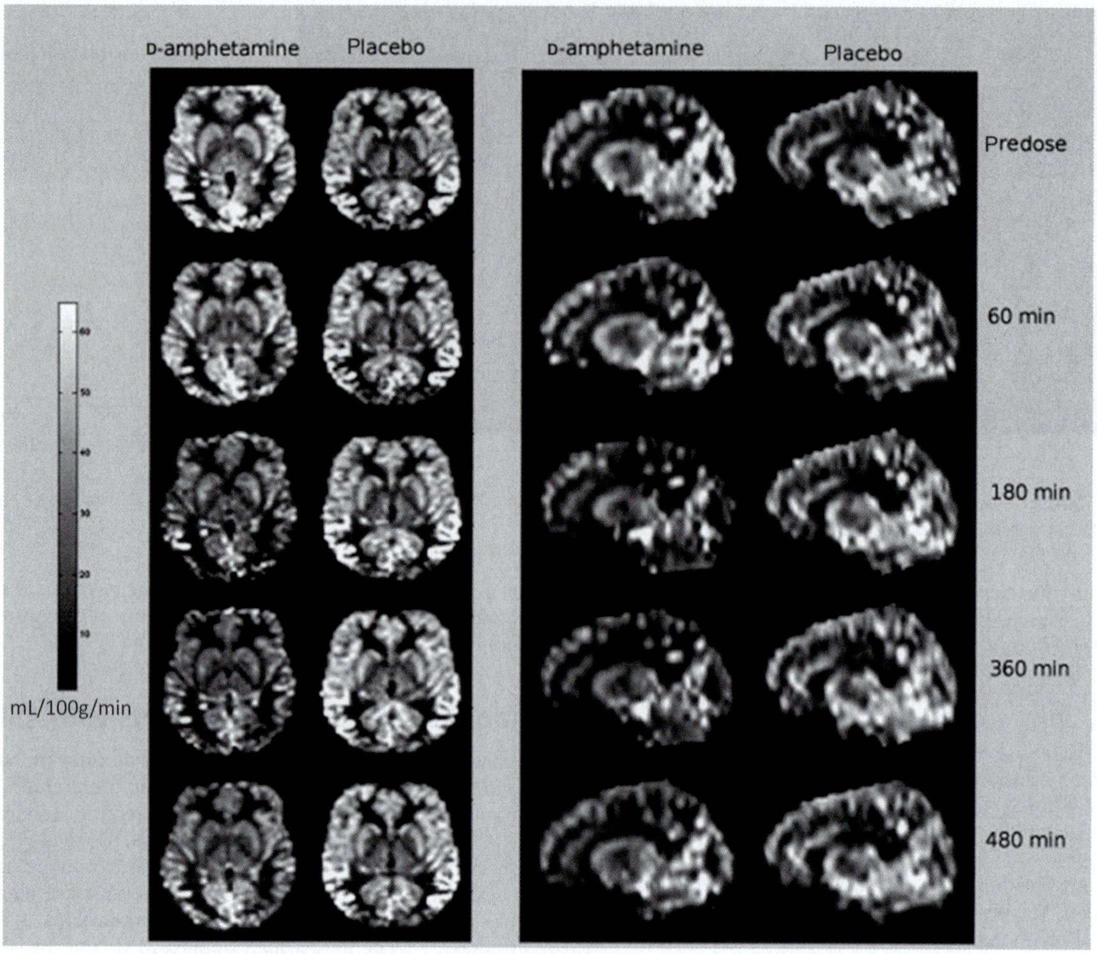

Figure 16-8. CBF maps of two subjects displaying the perfusion changes at several time points after oral administration of D-amphetamine as compared to placebo. A clear reduction of CBF can be seen as the result of the pharmacologic challenge highlighting the ability to use ASL to monitor pharmacodynamics of cerebral perfusion. (From Nordin LE, et al. Cortical responses to amphetamine exposure studied by pCASL MRI and pharmacokinetic/pharmacodynamic dose modeling. *Neuroimage* 2013;68:75–82.)

their affinity to dopamine and serotonin receptors. While both compounds decreased rCBF in frontal areas but increased CBF in anterior cingulate, first-generation antipsychotics (haloperidol) induced a decrease of CBF in the temporal lobe and second-generation drugs (aripiprazole) increased CBF in the superior temporal gyrus. Discriminatory effects have also been reported for stimulant (methylphenidate) versus nonstimulant (atomoxetine) medication used in ADHD.[112] These studies provide insight into the regional distribution and selectivity of brain modulatory effects of different classes of drugs. Since patients have been shown to present with different brain perfusion patterns (subgroups with different symptoms or responders vs. nonresponders), these insights can guide drug prescription for targeted normalization of brain metabolism.

Selective Targeting of Brain Areas/Networks

Novel neuromodulatory methods such as transcranial magnetic stimulation (TMS) or transcranial direct current stimulation (tDCS) can be used to manipulate brain function in healthy controls and have potential therapeutic applications (TMS[128] and tDCS[129,130]). TMS is based on the principle of electromagnetic induction of an electric field, and depending on the strength, it can depolarize neurons and evoke action potentials or alter brain excitability. Increased excitability can be achieved by single or paired pulsed TMS, whereas repetitive TMS can produce a reduction of excitability based on the intensity of frequency of stimulation. In contrast to TMS, tDCS applies low-amplitude direct currents via electrodes placed on the scalp. The time-invariant currents are thought to modulate the transmembrane neuronal potentials to influence the excitability and firing rate of neurons. Depending on the polarity of the applied currents, tDCS can increase (anode) or decrease (cathode) excitability of the brain areas beneath the electrodes.

The usefulness of ASL to monitor and understand TMS treatment effects has been demonstrated for the example of AVH in schizophrenia. In a series of papers, a group from Switzerland has found that inhibitory TMS can efficiently reverse CBF hyperperfusion in the language network associated with AVH,[79] specifically in the auditory cortex, Broca's area, and also the anterior cingulate that is thought to be related to malattribution of self-generated thoughts to an external agency. Furthermore, they identified regional CBF measured by ASL as a possible biologic marker for responsiveness to TMS therapy. CBF in the superior temporal gyrus was significantly higher in responders than in nonresponders and was able to predict treatment efficacy.[77] Of note, this area did not show a treatment effect itself but remained hyperperfused after treatment. Accordingly, this area might represent a trait marker of the disease symptom as it exhibits continuous aberrant activity, whereas the areas that followed the clinical course are regarded as state-dependent markers.[78] The same group also published a case study with similar treatment effects using tDCS with long-lasting symptom improvement over 6 weeks.[131]

Future Directions

Baseline function and stimulus responsiveness, as well as the integrity (connectedness) of brain networks, are important factors for proper functioning of the brain. Alterations in these properties certainly underlie cognitive and emotional impairments that manifest as clinical symptomatology. Because regional brain function, both at rest and following task, pharmacologic, or neuromodulatory intervention, is closely coupled to regional brain perfusion, ASL MRI represents an important tool for understanding of brain functionality and the mechanisms of disease. Furthermore, the increasing availability of ASL and its consistency over time and scanner hardware allow multisite studies and thus the assembly of large cohorts. This is a prerequisite to establish norms, identify brain areas that are specific for different disorders, and to develop trait and state-specific biomarkers. Because ASL MRI is sensitive to trait effects, it also has applications in exploring phenotype–genotype correlations in the brain. Such approaches will likely provide new insights into the brain endophenotype due to genetic variation and could be used to identify persons at risk for disease.[63,132] While ASL MRI is also capable of identifying correlated networks in the brain, its temporal resolution is inherently lower than that of BOLD contrast, and ASL in combination with BOLD together provide a powerful tool to fully characterize the spatiotemporal dynamics and metabolism of brain networks.[27,133]

Conclusion

This chapter provides an overview of the technical principals of ASL, its comparison with more established PET measurements, and representative applications of ASL for studying normal neurodevelopment as well as neuropsychiatric disorders. With the newly published ASL white paper,[11] which has been widely endorsed by the MR community, it is expected that ASL, especially with the recommended implementation of pCASL with background-suppressed 3D acquisitions, will be increasingly adopted for neuroimaging studies in neuropsychiatry. The literature so far has shown promising results but nonetheless heterogeneous findings across the wide spectrum of neuropsychiatric disorders, perhaps because neuropsychiatric disorders are complex diseases with multiple genetic and environmental factors often intertwined with developmental trajectories. The findings of ASL as well as other neuroimaging modalities need to be interpreted in the context of the subjects' subtype of psychiatric disorders and other factors like age and gender. In the dawn of the age of "personalized medicine," it is expected that modern neuroimaging techniques, including ASL, will contribute both to the accurate phenotyping of patient presenting with neuropsychiatric symptoms and provide an objective marker for evaluating treatment effects. With its capability for quantitative CBF measurements with high test–retest repeatability and the potential to perform concurrent FC analysis, ASL is poised to become an important neuroimaging tool in neuropsychiatry.

ACKNOWLEDGMENTS

The authors would like to acknowledge the following institutions that supported their work in this area of research. The US National Institutes of Health grants R01 MH080729, P41 EB015893, P50-HD055784, R01-MH080892, R01-NS081077, R01-EB014922 as well as the Garen and Shari Staglin and the International Mental Health Research Organization.

KJ has a fellowship of the Swiss National Science Foundation & Swiss Foundation for Grants in Biology and Medicine grant 142743.

REFERENCES

1. **Wolf RL, Detre JA.** Clinical neuroimaging using arterial spin-labeled perfusion magnetic resonance imaging. *Neurotherapeutics* 2007;4(3):346–359.
2. **Wu WC, et al.** Quantification issues in arterial spin labeling perfusion magnetic resonance imaging. *Top Magn Reson Imaging* 2010;21(2):65–73.
3. **Wu WC, et al.** A theoretical and experimental investigation of the tagging efficiency of pseudocontinuous arterial spin labeling. *Magn Reson Med* 2007;58(5):1020–1027.
4. **Dai W, et al.** Continuous flow-driven inversion for arterial spin labeling using pulsed radio frequency and gradient fields. *Magn Reson Med* 2008;60(6):1488–1497.
5. **Elison JT, et al.** Frontolimbic neural circuitry at 6 months predicts individual differences in joint attention at 9 months. *Dev Sci* 2013; 16(2):186–197.
6. **Wang J, et al.** Comparison of quantitative perfusion imaging using arterial spin labeling at 1.5 and 4.0 Tesla. *Magn Reson Med* 2002;48(2): 242–254.
7. **Wang Z, et al.** Continuous ASL perfusion MRI with an array coil and parallel imaging at 3T. *Magn Reson Med* 2005;54:732–737.
8. **Fernandez-Seara MA, et al.** Minimizing acquisition time of arterial spin labeling at 3T. *Magn Reson Med* 2008;59(6):1467–1471.
9. **Fernandez-Seara MA, et al.** Imaging mesial temporal lobe activation during scene encoding: comparison of fMRI using BOLD and arterial spin labeling. *Hum Brain Mapp* 2007;28(12):1391–1400.
10. **Vidorreta M, et al.** Comparison of 2D and 3D single-shot ASL perfusion fMRI sequences. *Neuroimage* 2012;66C:662–671.
11. **Alsop DC, et al.** Recommended implementation of arterial spin labeling perfusion MRI for clinical applications: a consensus of the ISMRM perfusion study group and the European ASL in dementia consortium. *Magn Reson Med* April 8, 2014. doi: 10.1002/mrm.25197.
12. **Ye FQ, et al.** H(2)(15)O PET validation of steady-state arterial spin tagging cerebral blood flow measurements in humans. *Magn Reson Med* 2000;44(3):450–456.
13. **Feng CM, et al.** CBF changes during brain activation: fMRI vs PET. *Neuroimage* 2004;22(1):443–446.
14. **Xu G, et al.** Reliability and precision of pseudo-continuous arterial spin labeling perfusion MRI on 3.0 T and comparison with (15)O-water PET in elderly subjects at risk for Alzheimer's disease. *NMR Biomed* 2010;23(3):286–293.
15. **Kilroy E, et al.** Reliability of two-dimensional and three-dimensional pseudo-continuous arterial spin labeling perfusion MRI in elderly populations: comparison with 15o-water positron emission tomography. *J Magn Reson Imaging* 2014;39(4):931–939.
16. **Heijtel DF, et al.** Accuracy and precision of pseudo-continuous arterial spin labeling perfusion during baseline and hypercapnia: a head-to-head comparison with O HO positron emission tomography. *Neuroimage* 2014;92C:182–192.
17. **Zhang K, et al.** Simultaneous arterial spin labelling MRI and H2O15 positron emission tomography. In: *ISMRM*. 2013. Salt Lake City, Utah.
18. **Newberg AB, et al.** Concurrent CBF and CMRGlc changes during human brain activation by combined fMRI-PET scanning. *Neuroimage* 2005;28(2):500–506.
19. **Cha YH, et al.** Regional correlation between resting state FDG PET and pCASL perfusion MRI. *J Cereb Blood Flow Metab* 2013;33(12): 1909–1914.
20. **Shulman RG, et al.** Energetic basis of brain activity: implications for neuroimaging. *Trends Neurosci* 2004;27(8):489–495.
21. **Hyder F, Rothman DL, Shulman RG.** Total neuroenergetics support localized brain activity: implications for the interpretation of fMRI. *Proc Natl Acad Sci U S A* 2002;99(16):10771–10776.
22. **Kastrup A, et al.** Relationship between cerebral blood flow changes during visual stimulation and baseline flow levels investigated with functional MRI. *Neuroreport* 1999;10(8):1751–1756.
23. **Liu J, et al.** Does baseline cerebral blood flow affect task-related blood oxygenation level dependent response in schizophrenia? *Schizophr Res* 2012;140(1–3):143–148.
24. **Beckmann CF, et al.** Investigations into resting-state connectivity using independent component analysis. *Philos Trans R Soc Lond B Biol Sci* 2005;360(1457):1001–1013.
25. **Cole DM, Smith SM, Beckmann CF.** Advances and pitfalls in the analysis and interpretation of resting-state FMRI data. *Front Syst Neurosci* 2010;4:8.

26. **Damoiseaux JS, et al.** Consistent resting-state networks across healthy subjects. *Proc Natl Acad Sci U S A* 2006;103(37):13848–13853.
27. **Jann K, et al.** Functional connectivity in BOLD and CBF data: similarity and reliability of resting brain networks. *Neuroimage* 2015;106:111–122.
28. **Jann K, et al.** Topographic electrophysiological signatures of FMRI Resting State Networks. *PLOS One* 2010;5(9):e12945.
29. **Raichle ME, et al.** A default mode of brain function. *Proc Natl Acad Sci U S A* 2001;98(2):676–682.
30. **Biswal B, et al.** Functional connectivity in the motor cortex of resting human brain using echo-planar MRI. *Magn Reson Med* 1995;34(4):537–541.
31. **Power JD, et al.** Methods to detect, characterize, and remove motion artifact in resting state fMRI. *Neuroimage* 2014;84:320–341.
32. **Buxton RB, et al.** Modeling the hemodynamic response to brain activation. *Neuroimage* 2004;23(suppl 1):S220–S233.
33. **Obata T, et al.** Discrepancies between BOLD and flow dynamics in primary and supplementary motor areas: application of the balloon model to the interpretation of BOLD transients. *Neuroimage* 2004;21(1):144–153.
34. **Ye FQ, et al.** H(2)(15)O PET validation of steady-state arterial spin tagging cerebral blood flow measurements in humans. *Magn Reson Med* 2000;44(3):450–456.
35. **Aguirre GK, et al.** Experimental design and the relative sensitivity of BOLD and perfusion fMRI. *Neuroimage* 2002;15(3):488–500.
36. **Chuang KH, et al.** Mapping resting-state functional connectivity using perfusion MRI. *Neuroimage* 2008;40(4):1595–1605.
37. **Jann K, et al.** Quantification of network perfusion in ASL cerebral blood flow data with seed based and ICA approaches. *Brain Topogr* 2013;26(4):569–580.
38. **Liang XY, et al.** A k-space sharing 3D GRASE pseudocontinuous ASL method for whole-brain resting-state functional connectivity. *Int J Imaging Syst Technol* 2012;22(1):37–43.
39. **Zou Q, et al.** Static and dynamic characteristics of cerebral blood flow during the resting state. *Neuroimage* 2009;48(3):515–524.
40. **Liang X, et al.** Coupling of functional connectivity and regional cerebral blood flow reveals a physiological basis for network hubs of the human brain. *Proc Natl Acad Sci U S A* 2013;110(5):1929–1934.
41. **Tomasi D, Wang GJ, Volkow ND.** Energetic cost of brain functional connectivity. *Proc Natl Acad Sci U S A* 2013;110(33):13642–13647.
42. **Giedd JN.** Structural magnetic resonance imaging of the adolescent brain. *Ann N Y Acad Sci* 2004;1021:77–85.
43. **Paus T, et al.** Structural maturation of neural pathways in children and adolescents: in vivo study. *Science* 1999;283(5409):1908–1911.
44. **Giedd JN, et al.** Brain development during childhood and adolescence: a longitudinal MRI study. *Nat Neurosci* 1999;2(10):861–863.
45. **Gogtay N, et al.** Dynamic mapping of human cortical development during childhood through early adulthood. *Proc Natl Acad Sci U S A* 2004;101(21):8174–8179.
46. **Wang J, et al.** Pediatric perfusion imaging using pulsed arterial spin labeling. *J Magn Reson Imaging* 2003;18(4):404–413.
47. **Miranda MJ, Olofsson K, Sidaros K.** Noninvasive measurements of regional cerebral perfusion in preterm and term neonates by magnetic resonance arterial spin labeling. *Pediatr Res* 2006;60(3):359–363.
48. **Biagi L, et al.** Age dependence of cerebral perfusion assessed by magnetic resonance continuous arterial spin labeling. *J Magn Reson Imaging* 2007;25(4):696–702.
49. **Wang J, Rao H, Detre JA.** Arterial spin labeling perfusion MRI in developmental neuroscience. In: Rumsey JM, Ernst M, eds. *Neuroimaging in developmental clinical neuroscience.* Cambridge, UK: Cambridge University Press; 2009:326–343.
50. **Chiron C, et al.** Changes in regional cerebral blood flow during brain maturation in children and adolescents. *J Nucl Med* 1992;33(5): 696–703.
51. **Chugani HT.** A critical period of brain development: studies of cerebral glucose utilization with PET. *Prev Med* 1998;27:184–188.
52. **Taki Y, et al.** Correlation between gray matter density-adjusted brain perfusion and age using brain MR images of 202 healthy children. *Hum Brain Mapp* 2011;32(11):1973–1985.
53. **Taki Y, et al.** Gender differences in partial-volume corrected brain perfusion using brain MRI in healthy children. *Neuroimage* 2011;58(3): 709–715.
54. **Jain V, et al.** Longitudinal reproducibility and accuracy of pseudo-continuous arterial spin-labeled perfusion MR imaging in typically developing children. *Radiology* 2012;263(2):527–536.
55. **Shi Y, et al.** Sex differences in cerebral perfusion during brain development. 20th annual meeting of OHBM, 2014: Abstract.
56. **Bench CJ, Frackowiak RS, Dolan RJ.** Changes in regional cerebral blood flow on recovery from depression. *Psychol Med* 1995;25(2):247–261.
57. **Duhameau B, et al.** Chronic and treatment-resistant depression: a study using arterial spin labeling perfusion MRI at 3Tesla. *Psychiatry Res* 2010;182(2):111–116.
58. **Ho TC, et al.** Altered cerebral perfusion in executive, affective, and motor networks during adolescent depression. *J Am Acad Child Adolesc Psychiatry* 2013;52(10):1076–1091. e2.
59. **Lui S, et al.** Depressive disorders: focally altered cerebral perfusion measured with arterial spin-labeling MR imaging. *Radiology* 2009; 251(2):476–484.
60. **Chen Y, et al.** Quantification of cerebral blood flow as biomarker of drug effect: arterial spin labeling phMRI after a single dose of oral citalopram. *Clin Pharmacol Ther* 2011;89(2):251–258.
61. **Jarnum H, et al.** Longitudinal MRI study of cortical thickness, perfusion, and metabolite levels in major depressive disorder. *Acta Psychiatr Scand* 2011;124(6):435–446.
62. **Weiduschat N, Dubin MJ.** Prefrontal cortical blood flow predicts response of depression to rTMS. *J Affect Disord* 2013;150(2):699–702.
63. **Rao H, et al.** Genetic variation in serotonin transporter alters resting brain function in healthy individuals. *Biol Psychiatry* 2007;62(6):600–606.
64. **Orosz A, et al.** Reduced cerebral blood flow within the default-mode network and within total gray matter in major depression. *Brain Connect* 2012;2(6):303–310.
65. **Greicius MD, et al.** Resting-state functional connectivity in major depression: abnormally increased contributions from subgenual cingulate cortex and thalamus. *Biol Psychiatry* 2007;62(5):429–437.
66. **Zhu X, et al.** Evidence of a dissociation pattern in resting-state default mode network connectivity in first-episode, treatment-naive major depression patients. *Biol Psychiatry* 2012;71(7):611–617.
67. **Pizzagalli DA.** Frontocingulate dysfunction in depression: toward biomarkers of treatment response. *Neuropsychopharmacology* 2011; 36(1):183–206.
68. **Bullmore E, et al.** Functional MR imaging of confounded hypofrontality. *Hum Brain Mapp* 1999;8(2–3):86–91.
69. **Ingvar DH, Franzen G.** Abnormalities of cerebral blood flow distribution in patients with chronic schizophrenia. *Acta Psychiatr Scand* 1974;50(4):425–462.
70. **Liddle PF, et al.** Patterns of cerebral blood flow in schizophrenia. *Br J Psychiatry* 1992;160:179–186.
71. **Ota M, et al.** Pseudo-continuous arterial spin labeling MRI study of schizophrenic patients. *Schizophr Res* 2014;154(1–3):113–118.
72. **Pinkham A, et al.** Resting quantitative cerebral blood flow in schizophrenia measured by pulsed arterial spin labeling perfusion MRI. *Psychiatry Res* 2011;194(1):64–72.
73. **Scheef L, et al.** Resting-state perfusion in nonmedicated schizophrenic patients: a continuous arterial spin-labeling 3.0-T MR study. *Radiology* 2010;256(1):253–260.
74. **Walther S, et al.** Neural correlates of disbalanced motor control in major depression. *J Affect Disord* 2012;136(1–2):124–133.
75. **Horn H, et al.** Structural and metabolic changes in language areas linked to formal thought disorder. *Br J Psychiatry* 2009;194(2):130–138.
76. **Horn H, et al.** Semantic network disconnection in formal thought disorder. *Neuropsychobiology* 2012;66(1):14–23.
77. **Homan P, et al.** Cerebral blood flow identifies responders to transcranial magnetic stimulation in auditory verbal hallucinations. *Transl Psychiatry* 2012;2:e189.
78. **Homan P, et al.** Repeated measurements of cerebral blood flow in the left superior temporal gyrus reveal tonic hyperactivity in patients with auditory verbal hallucinations: a possible trait marker. *Front Hum Neurosci* 2013;7:304.
79. **Kindler J, et al.** Reduced neuronal activity in language-related regions after transcranial magnetic stimulation therapy for auditory verbal hallucinations. *Biol Psychiatry* 2013;73(6):518–524.
80. **Whitfield-Gabrieli S, Ford JM.** Default mode network activity and connectivity in psychopathology. *Annu Rev Clin Psychol* 2012;8:49–76.
81. **Kindler J, et al.** Static and dynamic characteristics of cerebral blood flow during the resting state in schizophrenia. *Schizophr Bull* 2013:41(1); 163–170.
82. **Razavi N, et al.** ASL based functional connectivity in schizophrenia relates to disease severity. In *International Conference on Basic and Clinical Multimodal Imaging (BaCI).* 2013. Geneva, Switzerland.

83. **Engel K, et al.** Neuroimaging in anxiety disorders. *J Neural Transm* 2009;116(6):703–716.
84. **Andreescu C, et al.** Altered cerebral blood flow patterns associated with pathologic worry in the elderly. *Depress Anxiety* 2011;28(3):202–209.
85. **Orosz A, et al.** Changes in cerebral blood flow following successful psychotherapy combined with cortisol treatment in spider phobia. In *ISMRM*. Milan: *Proceedings of the International Society for Magnetic Resonance in Medicine* 2014.
86. **Johanson A, et al.** Changes in frontal lobe activity with cognitive therapy for spider phobia. *Appl Neuropsychol* 2006;13(1):34–41.
87. **Wang J, et al.** Perfusion functional MRI reveals cerebral blood flow pattern under psychological stress. *Proc Natl Acad Sci U S A* 2005; 102(49):17804–17809.
88. **Giardino ND, Friedman SD, Dager SR.** Anxiety, respiration, and cerebral blood flow: implications for functional brain imaging. *Compr Psychiatry* 2007;48(2):103–112.
89. **Costenla AR, Cunha RA, de Mendonca A.** Caffeine, adenosine receptors, and synaptic plasticity. *J Alzheimers Dis* 2010;20 (suppl 1): S25–S34.
90. **Fisone G, Borgkvist A, Usiello A.** Caffeine as a psychomotor stimulant: mechanism of action. *Cell Mol Life Sci* 2004;61(7–8):857–872.
91. **Field AS, et al.** Dietary caffeine consumption and withdrawal: confounding variables in quantitative cerebral perfusion studies? *Radiology* 2003;227(1):129–135.
92. **Grichisch Y, et al.** Differential effects of intranasal insulin and caffeine on cerebral blood flow. *Hum Brain Mapp* 2012;33(2):280–287.
93. **Haller S, et al.** Acute caffeine administration impact on working memory-related brain activation and functional connectivity in the elderly: a BOLD and perfusion MRI study. *Neuroscience* 2013;250:364–371.
94. **Chen Y, Parrish TB.** Caffeine dose effect on activation-induced BOLD and CBF responses. *Neuroimage* 2009;46(3):577–583.
95. **Chen Y, Parrish TB.** Caffeine's effects on cerebrovascular reactivity and coupling between cerebral blood flow and oxygen metabolism. *Neuroimage* 2009;44(3):647–652.
96. **Liu TT, et al.** Caffeine alters the temporal dynamics of the visual BOLD response. *Neuroimage* 2004;23(4):1402–1413.
97. **Perthen JE, et al.** Caffeine-induced uncoupling of cerebral blood flow and oxygen metabolism: a calibrated BOLD fMRI study. *Neuroimage* 2008;40(1):237–247.
98. **Wang Z, et al.** Neural substrates of abstinence-induced cigarette cravings in chronic smokers. *J Neurosci* 2007;27(51):14035–14040.
99. **Gazdzinski S, et al.** Effects of chronic alcohol dependence and chronic cigarette smoking on cerebral perfusion: a preliminary magnetic resonance study. *Alcohol Clin Exp Res* 2006;30(6):947–958.
100. **Mon A, et al.** The impact of chronic cigarette smoking on recovery from cortical gray matter perfusion deficits in alcohol dependence: longitudinal arterial spin labeling MRI. *Alcohol Clin Exp Res* 2009;33(8): 1314–1321.
101. **Koob GF, et al.** Neurocircuitry targets in ethanol reward and dependence. *Alcohol Clin Exp Res* 1998;22(1):3–9.
102. **Khalili-Mahani N, et al.** Pseudocontinuous arterial spin labeling reveals dissociable effects of morphine and alcohol on regional cerebral blood flow. *J Cereb Blood Flow Metab* 2011;31(5):1321–1333.
103. **Marxen M, et al.** Acute effects of alcohol on brain perfusion monitored with arterial spin labeling magnetic resonance imaging in young adults. *J Cereb Blood Flow Metab* 2014;34(3):472–479.
104. **Rickenbacher E, et al.** Effects of alcohol intoxication and gender on cerebral perfusion: an arterial spin labeling study. *Alcohol* 2011;45(8): 725–737.
105. **Tolentino NJ, et al.** Alcohol effects on cerebral blood flow in subjects with low and high responses to alcohol. *Alcohol Clin Exp Res* 2011;35(6):1034–1040.
106. **Clark CP, et al.** Decreased perfusion in young alcohol-dependent women as compared with age-matched controls. *Am J Drug Alcohol Abuse* 2007;33(1):13–19.
107. **Tutus A, et al.** Transient frontal hypoperfusion in Tc-99m hexamethylpropyleneamine oxime single photon emission computed tomography imaging during alcohol withdrawal. *Biol Psychiatry* 1998;43(12):923–928.
108. **Denier N, et al.** Reduction in cerebral perfusion after heroin administration: a resting state arterial spin labeling study. *PLoS One* 2013; 8(9):e71461.
109. **Denier N, et al.** Association of frontal gray matter volume and cerebral perfusion in heroin addiction: a multimodal neuroimaging study. *Front Psychiatry* 2013;4:135.
110. **van Hell HH, et al.** Evidence for involvement of the insula in the psychotropic effects of THC in humans: a double-blind, randomized pharmacological MRI study. *Int J Neuropsychopharmacol* 2011;14(10): 1377–1388.
111. **O'Gorman RL, et al.** Increased cerebral perfusion in adult attention deficit hyperactivity disorder is normalised by stimulant treatment: a non-invasive MRI pilot study. *Neuroimage* 2008;42(1):36–41.
112. **Marquand AF, et al.** Dissociable effects of methylphenidate, atomoxetine and placebo on regional cerebral blood flow in healthy volunteers at rest: a multi-class pattern recognition approach. *Neuroimage* 2012;60(2):1015–1024.
113. **Boddaert N, Zilbovicius M.** Functional neuroimaging and childhood autism. *Pediatr Radiol* 2002;32(1):1–7.
114. **Yang WH, et al.** Regional cerebral blood flow in children with autism spectrum disorders: a quantitative ^{99m}Tc-ECD brain SPECT study with statistical parametric mapping evaluation. *Chin Med J (Engl)* 2011;124(9):1362–1366.
115. **Vissers ME, Cohen MX, Geurts HM.** Brain connectivity and high functioning autism: a promising path of research that needs refined models, methodological convergence, and stronger behavioral links. *Neurosci Biobehav Rev* 2012;36(1):604–625.
116. **Jann K, et al.** Perfusion based functional connectivity in autism reveals hypo-perfusion and altered connectivity of the Default Mode Network associated with increased symptom severity. In: Proceedings of the International Society of Magnetic Resonance in Medicine 2014 (Abstract No 1965), Milan, Italy. 2014.
117. **Kilroy E, et al.** Precuneus hyper-perfusion related to symptom severity and hypoconnectivity in individuals with autism spectrum disorder. In International Meeting for Autism Research. 2014. Atlanta, GA.
118. **Greicius MD, Menon V.** Default-mode activity during a passive sensory task: uncoupled from deactivation but impacting activation. *J Cogn Neurosci* 2004;16(9):1484–1492.
119. **Spreng RN, Grady CL.** Patterns of brain activity supporting autobiographical memory, prospection, and theory of mind, and their relationship to the default mode network. *J Cogn Neurosci* 2010;22(6): 1112–1123.
120. **Iannetti GD, Wise RG.** BOLD functional MRI in disease and pharmacological studies: room for improvement? *Magn Reson Imaging* 2007;25(6):978–988.
121. **Wang DJ, et al.** Potentials and challenges for arterial spin labeling in pharmacological magnetic resonance imaging. *J Pharmacol Exp Ther* 2011;337(2):359–366.
122. **Parkes LM, et al.** Normal cerebral perfusion measurements using arterial spin labeling: reproducibility, stability, and age and gender effects. *Magn Reson Med* 2004;51(4):736–743.
123. **Wang J, et al.** Arterial spin labeling perfusion fMRI with very low task frequency. *Magn Reson Med* 2003;49(5):796–802.
124. **Wang J, et al.** Reduced susceptibility effects in perfusion fMRI with single-shot spin-echo EPI acquisitions at 1.5 Tesla. *Magn Reson Imaging* 2004;22(1):1–7.
125. **Black KJ, et al.** Quantification of indirect pathway inhibition by the adenosine A2a antagonist SYN115 in Parkinson disease. *J Neurosci* 2010;30(48):16284–16292.
126. **Nordin LE, et al.** Cortical responses to amphetamine exposure studied by pCASL MRI and pharmacokinetic/pharmacodynamic dose modeling. *Neuroimage* 2013;68:75–82.
127. **Handley R, et al.** Acute effects of single-dose aripiprazole and haloperidol on resting cerebral blood flow (rCBF) in the human brain. *Hum Brain Mapp* 2013;34(2):272–282.
128. **Kindler J, et al.** Theta burst transcranial magnetic stimulation for the treatment of auditory verbal hallucinations: results of a randomized controlled study. *Psychiatry Res* 2013;209(1):114–117.
129. **Nitsche MA, et al.** Transcranial direct current stimulation: state of the art 2008. *Brain Stimul* 2008;1(3):206–223.
130. **Webster BR, Celnik PA, Cohen LG.** Noninvasive brain stimulation in stroke rehabilitation. *NeuroRx* 2006;3(4):474–481.
131. **Homan P, et al.** Muting the voice: a case of arterial spin labeling-monitored transcranial direct current stimulation treatment of auditory verbal hallucinations. *Am J Psychiatry* 2011;168(8):853–854.
132. **Hariri AR, et al.** A susceptibility gene for affective disorders and the response of the human amygdala. *Arch Gen Psychiatry* 2005;62(2): 146–152.
133. **Zhu S, et al.** Resting state brain function analysis using concurrent BOLD in ASL perfusion fMRI. *PLoS One* 2013;8(6):e65884.

CHAPTER

17 Brain Perfusion Imaging with SPECT and PET

Heidi Wassef, MD

Introduction

Changes in cerebral blood flow (CBF) often precede anatomic changes. Therefore, evaluation of brain perfusion allows earlier diagnosis of many diseases compared to the evaluation of anatomy alone. Single photon emission computed tomography (SPECT) and PET can provide qualitative and quantitative perfusion data. The role of SPECT and PET in the diagnosis of chronic vascular disease, traumatic brain injury (TBI), dementia, and epilepsy is discussed in this chapter. These studies can also provide prognostic information that aids in the management of patients with cerebrovascular disease[1–3] or head trauma. Brain SPECT with an acetazolamide challenge allows for the evaluation of cerebrovascular reserve and with balloon occlusion allows prediction of neurologic sequelae after carotid artery sacrifice. Finally, brain perfusion may confirm the clinical diagnosis of brain death.

Radiopharmaceuticals for Brain SPECT

The ideal radiopharmaceutical for the evaluation of CBF would cross the blood–brain barrier (BBB), distribute according to blood flow, and remain there sufficiently long to allow for imaging. ^{99m}Tc-ethyl cysteine dimer (ECD, Neurolite) and Technetium ^{99m}Tc-exametazime (HMPAO, Ceretec) are lipophilic, cross the BBB, and are the most commonly used brain SPECT radiopharmaceuticals. The radioisotope, ^{99m}Tc, has the advantage of optimal keV and half-life. ^{99m}Tc-HMPAO becomes hydrophilic upon crossing the BBB and is then trapped in the brain. Maximal brain uptake is achieved by 20 seconds and represents 5% of injected dose.[4,5] HMPAO has stable binding in vivo and prolonged retention in the brain. The latter allows for SPECT in addition to planar imaging. ^{99m}Tc-HMPAO can be imaged 30 to 90 minutes after injection.[5] The ECD brain uptake is 6% of the injected dose. The advantages of ECD are in vitro stability for 6 hours, faster clearance from the blood, higher target-to-nontarget ratio, earlier imaging after intravenous injection, and better-quality SPECT brain images. ^{99m}Tc-ECD is imaged 30 to 60 minutes after injection.[5] The gray-to-white matter uptake is 4.5:1 for ^{99m}Tc-ECD versus 1.6:1 for ^{99m}Tc-HMPAO. Thus, the gray-to-white matter contrast is greater with ^{99m}Tc-ECD. Although washout is minimal, the disadvantage of ECD is significant regional brain variation in clearance.[6] The brain clearance is biexponential.

Typical doses of HMPAO and ECD are 10 to 20 mCi (370 to 740 MBq), and the effective doses are similar.[5] Table 17.1 compares HMPAO and ECD. If patients are imaged in the subacute phase (1 to 4 weeks after symptoms of stroke) at which time CBF and metabolism are uncoupled, ^{99m}Tc-ECD is preferred since it is reported to show absence of CBF at the site of "luxury perfusion" unlike ^{99m}Tc-HMPAO.[7] The phenomenon of "luxury perfusion" describes the postischemic return of CBF to normal or sometimes elevated levels compared to the metabolic requirement.

Technique

Brain SPECT involves the injection of a radiopharmaceutical that distributes in the brain according to CBF. For indications other than evaluation of suspected brain death, patients should abstain from large amounts of stimulants such as caffeine, alcohol, smoking, and other drugs that may affect cerebral perfusion. To avoid excessive sensory stimulation near the time of radiopharmaceutical injection, instructions should be given early and the intravenous cannula placed approximately 15 minutes prior to the injection.[5] The patient should be injected in a quiet room with minimal stimuli. The patient should void prior to the scan. Patient comfort is critical to ensure that the patient will not move during the approximately 20 minutes required for scanning. The angiographic phase and planar anterior and lateral images are performed if the indication is suspected brain death. Dynamic images during the angiographic phase and SPECT images of the brain are obtained for most other indications. A low-energy, high- or ultra–high-resolution collimator with a dual-head camera with 180-degree rotation with step-and-shoot mode and a matrix of 128 × 128 or higher is used. Dedicated brain cameras allow proximity to the head and facilitate less scatter and improved sensitivity and spatial resolution. Unprocessed data should be checked for motion or other artifacts prior to iterative reconstruction and the application of a low-pass filter. CT attenuation correction is superior to Chang attenuation correction.[8] Images are reformatted to three orthogonal planes.[5] With typically used techniques, HMPAO and ECD do not provide quantitative blood flow measurements. Quantitation would require an indwelling arterial line although alternative methods using the time–activity curves of the aorta or carotid artery and brain also exist.[9–12]

TABLE 17.1 **SPECT Cerebral Blood Flow Radiopharmaceuticals**

	^{99m}Tc-HMPAO	^{99m}Tc-ECD
Maximum time from constitution to injection	4 h (stabilized)	6 h
Percent localizes to the brain	5%	6%
Gray-to-white matter uptake	1.6:1	4.5:1
Time of imaging after injection	30–90 min	30–60 min
Effective dose (mSv/MBq)	0.0093	0.007
Peak activity in the brain	20 s	1 min
Luxury perfusion	Uptake commonly seen	Uptake rarely seen

Data from Kapuco OL, Nobili F, Varrone A, et al. EANM procedure guideline for brain perfusion SPECT using ^{99m}Tc-labelled radiopharmaceuticals, version 2. *Eur J Nucl Med Mol Imaging* 2009;36(12):2093–2102.

This method will be explained in more detail in the section on PET quantitation. In most clinical settings, relative regional blood flow data are obtained by comparing the counts to the contralateral brain counts. In some cases, the assumption that the contralateral brain has normal CBF can be made. Semiquantitative blood flow can also be obtained by comparing the cortical CBF to that of the cerebellum. The cerebellum has greater flow than the cerebral cortex and basal ganglia. Normal rCBF to the cortex or basal ganglia is greater than or equal to 70% of cerebellar flow and to the medial temporal cortex is greater than or equal to 50% of cerebellar flow. In acute cerebrovascular disease, SPECT can provide information on complications, outcome, and treatment. SPECT can also detect hypoperfusion due to vasospasm following subarachnoid hemorrhage and can predict severity of future neurologic sequelae.[13] An advantage of SPECT radiopharmaceuticals is the rapid uptake and prolonged retention in the brain, which allows injection during a seizure or other acute event and delayed imaging after the stabilization of the patient. The disadvantage is that the prepared radiopharmaceutical and a technologist need to be available at all times.

Brain Positron Emission Tomography Radiopharmaceuticals

Unlike SPECT tracers that emit gamma rays, PET tracers emit positrons. The PET tracers most commonly used for the measurement of CBF are $^{15}O_2$, $C^{15}O_2$, and $H_2{}^{15}O$. These radiopharmaceuticals are produced in a cyclotron. Their very short half-life limits their usage to centers that have an onsite cyclotron. The half-lives of ^{15}O, ^{13}N, and ^{11}C are 2, 10, and 20 minutes, respectively.[14]

Extensive research with these radiopharmaceuticals has provided a wealth of information about cerebral hemodynamics and function. ^{18}F-fluorodeoxyglucose (FDG) can provide cerebral metabolic information. Its 110-minute half-life allows sufficient time for delivery of the tracer to most imaging centers. For this reason, FDG PET has gained widespread clinical appeal. PET spatial resolution is 4 to 6 mm.[14]

Technique

Patients fast for 4 to 6 hours, and the blood glucose levels are checked prior to FDG administration to confirm that they are not elevated. Excessive stimulation is to be avoided following tracer injection and thus it is recommended that the cannula for intravenous administration be placed 10 minutes or more before tracer injection. The patient is injected with 5 to 20 mCi (185 to 740 MBq) in a dimly lit room, and the patient is instructed to rest comfortably and not to speak, read, or do other activities. If an FDG study is performed for evaluation of epilepsy, EEG monitoring is necessary prior to and at least 20 minutes after injection. EEG leads are removed prior to image acquisition since most will cause attenuation artifacts. Imaging is performed 30 to 60 minutes following injection. Most current scanners are hybrid PET-computed tomography (CT). CT provides attenuation correction data for PET as well as anatomic correlation of the PET functional data. Basal ganglia, hippocampal area, thalami, cerebellum, posterior cingulate gyrus, and visual cortex are relatively metabolically stable with advancing age. Decreased cortical metabolism, especially in the frontal lobes, is reported with normal aging.[15]

Better image quality is possible with longer ^{18}F-FDG imaging time (15 to 30 minutes) compared to shorter $^{15}O\text{-}H_2O$ imaging time (1 to 2 minutes). The longer imaging time is possible because the ^{18}F-FDG half-life is 110 minutes compared to 2 minutes for ^{15}O-water. On the other hand, the advantage of the shorter $^{15}O\text{-}H_2O$ half-life is that the study can be repeated immediately.

PET Quantitation

The various PET radiopharmaceuticals can provide hemodynamic (rCBF, oxygen extraction fraction [OEF], and regional cerebral metabolic rate of oxygen [$rCMRO_2$]), metabolic, cell proliferation, or neurotransmission data. PET regional CBF (rCBF) quantitation with $^{15}O\text{-}H_2O$ PET water is regarded as the gold standard.[16] Quantification of rCBF from $^{15}O\text{-}H_2O$ PET requires the knowledge of the arterial input function (AIF) into the brain typically acquired by arterial blood sampling. PET can also provide quantification of the OEF and $rCMRO_2$.[17] Due to the invasive nature of arterial sampling, research has focused on image-derived input function (IDIF). An example of this IDIF uses the common carotid arteries that can be localized by coregistered MRI.[16] This is the same technique that can be used with SPECT as was shown in Figure 17.1. A region of interest (ROI) has been drawn over the common carotid arteries and used as an IDIF. Comparison of right and left hemisphere ROI time activity curves demonstrate relative perfusion differences. Deconvolution of the perfusion curves with the AIF can give an estimate of absolute perfusion.

PET can provide semiquantitative regional metabolic data. The brain depends almost exclusively on glucose metabolism. Unlike other organs, the brain cannot store oxygen or glucose, and rCBF is continuously changing to meet the changing metabolic demands. Thus, in most cases, regional metabolism correlates with rCBF. Standard uptake value is a semiquantitative parameter used in ^{18}F-FDG PET.

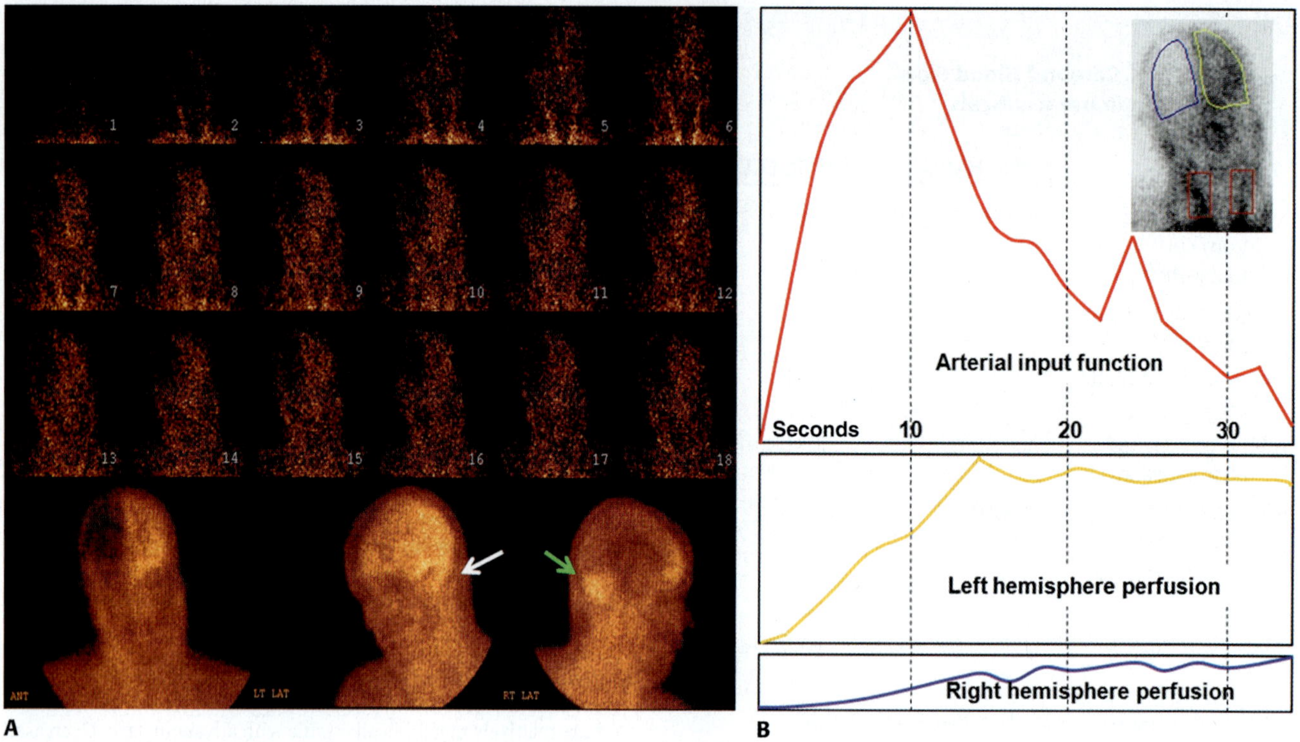

Figure 17-1. ^{99m}**Tc-exametazime cerebral perfusion images in a 34-year-old unresponsive man.** There is markedly decreased perfusion to the right cerebral hemisphere **(A)**. On the lateral views, note the apparent decreased flow to the left cerebellum (*white arrow*) with preserved right cerebellar activity (*green arrow*) demonstrating crossed cerebellar diaschisis on the delayed images. The measurable perfusion data include an estimate of the arterial input function (AIF) from the carotid regions of interest (ROI) in *red* **(B)**. Comparison of right (*blue*) and left hemisphere (*yellow*) ROI time–activity curves demonstrates relative perfusion differences. Deconvolution of the perfusion curves with the AIF can give an estimate of absolute perfusion. Images Courtesy of Patrick Colletti, M.D.

Pearls and Pitfalls

There are several differences between SPECT and PET to be noted. In general, the severity of hypometabolism seen on PET is greater than the severity of hypoperfusion on SPECT. Cerebellar metabolism is less than cortical metabolism in ^{18}F-FDG PET unlike SPECT (or ^{15}O-H_2O PET) where cerebellar blood flow is greater than CBF.[18] Cerebellar metabolism is approximately 85% of cortical metabolism while cortical blood flow is equal to or greater than 70% of cerebellar blood flow. Correlation with CT and/or MRI is essential to assess age-related and focal cerebral volume loss.[18] This will help avoid misinterpreting focal or global cerebral volume loss as hypometabolism or hypoperfusion.[18,19]

Clinical Applications

Acute Stroke

SPECT can help determine which patients with symptoms of acute stroke may benefit from thrombolysis to limit neurologic sequela and which patients are at high risk for hemorrhage. If initial CT excludes hemorrhage in a patient with symptoms of acute stroke, the next consideration is whether thrombolysis might be necessary. Pretherapy semiquantitative SPECT provides important information that helps select the patients who would benefit from thrombolysis.[2] A retrospective study of 30 patients who had SPECT prior to endovascular thrombolysis revealed that ischemic tissue with CBF greater than 55% of cerebellar blood flow can be spared with thrombolysis even if administered more than 6 hours after the onset of symptoms and tissue with CBF greater than 35% of cerebellar flow can be spared with thrombolysis within 5 hours. Ischemic tissue with CBF less than 35% of cerebellar flow is at risk for hemorrhage despite prompt initiation of thrombolysis.[2]

Not only does CBF information help determine patient management, but it also provides prognostic information as listed in Table 17.2. Severe hypoperfusion in the first 6 hours after symptom onset is highly correlated with poor neurologic outcome.

Ischemia may be divided into three phases. In the acute phase (hours—2 or 3 days) of ischemia, SPECT shows hypoperfusion in the tissue at risk. In the subacute phase (1 to 2 weeks), increased or "luxury" perfusion can occur while some cells may start dying. "Luxury perfusion," as previously noted, is the postischemic return of CBF to normal or high compared to the metabolic requirement.

TABLE 17.2 Cerebral Blood Blow Measurements and Neurologic Sequela

Cerebral Blood Flow (mL/100 g of tissue/min)	Sequela
Below 18–20	Neurologic dysfunction
Between 10 and 20	Infarction within minutes to hours
Below 10	Infarction within a few minutes

Cerebral blood volume (CBV) and CBF are normal or elevated in infarcted or nearly infarcted tissue and thus can be misinterpreted as nonischemic, and knowledge of OEF, mean transit time (MTT), and time to peak (TTP) derived from PET are necessary for correct interpretation. Hypoperfusion is present in the chronic phase (>1 month).

The "four tissue compartments concept" described by Lee clarifies the pathophysiology. The tissue compartments from peripheral to central are (a) nonischemic and unaffected tissue, (b) mildly hypoperfused but not at-risk tissue, (c) hypoperfused and at-risk tissue (the ischemic penumbra), and (d) irreversibly damaged tissue centrally.[19] Each of these four tissue compartments has characteristic parameters obtained by quantitative PET as seen in Figure 17.2.

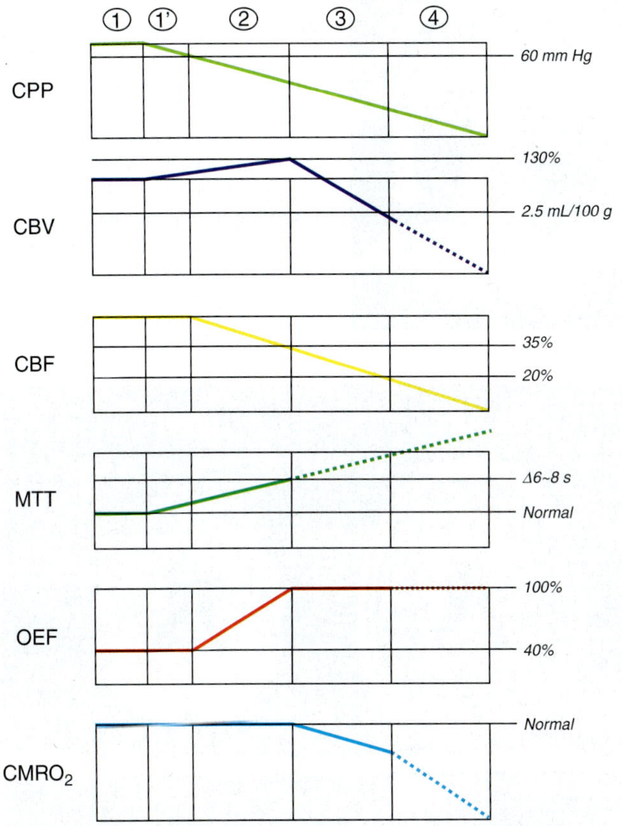

Figure 17-2. The *x*-axis is divided into four compartments, one to four, according to the four-compartment concept. Each *y*-axis represents the level of those parameters. Rough thresholds for the parameters are presented at the right side of each graph. Compartment 1 is the unaffected area (1′ is autoregulated), and compartment 2 is the benign oligemia. Tissue is mildly hypoperfused but not at risk. The initial decrease in regional cerebral blood flow (rCBF) and cerebral perfusion pressure (CPP) causes vascular dilatation. This results in increased cerebral blood volume (CBV) and OEF to maintain a normal $CMRO_2$. rCBF decreases below the cutoff of 10 to 12 mg/100 g/min in tissue compartment 3. The CPP has decreased to such an extent that the increase in OEF cannot maintain the $CMRO_2$. This is the ischemic penumbra. In the infarcted tissue (compartment 4), the $CMRO_2$ is markedly decreased. CBF, CBV, and OEF can vary. The MTT is prolonged in order of increasing severity in compartments 2, 3, and 4. (CPP, cerebral perfusion pressure; CBV, cerebral blood volume; rCBF, regional cerebral blood flow; MTT, mean transit time; OEF, oxygen extraction fraction; $CMRO_2$, cerebral metabolic rate of oxygen). (Lee DH, Kang DW, Ahn JS, et al. Imaging of the ischemic penumbra in acute stroke. *Korean J Radiol* 2005;6(2):64–74, with permission.)

The penumbra, compartment 3, is characterized by inadequate blood supply for the metabolic demands and by increased OEF.[20] There is abnormal decrease in CBF in compartments 2 through 4, being most severe in compartment 4 and least severe in compartment 2. Due to vascular dilatation, CBV increases in compartment 2 but subsequently decreases in 3 and further decreases in 4. OEF increases in compartment 2 and plateaus in 3 and 4. Figure 17.3 shows an example of the penumbra. In the periphery of the brain infarct, characterized by absent perfusion and metabolism, there are regions of viable but hypoperfused cortex consistent with the ischemic penumbra.

Increased OEF in patients with major arterial occlusive disease correlates with a high incidence of stroke.[20–23] Figure 17.4 shows a patient with absent cerebrovascular reserve (CVR) on $^{15}O-H_2O$ PET following acetazolamide, but OEF is still normal. Figure 17.5 shows $^{15}O-H_2O$ PET images of a patient with misery perfusion. CVR is absent, and now, the OEF is elevated.

SPECT can also detect hypoperfusion due to postvasospasm following subarachnoid hemorrhage and can predict severity of future neurologic sequelae.[13]

Hypoxia and Cellular Integrity Imaging

^{18}F-fluoromisonidazole (FMISO) is a PET hypoxia marker that localizes to the penumbra in acute stroke.[24,25] A rat study demonstrated elevated FMISO uptake in the stroke area only in the early phase of arterial occlusion but not after early reperfusion nor when tissue necrosis had developed.[26] ^{18}F FMISO PET may be able to identify true penumbral tissue that would be amenable to rescue interventions even beyond 12 to 24 hours after stroke onset.[25] A recent study found that FMISO uptake correlated not only with the penumbra but also with the core (compartment 4). Intense FMISO uptake was found when perfusion reached the penumbra threshold.[27]

[11C]flumazenil (FMZ), a benzodiazepine receptor ligand and a marker of cortical cellular integrity, can be used early after the onset of symptoms of stroke to differentiate between areas that are salvageable and areas that are already infarcted. In a small study, ^{15}O-water PET was performed immediately prior to and 24 hours after recombinant tissue plasminogen activator treatment, which was given within 3 hours of symptom onset. Eight of eleven patients had areas of critical perfusion using ^{15}O-water, but FMZ correctly identified the four patients who subsequently developed a stroke when imaged with MRI or CT 3 weeks later. The main limitation is that the cortex is the only cerebral tissue that has a sufficient number of benzodiazepine receptors to make this study helpful.[28]

Chronic Ischemia and Acetazolamide Challenge Test

The functional reserve capacity (FRC) in patients with chronic cerebrovascular disease is an important factor in determining the utility of vascular surgery. The normal response to decreased cerebral perfusion is compensatory vasodilatation. In a similar manner to cardiac perfusion scintigraphy, administering a vasodilator may show absent or decreased compensatory dilatation on the side of carotid or cerebral artery disease because the arteries are already maximally dilated. Cerebral perfusion to the affected brain therefore appears decreased in comparison to the contralateral hemisphere. One gram of acetazolamide (ACZ) is injected intravenously over 2 minutes. ACZ penetrates the BBB, inhibits carbonic anhydrase, and causes vasodilatation. The radiopharmaceutical is injected 15 to 20 minutes later at which time the effect of ACZ is at its peak. Imaging is performed up to an hour later.

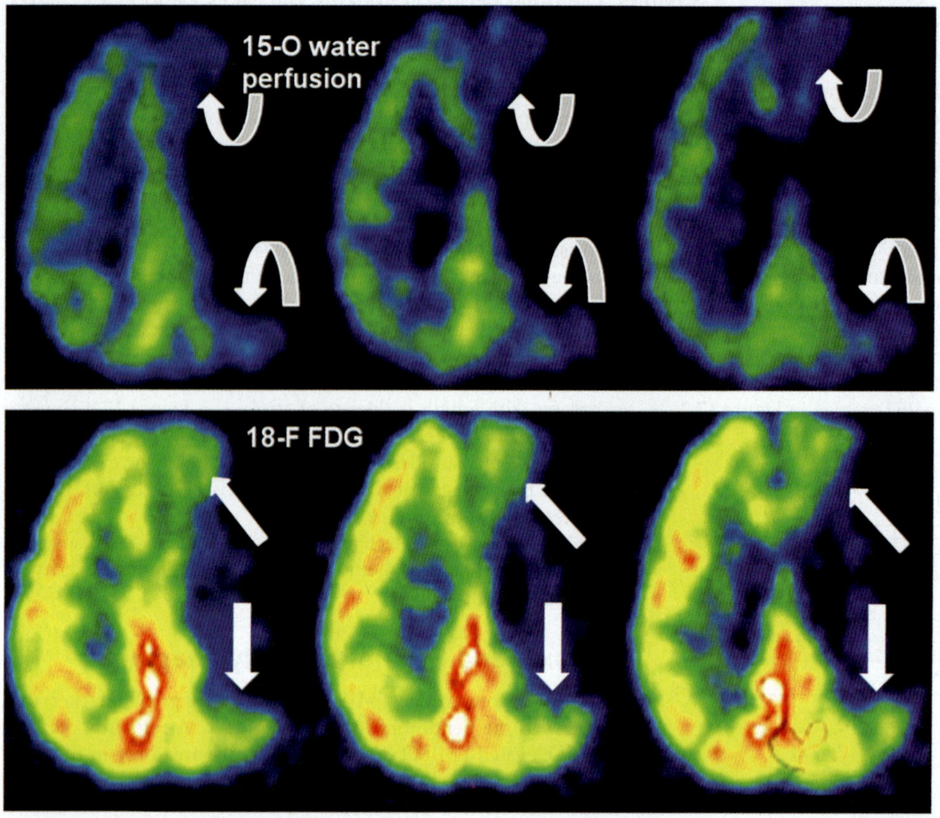

Figure 17-3. ^{15}O water and ^{18}F-FDG in a patient with acute left MCA infarction show areas of diminished perfusion (*curved arrows*) with preserved metabolism (*arrows*) in the left paramedian anterior frontal and posterior parietal lobes representing the penumbra. Regional perfusion is decreased relative to the regional metabolic demand for oxygen. The regional OEF in these areas would be expected to be increased.

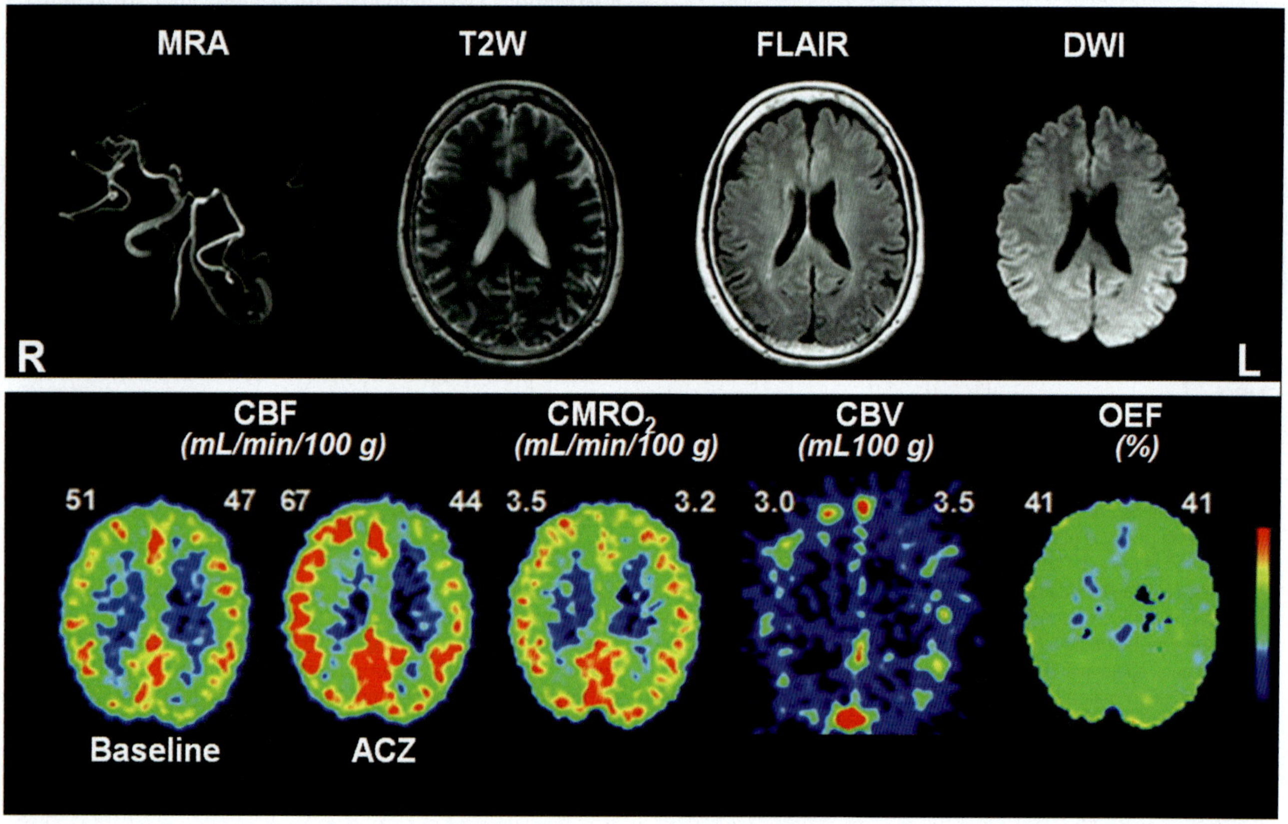

Figure 17-4. A patient with mild stenosis in the left MCA. Cerebral blood flow (CBF) and cerebral metabolic rate of oxygen ($CMRO_2$) did not show a significant decrease in the affected hemisphere, but cerebrovascular reserve (CVR) after acetazolamide (ACZ) administration showed the lack of vascular reactivity. Oxygen extraction fraction (OEF) is not elevated. Numbers are quantitative values for each hemisphere. (MRA, MR angiography.) (From Okazawa H, Kim YK. Cerebrovascular disease and PET (Fig 14.3 in Chapter 14). In: Kim EE, Lee MC, Inoue T, et al, eds. *Clinical PET and PET/CT*. 2nd ed. New York: Springer Science+Business Media 2004, 2013:175–185, with permission.)

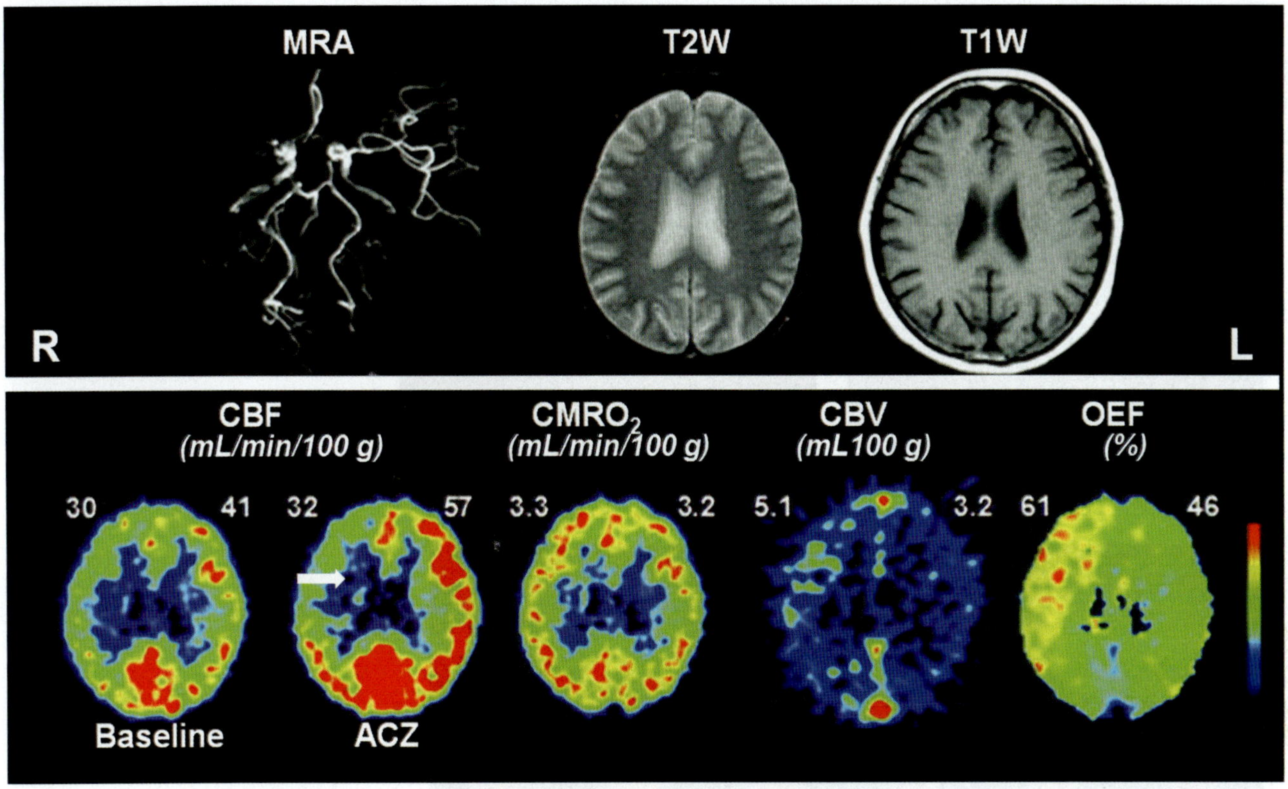

Figure 17-5. **Severe cerebrovascular disease (CVD) with misery perfusion in the right cerebral hemisphere as a result of right middle cerebral artery (MCA) occlusion (see MR angiography [MRA]).** Cerebrovascular reserve (CVR) is absent (*white arrows*) as seen in lack of increase in right frontoparietal perfusion between the baseline and postacetazolamide (ACZ) study. Elevated oxygen extraction fraction (OEF) (despite the increased cerebral blood volume [CBV]) indicates the presence of misery perfusion. Numbers are quantitative values for each hemisphere. (Okazawa H, Kim YK. Cerebrovascular disease and PET (Fig 14.3. in Chapter 14). In: Kim EE, Lee MC, Inoue T, et al, eds. *Clinical PET and PET/CT.* 2nd ed. New York: Springer Science+Business Media 2004, 2013:175–185.)

Patients without cerebrovascular disease will have normal CBF with a 30% to 60% increase after ACZ. A post-ACZ study is shown in Figure 17.6. Lack of compensatory dilatation in the left middle cerebral artery (MCA) territory results in relatively lower perfusion on the left compared to the right. Some patients may have decreased baseline flow and respond to ACZ challenge. Others may have normal baseline flow with no response to ACZ. The patients who benefit most from surgical revascularization are those with decreased CBF with further reduction following ACZ due to a steal phenomenon. The cerebrovascular reserve of the area of stroke, assessed by the ACZ challenge test, is a significant predictor of gross motor outcome in patients with initial cerebral infarction.[29]

If the challenge study is performed first, a normal study will not require the performance of a baseline study. Some have advocated for the performance of the baseline study first so that the challenge test is performed with caution in patients with large perfusion defects at baseline.[30]

Contraindications to acetazolamide include sulfa allergy, stroke within 3 days, or recent cerebral hemorrhage. It may cause headache in patients with history of migraine.[31]

Balloon Occlusion Studies

Preoperative evaluation for potential ischemia following carotid artery sacrifice in patients with tumors or aneurysms may be performed using balloon occlusion studies.

In the absence of balloon occlusion tests (BOT), carotid artery sacrifice had a stroke rate of 30% and mortality rate of 12%.[32] Up to 20% of patients who do not have neurologic symptoms during balloon occlusion testing will suffer postoperative neurologic sequelae.[33,34] SPECT scintigraphy with balloon occlusion is more sensitive than neurologic symptoms to identify patients who will suffer neurologic complications after carotid artery sacrifice. The technique involves balloon occlusion of the internal carotid artery for 30 minutes (less if neurologic symptoms develop) with injection of HMPAO or ECD 5 minutes before balloon deflation. The patient is then transferred to the nuclear medicine department for SPECT imaging. If there is inadequate collateral cerebral circulation, ipsilateral hypoperfusion results. A difference in perfusion, measured by using the counts, between the occluded side and the contralateral side of greater than 10% is considered significant.[35] An example of a BOT is shown in Figure 17.7. The predictive value of good clinical outcome after permanent carotid occlusion in patients with symmetric perfusion during BOT is reported to be between 90% and 100%.

Crossed Cerebellar Diaschisis

Patients who have a cerebral lesion such as neoplasm, stroke, or trauma will display hypoperfusion on SPECT and PET and hypometabolism on FDG PET in the contralateral cerebellum as seen in Figure 17.8. This is what is referred to as crossed cerebellar diaschisis (CCD). The decrease in CBF and metabolism is due to disruption of the corticopontocerebellar pathway causing decreased synaptic activity.[36–38] This is a unique finding on SPECT and PET. The cerebellum appears unremarkable on CT. The main determining factor for the presence of CCD is the location of the lesion and not the severity or size of the lesion.[39]

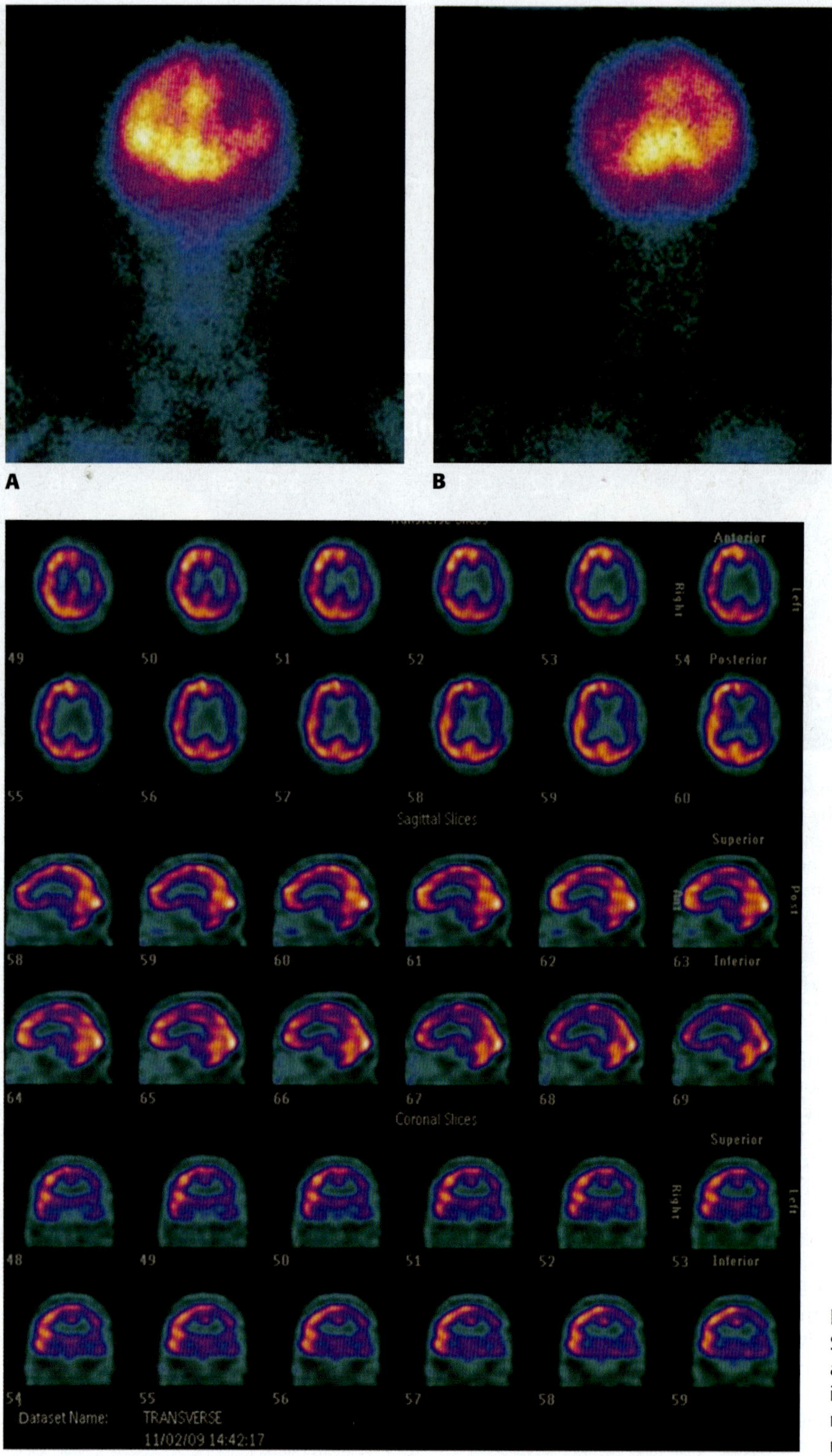

Figure 17-6. Anterior **(A)**, posterior **(B)**, and SPECT **(C)** from a ^{99m}Tc-ECD study with acetazolamide (ACZ) showed 30% less flow in the left MCA territory compared to the right indicating loss of CVR (cerebrovascular reserve). This patient has a high risk of stroke if carotid endarterectomy is not performed.

Traumatic Brain Injury

Of the estimated 1.5 million annual nonfatal brain injuries in the United States, 28% involve motor vehicles, 20% involve sports and physical activity, and 9% are a result of assaults.[40]

CT and MRI have a critical role in imaging TBI to diagnose hemorrhage or focal lesions. SPECT is helpful in patients with normal CT and MRI and persistent neurobehavioral symptoms following trauma. For mild head trauma, SPECT is more sensitive than CT and MRI in detecting TBI.[41,42]

In a prospective study of patients with mild-to-moderate brain injury, SPECT showed parenchymal lesions more often than CT. In addition, 83% of lesions detected by both modalities were larger on SPECT than on CT.[43] A study of 28 patients with mild TBI with normal CT or MRI studies and 20 controls revealed hypoperfusion

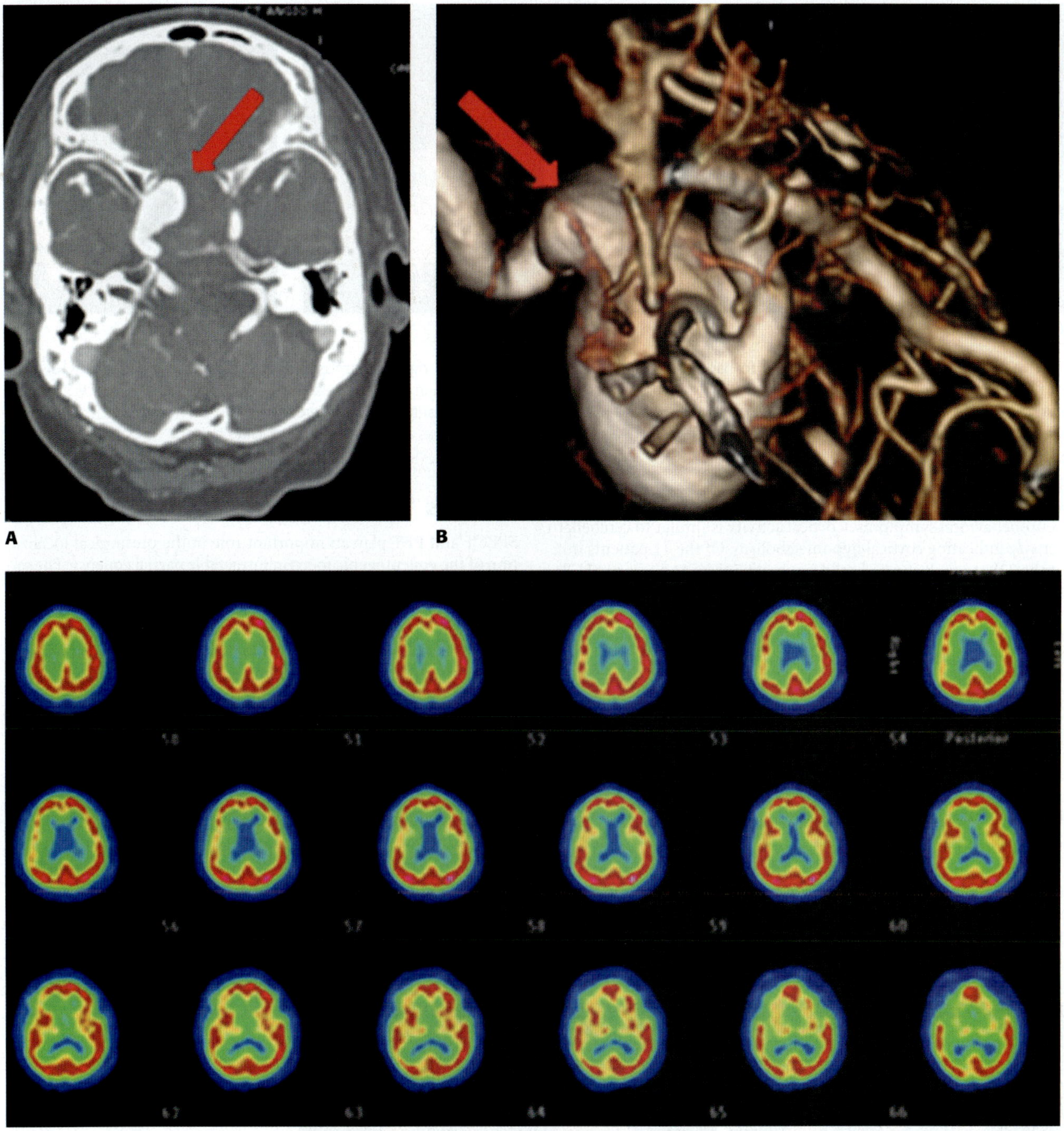

Figure 17-7. Three-centimeter multilobulated supraclinoid/cavernous carotid artery aneurysm is shown on CTA of the circle of Willis **(A)** and 3-D reconstruction **(B)** in a 57-year-old woman (*arrows*). ^{99m}Tc-ECD cerebral perfusion prior to sacrifice of the right internal carotid artery is shown **(C)**. The difference in counts in regions of interest in the right frontal and parietal cortex and the counts in the contralateral cortex were not significant. A difference of 10% is often regarded as significant.

in frontal, left posterior, and subcortical areas in the TBI patients with neuropsychologic symptoms corresponding to the site of hypoperfusion.[44]

In a study of 228 HMPAO SPECT scans in patients with mild-to-moderate TBI, the temporal lobe, frontal lobe, and basal ganglia were the most common sites of abnormal perfusion. Focal, well-circumscribed single or multiple areas of hypoperfusion were the most specific patterns for TBI. Bilateral diffuse cortical hypoperfusion can be seen following trauma but is more typically seen following hypovolemia/hypotension or hypoxic episode. Figure 17.9

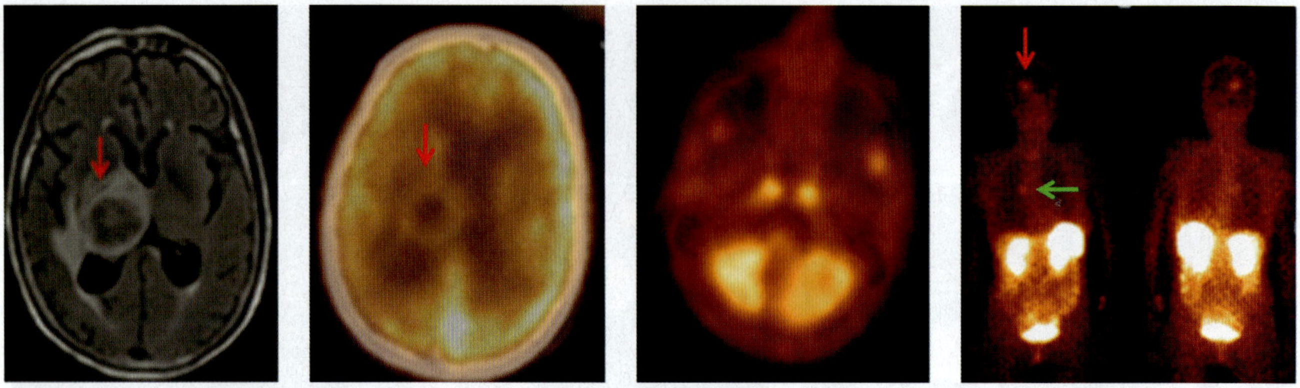

A B C D

Figure 17-8. **A 63-year-old male found to have a cerebral lesion centered on the right thalamus thought to represent metastatic disease or primary brain glioma (*red arrows*).** FDG-PET was ordered to search for a possible primary tumor elsewhere. T2W MRI, PET-CT, and PET images through the brain are shown **(A, B,** and **C)**. Note the diminished FDG PET uptake in the contralateral left cerebellum consistent with crossed cerebellar diaschisis **(C)**. **D:** A right pulmonary hilar mass (*green arrow*) was found on PET, which was a primary neuroendocrine tumor.

shows ^{18}F-FDG PET seen in a professional football player with neurobehavioral symptoms. Cortical activity is similar to cerebellar activity indicating cortical hypometabolism. Of the 41 patients out of the 228 studied who had mild traumatic injury and a normal CT, focal areas of hypoperfusion were present on SPECT in 77% with the most frequent locations in descending order: basal ganglia and thalami, 55.2%; frontal lobes, 23.8%; temporal lobes, 13%; parietal, 3.7%; and insular and occipital lobes together, 4.6%.[45]

In addition, SPECT and PET have a role uncovering the sequelae of trauma on the brain when CT and MRI are normal. The use of activation task studies with PET allows the study of the brain's plasticity and reorganizational capacity following TBI.[46]

CNS Tumors

Hypoxia in brain tumors can be measured by PET using ^{18}F-FMISO). The presence of hypoxia is an indicator of poor tumor response to therapy. Hypoxia cannot be predicted from the CBF as it has been shown that hypoxia is present in both hyperperfused and hypoperfused glioblastomas.[47]

Seizures

SPECT and PET play an important role in the presurgical localization of the epileptogenic focus in intractable partial epilepsy. The seizure focus is characterized by increased perfusion and metabolism during a seizure and decreased perfusion and metabolism between seizures. Epileptic foci in complex partial seizures are frequently in the temporal lobes. Partial temporal lobe resection in these patients results in improvement or resolution of seizures in 70% of cases. Ictal SPECT is superior to the interictal study in lateralizing and localizing the seizure focus.[48] Ictal SPECT has a sensitivity of 73% to 97% and interictal SPECT 50% in temporal lobe epilepsy. The sensitivity of ictal SPECT for extratemporal seizures is 66%.[49] Subtraction SPECT in a study of both temporal and extratemporal epilepsy had a sensitivity of 86% and a specificity of 75% compared to a sensitivity of intracranial EEG of 85% and ictal scalp EEG of 66%.[49]

In a study of 36 patients with temporal lobe seizures, 94% of those with mesial temporal FDG asymmetry of 15% or more became seizure free or much improved following surgery and only 6% did not improve.[48] Although greater asymmetry was seen in the lateral compared to mesial temporal cortex in all patients, asymmetry in

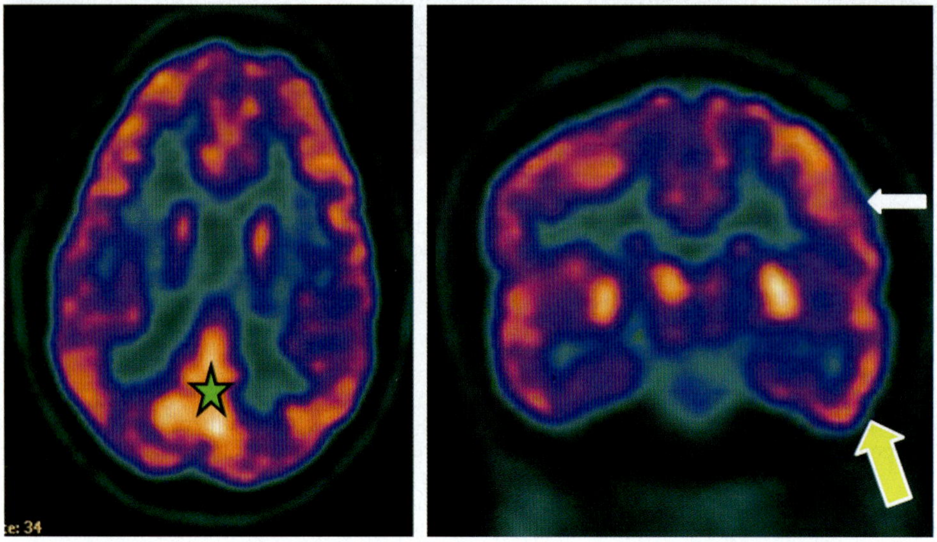

Figure 17-9. **^{18}F-FDG-PET scan in an ex professional football player with neurobehavioral symptoms revealed bilateral cortical hypometabolism.** Note most of the cerebral cortex (*white arrow*), with the exception of the visual cortex (*star*), has similar metabolism to cerebellum (*yellow arrow*) indicating relatively diffuse hypometabolism. A SPECT scan would likely show global hypoperfusion due to the close correlation of perfusion and metabolism.

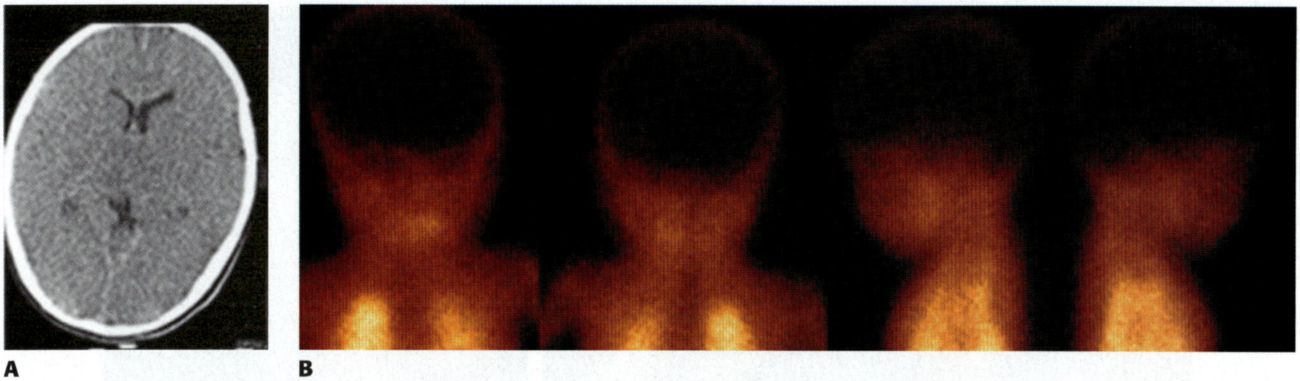

Figure 17-10. A 4-month-old presented to the hospital in pulmonary arrest. Head CT shows diffuse cerebral edema **(A)**. Anterior, posterior, left, and right lateral images **(B)** following the angiographic phase (not shown) from HMPAO cerebral perfusion reveal absence of cerebral perfusion.

the mesial cortex correlated with postsurgical improvement.[40] In a study of pediatric epilepsy, subtraction ictal SPECT (ictal minus interictal) coregistered to MRI (SISCOM) localized the seizure focus in 67% while ^{18}F-FDG FDG in 57%. Taken together, 76% of seizure foci could be localized. SISCOM and ^{18}F-FDG PET concordance with the epileptogenic zone proven by histopathology was significantly higher than MR imaging ($P < 0.05$).[51]

Evaluation of Dementia

Functional changes such as decreased neuronal activity precede anatomic changes such as atrophy. Regional perfusion (and metabolism) correlates with neuronal activity and thus decreased perfusion can detect neuronal dysfunction caused by degenerative dementias.[50] The pattern of cerebral perfusion and metabolism can aid in the diagnosis of dementia.

SPECT and PET can detect Alzheimer dementia prior to the onset of symptoms. Alzheimer disease commonly involves decreased temporal–parietal perfusion, which can be asymmetric early in the disease, with sparing of the basal ganglia, sensorimotor, and visual cortex. The Lewy body dementia pattern of hypoperfusion is similar to Alzheimer disease with sensorimotor cortex involvement and predominance of occipital involvement. Frontotemporal dementia (Pick disease) is characterized by frontal and anterior temporal hypoperfusion.[52] Huntington disease typically involves the caudate and lentiform nuclei. Parkinson disease has a similar pattern to Alzheimer disease with occipital involvement.

Brain Death

Brain death is a clinical diagnosis. Brain death scintigraphy is especially helpful in cases of hypothermia, intoxication with barbiturates, hypovolemic shock, or when EEG recording is not possible due to significant head injury or the clinical exam is inconclusive. Cerebral perfusion scintigraphy provides a rapid and reliable assessment of the presence or absence of brain perfusion in these cases. Prompt determination of brain death is critical in a patient who is a candidate for organ donation.

Dynamic images during the angiographic phase and planar images in the anterior and lateral projections 5 to 10 minutes after flow are preferred. Tissue edema associated with brain death causes increased intracranial pressure. When this pressure reaches or exceeds systemic arterial pressure or mean arterial pressure (diastolic pressure + one-third of pulse pressure), perfusion to the brain ceases. Images reveal blood flow in the common carotid arteries, which terminates at the base of the skull and absence of intracranial flow. Dural sinus activity is rarely seen since the amount of blood in the meningeal vessels is seldom enough to make the dural sinus activity visible. Pediatric and adult HMPAO studies confirming brain death are shown in Figures 17.10 and 17.11. HMPAO brain perfusion study in another patient with subdural hematoma and suspected brain death (Fig. 17.12) demonstrates cerebral perfusion. Photopenia is seen in the region of the right subdural hematoma. Thanks to Patrick Colletti, M.D. for his valuable guidance.

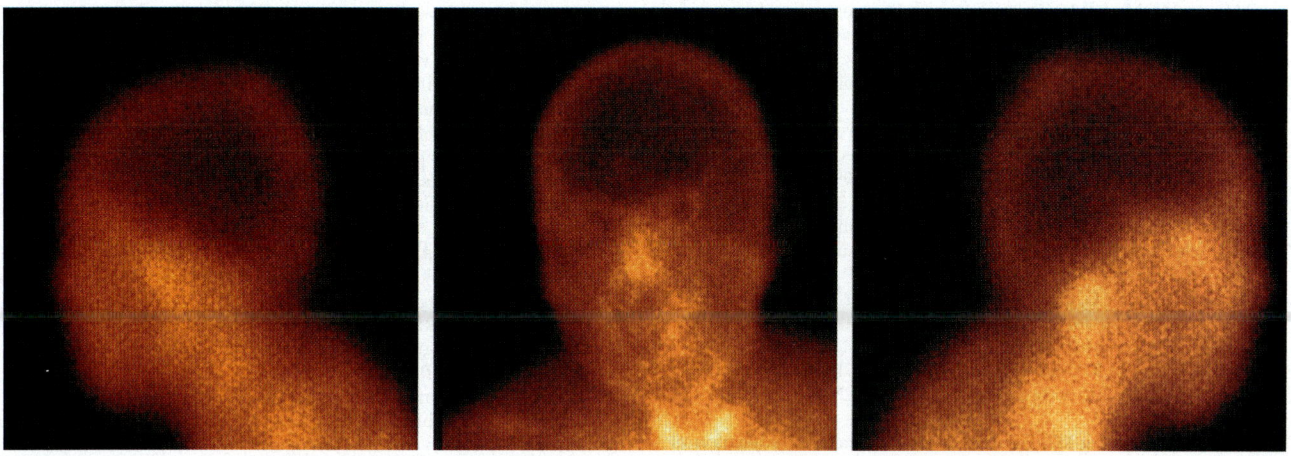

Figure 17-11. ^{99m}**Tc-HMPAO planar images reveal absent cerebral activity.**

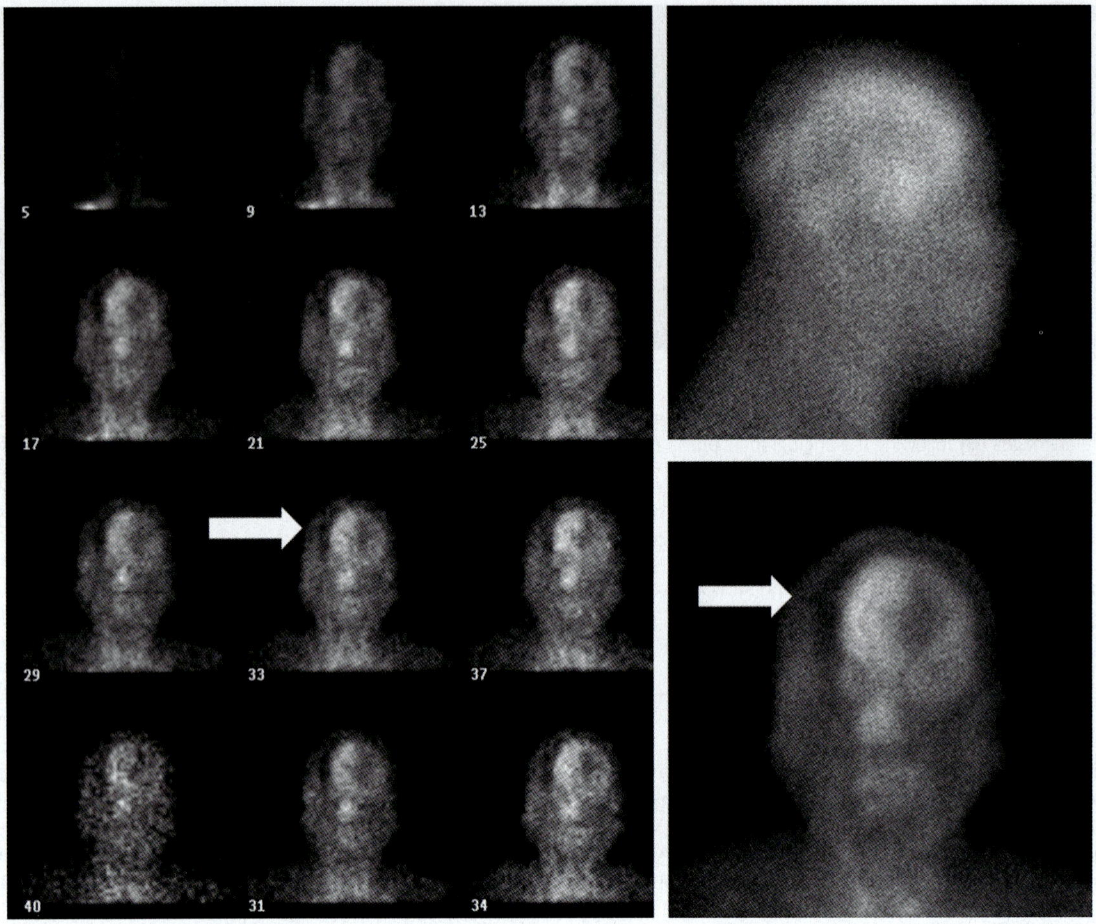

Figure 17-12. **HMPAO brain perfusion and anterior and right lateral planar images of a patient with subdural hematoma and suspected brain death reveal the presence of cerebral perfusion.** Photopenia is seen in the region of the right subdural hematoma (*arrow*).

REFERENCES

1. **Alexandrov AV, Ehrlich LE, Bladin CF, et al.** Simple visual analysis of brain perfusion on HMPAO SPECT predicts early outcome in acute stroke. *Stroke* 1996;27:1537–1542.
2. **Ueda T, Sakaki S, Kumon Y, et al.** Multivariable analysis of predictive factors related to outcome at 6 months after intra-arterial thrombolysis for acute ischemic stroke. *Stroke* 1999;30:2360–2365.
3. **Mountz JM, Modell JG, Foster NL, et al.** Prognostication of recovery following stroke using the comparison of CT and technetium-99m HMPAO SPECT. *J Nucl Med* 1990;31:61–66.
4. **Schaller B.** State-of-the-art imaging in stroke. Vol. 1. Hauppauge, NY: Nova; 2007.
5. **Kapuco OL, Nobili F, Varrone A, et al.** EANM procedure guideline for brain perfusion SPECT using 99mTc-labelled radiopharmaceuticals, version 2. *Eur J Nucl Med Mol Imaging* 2009;36:2093–2102. doi: 10.1007/s00259-009-1266-y.
6. **Ichise M, Golan H, Ballinger R, et al.** Regional differences in Tc-99m ECD clearance on brain SPECT in healthy subjects. *J Nucl Med* 1997;38(8):1253–1260.
7. **Moretti JL, Defer G, Cinotti L, et al.** "Luxury perfusion" with 99mTc-HMPAO and 123I-IMP SPECT imaging during the subacute phase of stroke. *Eur J Nucl Med* 1990;16(1):17–22.
8. **Ishii K, Hanoaka K, Okada Mi, et al.** Impact of CT attenuation correction by SPECT/CT in brain perfusion images. *Ann Nucl Med* 2012;26(3): 241–247.
9. **Patlak CS, Blasberg RG, Fenstermacher JD.** Graphical evaluation of blood-to-brain transfer constants from multiple-time uptake data. *J Cereb Blood Flow Metab* 1983;3(1):1–7.
10. **Matsuda H, Tsuji S, Shuke N, et al.** Noninvasive measurements of regional cerebral blood flow using technetium-technetium-99m hexamethylpropylene amine oxime. *Eur J Nucl Med* 1993;20:391–401.
11. **Ohnishi T, Yano T, Nakano S, et al.** The quantitative regional cerebral blood flow measurement with autoradiography method using 123I-IMP SPECT: evaluation of arterialized venous blood sampling as a substitute for arterial blood sampling. *Eur J Nucl Med* 1996;33:1105–1109.
12. **Ito H, Akaizawa T, Goto R, et al.** A simple method for measurement of cerebral blood flow using 123I-IMP SPECT with calibrated standard input function by one point blood sampling: validation of calibration by one point venous blood sampling as a substitute. *Kaku Igaku* 1994;31(9):1071–1076.
13. **Powsner RA, O'Tuama LA, Jabre A, et al.** SPECT imaging in cerebral vasospasm following subarachnoid hemorrhage. *J Nucl Med* 1998;39(5):765–769.
14. **Wintermark M, Sesay M, Barbier E.** Comments, opinions, and reviews: comparative overview of brain perfusion imaging techniques. *Stroke* 2005;36:e83–e99.
15. **Loessner A, Alavi A, Lewandrowski KU, et al.** Regional cerebral function determined by FDG-PET in healthy volunteers: normal patterns and changes with age. *J Nucl Med* 1995;36(7):1141–1149.
16. **Fung EK, Carson RE.** Cerebral blood flow with [15O] water PET studies using an image-derived input function and MR-defined carotid centerlines. *Phys Med Biol* 2013;58(6):1903.
17. **Frackowiak R, Lenzi GL, Jones T, et al.** Quantitative measurement of regional cerebral blood flow and oxygen metabolism in man using 15 O) and positron emission tomography: theory, procedure, and normal values. *J Comput Assist Tomogr* 1980;4(6):727–736.
18. **Lin EC, Alavi A.** PET and PET/CT: a clinical guide. New York: Thieme; 2011.

19. **Lee DH, Kang DW, Ahn JS, et al.** Imaging of the ischemic penumbra in acute stroke. *Korean J Radiol* 2005;6(2):64–74.
20. **Gupta A, Baradaran H, Schweitzer AD, et al.** Oxygen Extraction Fraction and Stroke Risk in Patients with Carotid Stenosis or Occlusion: A Systematic Review and Meta-Analysis. *AJNR* 2014;35:250–255.
21. **Yamauchi H, Fukuyama H, Nagahama Y, et al.** Evidence of misery perfusion and risk for recurrent stroke in major cerebral arterial occlusive diseases from PET. *J Neurol Neurosurg Psychiatry* 1996;61:18–25.
22. **Grubb Jr RL, Derdeyn CP, Fritsch SM, et al.** Importance of hemodynamic factors in the prognosis of symptomatic carotid occlusion. *JAMA* 1998;280(12):1055–1060.
23. **Yamauchi H, Higashi T, Kagawa S, et al.** Is misery perfusion still a predictor of stroke in symptomatic major cerebral artery disease? *Brain* 2012;135:2515–2526.
24. **Markus R, Donnan G, Kazui S, et al.** Penumbral topography in human stroke: methodology and validation of the "Penumbragram." *Neuroimage* 2004;21:1252–1259.
25. **Markus R, Reutens DC, Kazui S, et al.** Hypoxic tissue in ischaemic stroke: persistence and clinical consequences of spontaneous survival. *Brain* 2004;127:1427–1436.
26. **Takasawa M, Beech JS, Fryer TD, et al.** Imaging of brain hypoxia in permanent and temporary middle cerebral artery occlusion in the rat using (18)F-fluoromisonidazole and positron emission tomography: a pilot study. *J Cereb Blood Flow Metab* 2007;23:679–689.
27. **Alawneh JA, Moustafa RR, Marrapu ST, et al.** Diffusion and perfusion correlates of the 18F-MISO PET lesion in acute stroke: pilot study. *Eur J Nucl Med Mol Imaging* 2014;41(4):736–744.
28. **Wolf-Dieter H, Lutz K, Martin G, et al.** Early [11C] Flumazenil/H2O positron emission tomography predicts irreversible ischemic cortical damage in stroke patients receiving acute thrombolytic therapy. *Stroke* 2002;31(2):366–369.
29. **Park SA, Park HI, Kim D, et al.** The prediction of gross motor outcome using cerebrovascular reserve measured by acetazolamide-challenged SPECT. *NeuroRehabilitation* 2012;30:359–367.
30. **Saremi F, Jadvar H, Siegel ME.** Pharmacologic interventions in nuclear radiology: indications, imaging protocols, and clinical results. *Radiographics* 2002;(22):477–490.
31. **Kapucu OL, Nobili F, Varrone A, et al.** EANM procedure guideline for brain perfusion SPECT using 99mTc-labelled radiopharmaceuticals, version 2. *Eur J Nucl Med Mol Imaging* 2009;36:2093–2102. doi: 10.1007/s00259-009-1266-y.
32. **Linskey ME, Jungreis CA, Yonas H, et al.** Stroke risk after abrupt internal carotid artery sacrifice: accuracy of preoperative assessment with balloon test occlusion and stable xenon-enhanced CT. *AJNR Am J Neuroradiol* 1994;15(5):829–843.
33. **De Vries EJ, Sekhar LN, Horton JA, et al.** A new method to predict safe resection of the internal carotid artery. *Laryngoscope* 1990;100: 85–88.
34. **Hays RJ, Levinson SA, Wylie EJ.** Intraoperative measurement of carotid artery back pressure as a guide to operative management of carotid endarterectomy. *Surgery* 1972;72:953–960.
35. **Sugawara Y, Kikuchi T, Ueda T, et al.** Usefulness of brain SPECT to evaluate brain tolerance and hemodynamic changes during temporary balloon occlusion test and after permanent carotid occlusion. *J Nucl Med* 2002;43(12):1616–1623.
36. **Mettler F, Guiberteau M.** Essentials of nuclear medicine imaging. 6th ed. Philadelphia, PA: Elsevier; 2012.
37. **Baron JC, Bousser MG, Comar D, et al.** "Crossed cerebellar diaschisis": a remote functional suppression secondary to supratentorial infarction in man. *J Cereb Blood Flow Metab* 1981;1:s500.
38. **Pantano P, Baron JC, Samson Y, et al.** Crossed cerebellar diaschisis: further studies. *Brain* 1986;109:677–694.
39. **Komaba Y, Mishina M, Utsumi K, et al.** Crossed cerebellar diaschisis in patients with cortical infarction. Logistic regression analysis to control for confounding effects. *Stroke* 2004;35:472–476.
40. **Sosin DM, Sniezek JE, Thurman DJ.** Incidence of mild and moderate brain injury in the United States, 1991. *Brain Inj* 1996;10:47–54.
41. **Masdeu JC, Van Heertum RL, Kleiman A, et al.** Early single-photon emission computed tomography in mild head trauma. A controlled study. *J Neuroimaging* 1994;4(4):177–181.
42. **Warwick J.** Brain imaging with SPECT and PET. Continuing Medical Education. 2013;31(8):307–309. Retrieved from: http://www.cmej.org.za/index.php/cmej/article/view/2805/3140
43. **Nedd K, Sfakianakis G, Ganz W, et al.** ^{99m}Tc-HMPAO SPECT of the brain in mild to moderate traumatic brain injury patients: compared with CT—a prospective study. *Brain Inj* 1993;7(6):469–479.
44. **Bonne O, Gilboa A, Louzoun Y, et al.** Cerebral blood flow in chronic symptomatic mild traumatic brain injury. *Psychiatry Res* 2003;124(3):141–152.
45. **Abdel-Dayem H, Abu-Judeh H, Kumar M, et al.** SPECT brain perfusion abnormalities in mild or moderate traumatic brain injury. *Clin Nucl Med* 1998;23(5):309–317.
46. **Van Heertum R.** Traumatic brain injury: SPECT and PET. In: Functional cerebral SPECT and PET imaging. 4th ed. Philadelphia: Lippincott Williams & Wilkins; 2013.
47. **Bruehlmeier M, Roelcke U, Schubiger P, et al.** Assessment of hypoxia and perfusion in human brain tumors using PET with ^{18}F-Fluoromisonidazole and ^{15}O-H_2O. *J Nucl Med* 2004;45(11):1851–1859.
48. **Delbeke D, Lawrence, S, Abou-Khalil B, et al.** Postsurgical outcome of patients with uncontrolled complex partial seizures and temporal lobe hypometabolism on ^{18}FDG-positron emission tomography. *Invest Radiol* 1996;31(5):261–266.
49. **Spanaki MV, Spencer SS, Corsi M, et al.** Localization sensitivity and specificity of quantitative difference SPECT analysis in seizure. *J Nucl Med* 1999;40:730–736.
50. **la Fougère C, Rominger A, Förster S, et al.** PET and SPECT in epilepsy: a critical review. *Epilepsy Behav* 2009;15(1):50–55.
51. **Perissinotti A, Setoain X, Aparicio J, et al.** Clinical role of subtraction ictal SPECT coregistered to MR imaging and 18F-FDG PET in pediatric epilepsy. *J Nucl Med* 2014;55(7):1099–1105.
52. **Farid K MD, Caillat-Vigneron N, Sibon I.** Is brain SPECT useful in degenerative dementia. diagnosis. *J Comput Assist Tomogr* 2011;35:1–3.

CHAPTER 18

Perfusion Imaging in Maxillofacial Lesions

Hidenobu Matsuzaki, DDS, Yoshinobu Yanagi, DDS, Teruhisa Unetsubo, DDS, and Jun-ichi Asaumi, DDS

Introduction

The structures of the oral and maxillofacial regions are critical to functions such as facial expression, speech, chewing, and swallowing. These structures are highly complex, in very close proximity to each other, and are formed from soft and/or hard tissues. They include the oral cavity, tongue, jawbones, nasal cavity, paranasal sinuses, salivary glands, temporomandibular joints, facial muscles, and skin. Various conditions such as trauma, infections, cysts, tumors, and inflammatory processes affect this restricted area. These diseases can cause severe maxillofacial dysfunction and cosmetic disturbance. In most of these conditions, early detection and accurate diagnosis are vital in preventing and reducing functional and cosmetic problems.

For imaging diagnosis of oral and maxillofacial lesions, magnetic resonance imaging (MRI) is the preferred modality for analyzing the internal structure of the lesions and evaluating their extent. Given the diversity of pathologies in different tissues and organs of the oral and maxillofacial regions, characterization of these lesions with routine MRI based on the morphologic features and signal intensity (SI) differences can be very difficult. It is reported by several articles that dynamic contrast-enhanced magnetic resonance imaging (DCE-MRI) can improve diagnosis of benign and malignant lesions in oral and maxillofacial regions by providing hemodynamic information, including regional blood volume, flow, and vascular permeability.[1–15]

In this chapter, we review the clinical application of DCE-MRI in evaluating oral and maxillofacial lesions, with particular focus on benign and malignant neoplasms.

DCE-MRI for Oral and Maxillofacial Lesions

Extracellular gadolinium-DTPA contrast agents (at a dose of 0.1 to 0.2 mmol/kg body weight) are widely used in contrast-enhanced MRI, including DCE-MRI. Contrast agents delivered by intravenous injection distribute throughout the blood flow into the extravascular intercellular space by leaking between vascular endothelial cells. In tumoral lesions, blood flow is commonly increased by tumor angiogenesis/vasculogenesis, and contrast agent distribution into these lesions is enhanced further by the increased vascular permeability of these new blood vessels.[16] In MRI, contrast enhancement varies between tumors according to differences in their respective blood flow and vascular permeability.[17]

In DCE-MRI using contrast agents, the SIs of regions of interest (ROIs) within the lesions are measured over time on serial images after bolus injection of the contrast agent(s). These data can be used to produce a time–intensity curve (TIC) (or a contrast index curve), which holds information about tumor perfusion including regional blood volume, flow, and vascular permeability. The semiquantitative parameters, such as the gradient of the upslope of enhancement curves, the maximum enhancement, and the washout gradient indices, are not reliably reproducible and depend heavily on the SIs, which in turn are susceptible to scanning conditions such type of MRI equipment and the pulse sequences used.[17]

Recently, along with widespread use of high field magnets and the development of faster imaging sequences, it has become possible to perform DCE-MRI of tissues faster with better signal-to-noise ratio. The improved temporal resolution allows data analysis using pharmacokinetic modeling, which provides a quantitative approach to analyzing the distribution of contrast agents in relation to the vascularity of lesions.[18] Though this data analysis technique is complex, it is possible to acquire quantitative values associated with the hemodynamics of a tumor. Recently, DCE-MRI with post hoc pharmacokinetic modeling has been used clinically to determine the therapeutic effect of various cancer treatments including chemotherapy, antiangiogenic therapy, and radiotherapy.[19–21] However, there are only a few reports on its application in characterizing oral and maxillofacial lesions. In this chapter, we describe a traditional method of DCE-MRI that can be used for this type of characterization.

Choice of Pulse Sequence and DCE-MRI Protocol

The most commonly used pulse sequences for DCE-MRI in oral and maxillofacial lesions are fast spin-echo and gradient-echo sequences, both of which have merits and limitations. The optimal sequence for DCE-MRI is not well defined and varies depending on the MR machine and research protocols. At our institution, we use a

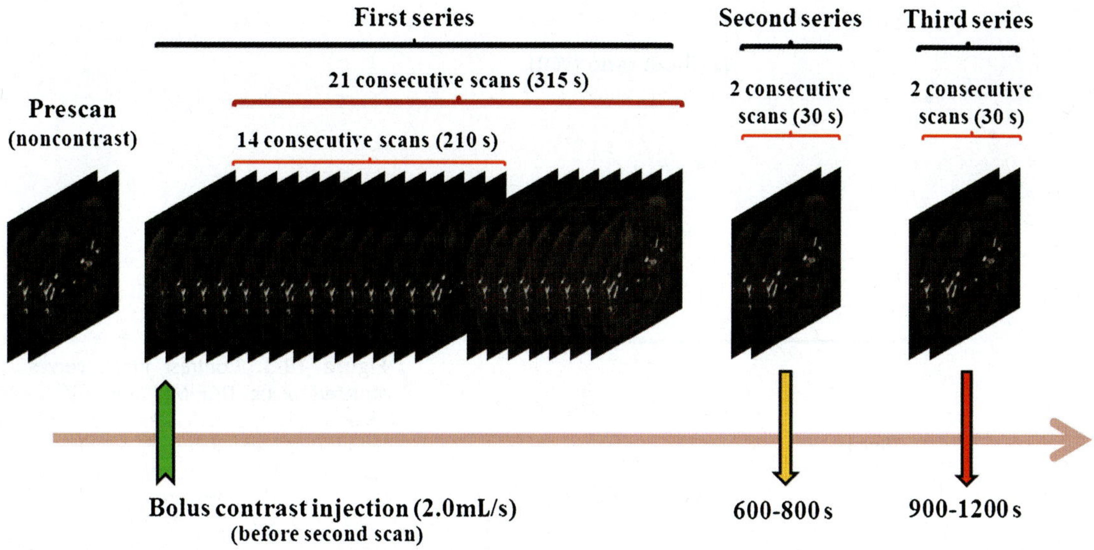

Figure 18-1. Representative schematic of a DCE-MRI protocol.

three-dimensional fast imaging sequence for DCE-MRI (Fig. 18.1). Two consecutive scans are performed initially as a prescan to check if the target lesion is within the imaging range and to confirm whether metal artifacts (e.g., dental metals) influence the resultant images. After this calibration, the first image series is captured, comprising 14 or 21 consecutive scans covering a total scan period of 210 or 315 seconds. Before the second scan of the first series, the contrast agent (0.2 mL/kg) is administered intravenously for 6 seconds at approximately 2.0 mL/s. The second and third image series of DCE-MRI are then acquired at approximately 600 to 800 seconds and 900 to 1,200 seconds, respectively, after bolus injection of contrast agent. These second and third series each comprise two consecutive DCE-MRI scans performed over a total scan time of 30 seconds.

Analysis of DCE-MRI

Region-of-Interest Setting

The ROIs for breast cancers are generally placed in the area showing maximum enhancement within the tumor portion and in the normal breast glands. However, no consensus has been reached on equivalent specific ROIs for oral and maxillofacial lesions. Therefore, observers place the ROIs subjectively in a discrete part of the lesion (e.g., the margins) or the entire lesion. However, large necrotic and/or inner fluid-filled areas that have no perfusion or vessels should not be included in the measurements (Fig. 18.2).

Creating TIC and Contrast Index Curve

The TIC is created by plotting the mean SI of the ROI against time. An analysis using a TIC is a simple clinical method for observing the time course of image enhancement within a lesion but is not suitable for comparing plurality of lesions with different baseline SIs. For comparing plurality of lesions, many investigators use calculated values, such as the contrast index (CI), enhancement ratio, and enhancement index, to observe the increase or decrease in SI within the lesion per unit of time after the bolus injection of contrast agent.[5,8,13] The CI is calculated using the formula

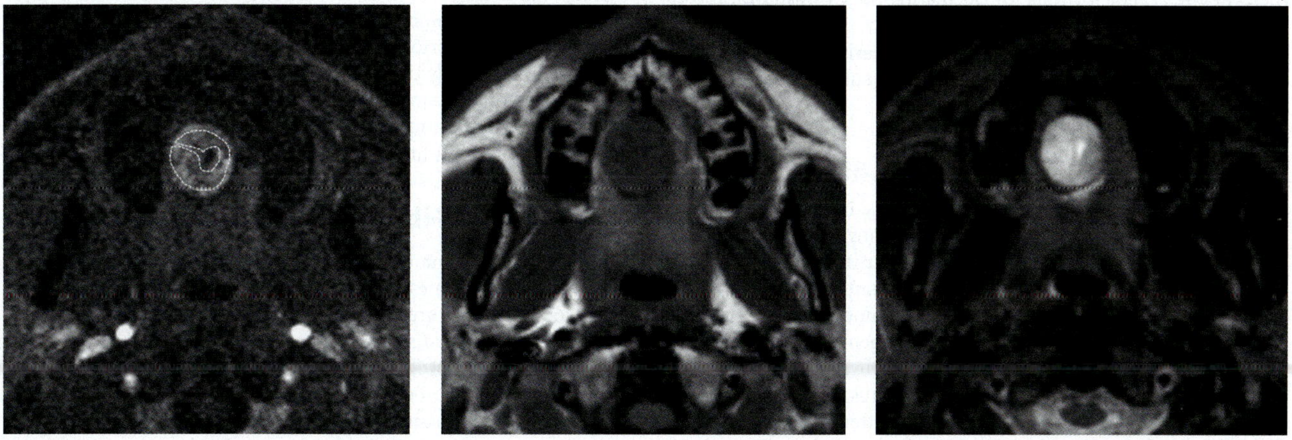

A B C

Figure 18-2. Example of ROI setting for a pleomorphic adenoma of the hard palate in a 29-year-old man. **A:** The region of interest (*dashed line*), which avoids the cystic parts of the tumor, is indicated on a transverse dynamic image. **B, C:** The corresponding T1W **(B)** and STIR T2W images **(C)**.

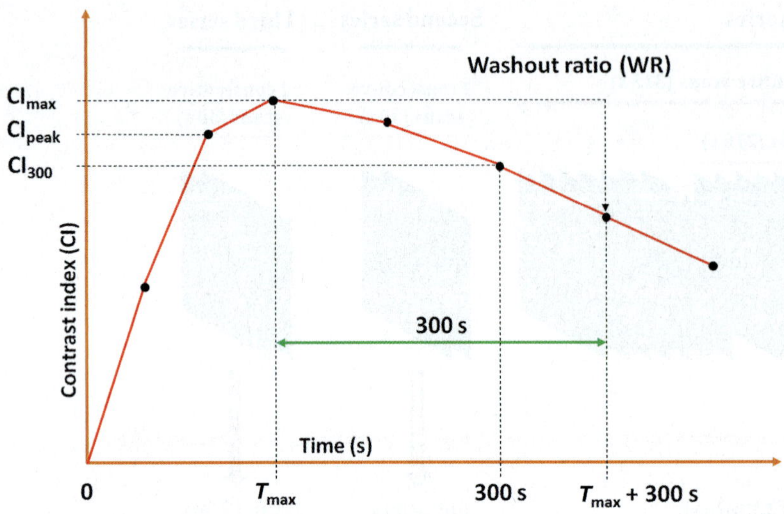

Figure 18-3. Contrast index curves (CICs) constructed using DCE-MRI and CIC parameters. To measure contrast index, signal intensity (SI) of the lesion before (pre-) and after (post-) contrast should be measured. $CI = (SI_{post} - SI_{pre})/SI_{pre}$, $CI_{peak} = CI_{max} \times 0.9$, and WR (in %) at 300 seconds $= (CI_{max} - CI_{wash})/CI_{max} \times 100$.

$$CI = \frac{(SI_{post} - SI_{pre})}{SI_{pre}},$$

where SI_{pre} and SI_{post} are the SIs within the ROI before and after the injection of contrast agent, respectively.

Analysis of DCE-MRI Parameters

In the analysis of TICs and CI curves (CICs), many investigators use simple quantification parameters. These include maximum SI or CI (SI_{max} or CI_{max}, at the maximum level of contrast enhancement), the time to maximum SI or CI (T_{max}, the time to reach SI_{max} or CI_{max}), the peak enhancement (SI_{peak} or CI_{peak}, defined as $SI_{max} \times 0.9$ or $CI_{max} \times 0.9$), the time to peak enhancement (T_{peak}, or the time to reach SI_{peak} or CI_{peak}), and the washout ratio (WR, or the ratio of SI or CI at an arbitrary time after T_{max}). The WR, expressed as a percentage, is defined as follows:

$$WR = \frac{SI_{max} - SI_{wash}}{SI_{max}} \times 100(\%),$$

where SI_{max} is the maximum value of SI, and SI_{wash} is the value of SI in the same ROI at an arbitrary time after SI_{max} is reached (i.e., after T_{max}). The formula for calculating the CI washout ratio is identical but instead uses "CI_{max}" and "CI_{wash}."

The TIC and CIC parameters are summarized in Figure 18.3. These parameters are commonly used for the subjective assessment of the patterns of TICs and CICs.

Application for Jawbone Lesions

The jawbones, which include the tooth germs, have several aspects that set them apart from other long bones. Many pathologic lesions, both odontogenic and nonodontogenic, occur in the jawbones and can be classified as: odontogenic cysts, nonodontogenic cysts, odontogenic tumors, and bone-related lesions (nonodontogenic tumors, giant cell lesions, and pseudocysts). Odontogenic tumors are neoplasms derived from the epithelial, ectomesenchymal, and/or mesenchymal elements of the tooth-forming apparatus.[22] The embryologic diversity of jawbone tumors influences the patterns (parameters) of their TIC/CIC.[15] We classified odontogenic tumors into five groups (types A–E) according to their DCE-MRI parameters (Fig. 18.4).[15] Furthermore, it became clear that a pseudocyst (simple bone cyst) also has characteristic and interesting enhancement patterns.[12]

Benign Odontogenic Tumors

Ameloblastoma

Ameloblastoma derived from odontogenic epithelium with mature and fibrous stroma but without odontogenic ectomesenchyme is one of the most common odontogenic tumors.[22] Ameloblastoma is categorized into four histologic types: solid/multicystic, extraosseous/peripheral, desmoplastic, and unicystic.[22] Our investigation found no characteristic relationship between the CIC patterns, the histopathologic type, and the lesion location (maxilla vs. mandible).[15] Nevertheless, although only few cases studied, two-thirds of CICs for ameloblastomas exhibited a relatively rapid increase ($T_{peak} < 200$ seconds) (Fig. 18.5), making them type A or type B according to the CIC pattern classification presented in Figure 18.4.

Odontogenic Myxoma

Odontogenic myxoma (odontogenic fibromyxoma) is a rare odontogenic tumor categorized as a neoplasm composed of mesenchyme and/or odontogenic ectomesenchyme with or without odontogenic epithelium.[22] Odontogenic myxoma contains stellate and spindle-shaped cells embedded in an abundant myxoid or mucoid extracellular matrix. The CICs of odontogenic myxomas have a unique pattern (type E), which shows a gradual weak increase and without washout for long periods (>600 seconds) (Fig. 18.6).[4,15] This minimal washout is likely due to histopathologic features of the odontogenic myxoma, namely that it contains connective tissue with scattered epithelia, and has abundant myxoid or mucoid extracellular matrix without lining epithelial cells.

Odontogenic Fibroma

Odontogenic fibroma is a rare nonepithelial benign tumor arising from odontogenic mesenchymal tissue in the jawbone.[22] Its histopathologic features are similar to odontogenic myxoma in that it contains connective tissue with scattered epithelia. Therefore, the CIC pattern of odontogenic fibromas also show absence of washout over long periods (>600 seconds) (Fig. 18.7).[23] However, the CIC for odontogenic fibroma is a type D, differing from that of odontogenic myxoma (type E) in the degree of enhancement, which is larger in the odontogenic fibroma.[15] These differences depend on the presence or absence of extracellular matrix consisting of myxoid or mucoid components within the lesion.

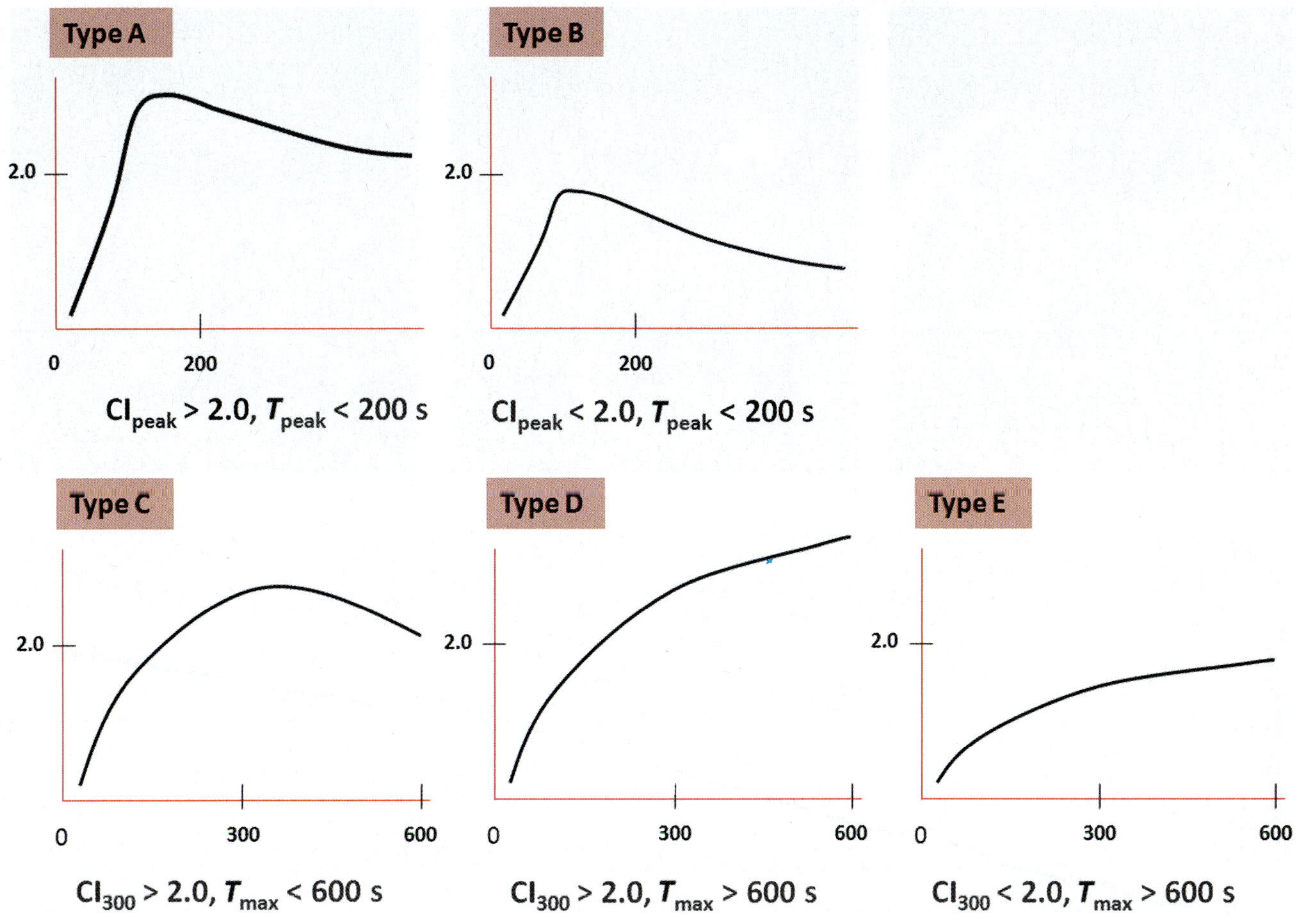

Figure 18-4. Classification of CIC patterns of odontogenic tumors. The CICs were classified into five patterns (types A–E). Type A: early peak and strong enhancement ($CI_{peak} > 2.0$ and $T_{peak} < 200$ seconds); type B: early peak and weak enhancement ($CI_{peak} < 2.0$ and $T_{peak} < 200$ seconds); type C: gradual strong enhancement with washout ($CI_{300} > 2.0$ and $T_{max} < 600$ seconds); type D: gradual strong enhancement without washout ($CI_{300} > 2.0$ and $T_{max} > 600$ seconds); and type E: gradual weak enhancement without washout ($CI_{300} < 2.0$ and $T_{max} > 600$ seconds).

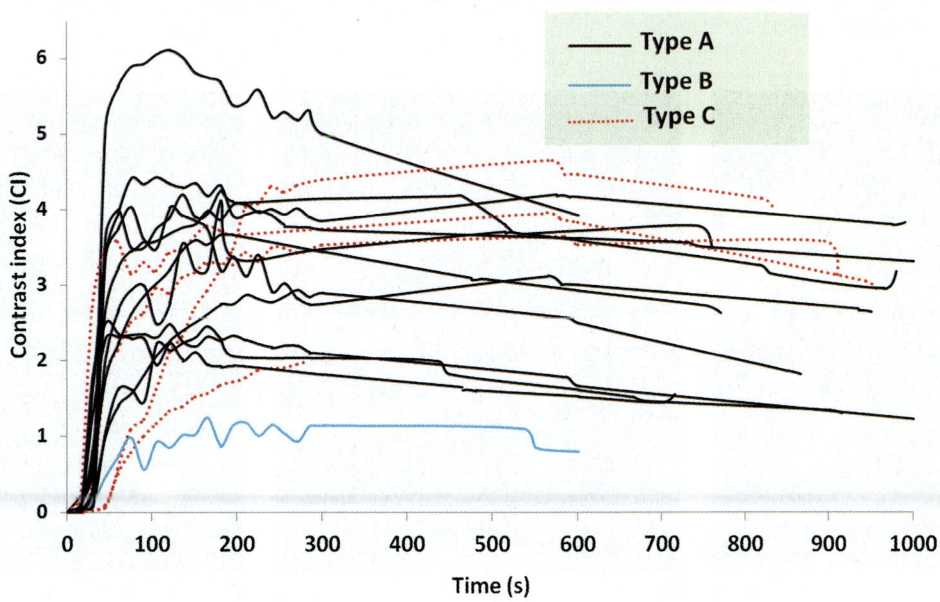

Figure 18-5. CIC patterns of 16 ameloblastomas (4 maxillary, 12 mandibular). Two-thirds of CICs show relatively rapid increase (11 type A and 1 type B, with remaining 4 cases being type C).

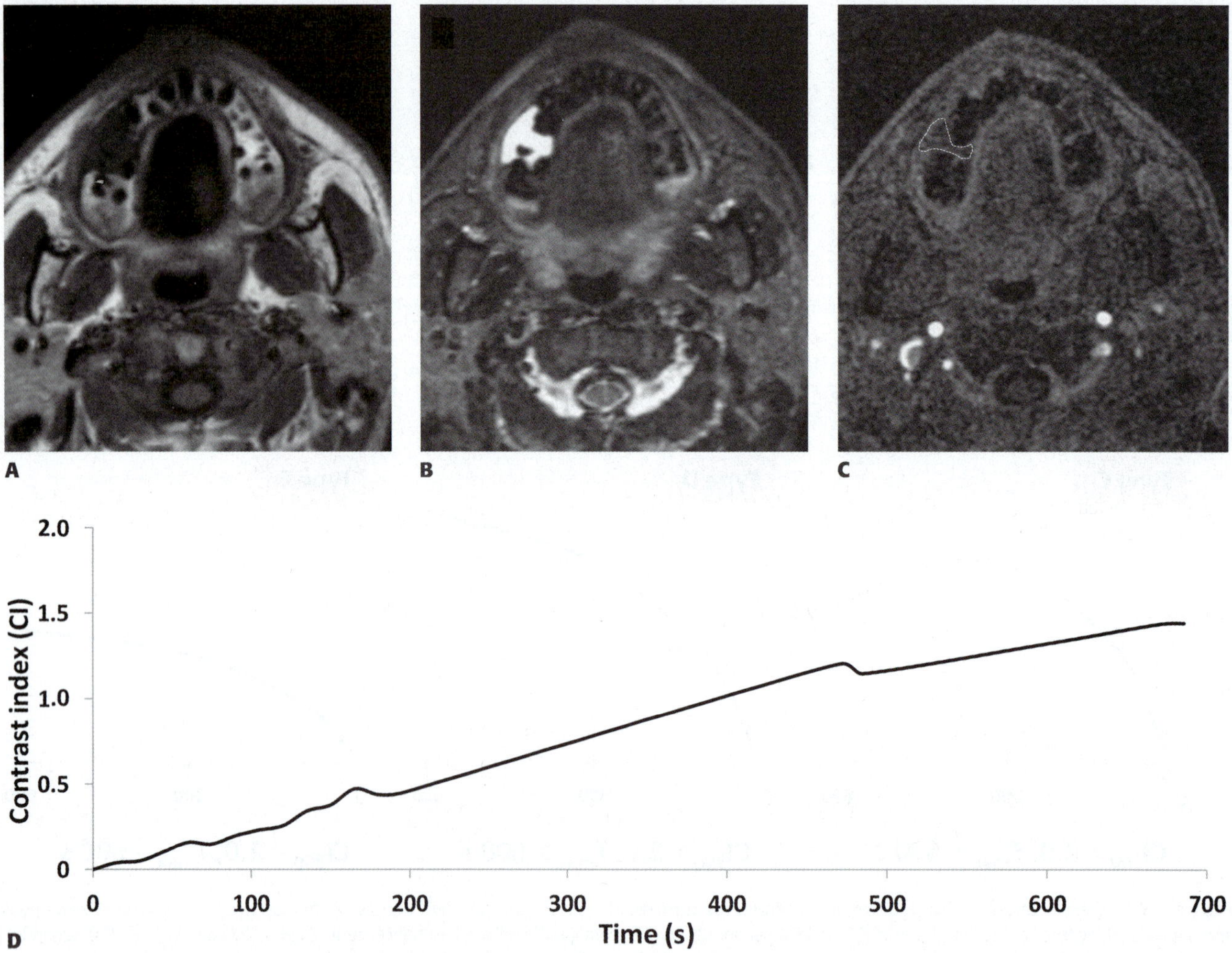

Figure 18-6. Odontogenic myxoma in the maxilla of a 23-year-old man. **A, B:** A mass in the right maxilla displays heterogeneous hypo-/isointensity on T1W image **(A)** and homogeneous hyperintensity on STIR T2W image **(B)**. **C:** The region of interest (*dashed line*) is indicated on a dynamic image. **D:** The unique pattern of CIC of an odontogenic myxoma, in which values increase gradually until approximately 700 seconds without washout of the contrast agent (type E).

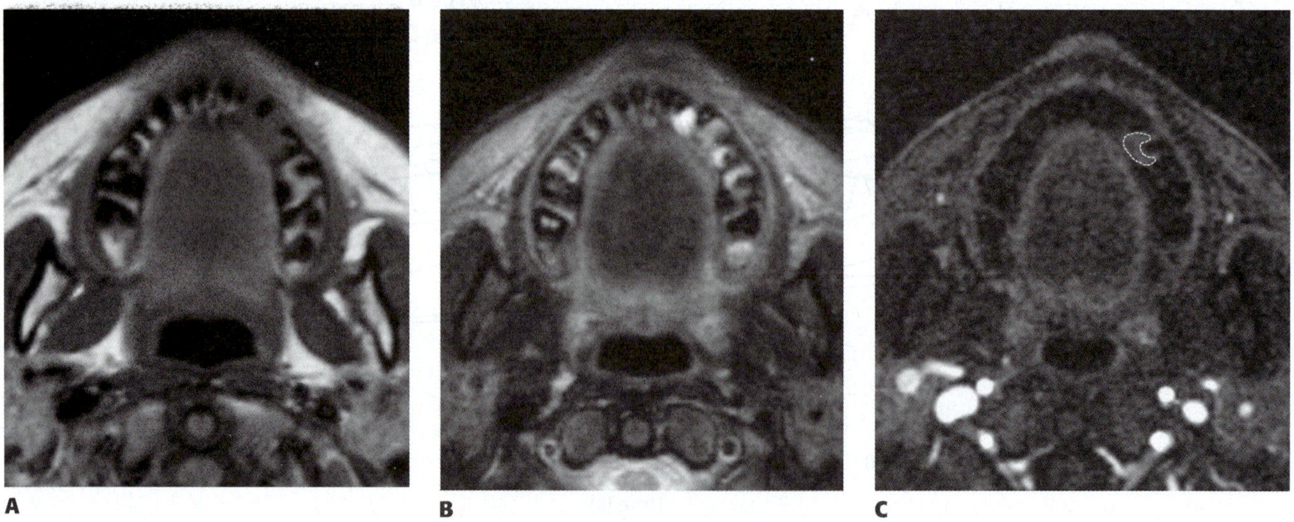

Figure 18-7. Odontogenic fibroma in the maxilla of a 24-year-old woman. **A, B:** A mass in the left maxilla displays homogeneous isointensity on T1W image **(A)** and heterogeneous iso- to hyperintensity on T2W image **(B)**. **C:** The region of interest (*dashed line*) is indicated on a dynamic image.

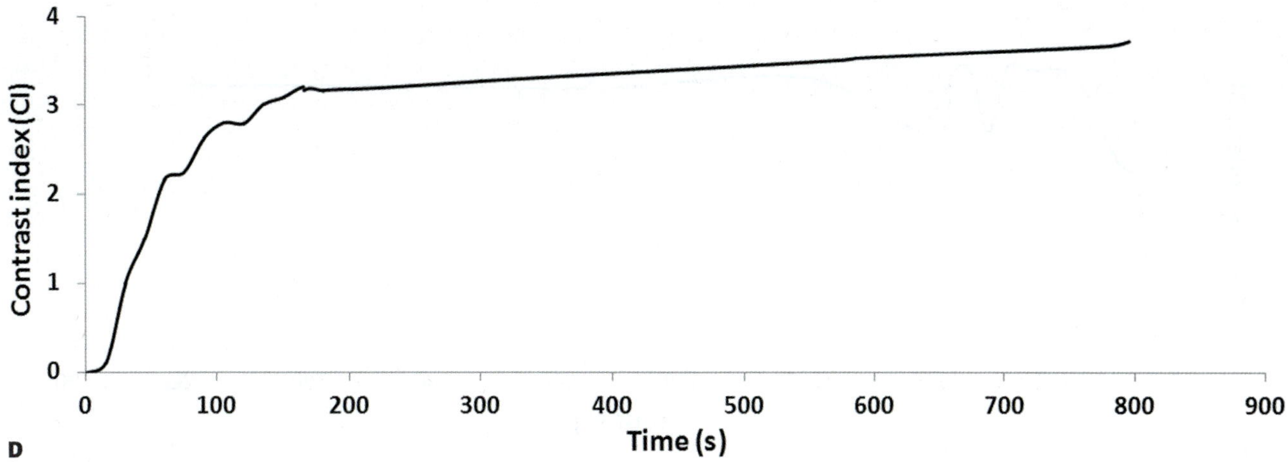

Figure 18-7. (*Continued*) **D:** The CIC of an odontogenic fibroma, in which values increase rapidly until approximately 200 seconds and then gradually continue to increase until approximately 800 seconds without washout of the contrast agent (type D). This pattern distinguishes it from odontogenic myxoma with type E CIC pattern.

Malignant Odontogenic Tumors

Malignant odontogenic tumors are subclassified as odontogenic carcinomas and odontogenic sarcomas.[22] Their incidence is extremely low (approximately 3% of all odontogenic tumors), and there are few reports about DCE-MRI findings in relation to these lesions.[24,25]

Ameloblastic Carcinoma

An ameloblastic carcinoma is a primary odontogenic malignancy.[22] Its CIC displays a relatively rapid increase (type B), similar to that of ameloblastomas (Fig. 18.8).[24]

Primary Intraosseous Squamous Cell Carcinoma

A primary intraosseous squamous cell carcinoma (SCC) is a central jawbone carcinoma arising from odontogenic epithelial remnants.[22] Its CIC also exhibits a relatively rapid increase (type A), similar to that of an ameloblastoma (Fig. 18.9).[25]

Distinguishing between Malignant and Benign Odontogenic Tumors

Among head and neck lesions, the TICs (or CICs) of malignant neoplasms commonly exhibit rapid increases followed by rapid decreases.[1,7,26] However, the CICs of both types of malignant odontogenic tumor have similar patterns to those of benign odontogenic tumors, so their DCE-MRI parameters are of little use in their differential diagnosis.[15,24,25]

Pseudocyst

Pseudocysts of jawbones are classified as bone-related lesions and exhibit a cyst-like appearance on radiographs.[22] However, pseudocysts differ from true cysts in that they have no epithelial lining. Because of the absence of this epithelial lining, pseudocysts have a characteristic TIC pattern on DCE-MRI.[12] Simple bone cysts in jawbones, as in the long bones, are intraosseous pseudocysts that contain serous or sanguineous fluid.[22] Despite the above recommendation regarding placement of ROIs on a solid part of the lesion, avoiding the internal fluid, the ROIs for this lesion should

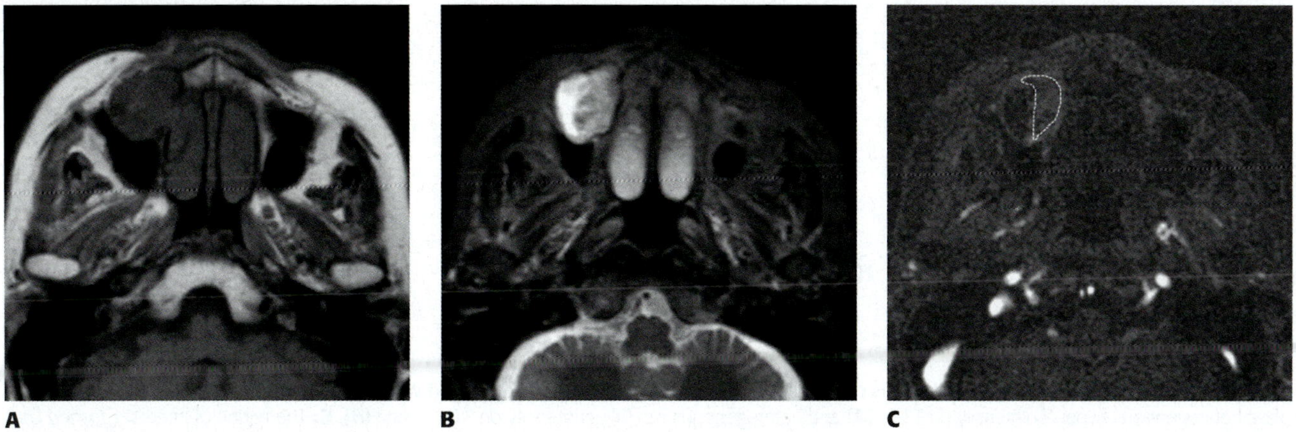

Figure 18-8. Ameloblastic carcinoma in the maxilla of a 73-year-old woman. **A, B:** A mass in the right maxilla displays heterogeneous hypo-/isointensity on T1W **(A)** and heterogeneous hyperintensity on STIR T2W **(B)** images. **C:** The region of interest (*dashed line*) is indicated on a dynamic image.

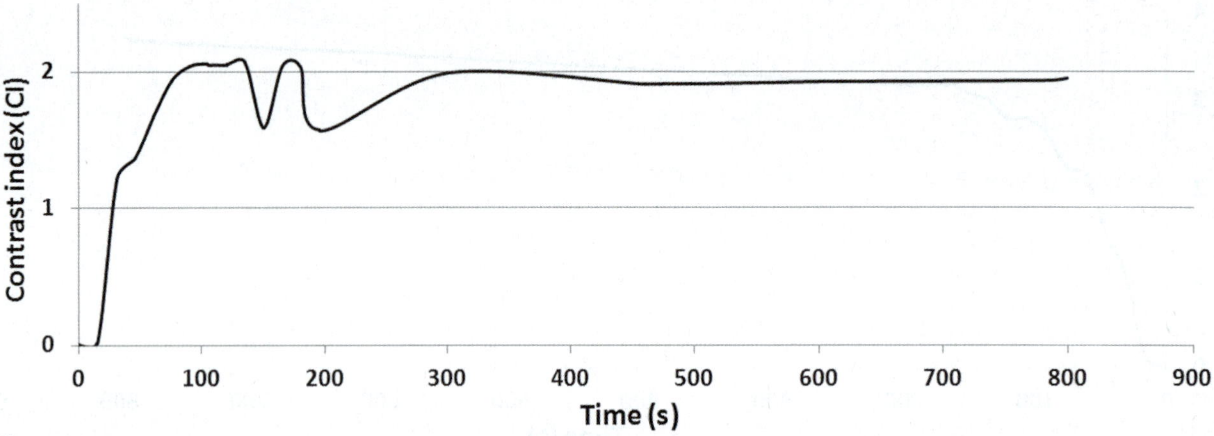

D

Figure 18-8. (*Continued*) **D:** The CIC of an ameloblastic carcinoma, in which values increase rapidly, reach a plateau at 90 to 120 seconds, and then nearly sustain this plateau to approximately 800 seconds (type B).

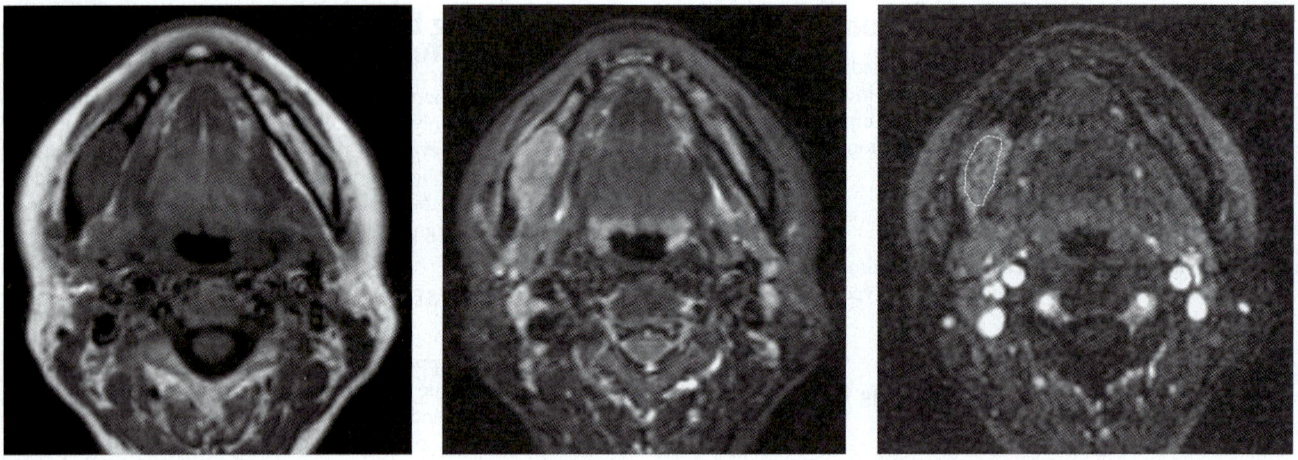

A B C

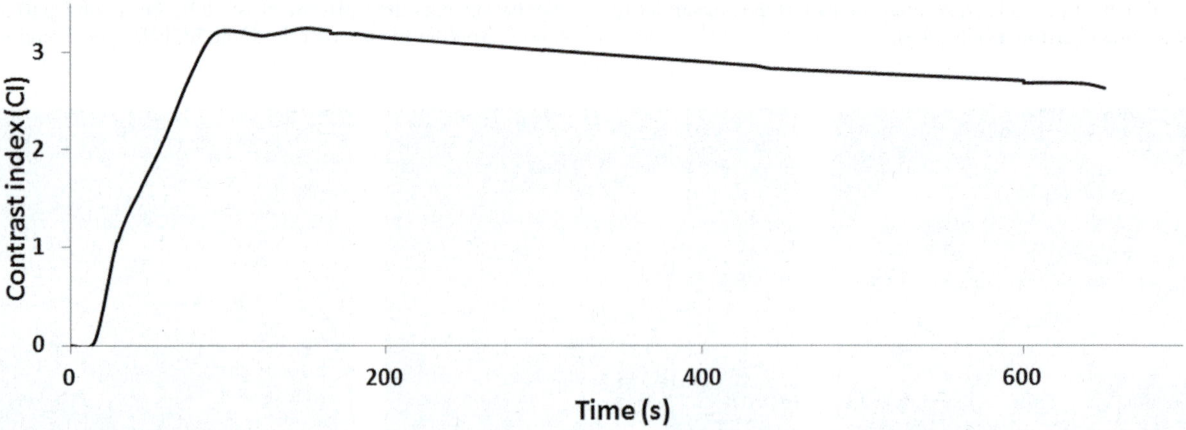

D

Figure 18-9. Primary intraosseous squamous cell carcinoma in the mandible of a 73-year-old woman. A, B: A mass in the right mandible displays heterogeneous hypo-/isointensity on T1WI **(A)** and heterogeneous iso-/hyperintensity on STIR image **(B)**. **C:** The region of interest (*dashed line*) is indicated on a dynamic image. **D:** The CIC of a primary intraosseous squamous cell carcinoma in which the values increase for 100 seconds and then gradually decrease until approximately 700 seconds (type A). Overall, it is not a distinguishing pattern from benign odontogenic tumors.

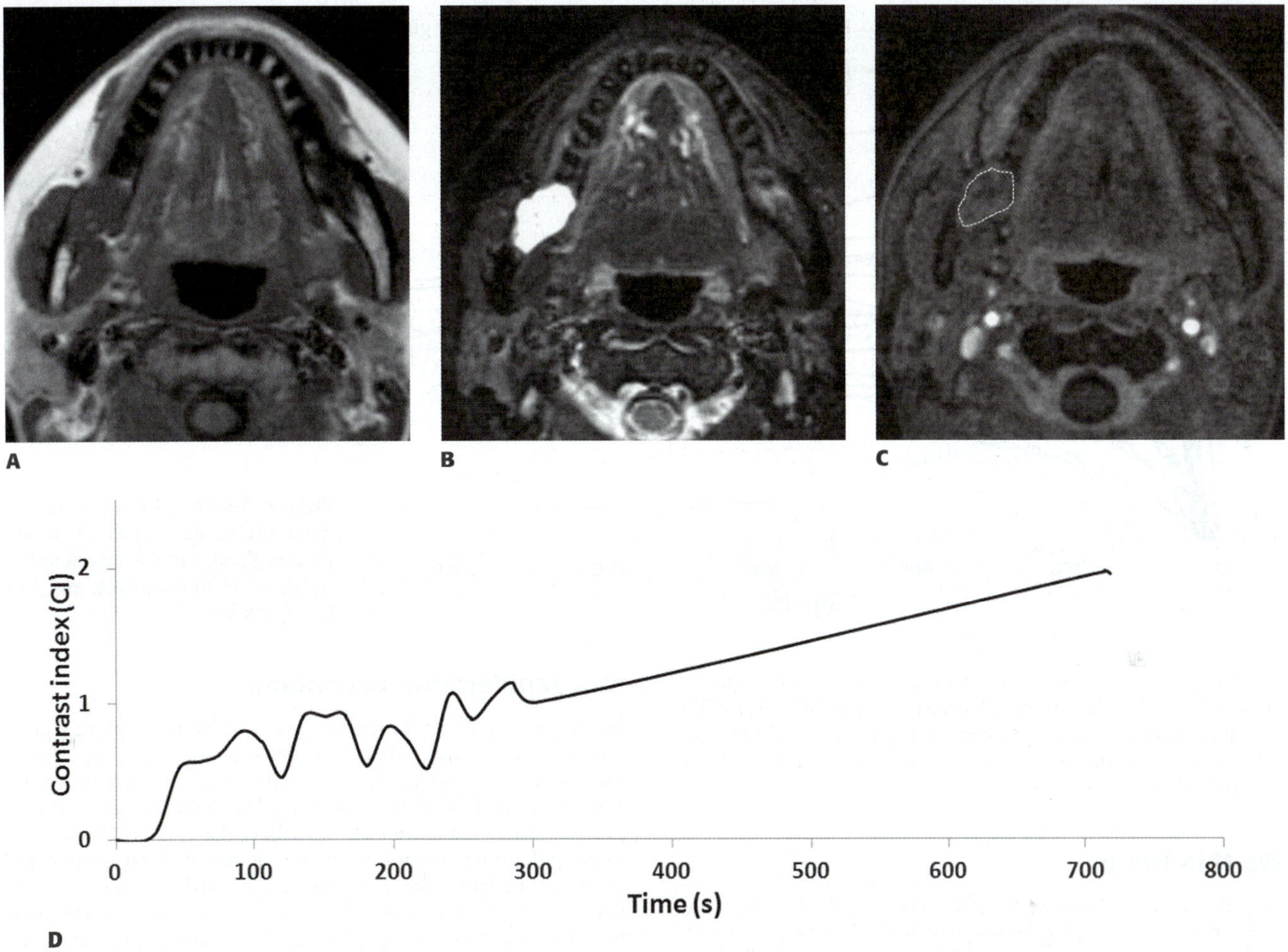

Figure 18-10. Simple bone cyst (pseudocyst) in the right mandible of a 40-year-old woman. **A, B:** A lesion in the right mandible displays homogeneous hypointensity on T1W image **(A)** and homogeneous hyperintensity on STIR T2W image **(B)**. **C:** The region of interest (*dashed line*) is indicated on a dynamic image. **D:** The CIC of a simple bone cyst in which values gradually increase until approximately 700 seconds. This finding is unique to simple bone cyst as true cysts show no such enhancement.

be placed on the fluid area because the fluid in a simple bone cyst shows a slow and gradual enhancement in SI after bolus injection of a contrast agent (Fig. 18.10).[12] This finding is unique to simple bone cysts, as true cysts show no such enhancement.

Application for Salivary Gland Tumors

Salivary gland tumors arise from the major (parotid, submandibular, and sublingual glands) and minor (within the oral mucosa) salivary glands and are neoplasms with morphologic and clinical diversity that present various diagnostic difficulties. Salivary gland tumors come in many histopathologic types (approximately 40 types), and over 50% of them are benign.[22] The most common salivary gland tumor is the benign pleomorphic adenoma, while the most frequent malignant salivary gland tumors are the mucoepidermoid carcinoma and adenoid cystic carcinoma.[22] Depending on the primary site of the tumor, the occurrence ratio of benign-to-malignant and the prevalence of each histopathologic tumor type are different.[22]

Major Salivary Gland

The major salivary glands include the parotid glands (which produce serous saliva) and the submandibular and sublingual glands (which produce seromucous saliva). Approximately 70% to 80% of all salivary gland tumors develop in the parotid gland.[22] The prevalence of malignant (as opposed to benign) neoplasms is 20% to 25% in the parotid, 35% to 40% in the submandibular gland, and greater than 90% in the sublingual gland.[22]

Minor Salivary Gland

Minor salivary glands are widely distributed throughout the oral mucosa, palate, uvula, floor of the mouth, posterior tongue, retromolar and peritonsillar area, pharynx, larynx, and paranasal sinuses.[22] Minor salivary gland tumors are unusual neoplasms (approximately 15% to 20% of all salivary gland tumors).[22] About 50% of minor gland tumors are malignant, and 80% to 90% of those that occur in the tongue, floor of the mouth, and retromolar areas are malignant.[22]

Pleomorphic Adenoma

Pleomorphic adenoma is a benign salivary gland tumor consisting of epithelial cells in a matrix of mucoid, myxomatous, or chondroid tissue and exhibits architectural diversity.[22] MR images of pleomorphic adenomas commonly (approximately 70%) show heterogeneous hyperintensity on T2-W images, reflecting the predominance

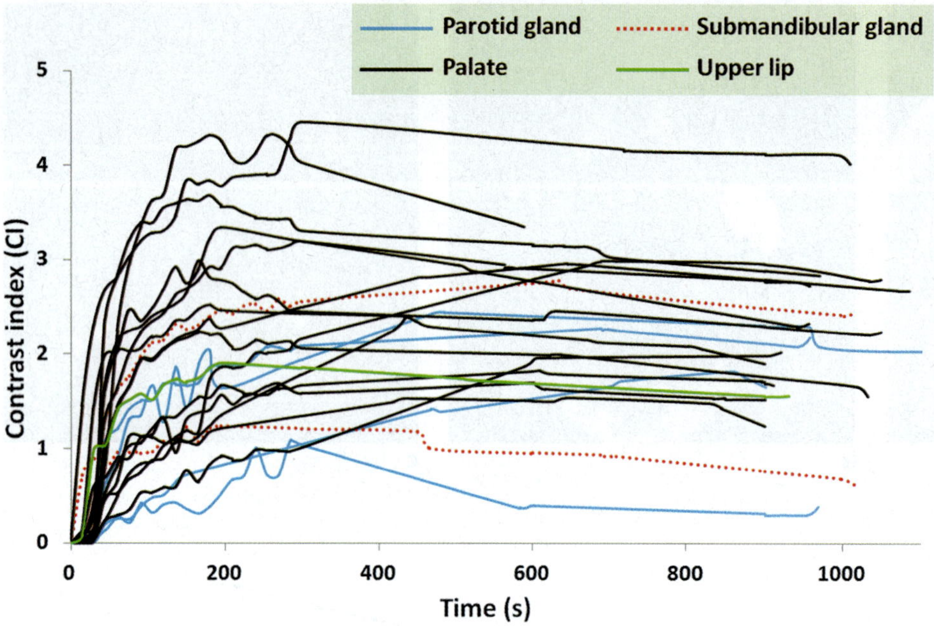

Figure 18-11. The CICs of 22 pleomorphic adenomas (4 in the parotid gland, 2 in the submandibular gland, 15 in the palate, and 1 in the upper lip).

of myxoid or chondroid components.[2,27,28] Many investigators, including ourselves, have reported that a pattern of TIC/CIC exhibits a gradual increase (T_{peak} > 120 seconds) (Fig. 18.11) with little washout of contrast agents before approximately 300 seconds (and even then only at a very low level).[2,3,5,10,11,13,14,27,29]

Warthin Tumor

Warthin tumor consists of an oncocytic epithelial cell component arranged in double layers (which develop into cysts and papillary projections) and a variable amount of lymphoid tissue, often with germinal centers.[22] Warthin tumor is the second most common benign lesion of the parotid gland but is extremely rare elsewhere.[22,30] Literature reports characteristic TIC/CIC patterns for Warthin tumors, comprising a rapid increase (T_{peak} < 120 seconds) and a rapid decrease (WR at 300 seconds [WR_{300}] ≥30%) (Fig. 18.12).[3,5,8,10]

Mucoepidermoid Carcinoma

Mucoepidermoid carcinomas represent a distinct type of tumor that contains three cellular elements in varying proportions: squamous cells, mucus-secreting cells, and intermediate cells.[22] Approximately half of these tumors (53%) occur in major salivary glands.[22] There are no reports describing the TIC/CIC patterns of mucoepidermoid carcinomas, mainly because their rarity has made them hard to define. Some articles have inferred that their TIC/CIC pattern is typified by a rapid increase (T_{peak} < 120 seconds) and a low washout ratio (WR_{300} < 30%).[3,5,9–11,13,14] Indeed, in our previous study of minor salivary gland tumors, two-thirds (4/6 cases) of mucoepidermoid carcinoma showed this pattern (Fig. 18.13).

Adenoid Cystic Carcinoma

ACCs arising from the salivary gland tissue are basaloid tumors consisting of epithelial and myoepithelial cells.[22] They account for

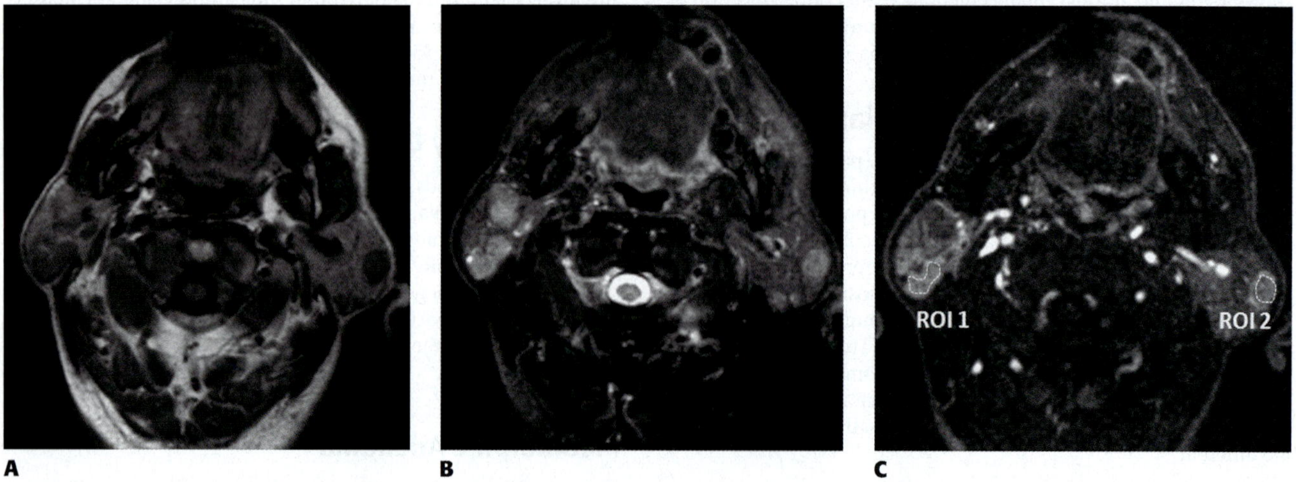

A B C

Figure 18-12. Warthin tumors in the both parotid glands of a 70-year-old man. **A, B:** Multiple masses present in the both parotid glands display heterogeneous hypo-/isointensity on T1W **(A)** and heterogeneous iso-/hyperintensity on STIR T2W **(B)** images. **C:** The regions of interest (*dashed line*), avoiding the vessels, are indicated on a dynamic image.

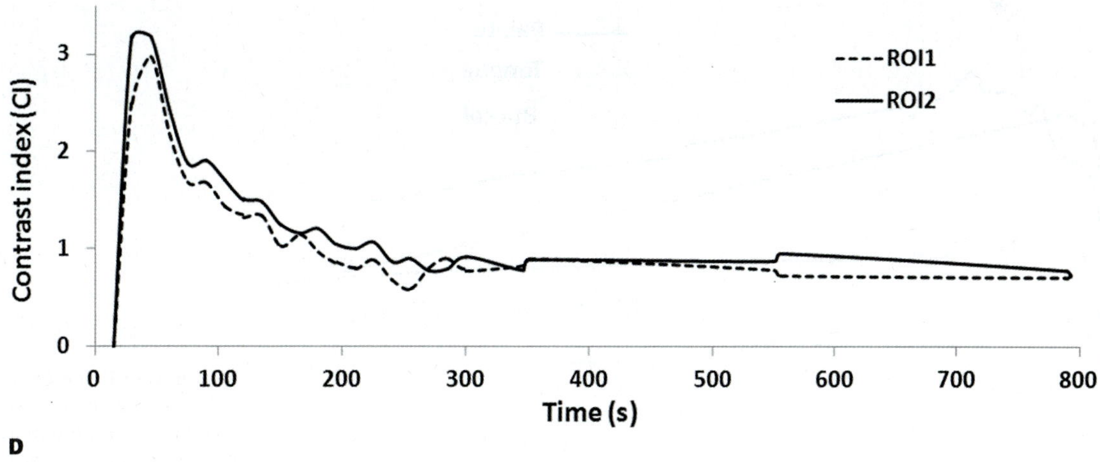

Figure 18-12. (*Continued*) **D:** The CICs of Warthin tumors in which values increase rapidly for 50 seconds and then rapidly decrease.

approximately 10% of all salivary gland neoplasms and commonly occur in the parotid, submandibular, and minor salivary glands.[22] Their TIC/CIC patterns are not clearly defined, for the same reasons as mucoepidermoid carcinomas, above. Some authors, including ourselves, have reported that the TIC/CIC patterns of ACCs are divided into two types: a gradually increasing type (T_{peak} > 120 seconds) without washout and a rapidly increasing type (T_{peak} < 120 seconds) with a low washout ratio (WR_{300} < 30%) (Fig. 18.14).[3,5,9–11,13,14]

Other Salivary Gland Tumors

Previous reports describing other benign and malignant salivary gland tumors such as myoepithelioma, acinic cell carcinoma, polymorphous low-grade adenocarcinoma, and carcinoma ex pleomorphic adenoma were case reports or comparison studies involving only one or a few histopathologic types.[3,5,9–11,13,14] Therefore, their patterns of TICs and CICs are also not clearly defined.

Differentiation of Salivary Gland Tumors Using DCE-MRI

Several authors, including ourselves, have reported the usefulness of DCE-MRI parameters and TICs/CICs in the differential diagnosis of salivary gland tumors.[1,3,5,8,10,11,27] In contrast, Tsushima et al.[2] reported that although DCE-MRI could help distinguish pleomorphic adenomas from Warthin tumors, it was not effective at differentiating between pleomorphic adenomas and adenoid cystic carcinomas or between Warthin tumors and other malignant tumors. Furthermore, in a previous study of minor salivary gland tumors, we reported that the DCE-MRI parameters of minor salivary gland tumors contributed little to their differential diagnosis compared with those for major salivary gland tumors.[13,14] These differences in results between investigators and/or subjects might be caused by the small numbers of subjects with malignant tumors, differences in tumor size/angiogenesis between major and minor salivary glands, and/or differences between major and minor glands in the amount of surrounding tissues (blood flow).

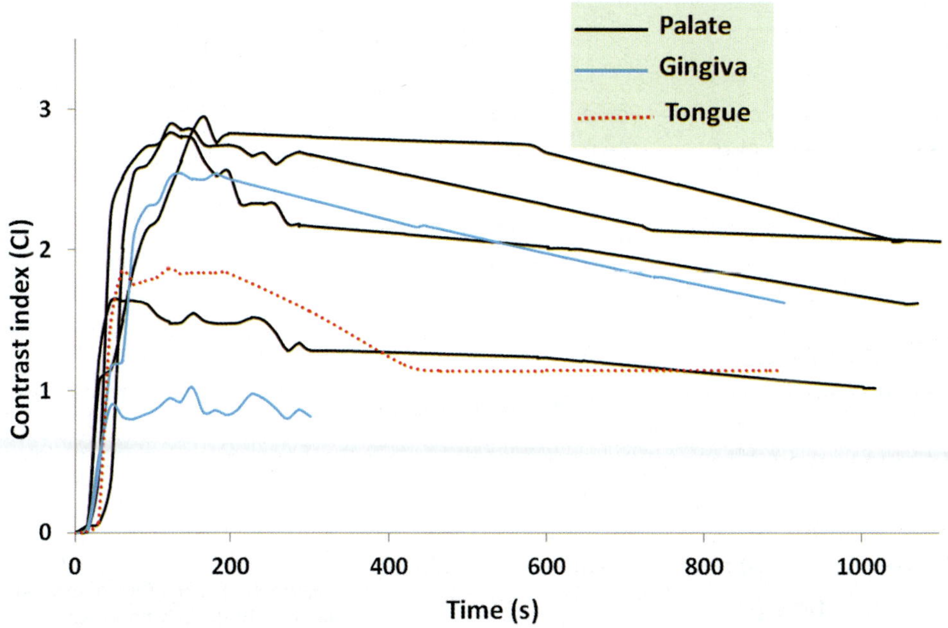

Figure 18-13. The CICs of seven mucoepidermoid carcinomas (four in the palate, two in the gingivae, and one in the tongue). The CICs of four cases show a rapid increase (T_{peak} < 120 seconds) and low washout ratio (WR at 300 seconds <30%).

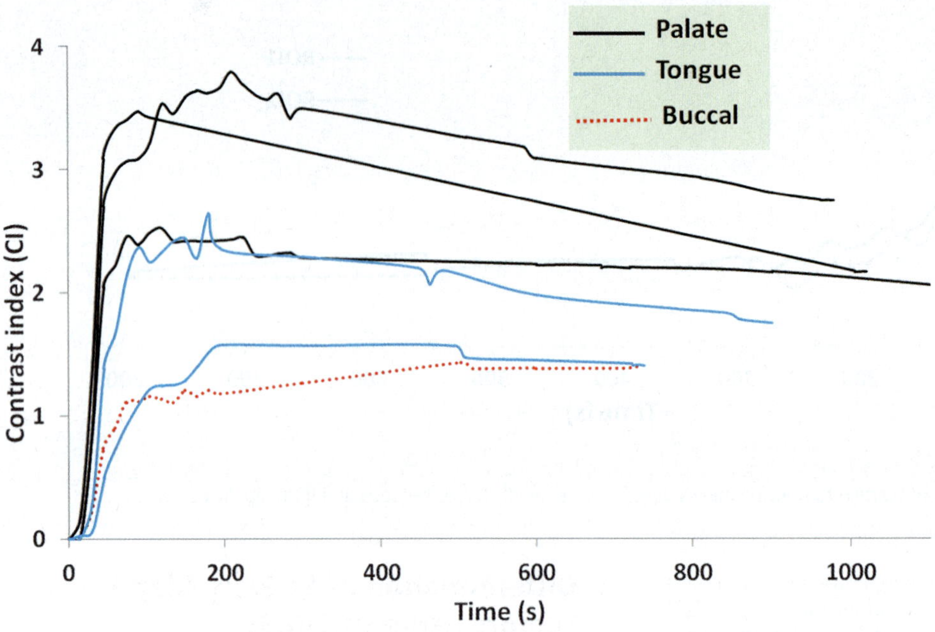

Figure 18-14. The CICs of six adenoid cystic carcinomas (three in the palate, two in the tongue, and one in the buccal mucosa). The CICs are equally divided into the "gradual increase" type (T_{peak} > 120 seconds) without washout, and the "rapid increase" type (T_{peak} < 120 seconds) and low washout ratio (WR at 300 seconds <30%).

Application for Squamous Cell Carcinomas

SCC is an invasive epithelial neoplasm with varying degrees of squamous differentiation. More than 90% of malignant neoplasms of the head and neck regions are SCCs.[22] It has been reported that the patterns of TIC/CIC for SCC commonly display a rapid increase and either a rapid or a gradual decrease.[1,7,26] For diagnosis of oral SCCs by imaging, DCE-MRI examination is of little relevance because most SCCs in this region can be identified as malignant by inspection and palpation. However, in some cases where SCCs arise at invisible sites or where inspection and biopsy are difficult (e.g., the paranasal sinus and salivary glands), DCE-MRI will be effective for differential diagnosis. Some investigators have attempted to predict local treatment response in SCCs using DCE-MRI.[31,32]

Application for Malignant Lymphomas

Malignant lymphoma is the second most common malignancy in the head and neck region, although its morbidity rate is not high.[33] There are two basic categories of lymphomas: Hodgkin lymphoma and non-Hodgkin lymphoma (NHL), with variable frequency depending on racial and geographical factors.[33–35] Lymphomas are also subdivided into nodal lymphomas (which arise from the lymph nodes) and extranodal lymphomas (which arise at outside the lymphoid system).

Extranodal Non-Hodgkin Lymphoma

The incidence of extranodal NHL is reported to be approximately 40%, and the most common site of presentation in the head and neck is Waldeyer ring.[33,35] Only 3.0% to 9.5% of extranodal NHL arises in the oral region, but those that do are commonly in the

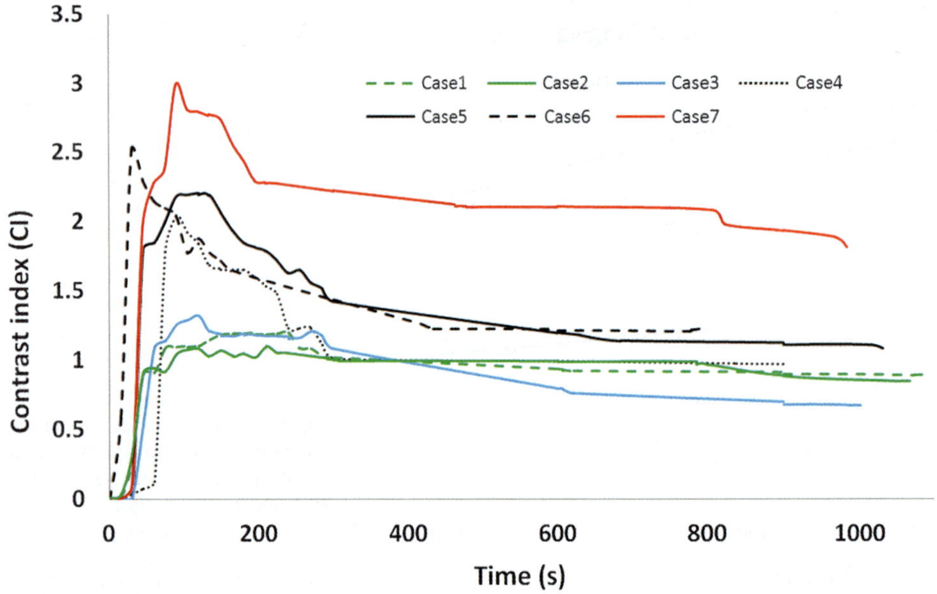

Figure 18-15. The CICs of extranodal non-Hodgkin lymphomas.

TABLE 18.1 **DCE-MRI Parameters in Seven Patients**

Location	Pathology	CI_{max}	T_{max} (s)	WR_{600} (%)	WR_{900} (%)
UG	DLBCL	1.19	165	21.5	23.6
Maxilla	DLBCL	1.08	120	8.4	18.1
MaxS	DLBCL	1.32	120	39.7	47.3
Palate	DLBCL	2.03	90	51.2	52.2
BM	MALT	2.21	120	45.7	49.3
BM	FL	2.51	30	51.3	–
Palate	DLBCL	2.99	90	29.6	35.1

CI_{max}, contrast index at maximum enhancement; T_{max}, time to maximum enhancement; WR, washout ratio; UG, upper gingiva; DLBCL, diffuse large B-cell lymphoma; MaxS, maxillary sinus; BM, buccal mucosa; MALT, mucosa-associated lymphoid tissue; FL, follicular lymphoma.

palate and maxilla.[33,34] MRI of extranodal lymphoma in the head and neck region has been reported to show variable homogeneity and SI in tumors on both T1W and T2W images.[36,37] The degree of enhancement in CE-T1W has been reported to be even more variable.[36,37] Regarding DCE-MRI, we have described nine cases of extranodal NHL and suggested that enhancement pattern of oral extranodal NHLs may be divided into at least four types based on CI_{max} and washout ratio: (1) CI_{max} ≥2.0 and WR_{900} ≥ 40%, (2) CI_{max} ≥2.0 and WR_{900} less than 40%, (3) CI_{max} less than 1.5 and WR_{900} ≥ 40%, and (4) CI_{max} less than 1.5 and WR_{900} less than 40% (Fig. 18.15 and Table 18.1).[38] These results indicated that the TIC/CIC of extranodal NHL does not have any lesion-specific pattern. However, this study included various primary sites (palate, buccal mucosa, gingiva, jawbones, and paranasal sinus) and various histopathologic types of NHL (diffuse large B-cell lymphoma, mucosa-associated lymphoid tissue, and follicular lymphoma). These differences in primary site and histologic type may have affected the DCE-MRI parameters and obscured any characteristic patterns.

REFERENCES

1. **Takashima S, Noguchi Y, Okumura T, et al.** Dynamic MR imaging in the head and neck. *Radiology* 1993;189(3):813–821.
2. **Tsushima Y, Matsumoto M, Endo K.** Parotid and parapharyngeal tumours: tissue characterization with dynamic magnetic resonance imaging. *Br J Radiol* 1994;67(796):342–345.
3. **Suenaga S, Indo H, Noikura T.** Diagnostic value of dynamic magnetic resonance imaging for salivary gland diseases: a preliminary study. *Dentomaxillofac Radiol* 2001;30(6):314–318.
4. **Asaumi J, Matsuzaki H, Hisatomi M, et al.** Application of dynamic MRI to differentiating odontogenic myxomas from ameloblastomas. *Eur J Radiol* 2002;43(1):37–41.
5. **Yabuuchi H, Fukuya T, Tajima T, et al.** Salivary gland tumors: diagnostic value of gadolinium-enhanced dynamic MR imaging with histopathologic correlation. *Radiology* 2003;226(2):345–354.
6. **Asaumi J, Yanagi Y, Hisatomi M, et al.** The value of dynamic contrast-enhanced MRI in diagnosis of malignant lymphoma of the head and neck. *Eur J Radiol* 2003;48(2):183–187.
7. **Asaumi J, Yanagi Y, Konouchi H, et al.** Application of dynamic contrast-enhanced MRI to differentiate malignant lymphoma from squamous cell carcinoma in the head and neck. *Oral Oncol* 2004;40(6):579–584.
8. **Ikeda M, Motoori K, Hanazawa T, et al.** Warthin tumor of the parotid gland: diagnostic value of MR imaging with histopathologic correlation. *AJNR Am J Neuroradiol* 2004;25(7):1256–1262.
9. **Ueda F, Suzuki M, Matsui O, et al.** MR findings of nine cases of palatal tumor. *Magn Reson Med Sci* 2005;4(2):61–67.
10. **Hisatomi M, Asaumi J, Yanagi Y, et al.** Diagnostic value of dynamic contrast-enhanced MRI in the salivary gland tumors. *Oral Oncol* 2007;43(9):940–947.
11. **Eida S, Ohki M, Sumi M, et al.** MR factor analysis: improved technology for the assessment of 2D dynamic structures of benign and malignant salivary gland tumors. *J Magn Reson Imaging* 2008;27(6):1256–1262.
12. **Yanagi Y, Asaumi J, Unetsubo T, et al.** Usefulness of MRI and dynamic contrast-enhanced MRI for differential diagnosis of simple bone cysts from true cysts in the jaw. *Oral Surg Oral Med Oral Pathol Oral Radiol Endod* 2010;110(3):364–369.
13. **Matsuzaki H, Yanagi Y, Hara M, et al.** Minor salivary gland tumors in the oral cavity: diagnostic value of dynamic contrast-enhanced MRI. *Eur J Radiol* 2011;81(10):2684–2691.
14. **Matsuzaki H, Yanagi Y, Hara M, et al.** Diagnostic value of dynamic contrast-enhanced MRI for submucosal palatal tumors. *Eur J Radiol* 2012;81(11):3306–3312.
15. **Fujita M, Matsuzaki H, Yanagi Y, et al.** Diagnostic value of MRI for odontogenic tumours. *Dentomaxillofac Radiol* 2013;42(5):20120265.
16. **Carmeliet P, Jain RK.** Angiogenesis in cancer and other diseases. *Nature* 2000;407(6801):249–257.
17. **Padhani AR.** MRI for assessing antivascular cancer treatments. *Br J Radiol* 2003;76(Spec No 1):S60–S80.
18. **Tofts PS.** Modeling tracer kinetics in dynamic Gd-DTPA MR imaging. *J Magn Reson Imaging* 1997;7(1):91–101.
19. **Cha S, Yang L, Johnson G, et al.** Comparison of microvascular permeability measurements, K(trans), determined with conventional steady-state T1-weighted and first-pass T2*-weighted MR imaging methods in gliomas and meningiomas. *AJNR Am J Neuroradiol* 2006;27(2):409–417.
20. **O'Connor JP, Jackson A, Parker GJ, et al.** DCE-MRI biomarkers in the clinical evaluation of antiangiogenic and vascular disrupting agents. *Br J Cancer* 2007;96(2):189–195.
21. **Haris M, Husain N, Singh A, et al.** Dynamic contrast enhanced (DCE) derived transfer coefficient (ktrans) is a surrogate marker of matrix metalloproteinase 9 (MMP-9) expression in brain tuberculomas. *J Magn Reson Imaging* 2008;28(3):588–597.
22. **Barnes L, Eveson JW, Reichart P, et al. International Agency for Research on Cancer.** *Pathology and genetics of head and neck tumours.* Lyon, France: IARC; 2005.
23. **Hara M, Matsuzaki H, Katase N, et al.** Central odontogenic fibroma of the jawbone: 2 case reports describing its imaging features and an analysis of its DCE-MRI findings. *Oral Surg Oral Med Oral Pathol Oral Radiol* 2012;113(6):e51–e58.
24. **Matsuzaki H, Katase N, Hara M, et al.** Ameloblastic carcinoma: a case report with radiological features of computed tomography and magnetic resonance imaging and positron emission tomography. *Oral Surg Oral Med Oral Pathol Oral Radiol Endod* 2011;112(1):e40–e47.
25. **Matsuzaki H, Katase N, Matsumura T, et al.** Solid type primary intraosseous squamous cell carcinoma of the mandible: a case report with imaging features. *Oral Surg Oral Med Oral Pathol Oral Radiol* 2012;114(5):e71–e77.
26. **Unetsubo T, Konouchi H, Yanagi Y, et al.** Dynamic contrast-enhanced magnetic resonance imaging for estimating tumor proliferation and microvessel density of oral squamous cell carcinomas. *Oral Oncol* 2009;45(7):621–626.
27. **Hisatomi M, Asaumi J, Yanagi Y, et al.** Assessment of pleomorphic adenomas using MRI and dynamic contrast enhanced MRI. *Oral Oncol* 2003;39(6):574–579.
28. **Kakimoto N, Gamoh S, Tamaki J, et al.** CT and MR images of pleomorphic adenoma in major and minor salivary glands. *Eur J Radiol* 2009;69(3):464–472.
29. **Motoori K, Yamamoto S, Ueda T, et al.** Inter- and intratumoral variability in magnetic resonance imaging of pleomorphic adenoma: an attempt to interpret the variable magnetic resonance findings. *J Comput Assist Tomogr* 2004;28(2):233–246.
30. **van der Wal JE, Davids JJ, van der Waal I.** Extraparotid Warthin's tumours—report of 10 cases. *Br J Oral Maxillofac Surg* 1993;31(1):43–44.

31. **Quon H, Brizel DM.** Predictive and prognostic role of functional imaging of head and neck squamous cell carcinomas. *Semin Radiat Oncol* 2012;22(3):220–232.
32. **Chawla S, Kim S, Dougherty L, et al.** Pretreatment diffusion-weighted and dynamic contrast-enhanced MRI for prediction of local treatment response in squamous cell carcinomas of the head and neck. *AJR Am J Roentgenol* 2013;200(1):35–43.
33. **Otter R, Gerrits WB, vd Sandt MM, et al.** Primary extranodal and nodal non-Hodgkin's lymphoma. A survey of a population-based registry. *Eur J Cancer Clin Oncol* 1989;25(8):1203–1210.
34. **Freeman C, Berg JW, Cutler SJ.** Occurrence and prognosis of extranodal lymphomas. *Cancer* 1972;29(1):252–260.
35. **Wong DS, Fuller LM, Butler JJ, et al.** Extranodal non-Hodgkin's lymphomas of the head and neck. *Am J Roentgenol Radium Ther Nucl Med* 1975;123(3):471–481.
36. **Yasumoto M, Shibuya H, Fukuda H, et al.** Malignant lymphoma of the gingiva: MR evaluation. *AJNR Am J Neuroradiol* 1998;19(4): 723–727.
37. **King AD, Lei KI, Ahuja AT.** MRI of neck nodes in non-Hodgkin's lymphoma of the head and neck. *Br J Radiol* 2004;77(914):111–115.
38. **Matsuzaki H, Hara M, Yanagi Y, et al.** Magnetic resonance imaging (MRI) and dynamic MRI evaluation of extranodal non-Hodgkin lymphoma in oral and maxillofacial regions. *Oral Surg Oral Med Oral Pathol Oral Radiol* 2012;113(1):126–133.

CHAPTER

19 Myocardial Perfusion Imaging: MR Techniques

Eike Nagel, MD, PhD, FACC, FESC, MRCR, Amedeo Chiribiri, MD, PhD, and Islam Z. Mahmoud, MD

Key Points

- Cardiac MRI perfusion, also known as stress CMR perfusion, is a clinical test performed on patients with chest pain who are known or suspected to have coronary artery disease to determine the myocardial perfusion status and the significance of coronary artery obstruction.
- Guidelines increasingly require the proof of ischemia before revascularization.
- CMR perfusion is increasingly used in imaging cardiology to test for inducible myocardial ischemia and has been well validated against other imaging modalities.
- CMR first-pass perfusion provides high spatial resolution images of myocardial ischemia, allowing regional myocardial perfusion assessment and separate visualization of subendo- and subepicardial layers.
- The absence of ionizing radiation and the noninvasive nature of the method make it the optimal clinical tool for repetitive evaluations of the patients during follow-up.
- CMR first-pass perfusion is more sensitive than is dobutamine stress test in the detection of ischemia, as it is aimed toward the imaging of blood flow, which is first reduced in the progression of the ischemic cascade.
- It is becoming increasingly established as a marker of prognosis in patients with coronary artery disease.
- It is a noninvasive test, is generally regarded as a safe procedure, and is usually well tolerated by patients.

Introduction

Myocardial perfusion imaging by first-pass contrast-enhanced cardiovascular magnetic resonance was introduced in 1990, when Atkinson et al. first used inversion recovery gradient-echo imaging after injection of a bolus of gadolinium-based contrast (Gd-DTPA) to observe contrast agent transit through the cardiac chambers and myocardium.[1] Myocardial perfusion CMR was examined in animal experiments during pharmacologic vasodilation and showed a good correlation with microspheres for the assessment of blood flow.[2–4] Early data from small studies showed that CMR can be a useful tool for the noninvasive assessment of myocardial perfusion reserve (MPR) and allows an accurate detection of significant myocardial ischemia when compared with x-ray coronary angiogram.[5,6] The technique has ongoing rapid development along with experimental validation and clinical evaluation. Recently, it has been validated in different large single and multicenter clinical trials against nuclear myocardial perfusion imaging.[7–9] Technical developments have also occurred in terms of gradient systems, field strength, radiofrequency coil arrays, pulse sequence design, contrast agents, and perfusion analysis methods.

With the advent and widespread availability of faster MRI scanners with very high spatial resolution (approximately 1 × 1 mm), CMR has become an established method for myocardial perfusion imaging. Compared with SPECT and PET, CMR perfusion offers the advantages of a noninvasive and radiation-free assessment, as well as higher spatial and temporal resolution images. In this chapter, we review the different CMR techniques used in myocardial perfusion imaging.

Myocardial Perfusion Pathophysiology

Myocardial blood flow (MBF) is controlled, during rest and stress, by an autoregulation mechanism mainly through the vascular resistance of precapillary arterioles (<100 μm in diameter) and prearterioles (diameter is between 100 and 500 μm). This autoregulatory mechanism is able to maintain a stable blood flow even with change of the perfusion pressure under normal myocardial oxygen demand. However, there are many factors such as arterial hypertension, increased myocardial workload, increased heart rate (HR), and raised left ventricular (LV) wall stress that increment myocardial oxygen demand and thus lead to increased resting blood flow. Exercise is an example of a situation where myocardial oxygen demand increases due to increased cardiac workload induced by the tachycardia, increased contractility, and blood pressure (BP). The precapillary vascular resistance decreases, allowing the MBF to increase in proportion and in response to the increased myocardial oxygen demand.

In normal subjects, resting blood flow is in the range of 0.8 to 1.2 mL/g/min. MBF can increase up to threefolds with peak exercise. The term coronary flow reserve (CFR) indicates the capability to increase blood flow of the myocardium in response to maximal exercise. Flow reserve is the ratio of the MBF at peak stress, or maximal vasodilatation, to the flow at rest. In normal adults, the flow reserve ratio is usually 1.5 or higher.

MBF impairment is not uniform across the LV myocardial wall thickness. When arteriolar perfusion pressure is decreased, perfusion is reduced earlier in the subendocardial than in the subepicardial layers. The subendocardium is even more susceptible to reduced perfusion if there is a shortening of the diastolic relaxation phase, as with stress-related tachycardia or in case of diastolic dysfunction.

Flow-Mediated Vasodilatation

Release of vasodilators, such as nitric oxide, endothelium-derived relaxation factor, and prostacyclin, by the endothelial cells causes flow-mediated vasodilatation. Thus, the MBF increases to meet an increase in myocardial oxygen demand. Adenosine is a potent vasodilator of arterioles by stimulating the A2 adenosine receptors on arteriolar smooth muscle. It is formed in the myocytes by the degradation of adenine nucleotides via ATP utilization. Hence, adenosine infusion can produce a near-maximal vasodilatation of the myocardial microcirculation. The existence of significant flow-limiting coronary stenosis reduces the ability of coronary circulation to increase MBF to meet the increased workload.

Maximal vasodilatation induced with adenosine can precipitate a reduction in MBF in the area supplied by a stenosed coronary artery with shunting of blood to the areas supplied by normal coronary arteries. Therefore, MBF decreases at peak stress or maximal vasodilatation in the affected segment. Resting blood flow is usually maintained at a normal level, even in segments supplied by stenotic arteries, due to the low resting myocardial oxygen demand, which can be met by the autoregulatory mechanism unless there is a severe flow-limiting stenosis. Therefore, an early decline of peak stress flow and CFR is often the first clue of early coronary artery disease. In other words, myocardial hypoperfusion is the first detectable event in the ischemic cascade (Fig. 19.1). Thus, perfusion evaluation is in principle the most sensitive test for ischemia, and flow quantification is a critical tool for characterization of patients at risk. In the absence of significant coronary artery disease, a reduction in CFR can reflect coronary microvascular dysfunction, which is often associated with systemic diseases like diabetes and hypertension. The main idea of CMR perfusion imaging is that the first myocardial passage of a contrast agent is visualized instantly every heartbeat. A vasodilator (e.g., adenosine, regadenoson, or dipyridamole) agent is used to induce myocardial hyperemia. With maximum hyperemia, wash-in of the contrast from the subepicardial layer to the subendocardial layer of the myocardium can be visualized and delineated with high sensitivity because of the high spatial resolution provided by CMR (Fig. 19.2). Detection of segments with hypoperfusion, where there is a delay and reduction in contrast wash-in means myocardial perfusion defect due to insufficient blood supply, as a result of coronary artery obstruction or microvascular dysfunction, to this segment. Currently, there are two main clinical indications of myocardial perfusion CMR, which are (a) detection of ischemia in patients who have chest pain and intermediate risk for coronary artery disease and (b) functional assessment of the significance of a stenosis in one or more of the coronary arteries that has been previously identified either by standard x-ray or by CT coronary angiography to determine the culprit lesions and guide revascularization either by angioplasty or by coronary bypass surgery.

How to Perform a Dynamic Contrast-Enhanced First-Pass Myocardial Perfusion

Requirements

MRI safe infusion pump, MRI safe noninvasive brachial BP, pulse oximetry, and single-lead ECG (vectrocardiogram or VCG), one advanced life support (ALS)-trained physician on site, basic life support–trained radiographer(s), regular MRI evacuation training, three members of staff at the scanner in total (one ALS trained, all trained in scanner evacuation).

Monitoring and Safety

For stress testing, careful monitoring of patients in CMR setting is vital. A physician experienced in cardiac resuscitation (holding a valid ALS certificate) should be present for all examinations. To ensure prompt recognition of adverse symptoms, the patient must be able to continuously communicate with the operators (e.g., via intercom) to report symptoms. Monitoring includes continuous BP, HR, and rhythm monitoring (single-lead ECG) (Table 19.1). It is easiest if BP monitoring is performed manually because automated inflated cuff may obstruct the delivery of the contrast into the vein with extravasation. Therefore, if automated BP monitoring is turned on, this must be switched off prior to starting imaging and contrast delivery. Vasodilator agent is delivered via infusion pump as a continuous infusion (i.e., adenosine or dipyridamole) or as a single bolus (i.e., regadenoson). The vasodilator agent should be connected to the side with no BP cuff. Contrast tubing is connected

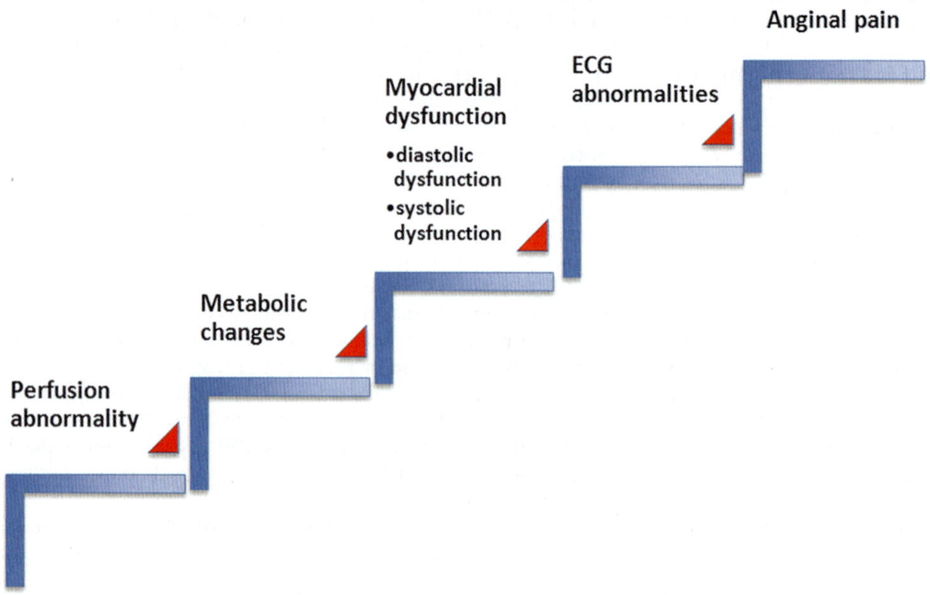

Figure 19-1. Ischemic cascade; myocardial hypoperfusion is the first detectable abnormality, followed by metabolic changes, then wall motion abnormality, then ECG changes, and finally chest pain.

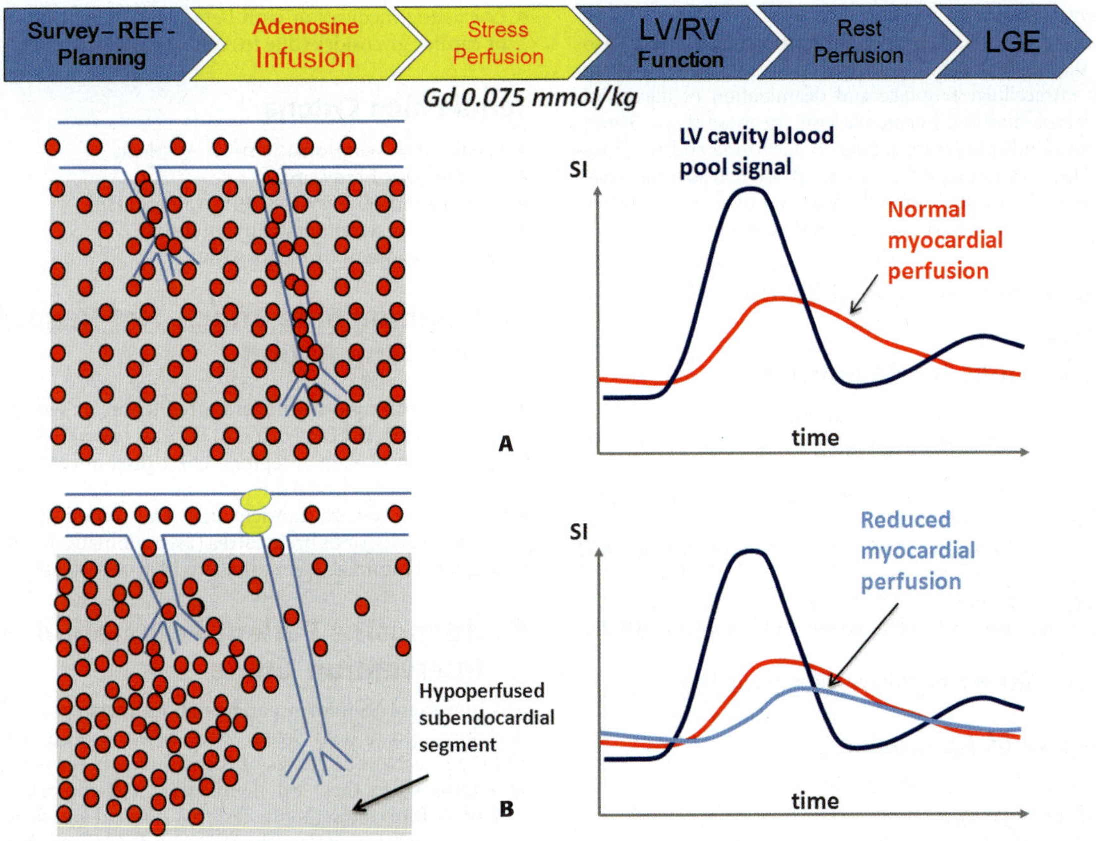

Figure 19-2. **The extracellular contrast agent reaches the myocardium and passes in the extracellular space with an amount and rate that is proportional to blood flow.** In normal conditions **(A)**, a certain amount of contrast agent diffuses into the interstitium, giving a strong myocardial signal (Myo) occurring later than the increment of signal in the left ventricle (LV); when regional coronary blood flow is impaired **(B)**, the amount and rate of wash-in of the contrast agent is reduced (upslope) and peak signal intensity is lower.

to the side with BP cuff. It is important that staff are familiar with the pump settings and the adjoining tubing, to be able to prepare, prime, and deliver the agent as well as to stop the agent timely. Emergency resuscitation policy must be in place including defibrillator and drugs for emergency treatment including aminophylline. In the emergency trolley, a full set of emergency drugs (including drugs such as epinephrine, beta-blockers, atropine, bronchodilators, and antiarrhythmic drugs) should be available.

Vasodilator Stress Agents

Adenosine (Most Commonly Used Vasodilator)

Concentration: Different concentrations are available (such as 1, 3, or 7 mg/mL) depending on the vendor and country.
Administration: Intravenous infusion
Dose: 140 to 210 µg/kg/min
Duration: Maximum of 6 minutes (see below for full protocol)

TABLE 19.1 Required Monitoring during Perfusion CMR

Heart rate and rhythm	Continuously
Blood pressure	Every minute
Symptoms	Continuously

Mode of Action: Adenosine is an endogenous nucleotide, causing vasodilation of most vascular beds, except for hepatic and renal arterioles. It exerts its pharmacologic effect through the activation of purine A1 and A2 cell surface adenosine receptors. Upon administration, a four to five fold hyperemia is seen in normal myocardial segments but not in regions subtended by obstructed coronary arteries. The differential perfusion changes are used to diagnose ischemic heart disease in the presence of significant coronary artery disease.

Regadenoson

Concentration: 5-mL vial contains 400 µg regadenoson (80 µg/mL)
Administration: Intravenous bolus
Dose: A single injection of 400 µg (5 mL) with no dose adjustment for body weight.
Duration: Rapid IV injection over 10 seconds using a 22-gauge or larger catheter or needle. Administer a 5 mL saline flush immediately after the injection of regadenoson. Administer the myocardial perfusion imaging contrast agent 10 to 20 seconds after the saline flush. The contrast may be injected directly into the same line as regadenoson (i.e., only one cannula can be inserted).
Mode of Action: Regadenoson is a selective A2 adenosine receptor agonist causing coronary vasodilator with a potential lower side effect profile than adenosine but with longer half-life.

Dipyridamole

Administration: Intravenous infusion
Dose: 0.56 mg/kg (142 µg/kg/min)

Duration: Over 4 minutes

Mode of Action: Dipyridamole is an indirect coronary artery vasodilator that increases the tissue levels of adenosine by preventing the intracellular reuptake and deamination of adenosine. Dipyridamole-induced hyperemia lasts for more than 15 minutes. Contraindications are similar to adenosine and more frequently requires aminophylline administration in adverse events.

As adenosine is the most commonly used vasodilator medication, the subsequent discussion focuses on this agent.

Contraindications and Termination Criteria

Contraindications for Adenosine

- Recent myocardial infarction less than 3 days
- Unstable angina pectoris (ongoing chest pain at rest, requiring glyceryl trinitrate)
- Asthma or severe chronic obstructive pulmonary disease requiring oral treatment or regular inhalers
- High-grade atrioventricular block (greater than AV block grade II Mobitz I)
- Sinus node dysfunction
- Severe arterial hypertension (BP systolic >220 mm Hg, BP diastolic >120 mm Hg)
- Severe arterial hypotension (BP systolic <90 mm Hg)

Cautious Use of Adenosine

- Preexisting AV block or bundle branch block
- Autonomic neuropathy
- Severe aortic and mitral stenosis
- Severe left ventricular outflow tract obstruction in hypertrophic cardiomyopathy
- Severe carotid stenosis
- Chronic obstructive pulmonary disease not requiring oral medication or regular inhaler therapy
- Coexisting medication with beta-blockers, calcium antagonists, or cardiac glycosides (due to AV/sinus node depression)

Termination Criteria

- Persistent or symptomatic II–III AV block
- Symptomatic bradycardia
- Significant drop in systolic BP (>20 mm Hg)
- Persistent or symptomatic hypotension
- Severe dyspnea or bronchospasm

Common Side Effects Not Requiring Test Termination

- Vasodilation: mild-to-moderate reduction in systolic, diastolic, and mean arterial BP (<10 mm Hg), increased HR (>100 bpm)
- Stimulation of pain receptors: chest discomfort, neck flushing, and angina-like chest pain
- Conduction system: transient first- and second-degree AV block (Wenckebach), sinus bradycardia (asymptomatic or HR > 45 bpm)
- Dyspnea (common approximately 14% of patients)

Adenosine Patient Preparation and Intervention Guide

It is important to inform patients about the steps of the test and that they need to hold breath when asked to do by the examiner and the possible side effects of the vasodilator agent and to report symptoms when they feel them. Also, it is important to notify patients before coming to the test that no food and drinks containing xanthines (tea, coffee, chocolate, and cola) may be consumed for at least 12 to 24 hours prior to the examination. Aminophylline, theophylline, and other xanthine medicines are competitive adenosine antagonists and should be avoided for 24 hours prior to the examination. Guide to intervention with adverse reactions (Table 19.2).

TABLE 19.2 Guide to Intervention with Adverse Reactions

Adverse reaction	Intervention
▪ Persistent or symptomatic II–III AV block ▪ Symptomatic bradycardia ▪ Significant drop in systolic BP (>20 mm Hg) ▪ Persistent or symptomatic hypotension ▪ Severe dyspnea or bronchospasm or any other deemed significant	▪ *Stop infusion!* ▪ High-flow oxygen
Persisting bradycardia	*Bradycardia algorithm (ALS). Atropine* 600 µg i.v. up to the total 1 mg. Consider *admission* for further monitoring. Adenosine antidote: *aminophylline* 250–500 mg (5 mg/kg) i.v. injection *25 mg/mL slowly over 20 minutes* under ECG monitoring—*requires admission to intensive care unit*
Persisting bronchospasm	*Short-acting beta2 agonist via oxygen-driven nebulizer (salbutamol 5 mg).* Consider hospital admission for further monitoring. Adenosine antidote: *aminophylline* 250–500 mg (5 mg/kg) i.v. injection *25 mg/mL slowly over 20 min* under ECG monitoring—*requires admission to high care unit e.g., CCU*

Dynamic Contrast-Enhanced First-Pass Perfusion Protocol

Dynamic contrast-enhanced first-pass perfusion is ideally acquired as dynamic series of images and displayed as a movie. It is a very challenging technical process to make this dynamic series of images demonstrating a motion-free cross section of cardiac muscle whose signal intensity rises and falls over time as the bolus of contrast agent passes through the myocardial tissue.

Standardized first-pass perfusion protocol has been proposed by the society of cardiac MRI (SCMR) as follows[10] (Fig. 19.3):

Scout imaging as per LV structure and function module aiming to plan a true short-axis (SA) view of the LV. For ischemia evaluation, data must be acquired for every heartbeat to visualize the flow of the contrast agent through the LV cavity and the myocardium. A minimum of three SA slices (apical, mid, and basal) should be acquired every heartbeat to ensure coverage of all except the most apical LV segment. Additional SA or long-axis slices may also be useful. The slice locations are timed to different points of time (i.e., phases) of the cardiac cycle, but each location is acquired repeatedly at the same phase. To obtain three SA, the four- and two-chamber views are used. First, align five slices on the four- and two-chamber views and adjust the slice gap so that the first slice is in the plane of the mitral valve and the last slice is at the apex. Then, remove the first and fifth slices by changing the number of slices from five to three. Slice thickness should be 8 mm, in-plane resolution ≤3 mm, and readout temporal resolution between 100 and 125 milliseconds or shorter as available (Fig. 19.4).

First-pass perfusion images must be T1 weighted in order to maximize the effect of the contrast agent on signal intensity. The fast (turbo-) gradient-echo and hybrid echo-planar imaging sequences described below employ small flip angles and very short time of repetition (TR), in order to reduce acquisition time, resulting in poor T1 contrast. While the balanced steady-state free precession sequence uses a higher flip, angle is weighted by the ratio of T2/T1. To overcome all of this, a preparation pulse is applied prior to the readout pulse sequence with an adequately long preparation pulse delay to establish a high T1 contrast prior to the readout sequence is employed.

How to Acquire T1-Weighted Images

A 90-degree prepulse is used to null the magnetization signal and then wait for signal recovery (Fig. 19.5). Saturation recovery pulse sequence signal depends on the amount of the contrast agent; thus good perfusion leads to high concentration of contrast agent and rapid recovery of signal giving a bright image, while reduced perfusion leads to low concentration and slow recovery of signal giving a dark image (Fig. 19.6). In comparison to inversion recovery sequences that are used for late gadolinium enhancement, saturation recovery pulse sequences have the advantages that the contrast is independent of heartbeat variations during ECG-triggered image acquisition, and it has shorter scan time.

T1 weighting is dependent on accurate selection of the saturation time (TS). Generally, each imaging slice is preceded by a preparation pulse; thus the number of preparation pulses is equal to the number of slices in a given R-R interval. This acquisition scheme ensures a constant level of contrast in adjacent slices. In order to maximize T1 contrast for visualization of perfusion defects within the myocardium, longer saturation times should be used. A common TS for cardiac perfusion imaging is around 100 milliseconds for 1.5 T, and 120 milliseconds is commonly used at 3 T, but a wide range of values have been employed due to the following reasons: shorter TS values are desirable for quantitative perfusion imaging analysis as it reduces the nonlinearity in the relationship between contrast

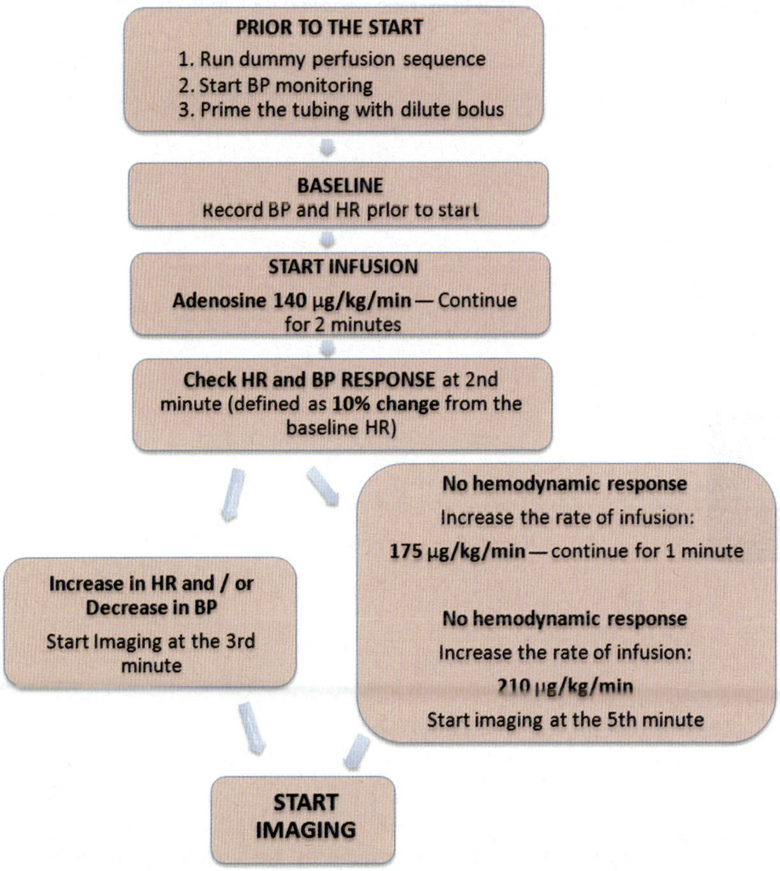

Figure 19-3. Adenosine stress protocol. BP, blood pressure; HR, heart rate.

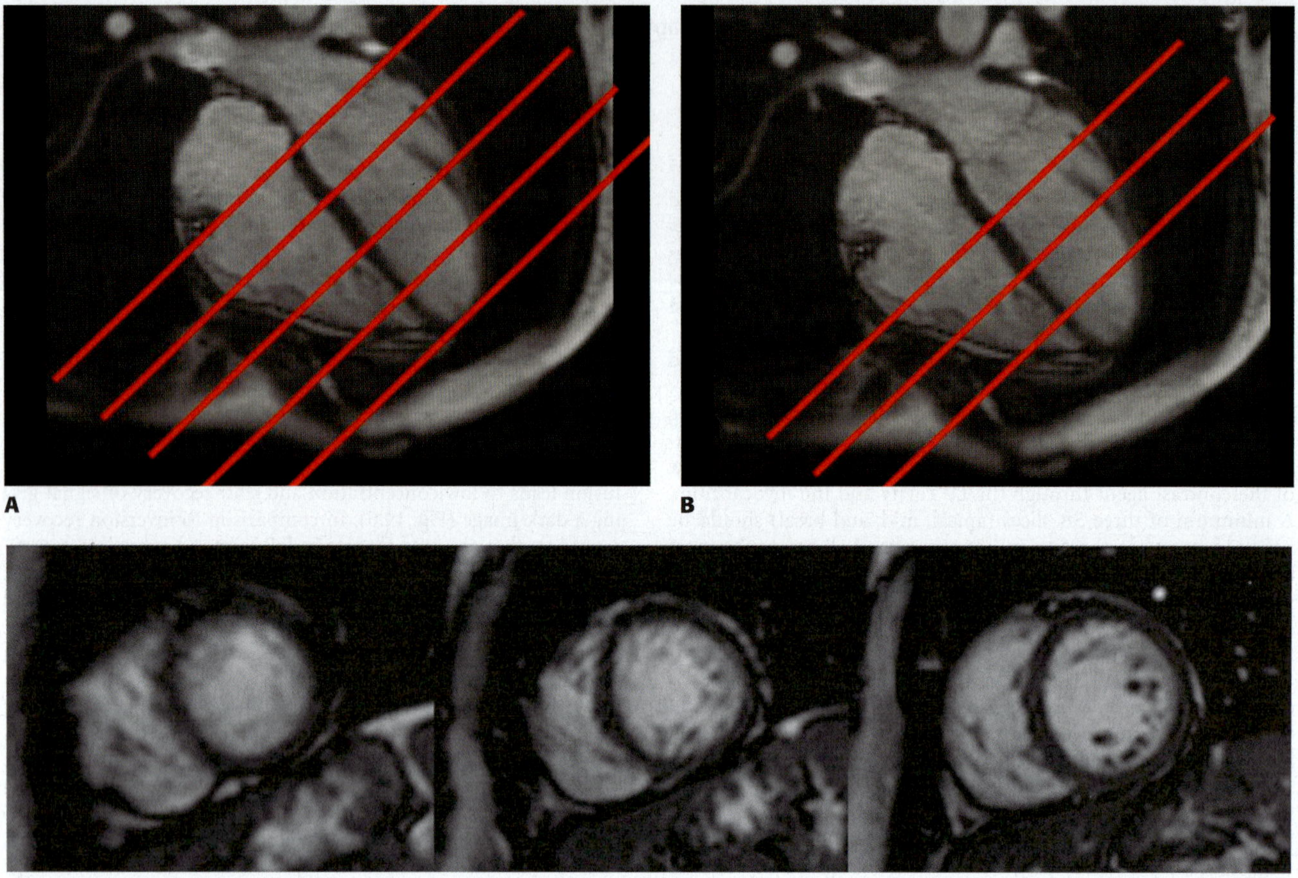

Figure 19-4. Illustrating planning of three SA slices. First, align five slices on the four-chamber view **(A)** and do the same in the two-chamber view (not shown). Ensure that the first slice is in the plane of the AV valves at end diastole and the last one is at the apex. Then, remove the first and the last slices by changing the number of slices from 5 to 3 **(B)**. Slice thickness should be 8 mm with in-plane resolution ≤3 mm to obtain three SA slices optimum for running the perfusion sequence **(C)**.

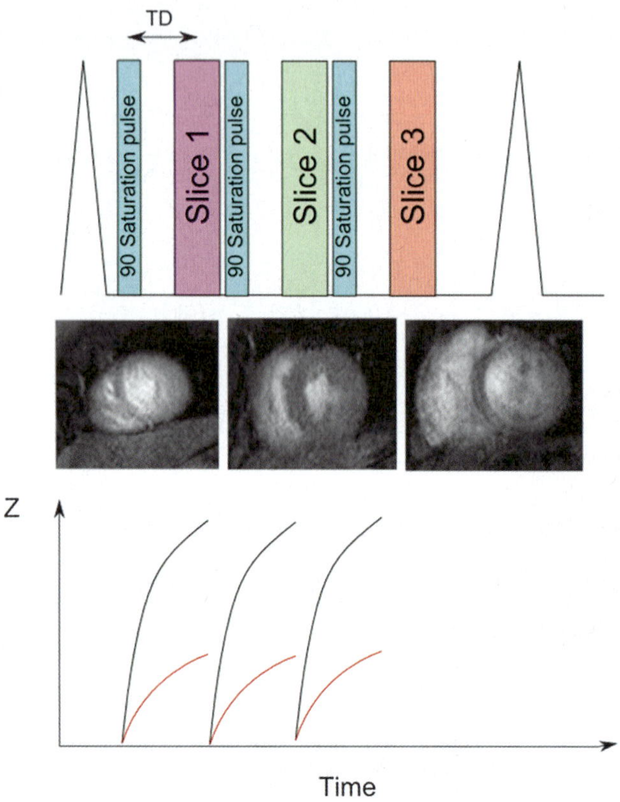

Figure 19-5. Perfusion sequences are usually generated with a 90-degree saturation pulse to produce the T1-weighted contrast.

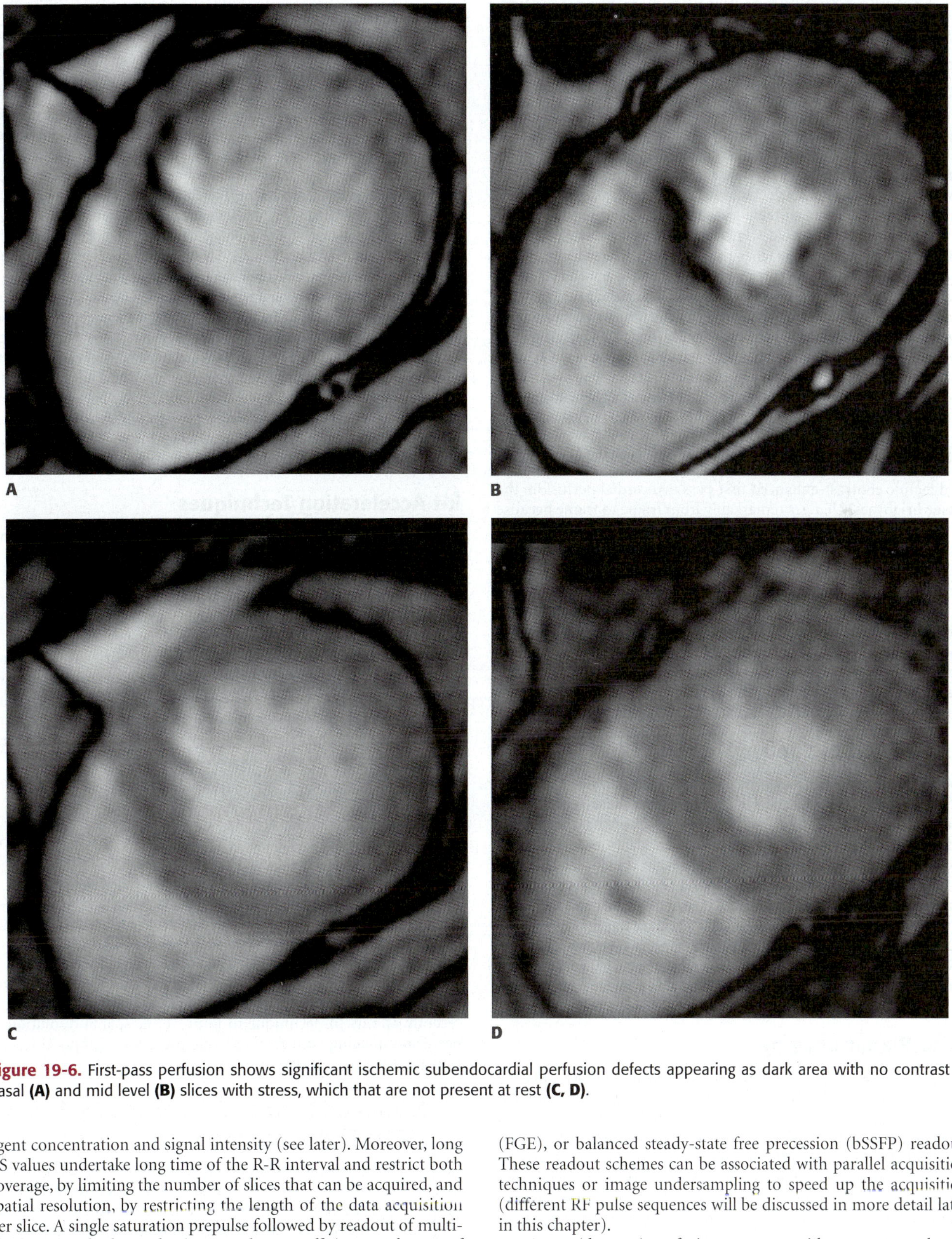

Figure 19-6. First-pass perfusion shows significant ischemic subendocardial perfusion defects appearing as dark area with no contrast in basal **(A)** and mid level **(B)** slices with stress, which that are not present at rest **(C, D)**.

agent concentration and signal intensity (see later). Moreover, long TS values undertake long time of the R-R interval and restrict both coverage, by limiting the number of slices that can be acquired, and spatial resolution, by restricting the length of the data acquisition per slice. A single saturation prepulse followed by readout of multiple slices can also be used to increase the scan efficiency at the cost of varying levels of image contrast between different slices. This is the preferred solution on slow scanners and can also be used in tachycardiac patients. However, full quantification becomes impossible.

Different imaging readout can be used; gradient-echo–echo-planar imaging (GRE-EPI) hybrid, fast or (turbo-) gradient-echo (FGE), or balanced steady-state free precession (bSSFP) readout. These readout schemes can be associated with parallel acquisition techniques or image undersampling to speed up the acquisition (different RF pulse sequences will be discussed in more detail later in this chapter).

A test (dummy) perfusion sequence without contrast should be run prior to starting the adenosine infusion in order to detect the presence of artifact, move or increase field of view if indicated, and ensure patient compliance with breath-holding commands. Patients are asked to hold their breath in end expiration during the injection of contrast as long as they can and are allowed to take shallow breaths thereafter until the end of the scan, and finally, the adequacy of VCG triggering is tested.

Gadolinium-containing contrast agents are given in a dose between 0.025 and 0.1 mmol/kg (4 mL/s) according to the local protocol followed by at least 25 mL saline flush (4 mL/s). The paramagnetic effect of gadolinium causes a shortening in T1 relaxation time thus resulting in more brightening of myocardial tissue with adequate perfusion. Higher doses (e.g., 0.1 mmol/kg body weight) are preferred for visual assessment but can result in more severe signal saturation effects; lower doses (e.g., 0.025 mmol/kg body weight) are more suitable for quantitative and semiquantitative evaluation. Breath-hold starts during early phases of contrast infusion before contrast reaches the LV cavity. Image for 40 to 50 heartbeats by which time contrast has passed through the LV myocardium. Rest perfusion is performed with the same protocol used for stress perfusion using identical slices and similar sequence settings but without vasodilator agent a minimum 10 to 15 minutes after the adenosine stress perfusion in order to compare stress with rest images. If regadenoson or dipyridamole is used, it may take longer than 15 minutes in order to be able to acquire the rest images, because both agents have a longer half-life than that of adenosine.

Different Acquisition RF Pulse Sequence

In dynamic contrast-enhanced first-pass myocardial perfusion, the image brightness changes remarkably from frame to frame because of the passage of the contrast agent through the heart so the ordinary multishot k-space imaging that fills k-space over multiple cardiac cycles is not applicable. Hence, in order to acquire images quickly, a single-shot technique with an FGE, EPI and hybrid EPI, or bSSFP pulse sequences are generally used to perform perfusion imaging. All three sequences are fast, having a very short TR since they avoid the need to wait for the remaining transverse magnetization to decay after readout of the MR signal echo. Several k-t acceleration techniques have been also developed for improving spatial resolution and temporal resolution of perfusion imaging.

Fast (or Turbo) Spoiled Gradient Echo

Spoiled gradient-echo sequence repeats rapidly the low flip angle RF pulse used in conventional gradient-echo pulse sequence to generate several gradient echoes. In order to avoid the interference that may occur between the transverse magnetization generated by each RF pulse with the signal generated from the consequent TR, a spoiler gradient at the end of each TR period, or alternatively a technique called RF spoiling,[11] is used to spoil this signal. Dynamic contrast-enhanced first-pass perfusion imaging requires fast imaging technique, so very short repetition time is used, for example, TR less than 10 milliseconds and time of echo (TE) less than 5 milliseconds, combined with a flip angle of around 30 degrees generating T1-weighted images.

Echo-Planar Imaging

EPI produces multiple gradient echoes following one RF pulse by changing the direction of frequency-encoding gradients quickly, generating an echo train. T2* decay throughout the echo train reduces the quality of images, relatively. Therefore, a hybrid EPI, also called segmented EPI, technique is typically employed in perfusion assessment where a number of shorter echo trains are obtained by applying multiple RF pulses. This reduces the harmful effect of T2* decay, enhancing the image quality while keeping the speeding advantage of the EPI technique.

Balanced Steady-State Free Precession

Compared to FGE, bSSFP gradient-echo sequence does not spoil the transverse magnetization, but instead, it reverses the signal dephased by the applied gradients by applying additional balancing gradients to rephase the MR signal before each subsequent RF pulse. After multiple repetitions, a steady-state condition arises, where the transverse magnetization from the successive repetitions accumulates to generate a much higher signal. The greater signal allows the use of higher receiver bandwidths, resulting in a shorter TE and TR compared to spoiled gradient-echo pulse sequences and therefore improved imaging efficiency. However, on the other hand, if the magnetic field is not homogenous, the transverse magnetization from several TRs can cancel each other rather than sum together in areas of magnetic field inhomogeneity, rendering the SSFP sequences susceptible to dark banding artifacts through the image.[12] Therefore, it is very important to ensure that the magnetic field is as uniform as possible over the region of interest (ROI). This can be achieved by a dynamic shimming process, which uses the magnetic field gradients to correct for patient-induced field inhomogeneity. The dark-rim artifacts can also be avoided by using TR as short as possible.

Dynamic contrast-enhanced first-pass perfusion requires very fast pulse sequence in order to acquire high spatial and temporal resolution, with optimum volume coverage, and high signal-to-noise ratio (SNR). Breath-holds required during perfusion test are relatively long and can be challenging for patients with heart failure or other breathing problems. Thus, several new acceleration techniques have been developed to overcome this problem.

k-t Acceleration Techniques

The raw data acquired from the scanner is typically plotted in a domain known as k-space and is converted mathematically to the final image by Fourier transformation. The central region of k-space defines the contrast in the image while the outer region of k-space defines the edges and structure boundaries (i.e., the high spatial frequencies).[13]

The most common k-space sampling trajectories are Cartesian, which means each data point is located in a Cartesian grid, with each echo filling an entire phase-encoded line. k-Space sampling can also have non-Cartesian trajectories, with the most common being spiral or radial. These facts have been exploited in different approaches aiming to reducing the scanning time as follows:

Parallel Imaging Approaches

To accelerate perfusion imaging and improve spatial resolution, parallel imaging approaches such as sensitivity encoding (SENSE) are used.[14,15] Parallel imaging depends on the spatial difference of radiofrequency coil sensitivities to fill the k-space and accelerate the image reconstruction process. Nevertheless, practically, this is limited to twofold acceleration due to associated artifact and noise drawback.[16] Another parallel k-t acceleration technique, known as kt-BLAST factor 5, with 11 training profiles has been shown to provide greater acceleration than SENSE and have been proposed more recently as a useful technique to improve the spatial resolution of perfusion imaging even further while preserving temporal resolution and cardiac coverage.[17]

Radial and Spiral Sequences Perfusion (SPIRIT) Approaches

Recently, novel techniques have been proposed for rapid acquisition of data. The main idea is to collect data in the k-space in radial spokes or spiral approach rather than the Cartesian approaches. A multislice "real-time" ungated data acquisition method is an example of the radial pulse sequence and has been proposed by Harrison et al.[18] The advantage of this method is the fast acquisition of data providing a number of perfusion images adequate for diagnosis without using ECG gating signals and during free breathing. Therefore, it can be potentially used in patients who have arrhythmias, have difficulties of gating, or are unable to perform adequate breath holding. In this method, a saturation recovery radial turboFLASH sequence is used, and 20 or 24 radial k-space radial rays in four subsets of five to six rays each are obtained for each slice. Four to five slices, according to the number of rays used, can be acquired after a single saturation pulse and a 40-millisecond delay. Each image is acquired in a few milliseconds (40 to 60 milliseconds) and is repeated continuously, roughly four times per second without gating and during free breathing. This means that each slice is acquired at different cardiac phases in every heartbeat. Image reconstruction from undersampled radial k-space data occurs by repetitive compressed sensing tool via spatial and temporal total variation constraints.[19] A retrospective image-based gating method is used, which is similar to a regional sum method applied to self-gate cardiac cine data.[20] Therefore, after reconstruction, the ungated images can be processed to self-gate into systole and diastole image sets. Subsequently, deformable image registration is used to correct for cardiac and respiratory motion remaining in systolic and diastolic images.[21] In comparison to conventional ECG-gated perfusion techniques, this method is efficient in terms of providing maximal information quickly enough for dynamic contrast-enhanced first-pass perfusion imaging; however, it has been assessed over a small number of patients, and larger trials on patients with ischemic heart disease are required to validate this technique for CMR perfusion. Linogram and PROPELLER are variable methods of radial acquisition. The explanation of these methods falls outside the scope of this chapter, but the interested reader is referred to the respective bibliographical references.[22,23]

Spiral k-space scanning is another fast data acquisition technique that allows a substantial speed of perfusion imaging compared to conventional techniques. In a spiral acquisition, each k-space line follows a spiral trajectory with variable number of interleaves (Fig. 19.7); this is valuable in terms of achieving more coverage of k-space with fewer shots than Cartesian. Spiral acquisition fills a circular area of k-space and neglects the corners of k-space, which are collected with a Cartesian acquisition. Simply, the technique consists of defining the required number of interleaves, sampling time, number of points per trajectory, nominal field of view, maximum gradient and slew rate parameters, and a function $w(t)$ describing the relative density as a function of time where (one corresponds to Nyquist sampling density) to determine the desired k-space trajectory. The details of this technique fall outside the scope of this chapter, but the interested reader is referred to the respective bibliographical references.[24,25] It is thought that spiral pulse sequences produce high-quality first-pass perfusion images with minimal dark-rim and off-resonance artifacts, high SNR and contrast-to-noise ratio (CNR), and good delineation of resting perfusion abnormalities.[26]

Furthermore, combining spiral sequence method with parallel imaging can reduce the scan time by a factor that is the product of the reduction factors for each of the techniques and therefore a very rapid imaging can be achieved. Variable techniques for performing image reconstruction are described, such as spiral partially parallel imaging with localized sensitivities, which is a simple image-domain approach that depends on localized coil sensitivities, and BOSCO, which is an approach relying on subsequent convolution operations in k-space.[24]

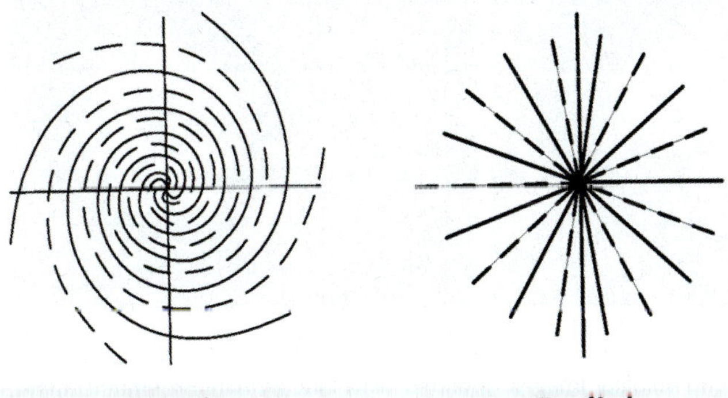

Figure 19-7. **Spiral and radial k-space filling.**

TABLE 19.3 **Comparison between the Three Sequences Commonly Used in Perfusion Imaging**

Sequence Type	Relative Acquisition Speed	Signal Intensity	Artifacts
FGE	Slow	Low	Prone to some artifacts
Hybrid EPI	Fastest	Medium	Less prone to artifacts
bSSFP	Fast	High	More prone to artifacts

Which Pulse Sequence to be Selected in Perfusion Imaging?

There is still no consensus on the optimal data acquisition pulse sequence for perfusion imaging despite several comparison studies. The ideal criteria of pulse sequence to be used include the acquisition speed, the lack of artifact, and two frequently used parameters of image quality: SNR and CNR. SNR is the ratio of the signal intensity of a specific tissue to the background image intensity in an area where signal is absent, while CNR is the ratio of the signal difference between two specific tissues and the background image intensity. Since FGE employs an RF pulse each readout line, it is less susceptible to variations in k-space, which should potentially make it less prone to ghosting artifacts.[27] Hybrid EPI is much faster, allowing more coverage and better resolution than FGE. On the other hand, bSSFP sequence generates the highest signal of the three methods via maintaining steady-state transverse magnetization.[28] The higher SNR and CNR of bSSFP images allow the detection of perfusion defects with greater sensitivity. In addition, a much higher bandwidth can be selected due to the higher SNR of bSSFP images, leading to shorter TE and TR, and subsequently making bSSFP a faster sequence than FGE. However, of the three sequences, SSFP is the most susceptible to artifacts caused by off resonance magnetization. It has a greater occurrence of susceptibility (i.e., dark rim) artifact and ghosting and is prone to Gibbs ringing in the endocardium because of the increased gap in signal intensity between the blood and the myocardium. Explanations of these artifacts are given elsewhere. Thus, bSSFP is capable of producing high-quality images in a relatively short time but prone to significant image artifacts. Table 19.3 summarizes the pros and cons of the three sequences.

Within one institution, the same perfusion sequence should be used until there are convincing arguments to change. This ensures consistency and avoids the learning curve related to new imaging approaches.

Data Analysis and Interpretation

Visual Assessment

Visual assessment relies on the detection of regions with lower signal (i.e., hypoperfusion) in comparison to normal myocardial segments. The speed of the contrast agent wash-in from the epicardial layer of the myocardium toward the endocardial surface is the best parameter for visual assessment. Visual assessment is usually performed comparing stress and rest images, and viability images obtained with late gadolinium enhancement techniques (Fig. 19.8).

How to Interpret Visual Assessment of Myocardial Perfusion Study, SCMR Guidelines[29]

Visual analysis of myocardial perfusion CMR images is often enough for most clinical indications. Rest and stress perfusion images should be displayed side by side. Displaying corresponding LGE images is also desirable. Image window and level adjustment is required in order to set a maximal window width without "overspilling" of the LV cavity signal into the myocardium. The way to adjust the window is as follows: ensure that myocardium before contrast arrival is nearly black and that signal in the RV and LV cavities is bright gray rather than a perfect white. Correct level and window settings may require review of both pre- and peak contrast images. Apply the same contrast, brightness, and window settings to all images of the dynamic series. Then, inspect series as cines and/or by scrolling through all the images. Some software packages allow the display of only dynamic images during the first myocardial passage bearing in mind that the key diagnostic feature is contrast arrival and first passage through the LV myocardium. Visual analysis relies on a comparison

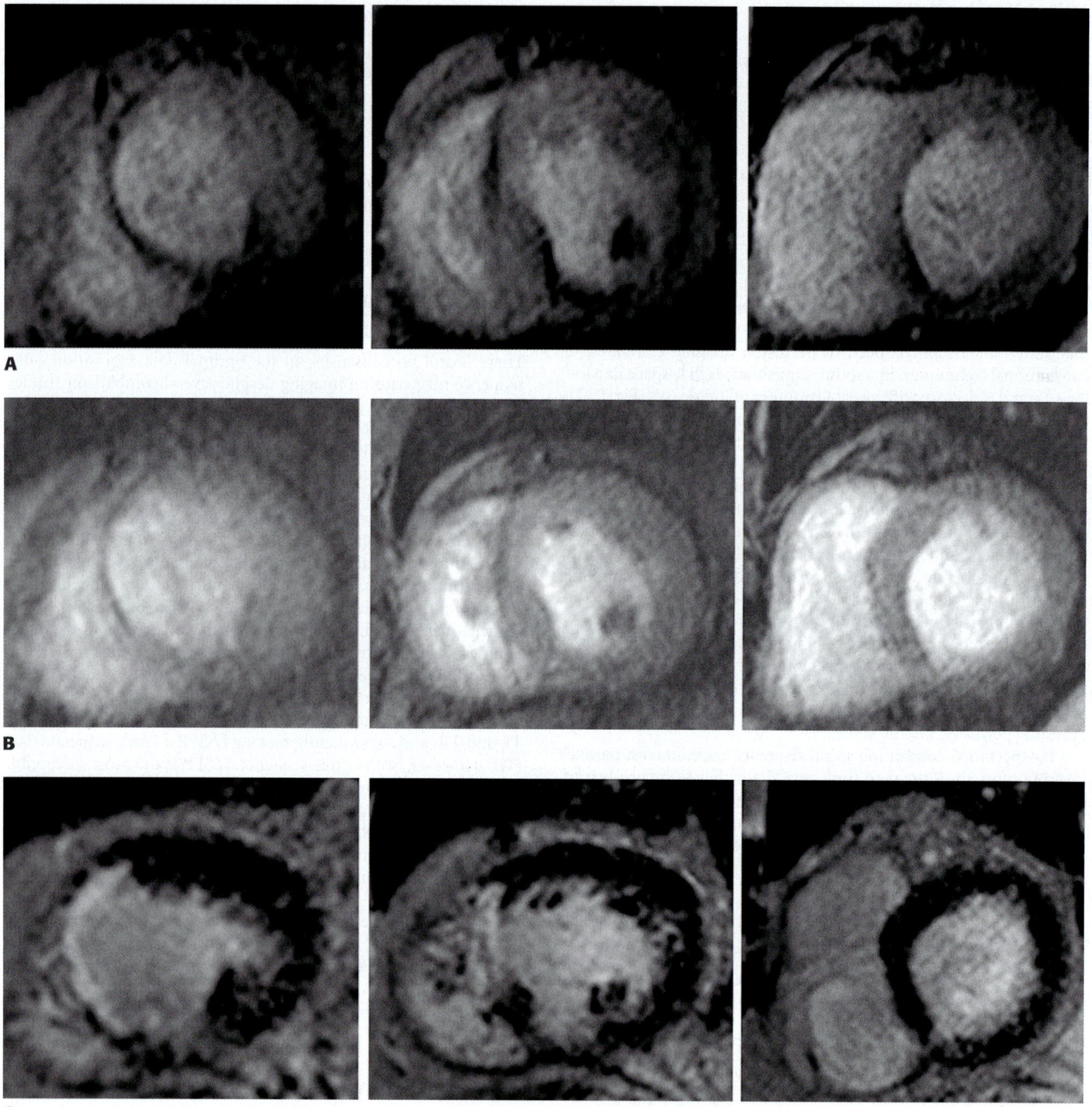

A

B

C

Figure 19-8. Visual assessment performed by comparing stress, rest, and viability images obtained with late gadolinium enhancement. Perfusion defects in stress **(A)** are extending beyond perfusion defects in rest images **(B)** and scar area in **(C)** indicating that there is periinfarct ischemia in both left anterior descending (LAD) artery and right coronary artery (RCA) territories.

TABLE 19.4 **Comparison between Criteria of True Inducible Perfusion Defect and Artifact**

Criteria	True Inducible Perfusion Defect	Artifact
1. Time of first appearance	When contrast arrives in LV myocardium	Before contrast arrives in LV myocardium (i.e., when contrast arrives in the LV blood pool)
2. Persistence	Persists beyond peak myocardial enhancement and for several R-R intervals (usually >4)	Often disappear before peak myocardial enhancement and lasts transiently for few R-R intervals (usually <6)
3. Number of pixels	More than one pixel wide	One pixel wide
4. Region of great intense	Usually most prominent in the subendocardial portion of the myocardium	May be prominent in the subendocardial portion of the myocardium
5. Transmural gradient	Often manifests as a transmural gradient across the wall thickness of the segment involved: densest in the endocardium and gradually becoming less dense toward the epicardium	Absence of transmural gradient
6. Dynamic change	Over time, defect regresses toward the subendocardium	No dynamic change
7. Comparison of stress and rest images[a]	Present at stress but not at rest	Present at stress and at rest without corresponding scar in LGE
8. Coronary artery territorial distribution	Follow the distribution territory of one or more coronary arteries except in microvascular dysfunction, it may be circumferential	Does not follow a territorial distribution

[a]Note that variations in HR and baseline contrast can change the appearance and presence of dark-rim defect between stress and rest perfusion images. Therefore, absence of dark-rim defect at rest with typical dark-rim artifact at stress should not on its own be considered diagnostic for an inducible perfusion defect.

between different regions to identify relative perfusion defects (i.e., hypoperfusion). Comparison can be made between endocardial and epicardial regions, between segments of the same slice, or between slices. Compare rest and stress images to identify stress inducible perfusion defects, and check for artifacts that can mimic hypoperfusion area in stress images but maintain the similar hypoperfusion appearance in rest images. It is worth to mention that in CMR, the presence of a "fixed perfusion defect" on rest and stress perfusion images to identify myocardial scar as done in nuclear perfusion imaging should not be used and may be misleading due to contrast accumulation masking a perfusion defect in the second scan. Instead, scar should be identified from LGE images so that it is preferable to display the late gadolinium images simultaneously with stress/rest perfusion images.

Comparison between criteria of true inducible perfusion defect and artifact is demonstrated in Table 19.4. Report location and extent of inducible perfusion defect(s) using the AHA segment model[30,31] including the following points:

1. Estimation of number of segments involved
2. Transmurality of perfusion defect
3. Extent of perfusion defect relative to scar on LGE images

Pitfalls of Visual Analysis

Dark-Rim Artifacts

A typical source of false-positive reports is small subendocardial dark-rim–like artifacts[32] since they are mimicking perfusion defects and should therefore be taken into consideration while assessing myocardial perfusion imaging (Fig. 19.9). Generally, in contrast to

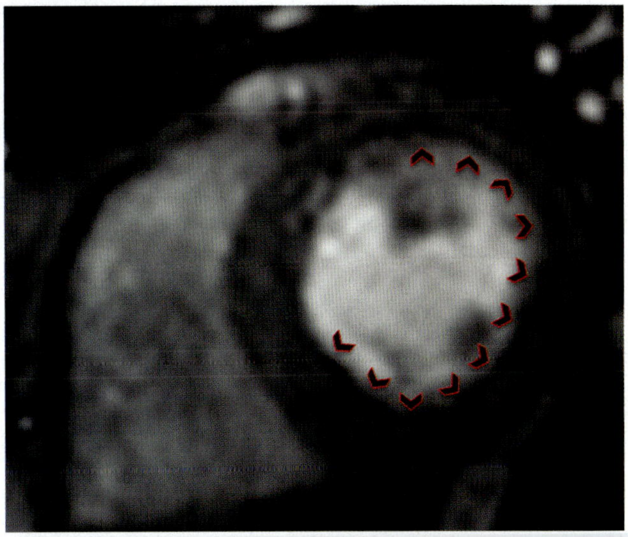

Figure 19-9. Dark-rim artifact (*arrowheads*): **The** ***black rim*** **starts to appear when the contrast enhances the LV cavity and before arriving to the myocardium.** It is a very thin band extending through the interphase between two tissues with different magnetic properties (i.e., blood pool in LV cavity and myocardium).

true inducible perfusion defects, dark-rim artifacts tend to be dark black and circumferential, often start with the first-pass contrast reaching the LV cavity and before the myocardial contrast wash-in, last for few heartbeats after the contrast agent has left the LV, and contain only 1 pixel in width (Table 19.4). They are usually due to susceptibility (i.e., artifacts due to strong differences of magnetization within a small area—e.g., one voxel) and manifest mainly in the phase-encoding direction. Theses artifacts lead to a reduction in signal intensity compared to baseline myocardial signal, while a true inducible perfusion defect, on the other hand, always shows an increase in signal intensity compared to the baseline although this rise of intensity is subtle. These tiny differences can be difficult to identify visually. It can therefore be useful to draw a ROI around the suspected artifact and display its signal intensity–time profile. Using smaller doses of contrast agent, FGE rather than bSSFP and higher spatial resolution can attenuate these artifacts.

Coil Bias

Distance of the myocardium from the surface coil can affect signal intensity (i.e., the remote part of myocardium from the surface coil may appear darker than the close part, which may misinterpreted as hypoperfusion). This issue can be avoided if acquisition is corrected for coil sensitivity.

Multivessel Disease

Multivessel disease can result in the presence of balanced ischemia, and thus the images can show a diffuse hypoperfusion, which is hard to be appreciated visually. This can lead to false-negative reporting and requires a great consideration in relevant clinical circumstances. On visual analysis, a definite signal gradient between the endocardial and epicardial layers may be visualized in multivessel disease.[33] In this particular situation, quantitative analysis of the dynamic perfusion data may be useful to detect globally reduced MPR.

Microvascular Disease

This phenomenon is due to pathology affecting the myocardial microvasculature such as diabetes mellitus and systemic hypertension, which may lead to circumferential reduction in perfusion.[34–37] This can lead to false-positive reporting relative to angiographic methods and needs to be considered in relevant clinical contexts. Features indicating microvascular disease are the presence of concentric LV hypertrophy and a circumferential perfusion defect overlapping coronary territories (Fig. 19.10). Discrimination between microvascular disease and multivessel disease can be very challenging. In this circumstance, quantitative analysis of the dynamic perfusion data may be useful to differentiate microvascular disease from multivessel disease.

Inadequate Vasodilation

Inadequate vasodilation during scanning may give rise to false-negative interpretation.[38] Quantitative analysis of the dynamic perfusion data can be useful in detecting globally myocardial hypoperfusion in case of inadequate vasodilation.

Presence of Scar

Perfusion defects in scarred area due to previous myocardial infarction should be reviewed carefully by comparing the location and extend of the defect in perfusion images with LGE images to detect whether there is inducible ischemia extending beyond the scarred myocardium.[39] High-resolution sequences can facilitate the identification of periinfarction ischemia.

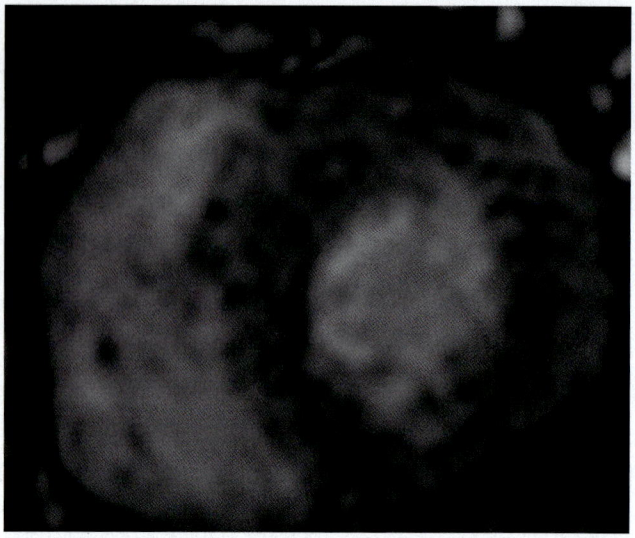

Figure 19-10. Microvascular disease, a circumferential perfusion defect with epicardial to endocardial contrast wash-in gradient in a patient with LV hypertrophy.

Semiquantitative Analysis Method

Similar to visual assessment, the rapidity of the wash-in of the contrast agent is the best parameter for semiquantification. Semiquantitative analysis measures the normalized upslope of signal intensity, that is, myocardium/ventricular blood pool—also known as arterial input function (AIF). This analysis approach relies on depicting the characteristics of the signal intensity profile of the contrast agent during myocardial perfusion, without estimating the MBF itself, and the upslope of signal intensity of the contrast agent wash-in is used as an index for blood flow; hence it is known as "semiquantitative analysis method."

Signal homogeneity is essential for accurate analysis. However, the signal acquired is usually inhomogeneous because of variation of the coil sensitivities used for data acquisition. The change of the upslope induced by the vasodilator agent, rather than the upslope itself, is used in order to correct for signal intensity variations. The simplest method is a linear fit of the time curve of the myocardial signal. Another challenge for the semiquantitative analysis is the variation in the arrival speeds of the different boluses during stress and rest. Therefore, the myocardial upslope is corrected for the upslope of the signal in the LV cavity.

How to Perform Semiquantitative Postprocessing

An image from the dynamic series with adequate contrast between the different cardiac chambers should be selected and then LV endocardial and epicardial contours shall be outlined manually or by using automated software option on this image (Fig. 19.11). Propagate contours to all other dynamic images. Correct the contour position for through-plane and in-plane motion. Care must be taken to avoid partial volume effect from blood, fat, or air to be involved in the ROI. Draw another ROI in the LV blood pool, excluding the papillary muscles, preferably in the basal slice. Then, select a reference point in the LV myocardium for segmentation (usually the RV insertion point) and segment LV myocardium according to AHA classification. Develop SI–time curves for myocardial segments +/− LV blood pool. Consider generating division into endocardial and epicardial layers and repeat the analysis.

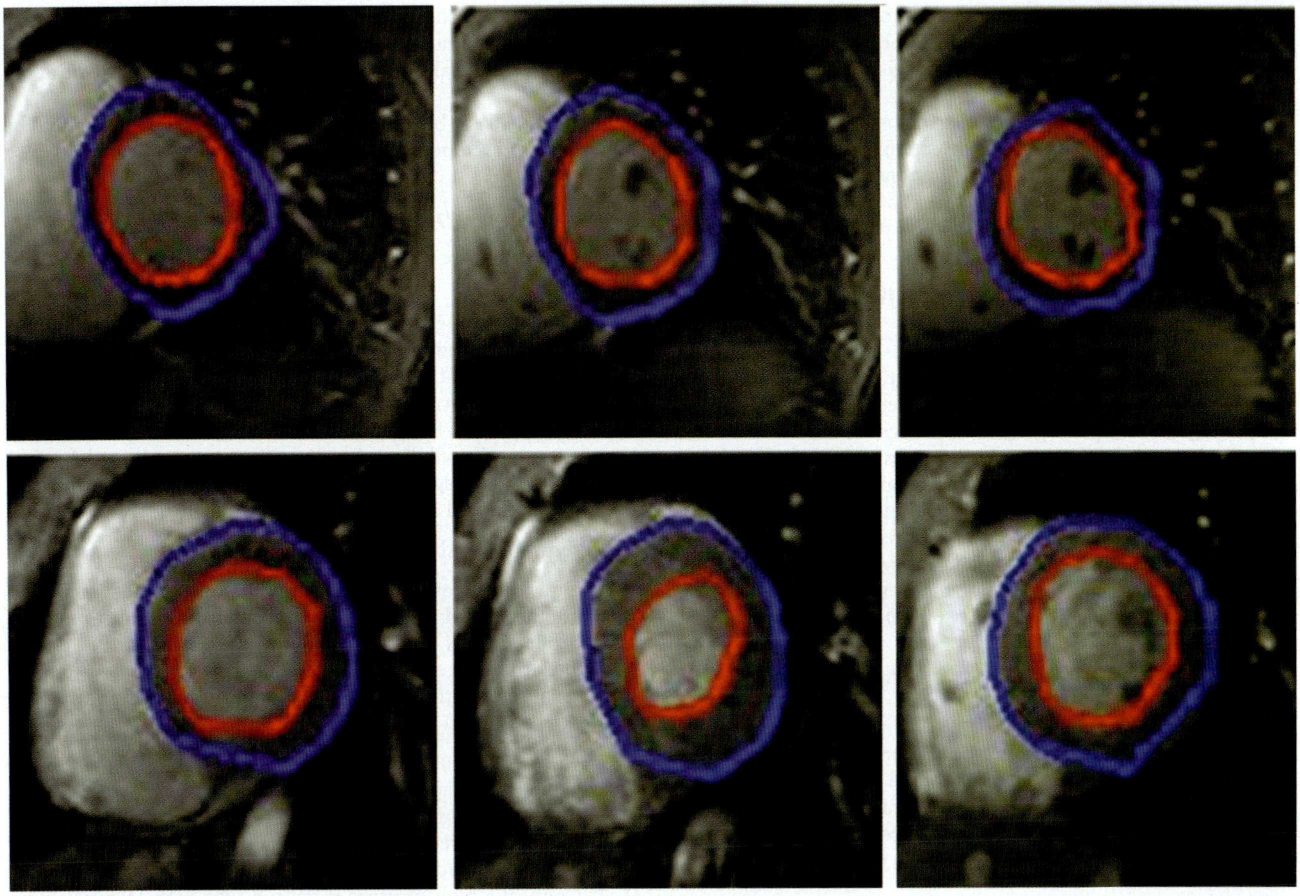

Figure 19-11. Segmentation of LV for semiquantitative analysis; select an image from the dynamic series with adequate contrast between the different cardiac chambers. Outline LV endocardial and epicardial contours manually or using automated software. Propagate contours to all other dynamic series. Avoid partial volume effect from blood, fat, or air to be involved in the ROI.

Commonly used semiquantitative analysis methods are as follows:

- Time-to-peak SI of the myocardial SI profile.[40]
- Maximal upslope of the myocardial SI profile may be normalized to LV upslope.[41]
- Ratio of stress/rest for the time-to-peak SI of the myocardial SI profile, also known as "myocardial perfusion reserve index."[42]
- The upslope integral (area under the SI–time curve).[2]

For more details about these methods, the reader is advised to review references.[43]

Pitfalls of Semiquantitative Analysis

Semiquantitative analysis is not linear with perfusion above 2 mL/g/min.[3] Therefore, the parameters acquired from semiquantification are called "myocardial perfusion reserve (MPR) index." Even though this approach is not fully quantitative and needs careful placement of the regions of interest, nevertheless, it has been shown to accurately discriminate between ischemic and normal segments and has been a highly reproducible yield among different centers. However, each sequence requires its own set of normal values.

Quantitative Analysis Methods

This means absolute quantification of MBF in mL/g/min of tissue by postprocessing of first-pass myocardial perfusion CMR data. In order to perform absolute quantification of MBF, a measurable relationship must exist between the signal intensity changes in the image and underlying blood flow. The vast majority of quantitative analysis methods require that the measured ventricular blood pool (AIF) and myocardial tissue (tissue function, TF) enhancement data are measured and mathematically deconvolved in order to estimate the system impulse response function, from which myocardial perfusion can be determined. Multiple fitting models have been suggested to deconvolve the myocardial signal and to account for the different compartments of contrast agent distribution.

There are two main deconvolution approaches: compartment kinetic modeling and Fermi function deconvolution. In compartmental kinetic models, the forward influx of contrast from the blood to the myocardium is taken to represent absolute MBF.[41,43] Fermi function method is based on the calculation of the amount of contrast present within a region of myocardium.[40] This approach is relatively robust to the effects of extracellular accumulation of the contrast agent during first pass of the contrast. Both of the approaches described above have been shown to correlate with myocardial perfusion over a wide range of flow. Several other approaches have been used for deconvolution and are currently under validation.[42]

All quantification models have in common that they anticipate linearity between signal intensity and contrast concentration. However, at higher contrast concentration, the curve loses its linearity. To overcome this problem, two techniques can be used, dual bolus where relatively low doses of contrast (0.03 to 0.05 mmol/kg) are given as a prebolus for data acquisition, followed by mean bolus or dual sequences (see below). Several analysis methods have been described, including model-based methods[44] and model-independent methods.[45]

Quantitative and semiquantitative methods of CMR perfusion data analysis may play a role in the detection of balanced multivessel ischemia, or suspected inadequate response to vasodilator agent as well as in research studies of therapeutic interventions, but are currently of minimal use in routine clinical practice.

Pitfalls of Quantitative Analysis

Dark-Rim Artifacts

The solutions for these artifacts at the stage of postprocessing are limited. Exclusion of the dark-rim band when the endocardial contour is delineated, by pulling the contour back toward the epicardial layer, can be used, but this may lead to missing a perfusion defect limited to the excluded subendocardial region. Another solution is to ignore the data points in the signal intensity curve where a significant drop of the signal beyond the precontrast baseline level occurs. Obviously, this is also a limited option, as it needs the signal intensity curve to be constrained by a model to estimate blood flow, and the missing data points make a model-independent analysis unfeasible.

Signal Intensity Artifacts

The regional signal intensity average at the endocardial border may include a mixture from the ventricular blood pool. Using the higher spatial resolution of MRI, to further optimize the image acquisition, and careful delineation of the endocardial border can reduce the signal intensity artifacts.

Arterial Signal Saturation

Quantitative analysis methods require measuring the contrast enhancement in the LV blood pool (i.e., AIF) as reference for the analysis of the myocardial contrast enhancement. Therefore, accurate estimation of the AIF is essential for quantitative analysis. However, the contrast enhancement in the LV cavity blood pool has a nonlinear pattern at high concentration due to arterial signal saturation, which can lead to underestimation of the arterial input. In order to avoid arterial signal saturation, two techniques have been developed, which are as follows

Dual-Contrast Bolus Technique

This technique consists of administrating a low dose of diluted contrast agent (dilute ratio is 1:10) as a prebolus followed by the main bolus of neat contrast agent. The dual-bolus technique enables accurate quantification of MBF by first-pass myocardial perfusion CMR using the high gadolinium concentration contrast of the main bolus, and in the same time, the lower diluted gadolinium concentration of the prebolus maintains the linearity of the LV signal intensity. In other words, the role of low-dose contrast bolus is to measure the AIF of contrast, which is then followed by a higher dosage bolus to acquire the myocardial contrast enhancement.[3]

The dual-bolus method allows accurate first-pass myocardial perfusion analysis by CMR.[46] However, the preparation of the dual-bolus method is complex and requires an injector with a programmed pause and suitable postprocessing software.

Pitfalls of the Dual-Bolus Technique

Both the main (neat) bolus of contrast agent and the diluted prebolus should have an equal volume and be administered with the same flow rate.[3]

A saline flush should be given immediately after each bolus to maintain a solid amount of contrast agent in the LV chamber. The saline flush should also be equal in volume and administered at the same rate.[46]

The time delay between each bolus of contrast agent should be adjusted to prevent temporal overlap and may require to be adapted to HR.[47]

How to Setup a Dual-Bolus Technique[48]

Preparation of the 10% diluted prebolus for rest and stress perfusion:

1. Draw 1 mL of gadolinium contrast agent into a 10-mL syringe (syringe 1) and dilute it to a 10% solution by adding 9 mL of saline. Repeat this process for rest injection (syringe 2)
2. Calculate the volume of the prebolus according to the weight of the patient, for example, if a 70-kg patient requires 7 mL of 1.0 mmol/L gadolinium contrast agent, then discard 3 mL of the contrast agent from the prepared 10-mL syringes (i.e., syringes 1 and 2 contain 10% dilute of contrast)

Preparation of the neat main bolus for rest and stress perfusion:

1. Draw the same volume of neat gadolinium contrast agent into another 10-mL syringes (i.e., syringes 3 and 4 thus contain the proper dose of neat gadolinium contrast agent).

Note: All syringes should be carefully labeled.

Preparation of the injector and tubing (Figs. 19.12 and 19.13):

1. Fill both the first (A) and second (B) power injector syringes with at least 60 mL of saline.
2. Connect Y-shaped long tube to the injector's syringes as per the manufacturer's instructions.
3. Connect a three-way stopcock (stopcock A) to the distal end of the Y-shaped long tube.
4. Connect a high-pressure extension tube with 15 mL volume to stopcock A.
5. Flush these tubes with saline.
6. Connect the distal end of the high-pressure extension tubes to a venous cannula in the patient's antecubital vein.

Programming the dual-head power injector:

1. Injector A (first phase): Set the flow rate to 4 mL/s and the volume of saline flush to 25 mL.

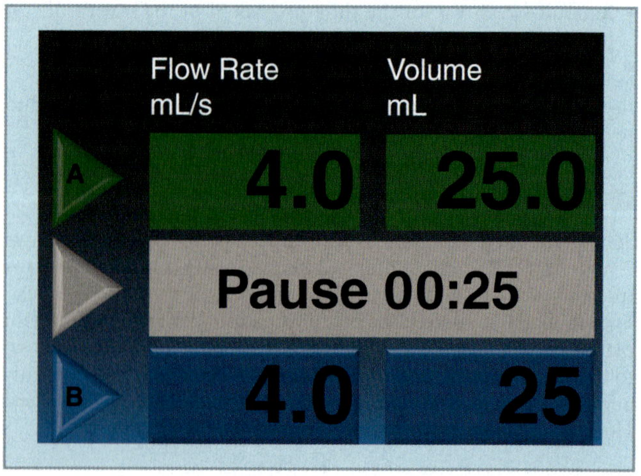

Figure 19-12. Programming the dual-head power injector with flow rate 4 mL/s and volume 25 mL for both injectors (*A*, *B*), and set a pause time between the two injections of 25 seconds.

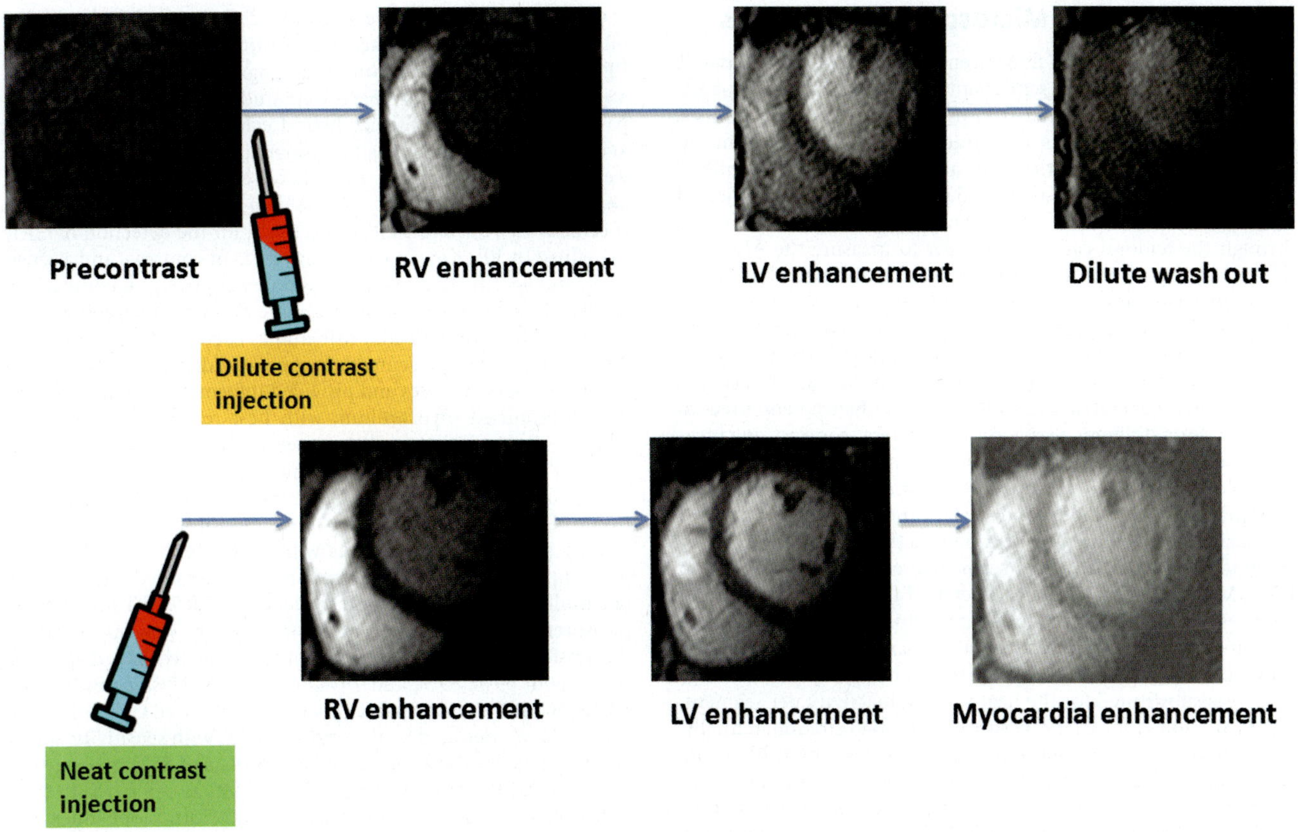

Figure 19-13. Dual bolus of first-pass perfusion technique in SA: the first image corresponds to the beginning of the sequence before intravenous injection of the contrast agent (baseline). Then, the contrast reaches the right ventricle, the left ventricle, and finally the myocardium. The dilute bolus is given at first followed by the neat bolus with a 25-second pause in between the two boluses. After 40 heartbeats, the redistribution of the contrast agent is complete. After 15 minutes, most of the contrast agent is washed out and the rest scan can be performed.

2. Injector A (second phase): Program the pause or the delay time between the prebolus and the main bolus, use the "pause" phase, and set the required time delay.
3. Injector B: Set the flow rate and volume of the saline injection similar to injector A.

Loading the gadolinium contrast agent and dual-bolus injection:

1. Connect the 10-mL syringe containing dilute prebolus (syringe 1) to stopcock A.
2. Once the setup for the perfusion scan is ready, arm the injector.
3. Just before the power injection, turn stopcock A and manually inject the entire volume of dilute prebolus (syringe 1) into the high-pressure extension tube.
4. Disconnect the syringe 1 (dilute prebolus) and connect the syringe containing neat main bolus (syringe 3) to stopcock A.
5. Start the perfusion scan and the power injection simultaneously.
6. During the delay time, turn stopcock A and manually inject the entire volume of neat bolus from the syringe 3 into the high-pressure extension tube.
7. After the programmed delay, injector B (saline) starts. This allows the contrast agent within the extension tube to be pushed into the patients.

Dual-Imaging Sequence Technique

The dual-imaging sequence involves low-resolution dynamic imaging of the contrast enhancement in the LV cavity and higher-resolution imaging of myocardial enhancement during the same heartbeat. The low-resolution sequence of the contrast enhancement in the ventricular cavity, yielding lower T1-weighting images than for the myocardium, is used to avoid saturation and to improve linearity at higher contrast concentrations, while the higher-resolution sequence acquires myocardial contrast enhancement with strong T1 weighting.[49]

Respiratory Artifacts

Respiratory artifacts due to inappropriate breath holding can also compromise study interpretation. Patients should be adequately trained to hold their breath before the study to avoid respiratory artifacts. A test (dummy) perfusion sequence without contrast should be run before starting the adenosine infusion in order to detect the presence of artifact and ensure patient compliance with breath-holding commands.

Recently proposed three-dimensional (3D) myocardial perfusion CMR methods and other fast techniques like SENSE can cover the whole heart within a single acquisition shot and may overcome the limitations of respiratory motion artifacts and selective cardiac coverage.

Validation Studies

Quantitative CMR perfusion imaging has been validated against microspheres in animals, more established noninvasive imaging modalities like SPECT and PET, and invasive catheter-based techniques for functional appreciation of coronary flow.

Validation against Microspheres in Animals

Christian et al.[3] compared fluorescent microsphere measurements of MBF with qualitative, semiquantitative, and absolute quantitative measurements of first-pass perfusion CMR in 16 canines. Coronary artery occlusion or intracoronary adenosine infusion at 20 μg/kg/min was performed, and approximately 5 million fluorescent-labeled microspheres 15 μm in diameter were injected into the left atrial catheter with simultaneous reference sampling through the femoral catheter. In order to measure the AIF from the LV blood pool and improve the SNR for myocardial enhancement, first-pass myocardial perfusion imaging was performed using a dual-bolus approach of gadopentetate dimeglumine (0.0025 mmol/kg followed by 0.10 mmol/kg). The first, small bolus was used to determine the LV blood pool AIF. The second, higher bolus generated high myocardial enhancement used to calculate four different perfusion parameters: contrast enhancement ratio—considered as a qualitative method, myocardial-to-LV upslope index ratio, upslope integral ratio—both considered as semiquantitative methods, and Fermi function deconvolution—considered as absolute quantification method. Saturation recovery gradient-echo MRI with a segmented echo-planar readout on 1.5-T MRI was performed to generate T1-weighted images and acquires contrast-enhanced first-pass perfusion data. Microsphere estimates of MBF were measured, after sacrificing the animals, by using conventional formulas where the number of spheres per segment was substituted for the degree of radioactivity per segment. The MBF values for each heart slice were plotted circumferentially. It was found that absolute quantitative analysis of MBF, using Fermi deconvolution, correlated with microsphere MBF measurement ($r = 0.95$, $p < 0.001$) over the whole spectrum of blood flow rates encountered (from 0 to >5.0 mL/min/g). On the other hand, both qualitative and semiquantitative measurements did not show correlation with MBF.

Another experimental study on dogs compared first-pass perfusion imaging with SPECT imaging and using microspheres performed, as a reference for MBF, on 1.5-T MRI with bSSFP inversion recovery sequence. The quantitative analysis was generated by measuring the areas under signal intensity–time curves from the onset of contrast appearance to the peak of the curve showing the most rapid upstroke where a curve was drawn for each radial 30-degree sector of the myocardial full thickness. The results of the areas under signal intensity–time curves represented the relative regional myocardial flows. They were consecutively normalized to the highest sector value and compared with relative regional concentrations of fluorescent microspheres normalized to their highest sector value. The endocardial-to-epicardial slope of the regression represented the transmural flow gradient across the wall. The study demonstrated the ability of perfusion MRI to determine regional reductions in full-thickness MBF across a wider range of coronary vasodilation than SPECT. Perfusion MRI was also correlated with reference microsphere relative regional myocardial flows over the full range of vasodilation.[4]

Validation against PET

PET is well established as a validated technique for noninvasive quantitative measurements of myocardial perfusion using either $^{15}O_2$-labeled water or $^{13}NH_3$. CMR has emerged as a potential tool for clinical quantitative perfusion imaging and may be a good alternative for noninvasive quantitative evaluation of the myocardial perfusion and detection of CAD.

Initial studies comparing CMR semiquantitative analysis methods with PET have shown good correlation in patients with CAD.[50,51]

In a pivotal prospective study by Schwitter et al.,[50] the quality of a multislice CMR approach was identified and compared to both PET and quantitative coronary angiography (QCA). A total of 48 patients and healthy subjects were studied by dipyridamole first-pass CMR using a multislice hybrid echo-planar pulse sequence, and segmental signal intensity upslope quantitative measurements were compared to $^{13}NH_3$ PET. Receiver–operator characteristic analysis of subendocardial upslope data revealed a sensitivity and specificity of 91% and 94%, respectively, for the detection of CAD as defined by PET (mean CFR minus 2 SD of controls) and a sensitivity and specificity of 87% and 85%, respectively, in comparison to QCA (diameter stenosis ≥50%). The number of pathologic sectors per patient on PET and MR studies correlated linearly (slope: 0.94; $r = 0.76$). The presented MR approach identified patients with coronary artery stenoses and provided information on the amount of compromised myocardium, with best results being obtained when perfusion indices were assessed in the subendocardial layer, which is most sensitive to an ischemic challenge.

In another study comparing semiquantitative adenosine perfusion CMR with quantitative measures of QCA and PET in healthy volunteers and patients with CAD, Ibrahim et al.[51] compared upslope and peak-intensity indices, measured with the use of a multislice ultra-fast hybrid sequence to $^{13}NH_3$ PET flow reserve measurements. Localization of coronary artery stenosis, based on the upslope index, yielded sensitivity, specificity, and diagnostic accuracy of 69%, 89%, and 79%, respectively. Upslope index correlated with PET flow reserve ($r = 0.70$). A reduced CFR (PET: 2.0, MRI: 1.3) was detected by the upslope index with sensitivity, specificity, and diagnostic accuracy of 86%, 84%, and 85%, respectively. Although MPR was underestimated by CMR as compared to PET, a close relationship was observed between MRI upslope index and PET estimates of flow reserve, yielding acceptable diagnostic performance for localization of CAD.

Improvement in imaging acquisition and postprocessing methods permitted the development of quantitative algorithms in perfusion CMR. Few studies have examined its accuracy and diagnostic value against PET perfusion. Parkka et al.[52] studied the accuracy of first-pass CMR and kinetic modeling for quantitative analysis of MBF and MPR during dipyridamole infusion, compared to PET, in 18 healthy subjects. Using a perfusion-related parameter, the unidirectional influx constant (K_i), MBF was computed in three coronary artery territories. There was a significant correlation for both dipyridamole-induced flow and MPR between CMR and PET. However, in accordance with previous studies, MPR values provided with MRI were lower compared to PET (2.5 ± 1.0 vs. 4.3 ± 1.8).

In the same concept, Fritz-Hansen et al.[53] assessed quantitative CMR with the K_i perfusion method in healthy volunteers, using $^{13}NH_3$ PET as a reference method. Ten healthy males were examined with combined PET and CMR dipyridamole perfusion imaging in order to determine absolute MPR. A two-compartment perfusion model used to fit CMR-derived myocardial and blood time concentration curves. A linear relationship was observed between CMR- and PET-derived MPR for regional and global data. A good agreement between the two methods to determine low or high perfusion reserves was found.

These studies, with the use of quantitative CMR methods in healthy humans, enforced previous evidence that K_i constant can identify myocardial regions of occluded infarct-related arteries. However, the method seems to underestimate perfusion at stress compared to PET.

Moreover, model-independent analysis methods tested at 3-T CMR have provided similar results. Pack et al.[54] applied in five normal subjects adenosine perfusion CMR imaging with the use of a saturation recovery turboFLASH sequence and subsequent PET perfusion imaging. Regional and pixel wise quantitative perfusion estimates correlated with dynamic $^{13}NH_3$ PET ($r = 0.85$) and were similar to results from other validated CMR studies. The authors demonstrated that a model-independent analysis method can be used to quantify myocardial perfusion with dynamic contrast-enhanced perfusion CMR.

More recently, Morton et al.[55] compared MBF and MPR with both CMR and PET in a cohort of 41 patients with known or suspected CAD. Patients underwent quantitative $^{13}NH_3$ PET and adenosine CMR perfusion imaging before coronary angiography. CMR-derived indices correlated well with PET-derived measurements ($r = 0.75$). MBF and MPR for the two lowest scoring segments in each coronary territory also correlated strongly between the two techniques ($r = 0.79$). Absolute CMR perfusion values correlated significantly, but weakly, with PET values both at rest ($r = 0.32$) and during stress ($r = 0.37$). An MPR by PET < 1.44 predicted significant CAD with 82% sensitivity and 87% specificity, and MPR by CMR < 1.45 predicted significant CAD with 82% sensitivity and 81% specificity. This has been the single study so far to compare fully quantitative CMR against PET perfusion imaging in patients with CAD. Quantitative indices derived by the two techniques correlated strongly, and both techniques proved comparable and accurate. However, the correlation between the absolute perfusion values from PET and CMR was relatively weak, suggesting that a single absolute stress perfusion cutoff value is not superior for the detection of CAD at the moment. Interestingly, there was not any incremental value in combining MPR data from both PET and CMR for the diagnosis of CAD.

Overall, although the number of studies is relatively small, a good correlation has been steadily confirmed for semi- and absolute quantitative perfusion CMR methods, when PET quantification techniques are considered as the reference standard. Both techniques have proven their usefulness for the detection and estimation of coronary artery stenosis. The tendency to measure lower stress perfusion with CMR than with PET, observed in all studies, could in part be explained by the different methods used in both the acquisition and the postprocessing of the exams. Different contrast agents with particular pharmacodynamic and pharmacokinetic properties, differences among stressors as well as differences in the mathematical models used for exam analysis, could also partially explain this difference. Further research in this area will be needed.

Validation against Fractional Flow Reserve

Pressure wire–derived fractional flow reserve (FFR) during coronary angiogram is considered the invasive gold standard reference for assessing the functional significance of coronary artery stenosis and a better comparator for ischemia assessment than anatomical coronary angiography. Multiple studies have recently compared perfusion CMR with FFR qualitatively, semiquantitatively, and/or quantitatively, in terms of diagnostic accuracy for detection of significant obstructive CAD.[7,42,56–58]

In a study over 43 patients with suspected or known CAD using FFR cutoff value of 0.75 and 1.5-T MRI system for perfusion imaging, first-pass perfusion CMR showed a sensitivity of 88% and specificity of 90% to discriminate hemodynamically significant coronary artery stenosis as defined by FFR values.[42] Kuhl et al.[56] studied 19 patients with known CAD and 9 normal subjects served as control with FFR cutoff value of 0.75 for determining significant coronary artery stenosis. MPR derived from perfusion CMR performed on 1.5-T MRI was compared to the FFR-derived data. MPR by CMR < 1.5 predicted significant CAD with 92% sensitivity and 92% specificity. Costa et al.[57] compared MPR and FFR prospectively on a cohort of 30 patients with suspected CAD using 1.5-T MRI scanner. MPR < 2.04 predicted significant CAD with 93% sensitivity and 57% specificity.

More recently, Lockie et al.[58] using a 3-T MR system with high resolution (1.2 × 1.2 × 10 mm) to perform quantitative perfusion CMR and calculate MPR using Fermi deconvolution and compare the results to angiographic coronary lesions with FFR cutoff value of 0.75 revealed the cutoff MPR to detect such lesions 1.58, with a sensitivity of 0.80, specificity of 0.89 ($p < 0.0001$), and area under the curve of 0.89 ($p < 0.0001$).

Validation Using Meta-analyses

In a meta-analysis by Nandalur et al.,[59] with pooled data from 24 studies using perfusion CMR on a total of 1,516 patients, comparing the results of perfusion CMR with coronary angiography. Perfusion CMR showed a sensitivity of 91% and specificity of 81% on a patient level and a sensitivity of 84% and specificity of 85% on a coronary territory–level analysis for the detection of ischemia. In another meta-analysis, data pooled from 26 studies on 2,125 patients comparing perfusion CMR to results of invasive assessment of ischemia by coronary angiogram. Overall, per patient analysis revealed that perfusion CMR had a sensitivity of 89% and specificity of 89% to detect CAD with 4.2 positive likelihood ratio and 0.15 negative likelihood ratio. Further comparison between the vasodilator agents used adenosine in 1658 patients pooled from 20 studies, while dipyridamole in 417 patients pooled from 5 studies. Adenosine perfusion CMR had a higher sensitivity and specificity than dipyridamole (sensitivity: 90% vs. 86%, respectively, and specificity: 81% vs. 77%, respectively). In the same meta-analysis, a comparison between 3-T and 1.5-T MRI scanners demonstrated that 3-T scanners had 92% sensitivity, 78% specificity, 3.96 positive likelihood ratio, and 0.12 negative likelihood ratio while 1.5-T scanner had 89% sensitivity, 80% specificity, 4.26 positive likelihood ratio, and 0.15 negative likelihood ratio. On a perterritory analysis, 2,709 coronary territories pooled from 17 studies, perfusion CMR showed a sensitivity of 82% and specificity of 84%.[60] In a more recent meta-analysis including 2,970 patients from 28 studies, perfusion CMR demonstrated a sensitivity of 91%, specificity of 80%, 4.43 positive likelihood ratio, and 0.12 negative likelihood ratio. In addition, comparing perfusion CMR with both stress perfusion contrast-enhanced echocardiogram and perfusion SPECT suggested that CMR is superior for the diagnosis of obstructive CAD than echo and SPECT.[61]

Validation Using Multicentre Clinical Trials

The MR-IMPACT (Magnetic Resonance Imaging for Myocardial Perfusion Assessment in Coronary Artery Disease) trial[8] enrolled 234 patients in 18 centers and compared the results of perfusion CMR with coronary artery angiography and SPECT. The trial outcomes proved the high diagnostic accuracy of first-pass perfusion CMR with 85% sensitivity and 67% specificity. The receiver operating characteristic curve showed that first-pass perfusion CMR is not inferior to SPECT for detecting CAD. MR-IMPACT II trial[62] enrolled 533 patients in 33 centers from the United States and Europe with the primary end point was noninferiority of CMR versus SPECT for the detection of CAD. The results of the trial showed that CMR had a higher sensitivity than SPECT (67% vs. 59%, respectively) but lower specificity than SPECT (61% vs. 72%, respectively). The most recent CE-MARC trial[7] was the largest prospective study that enrolled 742 patients and compared the diagnostic accuracy of multiparametric CMR, including adenosine stress and rest perfusion, cine imaging, late gadolinium enhancement, and MR coronary angiography imaging, with SPECT and using QCA as the standard reference in patients with suspected CAD. In comparison with QCA, the CMR yielded a sensitivity, specificity, positive predictive value, and negative predictive value of 86.5%, 83.4%, 77.2%, and 90.5%, respectively. In comparison with SPECT, CMR showed a higher sensitivity (86.3% vs. 66.5%; $p < 0.001$) and negative predictive value (90.3% vs. 79.1%; $p < 0.001$), and slightly higher specificity (83.2% vs. 82.6%; $p = 0.916$) and positive predictive value (77% vs. 71.4%; $p = 0.061$). CMR also showed a high diagnostic accuracy of single-vessel and multivessel CAD, regardless of the cutoff value used to define severity of significant angiographic stenosis (>50% or 70%). The MR-INFORM study[63] is a prospective, multicenter, randomized, controlled, noninferiority outcome trial. It is actively recruiting patients with stable angina within the United Kingdom, Germany, and Portugal. MR-INFORM will assess whether an initial strategy of perfusion CMR is noninferior to invasive angiography including FFR measurements to guide the management of patients with stable coronary artery disease. Patients presenting with stable angina are randomized into two arms: The FFR-INFORMED arm has the following clinical decisions guided by coronary angiography and FFR measurements, while the MR-INFORMED arm has clinical decisions guided by perfusion CMR. The primary end point is the occurrence of major adverse cardiac events (i.e., death, myocardial infarction, and repeat revascularization) at 1 year.

Conclusion

Dynamic first-pass perfusion CMR plays an increasing role in the diagnosis and prognostic assessment of CAD due to its high spatial resolution, tissue contrast, anatomical details, and the ability to provide reproducible quantitative data. Compared with the more frequently used SPECT and PET imaging, CMR provides the advantages of higher spatial resolution and lack of ionizing radiation. Ongoing technical developments in acceleration methods including 3D-perfusion CMR aiming to overcome the limitations of current techniques and cover the whole heart within a single acquisition shot rather than selective cardiac coverage would improve the robustness of the method in the future and facilitate quantification of MBF for the whole heart.

REFERENCES

1. **Atkinson DJ, Burstein D, Edelman RR.** First-pass cardiac perfusion: evaluation with ultrafast MR imaging. *Radiology* 1990;174(3 Pt 1): 757–762.
2. **Klocke FJ, Simonetti OP, Judd RM, et al.** Limits of detection of regional differences in vasodilated flow in viable myocardium by first-pass magnetic resonance perfusion imaging. *Circulation* 2001;104(20):2412–2416.
3. **Christian TF, Rettmann DW, Aletras AH, et al.** Absolute myocardial perfusion in canines measured by using dual-bolus first-pass MR imaging. *Radiology* 2004;232(3):677–684.
4. **Lee DC, Simonetti OP, Harris KR, et al.** Magnetic resonance versus radionuclide pharmacological stress perfusion imaging for flow-limiting stenoses of varying severity. *Circulation* 2004;110(1):58–65.
5. **Al-Saadi N, Nagel E, Gross M, et al.** Noninvasive detection of myocardial ischemia from perfusion reserve based on cardiovascular magnetic resonance. *Circulation* 2000;101(12):1379–1383.
6. **Nagel E, Klein C, Paetsch I, et al.** Magnetic resonance perfusion measurements for the noninvasive detection of coronary artery disease. *Circulation* 2003;108(4):432–437.
7. **Greenwood JP, Maredia N, Younger JF, et al.** Cardiovascular magnetic resonance and single-photon emission computed tomography for diagnosis of coronary heart disease (CE-MARC): a prospective trial. *Lancet* 2012;379(9814):453–460.
8. **Schwitter J, Wacker CM, van Rossum AC, et al.** MR-IMPACT: comparison of perfusion-cardiac magnetic resonance with single-photon emission computed tomography for the detection of coronary artery disease in a multicentre, multivendor, randomized trial. *Eur Heart J* 2008;29(4):480–489.
9. **Schwitter J, Wacker CM, Wilke N, et al.** Superior diagnostic performance of perfusion-cardiovascular magnetic resonance versus SPECT to detect coronary artery disease: the secondary endpoints of the multicenter multivendor MR-IMPACT II (Magnetic Resonance Imaging for Myocardial Perfusion Assessment in Coronary Artery Disease Trial). *J Cardiovasc Magn Reson* 2012;14:61.
10. **Kramer CM, Barkhausen J, Flamm SD, et al.** Society for Cardiovascular Magnetic Resonance Board of Trustees Task Force on Standardized P. Standardized cardiovascular magnetic resonance (CMR) protocols 2013 update. *J Cardiovasc Magn Reson* 2013;15:91.
11. **Zur Y, Wood ML, Neuringer LJ.** Spoiling of transverse magnetization in steady-state sequences. *Magn Reson Med* 1991;21(2):251–263.
12. **Scheffler K, Lehnhardt S.** Principles and applications of balanced SSFP techniques. *Eur Radiol* 2003;13(11):2409–2418.
13. **Ridgway JP.** Cardiovascular magnetic resonance physics for clinicians: part I. *J Cardiovasc Magn Reson* 2010;12:71.
14. **Maredia N, Radjenovic A, Kozerke S, et al.** Effect of improving spatial or temporal resolution on image quality and quantitative perfusion assessment with k-t SENSE acceleration in first-pass CMR myocardial perfusion imaging. *Magn Reson Med* 2010;64(6):1616–1624.
15. **Plein S, Schwitter J, Suerder D, et al.** k-Space and time sensitivity encoding-accelerated myocardial perfusion MR imaging at 3.0 T: comparison with 1.5 T. *Radiology* 2008;249(2):493–500.
16. **Pruessmann KP, Weiger M, Scheidegger MB, et al.** SENSE: sensitivity encoding for fast MRI. *Magn Reson Med* 1999;42(5):952–962.
17. **Morton G, Ishida M, Schuster A, et al.** Perfusion cardiovascular magnetic resonance: Comparison of an advanced, high-resolution and a standard sequence. *J Cardiovasc Magn Reson* 2012;14:34.
18. **Harrison A, Adluru G, Damal K, et al.** Rapid ungated myocardial perfusion cardiovascular magnetic resonance: preliminary diagnostic accuracy. *J Cardiovasc Magn Reson* 2013;15(1):26.
19. **Adluru G, McGann C, Speier P, et al.** Acquisition and reconstruction of undersampled radial data for myocardial perfusion magnetic resonance imaging. *J Magn Reson Imaging* 2009;29(2):466–473.
20. **Larson AC, White RD, Laub G, et al.** Self-gated cardiac cine MRI. *Magn Reson Med* 2004;51(1):93–102.
21. **Adluru G, DiBella EV, Schabel MC.** Model-based registration for dynamic cardiac perfusion MRI. *J Magn Reson Imaging* 2006;24(5):1062–1070.
22. **Axel L, Herman GT, Roberts DA, et al.** Linogram reconstruction for magnetic resonance imaging (MRI). *IEEE Trans Med Imaging* 1990;9(4):447–449.
23. **Pipe JG.** Motion correction with PROPELLER MRI: application to head motion and free-breathing cardiac imaging. *Magn Reson Med* 1999;42(5):963–969.
24. **Meyer CH, Hu P.** Spiral parallel magnetic resonance imaging. *Conf Proc IEEE Eng Med Biol Soc* 2006;1:369–371.
25. **Salerno M, Sica C, Kramer CM, et al.** Improved first-pass spiral myocardial perfusion imaging with variable density trajectories. *Magn Reson Med* 2013;70(5):1369–1379.
26. **Ferreira PF, Gatehouse PD, Mohiaddin RH, et al.** Cardiovascular magnetic resonance artefacts. *J Cardiovasc Magn Reson* 2013;15:41.
27. **Lyne JC, Gatehouse PD, Assomull RG, et al.** Direct comparison of myocardial perfusion cardiovascular magnetic resonance sequences with parallel acquisition. *J Magn Reson Imaging* 2007;26(6): 1444–1451.
28. **Wang Y, Moin K, Akinboboye O, et al.** Myocardial first pass perfusion: steady-state free precession versus spoiled gradient echo and segmented echo planar imaging. *Magn Reson Med* 2005;54(5):1123–1129.
29. **Schulz-Menger J, Bluemke DA, Bremerich J, et al.** Standardized image interpretation and post processing in cardiovascular magnetic resonance: Society for Cardiovascular Magnetic Resonance (SCMR) board of trustees task force on standardized post processing. *J Cardiovasc Magn Reson* 2013;15:35.
30. **Hundley WG, Bluemke D, Bogaert JG, et al.** Society for Cardiovascular Magnetic Resonance guidelines for reporting cardiovascular magnetic resonance examinations. *J Cardiovasc Magn Reson* 2009;11:5.
31. **Cerqueira MD, Weissman NJ, Dilsizian V, et al.** Standardized myocardial segmentation and nomenclature for tomographic imaging of the heart. A statement for healthcare professionals from the Cardiac Imaging Committee of the Council on Clinical Cardiology of the American Heart Association. *Circulation* 2002;105(4):539–542.

32. **Di Bella EV, Parker DL, Sinusas AJ.** On the dark rim artifact in dynamic contrast-enhanced MRI myocardial perfusion studies. *Magn Reson Med* 2005;54(5):1295–1299.
33. **Chung SY, Lee KY, Chun EJ, et al.** Comparison of stress perfusion MRI and SPECT for detection of myocardial ischemia in patients with angiographically proven three-vessel coronary artery disease. *AJR Am J Roentgenol* 2010;195(2):356–362.
34. **Stanton T, Marwick TH.** Assessment of subendocardial structure and function. *JACC Cardiovasc Imaging* 2010;3(8):867–875.
35. **Panting JR, Gatehouse PD, Yang GZ, et al.** Abnormal subendocardial perfusion in cardiac syndrome X detected by cardiovascular magnetic resonance imaging. *N Engl J Med* 2002;346(25):1948–1953.
36. **Pilz G, Klos M, Ali E, et al.** Angiographic correlations of patients with small vessel disease diagnosed by adenosine-stress cardiac magnetic resonance imaging. *J Cardiovasc Magn Reson* 2008;10:8.
37. **Kawecka-Jaszcz K, Czarnecka D, Olszanecka A, et al.** Myocardial perfusion in hypertensive patients with normal coronary angiograms. *J Hypertens* 2008;26(8):1686–1694.
38. **Karamitsos TD, Ntusi NA, Francis JM, et al.** Feasibility and safety of high-dose adenosine perfusion cardiovascular magnetic resonance. *J Cardiovasc Magn Reson* 2010;12:66.
39. **Klem I, Heitner JF, Shah DJ, et al.** Improved detection of coronary artery disease by stress perfusion cardiovascular magnetic resonance with the use of delayed enhancement infarction imaging. *J Am Coll Cardiol* 2006;47(8):1630–1638.
40. **Kelle S, Graf K, Dreysse S, et al.** Evaluation of contrast wash-in and peak enhancement in adenosine first pass perfusion CMR in patients post bypass surgery. *J Cardiovasc Magn Reson* 2010;12(1):28.
41. **Schwitter J, DeMarco T, Kneifel S, et al.** Magnetic resonance-based assessment of global coronary flow and flow reserve and its relation to left ventricular functional parameters: a comparison with positron emission tomography. *Circulation* 2000;101(23):2696–2702.
42. **Rieber J, Huber A, Erhard I, et al.** Cardiac magnetic resonance perfusion imaging for the functional assessment of coronary artery disease: a comparison with coronary angiography and fractional flow reserve. *Eur Heart J* 2006;27(12):1465–1471.
43. **Jerosch-Herold M.** Quantification of myocardial perfusion by cardiovascular magnetic resonance. *J Cardiovasc Magn Reson* 2010;12:57.
44. **Jerosch-Herold M, Wilke N, Wang Y, et al.** Direct comparison of an intravascular and an extracellular contrast agent for quantification of myocardial perfusion. Cardiac MRI Group. *Int J Card Imaging* 1999;15(6):453–464.
45. **Jerosch-Herold M, Swingen C, Seethamraju RT.** Myocardial blood flow quantification with MRI by model-independent deconvolution. *Med Phys* 2002;29(5):886–897.
46. **Utz W, Greiser A, Niendorf T, et al.** Single- or dual-bolus approach for the assessment of myocardial perfusion reserve in quantitative MR perfusion imaging. *Magn Reson Med* 2008;59(6):1373–1377.
47. **Christian TF, Aletras AH, Arai AE.** Estimation of absolute myocardial blood flow during first-pass MR perfusion imaging using a dual-bolus injection technique: comparison to single-bolus injection method. *J Magn Reson Imaging* 2008;27(6):1271–1277.
48. **Ishida M, Schuster A, Morton G, et al.** Development of a universal dual-bolus injection scheme for the quantitative assessment of myocardial perfusion cardiovascular magnetic resonance. *J Cardiovasc Magn Reson* 2011;13:28.
49. **Kim D AL.** Multislice, dual-imaging sequence for increasing the dynamic range of the contrast-enhanced blood signal and CNR of myocardial enhancement at 3T. *J Magn Reson Imaging* 2006; 23:81–86.
50. **Schwitter J, Nanz D, Kneifel S, et al.** Assessment of myocardial perfusion in coronary artery disease by magnetic resonance: a comparison with positron emission tomography and coronary angiography. *Circulation* 2001;103(18):2230–2235.
51. **Ibrahim T, Nekolla SG, Schreiber K, et al.** Assessment of coronary flow reserve: comparison between contrast-enhanced magnetic resonance imaging and positron emission tomography. *J Am Coll Cardiol* 2002;39(5):864–870.
52. **Parkka JP, Niemi P, Saraste A, et al.** Comparison of MRI and positron emission tomography for measuring myocardial perfusion reserve in healthy humans. *Magn Reson Med* 2006;55(4):772–779.
53. **Fritz-Hansen T, Hove JD, Kofoed KF, et al.** Quantification of MRI measured myocardial perfusion reserve in healthy humans: a comparison with positron emission tomography. *J Magn Reson Imaging* 2008;27(4):818–824.
54. **Pack NA, DiBella EV, Rust TC, et al.** Estimating myocardial perfusion from dynamic contrast-enhanced CMR with a model-independent deconvolution method. *J Cardiovasc Magn Reson* 2008;10:52.
55. **Morton G, Chiribiri A, Ishida M, et al.** Quantification of absolute myocardial perfusion in patients with coronary artery disease: comparison between cardiovascular magnetic resonance and positron emission tomography. *J Am Coll Cardiol* 2012;60(16):1546–1555.
56. **Kuhl HP, Katoh M, Buhr C, et al.** Comparison of magnetic resonance perfusion imaging versus invasive fractional flow reserve for assessment of the hemodynamic significance of epicardial coronary artery stenosis. *Am J Cardiol* 2007;99(8):1090–1095.
57. **Costa MA, Shoemaker S, Futamatsu H, et al.** Quantitative magnetic resonance perfusion imaging detects anatomic and physiologic coronary artery disease as measured by coronary angiography and fractional flow reserve. *J Am Coll Cardiol* 2007;50(6):514–522.
58. **Lockie T, Ishida M, Perera D, et al.** High-resolution magnetic resonance myocardial perfusion imaging at 3.0-Tesla to detect hemodynamically significant coronary stenoses as determined by fractional flow reserve. *J Am Coll Cardiol* 2011;57(1):70–75.
59. **Nandalur KR, Dwamena BA, Choudhri AF, et al.** Diagnostic performance of stress cardiac magnetic resonance imaging in the detection of coronary artery disease: a meta-analysis. *J Am Coll Cardiol* 2007;50(14):1343–1353.
60. **Hamon M, Fau G, Nee G, et al.** Meta-analysis of the diagnostic performance of stress perfusion cardiovascular magnetic resonance for detection of coronary artery disease. *J Cardiovasc Magn Reson*. 2010; 12(1):29.
61. **de Jong MC, Genders TS, van Geuns RJ, et al.** Diagnostic performance of stress myocardial perfusion imaging for coronary artery disease: a systematic review and meta-analysis. *Eur Radiol* 2012;22(9): 1881–1895.
62. **Schwitter J, Wacker CM, Wilke N, et al.** MR-IMPACT II: magnetic resonance imaging for myocardial perfusion assessment in coronary artery disease trial: perfusion-cardiac magnetic resonance vs. single-photon emission computed tomography for the detection of coronary artery disease: a comparative multicentre, multivendor trial. *Eur Heart J* 2013;34(10):775–781.
63. **Hussain ST, Paul M, Plein S, et al.** Design and rationale of the MR-INFORM study: stress perfusion cardiovascular magnetic resonance imaging to guide the management of patients with stable coronary artery disease. *J Cardiovasc Magn Reson* 2012;14:65.

CHAPTER

20 Myocardial Perfusion with MRI, Clinical Applications

Farhood Saremi, MD

Introduction

Coronary artery disease (CAD) has remained a major cause of death and public health expenses in spite of major advancement in treatment and diagnosis. Widespread implementation of preventive policies, newer therapeutic and interventional strategies, as well as availability of modern diagnostic modalities have contributed to a significant reduction in the mortality and morbidity in patients with CAD. A further reduction in morbidity would require a better characterization of subtle functional abnormalities of the coronary circulation at microvascular level in the preclinical stages of CAD by improvement in diagnostic strategies.[1] With the availability of noninvasive imaging technology that includes nuclear perfusion imaging, magnetic resonance imaging (MRI), and computed tomography (CT) myocardial perfusion imaging (MPI), as well as myocardial contrast echocardiography, microvascular dysfunction (MVD) has been increasingly diagnosed not only in those with ischemic heart disease but also in other clinical cases. Using these techniques, noninvasive identification and characterization of coronary macro- and microvascular abnormalities even in subclinical stages of CAD is possible.

Coronary macrovascular disease is mainly related to plaque formation and stenosis of the epicardial arteries. Its diagnosis is based either on the identification of the anatomic changes (stenosis) of the large epicardial coronary arteries or on the functional consequences of these stenotic lesions on coronary flow reserve (CFR) or regional left ventricle (LV) function. On the other hand, coronary microcirculation (small vessels, approximately 300 to 400 μm) dysfunction may occur in patients with normal coronary angiograms. Extensive research data in recent years have identified an important role for the coronary microcirculation in the clinical presentation and prognosis of patients who have typical chest pain despite a normal coronary angiogram and also in patients with other cardiac conditions.[2] Since direct visualization of the coronary microcirculation is not possible with available techniques, its assessment relies on the measurement of parameters that reflect its functional status, such as absolute myocardial blood flow (MBF) and CFR. Studies in patients who are asymptomatic but the presence of risk factors for CAD including hypercholesterolemia, essential hypertension, diabetes mellitus, and smoking can cause measurable damage to the coronary microcirculation even in the absence of significant stenosis of the epicardial arteries.[1]

In this chapter, we review the clinical applications of MPI with cardiac MR (CMR) mainly focused on first-pass dynamic contrast-enhanced MRI (DCE-MRI). CMR protocols, image findings, and potential diagnostic pitfalls are reviewed.

Coronary Blood Flow

The driving force for blood flow in coronary arteries is the pressure gradient between the aorta and the coronary sinus (or the right atrium). In stenotic epicardial coronary arteries, resting MBF and tissue oxygen supply will be maintained by autoregulatory reduction in resistance of distal microcirculation. Greater than 85% luminal stenosis is required before significant reductions in resting blood flow occur (Fig. 20.1). At this point, the stenosis can be called "critical."[3] In clinical practice, a narrowing of approximately 70% is used as the threshold of a significant stenosis that guides to interventions. However, under vasodilator stimulus, maximal coronary flow (CFR) may be decreased with stenosis of approximately 45% to 50%. This has been demonstrated clinically using quantitative positron emission tomography (PET) MPI.[4] Because perfusion abnormality is an early manifestation of ischemia, imaging of coronary perfusion reserve at stress has a higher sensitivity in detecting flow-limiting stenosis than analysis of stress-induced wall motion abnormalities.[5] The functional behavior of a coronary artery stenosis is difficult to estimate from morphologic changes in the images (angiography, MRI, and even CT). Therefore, interventions combined with measurements of pressure or pressure gradient and/or flow have been proposed to quantify the functional severity of a stenosis.[5]

MBF in healthy population has been studied by Chareonthaitawee et al.[6] They found that baseline and hyperemic MBFs are heterogeneous both within and between individuals. In their analysis, resting myocardial perfusion ranged from 0.59 to 2.05 mL/min/g (average, 0.98 ± 0.23 mL/min/g) and hyperemic perfusion ranged from 1.85 to 5.99 mL/min/g (average, 3.77 ± 0.85 mL/min/g). MBF was significantly higher in women than in men, and hyperemic MBF declined in individuals greater than 65 years old. In a number of patients who present with angina attacks, no apparent epicardial coronary artery stenosis or systemic disease can be found.[7–9] In these patients, coronary MVD has been suggested to be the cause of symptoms.[8,9] Diagnosis of coronary MVD as the cause of ischemic syndromes can be difficult. One of the reasons is that small coronary arteries cannot be visualized by angiography, and

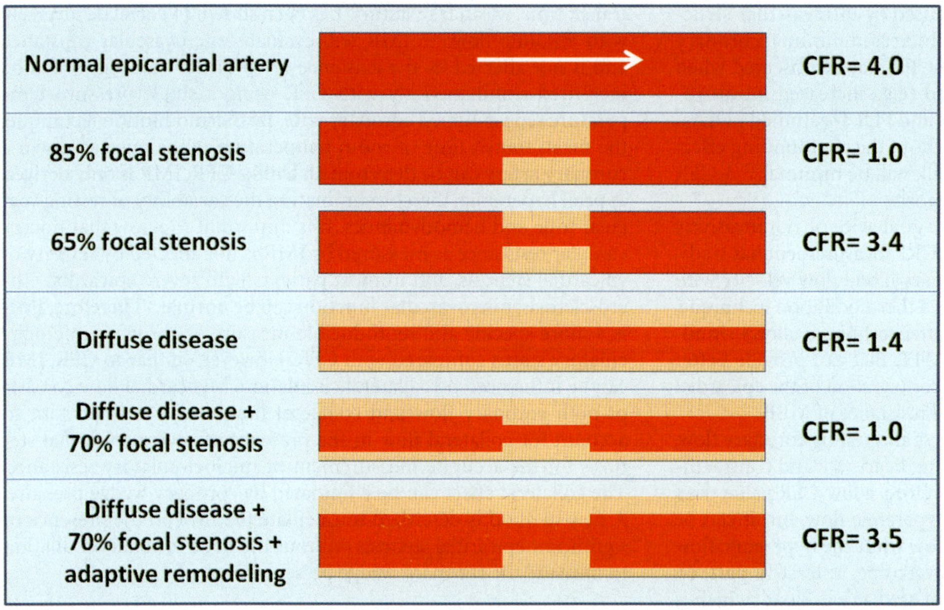

Figure 20-1. Schematic illustrations demonstrate limitations of anatomic measures of focal stenosis severity (by arteriogram or intravascular ultrasound) due to superimposed diffuse disease with and without remodeling compared to coronary flow reserve (CFR). (Gould KL. Does coronary flow trump coronary anatomy? *JACC Cardiovasc Imaging* 2009;2(8):1009–1023, with permission.)

in most cases, ischemic biomarkers are undetectable.[7] Additional invasive studies for diagnosis can be complex and time consuming. Therefore, the role of noninvasive imaging diagnosis in these cases could be critical.[9]

Indices of Microvascular Dysfunction

The state of coronary microcirculation is an important determinant of patient outcomes in a number of clinical settings, including acute coronary syndromes, percutaneous coronary interventions (PCIs), and post–cardiac transplantation vasculopathy. The measurement of fractional flow reserve (FFR) and CFR using invasive and noninvasive techniques is frequently used to test the integrity of microcirculation. Recent advances in different imaging modalities offer the possibility to quantify myocardial perfusion and resistance in absolute terms.[7]

Fractional Flow Reserve

FFR, is an accurate and specific index of epicardial stenosis severity; however, it does not account for increased microvascular resistance.[10,11] It is defined as the ratio of the maximal flow in the vascular bed perfused by a stenotic artery and the maximal flow in a territory supplied by a normal artery. In theory, if the coronary microcirculatory resistance is constant and minimal, coronary pressure will be linearly related to flow.[10] FFR can then be calculated from the ratio of absolute translesional pressures measured by a pressure wire during pharmacologically induced (usually adenosine) hyperemia required to achieve the necessary resistance condition. Therefore, FFR cannot be measured noninvasively using ultrasound Doppler or MRI. FFR is expressed as a fraction of 1. It has been agreed that for values less than 0.75, the stenosis is functionally significant that requires an intervention and evaluation of angioplasty or coronary stenting. For a segmented stenosis or tandem lesions, the decision making is more complicated.

Coronary Flow Reserve

CFR, is a quantitative marker of MVD. It is defined as the ratio of maximal MBF measured at peak stress (i.e., during vasodilator-induced hyperemia) and the resting or reference flow[11] (Fig. 20.2). Use of CFR to evaluate the microcirculation is limited because CFR involves the entire coronary system, including the epicardial artery and the microcirculation (Fig. 20.1). Therefore, a reduction of CFR can also be due to the narrowing of the epicardial coronary arteries. In the absence of obstructive epicardial CAD, it is frequently used as

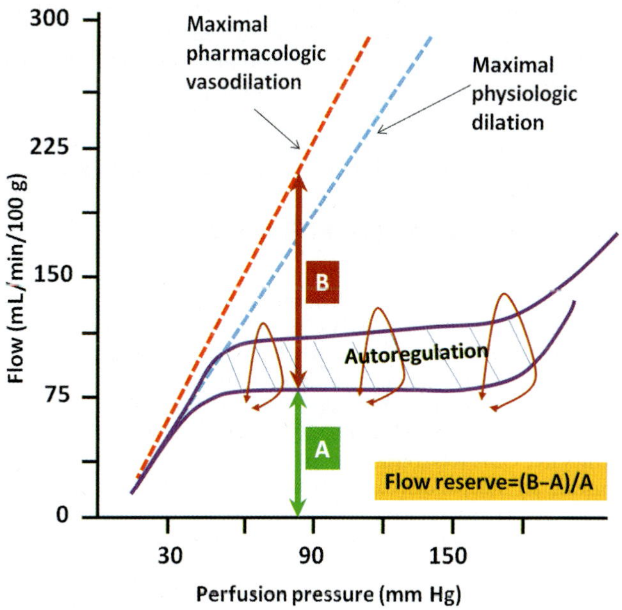

Figure 20-2. Autoregulation maintains flow during constant metabolism. Over the autoregulation range flow is rather constant for a range of perfusion pressures (plateau of the autoregulation curves between *circular arrows*). The level of the plateau is related to the metabolic state of the heart. The maximal pharmacologic vasodilation (*red dashed line*) is slightly larger than maximal physiologic dilation (*blue dashed line*). The flow reserve is given by the ratio (*B*–*A*)/*A*. Flow reserve is dependent on the basal level of myocardial metabolism (*A*), irrespective of minimum hyperemic coronary resistance. (Reprinted with permission from Westerhof N, Boer C, Lamberts RR, et al. Crosstalk between cardiac muscle and coronary vasculature. *Physiol Rev* 2006;86:1263–1308.)

an index of MVD. The latter can be caused by intravascular structural or functional abnormalities (e.g., increased minimal coronary resistance). Furthermore, an abnormal CFR may be observed when the extravascular resistance is increased (e.g., increased intramyocardial pressure/cross talk). When CFR and FFR are studied in diastole, the microcirculation is studied without the confounding effect of the cardiac contraction, and cross talk will be minimal.[12] A CFR of less than 2 indicates a functional stenosis.

CFR can be estimated invasively by guidewire or noninvasively with PET or MRI.[13–15] Guidewire-based CRF measurement has traditionally required measurement of coronary blood flow velocity with a Doppler wire and, more recently using a thermodilution technique, with a coronary pressure wire.[11] The latter technique allows simultaneous measurement of the CFR and FFR that can provide better information with respect to the relative contribution of the epicardial vessels and microvasculature to the total resistance of MBF.

Because CFR is the ratio of peak stress and resting coronary flow, factors that change resting flow, including heart rate and contractility, may affect its measurements.[16] Therefore, a low CFR value does not necessarily reflect a reduction of hyperemic flow, but it can be due to an abnormally elevated resting flow while the hyperemic flow can be normal. This problem can be overcome, at least in part, by normalizing resting flow for the external cardiac workload, which is generally measured using the "rate–pressure product."[14] Resting flow is also influenced by increasing myocardial thickness and a reduction of arterial oxygen content such as anemia.[9,17] It is shown that sudden increases in heart rate leads to a substantial reduction in maximal MBF.[16] Furthermore, CFR only gives global information, whereas microcirculation flow usually is heterogeneously distributed.[6,18]

In clinical practice, dividing absolute perfusion and CFR into normal or abnormal groups is not helpful because many people over 40 to 50 years of age have some degrees of nonobstructive coronary atherosclerosis or some other causes of reduced CFR compared with healthy young individuals. The threshold for a clinically significant flow-limiting stenosis to justify an invasive procedure requires an absolute maximum perfusion (after adenosine stress) below 1.0 to 1.2 mL/min/g and/or a CFR of 1.5 to 1.7 or lower plus a corresponding regional stress-induced abnormality on perfusion images.[19]

Coronary Microvascular Resistance

Coronary microvascular compartment is the site of major resistance (approximately 70% with normal vasomotor tone). Coronary microvascular resistance (CMVR) is affected not only by intrinsic characteristics of the microvessels but also by mechanical cross talk between contracting myocardium and the coronary vasculature such as diastolic perfusion time, cardiac contraction, and LV diastolic wall stress.[12] Given all limitations of CFR, minimum achievable CMVR is considered the preferred parameter that would provide an independent assessment of microcirculatory function. Microvascular resistance can be calculated by dividing the distal coronary pressure by absolute coronary flow.[19–21] For correct measurement of minimal CMVR, maximal vasodilatation is necessary while recording pressure distal to stenosis and quantifying flow. Correction for coronary back pressure is required, and in clinical studies many investigators, therefore, assume it to be zero or to be equivalent to right atrial pressure.[21] New techniques with single guidewires allow for the analysis of pressure and Doppler flow velocity simultaneously. Knowing the diameter and cross-sectional area of the vessel, CMVR is then calculated.

Index of Microcirculatory Resistance

Index of microcirculatory resistance (IMR) is a recently introduced parameter to measure minimum CMVR. It is defined as the distal coronary pressure divided by the inverse of the hyperemic mean transit time. Mean transit time has been shown to correlate inversely with absolute flow.[19,20] IMR will evaluate microvascular resistance and is not affected by the existence of epicardial stenosis. It can be measured simultaneously with CFR using a single pressure–temperature sensor-tipped coronary wire. By thermodilution technique, the mean transit time of room temperature saline injected down a coronary artery can be determined. Unlike CFR, IMR is only derived at peak hyperemia, thereby eliminating the variability of resting vascular tone and hemodynamics. It is important to know that microvascular resistance as measured by IMR is not affected by severity of epicardial stenosis, and in most patients with severe epicardial atherosclerosis, microvascular function can be normal.[9] Therefore, IMR is a more specific and reproducible measure of coronary microcirculatory status compared with CFR. However, similar to CFR, IMR can be influenced by collateral circulation. Myocardial flow consists of both coronary flow and collateral flow, and it is important to account for collateral flow in the presence of severe epicardial stenosis for the accurate measurement of microcirculatory resistance. The collateral effect can be eliminated by coronary wedge pressure. A new method is described to calculate the IMR in the presence of significant epicardial stenosis without the need for balloon dilation to measure the coronary wedge pressure.[20]

Invasive versus Noninvasive Quantification of Minimal CMVR

The major advantage of the catheter-based approach is that pressure and flow to calculate regional CMVR can be measured at the time of catheter angiography. Furthermore, the contribution of the epicardial stenosis to total coronary resistance can be evaluated by measuring the FFR (pressure drop at the level of epicardial stenosis). Although thermodilution flow measurement is a robust method, it is not without technical limitations. Doppler velocity measurement is accurate, but angiographic determination of the cross-sectional area of the vessel for subsequent conversion to absolute flow remains problematic, and intravascular ultrasound (IVUS) probe is also expensive. In the presence of an obstructive coronary lesion, IMR does not account for collateral flow and therefore overestimates actual microvascular resistance.[21,22]

Noninvasive measurement of CMVR can be obtained with positron PET, CMR, or echocardiography.[21] Each of these imaging modalities allows for the absolute quantification of perfusion using radiolabeled or contrast agents. The coronary driving pressure can simply be obtained by measuring mean arterial blood pressure with the use of a sphygmomanometer. Systemic vasodilatation is usually achieved by the infusion of adenosine. Using a high-resolution imaging method, perfusion and resistance can even be distinguished between the subendocardial and subepicardial layers.

Generally, noninvasive imaging techniques are not able to exclude the proximal pressure drop in obstructive epicardial CAD to distinguish microvascular from epicardial stenosis resistance. However, compared to a reference region with normal hyperemic perfusion in the same heart, markedly decreased perfusion in an area adjacent to it can be assumed to be caused by epicardial lesion. PET perfusion imaging is the noninvasive gold standard for assessing physiologic stenosis severity by absolute maximal myocardial perfusion in mL/min/g and CFR.[4] However, several limitations of this technique, including high cost, relatively low spatial resolution (approximately 5 mm), and lack of suitable anatomical information compared with CMR and echocardiography, have prevented its widespread clinical application.

First-Pass Myocardial Perfusion CMR

MPI assesses the blood supply to the myocardium and plays an increasing role in the diagnosis of ischemic heart disease. There are different approaches to evaluate myocardial perfusion with MRI. The most popular perfusion techniques are those that use intravenous contrast as tracer using a T1-weighted sequence. Contrast-enhanced first-pass MPI has been tested for years and proved to be a robust technique to quantify MBF. It is one of the most challenging applications of perfusion MRI because of the temporal and spatial constraints imposed by the cardiac physiology and the nature of DCE MR signal collection. Contrast-enhanced first-pass MPI was introduced by Atkinson et al. in 1990, using an inversion recovery gradient-echo sequence and after injection of a gadolinium-based contrast to demonstrate dynamic passage of contrast agent through the cardiac chambers and myocardium.[23] Since its first introduction, the technique has been continuously developed.[15,24] With rapid technical advancement in MR hardware and software as well as development of newer analytical methods, MPI can be routinely performed in most institutions, and many initial limitations such as poor anatomic coverage and low temporal resolution have been compensated.[25] Recent clinical studies show that CMR now compares quite favorably to single photon emission computed tomography (SPECT) and PET.[26,27]

Noncontrast MPI techniques include blood oxygen level–dependent (BOLD) and arterial spin labeling (ASL).[28–31] BOLD takes advantage of intrinsic contrast agent property of deoxygenated hemoglobin in blood, which will change proton signals in the MR sequence proportional to the level of blood oxygenation. Increases in O_2 saturation enhances the BOLD imaging signal (T2 or T2*), whereas decreases in O_2 saturation will diminish it. Steady-state free precession (SSFP) sequences have shown promising results, allowing for a simultaneous acquisition of morphologic, functional, and oxygenation-sensitive data of the heart.[28,29] ASL provides noninvasive measurement of tissue blood flow without intravenous contrast administration. Although popular in brain perfusion, high sensitivity to respiratory motions and low sensitivity to blood flow have limited its application for MPI.[30,31] A free-breathing myocardial ASL technique using a respiratory navigator–gated SSFP with the potential for reliable clinical application has been introduced.[31]

Contrast Material

Most CMR studies of myocardial perfusion are based on the first pass of a bolus of gadolinium-DTPA (Diethylene triamine pentaacetic acid) contrast agents. Extravascular, extracellular classes of gadolinium-based agents are the most common contrast material used for contrast-enhanced perfusion imaging. Two primary mechanisms of image contrast are relaxivity and susceptibility effects. Relaxivity effects result from dipolar enhancement of T1 and T2 rates. Because tissue T1 rates are intrinsically smaller, the dominant effect is shortening of T1 relaxation times.[32] Due to its seven unpaired electrons, gadolinium is an effective paramagnetic agent causing enhancement in T1-weighted (T1W) images by accelerating T1 relaxation of tissue. Therefore, areas that are well perfused will have a shorter T1 and appear bright on heavily T1-weighted images, whereas regions that are hypoperfused will have longer T1 and will appear hypointense.[33] After intravenous administration, extracellular contrast agent (such as gadopentetate dimeglumine, Gd-DTPA) enters the vascular compartment of the myocardium and extravasates into the interstitial space but remains extracellular in healthy myocardium. In healthy volunteers at rest, the vascular compartment (mostly venous) occupies approximately 10% of tissue volume.[34] Quantization of tissue perfusion requires a detailed understanding of the relation between contrast agent concentration and associated MR signal changes. Studies to date show a linear relationship between gadolinium contrast concentration and enhancement in most tissues on first-pass perfusion imaging.[34]

Intravascular blood pool contrast agents have been used for MPI. Gadofosveset trisodium (ABLAVAR, Lantheus Medical Imaging, North Billerica, MA) is approved by the Food and Drug Administration (FDA). These agents have the potential to visualize perfusion defect over a longer period of time compared to extracellular agents. At higher dose may overestimate MBF and the optimum dose for 1.5-T scanner is suggested at 0.00375 mmol/kg.[35]

Pharmacologic Stress Imaging

The diagnostic performance of the stress imaging may vary considerably, depending on the imaging modality or stress agent used. Common pharmacologic stress agents include adenosine or dipyridamole and the synthetic β-adrenergic agent dobutamine.[36] Regadenoson is a new agent recently approved by the FDA for stress testing.[37,38] Investigators have different opinions regarding the "optimal" stress agent to use. Stress CMR imaging is predominantly used in adults with structurally normal hearts for the assessment of CAD. CMR stress testing can be performed by two methods: (a) functional cine MRI using exercise or pharmacologic stress and (b) stress perfusion CMR with pharmacologic stress. Adenosine has a more favorable safety profile and is the preferred pharmacologic agent for stress MPI, whereas dobutamine is the pharmacologic stress agent of choice for the detection of stress-inducible wall motion abnormalities, and it is reserved for patients with contraindications for vasodilator testing.[36]

It is generally accepted that myocardial ischemia is the most effective stimulus for vasodilatation of coronary resistive vessels and that, under normal circumstances, reactive hyperemic peak flow represents the maximum flow available at a given coronary perfusion pressure. Values of coronary blood flow comparable to the peak flow of reactive hyperemia can be achieved using coronary vasodilators such as intravenous adenosine or dipyridamole, which induce a near-maximal vasodilatation of the coronary microcirculation. Adenosine is one of the key mediators of metabolic blood flow regulation. Its local production increases in the case of an imbalance in the supply or demand ratio of myocardial oxygen. Adenosine then diffuses from myocytes into interstitial fluid, where it exerts powerful arteriolar dilator effects through the stimulation of A2 adenosine receptors on smooth muscle cells. Adenosine nonselectively activates four cardiac receptor subtypes: A1, A2A, A2B, and A3.[37] The use of adenosine for stress MPI is primarily related to the activation of A2A receptors and the resultant increase in MBF. The activation of A1, A2B, and A3 receptors produces short-term undesirable side effects. A patient with a fixed coronary stenosis who is given an adenosine infusion will have a perfusion mismatch between the area of distribution of the affected coronary artery and other areas of myocardium. Adenosine has a very short half-life so it must be given as a continuous infusion (0.14 mg/kg/min). At most centers, adenosine is given for 2 to 4 minutes or until the patient experiences typical symptoms of flushing, tachycardia, chest discomfort, shortness of breath, dizziness, and headache. After 2 minutes of adenosine infusion, gadolinium is administered and the imaging sequence is initiated. It is suggested to use separate lines for the injection of adenosine and contrast. Adenosine is contraindicated in patients with reactive airway disease, second- or third-degree heart block, severe carotid stenosis, pregnancy, and in patients taking dipyridamole.[36] Caffeine and theophylline should also be avoided as they act as adenosine receptor antagonists. Dipyridamole has the same side effects, but it is cheaper than adenosine and provides longer vasodilation (half-life of approximately 30 minutes vs. <10 seconds for adenosine).

Regadenoson is the first selective A2A receptor agonist that is currently used clinically.[37,30] It seems to be an ideal stress perfusion agent. It is a potent coronary vasodilator with a rapid onset of action and a short half-life that can be administered as a fixed-dose bolus (0.4-mg bolus). Unlike adenosine, regadenoson could also be used in patients with mild-to-moderate reactive airway disease and obstructive lung disease.[37] If serious complications occur, intravenous aminophylline, an adenosine antagonist, should be administered.

Vasu et al.[38] tested the relative potency of regadenoson, dipyridamole, and adenosine by quantifying stress and rest myocardial perfusion MRI in humans. Rest perfusion was performed first and 20 minutes later stress imaging was performed at peak vasodilation, that is, 70 seconds after regadenoson, 4 minutes after dipyridamole infusion, and between 3 and 4 minutes of the adenosine infusion. MBF in mL/min/g and myocardial perfusion reserve (MPR) were quantified using a fully quantitative deconvolution method. Regadenoson produced higher stress MBF and faster heart rate than did dipyridamole and adenosine. However, after adjustment for the heart rate, values of MBF and MPR were similar for regadenoson and adenosine indicating similar vasodilator efficacy.[38] Myocardial infarction, ventricular arrhythmias, and cardiac arrest have been reported following injection of regadenoson. Its use should be avoided in unstable angina or cardiovascular instability.

Choice of Pulse Sequence

First-pass contrast-enhanced perfusion MRI is a robust technique to show myocardial ischemia, but the difficulty in optimizing all aspects of the acquisition sequence has resulted in compromised image quality or reduced anatomic coverage.[25]

In an ideal first-pass MPI pulse sequence, several issues should be addressed[39]: (a) strong T1 weighting to improve demonstration of T1-lowering effect of contrast, (b) coverage of the heart from apex to base, (c) high signal-to-noise ratio (SNR) and contrast-to-noise ratio (CNR) to show small areas of ischemia, (d) minimal artifacts, (e) rapid data acquisition and adequate temporal resolution to increase spatial coverage and to allow adequate sampling of the first pass of the contrast material bolus, and (f) a linear relationship between signal intensity and contrast material dose (input function). Another important consideration is that in an ideal first-pass MPI all image data must be obtained in one single heartbeat to demonstrate passage of the contrast and minimize breathing and cardiac motion artifacts between contiguous frames. Therefore, perfusion imaging is generally performed as a single-shot technique and multishot k-space filling strategies over multiple cardiac cycles is not desirable.

To serve the above goals, a variety of rapid readout techniques are introduced including fast low-angle shot (FLASH), echo-planar imaging (EPI), and balanced SSFP (b-SSFP).[39–43] T1-weighted fast gradient echo (FGE, FLASH) is the most commonly used sequence. Figure 20.3 contains a schematic of a typical first-pass imaging sequence.

The advantages of FLASH include reduced susceptibility-induced image artifacts, and disadvantages include lower achievable SNR and longer readout duration. The higher SNR of b-SSFP images allows a much higher bandwidth to be selected leading to shorter echo time (TE) and repetition time (TR) in b-SSFP that makes it a faster sequence than FGE. However, b-SSFP is the most prone to off resonance and susceptibility effects and commonly shows Gibbs ringing in the endocardium due to the increased difference in signal intensity between the blood and myocardium. b-SSFP is not suitable for greater than 1.5-T magnetic fields. EPI techniques have the highest temporal resolution (100 to 150 milliseconds compared to 150 to 200 milliseconds in FLASH); however, ghost artifacts (due to periodic fluctuations of the k-space signal) and T2* susceptibility signal loss are common.[44]

In all these sequences, preparation pulse is applied prior to the readout pulse to increase with a sufficiently long preparation pulse delay to establish T1 weighting. These preparation pulses include

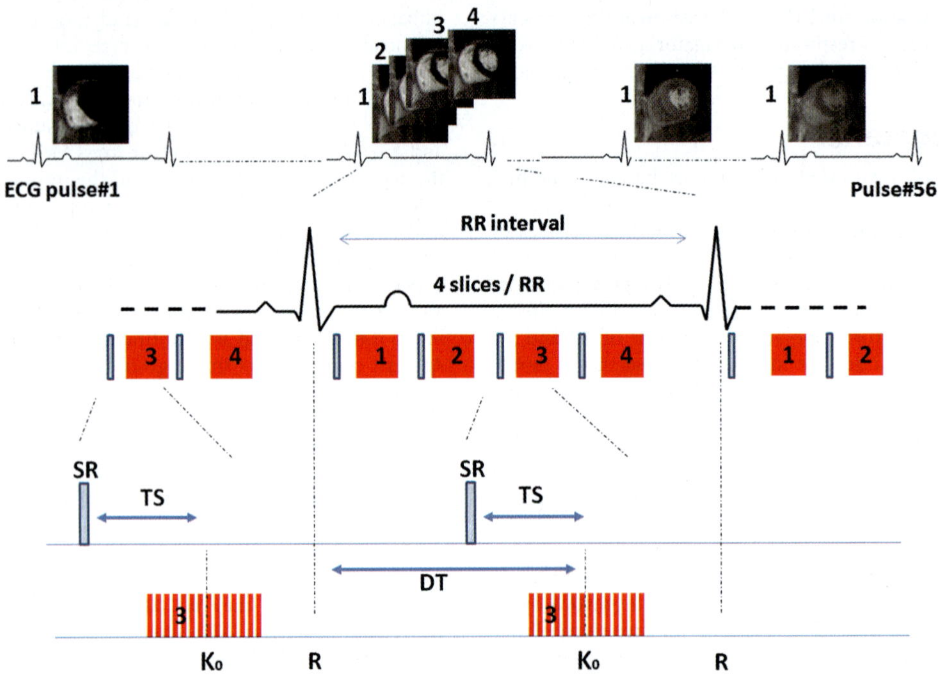

Figure 20-3. Schematic description of myocardial perfusion imaging data acquisition scheme. Choice of ECG-gated pulse sequence include fast gradient echo (FGE), balanced steady-state free precession (bSSFP), or echo-planar imaging (EPI). The chosen sequence is repeated for each slice in every R-R interval for approximately 60 to 70 heartbeats. Common to all these sequences is the presence of a saturation recovery (SR) preparation pulse to increase T1 weighting. T1 weighting is controlled by the saturation time (TS), which is the time between the saturation pulse (SR) and the centre of k-space (k0). The trigger delay (TD) is time delay from R in ECG pulse to the centre of k-space (k0). The number of slices that can be acquired (up to three in most scanners) is limited by the R-R interval, the saturation delay, and the length of data acquisition (*red lines and boxes*) period. Detail is shown for slice 3. The number of slices can be increased and distributed in two R-R intervals (i.e., three slices in each for a total of six) and repeated every other beat.

inversion recovery (IR), saturation recovery (SR), and partial saturation.[40] Preparatory pulses play a major role in determining contrast, SNR, and the maximum number of sections that can be acquired. A typical saturation time (TS) (from beginning of preparation pulse to the center of the readout pulse) for MPI is around 100 milliseconds. A shorter TS permit the acquisition of more sections per cardiac cycle, and the signal intensity is more linearly related to T1, but the SNR is generally lower. At longer TSs, the SNR is higher, but there is a loss of linearity, especially at higher contrast agent concentrations.[39] SR-prepared pulse scheme is well suited for most current multislice perfusion imaging. SR is typically implemented using a nonselective 90-degree radiofrequency (RF) excitation followed by a gradient crusher.[40] It is faster than are IR-prepared pulse sequences and appears to be insensitive to variations in heart rate.[39]

Faster acquisition can be obtained with short TR, small matrix (in phase-encoding direction), EPI, single-shot sequence, parallel imaging, or keyhole imaging, all at the expense of loss of SNR and contrast. Parallel imaging with acceleration factors of 2 is now routinely used in clinical practice. Higher acceleration factors are possible in new scanners.[45] One of the major limitations of parallel imaging techniques is reduction of SNR according to the square root of the acceleration factor. For this reason, parallel imaging should only be applied when the image SNR is relatively high. Therefore, it works better at higher fields (i.e., 3 T).

High spatial resolution to detect subendocardial lesions is important parameter in data acquisition. However, increasing spatial resolution is at the expense of increases in acquisition time, which in turn limits the left ventricle coverage and increases motion artifacts. In most conventional techniques, in plane spatial resolution of 1.5 to 3.5 mm, a voxel thickness of 6 to 10 mm can be achieved in 50 to 200 millisecond per slice. To make it faster, most sequences are designed to acquire images during different phases of cardiac cycle. Therefore, some images are obtained in systole and some in diastole (Fig. 20.3). However, for each slice location, data acquisition is performed at the same point of cardiac cycle in successive heartbeats to exclude cardiac motion when the dynamic images are viewed in a cine loop. Images obtained in late diastole are less susceptible to motion artifacts. Conversely, thicker myocardial wall in systole allows improved myocardial SNR in contrast uptake curves.

For qualitative perfusion imaging and demonstration of the location of ischemia, routine 2D technique with four to six slices will usually suffice. With the goal of characterizing the extent of disease, it may be necessary to cover the whole heart using either a large number of 2D slices or a special 3D encoding. More recent techniques that exploit the spatial–temporal correlations in the series of first-pass perfusion imaging using techniques such as SENSitivity Encoding are enabling true 3D coverage of the ventricle with high spatial resolution.[46] Compressed sensing techniques, which rely on the compressibility of image data (image sparsity), hold potential for even more acceleration of perfusion image acquisition.[47] While any of these techniques can be used for quantification of myocardial perfusion, care must be taken to make sure that the techniques used do not disrupt the temporal evolution of the signal intensities.

Perfusion MR Protocol

Perfusion MR study is generally performed as part of a comprehensive study that evaluates ventricular function, stress and rest perfusion, and viability/myocardial infarction. The MR examination typically takes approximately 45 to 60 minutes in experienced centers (Fig. 20.4). First, cine images are obtained to assess ventricular function. For function analysis, retrospectively ECG-gated b-SSFP cine MRI will be performed in short- and long-axis planes. The study is followed by stress/rest perfusion, and finally, late gadolinium-enhanced (LGE) images are obtained covering the heart by copying sample planes used for cine study.

A test run perfusion sequence will be obtained before injection of contrast to evaluate for artifacts. Stress perfusion images

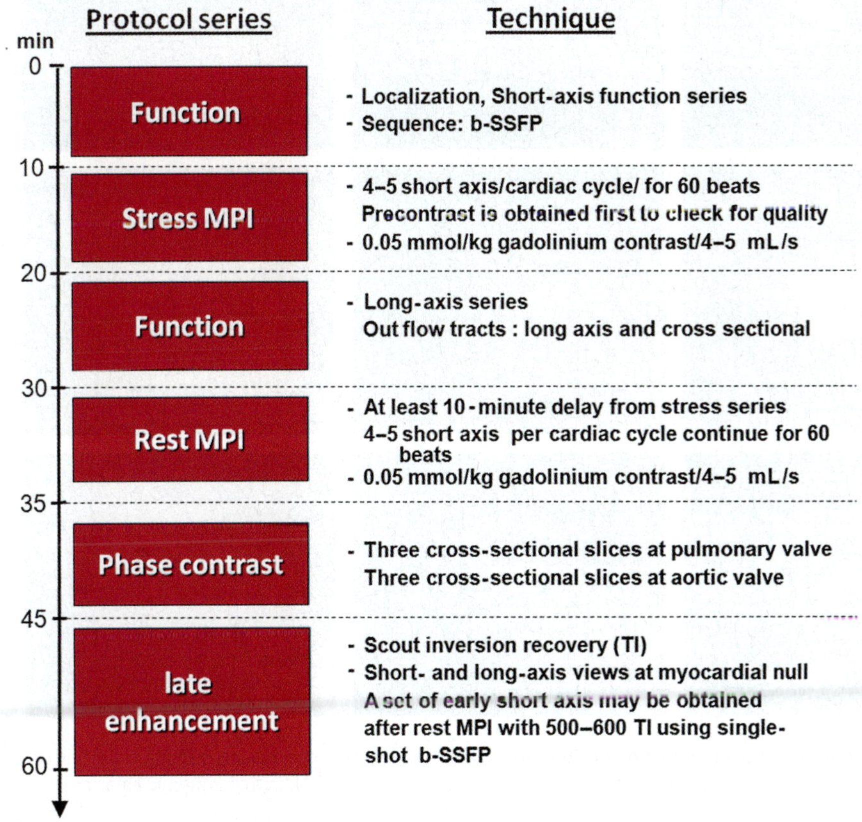

Figure 20-4. Typical CMR examination in perfusion studies. (MPI, myocardial perfusion imaging; b-SSFP, balanced steady-state free precession.)

are then acquired during the first pass of contrast and infusion of 140 μg/kg/min of adenosine for 3 to 4 minutes. Gadolinium-based contrast will be injected by a power injector at 4 to 5 mL/s followed immediately by a 20 mL of normal saline flush at 4 to 5 mL/s for both stress and rest perfusion MR images (0.05 mmol/kg each for both rest and stress MR imaging).

For SR-FLASH sequence, the following parameters are used: TR/TE 2.0 milliseconds/1.0 milliseconds, SR time 100 milliseconds, slice thickness 8 mm, voxel size 2.1 × 2.6 × 8 mm, and flip angle 18 degrees. For SR-SSFP sequence, scan parameters include TR/TE 2.4 milliseconds/1.0 milliseconds, SR time 180 milliseconds, flip angle 50 degrees, acquisition duration 150 milliseconds, and slice thickness 8 mm. Parallel imaging is included with an acceleration factor of 2.

Typically, short-axis images covering the entire LV are acquired, but one long-axis image is sometimes additionally acquired in order to cover the apex of the heart. Coverage of relevant myocardial segments is achieved using an interleaved acquisition of arbitrarily oriented slices. Most sequences enable five to six slices with a temporal resolution of two R-R intervals and 6 to 8 mm thickness. With single-shot FGE sequences, entire data readout can be obtained in a single R-R interval. The number of slices per R-R may need to be reduced if the heart rate is too fast. With faster imaging methods such as 3D SR FGE, it is possible to image the entire heart, and all images can be obtained in systole or diastole.[48] Using a dual-phase DCE MRI pulse sequence, signal readout can be timed to allow two identical single-shot acquisitions within each R-R interval. This way perfusion images can be obtained in both systole and diastole for same slice location.[49]

Patients breathe quietly during the first 15 seconds of scan and then hold their breath for as long as possible in end inspiration. Forty to sixty image frames are usually obtained (Fig. 20.5). Respiratory motion during free breathing can be corrected by

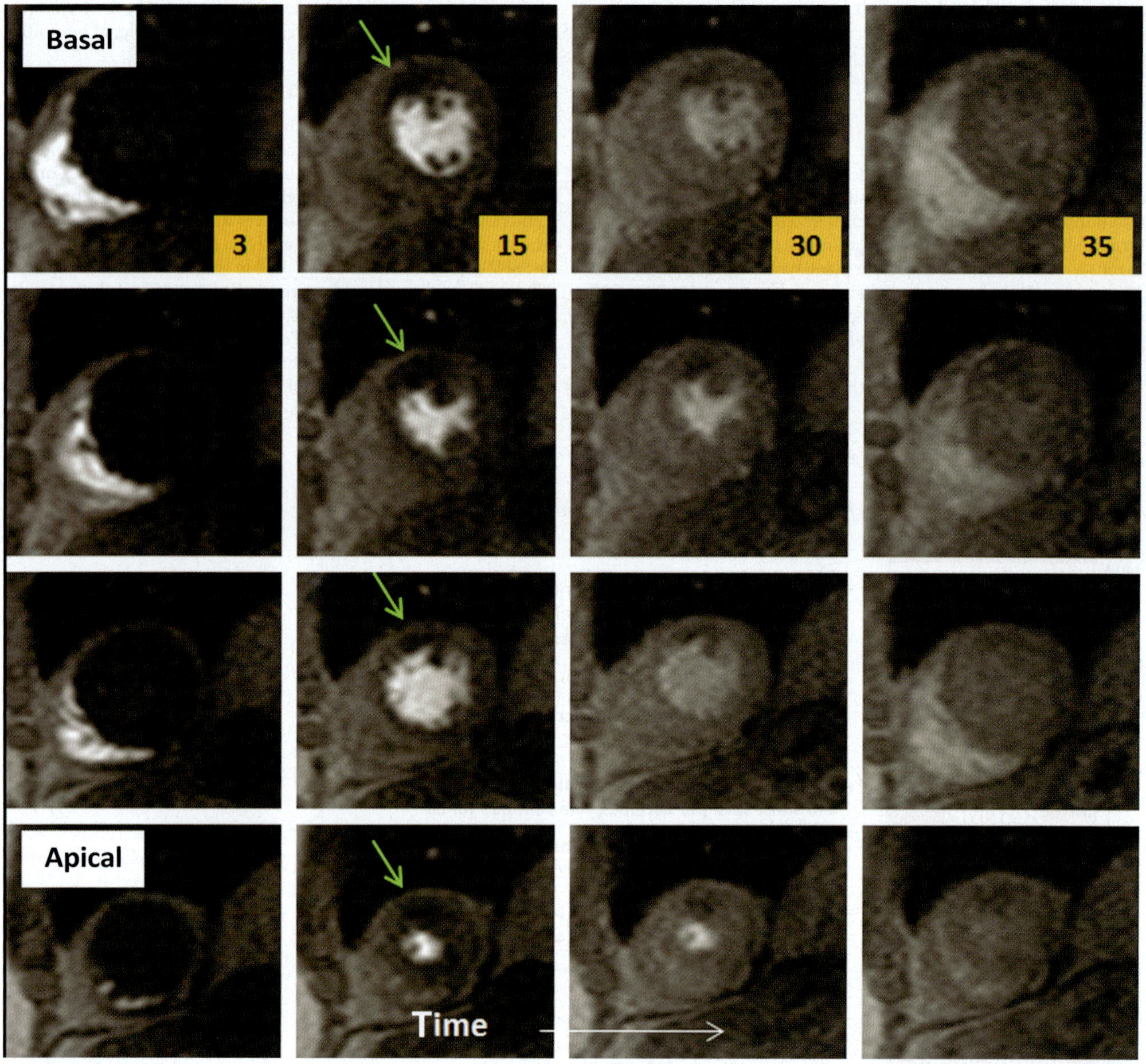

Figure 20-5. Typical images of stress myocardial perfusion in a patient with LAD ischemia. Subendocardial hypoperfusion (*arrows*) of the anterior wall extends from basal to apical obtained at four slice levels (*rows*). Columns show selected frames of these slices. Note that ischemic areas are best shown in frames between 15 and 30.

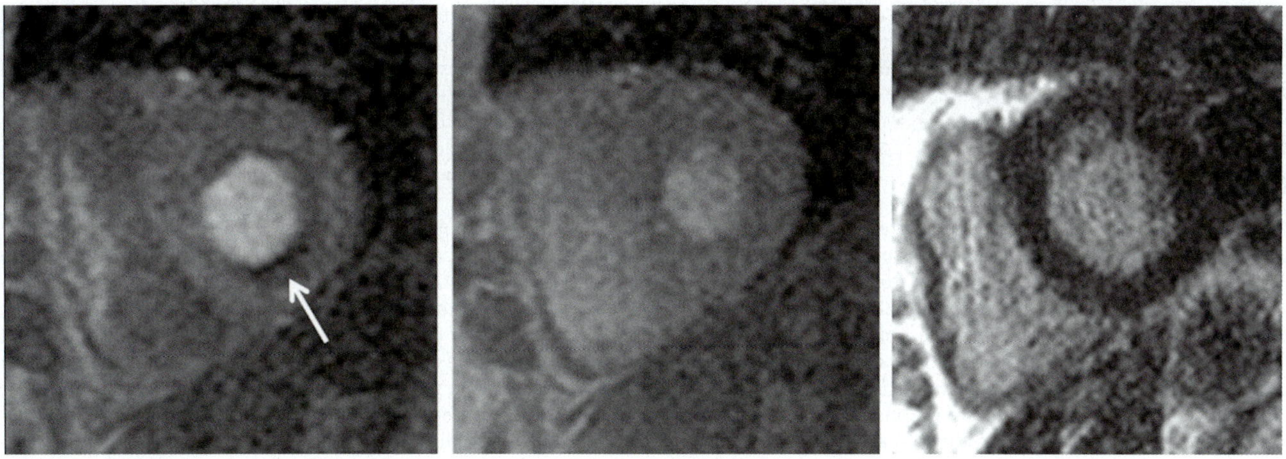

A B C

Figure 20-6. Typical case of inducible ischemia by adenosine in RCA (Right coronary artery) distribution. **A:** Stress perfusion shows subendocardial ischemic zone (*arrow*) in the inferior wall that recovers in rest image **(B)**. **C:** Delayed postcontrast image is normal.

navigator pulse placed over the diaphragm.[50] The same imaging sequence will be repeated 10 minutes later without adenosine to obtain perfusion images at rest. Following a delay of 10 minutes after rest perfusion imaging, late postcontrast IR-FGE is obtained (Fig. 20.6). Short-axis and long-axis images are acquired to cover the entire heart. Scan parameters per slice for the LGE MRI are TR/TE 5.4 milliseconds/3.0 milliseconds, flip angle 20 degrees, slice thickness 8 mm with 2-mm spacing between each slice.

Most protocols consist of adenosine stress series followed by rest perfusion studies, to allow distinction of perfusion defects from ischemia versus image artifacts.[26] Adenosine has a short half-life, and its effect has been disappeared by the time rest perfusion is performed. If resting perfusion is performed first, the injected gadolinium may enhance infarcted myocardium and in part mask the inducible ischemic areas on a subsequent stress perfusion images.[26] For correct quantitative perfusion analysis, at least 10-minute delay between stress and rest series is necessary.

Accurate Determination of the Arterial Input Function

If MPI is performed to quantify MBF, then additional technical modification may be necessary for image acquisition. To calculate regional MBF in mL/min/g using time–intensity curve deconvolution, accurate measurement of arterial input function (AIF) at stress and rest is required. The AIF is the time–intensity signal of blood pool, which is usually measured in the left ventricle cavity or within the ascending aorta lumen. High concentrations of passing blood pool contrast in these structures can affect measurement of the AIF by T1-induced MR signal saturation and T2* effects.[51] Therefore, higher concentrations of gadolinium contrast that might be ideal for visual assessment of myocardial tissue can cause nonlinearity in the blood pool and blunting of the AIF peak, leading to underestimates in MBF. Nonlinearity depends on the dose and injection rate of the administered contrast agent, the type of MR pulse (FLASH, EPI, SSFP), and the TS.[52] The simplest method to ensure linearity in AIF is to decrease the contrast dose to less than 0.01 mmol/kg. However, lower contrast concentration can reduce the change in myocardial signal (tissue input) to such an extent that MBF estimates become significantly affected by image noise. Approaches that try to overcome these issues include dual-bolus protocol that repeats the experiment using low-contrast and high-contrast doses,[53,54] and dual-sequence strategies that repeat the experiment using two pulse sequences optimized for the blood pool and myocardial curves.[55] In dual bolus, 0.005 mmol/kg of gadolinium-DTPA is administered during a first breath-hold (low-dose sequence), and 0.1 mmol/kg (high-dose bolus) is given during a second breath-hold sequence after the subject was allowed to take two to four large breaths between the two scans.[53] The low-dose data are used for analysis of the AIF and the high dose for myocardial tissue response computation and visual interpretation.

Clinical Benefits of High-Field MRI

High-field (3-T) MR has been used for cardiac imaging in the past decade with encouraging results. MR perfusion imaging is a signal-starved sequence especially for underperfused myocardium. The main advantage of 3 T compared to 1.5T is higher SNR, which results in improved spatial, contrast, and temporal resolution.[56,57] There is a linear relationship between Bo and SNR, and the SNR is predicted to double for every doubling of Bo.[56] An important advantage of 3 T over 1.5 T is increased in T1 for all tissues, which provides a wider dynamic range for contrast-induced T1 changes, compared with 1.5T. This wider dynamic range can increase the contrast-to-noise differences between tissues with different perfusion rates. Some limitations of 3-T scanners include suboptimal ECG signal, and increased chemical shift, T2*, and banding artifacts.[56] High-field myocardial perfusion can be performed with parallel imaging to speed acquisition.[58] 3D encoding methods have been combined with parallel imaging to improve spatial coverage of perfusion imaging using either 3D b-SSFP or 3D FGE. However, as explained earlier, perfusion imaging with b-SSFP might produce unacceptable artifacts at 3.0 T from banding artifacts and RF inhomogeneity.

Christian et al.[59] measured absolute MBF by first-pass perfusion imaging at both 1.5 and 3 T and showed similar accuracy but better SNR at 3 T. They showed lower noise and doubling of myocardial enhancement with a fixed concentration of gadolinium-based contrast at 3-T imaging. In a qualitative study, Cheng at al.[60] reported superiority of 3-T CMR perfusion imaging in the diagnosis of significant single-vessel and multivessel coronary disease and a significant increase in both SNR (17 ± 6 at 3 T vs. 11 ± 2 at 1.5 T; $p < 0.01$) and CNR (17 ± 10 at 3 T vs. 11 ± 4 at 1.5 T; $p < 0.01$) of 3 T compared with 1.5 T.

In regard to quantitative measurements, Bernhardt et al.[61] directly compared the performance of quantitative CMR at 1.5- and 3-T field strengths to detect FFR less than 0.8 in 34 patients with known or suspected CAD. This study demonstrated a higher receiver operating characteristic area under the curve (0.96 vs. 0.64, $p < 0.001$), sensitivity (90% vs. 62%), and specificity (100% vs. 77%) at 3 T versus 1.5 T.

Image Interpretation

Qualitative Evaluation

Although research studies often emphasize quantitative analysis, simple visual assessment of the first-pass perfusion images is the most common approach in clinical laboratories. A real myocardial perfusion defect associated with epicardial coronary stenosis or microvascular obstruction appears as a nonenhancing dark zone during the myocardial phase of contrast medium transit (Figs. 20.5 and 20.6). Perfusion defects cannot be distinguished from nonenhancing myocardium and are not visible during the luminal phase of contrast arrival into the LV cavity. A true perfusion defect due to significant CAD should persist for at least four to five heartbeats; it should extend into the myocardial muscle (i.e., it should not be just a dark line at the subendocardium–cavity interface) and should be more conspicuous during stress than at rest (inducible defect). Stress perfusion defect due to infarcted myocardium may also fade or completely normalize to myocardial signal on rest series performed after stress due to enhancement of infarcted myocardium (Fig. 20.7). In routine MR protocol containing rest perfusion–only series, the presence of dark rim is usually due to no reflow/hemorrhage or artifact. Comparison with delayed postcontrast image in this situation can help reach correct diagnosis.

A step-wise approach is suggested by Klem et al. to improve correct interpretation of the image findings.[62] The interpretation starts with review of LGE images, followed by stress and rest perfusion. This way, the interpreting physician can better determine whether perfusion defects match regions of scar versus those that extend beyond the scar (Table 20.1). A region of stress perfusion defect that is larger than corresponding enhancing scar in the same region can be interpreted as "infarct with periinfarct ischemia" (Fig. 20.8). Clinically, this is helpful to the referring physician when judging whether or not to revascularize a chronically occluded vessel (Fig. 20.9). Perfusion defects detected both at stress and rest (fixed defect) combined with no detection of infarcted areas on the LGE should be interpreted as a dark-rim artifact (DRA).

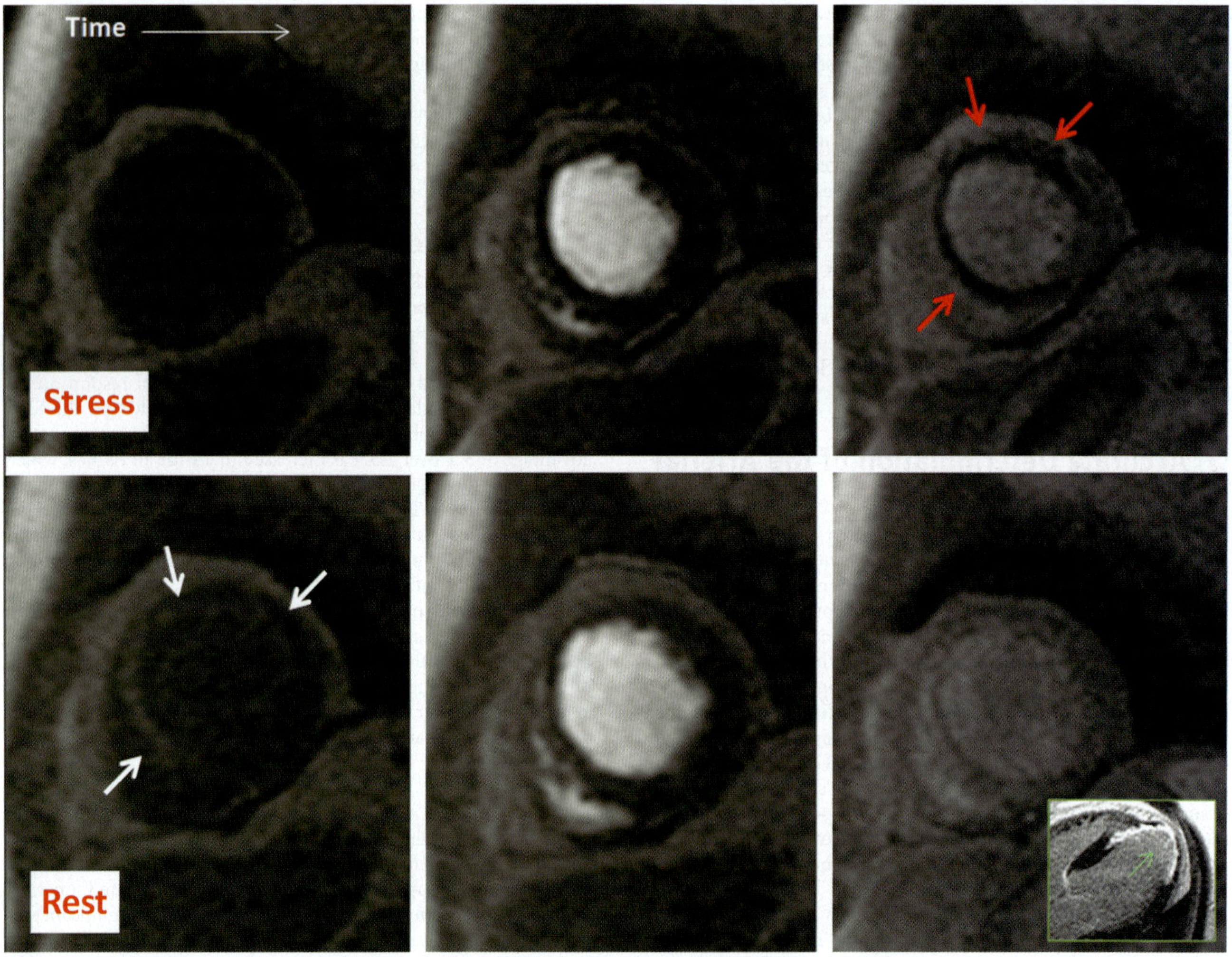

Figure 20-7. Early enhancement of infarcted tissue on rest perfusion. The perfusion defect due to infarction seen on stress (*red arrows*) disappears on rest image due to early enhancement (*white arrows*). Enhancement is clearly shown on first frame of rest perfusion (*arrows*) before arrival of contrast. As a result, infarcted tissue cannot be distinguished from the rest of the myocardium on myocardial phase of rest perfusion series (last image). Inlay image shows extensive myocardial infarct of apical zone of left ventricle (*green arrow*) on this long-axis view of late gadolinium enhancement.

TABLE 20.1 **Image Findings in MR Perfusion Imaging**

Underlying Problem	Stress	Rest	Delayed Postgadolinium	T2W
Ischemia due significant CAD stenosis	Dark (parenchymal phase)	Normal	Normal	Normal
Chronic infarction	Dark	Dark/normal	LGE	Normal
Acute infarction with no reflow	N/A (usually rest only)	Dark/normal	LGE + dark area	Dark
Acute infarction with hemorrhage	N/A (rest-only exam)	Normal or slightly dark	LGE + dark area	Normal or slightly bright
Dark-rim artifact	Dark (blood pool phase)	Dark (blood pool phase)	Normal	Normal
Calcification	Abnormal (dark)	Abnormal (dark)	Abnormal (dark)	Abnormal (dark)

However, care should be taken not to miss a small subendocardial infarction that can be isointense to blood pool contrast on delayed postcontrast studies. The later condition is more common when blood pool contrast washout is delayed especially in patients with decreased cardiac output and slow heart rate. In our institution, two sets of short-axis delayed series are routinely obtained, one at 10 to 15 minutes and the second after 20 to 25 minutes post–contrast administration. Attention to anatomic location of the lesions is important since most ischemic lesions due to epicardial arterial stenosis are limited to the anatomic distribution of the affected artery. This may not be the case in artifacts and microvascular lesions. Patients with late enhancement due to ischemic scar, history of coronary stent placement, or coronary artery bypass graft without stress-induced reversible perfusion deficit may be categorized as "significant large vessel disease without reversible ischemia."[63] Finally, patients with diffuse stress-induced subendocardial hypoperfusion (<1/2 of the myocardial wall thickness) in at least two different coronary artery territories or circumferentially lasting for up to six heartbeats after the time of maximal signal peak intensity in the left ventricle can be classified as having multivessel disease at epicardial level or diffuse MVD and need to be further investigated by coronary angiography and related hemodynamic indices measurement.

Quantitative Image Analysis

For each patient, left ventricular end-diastolic and -systolic volumes, ejection fraction, and mass will be calculated in the standard way by manually tracing the endocardial and epicardial contours in end-diastolic and -systolic images. Following visual assessment of perfusion images, data are transferred to a dedicated commercially available cardiac image analysis software for semiautomated image analysis. Endocardial and epicardial contours are traced manually and propagated throughout dynamic image series.

The AIF will be derived from a region of interest placed within the left ventricular cavity, avoiding the papillary muscles. Regions of interest are also drawn to define the myocardium. Abnormal myocardium can be separated from the normal part. The 17-segment model proposed by the American Heart Association is commonly used.[64] This segmentation model corresponds to the typical blood flow distributions of the coronary arteries.

Since the subendocardial portion of the heart wall is most vulnerable to ischemia, in addition to analyzing transmural MBF estimates from myocardial signal intensity curves derived from the entire area between the endocardial and epicardial borders, transmural distribution of MBF can be assessed by subdividing the LV wall into three concentric zones: subendocardial, middle,

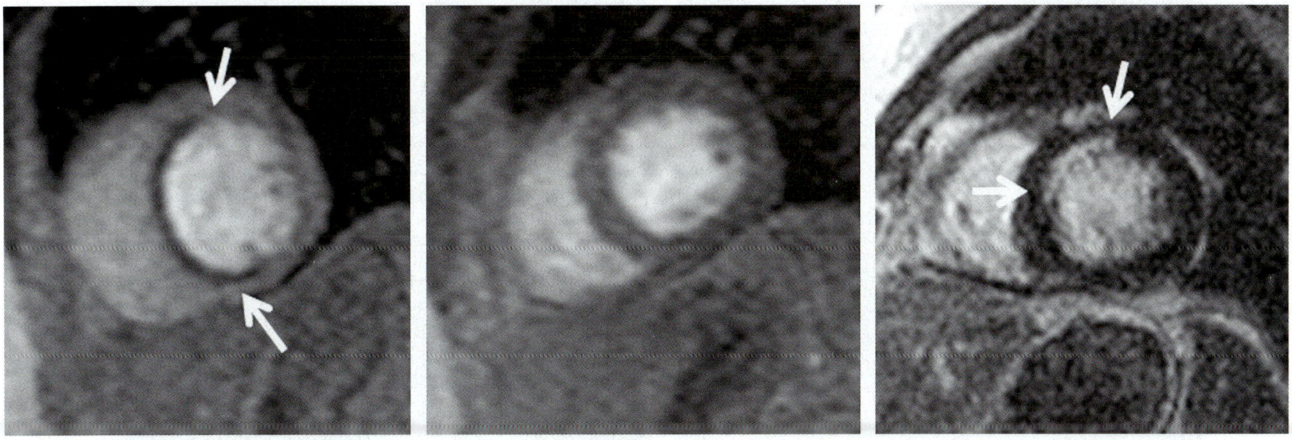

A B C

Figure 20-8. Larger perfusion defect (LAD and RCA distribution) compared with the infarct size. Not in this patient, large perfusion defect shown on stress perfusion image **(A)** involves the entire septum and parts of the anterior and inferior walls (*between arrows*). Rest perfusion **(B)** appears normal, and delayed postcontrast image **(C)** shows hyperenhancement of the subendocardial anteroseptal region (*between arrows in* **C**), which appears remarkably smaller than the stress-induced perfusion defect. This mismatch of hypoperfusion and myocardial infarction indicates that most myocardium is viable, and the patient may benefit from revascularization.

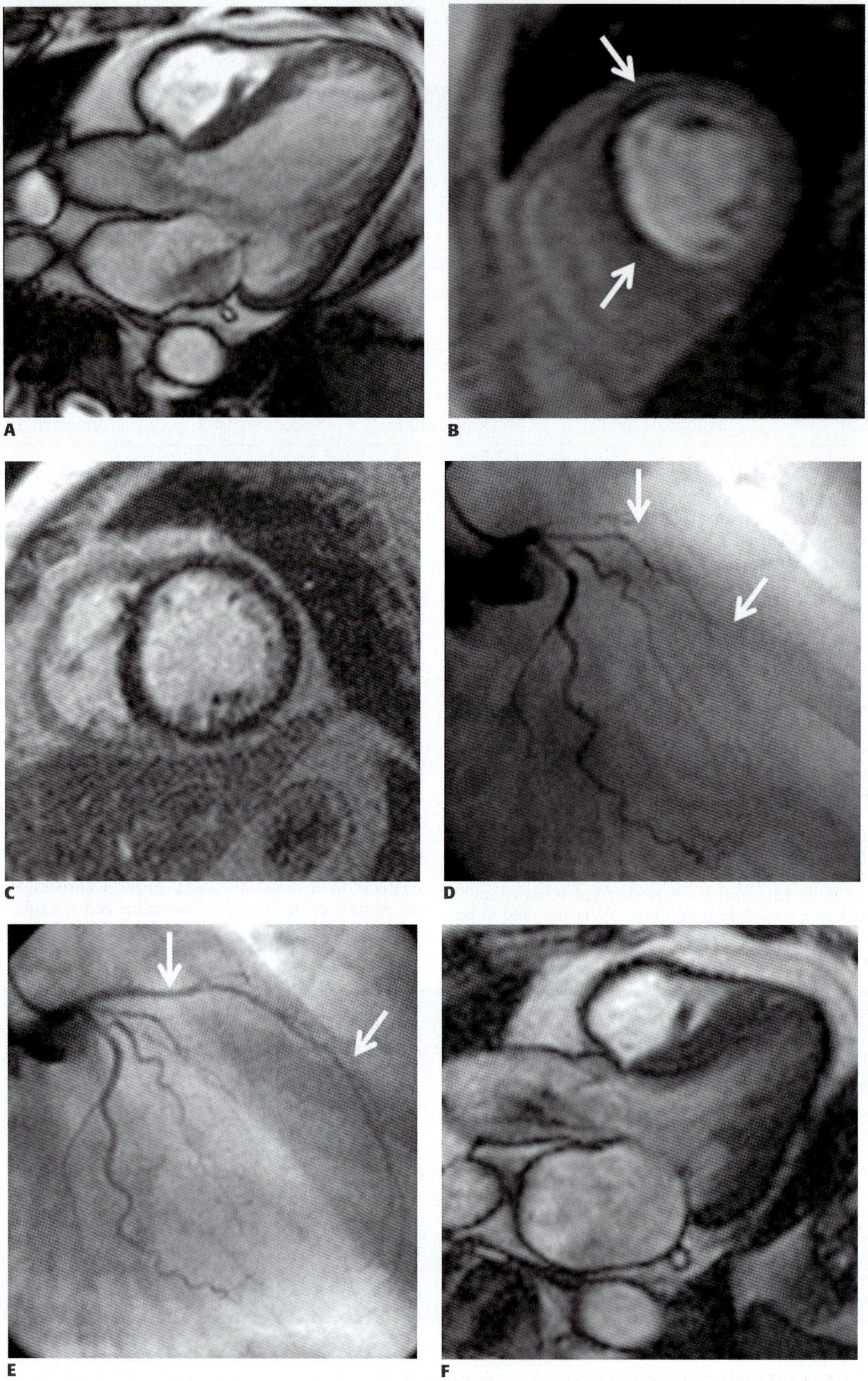

Figure 20-9. The significance of regional stress perfusion defect and negative late gadolinium enhancement (LGE). **A–C:** MR images before stenting showing dilated left ventricle and moderate mitral regurgitation on cine frame **(A)**, large defect in anteroseptal and septal walls (*arrows*) on stress perfusion image **(B)**, and lack of enhancement on delayed postcontrast sequence **(C)**. Ejection fraction was calculated at 20%. **D:** Left main angiogram showed severe LAD disease (*arrows*). Proximal LAD was stented, and postprocedure angiogram **(E)** showed restoration circulation (*arrows*) in LAD distribution. **F:** Follow-up MR after 6 months showed normal ejection fraction and improved functional mitral regurgitation. (LAD, left anterior descending artery).

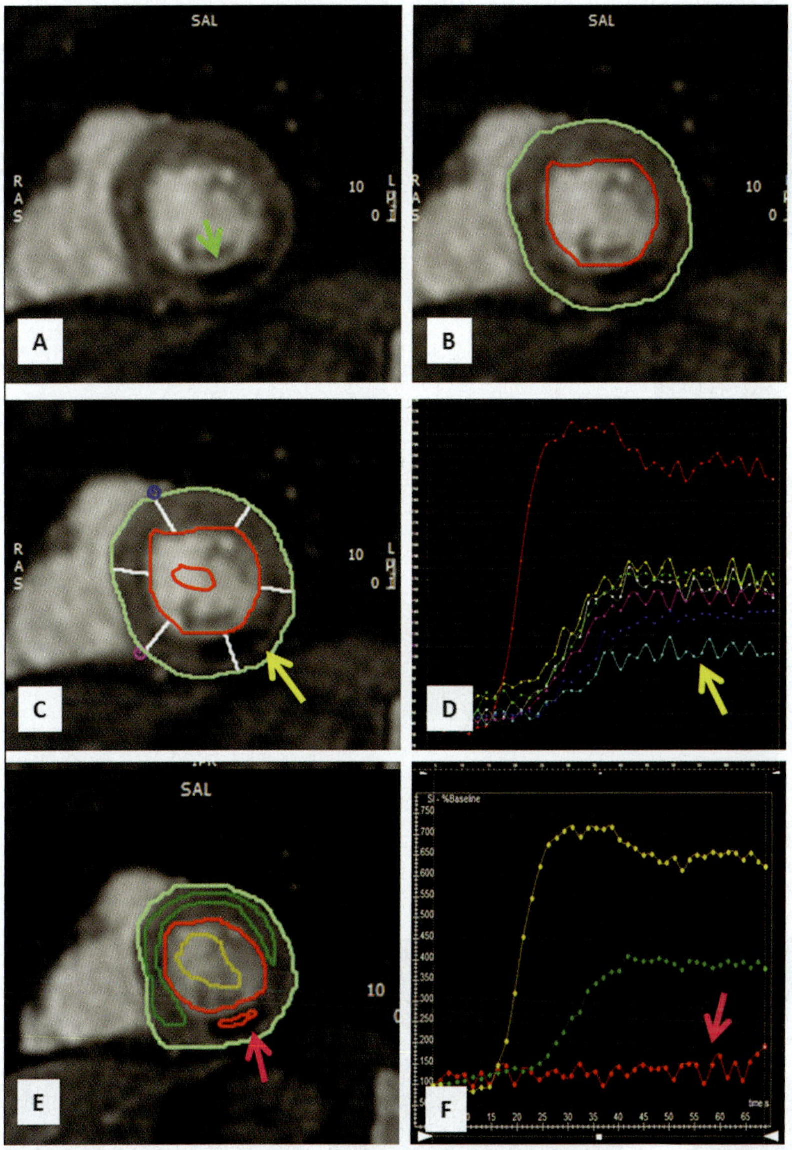

Figure 20-10. Data postprocessing in myocardial perfusion imaging. **A:** Short-axis frame of MPI shows focal dark area of abnormal perfusion (*green arrow*) in the inferior and inferolateral segments. **B:** Epicardial and endocardial borders are manually traced. **C, D:** Show segmentation method. First, anterior and inferior right ventricle insertion points to the septum are determined **(C)**. Then, automated segmentation will be performed and propagated through the entire perfusion frames in that slice, and time–signal curves will be automatically traced for all segments. The average signal for each segment is presented. Note that abnormal inferolateral segment shows the lowest perfusion (*yellow arrows*). **E, F:** Show targeted method of tracing. In this method, the abnormal perfusion area (*pink arrows*) is traced against the normal myocardium. As is obvious from tracings, the abnormal area (*red line*) shows markedly decreased perfusion compared to normal curve (*green*).

and subepicardial.[65] The entire series need to be reviewed visually (first-pass breath-hold and free breathing tail), and manual correction for respiratory motion will be applied when required, typically in dynamic frames acquired during the free-breathing part of the acquisition. When defining endocardial contours, care should be taken to exclude areas affected by endocardial banding artifacts. One has to be careful contaminating the myocardial signal with signal from the adjacent blood. Premature ventricular beats leading to variability of the size of the ventricular cavity can cause misplacement of the region of interest and need to be corrected.

Time–intensity curves are then obtained for both stress and rest images and analyzed in order to estimate MBF. A segmental-based approach can be used to demonstrate time–intensity curves for each myocardial segment. This requires manual tracings of the epicardial and endocardial borders. Mean signal intensity for each myocardial segment is then registered over time, and signal intensity–time curves will be calculated for each segment (Fig. 20.10). Alternatively, a pixel-based approach can be used to create color-coded parameter map of myocardial perfusion.[66] This technique has a better spatial resolution for showing MBF compared with sector-based mapping (Fig. 20.11). Pixels below or above a threshold for MBF are given different colors (Fig. 20.12). The rest of analysis can be derived without any further user intervention.

Semiquantitative analysis is based on the analysis of the signal intensity changes over the course of the first pass of the contrast through the myocardium. It uses a specific property of the time–intensity curve, such the maximum upslope, as an index of MBF and has been shown to be diagnostically effective.[67–69] The area under the myocardial signal curve, up to the time peak of AIF curve, is used to estimate the MPR at stress and rest (Fig. 20.13). The index of MPR is then calculated by ratio of stress/rest.[68,69] The accuracy of the upslope analysis may, however, be affected by differences in the contrast agent's pharmacodynamics and pharmacokinetic properties, which may be avoided by fully quantitative perfusion analysis.[67] Quantitative methods aim to calculate an absolute MBF value in mL/min/g by fitting the time–intensity curves to a mathematical model such as Fermi function deconvolution.[15,70] It describes the amount of gadolinium present within a region of myocardium and is relatively robust to the effects of extracellular accumulation of the injected contrast during the first pass of the contrast.[70]

Myocardial perfusion refers to coronary microcirculation blood volume flowing through a mass unit of myocardium, per

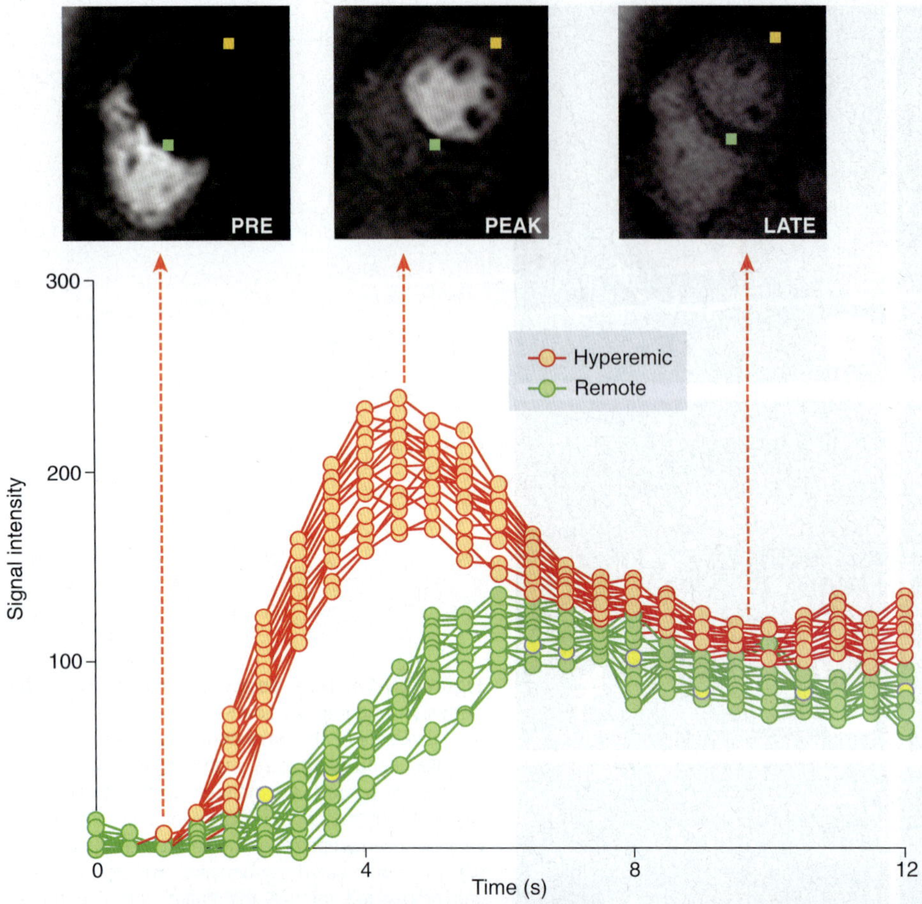

Figure 20-11. Time–signal intensity curves at a pixel level. (Adapted from Hsu LY, Groves DW, Aletras AH, et al. A quantitative pixel-wise measurement of myocardial blood flow by contrast-enhanced first-pass CMR perfusion imaging: microsphere validation in dogs and feasibility study in humans. *JACC Cardiovasc Imaging* 2012;5(2):154–66., with permission.)

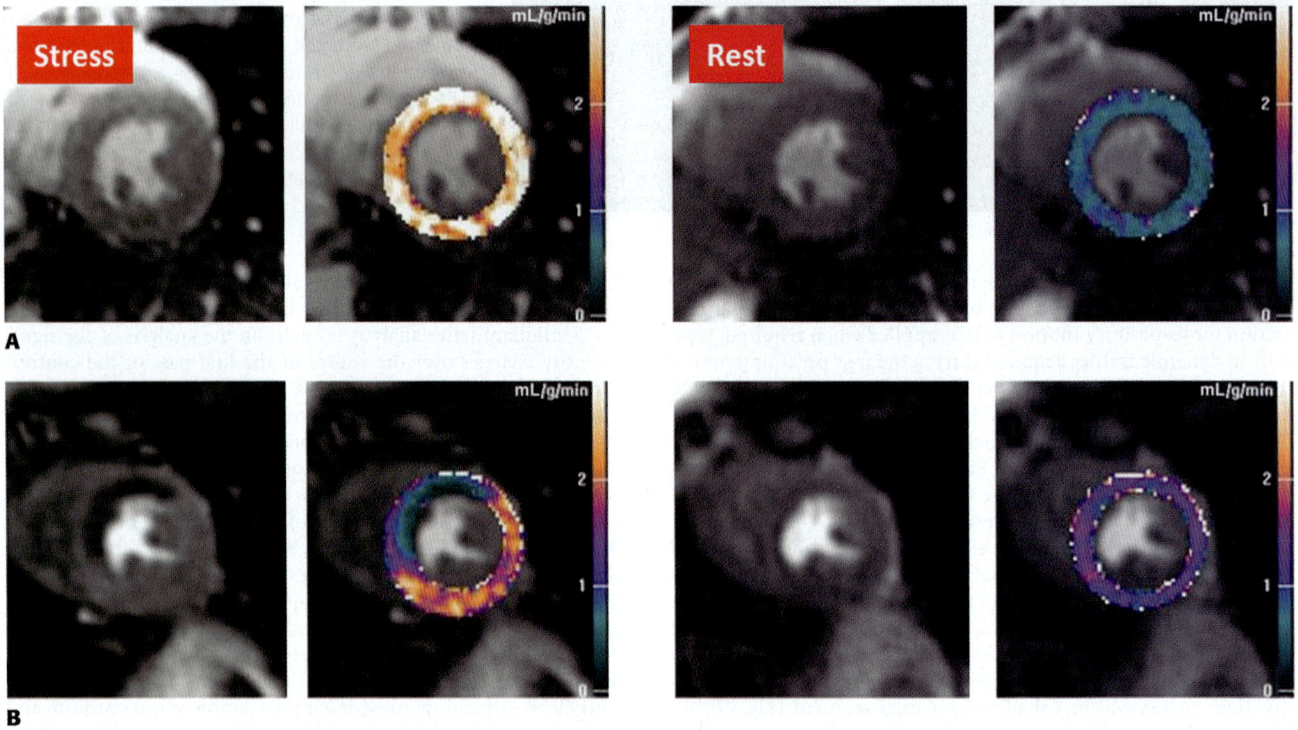

Figure 20-12. Quantitative visualization of first-pass gadolinium-enhanced perfusion MR using pixel-wise myocardial flow (MBF) parametrial maps. **A:** Normal patient shows MBF estimates in the range of 0.5 to 1.0 mL/g/min at rest and above 2.5 mL/g/min during stress. **B:** Transmural perfusion gradients in the LAD territory.

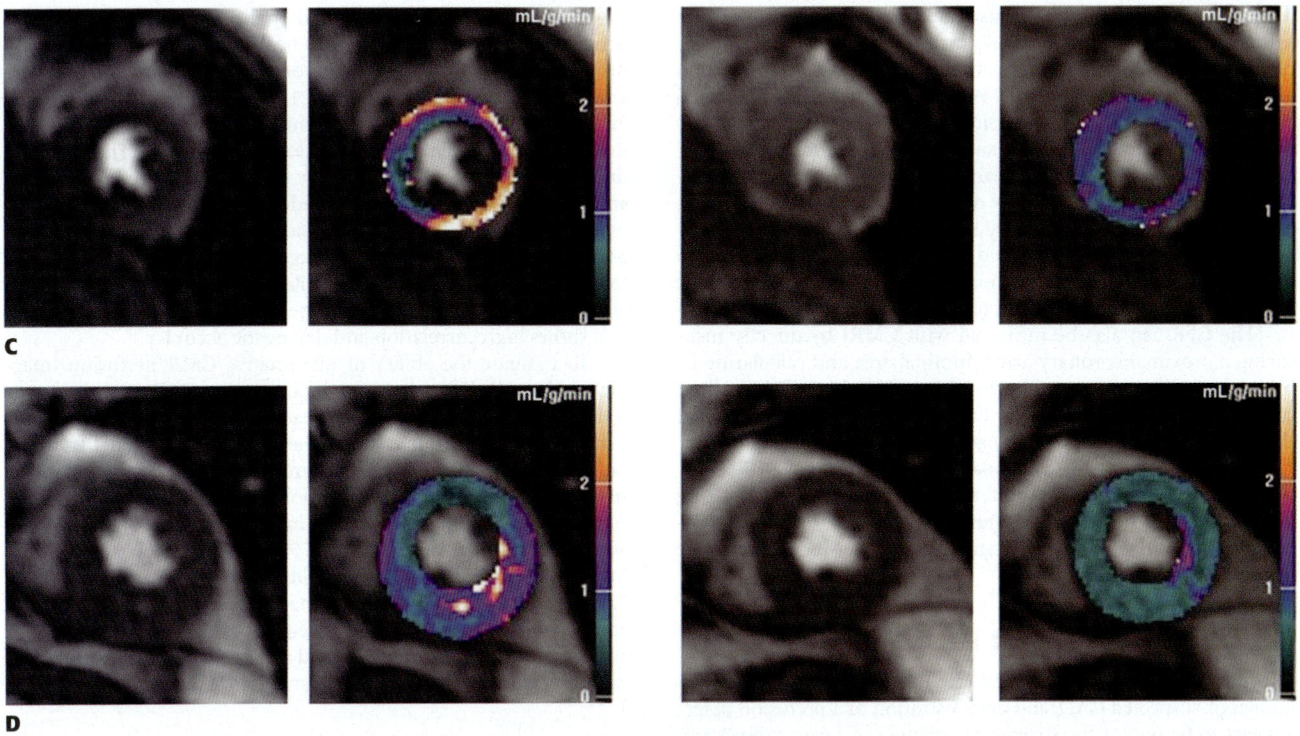

Figure 20-12. (*Continued*) **C:** Stress-induced perfusion defects mainly in the LAD and RCA territories. **D:** Reduced MBF in all myocardial regions on the stress perfusion map. Overall, perfusion maps are more homogeneous at rest compared to stress MR maps in all patients with coronary artery disease. (Adapted from Hsu LY, Groves DW, Aletras AH, et al. A quantitative pixel-wise measurement of myocardial blood flow by contrast-enhanced first-pass CMR perfusion imaging: microsphere validation in dogs and feasibility study in humans. *JACC Cardiovasc Imaging* 2012;5(2):154–166., with permission.)

unit of time. Assuming that myocardial perfusion can be quantified independently at rest and during maximal vasodilation, one can calculate the regional MPR, analogous to the CFR, as the ratio of hyperemic flow divided by the resting flow. Flow reserve can be determined at coronary arterial or at myocardial (perfusion) levels. In the presence of functional collateral circulation, CFR and MPR may differ.[69–72]

In a healthy coronary circulation, the CFR and the MPR agree in magnitude, but with epicardial CAD, the presence of coronary collaterals can result in an epicardial flow reserve, which is lower

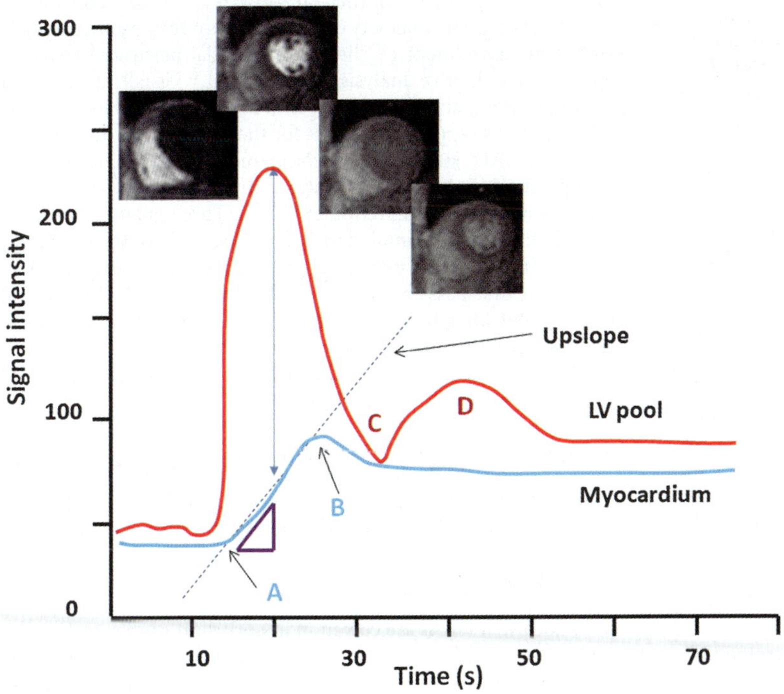

Figure 20-13. Demonstration of time-intensity curves in myocardial perfusion imaging (MPI). Arterial input function curve (*red*) of the left ventricle (LV) and myocardial tissue function curve (*blue*) of the septum are shown. Selected frames of MPI are shown on the top. The *dashed line* is defined to as the upslope parameter and gives the initial rate of contrast enhancement. It is often normalized by the upslope of the AIF, as an empirical correction factor to account for hemodynamic changes between rest and stress. The area under the myocardial curve (*triangle area*), from the foot (*point A*) up to the peak of the AIF, can be used as an alternative parameter to assess the perfusion reserve. The myocardial peak signal intensity (*point B*) is not a sensitive parameter to evaluate changes or differences in myocardial perfusion. (*A,* foot; B, myocardial peak signal; C, end of LV first pass; D, LV second-pass curve). (Jerosch-Herold M. Quantification of myocardial perfusion by cardiovascular magnetic resonance. *J Cardiovasc Magn Reson* 2010;12(1):57.)

than the MPR measured downstream from the lesion.[72,73] The MPR is probably a more accurate measure of the capacity of the coronary circulation to deliver sufficient oxygen to a given region of interest in the heart muscle. As stated earlier in this chapter, since coronary reserve or perfusion reserve are ratios, any factor that increases rest blood flow can cause underestimate ratio. For example, low perfusion reserve value in a hypertensive patient may be related to increasing rest flow not a decrease in stress flow. The minimum threshold of clinically significant ischemia for MPR is not well defined. A CFR threshold (2:1) has been used as cutoff to cause clinically significant ischemia that need to be treated.[74] Same index value is also used for MPR to indicate a significant MVD.

The CFR can also be measured with CMRI by directly measuring a proximal coronary artery luminal area and calculating its blood flow velocity using a phase-contrast technique. This method could be challenging due to cardiac and respiratory motions and the relatively small size of coronary artery lumen (approximately 1.5 to 3 mm).[75] Another way of analysis of CFR is to calculate coronary sinus flow at stress and rest, and the ratio will be CFR. Using phase-contrast MR, coronary sinus blood flow (mL/min) is calculated by summing the flow per cardiac phase over the cardiac cycle multiplied by heart rate.[76]

Validation of CMR Perfusion in Human

Imaging of ischemia has a pivotal role in workup of patients with known or suspected CAD, and demonstration of a perfusion defect appears to be one of the strongest predictors of cardiac death and nonfatal MI in large studies.[77] Abnormal MPR shown by noninvasive imaging in patient without obstructive CAD has been associated with adverse cardiovascular outcomes.[78] Among all noninvasive methods, SPECT is widely available and appears to be the most extensively validated method.[27,44] CMR has a number of advantages over other noninvasive techniques, including high spatial and temporal resolution, no exposure to ionizing radiation, and a similar diagnostic accuracy as PET. CMR also allows integration of MPI with a comprehensive assessment of biventricular function, regional function (wall thickening or strain imaging), and edema and infarction imaging. However, perfusion CMR is not without shortcomings and can be adversely affected by multiple potential factors during data acquisition as well as postprocessing. These factors are related to diverse methods of data acquisition, contrast administration, image analysis, and postprocessing as well as expertise of the MR personnel and image interpreters. No single quantitative perfusion analysis technique has been adopted in clinical practice at this time, and visual inspection remains the most common way of image reporting. Validation of CMR perfusion in humans has been performed in a number of clinical studies using different contrast agents, analysis techniques, and reference standards. In spite of this, it remains a challenge to introduce an easy, yet accurate and reproducible method to analyze myocardial perfusion.[79,80]

Conventional exercise testing has a sensitivity of 67% and specificity of 72% for correctly identifying patients with significant CAD who have not had a previous myocardial infarction.[81] Comparing diagnostic performance of CMR with SPECT for the detection of perfusion deficits in CAD (defined as ≥75% area reduction in coronary angiography), a large multicenter study emphasized CMR perfusion imaging as a valuable technique for CAD detection with higher sensitivity but lower specificity compared to SPECT.[27] In a recent meta-analysis comparing SPECT, CMR, and PET perfusion imaging techniques for the diagnosis of obstructive CAD, all showed a high sensitivity, while specificity was lowest for SPECT and highest for PET.[82] In another meta-analysis for CAD with greater than 50% coronary stenosis, MRI was shown to be superior compared with echocardiography and SPECT.[83] Echocardiography and SPECT demonstrated similar diagnostic performance.

CMR has also been validated in human subjects by direct comparison to PET. A study of 10 healthy males for absolute perfusion and MPR showed strong correlation between quantitative CMR using kinetic modeling and 13N-ammonia PET with mean perfusion values of 80 ± 20 mL/min/100 g at rest and 183 ± 56 mL/min/100 g at hyperemia as measured by CMR. There was an underestimate of peak perfusion by CMR as compared to PET.[84] In another study, analysis of the subendocardial upslope data showed a sensitivity and specificity of 91% and 94%, respectively, when compared to 13N-ammonia PET and greater than 85% when compared to quantitative angiography.[61] While PET with oxygen-15–labeled water is the gold standard technique for MBF quantification, CMR also shows high correlation and diagnostic accuracy.

To evaluate the ability of quantitative CMR perfusion imaging to assess the hemodynamic significance of CAD compared with well-established anatomic and physiologic techniques, Costa et al.[85] performed a comparative study. The MPR was calculated from the ratio between stress and rest myocardial flow based on signal intensity–time curves using deconvolution analysis. MPR cutoff of 2.04 was 93% sensitive and 57% specific in predicting a coronary segment with FFR less than or equal to 0.75. The study showed a reduced MPR of 1.54 for segments with FFR less than 0.75 and an MPR of 2.1 for segments with FFR greater than 0.75. In another study, Rieber et al.[86] compared the diagnostic accuracy of perfusion CMR versus angiographically measured FFR and reported good diagnostic accuracy of perfusion CMR to this invasive gold standard.

Quantitative versus Qualitative Assessment of Perfusion

Potential benefits of quantitative MPR measuring include reduced interpreter bias, quantification of treatment response, and improved detection of balanced ischemia. Patel et al.[87] showed similar diagnostic accuracies for detection of coronary stenosis greater than 50% for quantitative perfusion reserve measurement or by qualitative interpretation. However, improved assessment of severe and triple-vessel CAD with quantitative method was seen as compared with the visual assessment. Major limitations of quantitative perfusion analysis that prevent its widespread clinical use include lack of standardization, expensive commercial software, and time-consuming data processing. The majority of centers continue to use visual analysis for the assessment of clinical myocardial perfusion scans. In support of qualitative analysis, Watkins et al.[88] visually assessed all perfusion defects and compared it with FFR. They showed 91% sensitivity and 94% specificity of MR for the detection of functionally significant CAD. Husser et al.[89] compared quantitative assessment of contrast CMR with visual analysis in patients with ST-segment elevation myocardial infarction (STEMI). Three quantitative indices (initial slope, maximal signal intensity, and contrast delay in first-pass imaging) and two visual perfusion indices (hypoenhancement in the first-pass and microvascular obstruction [MVO] in late enhancement imaging) were evaluated. Quantification of the perfusion images was very time consuming and proved not superior to visual perfusion analysis to predict reduced ejection fraction and/or major adverse cardiac events (MACEs).

Myocardial Perfusion Imaging Artifacts

Several artifacts can occur in first-pass perfusion imaging that must be recognized in order to correctly interpret the images qualitatively.

Dark-Rim Artifacts

Subendocardial DRAs are common in perfusion studies and can be quite problematic as they can be confused with myocardial perfusion defects. These artifacts transiently appear as a dark line at the

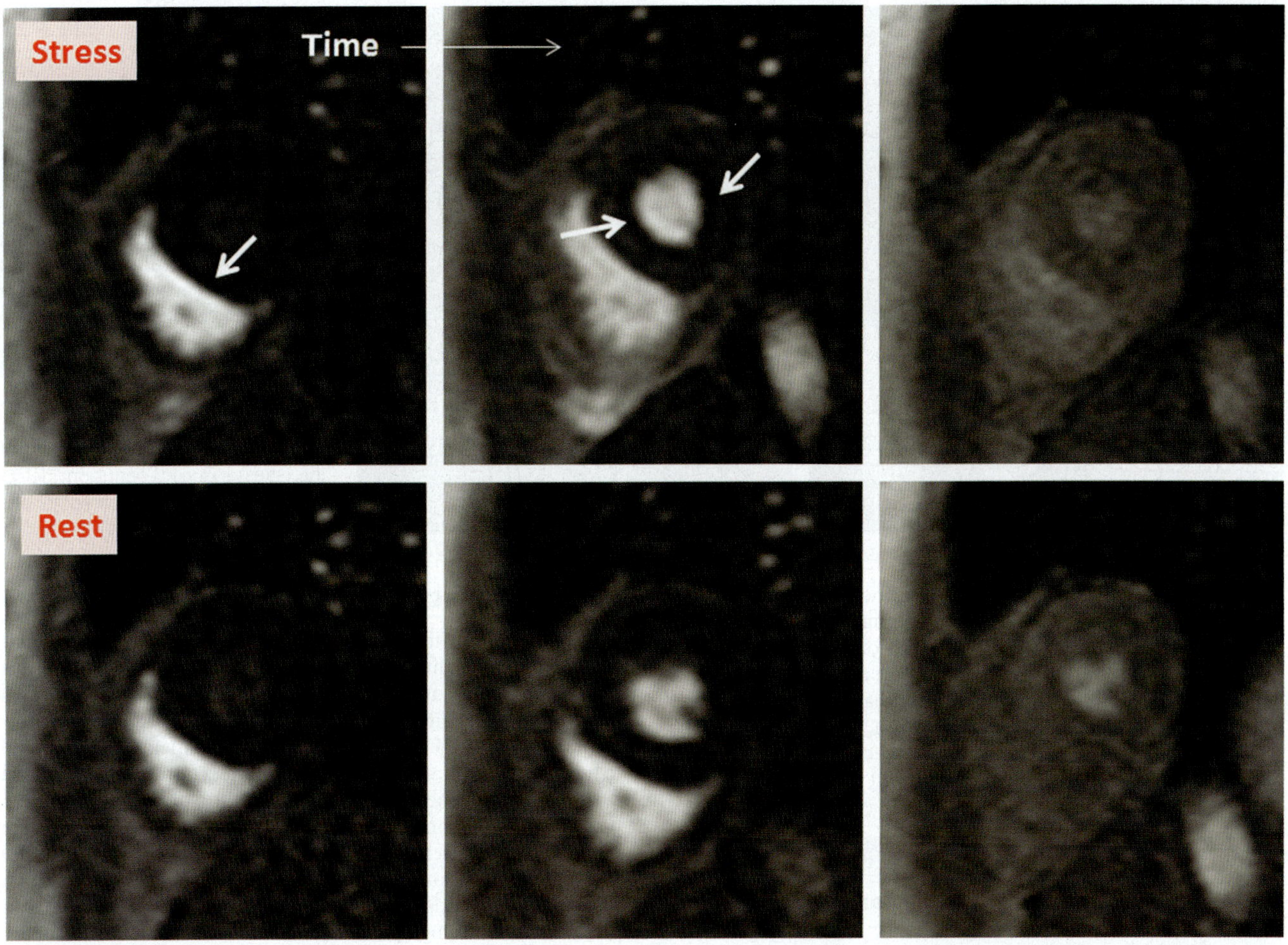

Figure 20-14. **Susceptibility effect shown as a dark-rim artifact (DRA) at myocardial–blood pool interfaces (*arrows*).** It is most pronounced when blood concentration is highest (*arrows*) and less apparent on late frames when the myocardial is enhanced and blood pool is washed out of contrast. Note that artifact is not as conspicuous on rest images as it is on stress images. The reason is likely due to relative increase in myocardial signal in rest series from pervious contrast administration during stress perfusion.

interface between the myocardium and LV cavity during the influx of high concentration bolus of contrast agent (Fig. 20.14) and typically last only a few heartbeats. In contrast, a real perfusion defect tends to be visible after myocardial enhancement and for a longer duration of the imaging. DRAs can be seen in both stress and rest perfusion phases. The extent of DRA is most prominent during stress and in systole (Fig. 20.15). Increased cardiac function at stress leads to increased LV blood pool signal and more artifact at the margin of the blood pool. DRAs can cause the myocardial signal intensity to drop below the baseline (precontrast) signal value.[42,88] b-SSFP sequence is more prone to DRAs than to other acquisition sequences.[91]

Several factors have been suggested as contributory to the production of DRAs such as partial volume averaging, susceptibility effects induced by the gadolinium bolus, myocardial motion, undersampling from low spatial resolution, or a combination of these factors[91–93] (Table 20.2). These effects will be reduced by the use of higher spatial and temporal resolution. Motion during image acquisition can generate abrupt discontinuities in k-space, which translate into banding artifacts at tissue boundaries in the image.

Magnetic susceptibility effects may also cause DRA due to increase magnetic field distortions at interfaces. Magnetic susceptibility will be increased on the arrival of contrast agent and with higher concentration of contrast agent.[43,90] b-SSFP sequence is even more sensitive to changes in magnetic susceptibility, which cause local changes to the Larmor frequency (off-resonance effect).[43]

In a recent study, it has been suggested that DRAs are actually truncation artifacts and may be largely due to limited spatial resolution rather than motion alone.[93] Therefore, Fourier transform is unable to accurately represent true high contrast boundaries in the image and to reconstruct sharp edges perfectly. This causes signal variations adjacent to these boundaries that appear as bright and dark bands. This effect is also more prominent at higher contrast concentrations and when using b-SSFP sequence.[94] Truncation ring artifacts (and DRA) tend to be most prominent next to the blood–myocardium interface perpendicular to the direction with the lowest spatial resolution (which is typically the phase-encoding direction). Increasing spatial resolution by increasing phase-encoding steps can obviate ring artifacts. This may not be feasible due to time constraints in cardiac imaging. The position of the bands changes with the phase-encoding direction.[90] Parallel acquisition schemes are the most efficient way to reduce acquisition time in conjunction with improving spatial resolution.[95] The greater SNR available on 3-T scanners can potentially offset the loss in SNR that results from incorporating parallel acquisition techniques. Lower concentrations of gadolinium dose can be used at 3 T (leading to less susceptibility problems) since the effective relaxivity of the contrast agents increases with Bo.[96]

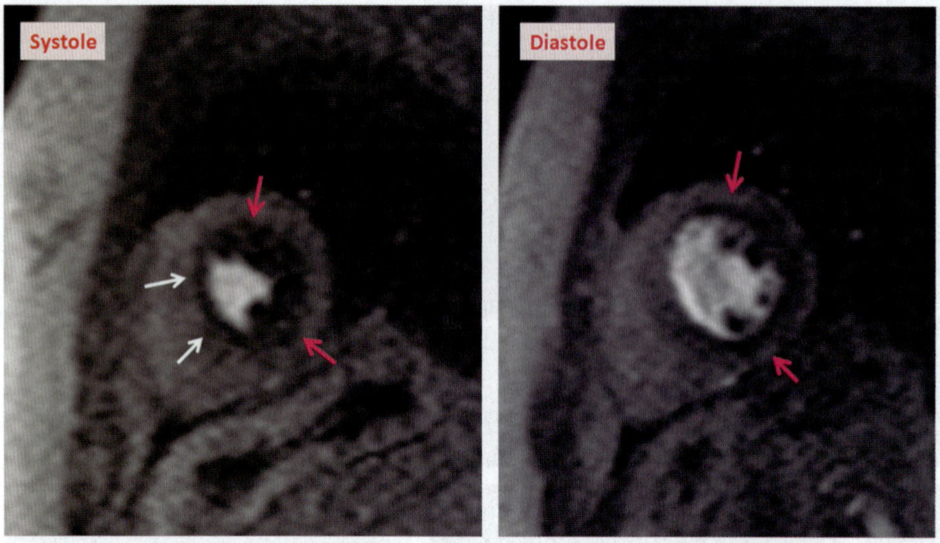

Figure 20-15. Stress perfusion defect in systole and diastole in a patient with severe left ventricular hypertrophy. Subendocardial dark rim of septum in systole (*white arrows*) is likely related to susceptibility and Gibbs along phase-encoding gradient, which is not seen on diastolic image. Also note the relative conspicuity of the stress-induced perfusion defect on systolic image compared to diastolic image (*pink arrows*).

Pseudo-DRA can occur in the presence of subendocardial calcification, a common finding in chronic myocardial infarction. Generally, calcifications appear dark of all pulse sequences (Fig. 20.16). Diagnosis of DRAs is important as those may interfere with correct diagnosis of ischemia and potentially affect the estimates of MBF. For correct perfusion quantification, endocardial contours should be carefully placed to exclude the affected areas. In this way, we may avoid potential contamination of MPI curves by DRAs.

TABLE 20.2 **Dark-Rim Artifact: Types, Reason, and Remedies**

Artifact	Reason	Remedy
Truncation	Undersampling of high-frequency data causes signal oscillations at high contrast boundaries	Increasing image resolution by (a) increasing number of phase-encoding lines, (b) adding parallel imaging
Susceptibility	Magnetic field distortions at blood–myocardium interface due to arrival of concentrated contrast	(a) Avoid b-SSFP, (b) decrease contrast concentration
Motion	Motion causes discontinuities in k-space and banding at boundaries	(a) Use sequential k-space ordering, (b) parallel imaging

b-SSFP, balanced steady-state at free precession.
Biglands JD, Radjenovic A, Ridgway JP. Cardiovascular magnetic resonance physics for clinicians: Part II. *J Cardiovasc Magn Reson* 2012;14:66.

Motion Artifacts

Ghost artifacts due to motion are one of the most common reasons for poor image quality when imaging the heart. Breath holding and ECG triggering are usually sufficient to account for these motions during short acquisition time of 10 to 15 seconds. Since data acquisition is much longer in perfusion imaging, patients are requested to hold their breath, starting 10 seconds after contrast injection, and keep it as long as they can and then breathe slowly. Unfortunately, problems with poor breath holding or poor ECG triggering are not uncommon. Technical problem with ECG gating is even more common in 3-T scanners. In some cases, it can be substituted with peripheral pulse gating/triggering. Obviously, these artifacts are less pronounced with single-shot sequences. Variation in position of the heart may limit correct analysis of myocardial perfusion particularly in semiautomated techniques. Frame-by-frame corrections may be needed to place the epicardial and endocardial tracings as well as the region of interests in correct locations.

In some patients, the problem is not the inability to breath-hold for 8 to 10 seconds, but the fact that "straining" occurs during breath holding, which leads to small motions that degrade image quality. To lessen these breathing artifacts, we coach the patient to relax during breath holding, which should usually take place after a normal expiration rather than after forced inspiration or expiration.

Aliasing

Like other MR sequences, wrap around artifacts are common in perfusion sequences. Solutions can be in-plane rotation of the phase/frequency encode direction or increasing the field of view along phase-encoding direction. Parallel imaging methods can accelerate imaging, but at the cost of reduction in SNR and increased propensity for artifacts. Aliasing can occur with the use of parallel imaging when the reconstructed field of view is smaller than the object being imaged. Aliasing is more common in sensitivity encoding (SENSE) than generalized autocalibrating partially parallel acquisition (GRAPPA). Contrary to conventional imaging, these artifacts are present not only at the edges of the field of view but also in the central portion of the image. To remove aliasing artifacts, one can increase the field of view, although at the expense of lower spatial resolution (Fig. 20.17). Another solution would be to increase the number of phase-encodings steps, which will reduce the effective acceleration factor while maintaining the same spatial resolution. Newer methods such as Dynamic Parallel Imaging with TSENSE or

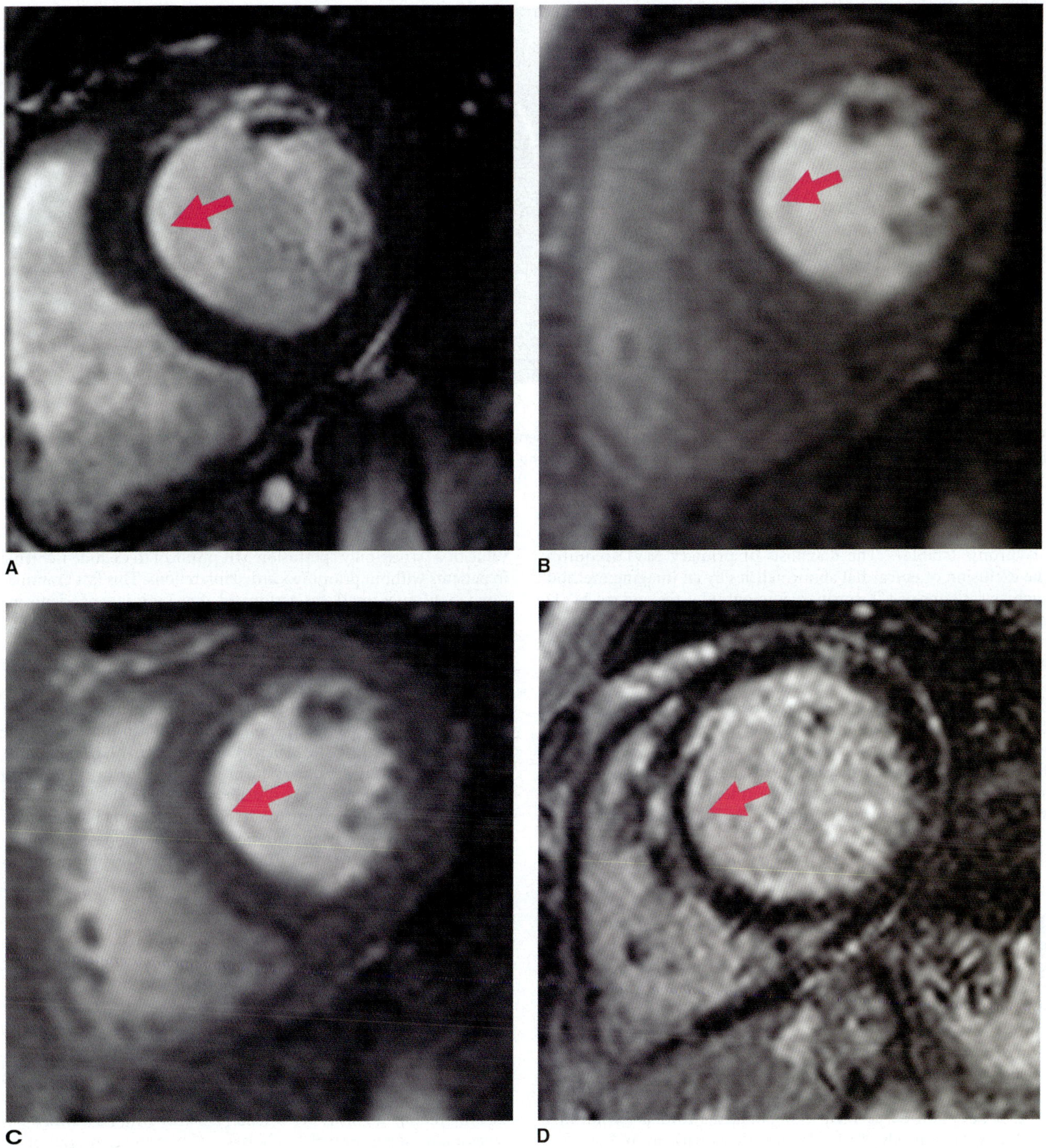

Figure 20-16. **Short-axis images of the heart demonstrate subendocardial rim calcification along the septal wall of the left myocardium.** Note that calcification appears relatively dark on all imaging sequences (*arrows*). Cine balanced steady-state free precession (b-SSFP) **(A)**, saturation recovery fast gradient-echo stress perfusion **(B)**, rest perfusion **(C)**, and inversion recovery fast gradient-echo postcontrast viability image **(D)**.

TGRAPPA may suppress coil-related residual aliasing artifacts and would be a better choice for perfusion studies.[97–99]

Clinical Applications of Perfusion CMR

Perfusion CMR can be used in two major categories of myocardial ischemia caused by (a) epicardial obstructive CAD and (b) coronary MVD. Epicardial CAD is more common, but several conditions may primarily involve microvascular. Coronary MVD can present clinically primarily associated with the syndrome of chest pain despite normal coronary arteriograms or in the context of cardiac disease processes. In the absence of any apparent cardiac or systemic disease, MVD may be the only cause of angina. This group of MVD is defined as "primary," and the resultant angina is known as microvascular angina (MVA). Clinical presentation of primary MVD can be acute (unstable)

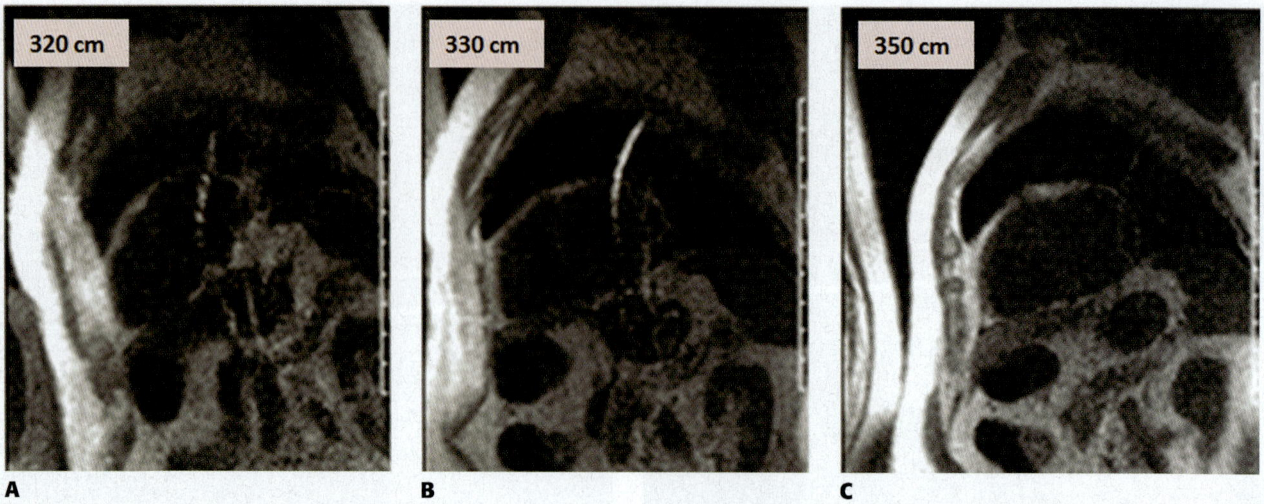

Figure 20-17. **Effect of field of view (FOV) on artifacts.** Precontrast perfusion images using saturation recovery fast gradient-echo sequence with TSENSE parallel imaging demonstrate inverse relation of severity of aliasing artifacts with the size FOV. Aliased ghosts are significantly reduced when phase FOV is increased from 320 cm **(A)** to 330 cm **(B)** and 350 cm **(C)**. The trade-offs for larger FOV are decreased spatial resolution and increased scan time.

or chronic (stable).[8] The diagnosis of primary MVD requires the exclusion of epicardial abnormalities by an imaging method such as catheter or CT coronary angiography. Secondary MVD can occur (a) in the presence of obstructive CAD (acute coronary syndrome), (b) after coronary interventions (reperfusion injury), (c) after heart transplantation, and (d) in the presence of cardiomyopathies.[1,100]

It is important to know that patients with epicardial CAD commonly have a higher microvascular resistance. In other word, when the two conditions coexist, it is possible that MVD started first before any epicardial disease.[101] This may explain persistence of symptoms in 20% of patients after treatment of hemodynamically significant epicardial coronary stenosis.[102]

Stratifying Patients Presenting with Chest Pain

The real challenge in initial triage of patients presented to emergency chest pain units is the identification of low-risk chest pain group who could safely be discharged. Several advances in noninvasive imaging techniques, such as dobutamine stress echocardiography, stress nuclear studies, CT coronary angiography, and, recently, stress CMR, have enhanced the accuracy and efficiency of evaluation of patients with acute chest pain.[103,104] Highly desirable features of such techniques include a high negative prognostic value. Fewer than 5% of patients presenting with chest pain have STEMI, and up to 25% have non–ST-segment elevation acute coronary syndrome (ACS). Approximately 2% to 5% of patients with an ACS are discharged from the emergency room with an erroneous diagnosis of noncardiac chest pain. Therefore, a negative study would allow the safe discharge of patients with low-risk chest pain. Adenosine stress CMR is a useful tool to rule out significant CAD in patients with chest pain, nondiagnostic electrocardiogram, and negative serum biomarkers for myocardial infarction. It has a negative predictive value of 100%.[105] Jahnke et al.[106] evaluated a combined sequential adenosine/dobutamine stress CMR imaging protocol and showed that in a moderate-risk population, myocardial ischemia detected by these tests can be used to identify patients at high risk for subsequent cardiac death or nonfatal myocardial infarction. For patients with normal adenosine/dobutamine stress MR, the 3-year event-free survival was 99.2%. Lubbers et al.[107] showed high diagnostic value of a "stress-only" perfusion MR protocol to exclude ischemia in patients without prior myocardial infarctions. This fast examination (15 minutes total) was performed after 3 minutes of adenosine infusion during the first pass of injection of 0.1 mmol/kg gadolinium contrast at a flow rate of 5 mL/s.

The American College of Cardiology Foundation Task Force on Expert Consensus Documents recently published a report regarding the significance of CMR perfusion imaging in evaluation of patients with chest pain suspicious for CAD.[108] In this report, the combination of CMR stress perfusion, function, and LGE allows the use of CMR as a primary form of testing for (a) identifying patients with ischemic heart disease when there are resting ECG abnormalities or an inability to exercise, (b) defining patients with large vessel CAD and its distribution who are candidates for interventional procedures, or (c) determining patients who are appropriate candidates for interventional procedures.

Microvascular Obstruction and Acute Myocardial Infarction

"No-reflow" Phenomenon

In patients diagnosed with STEMI, prompt restoration of CBF to the infarcted myocardium should be undertaken. Significant improvement in mortality and morbidity may be achieved even when reperfusion occurs up to 6 to 12 hours after acute myocardial infarction.[109] This is performed primarily with PCI, which has several advantages over thrombolysis. PCI improves overall prognosis by providing greater patency rates of the reopened arteries and infarct-related artery and higher coronary flow grades.[109,110] However, the restoration of the perfusion can paradoxically damage myocytes and endothelial cells. This phenomenon is called "reperfusion injury."[110] Therefore, in spite of patency of epicardial arteries after PCI, MVO can occur in up to 40% due to swelling of endothelial cells and microembolization of plaque debris and fibrin clots.[110] Rupture or erosion of epicardial coronary artery plaques, either spontaneously or induced by PCI, can lead to obstruction of the microvessels due to distal microembolization and secondary inflammatory response with the release of vasogenic and thrombogenic factors.[111] This condition is commonly referred to as the "no-reflow" phenomenon[112] (Fig. 20.18).

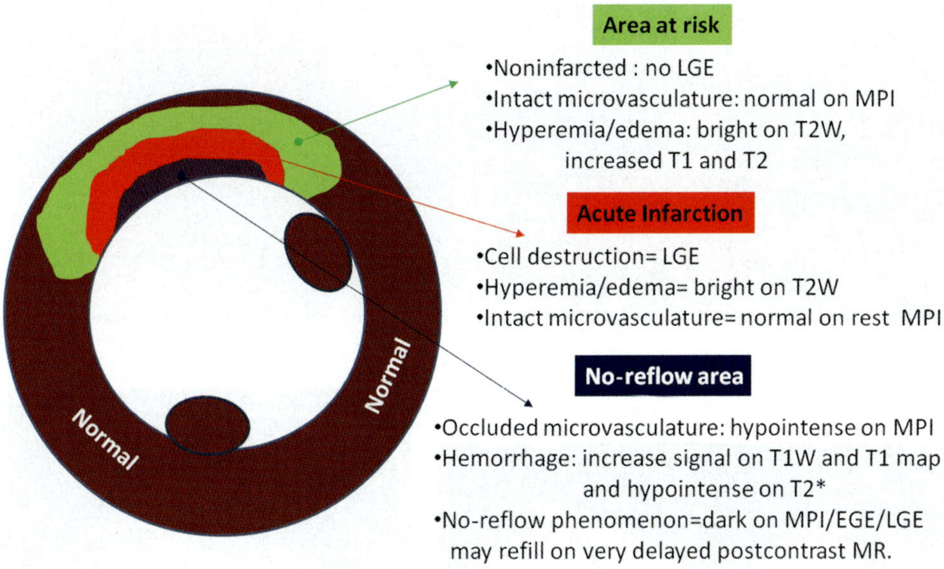

Figure 20-18. **Schematic presentation of the components of injured myocardium after reperfusion for STEMI.** LGE, late gadolinium enhancement; MPI, myocardial perfusion imaging, EGE, early gadolinium enhancement.

As a consequence, chest pain and ST-segment elevation can persist or recur despite the successful resolution of epicardial artery occlusion. Several factors determine the extent of anatomic no-reflow development. An important factor is the duration of myocardial ischemia; the extent of MVO worsens with longer durations of ischemia before reperfusion intervention.[112] The size of myocardial infarction is the major determinant of the amount of necrosis in no-reflow zone. The no-reflow zone is generally confined to the zone of infarction and tends to be slightly smaller in size. The size of no reflow and the amount of macroscopically visible hemorrhage in it correlate with each other. In a canine model of myocardial infarction used in the MRI investigations by Rochitte et al.,[113] the zone of MVO increased from 13% at 2 hours after reperfusion to 23% at 6 hours of reperfusion with a further increase to 30% at 48 hours of reperfusion. Therefore, most significant amount of microvascular deterioration occurs during the first hours after initiation of reperfusion, presenting a potential time window for therapeutic interventions.

Patients with "no reflow" exhibit a higher prevalence of early postinfarct complications, adverse left ventricular remodeling, and mortality.[109,110] Therefore, the diagnosis of "no-reflow" phenomenon is very important and any imaging method including myocardial perfusion MR should be able to estimate the size and location of the "no-reflow" area (zone). Using first-pass MPI, it is shown that in STEMI patients, a larger release of cardiac necrosis markers especially troponin markers soon after reperfusion therapy relates to abnormal perfusion.[114]

Diagnosis of "No Reflow"

The diagnosis of "no reflow" or "slow reflow" can be made using angiography, electrocardiography, nuclear scintigraphy, contrast echocardiography, CMR, and perfusion CT[115,116] (Figs. 20.19 to 20.21). Angiographic assessment of "no reflow" is routinely performed after PCI. Common methods include thrombolysis in myocardial infarction (TIMI) flow grades (TFG), TIMI myocardial perfusion grade (TMPG), myocardial blush grade, and corrected TIMI frame count (CTFC).[116]

TFG is a very simple practical method to use and graded from 0 to 3. TIMI grade 3 flow is regarded as equal rate of flow compared to non–culprit-related artery. However, this technique suffers from high interobserver variability, and it depends on the length and size of vessel. In CTFC method, the number of cine frames for contrast to reach standard distal landmarks will be counted (Figs. 20.19 and 20.20). Since the left anterior descending artery (LAD) is longer, the frame counts are corrected by dividing by 1.7.[117] In addition to assessing the epicardial blood flow, CTFC is dependent on resistive components within the microvasculature and is therefore a marker of microcirculatory function. In patients with TIMI grade 3 flow, CTFC can vary from 14 to 40, and if it is less than 14, the 30-day mortality is almost zero.[117] In TMPG technique, clearing of myocardial blush following contrast injection is categorically graded from 0 to 3. TMPG 0 represents minimal or no myocardial blush, and TMPG 3 represents normal entrance and exit of contrast in the myocardium. Impaired TMPG is associated with MACEs. Appelbaum et al. showed that impaired TMPG (<3) was associated with larger infarct size at baseline and follow-up.[118] Angiographic assessments of no reflow such as CTFC and TMPG are well validated but lack accuracy and do not allow direct visualization of the affected myocardium. Furthermore, the extent of MVO may continue to evolve over time following reperfusion therapy.

Gadolinium-enhanced CMR has been used extensively in the study of myocardial infarction and to evaluate the extent of microvascular obstruction. Since MVO has different appearances in perfusion and delayed postcontrast MRI, a comprehensive study is necessary. The routine protocol adopted in our institution includes T2W sequence to show myocardial edema, short-axis cine, rest perfusion, long-axis cine, and LGE series. Rest perfusion imaging is performed during bolus injection (4 to 5 mL/s) of half dose of gadolinium (0.05 to 0.1 mmol/kg). The rest of contrast is injected after rest perfusion. In order to image the extent of MVO/no reflow, the spatial coverage or rest perfusion sequence should be increased to cover entire left ventricle. The standard LGE sequence is usually obtained 15 to 30 minutes after the second contrast dose, and the inversion time is set to null the normal myocardium (TI, 220 to 280).

In MR study of MVO, it is important to image MVO soon after injection of contrast.[113] Diffusion of gadolinium into the area of MVO occurs causing decreased size of no reflow over time. In an animal study, Wu et al.[111] compared the size of no reflow in rest perfusion MRI with histopathologic specimens. They noticed good correlation between the two techniques but MRI underestimated the size of no-reflow. Therefore, high-resolution perfusion technique that covers the entire LV is necessary. With the recent advent of accelerated high-resolution perfusion sequences (1.5 mm × 1.5 mm spatial resolution, 8 slices acquired over 2 R-R intervals), it is

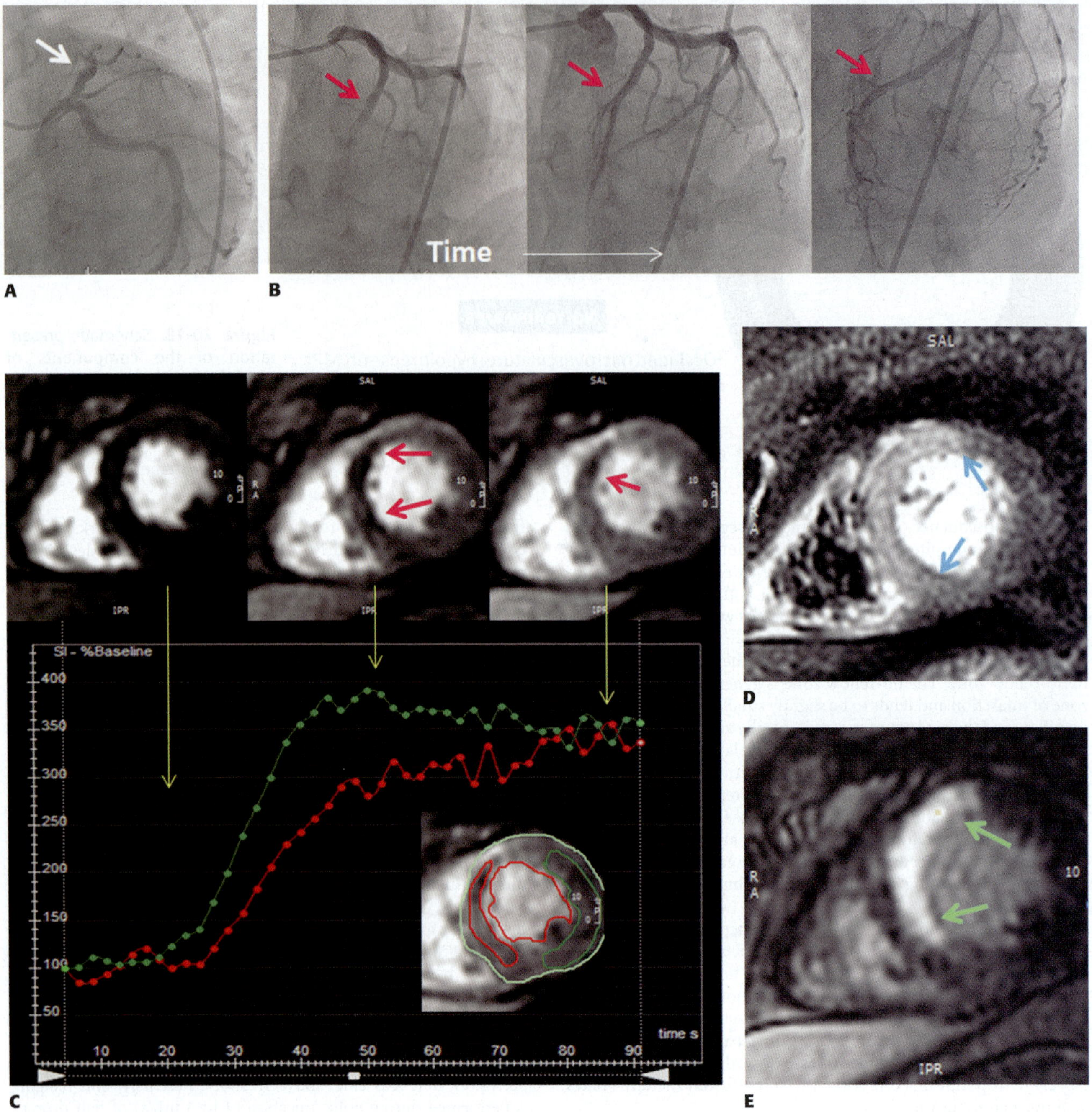

Figure 20-19. **STEMI patient due to left anterior descending artery (LAD) occlusion, status postreperfusion of LAD with proximal stenting, and mild microvascular impairment.** **A:** Caudal right anterior oblique (RAO) angiogram shows occluded LAD (*arrow*). **B:** Poststenting angiogram series show patent LAD (*pink arrows*) with mild decreased flow compared to left circumflex branches. TIMI grade improved from 0 before to 2 after stenting. Uncorrected TIMI frame count was 30 for LAD, which is upper limit of normal values. **C:** Rest perfusion MR time–intensity curves and corresponding MR images are shown. The curve obtained from diseased myocardium of septum (*red*) shows slight decreased perfusion compared to normal lateral wall (*green*). Corresponding images show decreased signal of the septum consistent with no-reflow area (NRA) (*pink arrows*). **D:** Short-axis T2-weighted image shows the extent of edema (*blue arrows*), and **(E)** delayed postcontrast image shows the extent of infarcted tissue (*green arrows*). Note that size of no reflow (or slow reflow) is markedly smaller than the infarcted zone. Absence of NRA and faster TIMI frame counts are good prognostic indicators.

now possible to detect true size of no reflow and quantify it for the entire LV.[119]

The importance of detecting MVO early after contrast injection is increasingly being recognized and has led to including additional postcontrast sequences. Whereas traditional LGE CMR (after 15 minutes) may underestimate the true extent of MVO, perfusion MRI and EGE may show the real extent of MVO (Fig. 20.21). For example, in a CMR study performed by Bekkers et al.,[120] it was shown that compared with "early no reflow," the "late no reflow" disappeared in 9% patients, and in almost all patients, the extent of MVO decreased significantly from early to late imaging.[120] For this reason, some institutions, including ours, also obtain an EGE 2 to

5 minutes after the second dose of contrast, and the inversion time is set to 450 to 600 milliseconds using single-shot IR b-SSFP or fast gradient-echo sequence to enhance the contrast for the detection of MVO. At 1.5-T field strength, the application of a 400 to 600 delay will null the signal of blood clot and the no-reflow region and makes these areas dark relative to the normal myocardium.[119] Therefore, infarcted myocardium appears hyperenhanced or "bright" compared to normal myocardial tissue while microvascular obstruction or hemorrhage appears as a central hypoenhanced region within the hyperenhanced region in both EGE and LGE studies[115] (Figs. 20.20 and 20.21).

MRI is typically performed 3 to 7 days after reperfusion in STEMI situation. Mather et al. observed significant changes in LV function, infarct size, MVO, and extent of myocardial edema during the 1st week after acute myocardial infarction.[121] The authors also observed that the extent of MVO on LGE imaging diminished significantly between day 2 and 1 week. Using first-pass rest perfusion in STEMI patients, Rogers et al.[122] described three patterns on MR images. (a) Decreased signal on first-pass only, (b) normal first-pass signal plus hyperenhanced signal on delayed images, and (c) low-signal lesions on first-pass enhancement plus delayed hyperenhancement. The second group with normal perfusion had partially reversible dysfunction and predominantly viable myocardium. Decreased signal on perfusion indicates little functional improvement at 7 weeks due to microvascular damage. It is important to know that superimposed myocardial hemorrhage in no-reflow zone after reperfusion can create confusing pattern on first-pass images (Fig. 20.20). Although hemorrhage may not be directly detected on first-pass series (low resolution and high noise), its presence can increase myocardial signal in the area of MVO and falsely obscure the low signal intensity of the no-reflow zone to become isosignal to normal myocardium. It is therefore necessary to carefully review all MR sequences. Adding sequences sensitive to intramyocardial hemorrhage (IMH) may prevent false interpretation.

Assessment of Reperfusion Hemorrhage

Recently, it has been shown that the presence of IMH is associated with adverse left ventricular remodeling and poor prognosis.[121] A noninvasive imaging modality capable of identifying IMH may provide further prognostic information. Hemorrhage usually occurs within the area of no reflow. Robbers et al.[123] demonstrated in pathology that at 1 week after reperfused STEMI, no reflow and hemorrhage are two manifestations of the same pathophysiologic process,

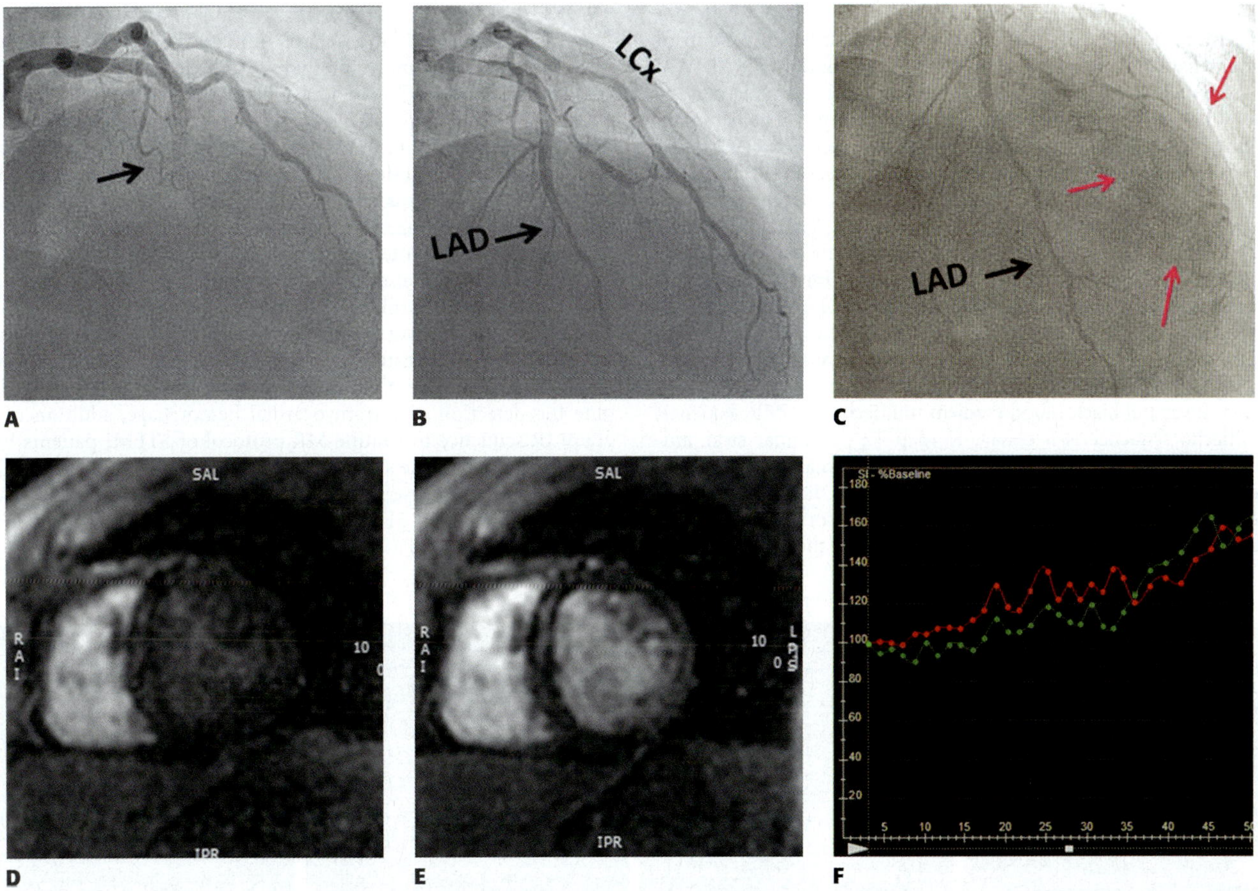

Figure 20-20. **False-negative appearance of no-reflow area (NRA) on rest perfusion due to hemorrhage within NRA in an STEMI patient 3 days after revascularization with stent for LAD occlusion and development of extensive microvascular impairment. A–C:** RAO cranial views show post-LAD stenting. **A:** Before reperfusion. TIMI flow grade of 0. **B, C:** After reperfusion. TIMI flow grade of 2. Corrected TIMI frame count was 85 divided by 1.7 for the LAD artery. Note delayed filling of the LAD. Normal myocardial blush seen in the left circumflex territory (*pink arrows*) is absent in the LAD distribution. **D, E:** Rest perfusion images before contrast arrival in left ventricle and **(E)** after arrival of contrast. **F:** Time–intensity curves of septal (*red*) and lateral (*green*) walls. Mild higher signal of the septal wall on initial frame **(D)** likely due to superimposed hemorrhage is shown, which falls below the lateral wall curve on late frames **(E)**. Late frame **(E)** does not show the expected low signal of NRA either due to the lack of NRA or due to superimposed hemorrhage.

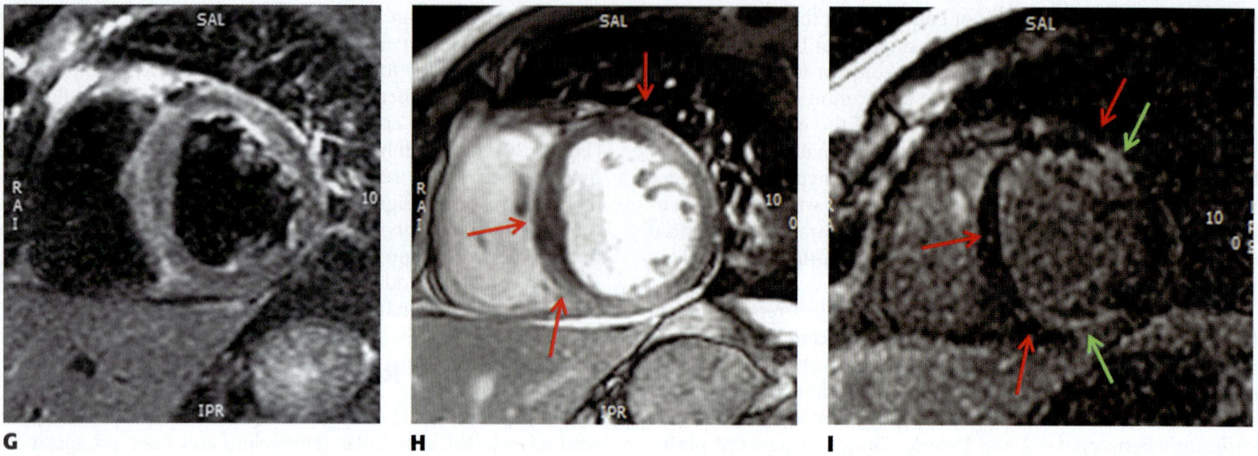

Figure 20-20. (*Continued*) **G:** T2W triple IR fast spin echo image obtained for edema assessment underestimates the size of edema in septum due to superimposed hemorrhage. **H:** On the other hand, the hemorrhagic extent of NRA (*red arrows* in **H**) is best shown in b-SSFP **(H)** image due to higher susceptibility effect in this gradient-echo sequence. **I:** LGE shows low signal of extensive NRA (+hemorrhage) involving entire septum and the anterior wall (*red arrows*), which is delimited by enhancing infarct at both ends (*green arrows*). The lateral wall is intact. b-SSFP, balanced steady state free precession. LAD, left anterior descending artery.

reflecting extensive coagulation necrosis with severe disruption of endothelial coherence and erythrocyte extravasation. Overall, MRI is great modality to detect blood products and to demonstrate the extent hemorrhage at different stages of evolution.[124] The paramagnetic effects of hemorrhage appear to predominate between 1 and 7 days after reperfusion. Signal voids have been observed within infarctions on gradient-echo MR images (T2 and T2* effect), which correspond to histologic evidence of hemorrhage.[125] Therefore, cardiac T2*-weighted mapping can quantify postreperfusion hemorrhage and compare it with other indexes of ischemic injury. It is important to know that susceptibility effect of hemorrhage can decrease the bright signal of edema on precontrast T2-weighted spin-echo images commonly used to assess the extent of myocardial at risk in STEMI patients (Fig. 20.20G). Myocardial hemorrhage can be detected with a dual-inversion black-blood gradient multiecho T2* MR sequence. Multiecho sequence is necessary to map T2*.[126] Kumar et al. animal study[127] showed that gross hemorrhage is smaller than area of no reflow and correlates with the size of infarct. It was also shown that size of hemorrhage detected pathologically correlated with that detected by T2* imaging but CMR overestimated the extent.

T2 and T2* techniques have limitations. MVO without or with hemorrhage can result in hypoenhanced regions seen on T2-weighted and LGE sequences. A certain amount of hemorrhage is needed before the paramagnetic effects are significant enough to cause signal loss on T2W images. Since the paramagnetic effects of hemoglobin by-products on T2* are stronger than are those on T2, T2*-weighted sequences should generally exhibit higher sensitivity for hemorrhage.[126] It is sometime difficult to separate the hypointense signal intensity associated with IMH from normal myocardium, which also appears dark on triple IR T2W sequence and T2*W images. In this case, T2 map can help distinguish hemorrhage for normal myocardium. Furthermore, hypointense signals attributable to other causes, for example, tissue interface or motion artifacts, may also be difficult to distinguish from IMH. To facilitate the detection of intramyocardial hemorrhage, addition of a T1W IR sequence to routine MR protocol of STEMI patients has been suggested.[128] The short T1 relaxation time of methemoglobin results in hyperintense signal intensity on T1W images. For T1W images, a double-IR 3D fast gradient-echo black blood sequence can be used.[128]

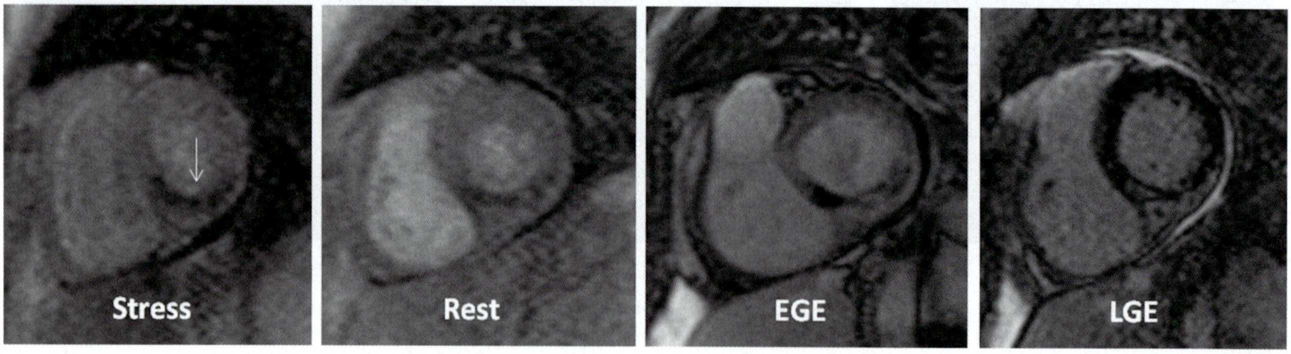

Figure 20-21. Effect of time on the size of no-reflow area (NRA). In adenosine stress image, abnormal low-signal area is seen in subendocardial region of inferior and inferoseptal walls (*arrow*). This area appears thinner on rest perfusion image obtained 7 minutes later. Early gadolinium enhancement (EGE) image using single-shot b-SSFP that was obtained 5 minutes after rest perfusion shows further enhancement of the inferior wall. Note that the signal of NRA appears very dark in EGE due to setting of inversion time around 600 milliseconds. Late gadolinium enhancement (LGE) image 10 minutes after EGE shows transmural enhancement of the inferior wall and smaller NRA. b-SSFP, balanced steady-state free precession.

Microvascular Angina with Normal Coronary Arteries

MVA with normal coronary arteries or "cardiac syndrome X" (CSX) is typically recognized by an effort-induced angina and ST-segment depression on stress electrocardiography despite normal or near-normal coronary arteries[129] (Table 20.3). Increased cardiac adrenergic activity can play a significant pathogenetic role in patients with stable (chronic) MVA.[129,130] An impairment of endothelium-dependent vasodilation due to reduced nitric oxide release is also a proposed mechanism of MVD in stable MVA patients and has been suggested mainly by reduced coronary flow response to acetylcholine.[131] Common cardiovascular risk factors including hypertension, hyperlipidemia, diabetes mellitus, and smoking are known causes of MVD and may therefore contribute to pathogenesis in at least a proportion of patients with CSX.[8] In contrast to territorial region of ischemia, which is typical of epicardial CAD stenosis, the MVD is not limited to one territory and often shows a patchy pattern of perfusion abnormalities. These patients often present with chronic stable angina and/or dyspnea. Compared with exertional chest pain, which is typically seen in obstructive epicardial CAD, MVD chest pain persists for several minutes after activity is stopped and usually presents with ischemic ECG changes during noninvasive testing, exertional dyspnea, and intermittent rest angina.[130] MVA shows poor or slow response to nitroglycerin. In contrast to Prinzmetal variant angina, ST-segment elevation is rare in patients with MVA.[100] MVA may present as an acute coronary syndrome in a small group of ACS patients admitted to hospital and found to have "normal" coronary angiograms.[132] Although exercise ECG and scintigraphic stress tests are usually unremarkable for the diagnosis, the induction of angina and ST-segment depression, but not left ventricular contractile abnormalities, during an echocardiographic dipyridamole or dobutamine stress test is strongly suggestive of a microvascular origin of symptoms.

Noninvasive tests are generally preferred for diagnosis. There have been conflicting data on CMR perfusion in CSX. Lanza et al.[133] demonstrated regional (LAD) perfusion defects on dobutamine stress MRI only in patients with CSX compared with a normal group. Panting et al.,[134] using semiquantitative perfusion analysis, showed global subendocardial ischemia in these patients. In Vermeltfoort et al. investigation[135], a myocardial perfusion index was calculated using the normalized upslope of myocardial signal enhancement. They found no evidence for subendocardial hypoperfusion in these patients. In a recent study by Karamitsos et al.[136] using 3-T magnet, combined assessment of regional perfusion and oxygenation was performed at adenosine stress and rest. MBF was measured by model-independent deconvolution contrast-enhanced MR, and myocardial oxygenation was assessed by BOLD sequence. Patients with syndrome X showed greater sensitivity to chest pain compared with controls but no evidence of deoxygenation or hypoperfusion during vasodilatory stress.[135] One reason for negative MR in these patients may be due to limited MR spatial resolution. For example, in Karamitsos's study, the voxel size for contrast perfusion MR was $2.1 \times 2.6 \times 8$ mm^3. Recently, high-resolution CMR perfusion techniques have been developed at 3T with $1.2 \times 1.2 \times 10$ mm^3 voxel size that will likely enable reliable assessment of subendocardial versus subepicardial perfusion.[137] In aortic stenosis with secondary left ventricle hypertrophy, reduced coronary vasodilator reserve occurs especially in subendocardial region despite angiographically normal coronary arteries (Fig. 20.22). Severity of MVD is more related to aortic valve area and diastolic perfusion rather than to left ventricle hypertrophy.[138]

TABLE

20.3 Diagnosis of Cardiac Syndrome X

1. Typical stable angina, exclusively or predominantly induced by effort
2. Evidence of myocardial ischemia on diagnostic tests in ≥1 of the following
   - *ST-segment depression (spontaneous or stress induced)*
   - *Reversible perfusion defects on stress perfusion imaging*
   - *Abnormal CBF by more advanced diagnostic techniques*
3. Normal or near-normal (irregularities and <20% narrowing) coronary angiograms
4. Absence of a specific underlying cardiac disease (e.g., cardiomyopathy, aortic stenosis)

Lanza GA. Cardiac syndrome X: a critical overview and future perspectives. *Heart* 2007;93:159–166.

Unstable Primary Microvascular Angina

In diagnosis of unstable (acute) MVD angina, absence of epicardial coronary spasm and transient coronary thrombosis are required.[8] Unstable microvascular angina should be considered in patients with prolonged chest pain typical enough to suggest non–ST-segment elevation acute coronary syndrome (NSTE-ACS) but in setting of a normal appearing coronary angiogram. The prevalence of patients presenting with NSTE-ACS and normal coronary arteries is probably less than 5% of all patients with NSTE-ACS.[132]

Cardiomyopathies

Cardiomyopathy is defined as a myocardial abnormality in which the heart muscle is structurally and functionally abnormal in the absence of significant CAD, hypertension, valvular heart disease, and congenital heart disease.[139] Cardiomyopathies are therefore grouped into specific morphologic and functional phenotypes and subclassified into familial and nonfamilial forms. In the investigative workup for a suspected cardiomyopathy, typically a considerable number of tests are performed, ranging from the more routine and straightforward tests, including ECG, echocardiogram, and exercise treadmill, to the more advanced studies such as MRI and endomyocardial biopsy. It is key to identify a potentially treatable substrate and then to risk stratify patients for treatment.

Myocardial ischemia is an established pathophysiologic feature in hypertrophic cardiomyopathy (HCM) causing important disease-related complications. MVD can be demonstrated in most patients with HCM mostly due to intimal and medial hyperplasia of the intramural coronary arteries and subsequent lumen reduction.[140,141] More recently, a number of studies using contemporary cardiovascular imaging modalities such as PET and CMR imaging have led to an enhanced understanding of the role that myocardial ischemia plays in this complex and heterogeneous genetic disease.[140,141] MRI has shown decreased stress MBF, particularly in the endocardium, and in proportion to the magnitude of hypertrophy.[140] It is also shown that areas of myocardium in which fibrosis was present (as shown by enhancement) are most often associated with reduced MBF. Therefore, abnormal MBF caused by MVD is responsible for myocardial ischemia–mediated myocyte death, and ultimately repair in the form of fibrosis.[142] Cardiomyopathy

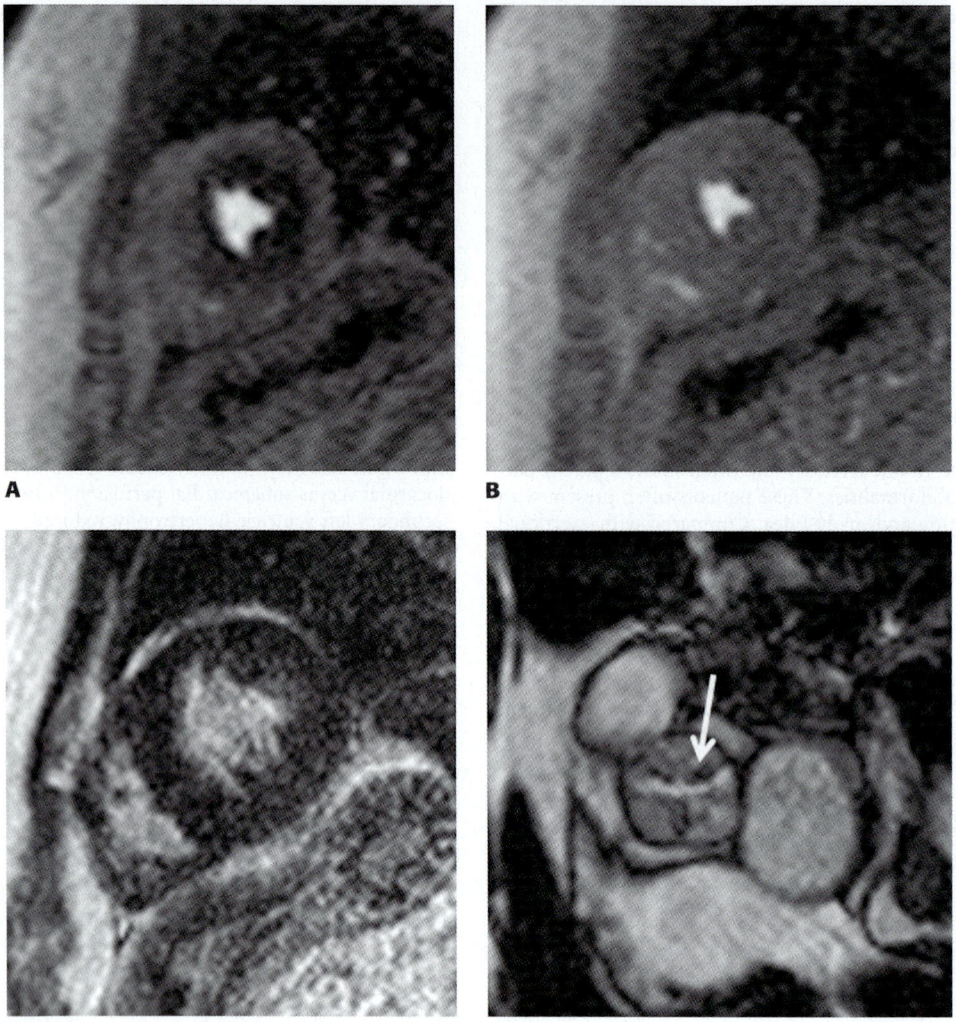

Figure 20-22. Adenosine stress/rest perfusion and delayed postcontrast images in a patient with left ventricular hypertrophy due to stenotic bicuspid aortic valve are shown. **A:** Stress perfusion shows extensive subendocardial hypoperfusion. **B:** Rest perfusion shows normal-appearing myocardium. **C**: Delayed postcontrast image shows no abnormal myocardial enhancement. **D:** Cine frame at aortic root shows bicuspid valve with severe stenosis (*arrow*).

produces significant mortality in patients with Friedreich ataxia, a genetic disorder that produces intramitochondrial iron accumulation. In these patients, CMR shows impaired perfusion reserve, and fibrosis occurs in the absence of significant hypertrophy and prior to clinical heart failure.[143]

Apical ballooning syndrome (Takotsubo) is a unique reversible cardiomyopathy that is frequently precipitated by a stressful event (stress induced) and has a clinical presentation that can be indistinguishable from a myocardial infarction.[144,145] The typical hallmark of Takotsubo is left ventricular apical akinesia but preserved function in basal segments. Catecholamines are postulated to play an important role in Takotsubo, but the precise pathophysiology is incompletely understood. Whether myocardial perfusion of the affected segments is impaired has been debated and remains unknown.[144] Some reports have shown temporary reduced CBF in the affected myocardial segments in the acute phase.[145] A recent report revealed apparently normal coronary perfusion in a rat model of stress-induced cardiomyopathy.[146] Coronary microcirculatory flow is also impaired in nonischemic dilated cardiomyopathy.[147] Reduced MPR and increased coronary resistance in dilated cardiomyopathy are shown and appear to be more severe in patients with superimposed atrial fibrillation.[148] Two potential applications of CMR MPI in pediatric patients are (a) detection of ischemia before medical therapy or revascularization and (b) detection of MVD in various congenital heart diseases.[72]

REFERENCES

1. **Camici PG, Crea F.** Coronary microvascular dysfunction. *N Engl J Med* 2007;356:830–840.
2. **Cecchi F, Olivotto I, Gistri R, et al.** Coronary microvascular dysfunction and prognosis in hypertrophic cardiomyopathy. *N Engl J Med* 2003;349:1027–1035.
3. **Gould KL, Lipscomb K, Hamilton GW.** Physiologic basis for assessing critical coronary stenosis. Instantaneous flow response and regional distribution during coronary hyperemia as measures of coronary flow reserve. *Am J Cardiol* 1974;33:87–94.
4. **Kaufmann PA, Camici PG.** Myocardial blood flow by PET: technical aspects and clinical applications. *J Nucl Med* 2005;46:75–88.
5. **Chilian WM.** Coronary microcirculation in health and disease: summary of an NHLBI workshop. *Circulation* 1997;95:522–528.

6. **Chareonthaitawee P, Kaufmann PA, Rimoldi O, et al.** Heterogeneity of resting and hyperemic myocardial blood flow in healthy humans. *Cardiovasc Res* 2001;50:151–161.
7. **Porto I, Hamilton-Craig C, Brancati M, et al.** Angiographic assessment of microvascular perfusion–myocardial blush in clinical practice. *Am Heart J* 2010;160:1015–1022.
8. **Lanza GA, Crea F.** Primary coronary microvascular dysfunction: clinical presentation, pathophysiology, and management. *Circulation* 2010;121:2317–2325.
9. **Knaapen P, Camici PG, Marques KM, et al.** Coronary microvascular resistance: methods for its quantification in humans. *Basic Res Cardiol* 2009;104:485–498.
10. **Pijls NHJ, van Son JAM, Kirkeeide RL, et al.** Experimental basis of determining maximum coronary, myocardial and collateral blood flow by pressure measurements for assessing functional stenosis severity before and after PTCA. *Circulation* 1993;87:1354–1367.
11. **Pijls NH, De Bruyne B, Smith L, et al.** Coronary thermodilution to assess flow reserve: validation in humans. *Circulation* 2002;105: 2482–2486.
12. **Westerhof N, Boer C, Lamberts RR, et al.** Crosstalk between cardiac muscle and coronary vasculature. *Physiol Rev* 2006;86:1263–1308.
13. **Gould KL, Schelbert HR, Phelps ME, et al.** Noninvasive assessment of coronary stenoses with myocardial perfusion imaging during pharmacologic coronary vasodilatation. V. Detection of 47 percent diameter coronary stenosis with intravenous nitrogen-13 ammonia and emission-computed tomography in intact dogs. *Am J Cardiol* 1979;43:200–208.
14. **Camici PG.** Myocardial blood flow measurement by PET: technical aspects and clinical applications. *J Nucl Med* 2005;46:75–88.
15. **Jerosch-Herold M, Swingen C, Seethamraju RT.** Myocardial blood flow quantification with MRI by model-independent deconvolution. *Med Phys* 2002;29:886–897.
16. **Rossen JD, Winniford MD.** Effect of increases in heart rate and arterial pressure on coronary flow reserve in humans. *J Am Coll Cardiol* 1993;21:343–348.
17. **Camici P, Marraccini P, Marzilli M, et al.** Coronary hemodynamics and myocardial metabolism during and after pacing stress in normal humans. *Am J Physiol* 1989;257:E309–E317.
18. **Austin RE Jr, Aldea GS, Coggins DL, et al.** Profound spatial heterogeneity of coronary reserve. Discordance between patterns of resting and maximal myocardial blood flow. *Circ Res* 1990;67:319–331.
19. **Gould KL.** Does coronary flow trump coronary anatomy? *JACC Cardiovasc Imaging* 2009;2(8):1009–1023.
20. **Ng MK, Yeung AC, Fearon WF.** Invasive assessment of the coronary microcirculation: superior reproducibility and less hemodynamic dependence of index of microcirculatory resistance compared with coronary flow reserve. *Circulation* 2006;113(17):2054–2061.
21. **Yong AS, Layland J, Fearon WF, et al.** Calculation of the index of microcirculatory resistance without coronary wedge pressure measurement in the presence of epicardial stenosis. *JACC Cardiovasc Interv* 2013;6(1):53–58.
22. **Aarnoudse W, Fearon WF, Manoharan G, et al.** Epicardial stenosis severity does not affect minimal microcirculatory resistance. *Circulation* 2004;110:2137–2142.
23. **Atkinson DJ, Burstein D, Edelman RR.** First-pass cardiac perfusion: evaluation with ultrafast MR imaging. *Radiology* 1990;174(3 Pt 1): 757–762.
24. **Kurita T, Sakuma H, Onishi K, et al.** Regional myocardial perfusion reserve determined using myocardial perfusion magnetic resonance imaging showed a direct correlation with coronary flow velocity reserve by Doppler flow wire. *Eur Heart J* 2009;30(4):444–452.
25. **Kellman P, Derbyshire JA, Agyeman KO, et al.** Extended coverage first-pass perfusion imaging using slice-interleaved TSENSE. *Magn Reson Med* 2004;51:200–204.
26. **Gerber BL, Raman SV, Nayak K, et al.** Myocardial first-pass perfusion cardiovascular magnetic resonance: history, theory, and current state of the art. *J Cardiovasc Magn Reson* 2008;10:18.
27. **Schwitter J, Wacker CM, van Rossum AC, et al.** MR-IMPACT: comparison of perfusion-cardiac magnetic resonance with single-photon emission computed tomography for the detection of coronary artery disease in a multicentre, multivendor, randomized trial. *Eur Heart J* 2008;29:480–489.
28. **Friedrich MG, Karamitsos TD.** Oxygenation-sensitive cardiovascular magnetic resonance. *J Cardiovasc Magn Reson* 2013;15(1):43.
29. **Fieno DS, Shea SM, Li Y, et al.** Myocardial perfusion imaging based on the blood oxygen level-dependent effect using T2-prepared steady-state free-precession magnetic resonance imaging. *Circulation* 2004;110:1284 –1290.
30. **Zun Z, Wong EC, Nayak KS.** Assessment of myocardial blood flow (MBF) in humans using arterial spin labeling (ASL): feasibility and noise analysis. *Magn Reson Med* 2009;62(4):975–983.
31. **Wang DJ, Bi X, et al.** Estimation of perfusion and arterial transit time in myocardium using free-breathing myocardial ASL with Navigator-echo. *Magn Reson Med* 2010;64(5):1289–1295.
32. **Rosen BR, Belliveau JW, Vevea JM, et al.** Perfusion imaging with NMR contrast agents. *Magn Reson Med* 1990;14(2):249–265.
33. **Donahue KM, Weisskoff RM, Burstein D.** Water diffusion and exchange as they influence contrast enhancement. *J Magn Reson Imaging* 1997;7(1):102–110.
34. **Larsson HBW, FritzHansen T, Rostrup E, et al.** Myocardial perfusion modeling using MRI. *Magn Reson Med* 1996;35:716–726.
35. **Niedermayer S, Sourbron S, Prompona M, et al.** Dose response of the intravascular contrast agent gadofosveset trisodium in MR perfusion imaging of the myocardium using a quantitative evaluation. *Int J Cardiovasc Imaging* 2013;29(7):1527–1536.
36. **Bokhari S, Ficaro EP, McCallister BD Jr.** Adenosine stress protocols for myocardial perfusion imaging. *J Nucl Cardiol* 2007;14(3):415–416.
37. **Al Jaroudi W, Iskandrian AE.** Regadenoson: a new myocardial stress agent. *J Am Coll Cardiol* 2009;54(13):1123–1130.
38. **Vasu S, Bandettini WP, Hsu LY, et al.** Regadenoson and adenosine are equivalent vasodilators and are superior than dipyridamole—a study of first pass quantitative perfusion cardiovascular magnetic resonance. *J Cardiovasc Magn Reson* 2013;15(1):85.
39. **Kellman P, Arai AE.** Imaging sequences for first pass perfusion: a review. *J Cardiovasc Magn Reson* 2007;9:525–537.
40. **Slavin GS, Wolff SD, Gupta SN, et al.** First-pass myocardial perfusion MR imaging with interleaved notched saturation: feasibility study. *Radiology* 2001;219(1):258–263.
41. **Epstein FH, Wolff SD, Arai AE.** Segmented k-space fast cardiac imaging using an echo-train readout. *Magn Reson Med* 1999;41(3):609–613.
42. **Epstein FH, Arai AE.** Optimization of fast cardiac imaging using an echo-train readout. *J Magn Reson Imaging* 2000;11:75–80.
43. **Schreiber WG, Schmitt M, Kalden P, et al.** Dynamic contrast-enhanced myocardial perfusion imaging using saturation-prepared True FISP. *J Magn Reson Imaging* 2002;16:641–652.
44. **Panting JR, Gatehouse PD, Yang GZ, et al.** Echo-planar magnetic resonance myocardial perfusion imaging: parametric map analysis and comparison with thallium SPECT. *J Magn Reson Imaging* 2001;13(2): 192–200.
45. **Lyne JC, Gatehouse PD, Assomull RG, et al.** Direct comparison of myocardial perfusion cardiovascular magnetic resonance sequences with parallel acquisition. *J Magn Reson Imaging* 2007;26(6):1444–1451.
46. **Manka R, Jahnke C, Kozerke S, et al.** Dynamic 3-dimensional stress cardiac magnetic resonance perfusion imaging: detection of coronary artery disease and volumetry of myocardial hypoenhancement before and after coronary stenting. *J Am Coll Cardiol* 2011;57:437–444.
47. **Otazo R, Kim D, Axel L, et al.** Combination of compressed sensing and parallel imaging for highly accelerated first-pass cardiac perfusion MRI. *Magn Reson Med* 2010;64:767–776.
48. **Shin T, Pohost GM, Nayak KS.** Systolic 3D first-pass myocardial perfusion MRI: comparison with diastolic imaging in healthy subjects. *Magn Reson Med* 2010;63(4):858–864.
49. **Motwani M, Fairbairn TA, Larghat A, et al.** Systolic versus diastolic acquisition in myocardial perfusion MR imaging. *Radiology* 2012;262(3):816–823.
50. **Pedersen H, Kelle S, Ringgaard S, et al.** Quantification of myocardial perfusion using free-breathing MRI and prospective slice tracking. *Magn Reson Med* 2009;61(3):734–738.
51. **Kellman P, Aletras AH, Hsu LY, et al.** T2* measurement during first-pass contrast-enhanced cardiac perfusion imaging. *Magn Reson Med* 2006;56(5):1132–1134.
52. **Biglands JD, Radjenovic A, Ridgway JP.** Cardiovascular magnetic resonance physics for clinicians: Part II. *J Cardiovasc Magn Reson* 2012;14:66.
53. **Hsu LY, Rhoads KL, Holly JE, et al.** Quantitative myocardial perfusion analysis with a dual-bolus contrast-enhanced first-pass MRI technique in humans. *J Magn Reson Imaging.* 2006;23(3):315–322.

54. **Ishida M, Schuster A, Morton G, et al.** Development of a universal dual-bolus injection scheme for the quantitative assessment of myocardial perfusion cardiovascular magnetic resonance. *J Cardiovasc Magn Reson* 2011;13:28.
55. **Gatehouse PD, Elkington AG, Ablitt N, et al.** Accurate assessment of the arterial input function during high-dose myocardial perfusion cardiovascular magnetic resonance. *J Magn Reson Imaging* 2004;20(1):39–45.
56. **Stanisz GJ, Odrobina EE, Pun J, et al.** T1, T2 relaxation and magnetization transfer in tissue at 3T. *Magn Reson Med* 2005;54:507–512.
57. **Klumpp BD, Seeger A, Doesch C, et al.** High resolution myocardial magnetic resonance stress perfusion imaging at 3 T using a 1 M contrast agent. *Eur Radiol* 2010;20(3):533–541.
58. **Ruan C, Yang SH, Cusi K, et al.** Contrast-enhanced first-pass myocardial perfusion magnetic resonance imaging with parallel acquisition at 3.0 Tesla. *Invest Radiol* 2007;42:352–360.
59. **Christian TF, Bell SP, Whitesell L, et al.** Accuracy of cardiac magnetic resonance of absolute myocardial blood flow with a high-field system: comparison with conventional field strength. *JACC Cardiovasc Imaging* 2009;2(9):1103–1110.
60. **Cheng AS, Pegg TJ, Karamitsos TD, et al.** Cardiovascular magnetic resonance perfusion imaging at 3-tesla for the detection of coronary artery disease: a comparison with 1.5-tesla. *J Am Coll Cardiol* 2007;49:2440–2449.
61. **Bernhardt P, Walcher T, Rottbauer W, et al.** Quantification of myocardial perfusion reserve at 1.5 and 3.0 Tesla: a comparison to fractional flow reserve. *Int J Cardiovasc Imaging* 2012;28:2049–2056.
62. **Klem I, Heitner JF, Shah DJ, et al.** Improved detection of coronary artery disease by stress perfusion cardiovascular magnetic resonance with the use of delayed enhancement infarction imaging. *J Am Coll Cardiol* 2006;47(8):1630–1638.
63. **Pilz G, Klos M, Ali E, et al.** Angiographic correlations of patients with small vessel disease diagnosed by adenosine-stress cardiac magnetic resonance imaging. *J Cardiovasc Magn Reson* 2008;10:8.
64. **Cerqueira MD, Weissman NJ, Dilsizian V, et al.** Standardized myocardial segmentation and nomenclature for tomographic imaging of the heart: a statement for healthcare professionals from the Cardiac Imaging Committee of the Council on Clinical Cardiology of the American Heart Association. *Circulation* 2002;105(4):539–542.
65. **Radjenovic A, Biglands JD, Larghat A, et al.** Estimates of systolic and diastolic myocardial blood flow by dynamic contrast-enhanced MRI. *Magn Reson Med* 2010;64(6):1696–1703.
66. **Hsu LY, Groves DW, Aletras AH, et al.** A quantitative pixel-wise measurement of myocardial blood flow by contrast-enhanced first-pass CMR perfusion imaging: microsphere validation in dogs and feasibility study in humans. *JACC Cardiovasc Imaging* 2012;5(2):154–166.
67. **Nagel E, Klein C, Paetsch I, et al.** Magnetic resonance perfusion measurements for the noninvasive detection of coronary artery disease. *Circulation* 2003;108(4):432–437.
68. **Schwitter J, Nanz D, Kneifel S, et al.** Assessment of myocardial perfusion in coronary artery disease by magnetic resonance: a comparison with positron emission tomography and coronary angiography. *Circulation* 2001;103(18):2230–2235.
69. **Ibrahim T, Nekolla SG, Schreiber K, et al.** Assessment of coronary flow reserve: comparison between contrast-enhanced magnetic resonance imaging and positron emission tomography. *J Am Coll Cardiol* 2002;39(5):864–870.
70. **Jerosch-Herold M, Wilke N, Stillman AE.** Magnetic resonance quantification of the myocardial perfusion reserve with a Fermi function model for constrained deconvolution. *Med Phys* 1998;25:73–84.
71. **Jerosch-Herold M.** Quantification of myocardial perfusion by cardiovascular magnetic resonance. *J Cardiovasc Magn Reson* 2010; 12(1):57.
72. **Coelho-Filho OR, Rickers C, Kwong RY, et al.** MR myocardial perfusion imaging. *Radiology* 2013;266(3):701–715.
73. **Geldof MJ, Schalij MJ, Manger Cats V, et al.** Comparison between regional myocardial perfusion reserve and coronary flow reserve in the canine heart. *Eur Heart J* 1995;16(12):1860–1871.
74. **Iwata S, Hozumi T, Matsumura Y, et al.** Cut-off value of coronary flow velocity reserve by transthoracic Doppler echocardiography for the assessment of significant donor left anterior descending artery stenosis in patients with spontaneously visible collaterals. *Am J Cardiol* 2006;98(3):298–302.
75. **Nagel E, Thouet T, Klein C, et al.** Noninvasive determination of coronary blood flow velocity with cardiovascular magnetic resonance in patients after stent deployment. *Circulation* 2003;107(13):1738–1743.
76. **Vogel-Claussen J, Skrok J, Dombroski D, et al.** Comprehensive adenosine stress perfusion MRI defines the etiology of chest pain in the emergency room: comparison with nuclear stress test. *J Magn Reson Imaging* 2009;30(4):753–762.
77. **Iskander S, Iskandrian AE.** Risk assessment using single-photon emission computed tomographic technetium-99m sestamibi imaging. *J Am Coll Cardiol* 1998;32:57–62.
78. **Murthy VL, Naya M, Foster CR, et al.** Association between coronary vascular dysfunction and cardiac mortality in patients with and without diabetes mellitus. *Circulation* 2012;127:1858–1868
79. **Bratis K, Nagel E.** Variability in quantitative cardiac magnetic resonance perfusion analysis. *J Thorac Dis* 2013;5(3):357–359.
80. **Nandalur KR, Dwamena BA, Choudhri AF, et al.** Diagnostic performance of stress cardiac magnetic resonance imaging in the detection of coronary artery disease: a meta-analysis. *J Am Coll Cardiol* 2007;50:1343–1353.
81. **Ashley EA, Myers J, Froelicher V.** Exercise testing in clinical medicine. *Lancet* 2000;356:1592–1597.
82. **Jaarsma C, Leiner T, Bekkers SC, et al.** Diagnostic performance of noninvasive myocardial perfusion imaging using single-photon emission computed tomography, cardiac magnetic resonance, and positron emission tomography imaging for the detection of obstructive coronary artery disease: a meta-analysis. *J Am Coll Cardiol* 2012;59(19):1719–1728.
83. **de Jong MC, Genders TS, van Geuns RJ, et al.** Diagnostic performance of stress myocardial perfusion imaging for coronary artery disease: a systematic review and meta-analysis. *Eur Radiol* 2012;22(9):1881–1895.
84. **Fritz-Hansen T, Hove JD, Kofoed KF, et al.** Quantification of MRI measured myocardial perfusion reserve in healthy humans: a comparison with positron emission tomography. *J Magn Reson Imaging* 2008;27:818–824.
85. **Costa MA, Shoemaker S, Futamatsu H, et al.** Quantitative magnetic resonance perfusion imaging detects anatomic and physiologic coronary artery disease as measured by coronary angiography and fractional flow reserve. *J Am Coll Cardiol* 2007;50(6):514–522.
86. **Rieber J, Huber A, Erhard I, et al.** Cardiac magnetic resonance perfusion imaging for the functional assessment of coronary artery disease: a comparison with coronary angiography and fractional flow reserve. *Eur Heart J* 2006;27(12):1465–1471.
87. **Patel AR, Antkowiak PF, Nandalur KR, et al.** Assessment of advanced coronary artery disease: advantages of quantitative cardiac magnetic resonance perfusion analysis. *J Am Coll Cardiol* 2010;56(7):561–569.
88. **Watkins S, McGeoch R, Lyne J, et al.** Validation of magnetic resonance myocardial perfusion imaging with fractional flow reserve for the detection of significant coronary heart disease. *Circulation* 2009;120(22):2207–2213.
89. **Husser O, Bodi V, Sanchis J, et al.** Head to head comparison of quantitative versus visual analysis of contrast CMR in the setting of myocardial stunning after STEMI: implications on late systolic function and patient outcome. *Int J Cardiovasc Imaging* 2010;26(5):559–569.
90. **Arai AE.** Magnetic resonance first-pass myocardial perfusion imaging. *Top Magn Reson Imaging* 2000;11(6):383–398.
91. **Storey P, Chen Q, Li W, et al.** Band artifacts due to bulk motion. *Magn Reson Med* 2002;48:1028–1036.
92. **Barkhausen J, Hunold P, Jochims M, et al.** Imaging of myocardial perfusion with magnetic resonance. *J Magn Reson Imaging* 2004;19: 750–757.
93. **Di Bella EV, Parker DL, Sinusas AJ.** On the dark rim artifact in dynamic contrast-enhanced MRI myocardial perfusion studies. *Magn Reson Med* 2005;54:1295–1299.
94. **Wang Y, Moin K, Akinboboye O, et al.** Myocardial first pass perfusion: steady-state free precession versus spoiled gradient echo and segmented echo planar imaging. *Magn Reson Med* 2005;54(5):1123–1129.
95. **Glockner JF, Hu HH, Stanley DW, et al.** Parallel MR imaging: a user's guide. *Radiographics* 2005; 25:1279–1297.
96. **Neimatallah MA, Chenevert TL, Carlos RC, et al.** Subclavian MR arteriography: reduction of susceptibility artifact with short echo time and dilute gadopentetate dimeglumine. *Radiology* 2000;217:581–586.
97. **Kellman P, Epstein FH, McVeigh ER.** Adaptive sensitivity encoding incorporating temporal filtering (TSENSE). *Magn Reson Med* 2001;45:846–852.
98. **Madore B, Glover GH, Pelc NJ.** Unaliasing by Fourier-encoding the overlaps using the temporal dimension (UNFOLD), applied to cardiac imaging and fMRI. *Magn Reson Med* 1999;42:813–828.
99. **Breuer FA, Kellman P, Griswold MA, et al.** Dynamic autocalibrated parallel imaging using temporal GRAPPA (TGRAPPA). *Magn Reson Med* 2005;53(4):981–985.

100. **Herrmann J, Kaski JC, Lerman A.** Coronary microvascular dysfunction in the clinical setting: from mystery to reality. *Eur Heart J* 2012;33(22):2771–2782b.
101. **Melikian N, Vercauteren S, Fearon WF, et al.** Quantitative assessment of coronary microvascular function in patients with and without epicardial atherosclerosis. *EuroIntervention* 2010;5:939–945.
102. **Tonino PA, De Bruyne B, Pijls NH, et al.** Fractional flow reserve versus angiography for guiding percutaneous coronary intervention. *N Engl J Med* 2009;360:213–224.
103. **Amsterdam EA, Kirk JD, Diercks DB, et al.** Exercise testing in chest pain units: rationale, implementation, and results. *Cardiol Clin* 2005;23: 503–516.
104. **Lerakis S, McLean SD, Anadiotis AV, et al.** Prognostic value of adenosine stress cardiovascular magnetic resonance in patients with low-risk chest pain. *J Cardiovasc Magn Reson* 2009;11(1):37.
105. **Ingkanisorn WP, Kwong RY, Bohme NS, et al.** Prognosis of negative adenosine stress magnetic resonance in patients presenting to an emergency department with chest pain. *J Am Coll Cardiol* 2006;47(7):1427–1432.
106. **Jahnke C, Nagel E, Gebker R, et al.** Prognostic value of cardiac magnetic resonance stress tests: adenosine stress perfusion and dobutamine stress wall motion imaging. *Circulation* 2007;115(13):1769–1776.
107. **Lubbers DD, Rijlaarsdam-Hermsen D, Kuijpers D.** Performance of adenosine "stress-only" perfusion MRI in patients without a history of myocardial infarction: a clinical outcome study. *Int J Cardiovasc Imaging* 2012;28(1):109–115.
108. **Hundley WG, Bluemke DA, Finn JP, et al.** ACCF/ACR/AHA/NASCI/SCMR 2010 expert consensus document on cardiovascular magnetic resonance: a report of the American College of Cardiology Foundation Task Force on Expert Consensus Documents. American College of Cardiology Foundation Task Force on Expert Consensus Documents. *Circulation* 2010;121(22):2462–2508.
109. **Stone GW, Grines CL, Browne KF, et al.** Predictors of in-hospital and 6-month outcome after acute myocardial infarction in the reperfusion era: the Primary Angioplasty in Myocardial Infarction (PAMI) trial. *J Am Coll Cardiol* 1995;25:370–377.
110. **Bekkers SC, Yazdani SK, Virmani R, et al.** Microvascular obstruction. underlying pathophysiology and clinical diagnosis. *J Am Coll Cardiol* 2010;55(16):1649–1660.
111. **Wu KC, Kim RJ, Bluemke DA, et al.** Quantification and time course of microvascular obstruction by contrast-enhanced echocardiography and magnetic resonance imaging following acute myocardial infarction and reperfusion. *J Am Coll Cardiol* 1998;32:1756–1764.
112. **Kloner RA, Ganote CE, Jennings RB.** The "No-Reflow" phenomenon after temporary coronary occlusion in dogs. *J Clin Invest* 1974;54: 1496–1508.
113. **Rochitte CE, Lima JA, Bluemke DA, et al.** Magnitude and time course of microvascular obstruction and tissue injury after acute myocardial infarction. *Circulation* 1998;98:1006–1014.
114. **Husser O, Bodi V, Sanchis J, et al.** Release of necrosis markers and cardiovascular magnetic resonance-derived microvascular perfusion in reperfused ST-elevation myocardial infarction. *Thromb Res* 2009;124(5):592–600.
115. **Wu KC.** CMR of microvascular obstruction and hemorrhage in myocardial infarction. *J Cardiovasc Magn Reson* 2012;14:68.
116. **Wong DT, Puri R, Richardson JD, et al.** Myocardial "no-reflow"—Diagnosis, pathophysiology and treatment. *Int J Cardiol* 2013;167(5): 1798–1806.
117. **Gibson CM, Murphy SA, Rizzo MJ, et al.** Relationship between TIMI frame count and clinical outcomes after thrombolytic administration. Thrombolysis In Myocardial Infarction (TIMI) Study Group. *Circulation* 1999;99:1945–1950.
118. **Appelbaum E, Abraham JM, Pride YB, et al.** Association of thrombolysis in myocardial infarction myocardial perfusion grade with cardiovascular magnetic resonance measures of infarct architecture after primary percutaneous coronary intervention for ST-segment elevation myocardial infarction. *Am Heart J* 2009;158:84–91.
119. **Mather AN, Fairbairn TA, Artis NJ, et al.** Timing of cardiovascular MR imaging after acute myocardial infarction: effect on estimates of infarct characteristics and prediction of late ventricular remodeling. *Radiology* 2011;261:116–126.
120. **Bekkers SC, Backes WH, Kim RJ, et al.** Detection and characteristics of microvascular obstruction in reperfused acute myocardial infarction using an optimized protocol for contrast-enhanced cardiovascular magnetic resonance imaging. *Eur Radiol* 2009;19(12):2904–2912.
121. **Mather AN, Fairbairn TA, Ball SG, et al.** Reperfusion hemorrhage as determined by cardiovascular MRI is a predictor of adverse left ventricular remodeling and markers of late arrhythmic risk. *Heart* 2011;97:453–459.
122. **Rogers WJ Jr, Kramer CM, Geskin G, et al.** Early contrast-enhanced MRI predicts late functional recovery after reperfused myocardial infarction. *Circulation* 1999;99(6):744–750.
123. **Robbers LF, Eerenberg ES, Teunissen PF, et al.** Magnetic resonance imaging-defined areas of microvascular obstruction after acute myocardial infarction represent microvascular destruction and haemorrhage. *Eur Heart J* 2013;34(30):2346–2353.
124. **Chavhan GB, Babyn PS, Thomas B, et al.** Principles, techniques, and applications of T2*-based MR imaging and its special applications. *Radiographics* 2009;29:1433–1449.
125. **van den Bos EJ, Baks T, Moelker AD, et al.** Magnetic resonance imaging of haemorrhage within reperfused myocardial infarcts: possible interference with iron oxide-labelled cell tracking? *Eur Heart J* 2006;27:1620–1626.
126. **O'Regan DP, Ahmed R, Karunanithy N, et al.** Reperfusion hemorrhage following acute myocardial infarction: assessment with T2* mapping and effect on measuring the area at risk. *Radiology* 2009;250:916–922.
127. **Kumar A, Green JD, Sykes JM, et al.** Detection and quantification of myocardial reperfusion hemorrhage using T2*-weighted CMR. *JACC Cardiovasc Imaging* 2011;4:1274–1283.
128. **Pedersen SF, Thrysøe SA, Robich MP, et al.** Assessment of intramyocardial hemorrhage by T1-weighted cardiovascular magnetic resonance in reperfused acute myocardial infarction. *J Cardiovasc Magn Reson* 2012;14:59.
129. **Lanza GA.** Cardiac syndrome X: a critical overview and future perspectives. *Heart* 2007;93:159–166.
130. **Cannon RO, Epstein SE.** "Microvascular angina" as a cause of chest pain with angiographically normal coronary arteries. *Am J Cardiol* 1988;61:1338–1343.
131. **Bøttcher M, Bøtker HE, Sonne H, et al.** Endothelium dependent and independent perfusion reserve and the effect of L-arginine on myocardial perfusion in patients with syndrome X. *Circulation* 1999;99:1795–1801.
132. **Germing A, Lindstaedt M, Ulrich S, et al.** Normal angiogram in acute coronary syndrome-preangiographic risk stratification, angiographic findings and follow up. *Int J Cardiol* 2005;99:19–23.
133. **Lanza GA, Buffon A, Sestito A, et al.** Relation between stress induced myocardial perfusion defects on cardiovascular magnetic resonance and coronary microvascular dysfunction in patients with cardiac syndrome X. *J Am Coll Cardiol* 2008;51:466–472.
134. **Panting JR, Gatehouse PD, Yang GZ, et al.** Abnormal subendocardial perfusion in cardiac syndrome X detected by cardiovascular magnetic resonance imaging. *N Engl J Med* 2002;346:1948–1953.
135. **Vermeltfoort IA, Bondarenko O, Raijmakers PG, et al.** Is subendocardial ischaemia present in patients with chest pain and normal coronary angiograms? A cardiovascular MR study. *Eur Heart J* 2007;28:1554–1558.
136. **Karamitsos TD, Arnold JR, Pegg TJ, et al.** Patients with syndrome X have normal transmural myocardial perfusion and oxygenation: a 3-T cardiovascular magnetic resonance imaging study. *Circ Cardiovasc Imaging* 2012;5(2):194–200.
137. **Lockie T, Ishida M, Perera D, et al.** High-resolution magnetic resonance myocardial perfusion imaging at 3.0-Tesla to detect hemodynamically significant coronary stenoses as determined by fractional flow reserve. *J Am Coll Cardiol* 2011;57:70–75.
138. **Rajappan K, Rimoldi OE, Dutka DP, et al.** Mechanisms of coronary microcirculatory dysfunction in patients with aortic stenosis and angiographically normal coronary arteries. *Circulation* 2002;105:470–476.
139. **Elliott P, Andersson B, Arbustini E, et al.** Classification of the cardiomyopathies: a position statement from the European Society Of Cardiology Working Group on Myocardial and Pericardial Diseases. *Eur Heart J* 2008;29(2):270–276.
140. **Choudhury L, Rosen SD, Patel D, et al.** Coronary vasodilator reserve in primary and secondary left ventricular hypertrophy. *A study with positron emission tomography. Eur Heart J* 1997;18(1):108–116.
141. **Petersen SE, Jerosch-Herold M, Hudsmith LE, et al.** Evidence for microvascular dysfunction in hypertrophic cardiomyopathy: new insights from multiparametric magnetic resonance imaging. *Circulation* 2007;115(18):2418–2425.

142. **Maron MS.** Clinical utility of cardiovascular magnetic resonance in hypertrophic cardiomyopathy. *J Cardiovasc Magn Reson* 2012; 14:13.
143. **Raman SV, Phatak K, Hoyle JC, et al.** Impaired myocardial perfusion reserve and fibrosis in Friedreich ataxia: a mitochondrial cardiomyopathy with metabolic syndrome. *Eur Heart J* 2011;32(5): 561–567.
144. **Abdelmoneim SS, Mankad SV, Bernier M, et al.** Microvascular function in Takotsubo cardiomyopathy with contrast echocardiography: prospective evaluation and review of literature. *J Am Soc Echocardiogr* 2009;22(11):1249–1255.
145. **Meimoun P, Malaquin D, Sayah S, et al.** The coronary flow reserve is transiently impaired in tako-tsubo cardiomyopathy: a prospective study using serial Doppler transthoracic echocardiography. *J Am Soc Echocardiogr* 2008;21:72–77.
146. **Redfors B, Shao Y, Wikström J, et al.** Contrast echocardiography reveals apparently normal coronary perfusion in a rat model of stress-induced (Takotsubo) cardiomyopathy. *Eur Heart J Cardiovasc Imaging* 2014;15(2):152–157.
147. **Watzinger N, Lund GK, Saeed M, et al.** Myocardial blood flow in patients with dilated cardiomyopathy: quantitative assessment with velocity-encoded cine magnetic resonance imaging of the coronary sinus. *J Magn Reson Imaging* 2005;21(4):347–353.
148. **Range FT, Paul M, Schäfers KP, et al.** Myocardial perfusion in non-ischemic dilated cardiomyopathy with and without atrial fibrillation. *J Nucl Med* 2009;50(3):390–396.

CHAPTER

21 Myocardial Perfusion Imaging: CT Applications

Brian S. H. Ko, BSc, MBBS, PhD, FRACP, James D. Cameron, MBBS, MD,
Dennis T. L. Wong, BSc, MBBS, PhD, FRACP, and
Sujith K. Seneviratne, MBBS, FRACP

Introduction

Coronary artery disease (CAD) remains a leading cause of morbidity and mortality worldwide.[1] The natural history of CAD is characterized by the silent accumulation of atherosclerotic plaque in the wall of coronary arteries, progression into obstructive disease as excess plaque accumulates beyond maladaptive positive remodeling, the development of stress-induced ischemia as a result of luminal encroachment, and ultimate plaque rupture resulting in unstable angina, myocardial infarction, and sudden cardiac death.[2]

Over the past decade, multiple studies have demonstrated that coronary CT angiography (CCTA) is a robust noninvasive method for detection of atherosclerotic plaque and obstructive CAD (defined as the presence of >50% stenosis on invasive angiography) with a high sensitivity and negative predictive value in patients with suspected CAD.[3-6] Accordingly, since 2010, CCTA has been recommended by the American College of Cardiology as an appropriate upfront investigation for symptomatic patients with low and intermediate risk of CAD.[7,8] The use of CCTA in this population is currently a class IIa recommendation according to European Society of Cardiology and American College of Cardiology guidelines.[9,10]

While CCTA accurately detects anatomical disease, in its current form, it is limited in predicting lesion-specific ischemia.[11,12] When compared with invasive fractional flow reserve (FFR), which is the current gold standard for determination of vessel- and lesion-specific ischemia, CCTA has been found to have a high sensitivity and negative predictive value for ischemia, yet the specificity and positive predictive value are significantly limited (Table 21.1). This is a notable limitation as myocardial ischemia represents an important factor that determines clinical outcomes[21] and benefits from revascularization.[22–25] For this reason, patients with identified significant stenoses on CCTA often require further functional assessment, which entails additional testing, radiation exposure, cost, and inconvenience.

Current assessment for myocardial ischemia is typically performed with noninvasive stress imaging including stress echocardiography, single photon emission computed tomography (SPECT), or magnetic resonance imaging (MRI) myocardial perfusion imaging (MPI). It should be noted that with the exception of MRI MPI, which is commonly available only in quaternary referral centers,[19,26] stress echocardiography and SPECT MPI have been demonstrated to have poor discrimination of vessel-specific ischemia.[27–29] Using invasive FFR as reference standard for vessel-specific ischemia, SPECT MPI identifies ischemia territory correctly less than 50% of the time, with underestimation and overestimation in 36% and 22% of cases, respectively.[27] Such data have evoked concerns for the ability of stress testing to effectively isolate coronary lesions that benefit from revascularization (Table 21.2).

Over the past 5 to 10 years, an important focus of CT research is the development of novel techniques to evaluate each step in the pathophysiology of CAD including the assessment of the hemodynamic significance of coronary artery lesions and associated myocardial ischemia (Fig. 21-1). These are aimed at enabling cardiac CT to act as a one-stop shop modality to assess the anatomical and physiologic sequelae of CAD. The novel CT techniques, which will be discussed in this book chapter, include CT stress myocardial perfusion imaging (CTP) to evaluate for the presence of myocardial ischemia, the use of noninvasive CT fractional flow reserve (FFR CT), and the study of transluminal attenuation gradient (TAG) across coronary lesions to assess the hemodynamic significance of coronary lesions.

CT Myocardial Perfusion Imaging

Fundamentals of CT Myocardial Perfusion Imaging

MPI on CT is facilitated by the use of iodinated contrast, which possesses the unique ability to attenuate x-rays proportional to its concentration. Imaging is acquired as contrast transits from the arteries into the myocardium and can be performed at rest and during vasodilator stress such as adenosine,[15,16,33] regadenoson,[34,35] or dipyridamole.[36] In the absence of artifacts, hypoattenuated areas in the myocardium on CT represent areas of reduced perfusion. George et al.[37] were among the first to describe the use of the technique using a canine model of LAD ischemia, which demonstrated the significant difference in contrast attenuation between ischemic tissue and remote nonischemic tissue (Fig. 21-2).

Static and Dynamic Imaging

Two basic techniques can be applied for stress CTP: static imaging and dynamic imaging (Fig. 21-3). Static stress CTP is analogous to static SPECT MPI, and dynamic stress CT MPI is analogous to

TABLE

21.1 Per-Vessel Diagnostic Performance of Multidetector CT in Prediction of Hemodynamically Significant Stenoses Compared with Invasive Fractional Flow Reserve

Author	Year	Pt no	Prevalence (Per Vessel %)	Sensitivity (%)	Specificity (%)	PPV (%)	NPV (%)
Meijboom et al.[12]	2008	79	18	94	48	49	93
Sarno et al.[13]	2009	81	31	79	64	46	88
Koo et al.[14]	2011	103	37	91	40	47	89
Bamberg et al.[15]	2011	33	30	100	51	47	100
B. Ko et al.[16]	2012	42	51	93	60	68	90
B. Ko et al.[17]	2012	40	33	95	68	77	93
Wong et al.[18]	2013	53	38	94	66	64	94
Bettencourt et al.[19]	2013	101	24	95	67	48	97
Norgaard et al.[20]	2014	254	21	83	60	33	92

TABLE

21.2 Per Vessel Diagnostic Accuracy of Noninvasive Stress Imaging Compared with Invasive Fractional Flow Reserve

Author	Year	Population	Patient Number	Sens/Spec (%)	PPV/NPV (%)
SPECT MPI					
Hacker et al.[29]	2005	Intermediate stenoses	50	80/76	92/53
Ragosta et al.[30]	2007	Multivessel disease	36	59/85	86/57
Forster et al.[31]	2009	Multivessel disease†	72	62/90	62/90
Melikian et al.[27]	2010	Angiographic multivessel disease	67	61/69	47/80
Stress echocardiography					
Rieber et al.[32]	2004	Intermediate lesions	48	67/77	Not reported
Jung et al.[28]	2008	Intermediate lesions	70	56/67	48/74
MRI-MPI					
Watkins et al.[26]	2009	Chest pain evaluation	103	91/94	91/94
Bettencourt et al.[19]	2013	Suspected coronary disease	101	79/93	79/93

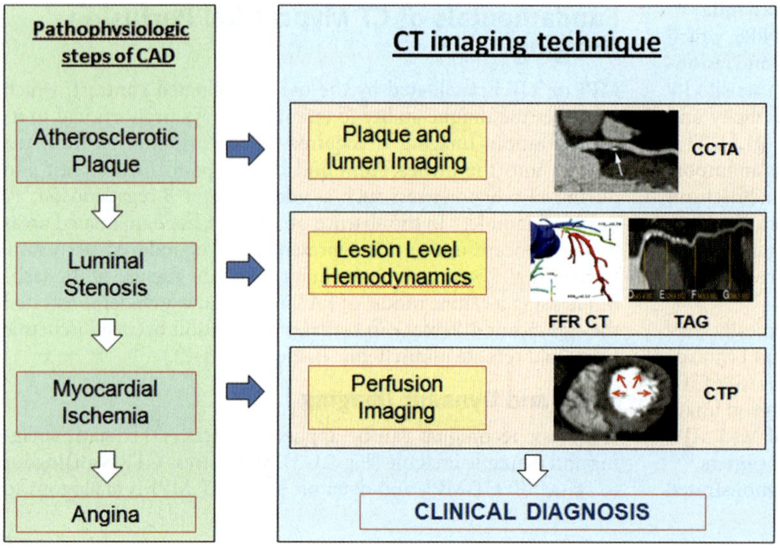

Figure 21-1. The "one-stop" anatomical and functional coronary assessment using cardiac CT.

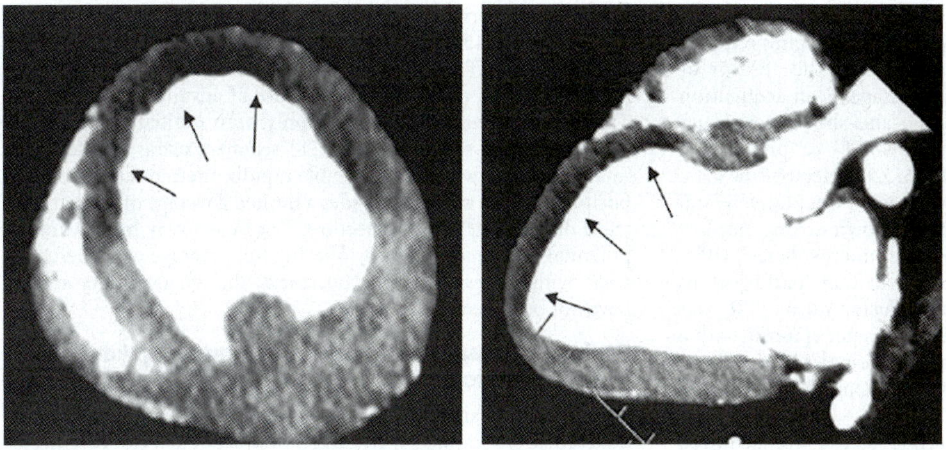

Figure 21-2. Perfusion defects (*arrows*) demonstrated using a canine model of LAD ischemia. (Adapted from George RT, Silva C, Cordeiro MA, et al. Multidetector computed tomography myocardial perfusion imaging during adenosine stress. *J Am Coll Cardiol* 2006;48:153–160, with permission from Elsevier.)

dynamic MRI MPI. Both static and dynamic CTP are performed during the first pass of contrast agent bolus passage through the myocardium. Differences in enhancement between normal and ischemic myocardium are maximal during the upslope of myocardial bolus passage, and the ability to distinguish enhancement differences is increased. During the downslope, the differences become less and disappear (Fig. 21-3). The timing of scan acquisition is hence paramount.

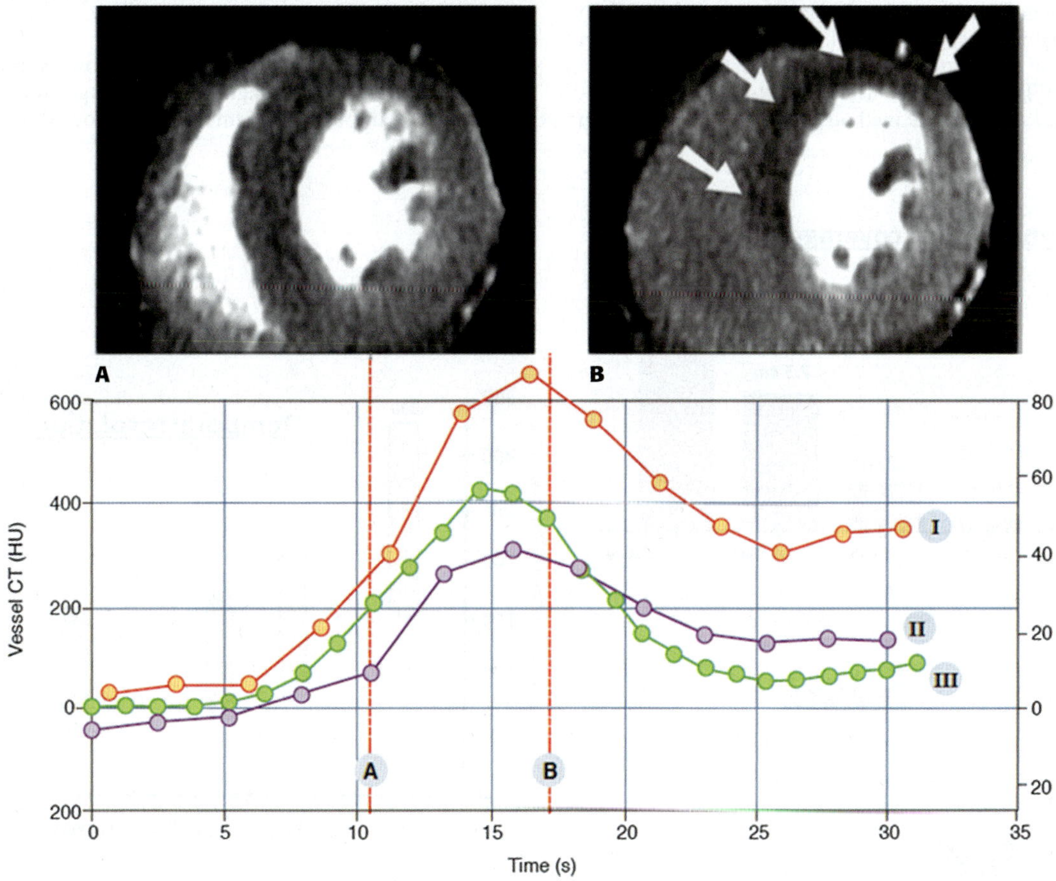

Figure 21-3. Dynamic and static CTP. This graph shows typical time–attenuation curve (TAC) acquired by dynamic CT MPI and two static images of the same midventricular slice, corresponding to different time points of CT MPI scan. The orange curve (*I*) in the graph represents the TAC in normal tissue, the purple curve (*II*) that of ischemic myocardium. The green curve (*III*) is the TAC of the ascending aorta. Differences in enhancement between normal and ischemic myocardium are maximal during upslope of myocardial bolus passage. Image **(A)** was taken at the time point indicated by line *A* in the graph during contrast upslope. Image **(B)** was taken 6 s later as indicated by line *B* during early contrast downslope. The variation between the images emphasizes that timing of CT image acquisition is paramount for MPI assessment. (Adapted from Ho KT, Chua KC, Klotz E, et al. Stress and rest dynamic myocardial perfusion imaging by evaluation of complete time-attenuation curves with dual-source CT. *JACC Cardiovasc Imaging* 2010;3:811–820, with permission from Elsevier.)

In static or "snapshot" CTP imaging, only a single image stack is acquired similar to CCTA acquisition. Static imaging requires exact scan timing at a single time point during the upslope or maximum of the contrast agent bolus passage. Scan acquisition can be performed using helical or step-and-shoot techniques using narrow detector (≤64-detector row CT) or prospective ECG gating using wide-detector CT (256/320-detector row CT). Myocardial blood flow (MBF) can be assessed qualitatively and semiquantitatively. Animal studies have shown strong nonlinear correlation between static CTP and microsphere MBF.[37] Subsequent human studies demonstrated that perfusion as assessed and quantified by transmural perfusion ratio (TPR) was inversely and linearly related to percent diameter stenosis with a correlation of $r = 0.63$.[33] Furthermore, abnormal TPR has been found to be significantly associated with ischemia demonstrated on invasive FFR.[17]

In dynamic CTP imaging, multiple stacks are acquired at multiple time points during the upslope of contrast passage through the myocardial tissue. From the series of images obtained, a time–contrast attenuation curve (TAC) can be derived (Fig. 21-3). The unique advantage of dynamic imaging is the ability to derive MBF and myocardial blood volume from TACs using various mathematical models including a model-based deconvolution method, upslope, and Patlak plot methods using available dedicated computer analysis software.[15,38,39] In one of the initial reports, George et al., using 64-detector CT in a canine model of moderate-to-severe LAD artery stenosis, demonstrated that CT-derived MBF using model-based deconvolution analysis and two upslope methods strongly correlated with microsphere-derived MBF ($R^2 = 0.91$, $p < 0.0001$) with a mean difference of 0.45 mL/g/min.[40]

Dynamic CTP when compared with static CTP requires a higher radiation exposure[39] and the use of advanced CT scanners. The technique has been thus far only been evaluated in second-generation dual-source CT (DSCT) scanners using shuttle mode imaging during which the CT table rapidly alternates between two positions and as a result provides a limited coverage of the left ventricle of 73 mm.[38] Wide-detector CT scanners may have a unique potential to overcome this by offering full coverage of the left ventricle without less than one heartbeat, though feasibility studies have not been performed as yet.

Perfusion Imaging Has Been Facilitated by Advances in CT Technology

Technologic advances over the past decade have equipped modern-day cardiac CT scanners with a larger number of detector rows, faster gantry rotation speed, dual x-ray source, and extended longitudinal coverage of the heart. While there is currently no one scanner that offers all of the above-mentioned technology, these advances have enabled contemporary imaging to occur with superior temporal and spatial resolution and to require shorter scan and breath hold times with reduced radiation exposure (Fig. 21-4). These advances have been particularly advantageous for perfusion imaging (Table 21.3).

Wide-Detector CT

Traditional narrow detector (64-detector row) scanners typically offer 3 to 4 cm of longitudinal coverage, and hence, the assessment of the entire volume of the myocardium can only

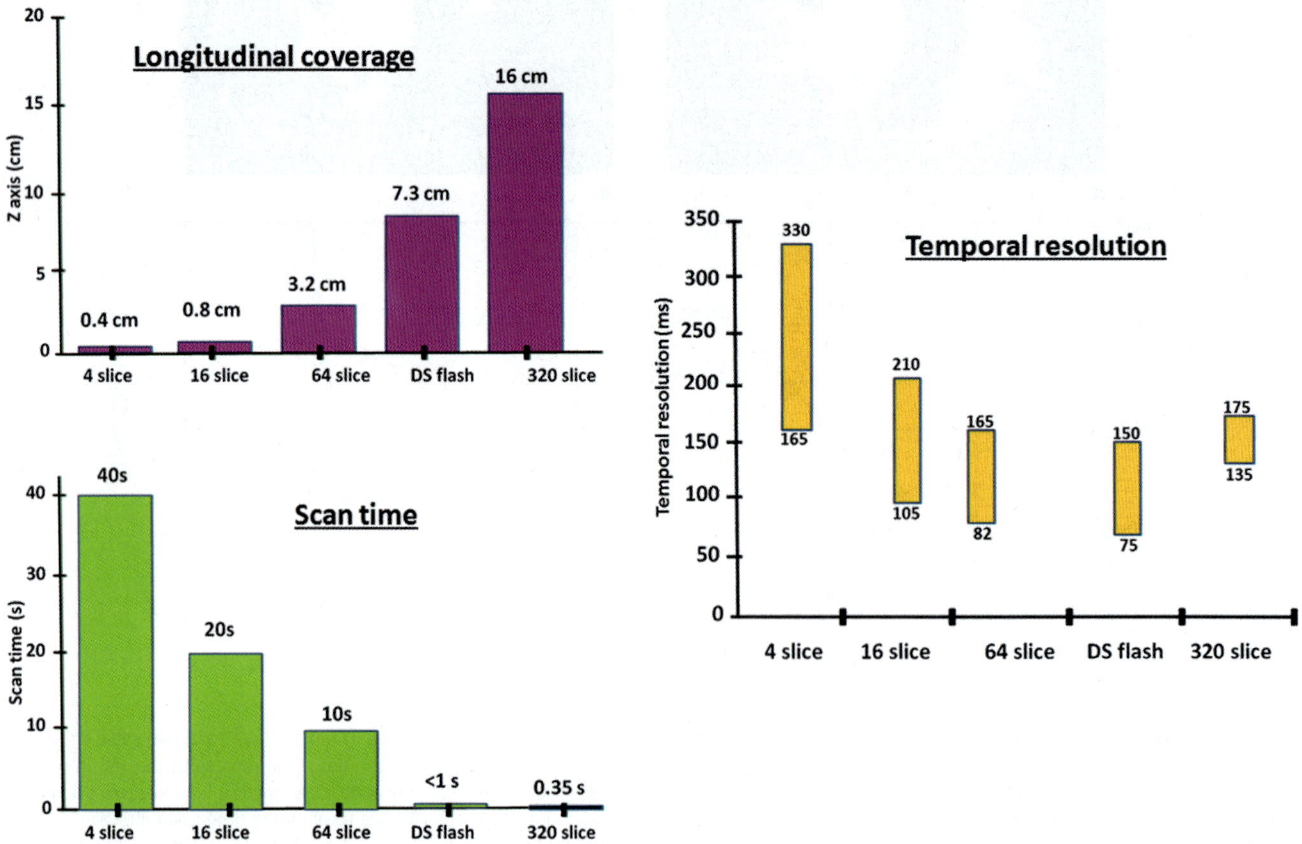

Figure 21-4. Advances in CT scanner technology. The advances, which have been most advantageous for perfusion imaging, include improvements in temporal resolution, increased longitudinal coverage, and decreased scan time.

TABLE 21.3 **CT Scanners Used in Myocardial Perfusion Imaging—Strengths and Limitations**

	Scanner/Mode of Acquisition	Strengths	Limitations
Narrow detector CT	64 detector helical CT	Readily available	Prolonged scan time/breath hold requirement Nonuniform temporal contrast enhancement in myocardium Slab misregistration artifacts High radiation dose
Wide-detector CT	320-detector CT using prospective ECG gating	Short scan time Temporal contrast distribution in entire myocardium No slab misregistration artifacts Low radiation dose	Low temporal resolution
Dual source CT (DSCT)	First-generation DSCT using retrospective ECG gating	High temporal resolution	Prolonged scan time Nonuniform temporal contrast enhancement in myocardium
	Second-generation DSCT using prospective dynamic shuttle mode	High temporal resolution Real-time imaging similar to MR perfusion	Limited z-axis coverage (73 cm) precluding assessment of some myocardial segments High radiation dose hence may not allow for complementary CCTA evaluation.
	Second-generation DSCT using prospective high-pitch spiral mode	High temporal resolution Short scan time Temporal contrast distribution in entire heart volume No slab misregistration artifacts Low radiation dose	
	Dual-energy CT using first- or second-generation DSCT	Offers additional information above contrast attenuation	Low temporal resolution

Adapted and revised from Ko BS, Cameron JD, Defrance T, et al. CT stress myocardial perfusion imaging using multidetector CT–A review. *J Cardiovasc Comput Tomogr* 2011;5:345–356, with permission from Elsevier.

be completed after multiple gantry rotations over three to four heartbeats. Myocardial contrast attenuation hence varies between the superior and inferior aspects of the heart due to the lack of temporal uniformity when image acquisition spans multiple cardiac cycles.

Wide-detector scanners (256- and 320-detector row CT) offer extended longitudinal coverage of 12 to 16 cm and hence the convenience of imaging the whole heart in one gantry rotation. This requires a shortened scan acquisition time of less than a heartbeat (0.35 milliseconds) and a short patient breath-hold time of 1 to 2 seconds without the need for table movement. The shortened scan time required is an asset in myocardial perfusion imaging (CTP) as there is only a narrow time period during the early portion of first-pass circulation when the iodinated contrast is predominantly intravascular and when the extravascular iodine concentration exceeds the intravascular iodine concentration.[41] In addition to this, because the entire volume is imaged at the same time, there is temporal contrast distribution across the entire volume of myocardium, which is ideal for myocardial perfusion assessment.[42]

Dual-Source CT

During vasodilator stress imaging, heart rates typically increase by 15 to 20 beats above the baseline heart rate at rest.[16,43] For this reason, improvements in temporal resolution are most welcome in stress CT perfusion imaging and may assist in the minimization of motion artifacts encountered during image acquisition in patient with higher heart rates. Single x-ray source CT scanners offer a temporal resolution between 135 and 175 milliseconds. Accordingly, images are optimized when acquired at heart rates of less than 65 to 70 bpm. DSCT scanners contain a single gantry with two x-ray tubes at an angle of 90 degrees and two corresponding x-ray detectors. This modification offers significant improvements in temporal resolution (75 to 83 milliseconds), which can more effectively freeze cardiac motion.[44] The latest generation of DSCT also offers the ability to image in shuttle and high-pitch spiral mode. During shuttle mode, images are acquired in two alternating table positions with the table shuttling back and forth to cover a 73-mm anatomic volume.[15,38] Alternatively, prospective ECG-synchronized high-pitch spiral mode allows acquisition of the entire myocardium within an ultrafast scan time of 0.25 to 0.27 seconds during one end-diastolic phase due to the fast table movement, which will also ensure temporal contrast enhancement throughout the entire myocardium.[45]

DSCT scanners have the added ability to operate in dual energy mode (DECT), in which one x-ray tube emits a high-energy spectra and the other, a low-energy spectra during a single scan. DECT exploits the principle that tissues in the body and intravascular iodinated contrast have unique spectral characteristics when irradiated with x-rays of different energy levels. Upon processing separate image reconstructions of the high- and low-energy data, the iodine content within the myocardium is determined based upon the unique x-ray absorption characteristics of iodine at different kV levels.[46] This provides color-coded iodine concentration myocardial maps, which offers additional information beyond the usual attenuation values and facilitates more specific tissue delineation that can be used for the detection of myocardial ischemia. DECT can be performed at a cost of increasing temporal resolution to 165 milliseconds.

Image Acquisition

CCTA/CTP Protocol

Patient Preparation

Before the scan, patients are advised to avoid caffeine, which is a nonselective competitive adenosine receptor antagonist. Intravenous access is obtained in both antecubital veins for the administration of contrast and vasodilator stress agent (Fig. 21-5). Given the importance of heart rate control to minimize motion artifacts, oral and/or intravenous beta-blockers are administered to aim for a heart rate of less than 60 bpm prior to CT acquisition. While beta-blockers have been described to mask ischemia in exercise MPI, such an effect has not been observed on coronary flow reserve,[47] vasodilator stress SPECT MPI,[48] or in CTP.[16]

Image Acquisition

Combined CCTA/CTP imaging requires two separate CT scan acquisitions during rest and vasodilator stress. During the procedure, the patient is closely monitored for heart rate, blood pressure, and ECG for ischemia. Both scans are performed using 50 to 75 mL of iodinated contrast (depending on patient size) aiming to achieve an iodine concentration of ≥320 mg I/mL.[43] The stress scan is performed during hyperemia, typically attained after 3 to 5 minutes of intravenous adenosine administration at 140 μg/kg/min. Real-time bolus tracking is encouraged, and CTP image acquisition is timed to occur in the late upslope, peak, or very early downslope of the contrast bolus. In our institution, this is timed to occur once the target threshold of 300 HU is achieved in the descending aorta, with full volumetric imaging occurring one to two heartbeats later.[16,33] In 64-row detector scanners, there is a longer delay between bolus tracking threshold detection and the onset of cardiac imaging, and triggering is recommended at a threshold of 100 to 180 HU.[43]

Depending on scanner type, images can be acquired using retrospective ECG gating or prospective ECG triggering with multicycle acquisition and reconstruction. Prospective ECG-gated image acquisition should ideally be timed to occur during mid- to late diastole. George et al.[33,49] noted that the best motion-free images were noted in mid- to end diastole in 79% of cases, which on average occurred during 86% of the R-R interval. In our institution, imaging is performed using the second-generation 320-detector row CT, with a tube voltage of 100 to 120 kV (depending on weight), tube current adjusted to weight, and a gantry rotation time of 270 ms (temporal resolution = 135 milliseconds). Prospective ECG gating targeting 70% to 90% of the R-R interval is used. Single heartbeat scans are acquired if the heart rate is ≤65 bpm. If the heart rate is greater than 65 bpm, a two-beat acquisition can be performed or alternatively a single-beat acquisition can be performed upon widening the window from 30% to 80% of the R-R interval.

The protocol can be performed with a rest/stress or a stress/rest protocol. The advantages and disadvantages of each imaging sequence are summarized in Table 21.4. When the time interval between the two scans is short, the contrast used during the first acquisition may still be present in the myocardium at the time of the second acquisition, which may decrease the sensitivity for detection of infracted and ischemic myocardium if the rest and

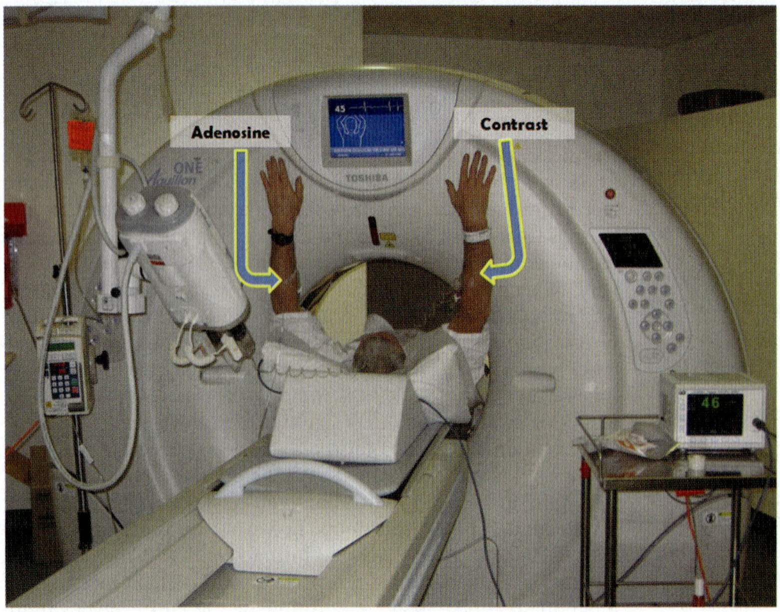

Figure 21-5. **Image acquisition during coronary CT angiography/CT stress myocardial perfusion imaging (CCTA/CTP).** Intravenous access is obtained in both antecubital veins for the administration of adenosine and iodinated contrast. The average time taken for the combined rest CCTA + stress CTP protocol on the CT table is 43 min. (From Ko BS, Cameron JD, Leung M, et al. Combined CT coronary angiography and stress myocardial perfusion imaging for hemodynamically significant stenoses in patients with suspected coronary artery disease: a comparison with fractional flow reserve. *JACC Cardiovasc Imaging* 2012;5:1097–1111.)

TABLE 21.4 CCTA/CTP imaging sequence

	Advantages	Disadvantages
Stress→ Rest	Better sensitivity during stress perfusion nitroglycerin (GTN) can be given for CTA.	Contrast contamination of rest CTA (detect infarct)
Rest→ Stress	Able to stop protocol after CTA of min DSC Better sensitivity of rest scan (detect infarct)	Late contrast enhancement during stress acquisition

Adapted from Techasith T, Cury RC. Stress myocardial CT perfusion: an update and future perspective. *JACC Cardiovasc Imaging* 2011;4:905–916, with permission from Elsevier.

stress scans, respectively, were performed as the second scan. The advantage of the stress followed by rest protocol is that the ability for the stress scan to detect ischemia is optimized. It will also allow the administration of nitrates for the subsequent rest scan, which may have otherwise been contraindicated if the rest scan was performed up front. On the contrary, initial rest-phase imaging more closely resembles clinical practice, where patients will only proceed to have CTP performed if a coronary stenosis of at least moderate severity is identified on resting CCTA. In our institution, we most often use a rest/stress sequence (Fig. 21-6).[95] Contrast contamination can be avoided in our experience by leaving an interval of at least 20 minutes between the two scans to allow wash-out of contrast from the myocardium.[17,50]

Image Interpretation

Systematic Approach for Image Interpretation

The use of a systematic approach for CCTA/CTP interpretation is vital in determining the diagnostic performance of the technique. A stepwise interpretation algorithm for CCTA/CTP interpretation has been described and outlined in Figure 21-7. The five main steps include (a) coronary CCTA interpretation, (b) CTP image reconstruction, (c) image quality assessment, (d) assessment of rest and stress CTP, and (e) correlation of coronary anatomy with perfusion defects.

Step 1: Coronary CTA Interpretation

Although blinded interpretations of coronary CTA and myocardial CTP are often devised in research studies, the clinical use of myocardial CTP should involve a combined reading of coronary CTA and myocardial CTP. Images of the coronary CTA should be interpreted first. Once a potential physiologically significant stenosis is identified (in general, a stenosis ≥50% severity), the role of myocardial CTP should be to (a) assess the functional significance of a stenosis (Fig. 21-8), (b) provide information about the presence of scar versus reversible perfusion abnormalities, and (c) assess the burden of myocardial ischemia.

Steps 2 and 3: CTP Image Reconstruction and Image Quality Assessment

CTP images are reconstructed from multiple phases at 3% intervals, and the cardiac phase with the least motion and artifacts is chosen for final interpretation as they can often mimic or hide perfusion abnormalities. The common causes of artifacts include motion, beam-hardening, cone-beam reconstruction, misalignment, and poor signal-to-noise ratio.

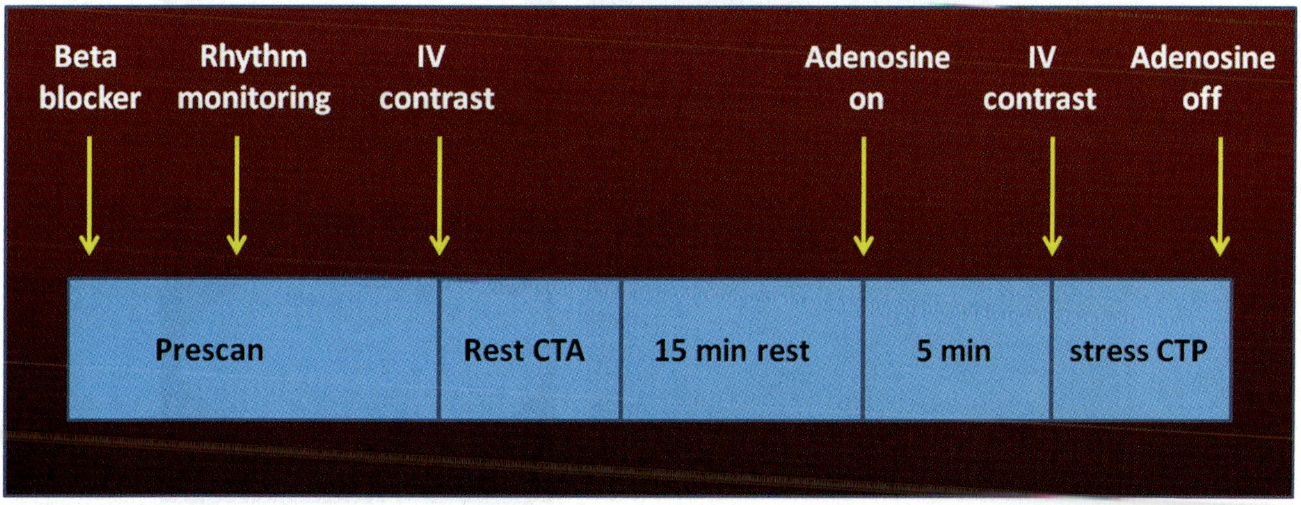

Figure 21-6. CCTA/CTP imaging protocol using 320-detector CT. (Adapted from Ko BS, Cameron JD, Defrance T, et al. CT stress myocardial perfusion imaging using multidetector CT–A review. *J Cardiovasc Comput Tomogr* 2011;5:345–356, with permission from Elsevier.)

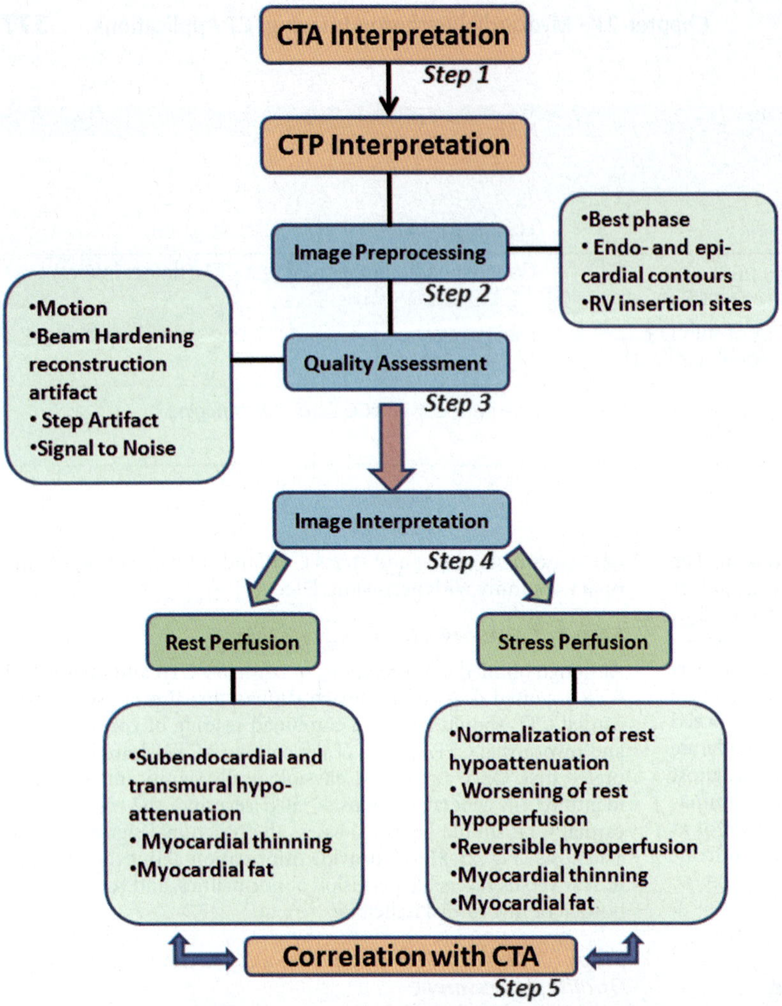

Figure 21-7. **Stepwise interpretation algorithm for CT-based anatomic/functional assessment.** This starts with evaluation of the coronary CCTA (*Step 1*) followed by myocardial CTP image reconstruction (*Step 2*) and evaluation of CTP image quality (*Step 3*). Serial rest and stress images are then analyzed and compared for perfusion defects and other abnormalities associated with ischemia and infarction (*Step 4*). Finally, these analyses are correlated with anatomic localization of coronary stenoses on CCTA (*Step 5*). (Adapted from Mehra VC, Valdiviezo C, Arbab-Zadeh A, et al. A stepwise approach to the visual interpretation of CT-based myocardial perfusion. *J Cardiovasc Comput Tomogr* 2011;5:357–369, with permission from Elsevier.)

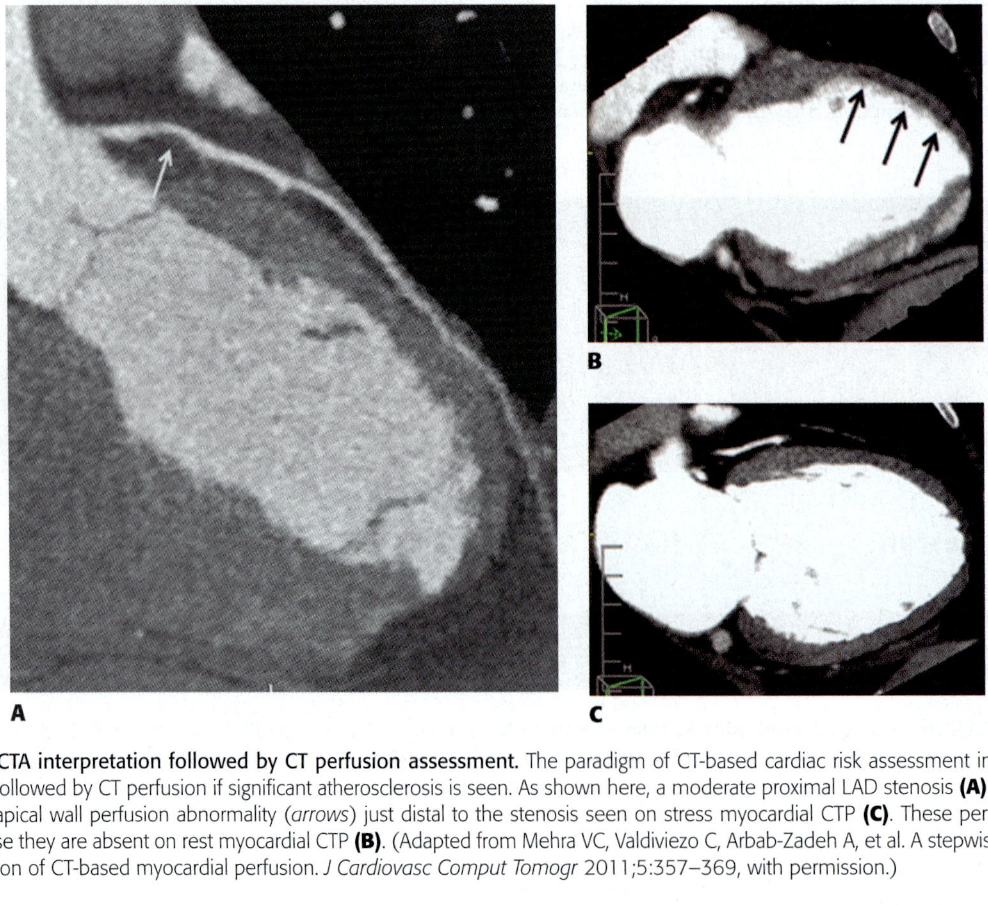

Figure 21-8. **CCTA interpretation followed by CT perfusion assessment.** The paradigm of CT-based cardiac risk assessment involves the use of CT angiography followed by CT perfusion if significant atherosclerosis is seen. As shown here, a moderate proximal LAD stenosis **(A)** is associated with an anterior and apical wall perfusion abnormality (*arrows*) just distal to the stenosis seen on stress myocardial CTP **(C)**. These perfusion defects are reversible because they are absent on rest myocardial CTP **(B)**. (Adapted from Mehra VC, Valdiviezo C, Arbab-Zadeh A, et al. A stepwise approach to the visual interpretation of CT-based myocardial perfusion. *J Cardiovasc Comput Tomogr* 2011;5:357–369, with permission.)

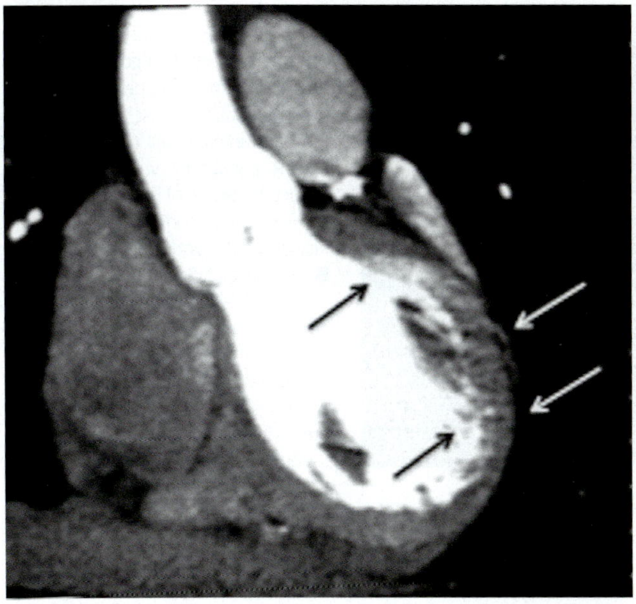

Figure 21-9. Example of images acquired during excessive cardiac motion. Cardiac motion during image acquisition can lead to ghosting of endocardial and epicardial edges and streaking (*arrows*). Presence of these features can make detection of perfusion abnormalities difficult and should mandate a search for alternative phases without motion. (Adapted from Mehra VC, Valdiviezo C, Arbab-Zadeh A, et al. A stepwise approach to the visual interpretation of CT-based myocardial perfusion. *J Cardiovasc Comput Tomogr* 2011;5:357–369, with permission.)

Motion Artifacts

Cardiac and respiratory motion during image acquisition can result in ghosting of endocardial and epicardial edges and streaking, and the presence of these features should mandate a search for alternative phases without motion (Figs. 21-9 and 21-10).[96] In our practice, the optimal phase chosen for interpretation is the one with the sharpest delineation of myocardial trabeculae.

Beam-Hardening Artifacts

Beam hardening occurs when x-rays pass through a radiodense or contrast-filled structure with high attenuation leading to absorption of low-energy photons, which results in a hypoattenuated shadowing artifact. The artifacts can occur in the context of bone (ribs, spine, sternum) or contrast-enhanced LV cavity or descending aorta. The areas most likely to be affected are the basal inferior wall secondary to the contrast-filled descending aorta and the anterior wall, which may be affected by the LV cavity and overlying ribs (Fig. 21-11). The artifacts are typically triangular and transmural and bear a hypoenhanced appearance emanating from a structure with high attenuation and for this reason do not necessarily follow the distribution of a coronary vascular bed. To minimize artifacts, CTP images are ideally reconstructed with a kernel that incorporates beam-hardening correction algorithms (FC03 in 320-detector CT).[51]

Cone-Beam Artifacts

Cone-beam artifacts typically occur in wide-detector CT acquisitions and arise from the fact that the scanner isocenter and projections from the x-ray source on to the multiple detectors do not lie in the same plane. The cone angle for a 320-detector CT is 15.2 degrees compared with 1.53 degrees for a 64-detector CT. The artifact presents as low and high attenuation bands in the image that most often affects the inferior wall and can mask or mimic hypoperfusion. The bands typically extend beyond the cardiac silhouette across the entire field of view (Fig. 21-2). Reconstruction algorithms that involve organ-specific reconstruction, such as combination-weighted reconstruction algorithm, can be effective at eliminating these artifacts.[52]

Misalignment Artifacts

Misalignment artifacts occur in images acquired using narrow detector CT scanners, when the entire volume of the heart is acquired over several heartbeats, using helical or step and shoot protocol. Accordingly, this may result in differences in contrast attenuation in the arterial bed and myocardium between the caudal and cranial portion of the z-axis, which may increase the difficulty in identifying perfusion defects.

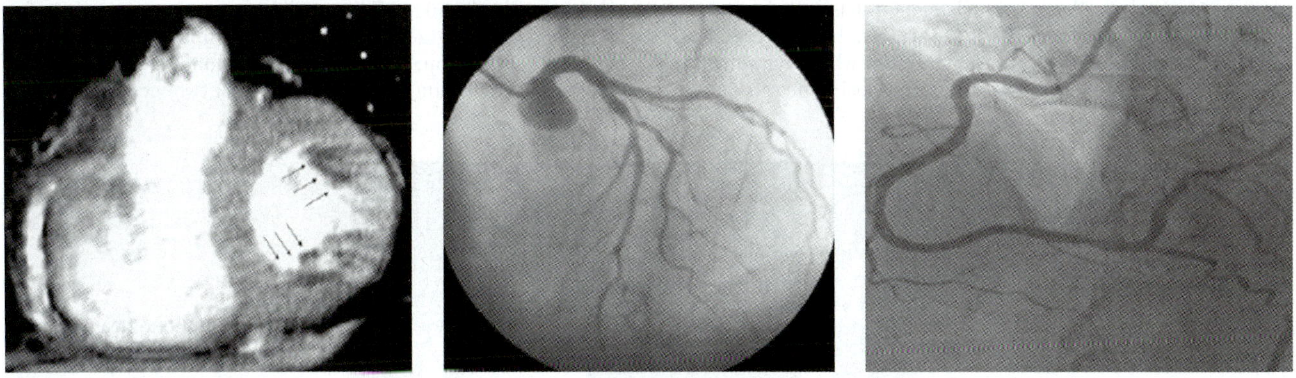

A **B** **C**

Figure 21-10. False-positive perfusion defect due to motion artifact in a patient who underwent adenosine perfusion scanning with a heart rate of 90 bpm. A: CT perfusion imaging showed apparent perfusion defects in the anterolateral and inferior walls (*black arrows*). **B:** Invasive coronary angiography (ICA) image of the LAD artery and large diagonal branch (which supplied the anterolateral wall) demonstrated no hemodynamically significant stenoses (fractional flow reserve [FFR] 0.92 in diagonal branch). **C:** ICA image of the right coronary artery also revealed no significant stenosis to account for apparent inferior ischemia. (Adapted from Nasis A, Seneviratne S, DeFrance T. Advances in contrast-enhanced cardiovascular CT for the evaluation of myocardial perfusion. *Curr Cardiovasc Imaging Rep* 2010;3:372–381, with permission.)

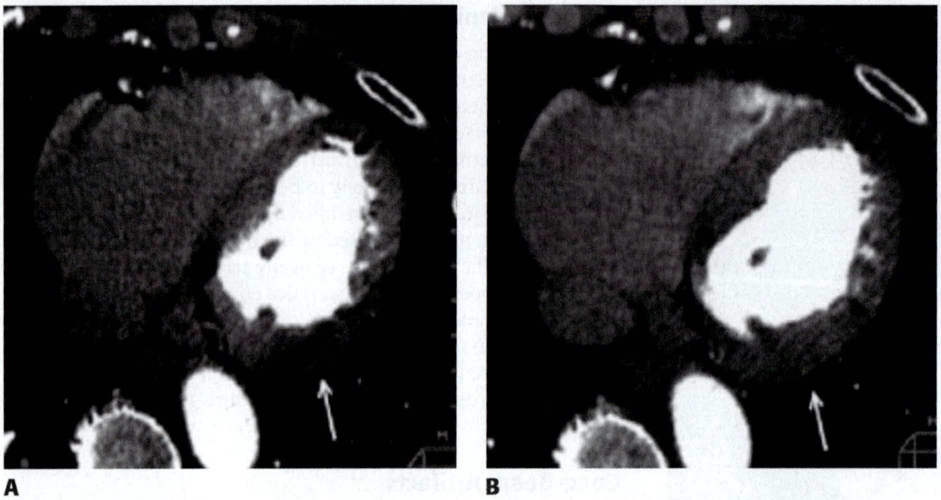

Figure 21-11. **Beam-hardening artifact correction algorithm.** Beam-hardening artifacts appear as areas of hypoattenuation most commonly in the basal inferior wall (*arrow*). **A:** This wall is particularly vulnerable to this artifact because of its location being between the contrast-rich left ventricular cavity and descending aorta. **B:** Reconstruction kernels that implement beam-hardening correction algorithm are effective in overcoming this artifact (*arrow*). (Adapted from Mehra VC, Valdiviezo C, Arbab-Zadeh A, et al. A stepwise approach to the visual interpretation of CT-based myocardial perfusion. *J Cardiovasc Comput Tomogr* 2011;5:357–369, with permission.)

Poor Signal-to-Noise Ratio

High noise and poor signal levels may degrade the entire image. To avoid high image noise, tube and current voltages are typically chosen based on weight or body mass index.

Maintenance of adequate signal-to-noise ratio depends on the timely triggering of the scan to avoid premature or delayed triggering. Images are best timed to occur in the late upslope, peak, or very early downslope of the contrast bolus. Premature triggering can lead to high amounts of contrast remaining in the right ventricle and inadequate contrast in the left heart and coronary circulation, which can lead to inadequate LV myocardial enhancement and significant beam hardening artifacts in the septal walls because of right ventricular contrast. Delayed triggering can lead to inadequate contrast in the cardiac chambers and coronary circulation, leading to poor myocardial enhancement and loss of the presence of perfusion deficits secondary to diffusion.[40]

Step 4: Assessment of Resting and Stress Myocardial Perfusion

Assessment of Rest Myocardial Perfusion on CT

Areas of prior infarction and scar can be first identified on the rest images. Studies have demonstrated that CT has a high sensitivity for identification of scar.[53–55] Rest images should be examined for stigmata of prior myocardial infarction, which may include the presence of subendocardial and transmural hypoattenuation, myocardial thinning, myocardial fat[56,57] and myocardial calcification, aneurysmal dilation, and mural thrombus.[43]

Methods to Assess Stress Myocardial Perfusion on CT

Recent guidelines for systematic myocardial perfusion assessment have detailed two main methods to assess myocardial perfusion including qualitative and quantitative assessment[43] (Fig. 21-13).

Qualitative assessment of CT myocardial perfusion based on visual inspection remains the most commonly used approach in clinical studies[58] (Fig. 21-13). Images are typically interpreted using axial, oblique, and orthogonal views using dedicated computer interpretation software (Fig. 21-14). This involves simultaneous visualization of rest and stress images for regions with hypoenhanced myocardium compared with normally enhanced remote myocardium. Images are typically interpreted using a narrow window width and level setting (W300/L150) and an averaged slice thickness of 3 to 5 mm, which optimizes the subtle differences in myocardial contrast attenuation.[43] Using the standard American Heart Association 17-segment model with apex excluded[33,59] or 13-segment model,[58] each myocardial segment is scored for the presence or absence of a perfusion defect and graded as transmural if it involved ≥50% of myocardium or nontransmural. Defect reversibility is also graded (0 = none, 1 = minimal, 2 = partial, 3 = complete) after comparing with the corresponding rest images. All defects should also be confirmed in at least two views and should

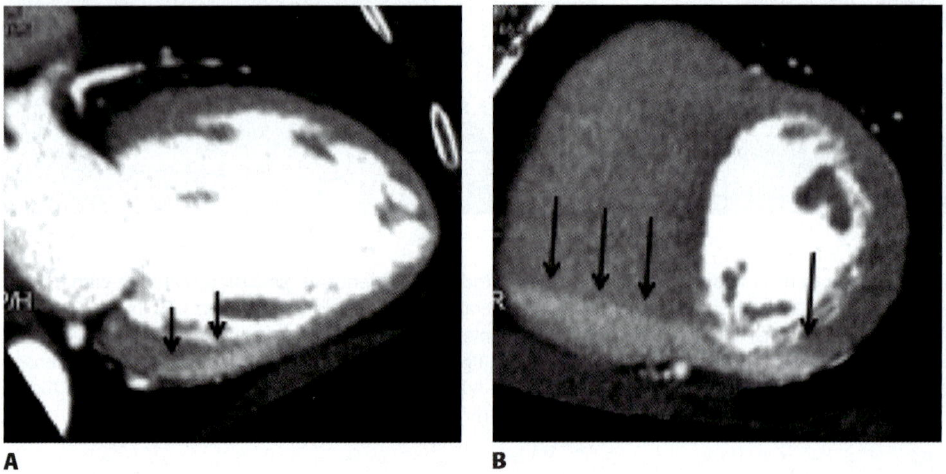

Figure 21-12. Cone-beam artifacts. They are seen here as a continuous linear hyperenhanced artefact (*arrows*) in the more caudal margins of the image appreciated on sagittal **(A)** and axial **(B)** views of the myocardium. (Adapted from Mehra VC, Valdiviezo C, Arbab-Zadeh A, et al. A stepwise approach to the visual interpretation of CT-based myocardial perfusion. *J Cardiovasc Comput Tomogr* 2011;5:357–369, with permission.)

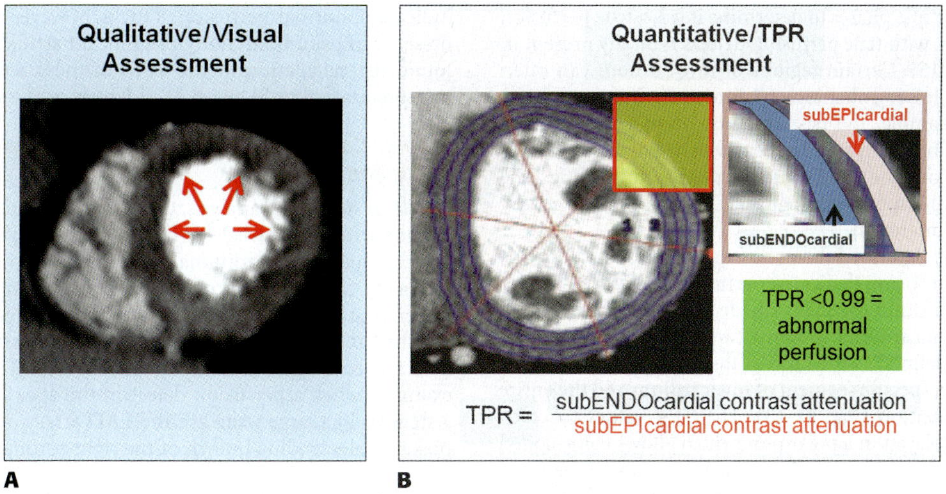

Figure 21-13. Qualitative and quantitative CTP interpretation on static CTP. **A:** Qualitative assessment is performed with visual inspection. **B:** Quantitative assessment is performed using transmural perfusion ration (TPR). (Adapted from George RT, Arbab-Zadeh A, Miller JM, et al. Computed tomography myocardial perfusion imaging with 320-row detector computed tomography accurately detects myocardial ischemia in patients with obstructive coronary artery disease. *Circ Cardiovasc Imaging* 2012;5:333–340 and Ko BS, Cameron JD, Defrance T, et al. CT stress myocardial perfusion imaging using multidetector CT—A review. *J Cardiovasc Comput Tomogr* 2011;5:345–356, with permission.)

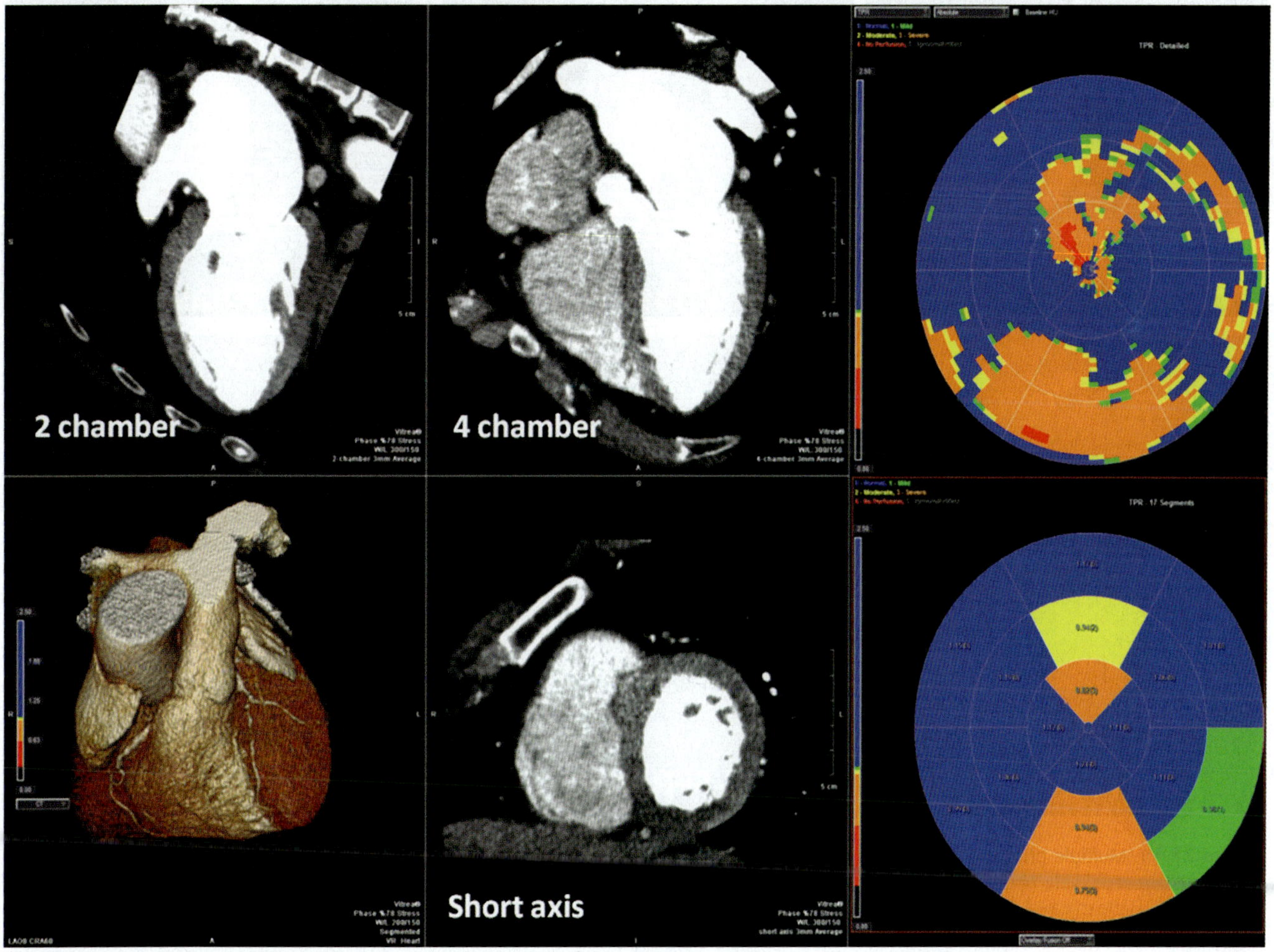

Figure 21-14. Dedicated CTP interpretation software. The myocardium is presented using standard echocardiographic interpretation views to facilitate confirmation of true perfusion defects on multiple views. There is also a polar plot for assessment of transmural perfusion ratio.

be examined in multiple phases to determine if it is a true perfusion defect or an artifact, with true perfusion defects typically present in all phases (Fig. 21-15). Certain regions of myocardium can often be associated with lower enhancement and could mimic a perfusion defect. For example, the basal anteroseptum (membranous septum) is more fibrous in consistency, which may result in the absence of photo counts on radionuclide perfusion imaging. The most distal part of the apex is also naturally thin and should not be mistaken for prior infarction.

George et al.[33,60] described the use of a semiautomated quantitative interpretation. Using dedicated perfusion analysis computer software, the myocardium is equally divided into three myocardial layers—the subendocardium, midmyocardium, and subepicardium. The TPR is defined as the ratio of the averaged subendocardial attenuation of a specific segment of myocardium and the entire subepicardial attenuation (Fig. 21-13). The TPR values for each segment can be displayed in a polar plot, which allows color-coded visualization of the variation of TPRs in each myocardial segment. In ischemic myocardium, contrast attenuation in the subendocardial layer has been demonstrated to be lower than in the subepicardial layer. Based on correlated studies using quantitative coronary angiography (QCA)[33] and invasive FFR[17] as reference standard, a threshold of less than 0.99 has been retrospectively derived to indicate abnormal perfusion. TPR is however not reliable in the presence of prior infarction or significant artifacts, which may confound the calculation of the TPR. In these settings, visual-based interpretation should be used to identify perfusion abnormalities.

Step 5: Correlating Coronary Anatomy with Perfusion Defects

As a final step to the analysis, the major epicardial vessels should be aligned with myocardial territories. Because of variation in coronary anatomy, the traditional assignment of vessels to myocardial segments can be enhanced by directly tracking vessels and their underlying territories on CT. It is recommended that the territory distal to an epicardial stenosis is tracked to assess for a perfusion defect occurring as a result of the stenosis. This will clarify, for example, when a perfusion defect in the apex is secondary to the a stenosis in a large wrap around LAD artery or a lesion in a large posterior descending branch of the right coronary artery.

Feasibility and Diagnostic Performance

CT perfusion imaging has been evaluated in numerous preclinical, single-center human studies and two multicenter studies to date (Tables 21.5 and 21.6). The overall clinical per vessel sensitivity

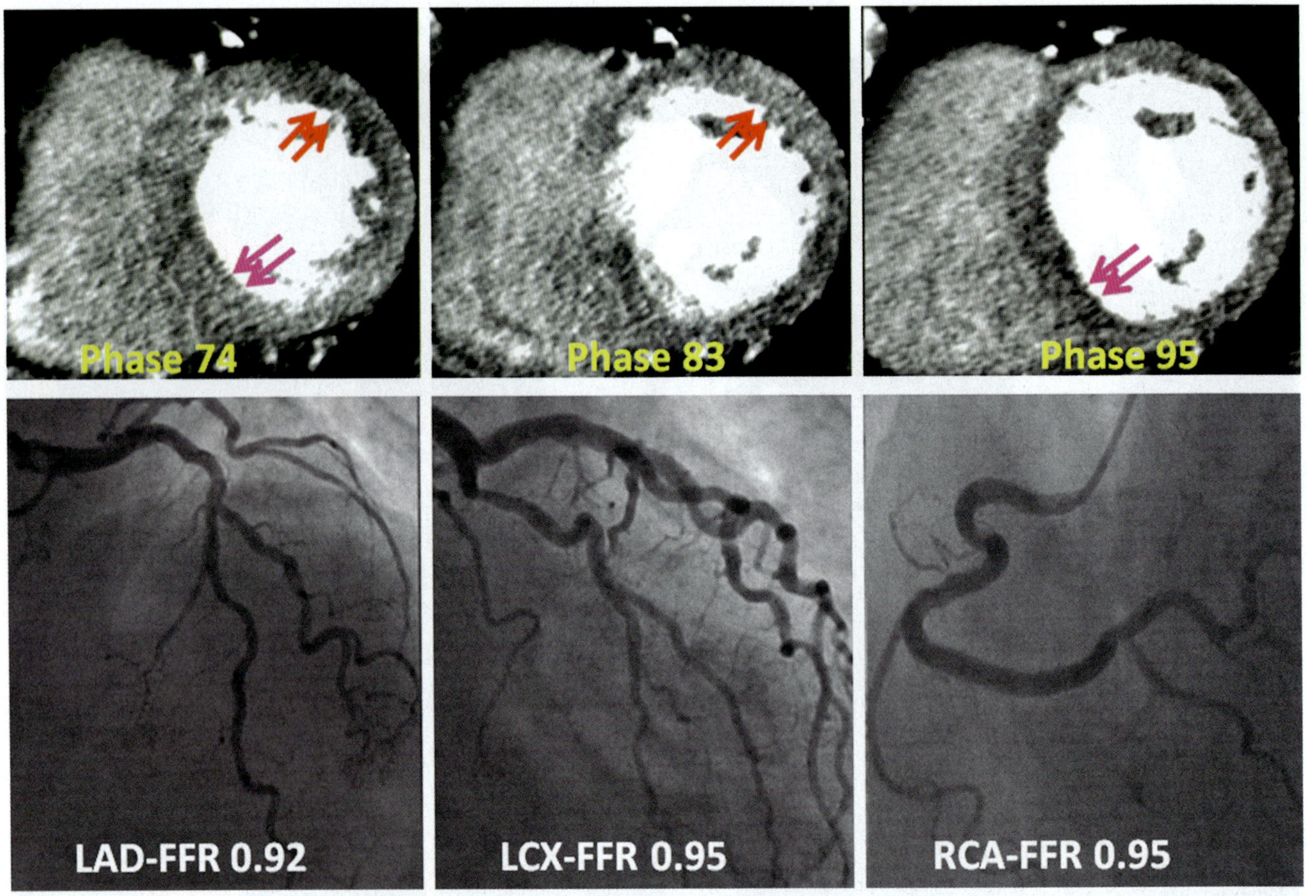

Figure 21-15. Multiple phases are examined to determine a true defect versus artifact. A true defect is typically present in all phases. This is a case of a 78-year-old lady who was investigated for chest pain on background of type 2 diabetes. FFR was not significant in all three major epicardial vessels. On CTP, the midaxial cuts demonstrate apparent perfusion abnormalities in the anterolateral wall in phase 74 (*red arrows*), not present in phase 83. Similarly, apparent perfusion abnormalities are present in the inferoseptal wall in phase 95 (*pink arrows*) yet absent in phase 74. Shifting perfusion abnormalities, which are not seen on all phases, are secondary to artifacts. In this case, this may be secondary to contrast enhancement of the left ventricle or motion. The heart rate during image acquisition was 80 bpm. (Adapted from Ko BS, Cameron JD, Meredith IT, et al. Computed tomography stress myocardial perfusion imaging in patients considered for revascularization: a comparison with fractional flow reserve. *Eur Heart J* 2012;33:67–77, with permission from Oxford Press.)

TABLE

21.5 Summary of Animal Studies Evaluating Myocardial Stress CTP.

First Author, Year (Ref. no.)	Animal Model	CTP Protocol	Reference Standard	Results	Conclusion
George et al., 2006[44]	Canine ($n = 8$) LAD stenosis	Adenosine stress 64-detector MDCT	Microsphere MBF	Linear relationship between myocardial signal density ratio (myocardial attenuation/left ventricular attenuation)	Adenosine stress MDCT provides semiquantitative measurements of myocardial perfusion in canine model of LAD stenosis
George et al., 2007[45]	Canine ($n = 6$) LAD stenosis	Adenosine stress 64-detector MDCT	Microsphere MBF	MDCT-derived MBF strongly correlated with microspheres ($r = 0.91$, $p < 0.0001$).	MDCT MBF measurements using upslope and model-based deconvolution methods correlate well with microsphere MBF.
Christain et al., 2010[46]	Porcine ($n = 8$)	Adenosine stress 64-detector MDCT	Microsphere MBF	Significant correlation between coronary flow reserve measurements between microsphere MBF and CT ($r = 0.94$, $p < 0.0001$)	CT first-pass myocardial perfusion imaging is feasible using a simple semiquantitative analysis, which provides reasonable estimates of MBF.
Mahnken et al., 2010[50]	Porcine ($n = 10$) LAD stenosis Normal control	Adenosine stress 128-detector DSCT dynamic scan mode	–	No significant differences in CT-based MBF between the stenotic and control group at rest; however, significant difference under adenosine stress ($p = 0.0024$)	DSCT permits quantitative whole heart perfusion imaging, with ability to show hemodynamic effect of high-grade coronary artery stenosis.

DSCT, dual-source computed tomography; LAD, left anterior descending coronary artery; MBF, myocardial blood flow; other abbreviations as in Tables 21.1 and 21.2.

Adapted from Rieber J, Jung P, Erhard I, et al. Comparison of pressure measurement, dobutamine contrast stress echocardiography and SPECT for the evaluation of intermediate coronary stenoses. The COMPRESS trial. *Int J Cardiovasc Intervent* 2004;6:142–147, with permission from Elsevier.

TABLE 21.6 **Clinical studies in CTP**

	Scanner Type	Imaging Protocol	Reference Standard	N[a]	Population	Radiation Dose (mSv)	Per Vessel Territory Sensitivity (%)	Per Vessel Territory Specificity (%)
Single-center studies								
Kurata et al.[61]	16 detector	Retrospective	SPECT MPI	12	Suspected CAD	Not reported	90	79
George et al.[33]	64 and 256 detector	Retrospective	QCA/SPECT MPI	27	Positive SPECT	16.8 (64 CT) 21.6 (256 CT)[b]	81	85
Blankstein et al.[59]	64 DSCT	Retrospective	QCA/SPECT MPI	33	Recent SPECT and ICA	9.1	93	74
Rocha-Filho et al.[62]	64 DSCT	Retrospective	QCA	34	Recent SPECT and ICA	9.8	91	91
Okada et al.[63]	64 DSCT	Retrospective	SPECT MPI	47	Recent SPECT and ICA or positive SPECT	10.0	Pearson $r = 0.56$ (rest) and 0.66 (stress)	
Cury et al.[36]	64 detector	Retrospective low resolution	QCA	26	Positive SPECT	3.4	88	79
Bastarrika et al.[38]	128 DSCT	Dynamic shuttle mode	MRI-MPI	10	Known or suspected CAD	21.9	86[c]	98[c]
Ho et al.[39]	128 DSCT	Dynamic shuttle mode	SPECT MPI	35	Positive SPECT	9.2	83	78
Ko S. et al.[64]	64 DSCT	Retrospective	MRI-MPI	41	Known CAD on CCTA scheduled for ICA	8.6	91	72
Tamarapoo et al.[65]	64 DSCT	Retrospective	SPECT MPI	30	Positive SPECT	15.7	92‡	86[c]
Weininger et al.[66]	128 DSCT	Dynamic shuttle mode (DSCT), retrospective (DECT)	MRI-MPI	20	Acute CP w known/ high likelihood CAD	12.8 (DSCT) 15.2 (DECT)	DSCT 86[c] DECT 93[c]	DSCT 98[c] DECT 99[c]
Feuchtner et al[45]	128 DSCT	Prospective high-pitch spiral mode	MRI-MPI	30	Known and suspected CAD	0.9	96	95

Bamberg et al[15]	128 DSCT	Dynamic shuttle mode	FFR	36	Known and suspected CAD	10.0	93	87
Ko B. et al[16]	320 detector	Prospective	FFR	42	Known CAD awaiting revascularization	5.3	76	84
George et al[60]	320 detector	Prospective	CCTA/SPECT MPI	50	Recent SPECT, known and suspected CAD	7.0	100	85
Nasis et al[67]	320 detector	Prospective	SPECT MPI	20	Suspected CAD	9.2	94	98
Bettencourt et al.[19]	64 detector	Retrospective	FFR	101	Suspected CAD	5.0 (including rest CCCTA)	71	90
Rief et al.[68]	320 detector	Prospective	QCA	91	Patients with previous coronary stenting	7.9	56	78
Multicenter studies								
Rochitte et al[58]	320 detector	Prospective	ICA/SPECT	381	Suspected or known CAD	9.3	80[d]	74[d]
Cury et al[69]	Multivendor	Prospective	SPECT	110	Suspected or known CAD	N/A	90[e]	84[e]

[a]Number of patients in the study who underwent both CTP and reference standard imaging modality. Radiation dose only for the stress perfusion acquisition.
[b]Only the radiation dose for both stress and rest perfusion was reported.
[c]Per segment has been reported.
[d]Assuming a summed stress score of 4.
[e]Per patient results available only.
Adapted from Ko BS, Cameron JD, Defrance T, et al. CT stress myocardial perfusion imaging using multidetector CT—A review. *J Cardiovasc Comput Tomogr* 2011;5:345–356, with permission from Elsevier.

ranges between 71% and 97% and specificity 72% and 98% in native lesions as demonstrated using various scanner types compared with different reference standards. SPECT MPI has been chosen as the reference standard in a large number of studies[33,58,59] as it provides incremental prognostic value when used in conjunction with coronary angiography.[23,70] Notably, in multivessel disease, its accuracy is limited as the technique relies on identifying relative differences in perfusion between adjacent myocardial territories,[27] and separate analyses have been performed to avoid penalizing CTP for detecting multivessel disease.[33] Accordingly, recent studies have chosen modalities that are less influenced by the presence of ischemia in adjacent territories such as MRI-MPI[19,38,64,66] and FFR[15–17,19] as an appropriate reference standard for lesion-specific ischemia.

Animal Studies

The first animal studies illustrating feasibility of myocardial CTP were performed by George et al.[37,40] in canine models (Table 21.5). These studies established the semiquantitative relationship between CT attenuation and blood flow based on microsphere MBF. Mahnken et al.[71] subsequently illustrated the ability of dynamic quantitative whole heart perfusion imagine to detect the hemodynamic effect of high-grade coronary artery stenosis in a canine model. Further work in a porcine model has confirmed that coronary flow reserve measurement by microsphere MBF and myocardial CTP correlate well with each other.[72]

Clinical Studies

Early Fundamental Studies

In 2005, Kurata et al.[61] were the first to demonstrate a high agreement (83%) between rest and stress adenosine CTP and stress thallium SPECT MPI in 12 patients with suspected CAD using 16-detector helical MDCT and retrospective ECG gating. Despite the favorable correlation, only 48% of coronary segments were evaluable under stress compared with 89% at rest, illustrating that myocardial CTP was not feasible at that time due to the limitations in the temporal resolution. In 2009, George et al. reported the feasibility and accuracy of CTP on 40 patients with a history of abnormal SPECT MPI who underwent adenosine stress CTP, using a 64 (n = 24) and 256 (n = 16) detector CT.[33] When considering an abnormal TPR to be less than 0.99, combined use of CCTA/CTP was found to be 81% sensitive and 85% specific for identifying vessel territories with a ≥50% stenosis on QCA, which were associated with a perfusion defect on SPECT MPI. Similar results were reported by Blankstein et al.[59] using dual-source CTP in 34 patients with a history of SPECT MPI and invasive angiography. The CTP protocol used included a rest, delayed phase acquisition, and stress MPI. Mean effective MDCT radiation exposure was 12.7 mSv, which was comparable to SPECT MPI alone. Combined CCTA and visual CTP assessment was demonstrated to have a per vessel sensitivity of 93% and specificity of 74% when compared against QCA and SPECT MPI. Based on this cohort, Okada et al.[63] further evaluated the ability to grade the severity of perfusion defects on CT using a score. When applied to vessel territories at rest and stress, the score was found to compare favorably against qualitatively derived summed rest (r = 0.66, $p < 0.0001$) and stress scores (r = 0.56, $p < 0.0001$) derived from SPECT MPI.[63] Rocha-Filho[62] demonstrated the incremental value of CTP in improving the accuracy of CCTA to detect a ≥50% stenosis on QCA, resulting in an increase in sensitivity from 83% to 91%, specificity from 71% to 91%, and the area under the receiver operating curve from 0.77 to 0.90 ($p < 0.005$). The addition of perfusion analysis also improved the reader confidence in stenosis classification and decreased interobserver variability (k value improved from 0.82 to 0.91).

64-Detector Row CTP

The feasibility and performance of CTP using standard 64-row detector CT has been evaluated in a number of single-center studies. Cury et al. demonstrated in the 36 patients, with history of abnormal SPECT MPI, that there was a moderate agreement between CTP and SPECT MPI on a per patient analysis ($k = 0.53$), and CT perfusion defects as qualitatively identified upon visual assessment had a sensitivity and specificity of 88% and 79% in identifying territories supplied by arteries with ≥50% stenosis on QCA albeit requiring a high radiation dose of 14.7 to 16.8 mSv.[36] Bettencourt et al.[19] demonstrated in 101 patients with suspected CAD that combined CCTA/CTP detected FFR ≤ 0.8 with 85% per vessel accuracy, which was comparable with MRI-MPI (88%). The rest CCTA and stress CTP were performed using prospective ECG gating and retrospective ECG gating with tube modulation, respectively, with a resultant decreased radiation exposure in the combined protocol of 5.0 ±0.96 mSv.[19]

Dual-Source CTP

The three techniques described to assess myocardial perfusion using DSCT include high-pitch spiral mode CTP, dual-energy CTP, and dynamic CTP using shuttle mode.

Feuchtner et al.[45] described the feasibility in the use of high-pitch prospectively ECG-synchronized spiral mode CTP using DSCT in 30 patients using MRI-MPI as reference standard (Fig. 21-16). The sensitivity and specificity was 96% and 95%, respectively. The main advantage of this technique is the low associated radiation dose of less than 1 mSv for the stress phase acquisition and 2.5 mSv for the combined CCTA and CTP.

Initial investigations by Ruzsics et al.[73] demonstrated that dual-energy CT had a sensitivity and specificity of 96% and 95% in detecting fixed perfusion defect on SPECT. Furthermore, DECT had a sensitivity and specificity of 88% and 89%, respectively, for the detection of reversible perfusion defect, although the physiologic mechanism behind such a concordance remains controversial as DECT was not performed under stress. S. Ko et al.[64] were among the first to describe the use of dual-energy CTP in 41 patients with known CAD scheduled to undergo coronary angiography using MRI-MPI as reference standard. Stress DECT had a 91% and 72% per vessel sensitivity and specificity, respectively. Using retrospective ECG gating with tube modulation, dual-energy myocardial computed tomography perfusion (DECTP) was achieved in 8.6 mSv.

Bastarrika[38] first described qualitative and quantitative assessment of MBF using dynamic CTP in 10 patients using MRI-MPI as reference standard. The presence of perfusion defects upon visual assessment on dynamic CTP had a sensitivity and specificity of 86% and 98%, respectively. Semiquantitative analysis demonstrated significant differences between ischemic and nonischemic myocardium using a CT-derived signal intensity upslope, which was comparable with MRI-derived values ($p < 0.05$). Overall, a moderate correlation was observed between semiquantitative CT measurements and absolute CT quantification of MBF for hypoperfused and normal myocardial segments. Similar work was performed by Ho et al.[39] who performed dynamic CTP using shuttle mode on 128 DSCT, over a course of 30 seconds, and demonstrated that the values for absolute MBF were similar to that seen in SPECT MPI. The required radiation is 9 mSv for the stress perfusion scan alone.

Bamberg et al.[15] extended upon this work by demonstrating that combined CCTA and dynamic CTP increased the accuracy of CCTA to predict hemodynamically significant coronary stenoses as assessed by FFR in a 36 patients with known and suspected CAD. The combination of an MBF below the threshold of 75 mL/100 mL/min together with a CCTA stenoses greater than 50% was 93% sensitive and 87% specific for detecting stenoses

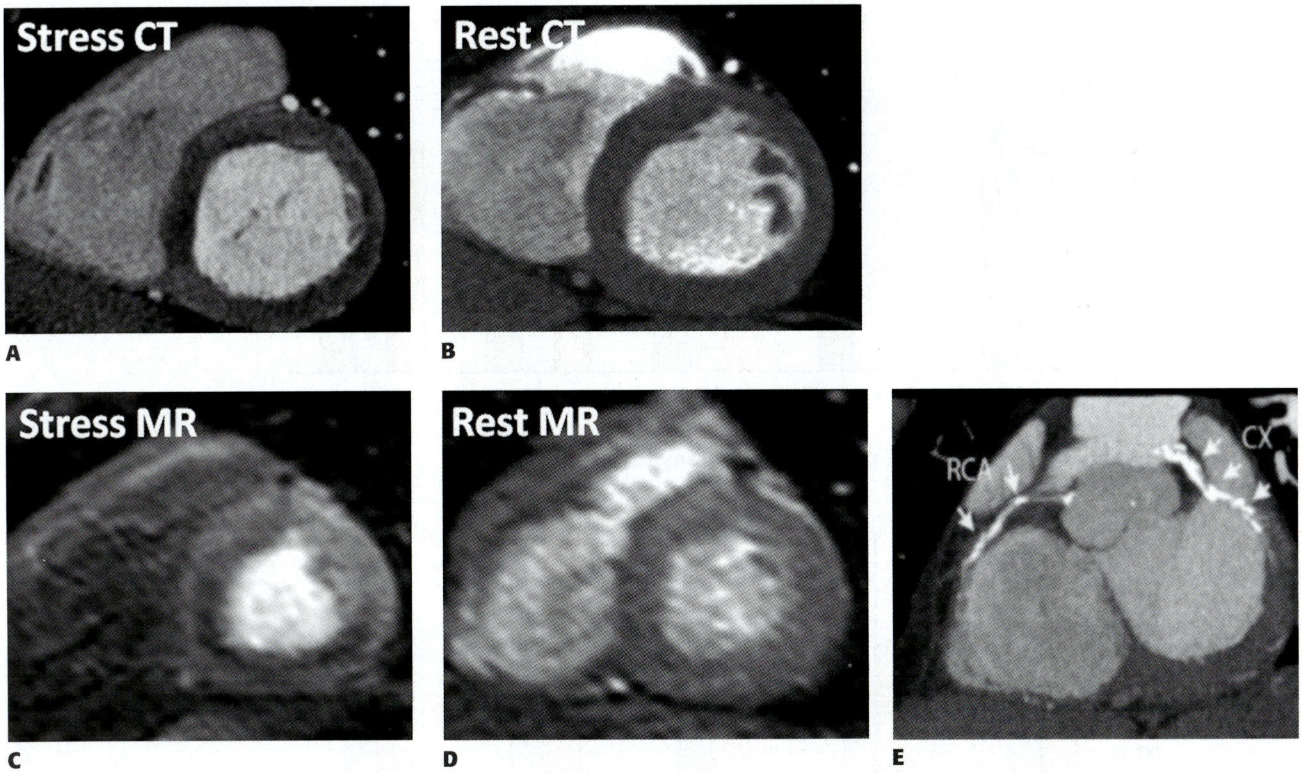

Figure 21-16. CT myocardial perfusion imaging using adenosine stress high-pitch 128-slice dual-source CT. Reversible myocardial ischemia in the inferior and inferoseptal wall demonstrated in stress CTP **(A, B)** and MRI-MPI **(C, D)**. The RCA had a 60% to 70% stenosis proximally **(E)**. There is also a reversible defect in the inferolateral wall on both CT and MRI, which correlates to a subtotal occlusion of the LCx **(E)**. (Adapted from Feuchtner G, Goetti R, Plass A, et al. Adenosine stress high-pitch 128-slice dual-source myocardial computed tomography perfusion for imaging of reversible myocardial ischemia: comparison with magnetic resonance imaging. *Circ Cardiovasc Imaging* 2011;4:540–549, with permission from LWW.)

with an FFR ≤ 0.75. A notable limitation of this technique is the short *z*-axis of 73 mm afforded by shuttle mode acquisition, which results in incomplete coverage of the entire myocardium in one-third of patients.

CTP Using Wide-Detector Coverage CT

B. Ko et al.[16] reported the initial experience of CTP using 320-detector CT in 42 patients with known CAD considered for nonurgent coronary revascularization using invasive FFR as reference standard. The median FFR value in territories with a perfusion defect on CTP was significantly lower than in territories with normal perfusion (FFR perfusion defect 0.72; normal myocardial 0.88, $p < 0.0001$) (Fig. 21-17). CTP had a per vessel territory sensitivity of 76% and specificity of 84%. Furthermore, the combination of a ≥50% stenosis on CCTA and perfusion defect on CTP was 98% specific for functionally significant stenoses as defined by FFR ≤0.8, while the presence of less than 50% stenosis on CCTA and normal perfusion on CTP was 100% specific for exclusion of ischemia. This demonstrated the complimentary role of CTP with CCTA when the two modalities are concordant. Importantly, the mean radiation for CTP and combined CT was 5.3 mSv and 11.3 mSv, respectively, which is much reduced from previous retrospective ECG-gated studies. B. Ko et al.[17] subsequently applied the same study design in 40 patients with suspected CAD. The addition of visual CTP assessment was found to significantly improve the diagnostic accuracy of CCTA (receiver operating characteristic [ROC] area under the curve [AUC] 0.93 vs. 0.85, $p = 0.0003$) and was superior to CCTA + TPR (0.93 vs. 0.79, $p = 0.0003$). This improvement is largely explained by a significant improvement in specificity and positive predictive values to detect FFR significant ischemia, which is in agreement with the results reported by Bettencourt et al.[19] using 64-detector row study (Fig. 21-18).

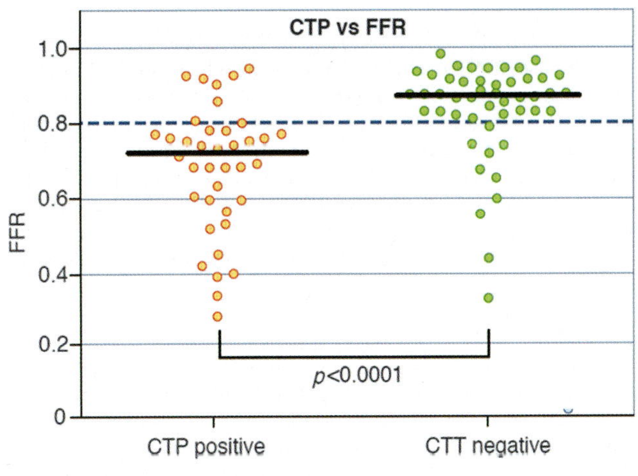

Figure 21-17. Relationship between CT myocardial perfusion imaging versus FFR. In the studied 86 vessel territories, the median FFR is marked with a *black line*, 0.72 with perfusion defect versus 0.88 with normal myocardial perfusion ($p < 0.0001$). (Adapted from Ko BS, Cameron JD, Meredith IT, et al. Computed tomography stress myocardial perfusion imaging in patients considered for revascularization: a comparison with fractional flow reserve. *Eur Heart J* 2012;33:67–77, with permission from Oxford Press.)

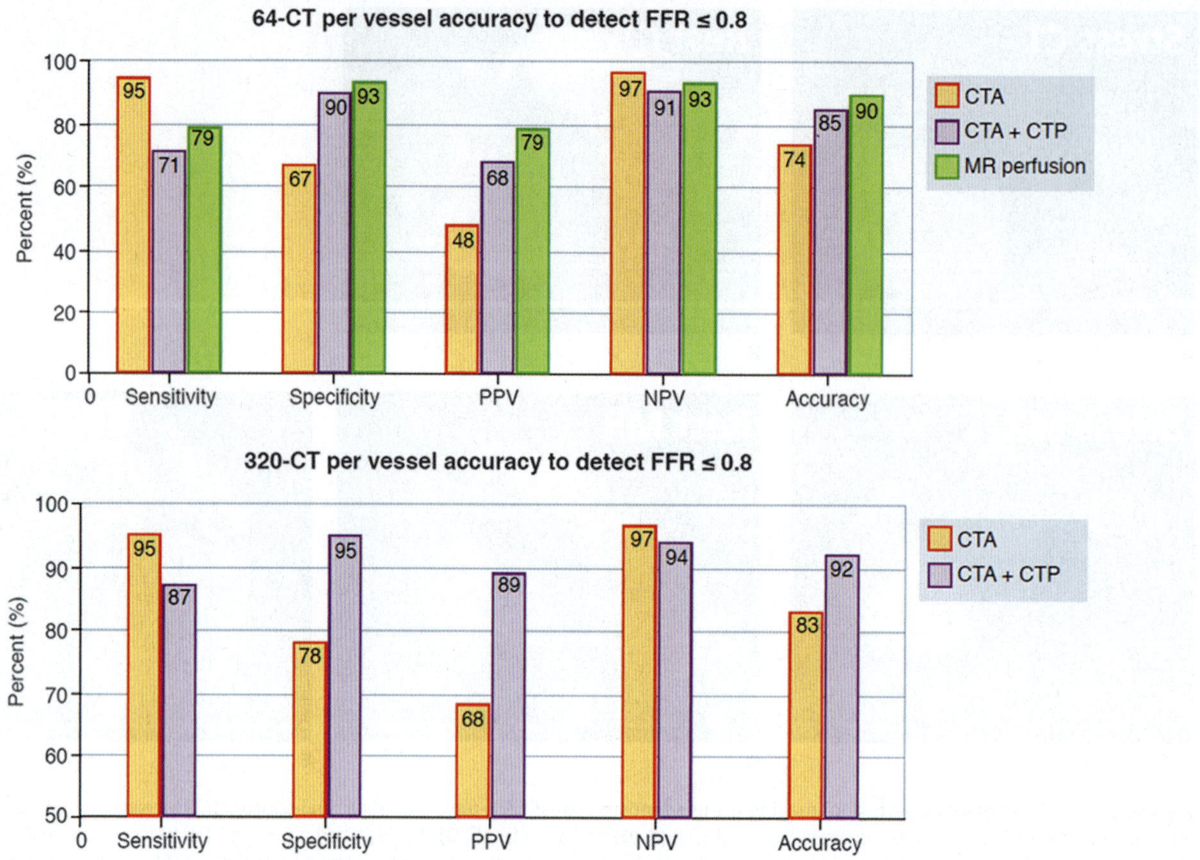

Figure 21-18. **Incremental per vessel accuracy of 64-detector row and 320-detector row CCTA/CTP when compared with CCTA alone to detect invasive FFR ≤0.8.** (Adapted from Bettencourt N, Chiribiri A, Schuster A, et al. Direct comparison of cardiac magnetic resonance and multidetector computed tomography stress-rest perfusion imaging for detection of coronary artery disease. *J Am Coll Cardiol* 2013;61:1099–1107 and Ko BS, Cameron JD, Leung M, et al. Combined CT coronary angiography and stress myocardial perfusion imaging for hemodynamically significant stenoses in patients with suspected coronary artery disease: a comparison with fractional flow reserve. *JACC Cardiovasc Imaging* 2012;5:1097–1111, with permission from Elsevier.)

The use of CT perfusion has been also been studied in evaluation for stents. CCTA of coronary stents has been limited by nondiagnostic studies caused by metallic stent material and coronary motion. Rief et al.[68] demonstrated in a cohort of 91 patients with stents that the addition of 320-CTP significantly improved diagnostic accuracy (ROC AUC 0.82 vs. 0.69, p <0.001) and nondiagnostic rate when compared with CCTA alone using quantitative invasive coronary angiography (ICA) as reference standard.

Multicenter Studies

The recently published CORE 320 study is the first prospective multicenter study that included 381 patients with suspected or known CAD from 16 centers across the globe. The aim was to evaluate the diagnostic accuracy of CCTA/CTP in detecting myocardial ischemia defined as the presence of a 50% stenosis on ICA causing a perfusion defect on SPECT MPI. The patient-based diagnostic accuracy defined by the area under the ROC curve (AUC) of CCTA/CTP for detecting or excluding myocardial ischemia was 0.87, which was statistically higher than when CCTA alone without CTP (0.82, $p \leq 0.001$) was used to predict ICA-SPECT MPI (Fig. 21-19). The improved diagnostic accuracy was consistently reported in all three major epicardial vessels (ROC AUC LAD 0.89 vs. 0.84, $p \leq 0.001$, LCx 0.86 vs. 0.81, $p = 0.002$, RCA 0.86 vs. 0.81, $p = 0.002$). The presence of stents prior to myocardial infarction likely influenced the diagnostic accuracy of the combined technique, and upon exclusion of patients with prior myocardial infarction and patients with known CAD, the diagnostic accuracy improved to 0.90 and 0.93, respectively[58] (Fig. 21-19). Notably, the Core 320 protocol acquired rest CCTA images before CTP. Due to the high sensitivity and negative predictive of CCTA for myocardial ischemia, the study findings support the use of stress CTP only in patients identified with intermediate degree of coronary stenosis within 1 hour of the initial CCTA diagnosis.

A multicenter multivendor study comparing regadenoson stress CTP and SPECT for visualization of myocardial ischemia is underway.[35] Patients with known or suspected CAD undergo both SPECT MPI and stress CTP, which is performed using multivendor CT scanners including 64-, 128-, 256-, and 320-detector row CT. Ischemia is defined as the presence of reversible defects in ≥2 myocardial segments. Preliminary results based on 110 patients from 11 US sites using six different CT scanners demonstrate an overall agreement rate of 87% between CTP and SPECT MPI, with a sensitivity of 90% and specificity of 84%[69] using SPECT MPI as reference standard. Compared to CCTA alone, the diagnostic accuracy of combined CCTA/CTP was superior to CCTA alone (ROC AUC 0.85 vs. 0.69, $p < 0.001$), which was driven primarily by improved specificity.

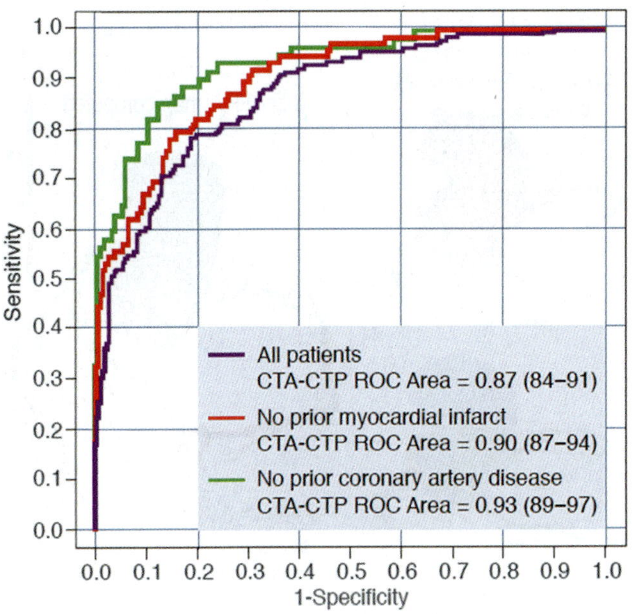

Figure 21-19. **Receiver operating characteristic (ROC) curve and corresponding area under the curve describing the diagnostic performance of combined CCTA and CTP to identify a ≥50% stenosis and a corresponding myocardial perfusion defect using the reference standard of invasive coronary angiography (ICA) and single-photon emission computed tomography myocardial perfusion imaging (SPECT MPI) at a patient level.** (Adapted from Rochitte CE, George RT, Chen MY, et al. Computed tomography angiography and perfusion to assess coronary artery stenosis causing perfusion defects by single photon emission computed tomography: the CORE320 study. *Eur Heart J* 2013. epub ahead of print November 21, 2013, with permission from Elsevier.)

Limitations

The three main limitations related to CTP are artifacts, radiation exposure, and contrast load. Artifacts can alter myocardial attenuation and interfere with myocardial perfusion analysis, which may result in the overestimation or underestimation of MBF and perfusion defects. Artifacts include those associated with motion and beam-hardening (Figs. 21-10, 21-11, and 21-15). Motion artifact can be minimized by the use of scanners with improved temporal resolution or wide-detector scanners with the capacity to perform multisegmented acquisition and reconstruction. Routine beta-blocker administration is also important to blunt vasodilator-induced tachycardia. The development and use of various myocardial-specific beam-hardening correction algorithms will help minimize these artifacts.[74,75]

As stress CTP is performed as a separate additional scan to rest imaging, this increases the radiation exposure, contrast load, and time required. On average, the entire CT protocol can be performed in 43 minutes and requires 120 mL of contrast.[17] For this reason, it needs to be used with caution in patients with abnormal renal function.

Lastly, the current evidence for CT perfusion is predominantly based on single-center studies with only one published multicenter study. The path of translation into clinical medicine will ultimately depend upon results of future multicenter studies, which will undoubtedly shape future guideline recommendations in the assessment of stable CAD. This will also determine the costs that future governments will spend to reimburse the technique.

Noninvasive or Computed Tomography Fractional Flow Reserve

Derivation of FFR CT

In the last 5 years, advances in computational fluid dynamics have enabled calculation of coronary flow and pressure fields from anatomic image data.[76] The focus of research has accordingly shifted to the application of this technique to CCTA images, which enables the calculation of a noninvasive FFR without additional imaging or medications (Fig. 21-20).[77,78]

A three dimensional model of the aortic root and coronary lumen is first constructed using CCTA images. Three key principles are then assumed and used to form boundary conditions: (a) coronary supply meets myocardial demand at rest, (b) the resistance of the microcirculation at rest is inversely but not linearly proportional to the size of the feeding vessel, and (c) the microcirculation reacts predictably to maximal hyperemic conditions in patients with normal coronary flow.[77] Blood is modeled as a Newtonian fluid with incompressible Navier-Stokes equations, and upon application of the physical laws of fluid dynamics on a parallel supercomputer, three dimensional models representing the pressure and flow along all points of the arteries are generated during rest and simulated maximal hyperemic conditions. Based on the approximated pressure measurements during hyperemia, a noninvasive FFR based on CT can be derived at any point in the coronary vascular tree (Fig. 21-21).

Feasibility and Diagnostic Performance

FFR CT (HeartFlow Redwood City, CA, USA) is the first noninvasive test to be validated from its inception by an outcome-based gold standard invasive FFR rather than one ultimately based on coronary stenosis measurement or noninvasive functional testing. A brief summary of the FFR CT trials is summarized in Table 21.7. In the DISCOVER FLOW multicenter, prospective study, Koo et al.[14] demonstrated in a cohort of 103 patients (159 vessels) with suspected or known CAD that FFR CT, using a threshold of ≤0.8, detected FFR-significant (≤0.8) stenoses with an accuracy, sensitivity, and specificity 84%, 88%, and 82%, respectively. The corresponding values for CCTA alone were 59%, 91%, and 40%, respectively. Overall, there was a good correlation between CT FFR and invasive FFR ($r = 0.72$, $p < 0.001$), and the area under the ROC curve (AUC) was 0.90, which was significantly higher than CCTA alone (0.70, $p < 0.0001$).

In the subsequent prospective DeFACTO (Determination of Fractional Flow Reserve by Anatomic Computed Tomographic Angiography) multicenter international trial, Min et al. reported the accuracy of FFR CT on a larger patient cohort (252 patients, 408 vessels) with suspected CAD. On a per-patient basis, FFR CT was superior to CCTA stenosis for diagnosis of ischemic lesions defined as invasive FFR ≤0.8 for accuracy (73% vs. 64%), sensitivity (90% vs. 84%), specificity (54% vs. 42%), positive predictive values (PPV) (67% vs. 61%), and negative predictive values (NPV) (84% vs. 72%).[79] It however did not meet the prespecified endpoint of a lower 95% confidence interval border for diagnostic accuracy of greater than 70%.[79] In patients with intermediate stenoses (30% to 70%), there was a more than twofold increase in sensitivity from 34% to 74% with the AUC increasing from 0.50 to 0.81 ($p = 0.0001$).[80]

The third multicenter study, An Analysis of Coronary Blood Flow Using CT Angiography: NeXt sTeps (NXT) Study, was performed to characterize the diagnostic accuracy of FFR CT in patients (254 patients, 484 vessels) with suspected CAD after substantial improvements in FFR CT technology including updated proprietary software with quantitative image quality analysis, improved image segmentation, refined physiologic models, and increased

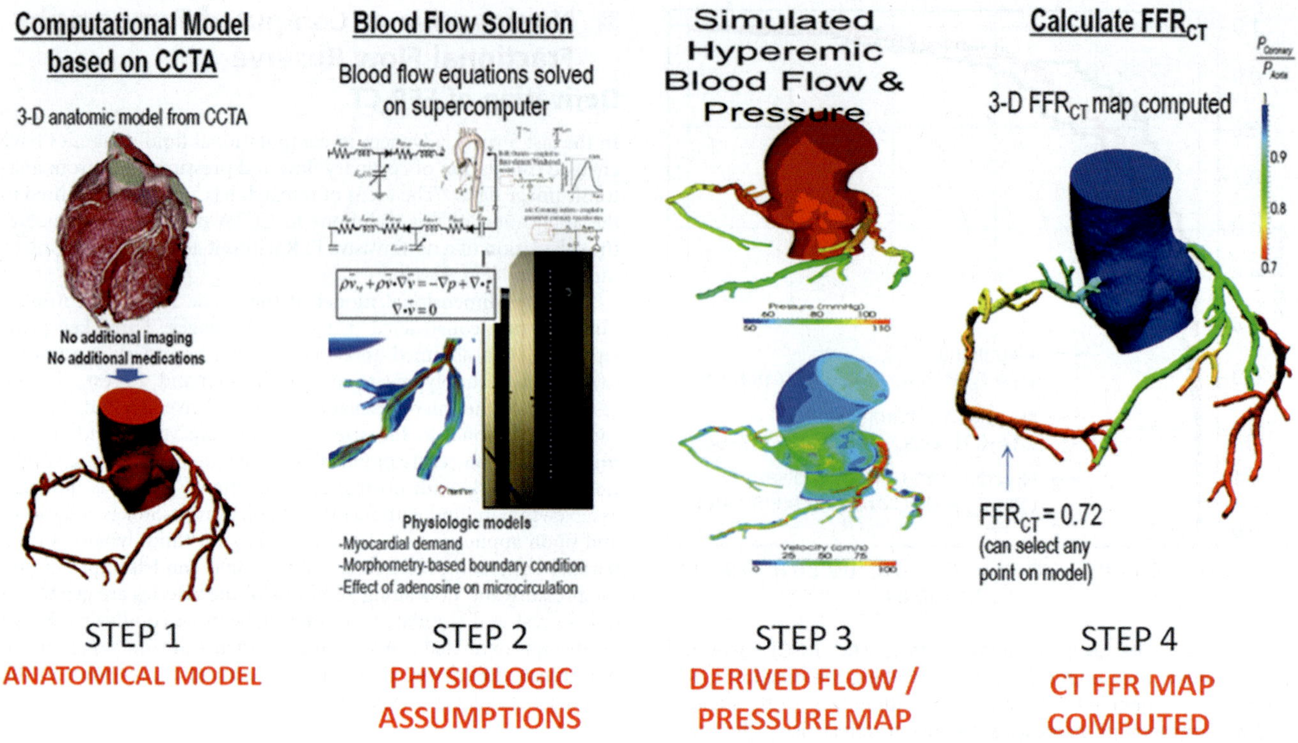

Figure 21-20. Technique in derivation of FFR CT. *STEP 1*: A three-dimensional model of the aortic root and coronary lumen is constructed using CCTA images. *STEP 2*: Assumptions are made regarding the properties of blood, basal total coronary flow, mean aortic pressure and total resistance coronary resistance. *STEP 3*: Using a supercomputer, three dimensional models throughout the cardiac cycle representing the pressure and flow along all points of the arteries are generated during rest and simulated maximal hyperemic conditions. *STEP 4*: Based on the approximated pressure measurements, a noninvasive FFR based on CT is derived. (Adapted from Min JK, Berman DS, Budoff MJ, et al. Rationale and design of the DeFACTO (Determination of Fractional Flow Reserve by Anatomic Computed Tomographic AngiOgraphy) study. *J Cardiovasc Comput Tomogr* 2011;5:301–309 and Koo BK, Erglis A, Doh JH, et al. Diagnosis of ischemia-causing coronary stenoses by noninvasive fractional flow reserve computed from coronary computed tomographic angiograms. Results from the prospective multicenter DISCOVER-FLOW (Diagnosis of Ischemia-Causing Stenoses Obtained Via Noninvasive Fractional Flow Reserve) study. *J Am Coll Cardiol* 2011;58:1989–1997, with permission from Elsevier.)

automation.[20] There was also strict adherence to pre-CCTA administration of beta blockers (99.6% of patients) and nitroglycerin (78% of patients) as per Society of Cardiac CT (SCCT) guidelines,[81] which was aimed to optimize image quality and interpretability. Per-patient sensitivity and specificity for FFR ≤0.8 were 86% and 79%, respectively. The area under the ROC for FFR CT was 0.90 versus 0.81 for coronary CCTA ($p = 0.0008$).

Kim et al.[82] assessed the accuracy of treatment planning using computational model to simulate a virtual stent and to determine with computation of anticipated poststent FFR CT could predict the success of stenting prior to the invasive procedure[82] (Fig. 21-22). In a prospective cohort of 44 patients (48 lesions), the mean difference between FFR CT and invasive FFR was 0.006 (95% limit of agreement −0.27 to 0.28) prior to intervention and 0.024 (−0.08 to 0.13) postintervention. Diagnostic accuracy to predict ischemia prior to stenting was 77% (sensitivity 85%, specificity 57%) and after stenting was 96% (sensitivity 100%, specificity 96%).

Strength and Limitations

The major advantage of FFR CT is that it can be performed without additional image reconstruction, acquisition, or administration of medications. Hence, it requires no additional contrast administration and radiation exposure.

The presence of artifacts on CCTA images including calcification, motion, and misregistration may limit the accuracy of FFR CT. Thus, adherence to protocols that ensure good quality data and facilitate accurate lumen boundary descriptions is essential.[81] Furthermore, the assumptions relating myocardial mass to total coronary flow, relative coronary microvascular resistance based on vessel size, or reductions in resistance in response to adenosine-induced hyperemia may vary among patients, such as in populations with microvascular disease and previous infarction. Finally, no published data exist for FFR CT in the evaluation of in-stent restenosis or for coronary artery bypass grafts.

In its current form, FFR CT analyses requires 5 hours per examination[79] using a parallel computer, though iterative improvements in automation are expected to reduce processing time. Therefore, it is a technology that requires offsite data analysis and attendant turnaround time.

Lastly, it remains unknown whether an FFR CT value of ≤0.8 is sufficient to proceed with intervention or whether this may require further confirmation using invasive FFR. Further refinements in the FFR CT technology or new algorithms from other vendors may improve upon the current reported positive predictive value of 54% to 82%, which may render confirmation with invasive FFR unnecessary.[14,20,79]

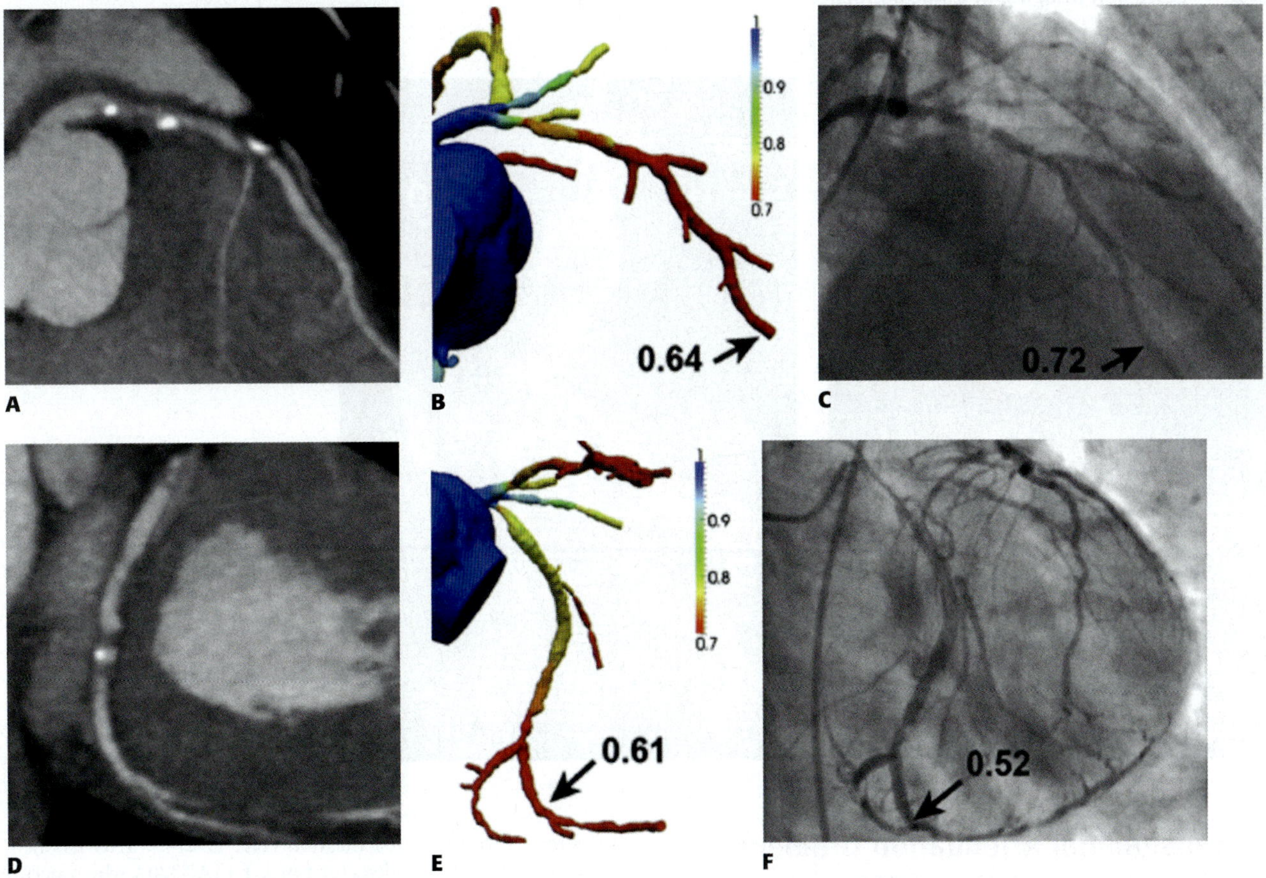

Figure 21-21. FFR CT results for 66-year-old man with multivessel CAD and lesion-specific ischemia. **A:** CCTA demonstrating stenosis in the LAD. **B:** FFR CT demonstrates ischemia in the LAD with a computed value of 0.64. **C:** Invasive coronary angiography (ICA) with FFR also demonstrates ischemia in the LAD with a measured value of 0.72. **D:** CCTA demonstrates stenosis in the LCx. **E:** FFR CT demonstrates ischemia in the LCx with a computed value of 0.61. **F:** ICA with FFR also demonstrates ischemia in the LCx with a measured value of 0.52. (Adapted from Taylor CA, Fonte TA, Min JK. Computational fluid dynamics applied to cardiac computed tomography for noninvasive quantification of fractional flow reserve: scientific basis. *J Am Coll Cardiol* 2013;61:2233–2241, with permission from Elsevier.)

TABLE **21.7** **Summary of FFR CT Trials for Per-Patient and Per-Vessel Detection of Invasive FFR ≤0.8**

	Koo et al. Discover Flow[14]	Min et al. DeFACTO[79]	Norgaard et al. NXT[20]
Year	2011	2012	2014
No. of patients	103	252	251
Design	Multicenter (4 centers)	Multicenter (17 centers)	Multicenter (10 centers)
Per patient			
Sensitivity (%)	93	90	86
Specificity (%)	82	54	79
PPV (%)	85	67	65
NPV (%)	91	84	93
Accuracy (%)	81	73	81
Per vessel			
Sensitivity (%)	88	80	84
Specificity (%)	82	63	86
PPV (%)	74	56	61
NPV (%)	92	84	95
Accuracy (%)	84	69	86

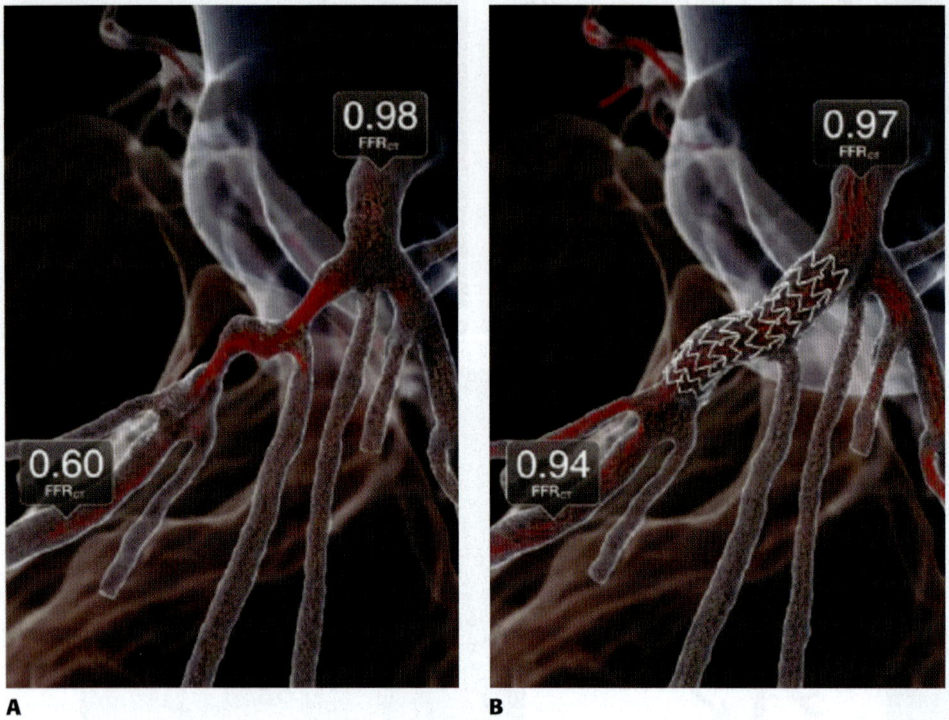

Figure 21-22. **Comparison of FFR CT results before (A) and after (B) simulated Percutaneous coronary intervention (PCI) with stent implantation.** (Adapted from Taylor CA, Fonte TA, Min JK. Computational fluid dynamics applied to cardiac computed tomography for noninvasive quantification of fractional flow reserve: scientific basis. *J Am Coll Cardiol* 2013;61:2233–2241, with permission from Elsevier.)

Transluminal Attenuation Gradient

Definition and Derivation of TAG

TAG defined as the gradient of intraluminal radiologic attenuation is a novel process that can evaluate the severity of coronary stenosis on CT.[83] It has been found to correlate linearly with the degree of coronary artery diameter stenosis in ex vivo studies and discern normal and obstructive coronary arteries in in vivo animal and human studies[84,85] (Fig. 21-23).

Using rest CCTA images, a centerline is determined for each major coronary artery and manually corrected if necessary. Cross-sectional images perpendicular to the vessel centerline are then reconstructed. The contrast attenuation as determined by the mean Hounsfield units (HU) in a region of interest positioned in the center of the cross-sectional images is recorded. The mean HU is measured at 5- to 10-mm intervals[18,83,86] from the ostium to a distal level where the cross-sectional area decreased to less than 2.0 mm^2. TAG is defined as the change in HU per 10 mm length of coronary artery and is calculated as the linear regression coefficient between intraluminal attenuation (HU) and axial distance typically taken from the ostium to the distal coronary vessel (Fig. 21-24).

Feasibility and Diagnostic Performance

Choi et al.[83] demonstrated, in a cohort of 127 patients (370 vessels) using 64-detector CT, that TAG64 was significantly lower in occluded vessels compared to those with lesions of 0% to 49% stenosis on QCA (−13.46 ±9.59 HU/10 mm vs. −2.37 ±4.67 HU/10 mm, p <0.001) (Fig. 21-23). Importantly, the addition of TAG64 to the interpretation of CCTA improved diagnostic accuracy for anatomical stenosis severity $p = 0.001$, especially in vessels with calcified lesions and provided a net reclassification improvement of 0.095.[83]

CCTA with 64-detector row CT requires multiple gantry rotations that are combined for image interpretations, which will result in temporal misalignment between subvolumes for determination of coronary contrast opacification (Fig. 21-25).[97] TAG has hence been studied with 320-detector row CT (TAG320), which permits quantification of the spatial variation of HU over the coronary artery at a single point in time. Similar to the results of Choi et al., Steigner et al.[84] demonstrated in a 36 patients cohort that TAG320 measured in vessels with obstructive lesions were significantly

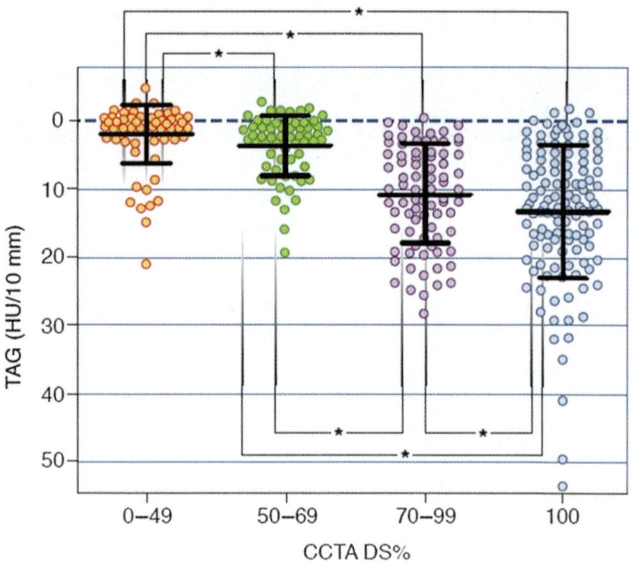

Figure 21-23. **Transluminal attenuation gradient versus diameter stenosis (DS) by coronary CTA.** DS 0% to 49%, −1.91 ±4.25 HU/10 mm; DS 50% to 69%, −3.54 ±4.43; DS 70% to 99%, −10.55 ±7.20; DS 100%, −13.37 ±9.81. $p < 0.0001$ by ANOVA analysis. (*, $p < 0.05$ by t test between two groups). (Adapted from Choi JH, Min JK, Labounty TM, et al. Intracoronary transluminal attenuation gradient in coronary CT angiography for determining coronary artery stenosis. *JACC Cardiovasc Imaging* 2011;4:1149–1157, with permission from Elsevier.)

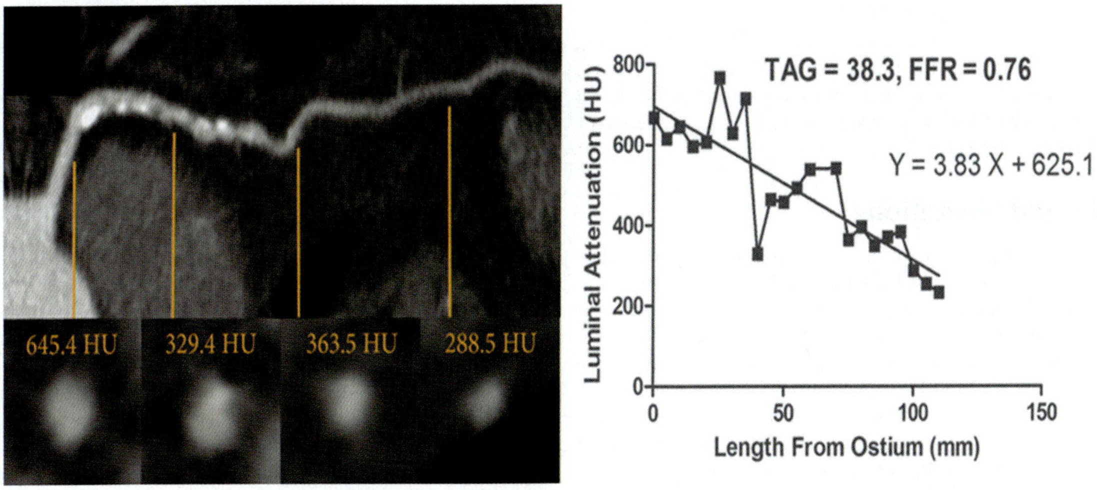

Figure 21-24. Transluminal attenuation gradient. LAD artery with significant obstructive plaque burden imaged by CCTA. Axial and representative cross-sectional views with corresponding luminal attenuation (HU) of CCTA. *Black square dots* represent 5-mm intervals at which intraluminal attenuation (HU) was measured. TAG was −38.3, and the FFR was 0.76. (Adapted from Wong DT, Ko BS, Cameron JD, et al. Transluminal attenuation gradient in coronary computed tomography angiography is a novel noninvasive approach to the identification of functionally significant coronary artery stenosis: a comparison with fractional flow reserve. *J Am Coll Cardiol* 2013;61:1271–1279, with permission from Elsevier.)

different than in vessels considered normal by CCTA ($p < 0.021$).[84] There was no significant difference in gradients obtained in varied cardiac phases, heart rates, and body mass index.

The diagnostic performance of TAG320 to predict the hemodynamic significance of CAD as assessed by invasive FFR has since been evaluated. Wong et al.[18] in a retrospective cohort of 53 stable CAD patients demonstrated that TAG assessed in FFR-significant vessels was significantly lower than that found in FFR nonsignificant vessels (−21 vs. −11 HU/10 mm, $p < 0.001$). Using a retrospectively determined TAG320 cutoff of −15.1 HU/10 mm, TAG320 was reported to predict FFR ≤0.8 with 77% sensitivity and 74% specificity. Importantly, the AUC for the combined use of TAG320 and CCTA was 0.88.

Over time, studies that aim to compare the diagnostic accuracy of novel CT techniques in assessment of hemodynamically significant coronary stenoses across various patient populations will be important to characterize the strength and weaknesses of each technique. There are currently two studies that have compared the use of TAG with FFR CT and CT stress perfusion imaging.[86,87]

Yoon et al. compared the diagnostic performance of FFR CT and TAG for the diagnosis of lesion-specific ischemia in 53 consecutive patients who underwent 64-detector CCTA and FFR. The retrospectively determined optimal TAG64 cutoff to predict significant FFR of −6.4 HU/10 mm was much higher than that reported for 320CT.[18] TAG64 was found to predict FFR ≤0.8 with 37.5% sensitivity and 88% specificity. The diagnostic performance of FFR CT was found to be superior to TAG64 and CCTA stenosis (0.93 vs. 0.63, $p < 0.001$ and 0.93 vs. 0.70, $p < 0.001$, respectively).

Wong et al[87] retrospectively compared the diagnostic accuracy of CCTA+ CTP with CCTA+ TAG320 in a 75 patient cohort using FFR as reference standard. Due to the presence of severe calcification in the coronary vessels, TAG320 was assessable in 76% of vessels, compared with visual assessment using CTP in 97% of vessels. In the vessels where both techniques could be performed, their diagnostic

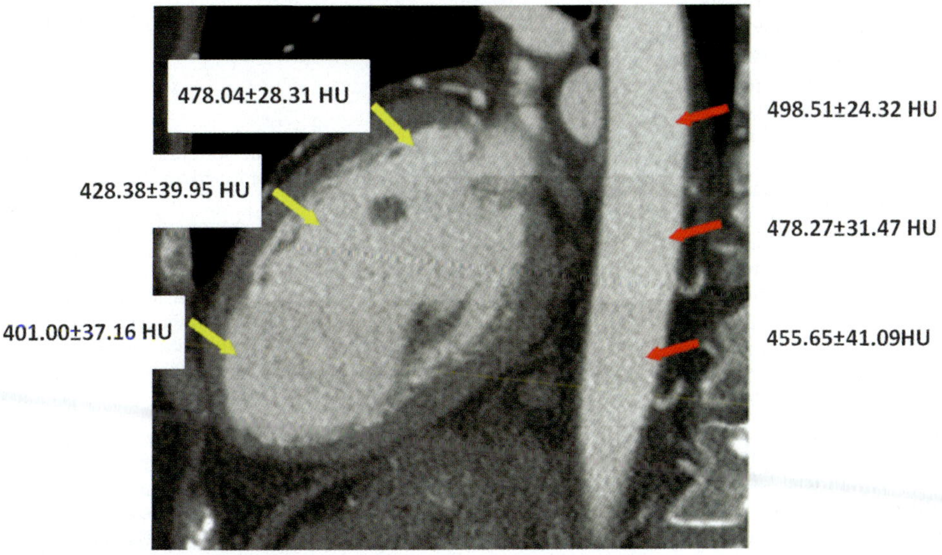

Figure 21-25. Contrast variability due to the lack of temporal uniformity of 64-slice CT. Contrast-enhanced ECG-gated cardiac computed tomography with varying contrast density (Hounsfield Units) in the aorta (*red arrows*) and left ventricle (*yellow arrows*) suggesting that the opacification of vascular structures is nonuniform when image acquisition spans multiple cardiac cycles. (Adapted from Chow BJ, Kass M, Gagne O, et al. Can differences in corrected coronary opacification measured with computed tomography predict resting coronary artery flow? *J Am Coll Cardiol* 2011;57:1280–1288, with permission from Elsevier.)

accuracy was comparable for CCTA+ CTP and CCTA+ TAG320 (0.85 vs. 0.84, $p = 0.98$). The diagnostic accuracy of combined CCTA, TAG320, and CTP, which defined positive vessels as the presence of ≥50% stenosis on CCTA associated with either a perfusion defect on CTP or significant TAG320, was superior to CCTA + TAG 320 or CCTA + CTP (AUC 0.91; $p = 0.01$).

Strengths and Limitations

TAG is a technique that has significant promise for the future. The advantage of the technique similar to FFR CT is that the information can be directly extracted from the resting CCTA images, without need for additional imaging, medications, radiation dose, and contrast administration. Furthermore, TAG evaluation does not require the need for a parallel supercomputer, but is rather performed using dedicated software at the point of care. In our experience, gradients can be derived within 10 minutes during CCTA interpretation. Future automated programs allowing instantaneous TAG320 analysis will be required for the methodology to be adopted in routine clinical practice.

Similar to FFR CT, the technique of TAG is highly dependent upon CCTA image quality, and the presence of extensive luminal calcification can limit its application.[87] TAG assessment has also been described to be not possible in short vessels and in the presence of significant intramyocardial bridging. This may limit the number of generated attenuation points, which is required for TAG to be processed using the current available manual derivation method. Furthermore, the value of TAG remains unknown in vessels with smaller luminal sizes, major epicardial vessels with severe distal vessel or branch disease, intracoronary stents, or coronary artery bypass graft surgery. While the feasibility and diagnostic accuracy of TAG320 to predict lesion-specific ischemia in native coronary disease appear to be promising in single-center studies, this will require further validation in future large multicenter trials.

Future Directions

The ultimate one-stop CT coronary anatomical and functional assessment technique will be not only one that improves the diagnostic performance of CCTA but one that can be performed conveniently with minimal added radiation exposure, contrast, and time. There are two important steps required in the future development of these techniques:

1. Large multicenter international registries and prospective studies aimed to evaluate the prognostic significance, cost-effectiveness, and downstream resource utilization of the three novel CT techniques will be crucial in determining their adoption into guideline and reimbursement recommendations, as had been evident historically in the case of established imaging techniques including CT coronary angiography[88–90] and noninvasive stress imaging such as SPECT MPI and stress echocardiography.[22,23,91,92] The ongoing multicenter "Prospective Longitudinal Trial of FFR CT: Outcome and Impact (PLATFORM) https://Clinicaltrials.gov Identifier NCT01943903 will seek to compare the effect of FFR CT-guided versus standard diagnostic evaluation on clinical outcomes, resource utilization, costs, and quality of life in patients with suspected CAD. In CT perfusion, the final results of the Regadenoson Crossover (A Study of Regadenoson in Subjects Undergoing Stress MPI Using Multidetector Computed Tomography Compared to SPECT) trial will be important to assess the diagnostic performance of the technique when applied in a multivendor trial.[35] Outcome studies are also underway including the PRECEPT registry, PeRfusion Evalution by ComputEd tomography Procedures and Techniques, a multicenter international study that is similar in concept as the CONFIRM registry performed for CT coronary angiography.[93] It currently has 14 centers participating worldwide and includes both retrospective and prospective registries of patients evaluated by CTP.
2. Technical refinements in CT scanner technology and image interpretation software remain much needed to improve the diagnostic performance and clinical application of these techniques. In CTP, the focus of future research will aim to improve CT scanner temporal resolution to facilitate image acquisition at high heart rates during vasodilator-induced hyperemia and to evaluate dose reduction strategies to lower radiation exposure. Furthermore, evaluation of dynamic wide-detector CTP, refinements in dual-energy CTP, and improvements in artifact correction algorithms will be important areas of research to improve diagnostic performance and reader confidence to identify perfusion defects. In the case of FFR CT, there remains a need to refine automated image processing methods[14,79] and to shorten the currently required processing time of 5 hours.[79] The current logistics requiring offsite data analysis and the attendant turnaround time[94] may limit the application of the technique especially in more symptomatic patients. Lastly, in the case of TAG, the development and validation of a semiautomated program to provide instantaneous TAG analysis is much anticipated[18] and may shorten TAG processing time.

Conclusions

Cardiac CT has been rapidly broadened to study the functional significance of CAD, which may enable CT to act as a one-stop shop to assess both coronary anatomy and associated lesion-specific ischemia. The techniques of CTP and CT FFR are rapidly validated by multicenter studies and have been demonstrated to detect lesion-specific ischemia with high accuracy, while TAG remains a promising technique based on single-center feasibility studies, which can be conveniently derived at point of care. Future large multicenter international registries and prospective studies, which aim to provide prognostic outcomes, downstream utilization, and cost-effectiveness of the three novel CT techniques, will ultimately determine their transition into clinical practice.

Acknowledgment

The authors wish to express their gratitude to the National Heart Foundation of Australia and the Robertson Family Research Scholarship for assistance in funding.

REFERENCES

1. **Roger VL, Go AS, Lloyd-Jones DM, et al.** Heart disease and stroke statistics—2012 update: a report from the American Heart Association. *Circulation* 2012;125:e2–e220.
2. **Stone GW, Maehara A, Lansky AJ, et al.** A prospective natural-history study of coronary atherosclerosis. *N Engl J Med* 2011;364:226–235.
3. **Budoff MJ, Dowe D, Jollis JG, et al.** Diagnostic performance of 64-multidetector row coronary computed tomographic angiography for evaluation of coronary artery stenosis in individuals without known coronary artery disease: results from the prospective multicenter ACCURACY (Assessment by Coronary Computed Tomographic Angiography of Individuals Undergoing Invasive Coronary Angiography) trial. *J Am Coll Cardiol* 2008;52:1724–1732.
4. **Miller JM, Rochitte CE, Dewey M, et al.** Diagnostic performance of coronary angiography by 64-row CT. *N Engl J Med* 2008;359:2324–2336.
5. **Meijboom WB, Meijs MF, Schuijf JD, et al.** Diagnostic accuracy of 64-slice computed tomography coronary angiography: a prospective, multicenter, multivendor study. *J Am Coll Cardiol* 2008;52:2135–2144.

6. **Schuetz GM, Zacharopoulou NM, Schlattmann P, et al.** Meta-analysis: noninvasive coronary angiography using computed tomography versus magnetic resonance imaging. *Ann Intern Med* 2010;152:167–177.
7. **Taylor AJ, Cerqueira M, Hodgson JM, et al.** ACCF/SCCT/ACR/AHA/ASE/ASNC/NASCI/SCAI/SCMR 2010 appropriate use criteria for cardiac computed tomography. A report of the American College of Cardiology Foundation Appropriate Use Criteria Task Force, the Society of Cardiovascular Computed Tomography, the American College of Radiology, the American Heart Association, the American Society of Echocardiography, the American Society of Nuclear Cardiology, the North American Society for Cardiovascular Imaging, the Society for Cardiovascular Angiography and Interventions, and the Society for Cardiovascular Magnetic Resonance. *J Am Coll Cardiol* 2010;56:1864–1894.
8. **Wolk MJ, Bailey SR, Doherty JU, et al.** ACCF/AHA/ASE/ASNC/HFSA/HRS/SCAI/SCCT/SCMR/STS 2013 Multimodality appropriate use criteria for the detection and risk assessment of stable ischemic heart disease: a report of the American college of cardiology foundation appropriate use criteria task force, American Heart Association, American Society of Echocardiography, American Society of Nuclear Cardiology, Heart Failure Society of America, Heart Rhythm Society, Society for Cardiovascular Angiography and Interventions, Society of Cardiovascular Computed Tomography, Society for Cardiovascular Magnetic Resonance, and Society of Thoracic Surgeons. *J Am Coll Cardiol* 2014;63:380–406.
9. **Montalescot G, Sechtem U, Achenbach S, et al.** 2013 ESC guidelines on the management of stable coronary artery disease: the Task Force on the management of stable coronary artery disease of the European Society of Cardiology. *Eur Heart J* 2013;34:2949–3003.
10. **Fihn SD, Gardin JM, Abrams J, et al.** 2012 ACCF/AHA/ACP/AATS/PCNA/SCAI/STS Guideline for the diagnosis and management of patients with stable ischemic heart disease: a report of the American College of Cardiology Foundation/American Heart Association Task Force on Practice Guidelines, and the American College of Physicians, American Association for Thoracic Surgery, Preventive Cardiovascular Nurses Association, Society for Cardiovascular Angiography and Interventions, and Society of Thoracic Surgeons. *J Am Coll Cardiol* 2012;60:e44–e164.
11. **Ko BS, Wong DT, Cameron JD, et al.** 320-row CT coronary angiography predicts freedom from revascularisation and acts as a gatekeeper to defer invasive angiography in stable coronary artery disease: a fractional flow reserve-correlated study. *Eur Radiol* 2013;24:738–747.
12. **Meijboom WB, Van Mieghem CA, van Pelt N, et al.** Comprehensive assessment of coronary artery stenoses: computed tomography coronary angiography versus conventional coronary angiography and correlation with fractional flow reserve in patients with stable angina. *J Am Coll Cardiol* 2008;52:636–643.
13. **Sarno G, Decraemer I, Vanhoenacker PK, et al.** On the inappropriateness of noninvasive multidetector computed tomography coronary angiography to trigger coronary revascularization: a comparison with invasive angiography. *JACC Cardiovasc Interv* 2009;2:550–557.
14. **Koo BK, Erglis A, Doh JH, et al.** Diagnosis of ischemia-causing coronary stenoses by noninvasive fractional flow reserve computed from coronary computed tomographic angiograms. Results from the prospective multicenter DISCOVER-FLOW (Diagnosis of Ischemia-Causing Stenoses Obtained Via Noninvasive Fractional Flow Reserve) study. *J Am Coll Cardiol* 2011;58:1989–1997.
15. **Bamberg F, Becker A, Schwarz F, et al.** Detection of hemodynamically significant coronary artery stenosis: incremental diagnostic value of dynamic CT-based myocardial perfusion imaging. *Radiology* 2011; 260:689–698.
16. **Ko BS, Cameron JD, Meredith IT, et al.** Computed tomography stress myocardial perfusion imaging in patients considered for revascularization: a comparison with fractional flow reserve. *Eur Heart J* 2012;33:67–77.
17. **Ko BS, Cameron JD, Leung M, et al.** Combined CT coronary angiography and stress myocardial perfusion imaging for hemodynamically significant stenoses in patients with suspected coronary artery disease: a comparison with fractional flow reserve. *JACC Cardiovasc Imaging* 2012;5:1097–1111.
18. **Wong DT, Ko BS, Cameron JD, et al.** Transluminal attenuation gradient in coronary computed tomography angiography is a novel noninvasive approach to the identification of functionally significant coronary artery stenosis: a comparison with fractional flow reserve. *J Am Coll Cardiol* 2013;61:1271–1279.
19. **Bettencourt N, Chiribiri A, Schuster A, et al.** Direct comparison of cardiac magnetic resonance and multidetector computed tomography stress-rest perfusion imaging for detection of coronary artery disease. *J Am Coll Cardiol* 2013;61:1099–1107.
20. **Norgaard BL, Leipsic J, Gaur S, et al.** Diagnostic performance of noninvasive fractional flow reserve derived from coronary CT angiography in suspected coronary artery disease: the NXT trial. *J Am Coll Cardiol* 2014;63(12):1145–1155.
21. **De Bruyne B, Pijls NH, Kalesan B, et al.** Fractional flow reserve-guided PCI versus medical therapy in stable coronary disease. *N Engl J Med* 2012;367:991–1001.
22. **Hachamovitch R, Rozanski A, Shaw LJ, et al.** Impact of ischaemia and scar on the therapeutic benefit derived from myocardial revascularization vs. medical therapy among patients undergoing stress-rest myocardial perfusion scintigraphy. *Eur Heart J* 2011;32:1012–1024.
23. **Hachamovitch R, Hayes SW, Friedman JD, et al.** Comparison of the short-term survival benefit associated with revascularization compared with medical therapy in patients with no prior coronary artery disease undergoing stress myocardial perfusion single photon emission computed tomography. *Circulation* 2003;107:2900–2907.
24. **Pijls NH, Fearon WF, Tonino PA, et al.** Fractional flow reserve versus angiography for guiding percutaneous coronary intervention in patients with multivessel coronary artery disease 2-year follow-up of the FAME (Fractional Flow Reserve Versus Angiography for Multivessel Evaluation) study. *J Am Coll Cardiol* 2010;56:177–184.
25. **Tonino PA, De Bruyne B, Pijls NH, et al.** Fractional flow reserve versus angiography for guiding percutaneous coronary intervention. *N Engl J Med* 2009;360:213–224.
26. **Watkins S, McGeoch R, Lyne J, et al.** Validation of magnetic resonance myocardial perfusion imaging with fractional flow reserve for the detection of significant coronary heart disease. *Circulation* 2009; 120:2207–2213.
27. **Melikian N, De Bondt P, Tonino P, et al.** Fractional flow reserve and myocardial perfusion imaging in patients with angiographic multivessel coronary artery disease. *JACC Cardiovasc Interv* 2010;3:307–314.
28. **Jung PH, Rieber J, Stork S, et al.** Effect of contrast application on interpretability and diagnostic value of dobutamine stress echocardiography in patients with intermediate coronary lesions: comparison with myocardial fractional flow reserve. *Eur Heart J* 2008;29:2536–2543.
29. **Hacker M, Rieber J, Schmid R, et al.** Comparison of Tc-99m sestamibi SPECT with fractional flow reserve in patients with intermediate coronary artery stenoses. *J Nucl Cardiol* 2005;12:645–654.
30. **Ragosta M, Bishop AH, Lipson LC, et al.** Comparison between angiography and fractional flow reserve versus single-photon emission computed tomographic myocardial perfusion imaging for determining lesion significance in patients with multivessel coronary disease. *Am J Cardiol* 2007;99:896–902.
31. **Forster S, Rieber J, Ubleis C, et al.** Tc-99m sestamibi single photon emission computed tomography for guiding percutaneous coronary intervention in patients with multivessel disease: a comparison with quantitative coronary angiography and fractional flow reserve. *Int J Cardiovasc Imaging* 2010;26:203–213.
32. **Rieber J, Jung P, Erhard I, et al.** Comparison of pressure measurement, dobutamine contrast stress echocardiography and SPECT for the evaluation of intermediate coronary stenoses. The COMPRESS trial. *Int J Cardiovasc Intervent* 2004;6:142–147.
33. **George RT, Arbab-Zadeh A, Miller JM, et al.** Adenosine stress 64- and 256-row detector computed tomography angiography and perfusion imaging: a pilot study evaluating the transmural extent of perfusion abnormalities to predict atherosclerosis causing myocardial ischemia. *Circ Cardiovasc Imaging* 2009;2:174–182.
34. **Patel AR, Lodato JA, Chandra S, et al.** Detection of myocardial perfusion abnormalities using ultra-low radiation dose regadenoson stress multidetector computed tomography. *J Cardiovasc Comput Tomogr* 2011;5:247–254.
35. **Cury RC, Kitt TM, Feaheny K, et al.** Regadenoson-stress myocardial CT perfusion and single-photon emission CT: rationale, design, and acquisition methods of a prospective, multicenter, multivendor comparison. *J Cardiovasc Comput Tomogr* 2014;8:2–12.
36. **Cury RC, Magalhaes TA, Borges AC, et al.** Dipyridamole stress and rest myocardial perfusion by 64-detector row computed tomography in patients with suspected coronary artery disease. *Am J Cardiol* 2010;106:310–315.

37. **George RT, Silva C, Cordeiro MA, et al.** Multidetector computed tomography myocardial perfusion imaging during adenosine stress. *J Am Coll Cardiol* 2006;48:153–160.
38. **Bastarrika G, Ramos-Duran L, Rosenblum MA, et al.** Adenosine-stress dynamic myocardial CT perfusion imaging: initial clinical experience. *Invest Radiol* 2010;45:306–313.
39. **Ho KT, Chua KC, Klotz E, et al.** Stress and rest dynamic myocardial perfusion imaging by evaluation of complete time-attenuation curves with dual-source CT. *JACC Cardiovasc Imaging* 2010;3:811–820.
40. **George RT, Jerosch-Herold M, Silva C, et al.** Quantification of myocardial perfusion using dynamic 64-detector computed tomography. *Invest Radiol* 2007;42:815–822.
41. **Newhouse JH, Murphy RX Jr.** Tissue distribution of soluble contrast: effect of dose variation and changes with time. *AJR Am J Roentgenol* 1981;136:463–467.
42. **Dewey M, Zimmermann E, Deissenrieder F, et al.** Noninvasive coronary angiography by 320-row computed tomography with lower radiation exposure and maintained diagnostic accuracy: comparison of results with cardiac catheterization in a head-to-head pilot investigation. *Circulation* 2009;120:867–875.
43. **Mehra VC, Valdiviezo C, Arbab-Zadeh A, et al.** A stepwise approach to the visual interpretation of CT-based myocardial perfusion. *J Cardiovasc Comput Tomogr* 2011;5:357–369.
44. **Achenbach S, Marwan M, Ropers D, et al.** Coronary computed tomography angiography with a consistent dose below 1 mSv using prospectively electrocardiogram-triggered high-pitch spiral acquisition. *Eur Heart J* 2010;31:340–346.
45. **Feuchtner G, Goetti R, Plass A, et al.** Adenosine stress high-pitch 128-slice dual-source myocardial computed tomography perfusion for imaging of reversible myocardial ischemia: comparison with magnetic resonance imaging. *Circ Cardiovasc Imaging* 2011;4:540–549.
46. **Douglas PS, Chen J, Gillam L, et al.** Achieving Quality in Cardiovascular Imaging II: proceedings from the Second American College of Cardiology—Duke University Medical Center Think Tank on Quality in Cardiovascular Imaging. *JACC Cardiovasc Imaging* 2009;2:231–240.
47. **Bottcher M, Refsgaard J, Madsen MM, et al.** Effect of antianginal medication on resting myocardial perfusion and pharmacologically induced hyperemia. *J Nucl Cardiol* 2003;10:345–352.
48. **Yoon AJ, Melduni RM, Duncan SA, et al.** The effect of beta-blockers on the diagnostic accuracy of vasodilator pharmacologic SPECT myocardial perfusion imaging. *J Nucl Cardiol* 2009;16:358–367.
49. **George RT, Arbab-Zadeh A, Cerci RJ, et al.** Diagnostic performance of combined noninvasive coronary angiography and myocardial perfusion imaging using 320-MDCT: the CT angiography and perfusion methods of the CORE320 multicenter multinational diagnostic study. *AJR Am J Roentgenol* 2011;197:829–837.
50. **Techasith T, Cury RC.** Stress myocardial CT perfusion: an update and future perspective. *JACC Cardiovasc Imaging* 2011;4:905–916.
51. **Kitagawa K, George RT, Arbab-Zadeh A, et al.** Characterization and correction of beam-hardening artifacts during dynamic volume CT assessment of myocardial perfusion. *Radiology* 2010;256:111–118.
52. **Mori S, Endo M, Komatsu S, et al.** A combination-weighted Feldkamp-based reconstruction algorithm for cone-beam CT. *Phys Med Biol* 2006;51:3953–3965.
53. **Gerber BL, Belge B, Legros GJ, et al.** Characterization of acute and chronic myocardial infarcts by multidetector computed tomography: comparison with contrast-enhanced magnetic resonance. *Circulation* 2006;113:823–833.
54. **Kachenoura N, Veronesi F, Lodato JA, et al.** Volumetric quantification of myocardial perfusion using analysis of multi-detector computed tomography 3D datasets: comparison with nuclear perfusion imaging. *Eur Radiol* 2010;20:337–347.
55. **Busch JL, Alessio AM, Caldwell JH, et al.** Myocardial hypo-enhancement on resting computed tomography angiography images accurately identifies myocardial hypoperfusion. *J Cardiovasc Comput Tomogr* 2011;5:412–420.
56. **Rodriguez-Granillo GA, Rosales MA, Renes P, et al.** Chronic myocardial infarction detection and characterization during coronary artery calcium scoring acquisitions. *J Cardiovasc Comput Tomogr* 2010; 4:99–107.
57. **George RT, Lardo AC.** Infarct detection or infarct characterization? Noncontrast CT and its implications for characterizing chronic myocardial scar. *J Cardiovasc Comput Tomogr* 2010;4:108–109.
58. **Rochitte CE, George RT, Chen MY, et al.** Computed tomography angiography and perfusion to assess coronary artery stenosis causing perfusion defects by single photon emission computed tomography: the CORE320 study. *Eur Heart J* 2014;35(17):1120–1130.
59. **Blankstein R, Shturman LD, Rogers IS, et al.** Adenosine-induced stress myocardial perfusion imaging using dual-source cardiac computed tomography. *J Am Coll Cardiol* 2009;54:1072–1084.
60. **George RT, Arbab-Zadeh A, Miller JM, et al.** Computed tomography myocardial perfusion imaging with 320-row detector computed tomography accurately detects myocardial ischemia in patients with obstructive coronary artery disease. *Circ Cardiovasc Imaging* 2012;5:333–340.
61. **Kurata A, Mochizuki T, Koyama Y, et al.** Myocardial perfusion imaging using adenosine triphosphate stress multi-slice spiral computed tomography: alternative to stress myocardial perfusion scintigraphy. *Circ J* 2005;69:550–557.
62. **Rocha-Filho JA, Blankstein R, Shturman LD, et al.** Incremental value of adenosine-induced stress myocardial perfusion imaging with dual-source CT at cardiac CT angiography. *Radiology* 2010;254:410–419.
63. **Okada DR, Ghoshhajra BB, Blankstein R, et al.** Direct comparison of rest and adenosine stress myocardial perfusion CT with rest and stress SPECT. *J Nucl Cardiol* 2010;17:27–37.
64. **Ko SM, Choi JW, Song MG, et al.** Myocardial perfusion imaging using adenosine-induced stress dual-energy computed tomography of the heart: comparison with cardiac magnetic resonance imaging and conventional coronary angiography. *Eur Radiol* 2011;21:26–35.
65. **Tamarappoo BK, Dey D, Nakazato R, et al.** Comparison of the extent and severity of myocardial perfusion defects measured by CT coronary angiography and SPECT myocardial perfusion imaging. *JACC Cardiovasc Imaging* 2010;3:1010–1019.
66. **Weininger M, Schoepf UJ, Ramachandra A, et al.** Adenosine-stress dynamic real-time myocardial perfusion CT and adenosine-stress first-pass dual-energy myocardial perfusion CT for the assessment of acute chest pain: Initial results. *Eur J Radiol* 2012;81:3703–3710.
67. **Nasis A, Ko BS, Leung MC, et al.** Diagnostic accuracy of combined coronary angiography and adenosine stress myocardial perfusion imaging using 320-detector computed tomography: pilot study. *Eur Radiol* 2013;23:1812–1821.
68. **Rief M, Zimmermann E, Stenzel F, et al.** Computed tomography angiography and myocardial computed tomography perfusion in patients with coronary stents: prospective intraindividual comparison with conventional coronary angiography. *J Am Coll Cardiol* 2013;62:1476–1485.
69. **Cury R, Kitt TM, Feaheny K, et al.** A randomized, multi-center, multivendor study comparing myocardial perfusion imaging with regadenoson stress computed tomography perfusion and single photon emission computed tomography. *J Cardiovasc Comput Tomogr* 2013;7:S42.
70. **Iskandrian AS, Chae SC, Heo J, et al.** Independent and incremental prognostic value of exercise single-photon emission computed tomographic (SPECT) thallium imaging in coronary artery disease. *J Am Coll Cardiol* 1993;22:665–670.
71. **Mahnken AH, Klotz E, Pietsch H, et al.** Quantitative whole heart stress perfusion CT imaging as noninvasive assessment of hemodynamics in coronary artery stenosis: preliminary animal experience. *Invest Radiol* 2010;45:298–305.
72. **Christian TF, Frankish ML, Sisemoore JH, et al.** Myocardial perfusion imaging with first-pass computed tomographic imaging: measurement of coronary flow reserve in an animal model of regional hyperemia. *J Nucl Cardiol* 2010;17:625–630.
73. **Ruzsics B, Schwarz F, Schoepf UJ, et al.** Comparison of dual-energy computed tomography of the heart with single photon emission computed tomography for assessment of coronary artery stenosis and of the myocardial blood supply. *Am J Cardiol* 2009;104:318–326.
74. **Perkins J, Field T, Kim J, et al.** Pharmacokinetic targeting of i.v. BU with fludarabine as conditioning before hematopoietic cell transplant: the effect of first-dose area under the concentration time curve on transplant-related outcomes. *Bone Marrow Transplant* 2011;46:1418–1425.
75. **So A, Hsieh J, Li JY, et al.** Beam hardening correction in CT myocardial perfusion measurement. *Phys Med Biol* 2009;54:3031–3050.
76. **Kim HJ, Vignon-Clementel IE, Coogan JS, et al.** Patient-specific modeling of blood flow and pressure in human coronary arteries. *Ann Biomed Eng* 2010;38:3195–3209.
77. **Taylor CA, Fonte TA, Min JK.** Computational fluid dynamics applied to cardiac computed tomography for noninvasive quantification of fractional flow reserve: scientific basis. *J Am Coll Cardiol* 2013;61:2233–2241.

78. **Min JK, Berman DS, Budoff MJ, et al.** Rationale and design of the DeFACTO (Determination of Fractional Flow Reserve by Anatomic Computed Tomographic AngiOgraphy) study. *J Cardiovasc Comput Tomogr* 2011;5:301–309.
79. **Min JK, Leipsic J, Pencina MJ, et al.** Diagnostic accuracy of fractional flow reserve from anatomic CT angiography. *JAMA* 2012:1–9.
80. **Nakazato R, Park HB, Berman DS, et al.** Noninvasive fractional flow reserve derived from computed tomography angiography for coronary lesions of intermediate stenosis severity: results from the DeFACTO study. *Circ Cardiovasc Imaging* 2013;6:881–889.
81. **Abbara S, Arbab-Zadeh A, Callister TQ, et al.** SCCT guidelines for performance of coronary computed tomographic angiography: a report of the Society of Cardiovascular Computed Tomography Guidelines Committee. *J Cardiovasc Comput Tomogr* 2009;3:190–204.
82. **Kim KH, Doh JH, Koo BK, et al.** A novel noninvasive technology for treatment planning using virtual coronary stenting and computed tomography-derived computed fractional flow reserve. *JACC Cardiovasc Interv* 2014;7:72–78.
83. **Choi JH, Min JK, Labounty TM, et al.** Intracoronary transluminal attenuation gradient in coronary CT angiography for determining coronary artery stenosis. *JACC Cardiovasc Imaging* 2011;4:1149–1157.
84. **Steigner ML, Mitsouras D, Whitmore AG, et al.** Iodinated contrast opacification gradients in normal coronary arteries imaged with prospectively ECG-gated single heart beat 320-detector row computed tomography. *Circ Cardiovasc Imaging* 2010;3:179–186.
85. **Lackner K, Bovenschulte H, Stutzer H, et al.** In vitro measurements of flow using multislice computed tomography (MSCT). *Int J Cardiovasc Imaging* 2011;27:795–804.
86. **Yoon YE, Choi JH, Kim JH, et al.** Noninvasive diagnosis of ischemia-causing coronary stenosis using CT angiography: diagnostic value of transluminal attenuation gradient and fractional flow reserve computed from coronary CT angiography compared to invasively measured fractional flow reserve. *JACC Cardiovasc Imaging* 2012;5:1088–1096.
87. **Wong DT, Ko BS, Cameron JD, et al.** Comparison of diagnostic accuracy of combined assessment using adenosine stress CT perfusion (CTP) + computed tomography angiography (CTA) with transluminal attenuation gradient (TAG320) + CTA against invasive fractional flow reserve (FFR). *J Am Coll Cardiol* 2014;63(18):1904–1912.
88. **Min JK, Dunning A, Lin FY, et al.** Age- and sex-related differences in all-cause mortality risk based on coronary computed tomography angiography findings results from the International Multicenter CONFIRM (Coronary CT Angiography Evaluation for Clinical Outcomes: An International Multicenter Registry) of 23,854 patients without known coronary artery disease. *J Am Coll Cardiol* 2011;58:849–860.
89. **Hadamitzky M, Achenbach S, Al-Mallah M, et al.** Optimized prognostic score for coronary computed tomographic angiography: results from the CONFIRM Registry (COronary CT Angiography EvaluatioN For Clinical Outcomes: An InteRnational Multicenter Registry). *J Am Coll Cardiol* 2013;62:468–476.
90. **Chow BJ, Small G, Yam Y, et al.** Incremental prognostic value of cardiac computed tomography in coronary artery disease using CONFIRM: COroNary computed tomography angiography evaluation for clinical outcomes: an InteRnational Multicenter registry. *Circ Cardiovasc Imaging* 2011;4:463–472.
91. **Marwick TH, Case C, Vasey C, et al.** Prediction of mortality by exercise echocardiography: a strategy for combination with the duke treadmill score. *Circulation* 2001;103:2566–2571.
92. **McCully RB, Roger VL, Mahoney DW, et al.** Outcome after abnormal exercise echocardiography for patients with good exercise capacity: prognostic importance of the extent and severity of exercise-related left ventricular dysfunction. *J Am Coll Cardiol* 2002;39:1345–1352.
93. **Min JK, Dunning A, Lin FY, et al.** Rationale and design of the CONFIRM (COronary CT Angiography EvaluatioN For Clinical Outcomes: an InteRnational Multicenter) Registry. *J Cardiovasc Comput Tomogr* 2011;5:84–92.
94. **Hecht HS.** The game changer? *J Am Coll Cardiol* 2014;63(12):1156–1158.
95. **Ko BS, Cameron JD, Defrance T, et al.** CT stress myocardial perfusion imaging using multidetector CT—a review. *J Cardiovasc Comput Tomogr* 2011;5:345–356.
96. **Nasis A, Seneviratne S, DeFrance T.** Advances in contrast-enhanced cardiovascular CT for the evaluation of myocardial perfusion. *Curr Cardiovasc Imaging Rep* 2010;3:372–381.
97. **Chow BJ, Kass M, Gagne O, et al.** Can differences in corrected coronary opacification measured with computed tomography predict resting coronary artery flow? *J Am Coll Cardiol* 2011;57:1280–1288.

CHAPTER

22 Myocardial Perfusion Imaging with PET, PET/CT, PET/MRI: Technical Advances and Future Applications

Vikas Veeranna, MD and Sharmila Dorbala, MD, MPH

Introduction

Radionuclide myocardial perfusion imaging (MPI) remains the mainstay for the diagnosis, risk assessment, and management of patients with known or suspected coronary artery disease (CAD).[1] MPI with radionuclide techniques can be accomplished with either single photon emission computed tomography (SPECT) or positron emission tomography (PET). With the improved image quality from higher spatial and temporal resolution, increased availability of PET scanners and radiotracers, and the ability to assess myocardial blood flow (MBF), PET MPI makes for an attractive alternative to SPECT MPI.[2–6]

PET is a noninvasive imaging modality that can be used to quantitatively assess minute biochemical pathways using radiotracers containing naturally occurring elements such as carbon, nitrogen, oxygen, and fluorine. Since its first use more than 50 years ago, PET has considerably evolved in terms of hardware, software, radiotracers, and clinical applications. Apart from relative and absolute quantitation of MBF, PET allows for the evaluation of myocardial metabolism and identification of ruptured or high-risk atherosclerotic plaques.[2,3,7–9] Further, cardiac PET has been used for imaging inflammation, sympathetic innervation, and infiltrative diseases of the heart.[3,10–12] With these technologic and clinical developments, PET may soon become the diagnostic modality of choice for the assessment of several cardiovascular diseases.[2,3,5,10,13–15] Furthermore, hybrid imaging using separate scanners or integrated hybrid scanners provides an opportunity for advanced imaging combining anatomical, physiologic, and functional information. In this chapter, we will focus on the recent advances in radiotracers, technology, and some of the novel clinical applications for PET MPI.

Advances in PET MPI

Myocardial Perfusion Radiotracers

Rubidium 82 or N-13 ammonia is used for clinical applications of PET MPI, while O-15 water is used for research applications.[2,9,16] Rubidium 82 is generator produced increasing its availability for sites without a cyclotron, but is expensive and in limited supply. N-13 ammonia, due to its 9.96-minute half-life, requires a cyclotron in close proximity to the imaging center. Conventional cyclotrons require a large space (which may be limited in medical centers with space constraints) and capital investment. Thus, PET radiotracer availability is a major limitation for more widespread use of PET MPI and had led to the development of novel cyclotrons and novel radiotracers. The development of novel compact cyclotrons solely for the production of N-13 ammonia circumvents some of these issues. A compact (room size 150 square feet), point-of-care, 12-MeV, self-shielded superconducting cyclotron, ION-12[sc], was developed by Ionetix Corporation.[17] Also, table-top cyclotron was developed by the University of Michigan,[18] and a laser plasma accelerator developed by Berkeley National Laboratory[19] will make N-13 ammonia more accessible for medical imaging.

Also, unlike O-15 water, rubidium 82 and N-13 ammonia are not completely extracted during first-pass circulation throughout the heart and not linearly taken up by the myocardium in relation to blood flow particularly during hyperemia. Further, the exercise stress is challenging with short-acting radiotracers such as rubidium 82 and N-13 ammonia PET MPI, limiting greater clinical applicability. These limitations have led to an interest in the development of perfusion tracers with superior extraction characteristics and tagged with F-18 for a longer half-life (110 minutes). These fluorinated radiotracers could be used for exercise PET perfusion imaging and shipped to various sites as unit doses, allowing for greater accessibility to a PET perfusion tracer. Several fluorinated PET perfusion tracers are under evaluation: (a) F-18-BMS-747158-02 (2-tert-butyl-4-chloro-5-[4-(2-(18F)fluoroethoxymethyl)-benzyloxy]-2H-pyridazin-3-one); (b) 2-tert-butyl-4-chloro-5-{6-[2-(2-18F-fluoroethoxy)-ethoxy]-pyridin-3-ylmethoxy}-2H-pyridazin-3-one(18F-BCPP-EF); and (c) 2-tert-butyl-4-chloro-5-[6-(4-18F-fluorobutoxy)-pyridin-3-ylmethoxy]-2H-pyridazin-3-one (18F-BCPP-BF).[20] Of these, F-18 BMS compound now known as F-18 flurpiridaz has been most extensively evaluated.

Fluorine 18 flurpiridaz (F-18 flurpiridaz) is a novel cyclotron-produced radiotracer with a long half-life of 110 minutes. Although, produced by a cyclotron, due to its long half-life, it can be produced at regional cyclotrons and delivered to imaging centers as unit doses (similar to F-18 FDG). It binds to the mitochondrial complex I of the electron transport chain[21] and is taken up by the heart due to high mitochondrial densities in the myocardium.[2,22] Phase 1 clinical trials established safety and biodistribution of F-18 flurpiridaz in humans.[23] This tracer has a short positron range, high first-pass extraction (>90% even at high flow rates), slow wash-out, and a

TABLE 22.1 **PET Radiotracers**

Perfusion	Half-life	Mechanism of Uptake
Rubidium 82*	78 s	Na/K-ATPase
Nitrogen 13–ammonia*	9.96 min	Diffusion with intracellular metabolic trapping
Oxygen 15–water	2 min	Free diffusion
Fluorine 18–flurpiridaz	110 min	Mitochondrial binding
Copper 62–pyruvaldehyde-bis (N4 methylthiosemicarbazone)	9.7 min	Free diffusion with intracellular binding
Metabolic and Molecular Imaging	**Half-life**	**Mechanism of Uptake**
Fluorine 18–fluorodeoxyglucose	110 min	Glucose transport and intracellular trapping by phosphorylation
Carbon 11–glucose	20 min	Glucose metabolism
Carbon 11–acetate	20 min	Oxidative metabolism
Carbon 11–palmitate	20 min	Fatty acid metabolism
Fluorine 18–sodium fluoride	110 min	Fluoride ion incorporating into hydroxyapatite
Carbon 11–meta-hydroxyephedrine	20 min	Transporter binding and storage in the sympathetic nervous system
Fluorine 18–galacto–arginine-glycine-aspartate	110 min	Binds to integrin αvβ3 receptors
Carbon 11–choline	20 min	Active transport and intracellular phosphorylation

*FDA approved for clinical use.

From Bengel FM, Higuchi T, Javadi MS, et al. Cardiac positron emission tomography. *J Am Coll Cardiol* 2009;54:1–15; Orbay H, Hong H, Zhang Y, et al. Positron emission tomography imaging of atherosclerosis. *Theranostics* 2013;3:894–902; Di Carli MF, Murthy VL. Cardiac PET/CT for the evaluation of known or suspected coronary artery disease. *Radiographics* 2011;31:1239–1254.

low background uptake.[22] These properties provide for a higher spatial resolution and make F-18 flurpiridaz an excellent tracer for flow quantitation. Indeed, in pig models, when compared to N-13 ammonia, F-18 flurpiridaz showed higher target-to-background activity ratios between the myocardium and the blood pool, lungs, and liver both at stress and rest accounting for the higher-quality images.[22] Further, regional MBF and defect extent correlated closely with radioactive microspheres.[22] F-18 flurpiridaz is also well suited for use with exercise stress testing due to its longer half-life.[16]

Results from a phase 2 trial showed F-18 flurpiridaz to be safe with superior image quality, improved diagnostic certainty, and more sensitivity compared to technetium (Tc)-99m SPECT MPI.[24] This multicenter study included 143 patients who underwent Tc-99m SPECT MPI as well as F-18 flurpiridaz PET MPI and invasive coronary angiography ($N = 86$).[24] For the detection of obstructive CAD by coronary angiography, when compared to SPECT MPI, PET MPI showed a significantly higher sensitivity (78.8% vs. 61.5%, $p < 0.05$) with no significant difference in specificity (76.5% vs. 73.5%, p = nonsignificant).[24] Furthermore, in patients with angiographic CAD, when compared to SPECT MPI, PET MPI demonstrated a greater magnitude of reversible perfusion defects (90.8% vs. 70.9%, $p < 0.01$). These improved characteristics may be attributable to the physical characteristics of F-18-flurpiridaz including a higher extraction even at higher flow rates compared to traditional SPECT tracers.[24]

Compared to the available PET perfusion tracers, F-18 flurpiridaz has high target-to-background ratio, higher myocardial extraction and uptake, accurate MBF quantitation, low positron range, and longer half life, allowing the tracer to be delivered in unit doses from regional cyclotrons. These features make this tracer an almost ideal PET tracer. However, the preliminary results of a phase 3 trial have shown similar high sensitivity but potentially lower specificity for the detection of CAD compared to SPECT MPI.[25] More large-scale clinical trials will be performed before it is FDA approved for clinical use (Table 1).

Technical Advances of PET, PET/CT, and PET/MR Systems

Several key technologic advances in software, hardware, and newer hybrid PET/CT and PET/MR systems have contributed to significant improvements in the performance characteristics of the present-day PET scanners.[3,5] Figures 22-1 to 22-3 illustrate some of the important technical advances in PET imaging.

Software Advances

Software advances in PET MPI include iterative reconstruction algorithms, high-definition PET, and cardiac "motion freeze" imaging. Conventional PET systems used filtered back projection algorithms for image reconstruction along with corrections for randoms, scatter, dead time, attenuation, and decay. The drawback of filtered back projection is streak artifacts, which affect the visual interpretation, especially in patients with large body size.[3] Iterative reconstruction algorithms improve image noise. These algorithms weigh the data based on their statistical quality and model the geometry of the imaging system such as intercrystal scatter and depth of interaction effects and nonuniform sensitivity along a line of response. These algorithms nearly eliminate streak artifacts and greatly improve the visual appearance of the image. However, these algorithms need high computational power to perform sufficient

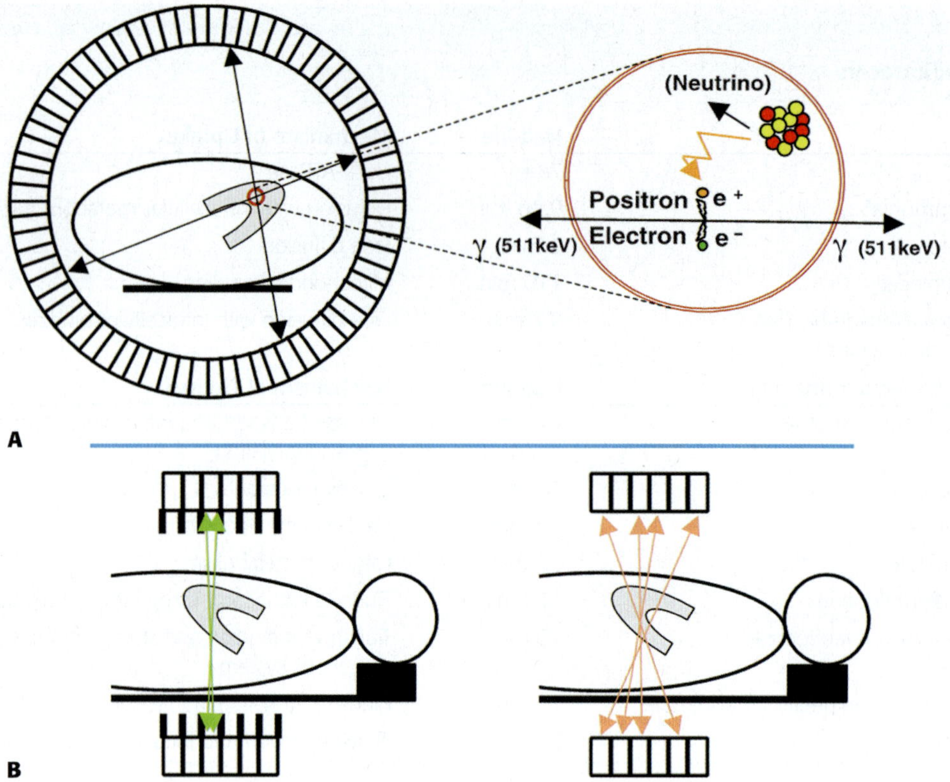

Figure 22-1. **Advances in PET technology. A:** Basic positron emission tomography (PET) principle: a positron (e+) is emitted from the atomic nucleus together with a neutrino. The positron moves randomly through the surrounding matter, where it hits electrons (e–) until it finally loses enough energy to interact with a single electron. This process, called "annihilation," results in two diametrically emitted photons with energy of 511 keV each. These photons are detected as coincidences in the detector ring of the PET camera. **B:** Traditional two-dimensional imaging **(left)** uses only coincidences that occur within the same axial detector ring. Adjacent detector rings are separated by septa. Advanced three-dimensional imaging **(right)** uses coincidences from all possible detector pairs. This increases sensitivity and count density but is demanding and requires correction for the higher amount of scatter and inhomogeneity at the axial edge of the field of view. (Reproduced with permission from Bengel FM, Higuchi T, Javadi MS, et al. Cardiac positron emission tomography. *J Am Coll Cardiol* 2009;54:1–15.)

iterations particularly to avoid artifacts in regions with low radiotracer uptake.[3] With the increased computer power of the current generation PET systems, iterative reconstruction is now the most commonly employed reconstruction protocol. Another improvement in image reconstruction is the introduction of high-definition PET with spatially variant 3D-specific point spread function (PSF), which can significantly improve spatial resolution of the images and signal-to-noise ratio providing high-quality images.[26,27] Cardiac motion freeze (CMF) technique, which addresses loss of image resolution from cardiac motion on the static images, is another recent advancement. Initially developed for SPECT imaging, it can be applied to PET as well. CMF processing involves the

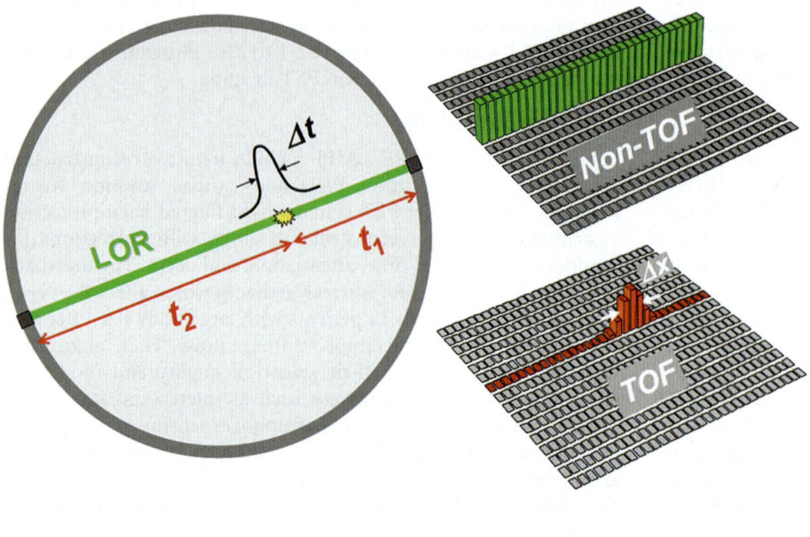

Figure 22-2. **Schematic showing the potential added value of time-of-flight (TOF) PET for localization of the event.** With conventional (non–time-of-flight) imaging, the precise position of the emission event between the two opposing detectors is not known. All the pixels along the line of response must by incremented during reconstruction **(right top)**. With TOF PET, the precise location of the event is better identified and the image can be accordingly reconstructed **(right bottom)**. (Reproduced with permission from Lecomte R. Novel detector technology for clinical PET. *Eur J Nucl Med Mol Imaging* 2009;36(suppl 1):S69–S85.)

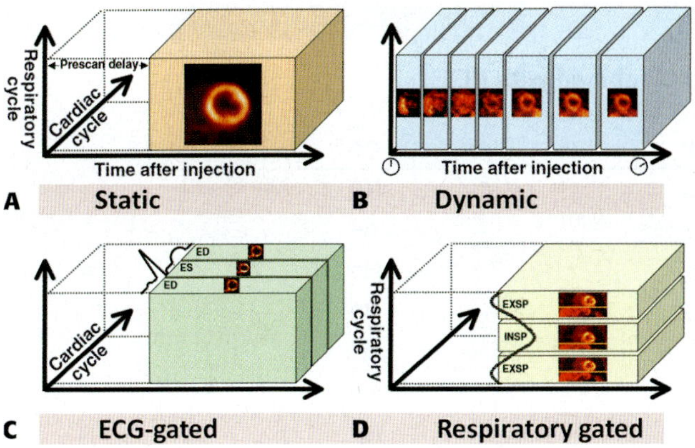

Figure 22-3. Multidimensional list-mode PET acquisition. Scanner coincidences are continuously recorded along with information about the time after the start of acquisition, the electrocardiographic signal, and the signal about breathing position (optional). Data can then be resampled in multiple formats at any time of the acquisition. **A:** High-count static images are reconstructed by summing all information after a predefined prescan delay (delay time after tracer injection). **B:** Dynamic imaging sequences are obtained by serial temporal sampling at different times after injection. This is used for tracer kinetic analysis. **C:** Electrocardiographically gated images are obtained at multiple phases of the cardiac cycle to assess ventricular function. **D:** Respiratory gated images can be obtained at different phases of the breathing cycle in order to correct for respiratory motion. (ED, end diastole; ES, end systole; EXSP, expiratory phase; INSP, inspiratory phase; PET, positron emission tomography). (Reproduced with permission. from Bengel FM, Higuchi T, Javadi MS, et al. Cardiac positron emission tomography. *J Am Coll Cardiol* 2009;54:1–15.)

tracking of left ventricular endo- and epicardial motion on the gated images and projecting the counts from all the cardiac phases to one single phase, usually end diastole. This resultant image has higher count statistics with spatial resolution similar to that of the end-diastolic image, and when applied with 3D-PSF, reconstruction algorithm provides a high-quality image free of blurring due to cardiac motion.[28]

Scintillation Crystals

At present, several different crystals—bismuth germanate (BGO); the newer gadolinium oxyorthosilicate (GSO), lutetium oxyorthosilicate (LSO), and lutetium yttrium orthosilicate (LYSO); and others—are used commonly in PET imaging.[29] Although BGO has high stopping power and provides good detector efficiency at 511 keV, the slow decay time and low light output of BGO leads to relatively poor timing and energy resolution.[3,5,30–32] Despite the lower stopping power, the main advantage of the newer crystals (GSO, LSO, and LYSO) is their significantly reduced dead time enabling 3D dynamic imaging for MBF quantitation. By their higher light output compared to BGO, these new scintillators also permit more crystal elements to be decoded per photomultiplier tube. These features have in turn contributed to development of higher quality images with PET MPI.[3,5,30,32]

Imaging Modes

Conventional PET scanners allow for imaging in a static mode, in an ECG-gated mode, or in a dynamic mode (Figure 22-3). The dynamic images are multiframe time sequence high temporal resolution images that enable assessment of radiotracer transit through the various cardiac chambers. Using a dynamic imaging sequence and tracer kinetic modeling techniques, absolute MBF, and physiologic or biochemical function can be estimated.[3,33] Using conventional scanners, if MBF assessment is desired, the protocols are tailored such that the dynamic images are obtained over the first few minutes of the scan and a separate gated or static image acquisition is started. A recent advance in PET scanners is greater computer memory allowing for the option of list mode acquisition. List mode acquisition is a multiframe acquisition in relation to time and ECG. The advantage of list mode data acquisition is ability to reconstruct the data acquired during a single image acquisition into static images for perfusion assessment, gated images for function assessment, and dynamic images for MBF assessment.[3,33] The ability to acquire images in a list mode has significantly enhanced PET MPI and has allowed for routine quantitation of MBF in all patients.

Semiconductor Detectors and Silicon Photomultiplier Tubes

Pixelated semiconductor detectors have been a recent advance in SPECT. Semiconductors directly convert the electronic signal into an image (allowing a compact system) and have a high sensitivity allowing for low radiation dose imaging. Their use is expanding to PET, and some of the next-generation PET scanners will incorporate semiconductor detector material cadmium telluride (CdTe). These detectors are compact and can be tightly packed and coupled one to one with the PET scintillation crystals.[34] These semiconductor detectors appear to have slightly better spatial resolution and significantly better energy resolution and lower scatter compared to conventional PET.[35,36] Also, conventional photomultiplier tubes are extremely sensitive to magnetic fields and limit the MR signal. For this reason, novel silicon-based solid-state sensors called avalanche photodiodes, which are insensitive to magnetic fields, have been developed for hybrid PET/MR systems. The silicon-based photomultiplier tubes also offer advantages of improved signal to noise and timing resolution allowing for time-of-flight (TOF) imaging.[37]

Time-of-Flight Imaging

TOF is the time difference between the two annihilation photons reaching their respective detectors 180 degrees apart.[3,32] The coincidence electronics in the new advanced PET scanners with TOF electronics are capable of measuring the exact time interval between the two annihilation photons reaching the opposing detectors. The exact location of the annihilation is estimated by multiplying the difference in time with the speed of light along the coincidence ray between the two opposing detectors.[32] This allows for the PET scanners with TOF to localize an annihilation event to a much smaller directional ray than conventional scanners, which results in an increased spatial resolution (Fig. 22-2).[32] However, the major limitation in its application in cardiac PET may be the presence of cardiac and respiratory motion. Advances in respiratory gating and freeze motion correction might improve the applicability of TOF in cardiac PET imaging.[29] Furthermore, with the advent of newer crystals, which have better timing resolution without a compromise on their stopping power, a further improvement in detector efficiency and signal-to-noise ratio can be expected.[5,32] This may be helpful in imaging obese patient where limited image quality from higher scattered counts has always been a concern.

Hybrid Radionuclide Imaging Systems: PET/CT and PET/MRI

Radionuclide imaging has the distinct advantage of high sensitivity to detect minute physiologic processes. However, the anatomical image resolution is limited. Hybrid imaging systems of PET/CT and PET/MR overcome these limitations. CT offers high-resolution anatomical images, and MR offers high resolution anatomical and

TABLE 22.2 **Key Characteristics of Imaging Systems Combined with PET**

Characteristic	MR	CT
Technically challenging	Yes	No
Increased radiation dose	No	Yes
Simultaneous imaging	Yes	No
Motion correction	Yes	No
Better spatial resolution	Yes	Yes
Better soft tissue contrast	Yes	No
Structure and function analysis	Yes	No
Scar assessment	Yes	No
Coronary angiography	Yes	Yes
Coronary calcium assessment	No	Yes
Molecular imaging	Yes	No
Renal dysfunction	No	No
Image with metallic implants	Yes/No	Yes

MR, magnetic resonance; CT, computed tomography.
From Rischpler C, Nekolla SG, Dregely I, et al. Hybrid PET/MR imaging of the heart: potential, initial experiences, and future prospects. *J Nucl Med* 2013;54:402–415; Adenaw N, Salerno M. PET/MRI: current state of the art and future potential for cardiovascular applications. *J Nucl Cardiol* 2013;20:976–989; Nuyts J, Dupont P, Strobants S, et al. Simultaneous maximum a posteriori reconstruction of attenuation and activity distributions from emission sinograms. *IEEE Trans Med Imaging* 1999;18:393–403.

functional assessments. Hybrid PET/CT and PET/MR images can be performed as images on separate scanners and fused using software or acquired at the same setting sequentially (PET/CT) or simultaneously (PET/MR). Sequential and simultaneous acquisition of hybrid images offers distinct advantages, which are discussed in a later section. Table 2 lists the key characteristics of integrated PET/CT and PET/MR systems.

PET/CT

The emergence of integrated PET/CT technology has gained great popularity over the past decade. With greater availability of scanners, especially in oncology, the use of hybrid scanners has permeated to cardiac imaging as well. Further, with increased use and development CT in cardiology, the newer hybrid scanners boast multislice CT scanners including 128-slice CT systems.[30] The CT scan in hybrid scanners is used for transmission imaging (ungated, free breathing, 10 mA at least 6-slice multidetector CT [MDCT]) and for hybrid imaging applications of MPI with calcium score (prospectively ECG triggered, end diastolic, 300 mA, breath hold, at least 64-slice MDCT) and/or CT coronary angiography (prospectively ECG triggered, 300 mA, breath hold, at least 64-slice MDCT).[38]

Attenuation Correction Using CT

With dedicated PET scanners, radionuclide line source sources (germanium 68 or caesium 137) are used for transmission imaging. However, it is expensive, transmission imaging takes time, and the line source decays over time, degrading images.[3,32] Hybrid PET/CT systems overcome these concerns as CT is quick (15 to 30 seconds) and of high quality.[3,30,32] However, due to the rapid transmission imaging (15- to 30-second CT), as opposed to the slower emission imaging (7 to 15 minutes), cardiac motion and breathing motion differences may cause misregistration between the transmission and emission images and artifacts. Also, due to the high spatial resolution of the CT images, there may be inherent spatial misregistration of the CT transmission with the lower resolution radionuclide emission images.[39] Hence, misregistration of the emission and transmission images remained a clinical challenge until recently. Several approaches to the CT transmission imaging have been tried: (a) reducing CT tube current with slowing of the rotational speed, (b) increasing the duration CT acquisition to better match the temporal resolution between the attenuation and emission maps, and (c) respiratory gating of the CT images and PET images.[38–41] A free tidal breathing CT scan remains the method of choice for the attenuation correction CT scan.[38] Also, several software advances have been developed to identify and successfully address misregistration artifacts. Software correction for misregistration artifacts has been a significant clinical advance, as more than a third of cardiac PET MPI cases have artifacts from misregistration of the transmission and emission images.[3,9]

Hybrid PET MPI and CT Imaging

With the integration of multislice CT scanners with PET, present-day scanners allow for hybrid PET/CT imaging with MPI combined with coronary artery calcium scoring and/or coronary angiography. Hybrid PET MPI and CT imaging can be performed on a single integrated scanner (PET and CT scanners located in the same gantry) or on separate scanners (using a common table that is coregistered to both scanners or as entirely separate scans) and fused using software. With either the integrated or the separate scanner technique, anatomical evaluation of calcified and noncalcified coronary artery atherosclerosis with MDCT and their functional status with PET MPI sequentially, within a single scanning session of less than 45 minutes, is feasible (Fig. 22-4).[9]

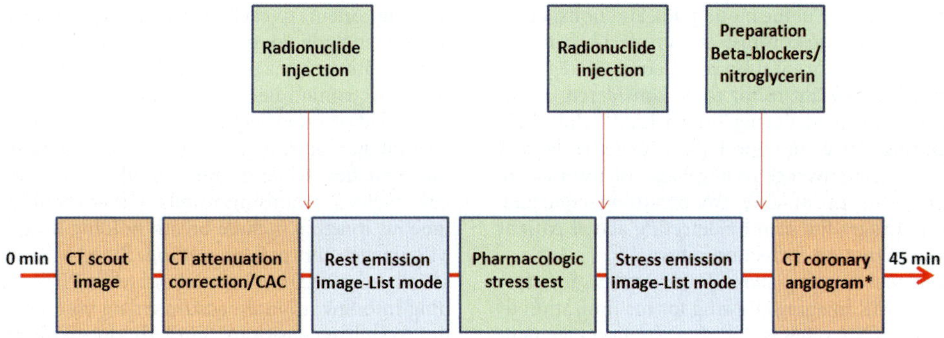

Figure 22-4. **Hybrid PET/CT imaging protocol with list-mode acquisition with pharmacologic/exercise stress and CT coronary angiography/calcium score.** This protocol allows for delineation of the anatomic as well as physiologic significance of coronary artery disease (CAD) in a single setting. (*, Only when clinically indicated after review of the PET MPI results; CT, computed tomography; coronary artery calcium score (CAC), coronary artery calcium score).

Despite these major advances and advantages, a significant limitation of hybrid PET/CT imaging is that data are acquired sequentially rather than simultaneously. Sequential scanning necessitates accurate coregistration of the images, and temporal correlation of nonrepeatable functional in vivo processes is not possible. Hybrid PET/MR imaging offers an advantage in this regard due to simultaneous PET and MR imaging.

Hybrid PET/MR

Cardiac magnetic resonance imaging (CMR) has evolved as a versatile imaging modality over the past decade. CMR offers significant advantages compared to MDCT imaging of the heart: high anatomic detail, excellent soft tissue contrast, and superior functional assessment. CMR is widely used for the assessment of structure, function, perfusion, soft tissue characterization, and myocardial scarring.[15,42] At present, CMR is the standard for quantification of myocardial volumes, mass, and function. It also provides an accurate assessment of myocardial scarring or fibrosis based on late gadolinium enhancement (LGE).[42]

PET/MRI is a rapidly evolving imaging modality with an enormous potential for extensive cardiovascular applications. A clear synergy exists between MR and PET, because each imaging modality can provide unique information, which is not attainable with the other.[37,43] Also, due to simultaneous imaging, there exists the potential for improving the PET image quality due to accurate corrections for partial volume averaging of counts and compensation for motion. Also, transmission maps and morphologic information necessary for interpretation of PET perfusion images can be acquired with MR.[15,44] However, the optimal design for hybrid PET/MR scanners has been a formidable technical challenge primarily due to the interference between the two systems and the generation of the transmission map for PET reconstruction. Hybrid PET/MR systems with various configurations have been developed: a tandem design (the two scanning systems mounted back to back in the same room or as distinct systems in separate rooms), an insert design (the PET detector ring is an insert within the MR system), and an integrated design (the systems are both fully integrated).[37]

Interference between PET and MR

The MR magnetic field interferes with the traditional photomultiplier tubes, which generate electric signals from light. This can lead to major artifacts and image distortion on both PET and MR images.[15,45,46] In order to overcome this interference between the systems, the current approaches used include shielding of PET detector components to effectively prevent the mutual interference between the PET and MR systems or modifications in photo multiplier tubes by the use of extended fiber optic cables or newer photo multiplier tubes made of silicone or the use of avalanche photodiode devices, which are resistant to magnetic field.[15,43]

Attenuation Correction in PET/MR

Derivation of transmission scan using MR has been challenging. Various processing techniques have been tested to overcome the challenges with image truncation (smaller MR field of view) and the need for repeat scans for soft tissue characterization and difficulty with bone imaging.[15] In a segmentation-based method, a transmission scan is used to generate an attenuation map, which is coregistered to the MRI images. Subsequently, the MR image is segmented into areas with different attenuation values based on tissues and then the attenuation map is applied to the PET images.[47] In emission-based attenuation correction, the recorded PET data provide the information needed to calculate an attenuation map, especially in truncated MR images, but may be limited by photon scatter.[48,49] Another approach is integration of hardware where previously measured attenuation maps, such as from prior CT, can be added.[15] Atlas- or template-based approach where the patient's image data are matched to a template derived from an atlas created from multiple patients associated attenuation values, but this has not been widely implemented.[50]

Present-day scanners use one or more of these approaches for deriving the attenuation maps. Although the correlation appears to be comparable to CT based attenuation correction, artifacts in MR can arise from respiratory and cardiac motion, truncation errors due to different fields of view, and partial MR signal loss due to metal implants.[15] Approach to motion correction with hybrid PET/MR by using real-time MR or 4-D MR data (such as tagged MRI) has been described, which have shown to reduce noise and improve image quality compared to just cardiac and respiratory gating techniques. This represents a significant advantage over PET/CT where CT images are static.[51,52]

Hybrid Imaging with PET/MR

Fusion versus Sequential versus Concurrent Imaging

Initial PET/MR imaging comprised of data obtained from individual MR and PET scanners. The images thus acquired were coregistered using image registration software.[53] Although this has been successful with neuroimaging, its utility in cardiac imaging has been not established. To achieve a high degree of registration accuracy between the image sets can be challenging. Individuals' physical and biologic factors such as noise, attenuation, scatter, partial volume effect, persistent activity in the blood pool, and nonspecific radiotracer uptake may decrease contrast and create blurring on images, making the landmark localization for accurate coregistration difficult.[46] Another important factor to be considered is that MR images are usually obtained during breath hold, while PET data are acquired during longer time periods so that the derived reconstructed image set is an average of all phases of respiration. This may be overcome by the use of newer free breathing sequences, where motion sensors trigger the scan by detecting actual patient motion or application of motion correction software.[15]

Sequential or coplanar imaging allows for a more straightforward approach for PET/MR imaging allowing for maximization of image quality with each of the systems. This is a serial arrangement in which both PET and MR are used sequentially end-to-end on two distinct systems but as part of a single examination, sometimes using a shuttle board. Another modification to the coplanar imaging is the option of trimodality imaging with PET/CT system and MR in two different rooms and the individual moved on a shuttle board between the two imaging systems.[54] In these cases, attenuation correction of the PET data is performed based on the CT transmission map. However, since serial rather than parallel image acquisition is done, there can be an increased predisposition to motion artifact. However, considering the workflow and cost-effectiveness, these models may be a more attractive option where each of the scanners can function as independent imaging systems.[37]

A fully integrated PET/MR system allows for simultaneous imaging that can be critical for evaluating some neurologic processes. Likewise, for pediatric applications, simultaneous imaging offers significant advantages due to the need for a single anesthesia session. Also, imaging of small moving structures (such as coronary arteries) may be significantly superior with integrated systems, as MR motion correction algorithms can be applied to the PET images and the images are inherently registered. However, combining the two imaging systems in a single gantry poses significant technical challenges. As described earlier, these systems will have to integrate technology such that there is no interference among the components of each, which can impair the image quality. Some of these include use of newer generation photomultipliers that are not sensitive to magnetic field or use of walled screens so there is no electronic interference from PET components on the magnetic field or radiofrequency. The preliminary data on these newer technologies such as using silicon photomultiplier tubes inside a magnetic field while running simultaneously running MR imaging have yielded promising results. Other considerations with simultaneous imaging include breath holding needed for acquisition of MR images and patient motion. Since MR images are still being serially acquired over breath hold while PET image acquisition running into few minutes, accurate data volumes cannot be achieved due to shifting positions. Similarly, due to different amount of time needed for imaging, there can be variability in assessment of function, especially based on patient heart rate variation during the imaging.[37,46] However, newer motion correction techniques may circumvent these shortcomings.[52] Another proposed approach is that of parallel imaging, as an alternative to simultaneous imaging, which is optimal in terms of workflow, patient compliance, and cost-effectiveness.[15]

Although there are many different designs in integrating PET and MR, further research needs to be performed in comparing each of the designs. Developing and testing free breathing sequences for better alignment between PET and MR, and also the feasibility of real-time MR-based motion correction and partial-volume correction, needs to be further investigated.[15,46] Figure 22-5 illustrates a potential hybrid PET/MR cardiac imaging protocol. Figure 22-6 illustrates the differences between fusion, sequential, and concurrent imaging.

Despite the present-day shortcomings, PET/MR systems hold promise by their potential advantages in the improved assessment of left ventricle (LV) function, morphology, ischemia, infarction and viability, and in cardiac molecular imaging. Hybrid PET/MR imaging allows for integration of function and perfusion or inflammation and scarring, providing for the most sophisticated "one-stop" imaging modality in cardiology.

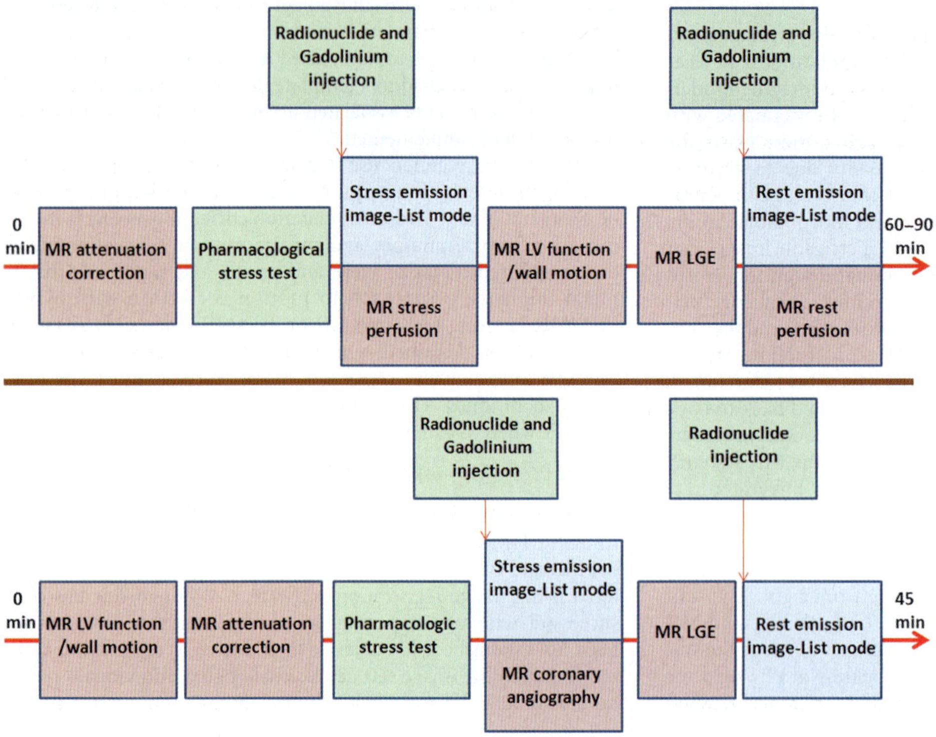

Figure 22-5. Two potential schemes for hybrid PET/MR stress. Hybrid imaging with PET/MR allows for accurate estimation of left ventricular systolic function, the ischemic burden with first-pass perfusion with magnetic resonance (MR) as well as PET perfusion imaging and evaluate viability by assessing late gadolinium enhancement of myocardium. The second dose of gadolinium can be utilized for either a coronary magnetic resonance angiogram (MRA) or rest perfusion. (Adapted from Rischpler C, Nekolla SG, Dregely I, et al. Hybrid PET/MR imaging of the heart: potential, initial experiences, and future prospects. *J Nucl Med* 2013;54:402–415. (LGE, late gadolinium enhancement).

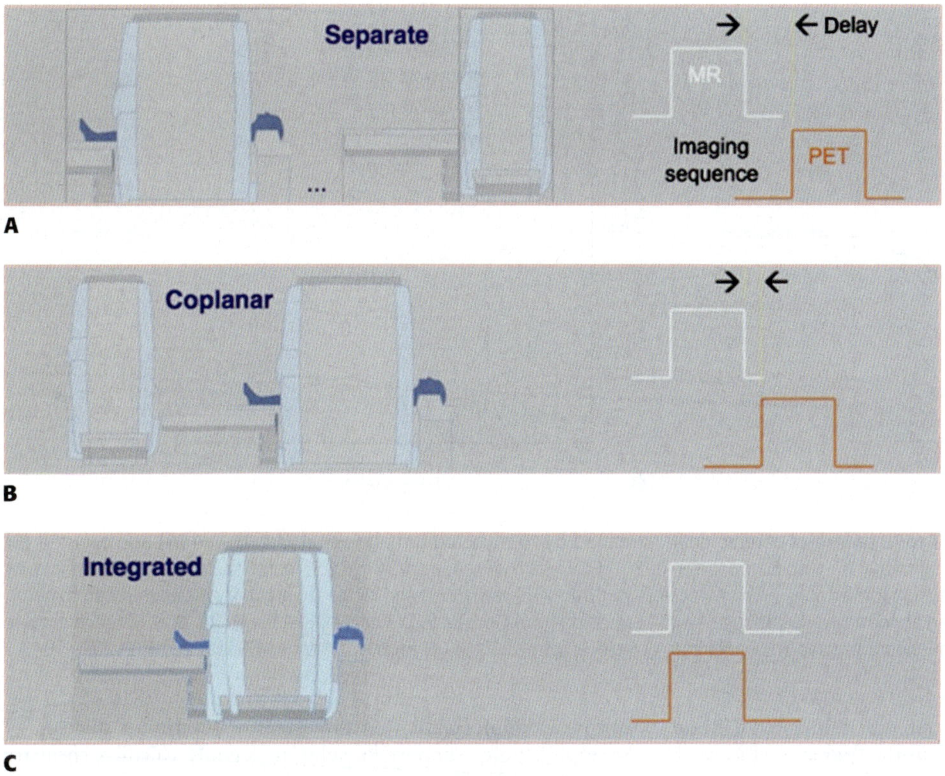

Figure 22-6. Designs for clinical PET/MR systems. **A:** Patients can be shuttled between separate magnetic resonance (MR) and positron emission tomography (PET)/computed tomography (CT) systems operated in different rooms, **(B)** patients are positioned on a common table platform between stationary PET and MR systems; the delay between the MR and PET examination is reduced (Philips Health-care), and **(C)** patients are positioned inside an integrated PET/MR gantry (Siemens Healthcare) with a PET insert that is mounted within a whole-body MR offering simultaneous PET/MR acquisitions. (Reproduced with permission from Beyer T, Freudenberg LS, Czernin J, et al. The future of hybrid imaging-part 3: PET/MR, small-animal imaging and beyond. *Insights Imaging* 2011;2:235–246.)

Clinical Advances: Myocardial Perfusion Imaging with Cardiac PET, PET/CT, and PET/MRI: Present and Future Applications

Myocardial Perfusion Imaging with PET-Only Imaging

The diagnostic accuracy of MPI with PET for detecting obstructive CAD surpasses that of MPI with SPECT. However, owing to its limited availability and higher costs, PET MPI is predominantly confined to larger clinical centers. In a weighted summary including nine studies, PET MPI had an average sensitivity of 90%, specificity of 89%, positive predictive value (PPV) of 94%, negative predictive value (NPV) of 73%, and accuracy of 90% for detecting a stenosis of greater than 50% in at least one coronary artery.[14] When compared to SPECT (thallium 201 or Tc-99m sestamibi), PET MPI demonstrated similar sensitivity (81% vs. 86%, SPECT vs. PET) but higher specificity (66% vs. 100%, $p = 0.00008$, SPECT vs. PET).[55] The above study compared separate groups of patients undergoing PET and non–attenuation-corrected SPECT MPI. In order to definitively establish superior diagnostic accuracy of PET MPI to diagnose obstructive coronary atherosclerosis, a study wherein the same patient undergoes SPECT MPI, PET MPI and invasive coronary angiography would be ideal. In one such study of 86 patients who underwent F-18 flurpiridaz, Tc-99m SPECT MPI, and invasive coronary angiography, PET MPI was more sensitive (78.8% vs. 61.5%, $p = 0.02$) but equally specific (76.5% vs. 73.5%, $p =$ NS) as SPECT MPI for the detection of obstructive epicardial CAD.[24] Also, two recent meta-analyses comparing PET and SPECT imaging showed that PET offered a greater diagnostic accuracy for detection of CAD.[56,57] In one of the analyses, specificity improved significantly when low-likelihood patients were excluded from the analysis.[57]

The prognostic value of perfusion defects noted on PET MPI has been well established. In a study from our lab, which included close to 1,500 patients who underwent vasodilator rubidium 82 MPI and over a mean follow-up of 1.7 years, the percentage of ischemic myocardium correlated closely with the risk of cardiac death or nonfatal MI.[58] While patients without ischemia had a low annualized event rate of 0.7%, those with greater than 20% ischemia had an annualized event rate of 11%. The percentage of ischemic myocardium added a significant incremental prognostic value for both cardiac events and for all-cause mortality independent of rest left ventricular ejection fraction.[58] Furthermore, patients who increased their left ventricular ejection fraction from rest to peak vasodilator stress demonstrated significantly better event-free survival compared to those with no change or a decline in left ventricular ejection fraction.

A multicenter study of rubidium 82 MPI including 7,061 patients from four medical centers in North America, the PET Prognosis Multicenter Registry,[59] has validated the powerful and incremental prognostic value of the extent and severity of PET MPI defects over clinical factors and rest ejection fraction. The hazard of cardiac death and all-cause death was significantly higher in patients with severely abnormal scans compared to those with normal PET MPI (Fig. 22-7). The results of this study have established the value of perfusion defects in appropriately reclassifying risk of one in nine patients with known or suspected CAD. Data from this large PET registry have confirmed the prognostic value of PET MPI in women compared to men,[60] obese compared to nonobese individuals,[61] and in individuals with prior CABG.[62]

Myocardial Blood Flow Quantification with PET

A major advantage of PET MPI is quantification of absolute MBF in milliliters/gram/minute. Quantification of MBF allows for the calculation of the coronary flow reserve (CFR), which is the ratio of MBF at peak hyperemic stress to MBF at rest.[3] The use of list-mode acquisition in the PET scanners now enables routine MBF quantification in conjunction with perfusion and gated LV and regional function. Estimates of MBF in milliliters of blood per minute per grams of myocardium are obtained by fitting time–activity curves with a validated tracer kinetic model, with additional corrections for tracer spillover and radioactive decay.[3]

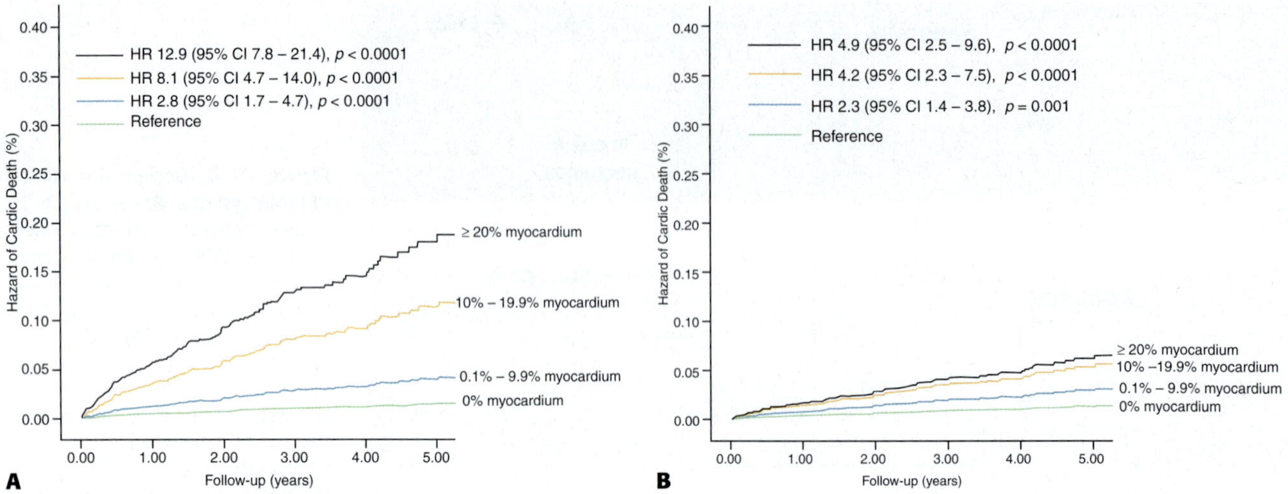

Figure 22-7. Risk stratification with PET MPI: hazard of cardiac death stratified by % myocardium abnormal. Unadjusted **(A)** and adjusted **(B)** hazard of events by percent myocardium abnormal on vasodilator stress Rb-82 PET. Hazard of cardiac death (6,037 patients, 169 cardiac deaths) was lowest in patients with normal positron emission tomography (PET) myocardial perfusion imaging (MPI) and increased gradually in patients with minimal, mild, moderate, and severe degrees of scan abnormality. (Reproduced with permission from Dorbala S, Di Carli MF, Beanlands RS, et al. Prognostic value of stress myocardial perfusion positron emission tomography: results from a multicenter observational registry. *J Am Coll Cardiol* 2013;61:176–184.)

Several investigators have demonstrated that impaired CFR or peak hyperemic MBF relates inversely to the degree of epicardial coronary artery stenosis.[63–66] However, among patients with no or minimal angiographic obstructive CAD, there is a wide variation in stress MBF and CFR values with lower values likely representing coronary microvascular dysfunction. Impaired CFR is thus challenging to interpret—it may represent severe microvascular dysfunction, balanced flow reduction from multivessel epicardial CAD, or rarely inadequate vasodilator response from caffeine intake or in caffeine nonresponders (individuals with innate inadequate vasodilator response to vasodilator stress agents).[9] In patients with impaired CFR, there is no threshold value of CFR below that we could identify multivessel epicardial CAD versus severe coronary microvascular dysfunction and coronary angiography is typically required. A hybrid PET–coronary CT angiography (CTA) may be particularly helpful in answering this question.[9] In contrast, preserved CFR (>1.93) identifies intact coronary vasodilator function and effectively excludes high-risk CAD.[67,68]

The prognostic value of CFR with N-13 ammonia PET or rubidium 82 is under active investigation. Quantitative PET and CFR provide incremental prognostic value at predicting adverse clinical outcomes when compared to clinical parameters and to perfusion defects. Murthy et al.[69] included 2,783 patients undergoing rubidium PET, followed them for a median of 1.4 years and found a 5.6-fold increase in the risk of cardiac death for those with a CFR < 1.5 and additionally close to 35% patients in the intermediate-risk category were reclassified correctly (Fig. 22-8 A-C). The incremental prognostic value of CFR, with normal CFR representing excellent prognosis, has been demonstrated in various subgroups of patients including those with renal failure,[70] with calcified coronary atherosclerosis,[71] and with diabetes.[72] The recurring message from most of these studies is the significant protective value afforded by preserved CFR independent of coexisting comorbid conditions.

Hybrid PET/CT Imaging

PET MPI with Coronary Artery Calcium Scoring

The integration of PET with multidetector CT provides an opportunity to obtain functional as well as anatomic information during the same test.[14] Although coronary artery calcium score does not provide information on the extent or severity of stenosis,[73,74] multiple studies support its value to identify calcified coronary atherosclerosis (albeit nonobstructive), particularly in the context of normal MPI.[73,74] While patients with coronary artery calcium score ≥400 had an annualized event rate from 3% to 11%, the event rate for those with coronary artery calcium score of zero was much lower and ranged from 0.7% to 2.4%.[74,75] Similar results have been also found in patients who have ischemia, with presence of coronary artery calcium score ≥1,000 having an annualized event rate of greater than 22% compared to those with coronary artery calcium score of zero having an event rate of 8.2% (Fig. 22-9).[74] A high coronary artery calcium score in the context of normal PET MPI may indicate a low short-term risk, but a higher long-term risk and thus be used to more aggressively manage coronary risk factors. Hence, most practices perform a CT calcium score study along with PET MPI in patients without known CAD. Also, the CT transmission scan can be routinely evaluated for the presence of coronary artery calcification and may help identify extensive or dense coronary artery calcification, despite being a nongated, low-dose, and free breathing scan.[76]

PET MPI with CCTA

The addition of CT coronary angiogram with PET MPI further allows for quantification of noncalcified plaques, identification of flow-limiting coronary stenoses, and identification of high-risk plaques by targeted molecular imaging.[9] PET MPI provides added value in determining the functional significance of an apparent stenosis on CT coronary angiogram. This may especially be helpful while assessing the severity of stenosis in calcified lesions.[9] Hybrid PET–CT angiography may be particularly helpful in patients with reduced CFR to differentiate flow-limiting coronary artery stenosis from microvascular disease. Initial data from Kajander et al.[77] showed accurate diagnosis of CAD by quantitative PET MPI in symptomatic patients when compared with invasive coronary angiography with or without fractional flow reserve (FFR) assessment (Table 3). Further, pooled data show that hybrid imaging had the greatest effect on specificity (91% for PET/CT compared to 61% for CTA and 87% for PET) and PPV (87% for PET/CT compared to 65% for CTA and 83% for PET).[77,78] A potential additional

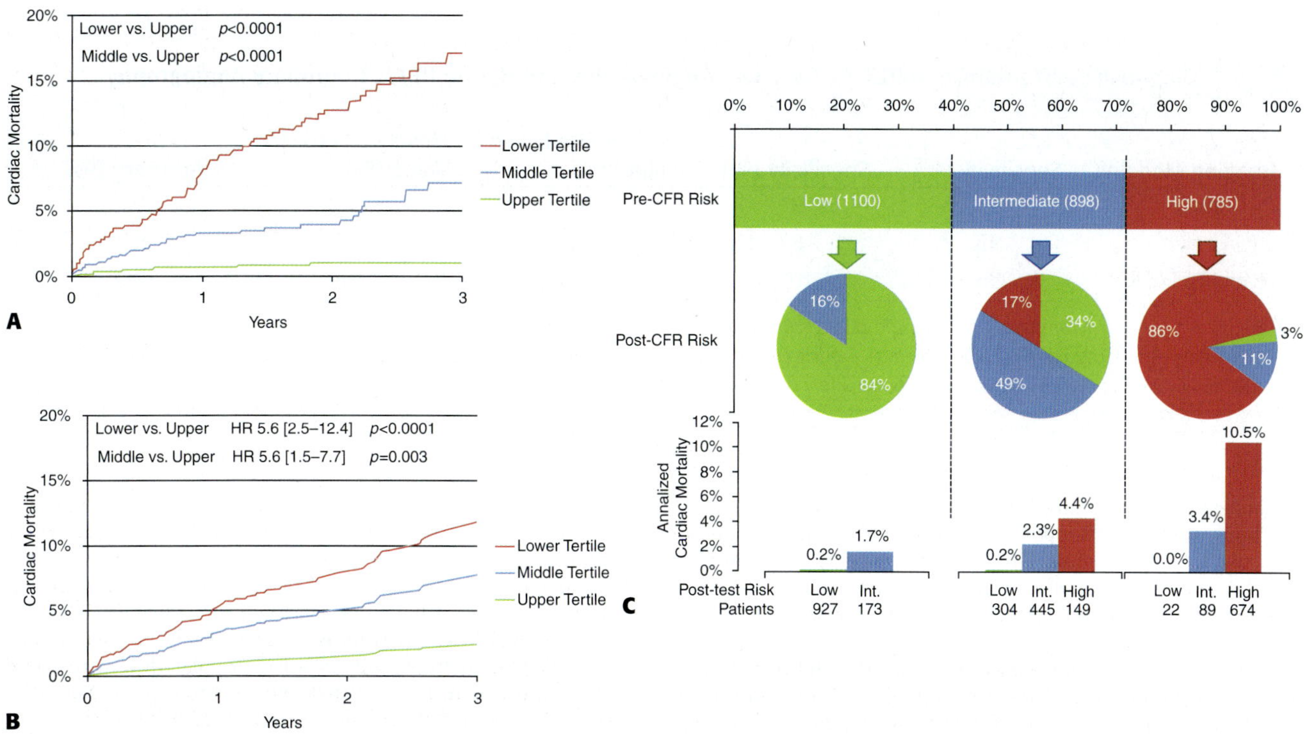

Figure 22-8. **Incremental prognostic value of coronary flow reserve on PET MPI.** Cumulative incidence of cardiac mortality for tertiles of coronary flow reserve (CFR) presented in Kaplan-Meier format **(A)** and after adjustment for age, sex, body mass index, hypertension, dyslipidemia, diabetes mellitus, family history of coronary artery disease (CAD), tobacco use, prior CAD, chest pain, dyspnea, early revascularization, rest left ventricular ejection fraction (LVEF), summed stress score, and LVEF reserve **(B)**, showing a significant association between CFR and cardiac mortality. **C:** Risk reclassification by addition of CFR to a model containing clinical risk factors, LVEF, LVEF reserve, and combined extent of myocardial scar and ischemia. The upper horizontal bar graph represents the distribution of risk across categories of less than 1 (*green*), 1 to 3 (*blue*), and greater than 3% (*red*) per year risk of cardiac death as estimated by a model containing clinical risk factors, rest LVEF, LVEF reserve, and the combination of myocardial scar and ischemia. The pie graphs represent the proportions of patients in each pre-CFR category reassigned to each risk category after the addition of CFR to the risk model. The vertical bar charts at the bottom represent the annualized rates of cardiac mortality in each of the post-CFR risk categories. (Reproduced with permission from Murthy VL, Naya M, Foster CR, et al. Improved cardiac risk assessment with noninvasive measures of coronary flow reserve. *Circulation* 2011;124:2215–2224.)

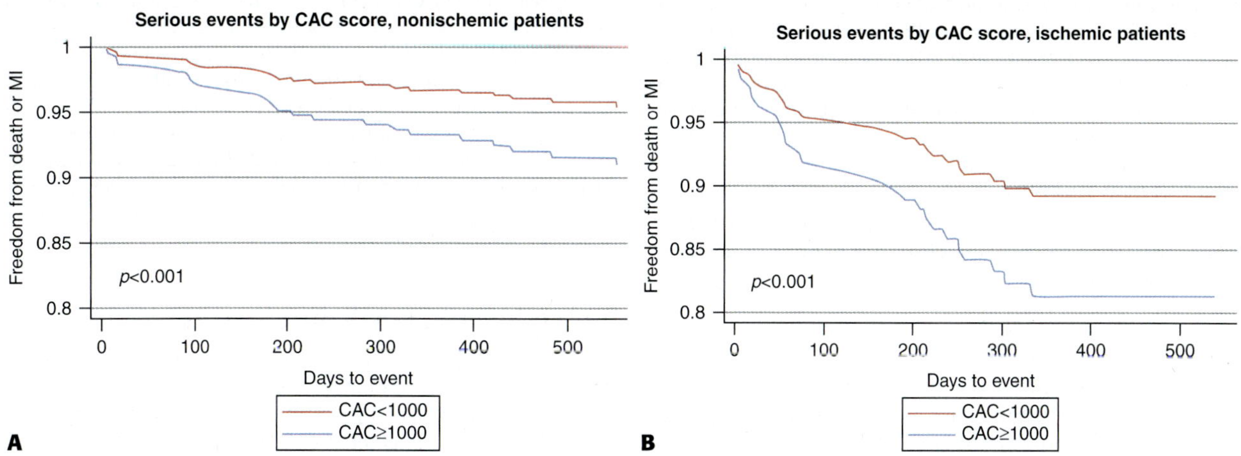

Figure 22-9. **Prognostic value of calcium score greater than 1,000 and less than 1,000 in patients with normal and abnormal PET MPI.** Cox proportional hazards regression model for freedom from death or MI adjusted for age, sex, symptoms, and conventional CAD risk factors in patients without ischemia **(A)** and with ischemia **(B)**. (Reproduced with permission from Schenker MP, Dorbala S, Hong EC, et al. Interrelation of coronary calcification, myocardial ischemia, and outcomes in patients with intermediate likelihood of coronary artery disease: a combined positron emission tomography/computed tomography study. *Circulation* 2008;117:1693–1700.)

TABLE 22.3 **Diagnostic Performance of PET, CT Coronary Angiography, and Hybrid PET/CT Coronary Angiography**

Imaging Modality	Sensitivity (%)	Specificity (%)	Positive Predictive Value (%)	Negative Predictive Value (%)	Accuracy (%)
PET only	95	91	86	97	92
CTCA only	95	87	81	97	90
Hybrid PET/CTCA	95	100	100	98	98

PET, positron emission tomography; CTCA, computed tomography coronary angiography.
From Kajander S, Joutsiniemi E, Saraste M, et al. Cardiac positron emission tomography/computed tomography imaging accurately detects anatomically and functionally significant coronary artery disease. *Circulation* 2010;122:603–613.

advantage of PET/CT angiography over PET alone is the growing body of evidence supporting the prognostic value of nonobstructive CAD detected on CT coronary angiography.[79] However, whether the identification of anatomic nonobstructive coronary atherosclerosis is of incremental value to CFR assessment is not known.

Advances in CT technology also offer the ability to assess myocardial perfusion and quantitation of MBF in addition to morphologic imaging by CT coronary angiography.[80] Emerging data suggest that the combined tests may offer complementary information in patients who are being evaluated for CAD, and detection of coronary atherosclerosis may help clinicians more aggressively manage their risk factors.[81,82] The combination of quantitative MBF assessment by PET MPI and visualization of coronary artery on CT angiogram has demonstrated greater diagnostic accuracy in the detection of hemodynamically significant obstructive CAD than each modality on its own.[9,77] Investigators have evaluated a CT coronary angiogram followed by a stress-only SPECT MPI and a rest MPI as needed as a comprehensive hybrid evaluation of anatomy and function with low radiation dose (4.8 ± 3.4 mSv vs. 8.1 ± 1.5 mSv for a conventional protocol).[83] A similar protocol could be applied to CT coronary angiogram and PET MPI as well. Despite the promising results from small studies, compared with invasive angiography or nuclear imaging, current literature does not support the broad clinical application of this technique. Combined hybrid PET/MPI and CTA imaging protocol offers higher radiation burden than either study alone, and combined studies are selectively used in a sequential fashion when the information from each study is necessary for clinical management.

Hybrid PET/MR Imaging

Despite the technical design and operation challenges of hybrid PET/MR systems, the potential for integration of function and perfusion or inflammation and scarring is attractive.[15]

Myocardial Perfusion Imaging and Blood Flow Quantitation with PET/MRI

Presently, PET and CMR have both established roles in perfusion assessment. PET MPI provides both information on perfusion at stress and at rest, and additional information on CFR can be obtained as described earlier.[3] First-pass contrast-enhanced CMR MPI has emerged as a method that can measure the presence and extent of hypoperfusion caused by flow-limiting CAD. Furthermore, CMR MPI provides assessment of myocardial ischemia with high spatial resolution and tissue contrast.[43,84] A recent meta-analysis comparing PET and CMR MPI found the diagnostic performance to be similar (sensitivity 84% vs. 89% and specificity of 81% vs. 76%, respectively).[85] Additionally, quantitative evaluation of MBF and in turn CFR with myocardial perfusion MRI may provide a more objective evaluation of CAD and has been validated against invasive measurements. Kurita et al.[86] compared regional MRI-based measurement of CFR, as determined by Patlak plot method, with invasive Doppler flow wire–based CFR measurement. In the Patlak plot method, the quantitative analysis of myocardial perfusion is performed using a blood time–intensity curve as an input function and a regional myocardial time–intensity curve as an output function. In this study for both culprit and nonculprit vessel groups, significant direct correlations were observed between MRI-based CFR and Doppler assessment of CFR ($r \geq 0.8$ for both). A reduced MRI-based CFR < 2.0 had a sensitivity of 88%, a specificity of 90%, a PPV of 88%, and a NPV of 90% in predicting a significant reduction of CFR on invasive flow wire–based measurements.[86] Similarly, in another study assessing the relation between CMR CFR and FFR in patients with suspected CAD, MRI-based CFR of ≤2.04 has a sensitivity of 93% and a specificity of 57% in predicting a coronary segment with FFR ≤0.75.[87] However, the correlation between MRI-based CFR and FFR although significant is at best moderate ($r = 0.41$).[88] Furthermore, CMR-based CFR has been compared with PET-based quantitation with good correlation in both healthy and diseased individuals (Fig. 22-10).[89,90] A combined simultaneous PET/MRI has the potential advantage of a direct comparison between the two modalities during stress and rest perfusion imaging and provides an opportunity for cross-validation in regard to the performance of each modality. The addition of PET perfusion imaging compensates for the limitations of stress CMR such as dark rim artifacts or the limited spatial coverage, whereas excellent morphologic information gathered from MR, such as coronary angiography and LGE, would further help in evaluation and characterization of CAD.[43]

Hybrid PET/MR Applications

The value of PET for molecular imaging application when combined with the soft tissue resolution and functional imaging advances offered by CMR makes a powerful molecular imaging tool. A few examples include imaging coronary atherosclerosis (combining plaque vulnerability imaging on MR with targeted PET radiotracers), vasculitis (imaging vessel wall abnormalities on MR and correlating with active inflammation by F-18 fluorodeoxyglucose or specific targeted PET tracers), stem cell imaging, gene therapy, imaging structure, and function and molecular processes in patients with cardiomyopathy. Hybrid PET/MR imaging offers great potential for

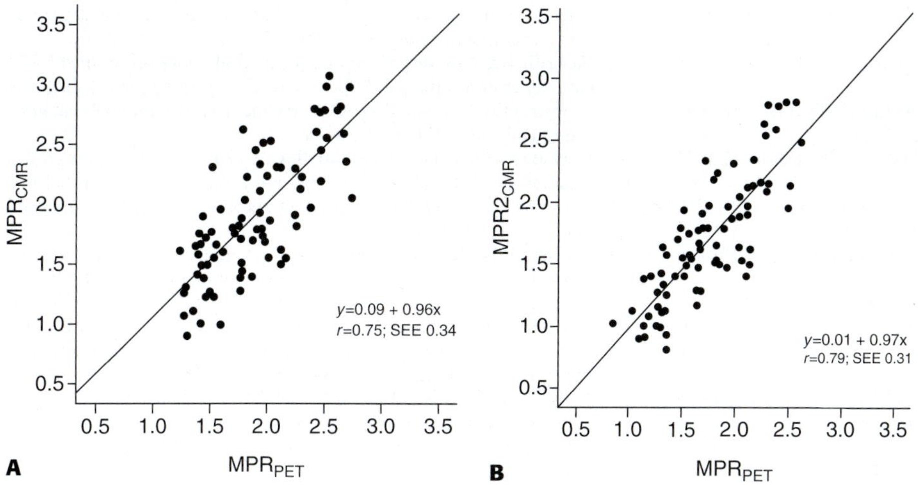

Figure 22-10. Scatter plots with fit lines comparing myocardial perfusion reserve (MPR) values from cardiac magnetic resonance (MPR_{CMR}) and positron emission tomography (MPR_{PET}) for the entire myocardial territory **(A)** and the mean of the lowest two segments in each territory (MPR2) **(B)**. (Reproduced with permission from Morton G, Chiribiri A, Ishida M, et al. Quantification of absolute myocardial perfusion in patients with coronary artery disease: comparison between cardiovascular magnetic resonance and positron emission tomography. *J Am Coll Cardiol* 2012;60:1546–1555.)

research in cardiovascular imaging. However, for a clinical cardiovascular imaging application, which patients would derive the most clinical benefit from hybrid PET/MR imaging techniques remains uncertain.

Conclusions

Modern-day PET has considerably evolved with new hardware, software, radiotracers, and clinical applications. With increasing clinical use, accumulating evidence base, and excellent image quality, PET has potential to become the test of choice for radionuclide MPI. The use of PET MPI is projected to increase further when unit dose F-18–labeled perfusion tracers become clinically available. PET/CT and PET/MR applications are evolving and pave the way for several advanced applications that combine anatomical, physiologic, and functional information into a single test. Integrated PET/MR image acquisition and processing and clinical application in the heart are presently challenging and will continue to evolve over time. More research is needed to better understand the optimal clinical and investigational role of hybrid PET/CT and PET/MR imaging.

REFERENCES

1. **Hendel RC, Abbott BG, Bateman TM, et al.** The role of radionuclide myocardial perfusion imaging for asymptomatic individuals. *J Nucl Cardiol* 2011;18:3–15.
2. **Nakazato R, Berman DS, Alexanderson E, et al.** Myocardial perfusion imaging with PET. *Imaging Med* 2013;5:35–46.
3. **Dilsizian V, Bacharach SL, Beanlands RS et al.** PET myocardial perfusion and metabolism clinical imaging. *J Nucl Cardiol* 2009;16:651.
4. **Rahmim A, Zaidi H.** PET versus SPECT: strengths, limitations and challenges *Nucl Med Commun* 2008;29:193–207.
5. **Cherry SR.** The 2006 Henry N. Wagner Lecture: of mice and men (and positrons)—advances in PET imaging technology. *J Nucl Med* 2006;47: 1735–1745.
6. **Bengel FM, Higuchi T, Javadi MS, et al.** Cardiac positron emission tomography. *J Am Coll Cardiol* 2009;54:1–15.
7. **Orbay H, Hong H, Zhang Y, et al.** Positron emission tomography imaging of atherosclerosis. *Theranostics* 2013;3:894–902.
8. **Joshi NV, Vesey AT, Williams MC, et al.** 18F-fluoride positron emission tomography for identification of ruptured and high-risk coronary atherosclerotic plaques: a prospective clinical trial. *Lancet* 2014;383: 705–713.
9. **Di Carli MF, Murthy VL.** Cardiac PET/CT for the evaluation of known or suspected coronary artery disease. *Radiographics* 2011;31:1239–1254.
10. **Ohira H, McArdle B, Cocker MS, et al.** Current and future clinical applications of cardiac positron emission tomography. *Circ J* 2013;77: 836–848.
11. **Thackeray JT, Bengel FM.** Assessment of cardiac autonomic neuronal function using PET imaging. *J Nucl Cardiol* 2013;20:150–165.
12. **Youssef G, Leung E, Mylonas I, et al.** The use of 18F-FDG PET in the diagnosis of cardiac sarcoidosis: a systematic review and metaanalysis including the Ontario experience. *J Nucl Med* 2012;53:241–248.
13. **Slomka PJ, Dey D, Duvall WL, et al.** Advances in nuclear cardiac instrumentation with a view towards reduced radiation exposure. *Curr Cardiol Rep* 2012;14:208–216.
14. **Di Carli MF, Hachamovitch R.** New technology for noninvasive evaluation of coronary artery disease. *Circulation* 2007;115:1464–1480.
15. **Rischpler C, Nekolla SG, Dregely I, et al.** Hybrid PET/MR imaging of the heart: potential, initial experiences, and future prospects. *J Nucl Med* 2013;54:402–415.
16. **Maddahi J.** Properties of an ideal PET perfusion tracer: new PET tracer cases and data. *J Nucl Cardiol* 2012;19(suppl 1):S30–S37.
17. **Ionetix Corporation.** http://www.ionetix.com/wp-content/uploads/2013/06/ION12SC-Datasheet.pdf Accessed August 1, 2014.
18. **University of Michigan.** http://ns.umich.edu/new/releases/2980 Accessed August 1, 2014.
19. **Berkeley National Laboratory.** http://loasis.lbl.gov Accessed August 1, 2014.
20. **Nekolla SG, Saraste A.** Novel F-18-labeled PET myocardial perfusion tracers: bench to bedside. *Curr Cardiol Rep* 2011;13:145–150.
21. **Yalamanchili P, Wexler E, Hayes M, et al.** Mechanism of uptake and retention of F-18 BMS-747158-02 in cardiomyocytes: a novel PET myocardial imaging agent. *J Nucl Cardiol* 2007;14:782–788.
22. **Nekolla SG, Reder S, Saraste A, et al.** Evaluation of the novel myocardial perfusion positron-emission tomography tracer 18F-BMS-747158-02: comparison to 13N-ammonia and validation with microspheres in a pig model. *Circulation* 2009;119:2333–2342.
23. **Maddahi J, Czernin J, Lazewatsky J, et al.** Phase I, first-in-human study of BMS747158, a novel 18F-labeled tracer for myocardial perfusion PET: dosimetry, biodistribution, safety, and imaging characteristics after a single injection at rest. *J Nucl Med* 2011;52:1490–1498.
24. **Berman DS, Maddahi J, Tamarappoo BK, et al.** Phase II safety and clinical comparison with single-photon emission computed tomography myocardial perfusion imaging for detection of coronary artery disease: flurpiridaz F 18 positron emission tomography. *J Am Coll Cardiol* 2013;61:469–477.
25. **Lantheus Medical Imaging, Inc.** http://investor.lantheus.com/phoenix.zhtml?c=241435&p=irol-newsArticle&ID=1869863&highlight= Accessed February 24, 2014.
26. **Panin VY, Kehren F, Michel C, et al.** Fully 3-D PET reconstruction with system matrix derived from point source measurements. *IEEE Trans Med Imaging* 2006;25:907–921.
27. **Le Meunier L, Slomka PJ, Dey D, et al.** Enhanced definition PET for cardiac imaging. *J Nucl Cardiol* 2010;17:414–426.

28. **Le Meunier L, Slomka PJ, Dey D, et al.** Motion frozen (18)F-FDG cardiac PET. *J Nucl Cardiol* 2011;18:259–266.
29. **Lecomte R.** Novel detector technology for clinical PET. *Eur J Nucl Med Mol Imaging* 2009;36(suppl 1):S69–S85.
30. **Beyer T, Townsend DW, Czernin J, et al.** The future of hybrid imaging-part 2: PET/CT. *Insights Imaging* 2011;2:225–234.
31. **Humm JL, Rosenfeld A, Del Guerra A.** From PET detectors to PET scanners. *Eur J Nucl Med Mol Imaging* 2003;30:1574–1597.
32. **Garcia EV.** Physical attributes, limitations, and future potential for PET and SPECT. *J Nucl Cardiol* 2012;19(suppl 1):S19–S29.
33. **Di Carli MF, Dorbala S, Meserve J, et al.** Clinical myocardial perfusion PET/CT. *J Nucl Med* 2007;48:783–793.
34. **Mikhaylova E, De Lorenzo G, Chmeissani M, et al.** Simulation of the expected performance of a seamless scanner for brain PET based on highly pixelated CdTe detectors. *IEEE Trans Med Imaging* 2014;33: 332–339.
35. **Arino G, Chmeissani M, De Lorenzo G, et al.** Energy and coincidence time resolution measurements of CdTe detectors for PET. *J Instrum* 2013;8:C02015.
36. **Takei T, Shiga T, Morimoto Y, et al.** A novel PET scanner with semiconductor detectors may improve diagnostic accuracy in the metastatic survey of head and neck cancer patients. *Ann Nucl Med* 2013;27:17–24.
37. **Torigian DA, Zaidi H, Kwee TC, et al.** PET/MR imaging: technical aspects and potential clinical applications. *Radiology* 2013;267:26–44.
38. **Dorbala S, Di Carli MF, Delbeke D, et al.** SNMMI/ASNC/SCCT guideline for cardiac SPECT/CT and PET/CT 1.0. *J Nucl Med* 2013;54: 1485–1507.
39. **Bacharach SL.** PET/CT attenuation correction: breathing lessons. *J Nucl Med* 2007;48:677–679.
40. **Pan T, Mawlawi O, Nehmeh SA, et al.** Attenuation correction of PET images with respiration-averaged CT images in PET/CT. *J Nucl Med* 2005;46:1481–1487.
41. **Nehmeh SA, Erdi YE, Pan T, et al.** Four-dimensional (4D) PET/CT imaging of the thorax. *Med Phys* 2004;31:3179–3186.
42. **Pennell DJ.** Cardiovascular magnetic resonance. *Circulation* 2010;121: 692–705.
43. **Adenaw N, Salerno M.** PET/MRI: current state of the art and future potential for cardiovascular applications. *J Nucl Cardiol* 2013;20: 976–989.
44. **Saraste A, Knuuti J.** Cardiac PET, CT, and MR: what are the advantages of hybrid imaging? *Curr Cardiol Rep* 2012;14:24–31.
45. **Beyer T, Freudenberg LS, Czernin J, et al.** The future of hybrid imaging-part 3: PET/MR, small-animal imaging and beyond. *Insights Imaging* 2011;2:235–246.
46. **Bolus NE, George R, Washington J, et al.** PET/MRI: the blended-modality choice of the future? *J Nucl Med Technol* 2009;37:63–71; quiz 72–73.
47. **Martinez-Moller A, Souvatzoglou M, Delso G, et al.** Tissue classification as a potential approach for attenuation correction in whole-body PET/MRI: evaluation with PET/CT data. *J Nucl Med* 2009;50:520–526.
48. **Nuyts J, Dupont P, Stroobants S, et al.** Simultaneous maximum a posteriori reconstruction of attenuation and activity distributions from emission sinograms. *IEEE Trans Med Imaging* 1999;18:393–403.
49. **Nuyts J, Bal G, Kehren F, et al.** Completion of a truncated attenuation image from the attenuated PET emission data. *IEEE Trans Med Imaging* 2013;32:237–246.
50. **Hofmann M, Bezrukov I, Mantlik F, et al.** MRI-based attenuation correction for whole-body PET/MRI: quantitative evaluation of segmentation- and atlas-based methods. *J Nucl Med* 2011;52:1392–1399.
51. **Nappi C, El Fakhri G.** State of the art in cardiac hybrid technology: PET/MR. *Curr Cardiovasc Imaging Rep* 2013;6:338–345.
52. **Quick HH.** Integrated PET/MR. *J Magn Reson Imaging* 2014;39: 243–258.
53. **Hill DL, Batchelor PG, Holden M, et al.** Medical image registration. *Phys Med Biol* 2001;46:R1–R45.
54. **Bailey DL, Barthel H, Beuthin-Baumann B, et al.** Combined PET/MR: where are we now? Summary report of the second international workshop on PET/MR imaging April 8–12, 2013, Tubingen, Germany. *Mol Imaging Biol* 2014;16:295–310.
55. **Bateman TM, Heller GV, McGhie AI, et al.** Diagnostic accuracy of rest/stress ECG-gated Rb-82 myocardial perfusion PET: comparison with ECG-gated Tc-99m sestamibi SPECT. *J Nucl Cardiol* 2006;13:24–33.
56. **Parker MW, Iskandar A, Limone B, et al.** Diagnostic accuracy of cardiac positron emission tomography versus single photon emission computed tomography for coronary artery disease: a bivariate meta-analysis. *Circ Cardiovasc Imaging* 2012;5:700–707.
57. **McArdle BA, Dowsley TF, deKemp RA, et al.** Does rubidium-82 PET have superior accuracy to SPECT perfusion imaging for the diagnosis of obstructive coronary disease?: a systematic review and meta-analysis. *J Am Coll Cardiol* 2012;60:1828–1837.
58. **Dorbala S, Hachamovitch R, Curillova Z, et al.** Incremental prognostic value of gated Rb-82 positron emission tomography myocardial perfusion imaging over clinical variables and rest LVEF. *JACC Cardiovasc Imaging* 2009;2:846–854.
59. **Dorbala S, Di Carli MF, Beanlands RS, et al.** Prognostic value of stress myocardial perfusion positron emission tomography: results from a multicenter observational registry. *J Am Coll Cardiol* 2013;61:176–184.
60. **Kay J, Dorbala S, Goyal A, et al.** Influence of sex on risk stratification with stress myocardial perfusion Rb-82 positron emission tomography: results from the PET (Positron Emission Tomography) Prognosis Multicenter Registry. *J Am Coll Cardiol* 2013;62:1866–1876.
61. **Chow BJ, Dorbala S, Di Carli MF, et al.** Prognostic value of PET myocardial perfusion imaging in obese patients. *JACC Cardiovasc Imaging* 2014;7:278–287.
62. **Pen A, Yam Y, Chen L, et al.** Prognostic value of Rb-82 positron emission tomography myocardial perfusion imaging in coronary artery bypass patients. *Eur Heart J Cardiovasc Imaging* 2014;15:787–792.
63. **Uren NG, Crake T, Lefroy DC, et al.** Reduced coronary vasodilator function in infarcted and normal myocardium after myocardial infarction. *N Engl J Med* 1994;331:222–227.
64. **Anagnostopoulos C, Almonacid A, El Fakhri G, et al.** Quantitative relationship between coronary vasodilator reserve assessed by 82Rb PET imaging and coronary artery stenosis severity. *Eur J Nucl Med Mol Imaging* 2008;35:1593–1601.
65. **Beanlands RS, Muzik O, Melon P, et al.** Noninvasive quantification of regional myocardial flow reserve in patients with coronary atherosclerosis using nitrogen-13 ammonia positron emission tomography. Determination of extent of altered vascular reactivity. *J Am Coll Cardiol* 1995;26:1465–1475.
66. **Di Carli M, Czernin J, Hoh CK, et al.** Relation among stenosis severity, myocardial blood flow, and flow reserve in patients with coronary artery disease. *Circulation* 1995;91:1944–1951.
67. **Naya M, Murthy VL, Taqueti VR, et al.** Preserved coronary flow reserve effectively excludes high-risk coronary artery disease on angiography. *J Nucl Med* 2014;55:248–255.
68. **Ziadi MC, Dekemp RA, Williams K, et al.** Does quantification of myocardial flow reserve using rubidium-82 positron emission tomography facilitate detection of multivessel coronary artery disease? *J Nucl Cardiol* 2012;19:670–680.
69. **Murthy VL, Naya M, Foster CR, et al.** Improved cardiac risk assessment with noninvasive measures of coronary flow reserve. *Circulation* 2011;124:2215–2224.
70. **Murthy VL, Naya M, Foster CR, et al.** Coronary vascular dysfunction and prognosis in patients with chronic kidney disease. *JACC Cardiovasc Imaging* 2012;5:1025–1034.
71. **Naya M, Murthy VL, Foster CR, et al.** Prognostic interplay of coronary artery calcification and underlying vascular dysfunction in patients with suspected coronary artery disease. *J Am Coll Cardiol* 2013;61: 2098–2106.
72. **Murthy VL, Naya M, Foster CR, et al.** Association between coronary vascular dysfunction and cardiac mortality in patients with and without diabetes mellitus. *Circulation* 2012;126:1858–1868.
73. **Berman DS, Wong ND, Gransar H, et al.** Relationship between stress-induced myocardial ischemia and atherosclerosis measured by coronary calcium tomography. *J Am Coll Cardiol* 2004;44:923–930.
74. **Schenker MP, Dorbala S, Hong EC, et al.** Interrelation of coronary calcification, myocardial ischemia, and outcomes in patients with intermediate likelihood of coronary artery disease: a combined positron emission tomography/computed tomography study. *Circulation* 2008;117:1693–1700.
75. **Chang SM, Nabi F, Xu J, et al.** The coronary artery calcium score and stress myocardial perfusion imaging provide independent and complementary prediction of cardiac risk. *J Am Coll Cardiol* 2009;54:1872–1882.
76. **Einstein AJ, Johnson LL, Bokhari S, et al.** Agreement of visual estimation of coronary artery calcium from low-dose CT attenuation correction scans in hybrid PET/CT and SPECT/CT with standard Agatston score. *J Am Coll Cardiol* 2010;56:1914–1921.

77. **Kajander S, Joutsiniemi E, Saraste M, et al.** Cardiac positron emission tomography/computed tomography imaging accurately detects anatomically and functionally significant coronary artery disease. *Circulation* 2010;122:603–613.
78. **Gaemperli O, Bengel FM, Kaufmann PA.** Cardiac hybrid imaging. *Eur Heart J* 2011;32:2100–2108.
79. **Bittencourt MS, Hulten E, Ghoshhajra B, et al.** Prognostic value of nonobstructive and obstructive coronary artery disease detected by coronary computed tomography angiography to identify cardiovascular events. *Circ Cardiovasc Imaging* 2014;7:282–291.
80. **Becker A, Becker C.** CT imaging of myocardial perfusion: possibilities and perspectives. *J Nucl Cardiol* 2013;20:289–296.
81. **Miedema MD, Duprez DA, Misialek JR, et al.** Use of coronary artery calcium testing to guide aspirin utilization for primary prevention: estimates from the multi-ethnic study of atherosclerosis. *Circ Cardiovasc Qual Outcomes* 2014;7:453–460.
82. **Hulten E, Bittencourt MS, Singh A, et al.** Coronary artery disease detected by coronary computed tomographic angiography is associated with intensification of preventive medical therapy and lower low-density lipoprotein cholesterol. *Circ Cardiovasc Imaging* 2014;7:629–638.
83. **Pazhenkottil AP, Herzog BA, Husmann L, et al.** Non-invasive assessment of coronary artery disease with CT coronary angiography and SPECT: a novel dose-saving fast-track algorithm. *Eur J Nucl Med Mol Imaging* 2010;37:522–527.
84. **Salerno M, Beller GA.** Noninvasive assessment of myocardial perfusion. *Circ Cardiovasc Imaging* 2009;2:412–424.
85. **Jaarsma C, Leiner T, Bekkers SC, et al.** Diagnostic performance of noninvasive myocardial perfusion imaging using single-photon emission computed tomography, cardiac magnetic resonance, and positron emission tomography imaging for the detection of obstructive coronary artery disease: a meta-analysis. *J Am Coll Cardiol* 2012;59:1719–1728.
86. **Kurita T, Sakuma H, Onishi K, et al.** Regional myocardial perfusion reserve determined using myocardial perfusion magnetic resonance imaging showed a direct correlation with coronary flow velocity reserve by Doppler flow wire. *Eur Heart J* 2009;30:444–452.
87. **Costa MA, Shoemaker S, Futamatsu H, et al.** Quantitative magnetic resonance perfusion imaging detects anatomic and physiologic coronary artery disease as measured by coronary angiography and fractional flow reserve. *J Am Coll Cardiol* 2007;50:514–522.
88. **Futamatsu H, Wilke N, Klassen C, et al.** Evaluation of cardiac magnetic resonance imaging parameters to detect anatomically and hemodynamically significant coronary artery disease. *Am Heart J* 2007;154:298–305.
89. **Fritz-Hansen T, Hove JD, Kofoed KF, et al.** Quantification of MRI measured myocardial perfusion reserve in healthy humans: a comparison with positron emission tomography. *J Magn Reson Imaging* 2008;27:818–824.
90. **Morton G, Chiribiri A, Ishida M, et al.** Quantification of absolute myocardial perfusion in patients with coronary artery disease: comparison between cardiovascular magnetic resonance and positron emission tomography. *J Am Coll Cardiol* 2012;60:1546–1555.

CHAPTER

23 Myocardial Perfusion Imaging with PET/SPECT: Techniques and Clinical Applications

Constantinos D. Anagnostopoulos, MD, PhD, FRCP, FRCR, FESC, Alexandros Georgakopoulos, MD, Nicolleta Pianou, MD, and Stephan G. Nekolla, FESC

Introduction

This chapter considers the fundamental principles, techniques, and applications of radionuclide myocardial perfusion imaging (MPI). It discusses briefly the main mechanisms involved in regulating myocardial perfusion and the pathophysiologic changes observed during myocardial ischemia. It covers issues related to instrumentation, software, imaging protocols, and stress regimes as well as the applications of single photon emission computed tomography (SPECT) and positron emission tomography (PET) in clinical practice with an emphasis on their role in the diagnosis and management of coronary artery disease (CAD).

Fundamental Principles and Techniques

Imaging Systems

There are two systems that are used in clinical practice for performing radionuclide MPI: (a) gamma camera (γ camera) that detects photons (70 to 150 keV) generated after administration of single photon emission tracers (single photon emitters) and (b) imaging systems based on the detection of high-energy 511-keV photons created as a result of interaction of positrons with electrons (PET scanners).

γ Camera

Most tests are performed using γ (or Anger) camera connected to a computer. The camera consists of a scintillation detector made of a single sodium iodide (NaI) crystal. Behind the crystal is an array of photomultiplier tubes that are optically coupled to the crystal, and that sense the scintillations produced by absorption of gamma photons by the crystal. The location of each scintillation is computed from the relative responses in each tube. In front of the crystal is a collimator, which consists of a disc of lead penetrated by a honeycomb of holes. The holes allow only photons that travel perpendicularly to the crystal face to enter the crystal and in this way the photons absorbed by the crystal form an image of the distribution of radionuclide in front of the camera. SPECT is an extension of the multiprojection method of acquiring planar images. A number of planar projections are acquired as the camera rotates around the patient. These are then reconstructed using special mathematical algorithms into tomograms, which are reoriented into orthogonal planes that are parallel and perpendicular to the long axis of the left ventricle. SPECT is now used routinely for myocardial perfusion studies. Its advantages include a true three-dimensional display of the distribution of the radionuclide within the myocardium, improved image contrast because of the elimination of overlying structures, and the potential for quantification of tracer uptake. Conventional gamma cameras used to have one rotating detector, but modern systems have multiple detectors (normally two), and this increases the speed of acquisition or provides more counts in the same time. A new generation of cameras has been developed in recent years, which use detectors based on cadmium, zinc, and telluride (cadmium zinc telluride, CZT). In contrast to traditional NaI detectors, CZT detectors can directly translate the photon energy and location into electronic signals without the need for photomultiplication of scintillation events. These imaging systems are more expensive compared to those with crystals of NaI, but the detector and microelectronic systems that characterize this type of CZT detectors allow more sensitive and precise measurement of counts that are important for performing myocardial perfusion studies (see below).[1]

Positron Emission Tomography

These studies are based on the use of tracers labeled with isotopes emitting positrons, which are particles with the mass of an electron but with a positive charge. Being basically antimatter, positrons travel only a very short distance within matter. After absorption of their kinetic energy, they undergo an annihilation reaction with an electron, the result of which is the creation of two gamma photons of 511 keV emitted in almost opposite directions. These are sensed by a ring of detectors, and, if an event is sensed in opposing detectors at the same time, they are presumed to have come from annihilation somewhere along the line between the detectors. PET has better spatial resolution (4 to 7 mm) than does SPECT (>10 mm), higher sensitivity, and ability to measure tracer distribution in absolute terms as a function of time. Contemporary SPECT and PET scanners are combined also with computed tomography (CT) capabilities and more recently with magnetic resonance imaging (MRI) creating hybrid systems (SPECT/CT, PET/CT, and PET/MRI, respectively), thus allowing a comprehensive functional and anatomical assessment of the cardiovascular system. The PET camera is more expensive compared to γ camera and not as widely available as the latter. In addition, because of the short half-life of the radiotracers that are used, it requires the presence of cyclotron within short distance from the laboratory for studies based on short-lived isotopes (see below).[2]

Imaging Techniques of Myocardial Perfusion

Physiology of Myocardial Perfusion

The arterioles and prearteriolar vessels constitute the major resistance vessels in the coronary system. The balance between vasodilator and vasoconstrictor tone at this level determines myocardial perfusion. When myocardial oxygen demand increases or coronary blood flow falls, autoregulatory and metabolic regulatory mechanisms become active to try to maintain myocardial perfusion at a normal level.[3–5] In patients with atherosclerotic coronary disease, compensatory mechanisms to preserve myocardial perfusion in the presence of significant epicardial stenoses are already active. There is vasodilatation of the distal vascular bed resulting in insufficient increase of myocardial perfusion when demand is higher, but in addition, there is abnormal endothelial function and impaired endothelium-derived vasodilator mechanisms. The first abnormality to be apparent during ischemia is, therefore, reduced perfusion to the affected supply territory. It is not until a diameter stenosis of around 80% that resting perfusion is finally reduced, and as a rule of thumb, any stenosis less than 40% diameter is unlikely to have any hemodynamic consequences even during maximum coronary dilatation with vasodilators such as adenosine, regadenoson, or dipyridamole (see below).[6]

In patients with stenotic plaques but no reduction in flow at rest due to the above compensatory mechanisms, perfusion abnormalities can be induced by stressing the perfusion system. Any further increase in myocardial oxygen demand will result in ischemia, as compensatory mechanisms are already maximally activated. Physical exercise combined with myocardial perfusion imaging (SPECT MPI) is the commonest way of demonstrating this in clinical practice. The radionuclide involved (either technetium 99m(^{99m}Tc)–labeled tracers or thallium 201 (^{201}Tl)) is extracted by the myocardium in a flow-dependent way. During exercise, myocardial perfusion increases in areas supplied by relatively normal coronary vessels, but there is no increase in the areas supplied by stenotic arteries. Tracer uptake in ischemic areas is therefore reduced compared with areas of normal perfusion.

Perfusion abnormalities secondary to stenotic coronary plaques can also be demonstrated using pharmacologic stress agents. Adenosine can be infused intravenously and will cause a significant increase in (at least fourfold) coronary blood flow (CBF) in normal arteries. As endogenous vasodilators are already active to compensate for coronary stenoses, there will not be a significant increase in CBF (or none at all) in these territories, thus creating flow heterogeneity between areas subtended by normal vessels and those supplied by stenotic ones. Dipyridamole acts via the adenosine pathway and has similar effects. It is important to appreciate that pharmacologic stress with the vasodilators unveils flow heterogeneity rather than ischemia, though the latter may occur if collateral circulation is present. Injection of a suitable tracer during pharmacologic stress will therefore allow the identification of territories subtended by stenotic arteries, in a similar way to dynamic exercise. As with exercise, both (^{99m}Tc) and (^{201}Tl) radiotracers can be used with pharmacologic stress. The regional uptake of the radiopharmaceutical also depends on the roll-off phenomenon; according to which, the first pass of most radiopharmaceuticals decreases when blood flow increases above 2.5-fold compared to baseline levels, leading to an underestimation of the flow in relation to the concentration of the radiopharmaceutical in the myocardium. This roll-off phenomenon is relevant in the setting of pharmacologic stress with vasodilators where coronary flow rates are higher compared to exercise, thereby limiting the ability of SPECT MPI when combined with vasodilators to detect coronary artery stenoses of mild-to-moderate severity. The effect of the roll-off phenomenon is greater in ^{99m}Tc tracers (see below) than it is in the ^{201}Tl. It is also greater in rubidium 82 (^{82}Rb) compared with other PET myocardial perfusion radiopharmaceuticals (see below).

Assessment of Myocardial Perfusion with SPECT MPI

Patient Preparation for SPECT MPI

Each patient and/or their attendants should be informed in writing about the purpose of the examination, duration, possible side effects that may occur during the process, and the radiation exposure of the examination. The patient should be informed by the cardiologist for possible discontinuation of his medication and refrain from foods and beverages that may contain caffeine.[7]

Radiotracers

Thallium 201 (^{201}Tl) has been used for more than 40 years for MPI. It is administered by intravenous injection (usual dose of 80 to 110 MBq). The myocardial uptake is proportional to perfusion and in absolute terms amounts to 4% of the injected dose.[8] After intravenous administration, approximately 88% is cleared from the blood after the first circulation.[9] ^{201}Tl is a monovalent cation, similar in size to the hydrated potassium ion (K^+). Approximately 60% enters the cardiac myocytes using the sodium–potassium ATPase-dependent exchange mechanism, and the remainder enters passively along an electropotential gradient. The extraction efficiency is maintained under conditions of acidosis and hypoxemia and only when myocytes are irreversibly damaged is extraction reduced.[10] The biologic half-life during extraction of the myocardium is 60 to 90 minutes, when it is injected directly into the coronary arteries, but it is much higher (4 to 5 hours) in the case of intravenous administration, because of the balance that develops between ^{201}Tl located intracellularly and ^{201}Tl present in the intravascular space.

Although significant experience has been gained over time with this tracer, it has some limitations. First, it has a relatively long physical half-life (72 hours), which results in a high radiation burden for the patient. Eighty MBq deliver an effective dose of 11 mSv.[11] This is greater than the average dose received by the patient during angiography (8 to 10 mSv). Second, the relatively low injected dose of 80 to 110 MBq results in a low signal-to-noise ratio and images can be suboptimal, especially in obese patients. Third, the relatively low-energy emission leads to low-resolution images and significant attenuation by soft tissue. Electrocardiographic (ECG)-gated imaging is possible, but the low count statistics may be a cause for concern. For these reasons, ^{201}Tl has mainly been superseded by technetium-based radiopharmaceuticals except for viability studies. With the use of novel CZT detector technology, smaller doses of tracer can be used to minimize radiation exposure, and this can be achieved without prolonging image acquisition and without loss of image quality, while technetium dose could be substantially lower than the standard dose (see below).

Two technetium (^{99m}Tc)-labeled perfusion tracers are commercially available: Tc-99m-2-methoxy-isobutyl-isonitrile (MIBI) or sestamibi and Tc-99m-1,2-bis[bis(2-ethoxyethyl) phosphino] ethane (tetrofosmin). MIBI is a cationic complex that diffuses passively through the capillary and cell membrane. Roughly 2.8% of MIBI injected at rest and 3.2% of the dose during dynamic exercise are concentrated in the myocardium, which is smaller than that of ^{201}Tl (4%). MIBI is mainly trapped in mitochondria and shows no significant redistribution for at least 2 to 3 hours after administration. Its elimination from the circulation is rapid, and its clearance occurs through the liver and kidneys.[12] Tetrofosmin is rapidly cleared from the blood, and the ultimate myocardial uptake is slightly less than that of MIBI.[13] The retention of the myocardium is satisfactory and in combination with rapid hepatic clearance makes it possible to obtain an image 20 minutes after the injection. The myocardial uptake mechanism is similar to that of MIBI (Table 23.1).

TABLE 23.1 **Common Radiopharmaceuticals for Myocardial Perfusion Scan**

	Tl 201	Tc 99m (Tetrofosmin-MIBI)
Main uptake mechanism	Na^+/K^+ATPase Pump (60%)–Passive diffusion (40%)	Passive diffusion
Product	Cyclotron	Generator
Photon energy	79 keV	140 keV
Resolution	+	++
Myocardial ejection fraction	++	++
Postinjection imaging	5–10 min	45–60 min (potentially less for tetrofosmin)
Redistribution	Yes	Not clinically significant
Extracardiac uptake	Stomach	Stomach, hepatobiliary, gut
Half time	72 h	6 h
Excretion	Renal	Hepatobiliary
Usual radiation exposure	11 mSv for 80 MBq, less with solid-state cameras and resolution recovery reconstruction	8–10 mSv for 1,000 MBq, less with solid-state cameras and resolution recovery reconstruction

Stress Tests

The response to the stress has a central role in assessing the function of the cardiovascular system. This is especially important in case of CAD, because flow at rest is normal until a diameter stenosis of around 80% of the lumen occurs. Most of these techniques use some type of stress of the cardiovascular system seeking to reveal differences in coronary flow reserve (CFR) between different arteries. Some of them cause myocardial ischemia due to the increased oxygen consumption by the myocardium, while others, such as, for example, the pharmacologic test with adenosine, alter blood flow levels without necessarily leading to ischemia. The most frequently used method is dynamic exercise, but in many patients, it is not feasible usually due to peripheral vascular disease and musculoskeletal diseases. Dynamic exercise is the method of choice and is applicable to patients who are able to achieve satisfactory load (at least 85% of their maximum heart rate appropriate to the age and sex of the patient). If the test is performed for diagnostic purposes, preparation of patients includes discontinuation of medications with anti-ischemic effect, ideally for five half-lives, provided that this is approved by the referring physician (the same applies also for pharmacologic stress with vasodilators). In addition, patients should avoid foods, liquids, and medicines that contain caffeine, while specific diet is not necessary. The aim is to perform a symptom-limited exercise test (see Table 23.2). However, there are patients who are unable to undergo dynamic exercise, absolute contraindications of which are the following: a recent acute coronary syndrome (ACS) (the patient should be hemodynamically stable for at least 24 to 72 hours, after chest pain depending upon clinically assessed risk), left main stem stenosis that is likely to be hemodynamically significant, symptoms of heart failure (HF) at rest, a recent history of severe arrhythmia, aortic stenosis, hypertrophic cardiomyopathy (HCM), severe hypertension (systolic blood pressure >220 mm Hg or diastolic blood pressure >120 mm Hg), recent pulmonary embolism or infarction, thrombophlebitis or active deep vein thrombosis, active endocarditis, myocarditis, or pericarditis. Relative contraindications to the dynamic stress are left bundle branch block (LBBB), paced rhythm, movement disorders, and inability to complete a recent exercise test.[14] In these cases, administration of drugs that alter the coronary flow or myocardial oxygen consumption is the only option. There are currently four pharmacologic stressors: dipyridamole, adenosine, regadenoson, and dobutamine.

Dipyridamole dilates arteriolar coronary circulation by increasing adenosine levels in the plasma, which is a strong vasodilator substance, acting via the purinergic receptors. The increase of flow in the coronary circulation in normal subjects is about 250% to 600% of flow at rest. In patients with CAD, the administration of dipyridamole causes uneven increase in the flow and deficits in SPECT MPI. Dipyridamole is administered intravenously at a dose of 140 μg/kg/min for 4 minutes. The time required to achieve maximal vasodilation is about 4 minutes, and therefore, the radiopharmaceutical should be injected in the 8th minute of the test. The maximum increase of flow in the coronary circulation is maintained for 10 min and then returns to baseline levels within half and hour. The administration of dipyridamole is indicated as stress test to patients who cannot exercise to an adequate level as well as for those with LBBB or paced rhythm. Chest pain (not necessarily ischemic) appears in 20% of patients and significant arrhythmias in less than 2% of patients. Extracardiac effects (headache, dizziness, nausea, epigastric pain, flushing) are observed in 30% to 40% of patients treated by slow intravenous aminophylline (up to 250 mg), which is a specific antagonist.[15]

Adenosine dilates coronary vessels, and the main advantage is the very short half-life time in plasma, which is estimated at less than 10 seconds. This has the effect of reducing the duration of side effects, and this is the main reason why, while it is more expensive than is dipyridamole, many nuclear medicine laboratories prefer to use adenosine. It causes arterial vasodilation in most networks by acting on A2a receptors and increasing the level of intracellular cyclic adenosine monophosphate. This results in relaxation of smooth muscle fibers of small vessels and consequently vasodilation. Adenosine has negative chronotropic and inotropic effect by its action on the A1 receptors. Intravenous administration at a rate of 140 μg/kg/min results in maximal or near-maximal hyperemia in 92% of patients, with an average increase of the flow in normal coronary vessels by 4.4 times compared to the resting value. The time required to achieve maximum vasodilatation is about 2 minutes,

TABLE 23.2 **Stress Test Protocols**

	Exercise Stress Test	Adenosine	Dipyridamole	Dobutamine	Regadenoson
Mechanism of action	Coronary vasodilatation secondary to increased myocardial oxygen demands—inducible ischemia	Direct coronary vasodilatation by nonselective stimulation of adenosine receptors	Direct coronary vasodilatation by inhibiting the reuptake of endogenous adenosine	(a)Vasodilatation through direct action into β-2 receptors and (b) increase of oxygen consumption due to an increase in heart rate and myocardial contractility	Coronary vasodilatation by selective stimulation of adenosine A_{2a} receptors
Protocol	Dynamic exercise	140 μg/kg/min intravenously for 6 min	140 μg/kg/min intravenously for 4 min	5–10 μg/kg/min gradually increasing every 3–5 min until 40 μg/kg/min	Single injection of 400 μg intravenously
Duration	Varies	6 min	8 min	Varies	30 s
Radiotracer injection time	At the peak of exercise (the exercise should be continued for 2 more min)	3–4 min after the beginning of the adenosine injection	4 min after the end of the dipyridamole injection	At ≥85% of the maximum target heart rate or after 3 min in 40 μg/kg/min	30 s after the end of regadenoson injection
Reason for discontinuation	Progressively increasing angina, dyspnea, dizziness, fatigue, severe hypo-/hypertension, severe heart rate reduction, peripheral hypoperfusion, ventricular arrhythmias or tachycardia, progressive ST segment depression or elevation >1 mm in non-Q wave leads	Severe dyspnea or angina, hypotension (<80 mmHg), persisting atrioventricular block	The same as for adenosine	The same as for dynamic exercise	

and therefore, the radiopharmaceutical may be given in the second to third minute of the test, and the test may be finished over 2.5 to 3 minutes later. Like dipyridamole, adenosine can be coupled with submaximal dynamic exercise when tolerated to reduce the frequency and severity of adverse effects associated with vasodilator infusion.[14] A bicycle ergometer, allowing a semirecumbent patient's position, may be preferable to a treadmill, because intravenous infusions are easily managed when the patient is relatively steady. Heart rate, blood pressure, and ECG should be measured and recorded at baseline and every 2 minutes during the infusion. The tracer is injected between the 3rd and 4th minutes of the adenosine infusion or sooner if symptoms or other complications require.

As with dipyridamole, most of the perfusion defects are created by flow heterogeneity between normal arteries and arteries with stenotic lesions. Ischemia is uncommon but may be caused by coronary steal, when collateral circulation is present. ST segment depression is observed in 15% of patients being investigated for CAD and in 25% of patients with known CAD, which is less than that observed during dynamic stress. Side effects are present in 80% of patients. Chest pain (not necessarily ischemic) is common seen in up to 40% of patients.[14,16] Other side effects are headache, facial redness, and atrioventricular (AV) block. Because the half-life of the drug in plasma is very short (10 seconds), side effects disappear rapidly. Contraindications and preparation for testing with adenosine are similar to those of dipyridamole and regadenoson.

To avoid the side effects of vasodilator stress, agonists with a high selectivity for the adenosine A_{2A} receptor responsible for the coronary vasodilator effect of adenosine have been developed. Of all compounds, regadenoson (Rapiscan, United Kingdom, or Lexiscan, United States) is the most commonly available for use in Europe and United States. Regadenoson has a rapid onset of action with peak coronary vasodilation by 30 seconds after administration and a short-lasting vasodilator effect of 2.30 minutes that is sufficient for adequate myocardial tracer extraction. Regadenoson was tested in two randomized double-blind studies of over 2,000 patients, and the results demonstrated that beyond its appealing features for clinical use, such as ease of administration as a rapid injection over 10 seconds and single non–weight-adjusted dose of 400 μg, regadenoson has comparable efficacy to adenosine and a similar side effect profile but better tolerability compared to the latter.[17,18] Moreover, regadenoson can be used safely in patients with mild-to-moderate reactive airway disease and obstructive lung disease.[19,20] Like adenosine and dipyridamole, regadenoson can also be combined with submaximal exercise when tolerated. Regadenoson has also been used during dynamic exercise when maximal exercise is not achieved, but there is little evidence for the effectiveness and safety of this approach.

Absolute contraindications for the administration of the above vasodilators are known bronchospasm requiring treatment with steroids, second- and third-degree AV block in the absence of functioning pacemaker, hypotension (systolic pressure <90 mm Hg), taking xanthine or dipyridamole during the last 24 hours, known or suspected sinoatrial disease, and any other cases in which a stress test is contraindicated (e.g., acute HF, hemodynamic instability). Relative contraindications are recent cerebral ischemia or infarction.[14] Patients with well-controlled or mild asthma or chronic obstructive pulmonary disease (COPD) can be stressed with adenosine. The latter can be given as a titrated protocol starting at a low dose of 70 or 100 μg/kg/min for a minute and increasing if tolerated up to 140 μg/kg/min with tracer injection two minutes after the maximal dose of 140 μg/kg/min. Patients who are already on a β_2-adrenergic agonist such as salbutamol can be given two puffs of the inhaler prior to starting the adenosine infusion.

In patients stressed with the vasodilators, dipyridamole should be withheld for at least 24 hours prior to adenosine or 48 hours before regadenoson administration. Patients must also avoid aminophylline and theophylline as well as consumption of any foods and drinks containing caffeine (coffee, tea, chocolate) or caffeine-containing medications, for a minimum of 24 hours prior to the test.[7] Caffeine ingestion may attenuate the normal vasodilator response to adenosine, dipyridamole, and regadenoson. Attenuation of adenosine-induced perfusion abnormality by caffeine (in patients who have consumed caffeine within 12 hours prior to the test) can be overcome by increasing the adenosine dose to 210 μg/kg/min.

Dobutamine is used in patients with asthma or COPD, where vasodilators cannot be administered and a dynamic stress test is not feasible. Dobutamine increases myocardial perfusion in two ways: (a) causing vasodilatation through direct action into β_2 receptors and (b) increasing the oxygen consumption due to an increase in heart rate and myocardial contractility. The increase of coronary flow due to dobutamine is greater than that induced by dynamic exercise, but lower than that with dipyridamole or adenosine.[21] The half-life in the plasma is approximately 90 seconds. Dobutamine is administered intravenously by a peripheral vein (initial dose of 5 to 10 μg/kg/min and then the dose is increased to 15, 20, 30, and 40 μg/kg/min every 3 to 5 minutes). The preparation of patients includes discontinuation of β-adrenergic antagonists for five half-lives, if possible, or at least for 24 hours. When dobutamine is used in echocardiography stress studies (stress echo), the additional intravenous atropine administration is useful (if there are no contraindications) when there is no satisfactory increase in heart rate. However, the use of atropine is less frequent in scintigraphic imaging, for the reason that the main mechanism of action of dobutamine is vasodilation, and therefore, the creation of perfusion deficits in patients with CAD is the result of inhomogeneous flow increase in coronary vessels. Intravenous administration of dobutamine in patients with CAD is safe, and serious complications occur rarely. Chest pain occurs in one-third of the patients, palpitation in 10%, and transient ventricular tachycardia, causing no hemodynamic changes, in 4% of patients. The effects of dobutamine are resolved by the administration of β-blockers. Given the positive chronotropic and inotropic action, dobutamine should not be used as a stress test in patients with contraindications to dynamic exercise as well as known hypokalemia. Relative contraindications are LBBB and paced rhythm, because dobutamine, like dynamic exercise, can cause septal perfusion defects even in the absence of epicardial CAD.

Imaging Protocols

Imaging with ^{201}Tl

^{201}Tl is usually administered at peak stress test, which is continued for about 2 minutes after the injection in order to maintain constant conditions during the uptake of the tracer from the myocardium. Imaging begins 5 to 10 minutes after injection and must be completed within 30 minutes. During this period, the distribution of the radiotracer in the myocardium is relatively stable, and the obtained images correspond to myocardial perfusion at the time of maximum stress. In areas with reduced perfusion, the concentration of ^{201}Tl is reduced, resulting in the creation of perfusion defects. Then, ^{201}Tl exits the myocardium with a washout rate that differs in regions with normal compared to those with reduced perfusion. The result of the different washout rates is the relative increase in uptake of ^{201}Tl after 2 to 4 hours in areas that initially showed reduced intake. The effect of improving or "filling" of a perfusion deficit over time is called redistribution. Comparison of images of stress with those of redistribution allows differentiation of inducible ischemia from permanent necrosis (partial or transmural). In some cases, it is likely that redistribution is incomplete at 4 hours. Therefore, for a more complete imaging, ^{201}Tl (40 MBq) is reinjected (ideally after sublingual nitrates) followed by a third set of images obtained at 45 to 60 minutes after injection.[22]

Imaging with ^{99m}*Tc*

For stress and rest imaging with ^{99m}Tc-labeled tracers, two separate injections are necessary, and these can be given on the same or different days. Different imaging protocols can be followed, depending on clinical indication and local practices: (a) 1-day stress–rest, (b) 1-day rest–stress, and (c) 2-day protocol. The latter is recommended on the grounds of image quality (it is ideal for obese patients), but it may be less convenient for the patient. In the United States, the 2-day protocol includes an initial study in which 888 to 1,332 MBq (this is lower in Europe, for instance, 800 MBq per study is used in the United Kingdom, www.arsac.org.uk) of the tracer are administered during stress followed by a resting study performed on a different day after administering the same tracer activity.[23] Imaging begins 30 to 60 minutes after injection to allow for hepatobiliary clearance with longer delays required for resting images and for stress with vasodilators alone because of the higher liver uptake. The two studies can also be performed on the same day if the second study is obtained after administration of a higher (usually three times compared with the first) tracer activity, in order to reduce significantly the influence of the residual activity of the first injection.[24] A count density of 1:3 or 4 between the two studies is recommended. The 1-day protocol of tetrofosmin or MIBI involves administration of 296 to 444 MBq (in the USA) at stress and, 3 hours later, injection of 888 to 1,332 MBq at rest.[23] Higher doses can be considered on an individual basis by the practitioner, for instance, in obese patients. The levels of activity can be reduced considerably when using modern imaging systems (see below). If a 1-day protocol is performed, a rest-first study has advantages including better contrast between normal and ischemic segments and lesser time interval between the two studies. However, in patients with low pretest likelihood of obstructive coronary disease, one could consider a stress-first study, especially with ECG gating and attenuation correction (AC) to obviate the need for a rest study.

The effective dose of SPECT MPI for the 2-day protocol with MIBI and tetrofosmin is 8.1 and 7.2 mSv, respectively, while for ^{201}Tl, it is 11 mSv. The effective dose is increased when the 1-day protocol with ^{99m}Tc is performed as the dose in the second study is usually three times higher than the first. The effective dose is also increased in ^{201}Tl studies when it is reinjected for viability assessment. When SPECT MPI with MIBI or tetrofosmin is performed for diagnostic purposes and the stress scan is normal, the effective dose is significantly reduced.[7]

An important consequence of the lack of redistribution of the ^{99m}Tc-labeled tracers is that stress imaging can be delayed for sometime after injection, and there is no need to inject close to the γ camera. Injections can be given during treadmill exercise testing, in the catheter laboratory, or in the coronary care unit immediately before thrombolysis. In addition, because of the higher activity that can be used with ^{99m}Tc, ventricular function can be assessed either by first-pass imaging of the tracer as it passes through the central circulation or by ECG-gated acquisition of the myocardial perfusion images (see below).

Imaging with Two Radiopharmaceuticals

This is designed to overcome the disadvantages of the time-consuming imaging protocol, which uses two injections of MIBI or tetrofosmin. However, it has the disadvantage of increasing the total radiation dose received by the patient. ^{201}Tl is initially administered at rest, and images are obtained 30 to 120 minutes after tracer injection. Following completion of the rest scans, stress images following a tracer injection of MIBI or tetrofosmin are obtained. The interval between injection and image acquisition for ^{201}Tl depends on the clinical indication for carrying out the study. Thus, if the study is performed in patients with significant CAD and impaired ventricular function wherein detection of viable myocardium is important, late imaging (120 minutes after injection) is recommended, whereas if the examination is performed for diagnostic purposes, imaging can begin much earlier.[25] The advent of the solid-state detector (such as CZT)–based technology enables the execution of such studies with a total radiation exposure comparable to that of high-dose 1-day stress/rest technetium-99m–MIBI SPECT MPI but lower than dual thallium-201/technetium-99m imaging using a conventional camera. With such scanners, a strong correlation for several variables including image quality and the extent and depth of perfusion abnormality was found between simultaneous acquisition of thallium-201 and technetium-99m images and sequential acquisition with conventional SPECT (see immediately below).

Acquisition and Image processing

Single photon emission computed tomography. This technique uses γ camera with a rotating head for the collection of data. Nowadays, in many nuclear cardiology departments, dual head tomographic imaging is performed over a 180-degree rotation from right anterior oblique (RAO) 45 degrees to left posterior oblique (LPO) 45 degrees. For ^{201}Tl, imaging general purpose collimators are used, while for ^{99m}Tc, high-resolution collimators are used, unless resolution recovery software is available, in which case, the use of low-energy general purpose should also be considered in order to reduce either the acquisition time or the administered dose. A 15% to 20% energy window at 72 and 167 keV for thallium-201 and 140 keV for technetium-99m–labeled radiopharmaceuticals should be selected. The acquired pixel size should be in the region of 6 mm. A step-and-shoot acquisition with 32 or 64 stops separated by 3 to 6 degrees or a continuous acquisition can be used. The duration of acquisition at each stop depends partly on the equipment, protocol, dose of radiopharmaceutical, patient size, and reconstruction algorithm. Total acquisition times of longer than 20 to 30 minutes can be counterproductive as they increase the likelihood of patient motion. ECG gating can be performed, particularly with technetium-99m–labeled radiopharmaceuticals.[26]

In recent years, there have been significant developments in terms of the image reconstruction algorithms, which, in combination with improvements in collimators, have resulted in resolution and signal-to-noise ratio improvement. The result is a reduction of the acquisition time to half the standard, or alternatively, administration of half the dose in standard time.[27–29] Reconstruction with the resolution recovery approach is the recommended option, but if resolution recovery is not available, then reconstruction is performed with iterative reconstruction. With the evolution of imaging systems (CZT camera), the administered radioactivity can be greatly reduced (e.g., 185 MBq at rest and 555 MBq at stress for ^{99m}Tc tracers), thereby reducing the effective dose to the patient by 50% to 70% compared with the conventional protocols. Reduction of imaging time is also feasible to 2 and 4 minutes, respectively, for stress and rest compared to 16 and 12 minutes, respectively, for a standard stress/rest SPECT study in a technetium-99m protocol. This shorter acquisition time has multiple benefits including a better tolerated examination by the patients, reduction of motion artifacts, and the ability to scan a higher number of patients without compromising the diagnostic accuracy or the predictive value of SPECT MPI.[1,25,30–35]

Modern systems also offer motion correction software. This can correct certain forms of motion such as movement in the longitudinal axis and vertically. Patient motion should be corrected only when it is greater than 2 pixels, since less significant motion does not create serious artifacts.[7] Another parameter that can affect image quality is photon scattering by the patient's body and the detectors, which can be corrected by the use of additional energy windows or by reducing the width of the selected energy window.[7] Photon attenuation by the patient's body is yet another source of artifacts. These are created by an unevenly reduced tracer uptake by

TABLE

23.3 Possible Causes of "Artifacts" during Imaging

- Patient motion
- Upward creep (caused by increase in lung volume during exercise leading to depression of the diaphragm and slow return of the heart to its original position during acquisition)
- Attenuation by soft tissue (diaphragmatic muscle and breast)
- External objects
- High radiopharmaceutical uptake in a structure adjacent to the heart (liver, intestine)

the myocardium, which depends on the type of tissue (soft tissue, bone, or lungs), the activity of the radiopharmaceutical, and the body type of the patient. The most common artifact is the appearance of an inferior defect in men due to attenuation of photons by the diaphragm or an anterior wall defect in women due to photon attenuation from the breast tissue[7] (Table 23.3).

AC of the tomographic images can be performed either using a radionuclide line source (e.g., gadolinium 153) or more commonly now by using a CT detector integrated into the gamma camera gantry. However, it may itself introduce artifacts of its own. Misalignment between emission and transmission data can risk incomplete correction and create artificial perfusion defects. Misregistration of just 1 pixel can cause a diagnostically significant artifact.[7] Both European and American guidelines recommend careful use of AC for myocardial perfusion SPECT studies.[36] The corrected images (AC) should be considered together with the uncorrected (non-AC) ones, because overcorrection can occasionally occur resulting in reduced sensitivity. CT-AC can improve the specificity of the test, but at the expense of sensitivity. Also, it can underestimate the size and severity of a perfusion defect, particularly in the inferior wall.[37]

Interpretation of the Images

Myocardial perfusion and hence tracer distribution is uniform in normal myocardium (Fig. 23-1). A regional defect indicates reduced perfusion in viable myocardium, a reduced amount of viable myocardium, or a combination of both. If a stress defect returns to normal in the resting images, this indicates an inducible perfusion abnormality that is sometimes referred to as inducible ischemia. Strictly, the term "ischemia" is not always correct, particularly if stress is performed with the vasodilators, in which case, the image indicates heterogeneity of perfusion rather than an absolute reduction. Areas of infarction are depicted as a defect in both stress and rest images, and the depth of the defect indicates the amount of myocardial loss. Ischemia can be superimposed upon partial thickness infarction, and in this case, a stress defect may be only partially reversible at rest (Fig. 23-2). Reverse redistribution is the term used to describe a defect in redistribution thallium images that is less apparent in the stress images. When the phenomenon is seen, it is often the result of artifact or other technical differences between images, and, in this case, it is not strictly speaking reverse redistribution. When true reverse redistribution is seen, it is the result of rapid washout of tracer as might occur in an area of partial thickness infarction supplied by a patent artery after angioplasty or thrombolysis. In addition to regional myocardial uptake, other features of the images are important. Ventricular dilation is best judged from the planar images although it is also apparent in the tomograms. Of particular significance is left ventricular dilatation in stress images that is less marked on the resting ones, since this implies extensive inducible ischemia and is associated with an adverse prognosis. The dilatation may be partly real, but it may also be the result of widespread subendocardial ischemia that simulates cavity enlargement. The normal right ventricular myocardium is much thinner than the left, but it is not unusual to see right ventricular uptake. Hypertrophy in either ventricle can be seen as myocardial thickening and an increase in counts. When a relative defect is seen, care must be taken to distinguish between reduced uptake in an area of reduced perfusion and increased uptake in a neighboring area of hypertrophy. Because the myocardial images are not of high spatial resolution, it is often necessary to make this distinction only after echocardiography or MRI has been used to define myocardial thickness.[38–41] Increased ^{201}Tl uptake of the lungs is caused by increased pulmonary capillary pressure and is accompanied by an

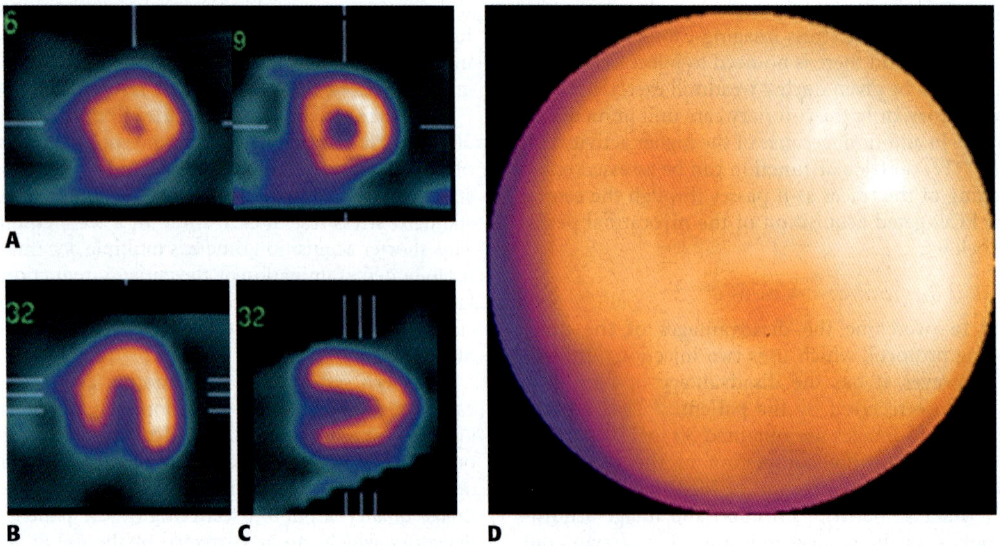

Figure 23-1. Normal myocardial perfusion scintigraphy (MPS). Homogeneous radiotracer uptake in the walls of the left ventricle are shown. **A:** Apical **(left)** and basal **(right)** short axis slices. **B:** Horizontal long axis. **C:** Vertical long axis. **D:** Polar mapping of the same patient demonstrating normal myocardial perfusion.

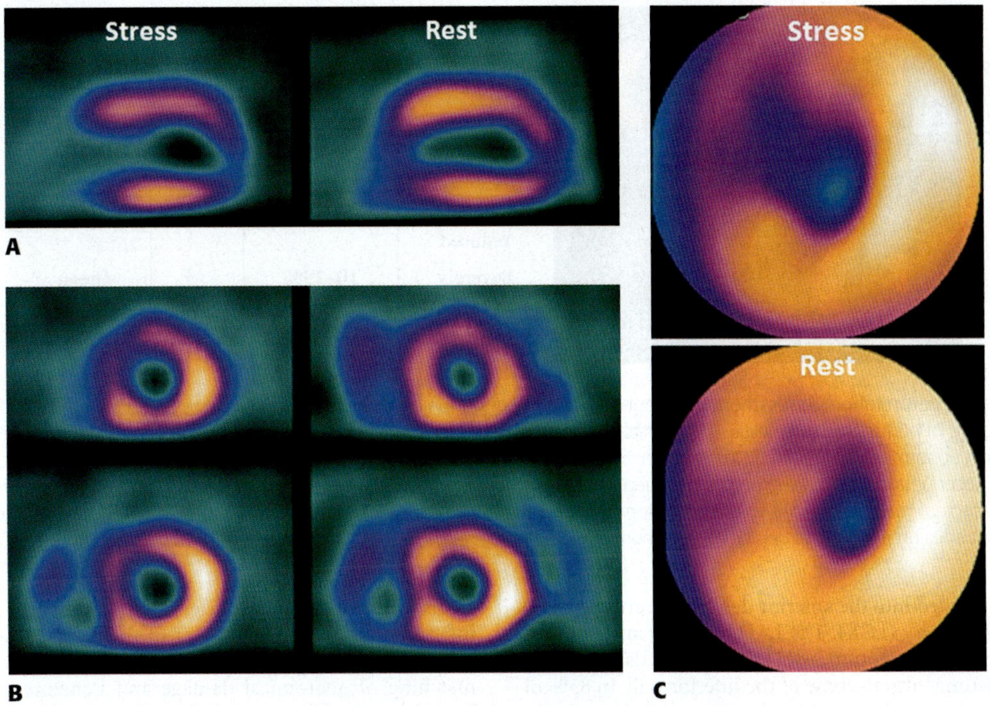

Figure 23-2. Reversible perfusion abnormality in the anteroapical region and the septum superimposed upon minor partial thickness damage at the apex. The perfusion defect is more pronounced towards the apex. The overall appearances are compatible with left anterior descending (LAD) disease. **A:** Long axis. **B:** Short axis. **C:** Polar maps.

increased incidence of future cardiac events in patients with CAD. Lung uptake is a marker of impaired left ventricular function at rest or induced by ischemia during exercise. It is expressed as a ratio between uptake in the lungs and the myocardium, even though myocardial uptake depends upon viability and perfusion. The measurements are obtained either from an initial anterior planar image or from the appropriate image of the tomographic acquisition, and a normal lung:heart ratio is less than 0.55 ± 0.11.[42] In a mechanism similar to that of ^{201}Tl, the increased uptake of MIBI or tetrofosmin by the lungs and an LHR more than 0.35 ± 0.08 is associated with LV dysfunction and is a predictor of adverse prognosis in patients with known or suspected CAD.[43,44] Perfusion defects are not always the result of CAD (see below). Abnormalities can be seen with coronary spasm, anomalous arteries, muscle bridges, small vessel disease as may occur in diabetes or syndrome X, the dilated and hypertrophic cardiomyopathies, hypertrophy caused by outflow obstruction or hypertension, infiltrative disorders such as sarcoidosis and amyloidosis, connective tissue disorders, and conduction defects such as LBBB.

Semiquantitative Assessment of Myocardial Tracer Distribution

Several methods have been used to quantify myocardial uptake, and these are all relative rather than absolute techniques in which uptake is expressed relative to the "hottest" voxel (i.e., highest uptake value) within the myocardium. The techniques include linear profiles, circumferential profiles, and analysis of count histograms, but a method that is popular for tomographic imaging is to display the whole myocardium as a polar map or "bull's-eye" image (Figs. 23-1 and 23-2). Individual polar maps can be compared with a normal database and abnormalities detected automatically as areas with counts less than two standard deviations (or other threshold) from the mean. The normal database should be gender and radionuclide specific and may also be institute specific. The polar mapping is usually visualized with a color scale, where the corresponding pixels below the normal range are displayed with different colors. The extent of myocardial perfusion deficit may be determined as a percentage of the pixels of the polar mapping in which the uptake of the radiopharmaceutical is less than the statistically predetermined threshold. Polar maps with quantification are probably most helpful to assess the depth and extent of defects, but they should not be used as sole basis. However, they can be helpful to assess changes posttreatment. Most experienced nuclear cardiologists prefer to assess the presence of a defect from the tomograms initially and to use quantification to assess depth and extent of an abnormality. The three-dimensional display of LV (3D display) is another option, helping to determine the presence, extent, and location of perfusion defects, while giving information for the size and configuration of LV. Additionally, it can help in correlating SPECT MPI findings with those of other imaging studies, such as those of angiography.[7] Segmental analysis can be performed by visual analysis or automated using a number of models of the left ventricular myocardium. A 17-segment model is recommended by several professional societies, and in each segment, tracer uptake is classified semiquantitatively on a five-point scale where 0 = normal (uptake >70%), 1 = mild deficit (uptake 50% to 69%), 2 = moderate deficit (uptake 30% to 49%), 3 = severe deficit (uptake 10% to 29%), and 4 = absence of perfusion (uptake <10%). By adding those numbers together, the sum of the stress scores (SSS), the sum of the rest scores (SRS), or the sum of the difference scores (SDS)[45,46] can be calculated (Figs. 23-3 and 23-4).

Because automated analysis has the drawback of being susceptible to artifacts leading sometimes to false-positive results, the findings must not be reported in isolation and without expert review of the images from which the results are derived.[7,47] Caution is also required in relating perfusion findings with coronary artery anatomy (Fig. 23-5). Usually, the right feeds the bulk of the inferior wall of the LV and the adjacent portion of the septum. The left after

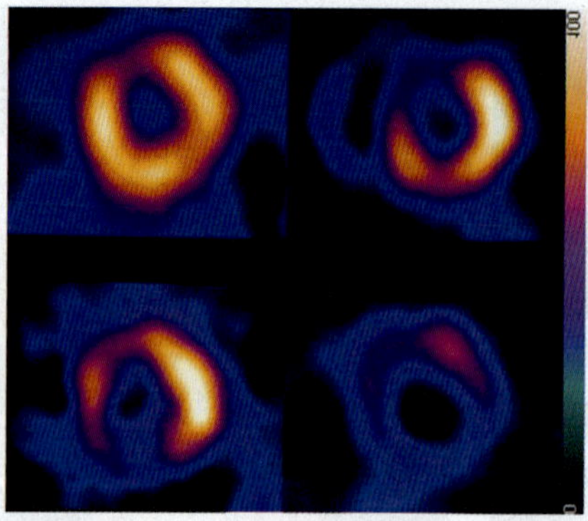

Severity	Percentage uptake	Score	Color scale
Normal	70–100%	0	Orange to white
Mildly reduced	50–69%	1	Purple
Moderately reduced	30–49%	2	Blue
Severely reduced	10–29%	3	Green
Absent	0–9%	4	Black

Figure 23-3. **Image interpretation: Assessment of extent and severity of perfusion defects.** Short-axis views of four different patients are presented demonstrating a range of perfusion abnormalities (from mild and limited at the left upper corner to extensive and severe at the right lower corner). The extent of a perfusion abnormality is defined by the number of abnormal segments involved, while the severity is determined by the reduction of uptake in each segment. Tracer uptake within a segment is classified as normal; mildly, moderately, or severely reduced; or absent. These categories reflect the counts as a percentage of maximum in the whole set of tomograms. For each category, a score is given, so that SSS, SRS, and SDS can be calculated. Based on the SSS, perfusion images can be classified as normal (SSS 0–3), mildly abnormal (SSS 4–8), or moderate–severely abnormal (SSS ≥ 9).

a short course is divided into the anterior descending artery (LAD) and the circumflex artery (LCX). The LAD feeds the anterior wall and the upper 2/3 of the septum, while the LCX feeds the lateral LV wall and sometimes also the base of the inferior wall. In 85% of cases, the right is the dominant (right dominance), giving rise to the posterior descending artery (PDA). In the rest of the cases, PDA stems from the circumflex artery (left dominance) and perfuses the inferior wall and the lower part of the intraventricular septum or (rarely) from both the LCX and the RCA (codominance).[48] Exact matching of anatomical damage and ischemia may be achieved by hybrid imaging, combining CT coronary angiography with SPECT MPI[49,50]

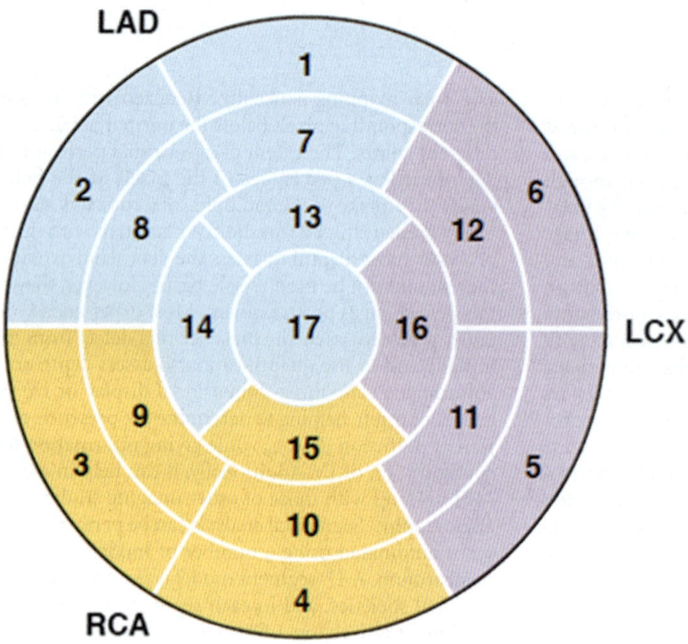

1. Basal anterior	7. Mid anterior	13. Apical anterior
2. Basal anteroseptal	8. Mid anteroseptal	14. Apical septal
3. Basal inferoseptal	9. Mid inferoseptal	15. Apical inferior
4. Basal inferior	10. Mid inferior	16. Apical lateral
5. Basal inferolateral	11. Mid inferolateral	17. Apical
6. Basal anterolateral	12. Mid anterolateral	

Figure 23-4. **Seventeen-segment model as per American College of Cardiology/American Heart Association (ACC/AHA) recommendations.** The left ventricle (LV) has four walls (anterior, septum, inferior, and lateral) and an apex. The LV myocardium can be divided into a certain number of segments, for example, 9, 12, 14, 17 (as it is shown here and recommended by the ACC/AHA), or twenty.

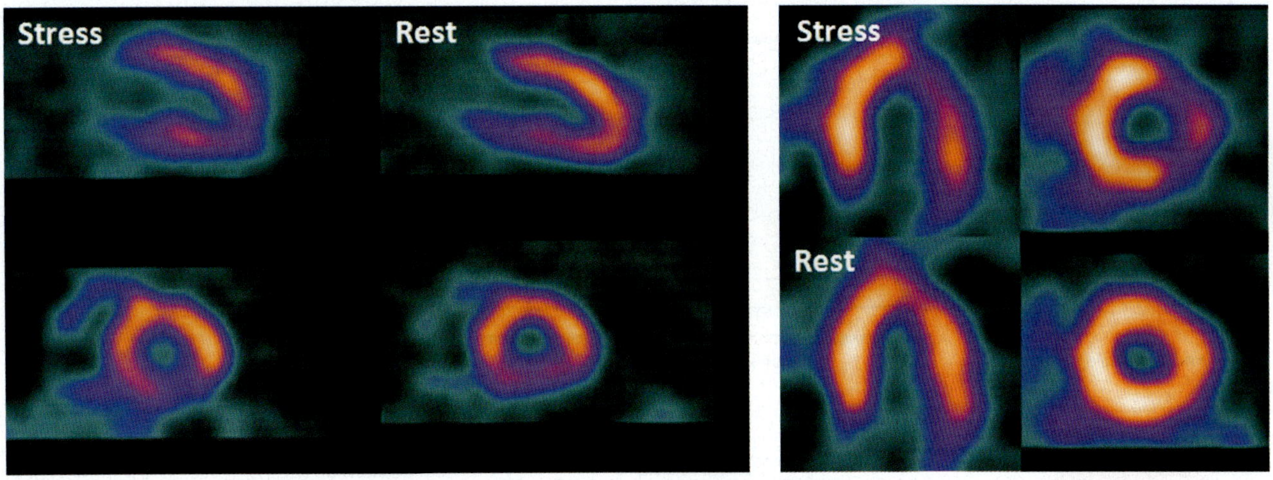

A B

Figure 23-5. Examples of myocardial ischemia **(A)** of the inferior wall and **(B)** the lateral wall.

Myocardial Perfusion Studies with Electrocardiographic Synchronization (ECG gated)

During the perfusion study, for assessment of myocardial function, the ECG is recorded while the R wave is used to identify the beginning of the cardiac cycle, as in conventional radionuclide equilibrium ventriculography. This method is used for calculating the ejection fraction (EF) and assessment of segmental contractility disorders of LV (Fig. 23-6). Eight frames per cardiac cycle are commonly used, but sixteen frames per cardiac cycle provide more accurate measurement of left ventricular EF or parameters of diastolic function. By this method, the lower limits of normal left ventricular ejection fraction (LVEF) are calculated around 45% to 50% (in male and female patients, respectively), while regarding the end systolic volume (ESV) and end diastolic volume (EDV), the corresponding values are 45 to 75 and 100 to 150 mL (in female and male patients, respectively).

The segmental movement and systolic thickening are usually studied subjectively, but recent software programs allow the automatic assessment of segmental contractility. Wall motion is best evaluated in linear gray scale without computer-derived edges and can be classified as normal, hypokinetic, akinetic, or dyskinetic (paradoxical). Because of the relatively low spatial resolution of the γ camera, the estimated systolic thickening is done by the periodic variation of scintillations (or counts) between diastole and systole. During the diastolic thinning, a decrease in density of the obtained scintillations is observed, while as the myocardium becomes thickened during systole, the number of scintillations increases. Wall thickening is best evaluated in a continuous color scale without computer-derived edges. Recent software advances permit also assessment of diastolic function and prediction of response to cardiac resynchronization therapy (CRT) using quantitative ECG-gated MPI.[51] The timing or phase of contraction of myocardial segments is calculated automatically (phase analysis) and presented in a polar map or phase histogram format. The phase analysis is a parametric image where the regional differences reflect the time difference between the start of contraction of the walls of LV (asynchronous). In normal volunteers, phase analysis values between the RV and LV

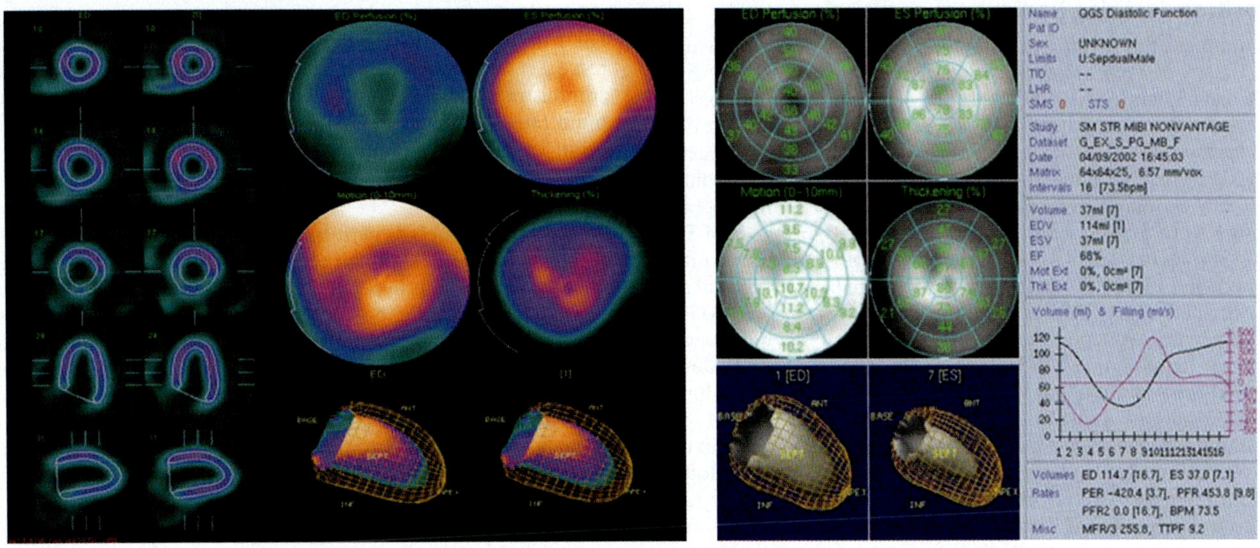

A B

Figure 23-6. Myocardial perfusion scintigraphy (MPS) with ECG-gated SPECT. End-diastolic and end-systolic images, representative images of polar mapping, and 3D images of regional wall motion **(A)**. Normal EF and normal end-diastolic and end-systolic volumes **(B)**.

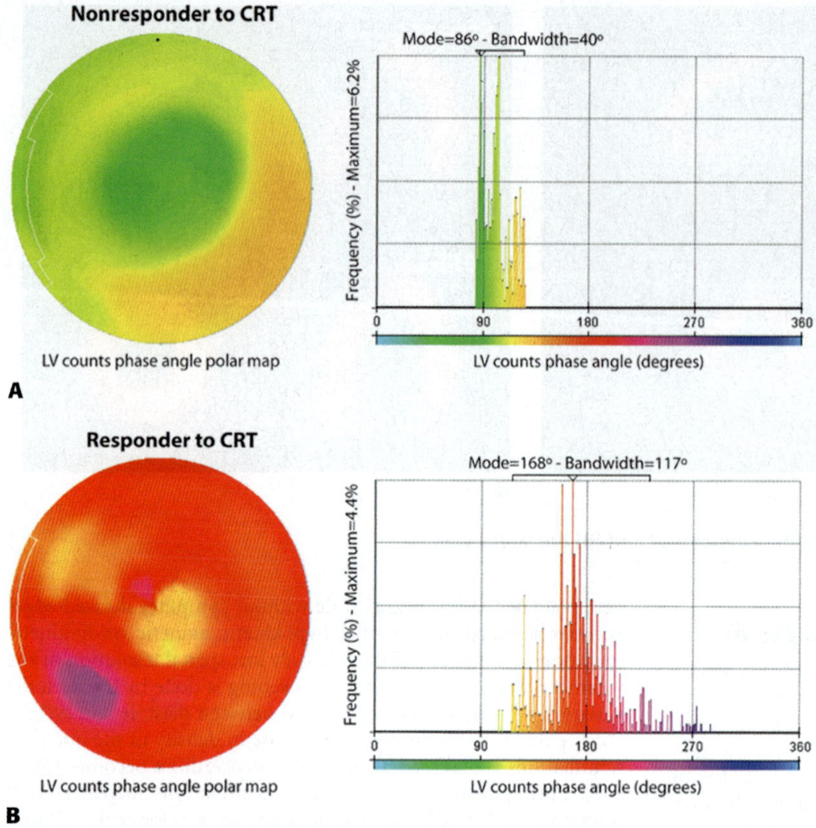

Figure 23-7. **A:** Example of a patient without LV dyssynchrony on ECG-gated SPECT MPI. Synchronous contraction pattern is reflected by homogeneous phase angle distribution of polar map **(left)** and narrow highly peaked histogram **(right)**. **B:** Example of a patient with extensive LV dyssynchrony on ECG-gated SPECT MPI. LV dyssynchrony is indicated by heterogeneous phase angle distribution of polar map **(left)** and wide histogram **(right)**. (Reprinted by permission of the Society of Nuclear Medicine, Boogers MM, Van Kriekinge SD, Henneman MM, et al. Quantitative gated SPECT-derived phase analysis on gated myocardial perfusion SPECT defects left ventricular dyssynchrony and predicts response to cardiac resynchronization therapy. *J Nucl Med* 2009;50:718–725.)

are similar while the phase histogram of the ventricles consists of a small amplitude peak. In cases of myocardial ischemia, fibrosis, or conduction disorders, there is enlargement of the histogram.[25] The imaging parameters most helpful for predicting response to CRT are histogram bandwidth and phase SD (Fig. 23-7).

Assessment of Myocardial Perfusion by Positron Emission Tomography

Positron-Emitting Radiopharmaceuticals

A number of positron-emitting radiopharmaceuticals can be used as tracers of myocardial perfusion. The most common are ^{82}Rb, nitrogen-13 ammonia (^{13}N-ammonia) (Fig. 23-8), and oxygen-15–labeled water (^{15}O-water). ^{82}Rb is a potassium analogue like ^{201}Tl and is the most widely used radiopharmaceutical in clinical practice for MPI with PET. It has a very short physical half-life (76 seconds), but it is produced by a commercially available elution generator with a 4- to 5-week shelf life, thus allowing performance of PET MPI studies in centers without access to cyclotron.[52] After an intravenous injection, ^{82}Rb rapidly crosses the capillary membrane and is extracted from plasma by myocardial cells via the Na^+/K^+ ATPase pump, by an extraction that is similar to that of ^{201}Tl but lower to that of ^{13}N-ammonia and ^{15}O-water. ^{13}N-ammonia is also administered intravenously and has a physical half-life of 9.96 minutes. Once inside the myocyte, ^{13}N-ammonia is incorporated into the glutamine pool and becomes metabolically trapped. The main disadvantage of ^{13}N-ammonia is that it requires an on-site cyclotron and a radiochemistry synthesis capability as well. ^{15}O-water (also a cyclotron produced tracer) can be administered either intravenously or by inhalation of $^{15}CO_2$ with rapid transformation to water by carbonic anhydrase in the lungs. More recently, a novel MPI tracer has been developed (^{18}F-labeled flurpiridaz). This agent is a structural analogue of pyridaben and binds to mitochondrial complex 1 with high affinity.[53] It has a high first-pass extraction fraction of 94% and is currently being evaluated in phase 3 clinical studies. Beyond the tracer kinetics that allows very accurate and reproducible quantification of myocardial perfusion, at least in the experimental setting, the 110-minute half-life of ^{18}F is an additional benefit as it permits a radiopharmaceutical distribution as a single-unit dose on a daily basis. It is estimated that a total administered activity of approximately 520 MBq, for a 2-day protocol, both for stress and rest, provides very satisfactory image quality with acceptable radiation exposure (mean effective dose 0.019 mSv/MBq). For 1-day protocol with adenosine, a minimum dose ratio stress/rest 2.2 is satisfactory, with a half an hour interval between the two administrations. For 1-day protocol with dynamic exercise, a minimum ratio dose stress/rest 3.0 is required, with a time interval of about 1 hour between the two administrations.[54]

Stress Tests

Pharmacologic stress is performed using the same agents, as with the SPECT studies. Although pharmacologic stress is the preferred method of inducing hyperemia, exercise testing can also be performed when ^{13}N-ammonia is used as a perfusion tracer (because of the relatively long physical half-life) but is rarely used in practice. In general, both stress and resting injections are administered while the patient is on the scanner's couch. For assessment of vascular endothelium function, a cold pressor test (CPT) can also be performed, where the patients immerse their left hand in ice water usually for 60 seconds and the tracer is injected while the test continues for another 60 seconds to permit trapping of tracer in the myocardium. CPT is used to assess the health of the vascular endothelium alone as opposed to the stress test performed with the vasodilators, which provides information on the vasomotor function that combines both the endothelial and the smooth muscle cell vasodilator function. CPT has a different action compared to vasodilators as

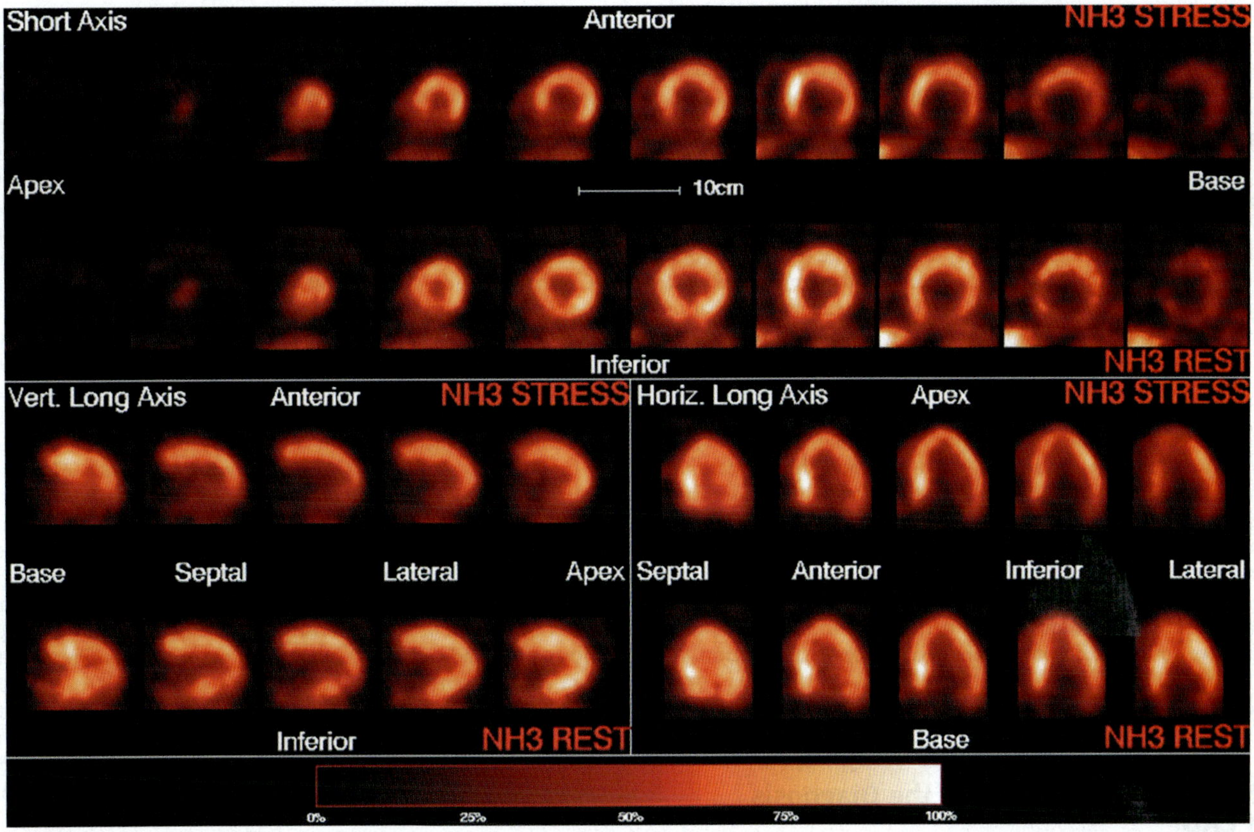

Figure 23-8. Qualitative assessment of myocardial perfusion by stress/rest ^{13}N-ammonia PET. Stress and rest images from a 69-year-old man demonstrating a small area of myocardial infarction at the basal inferior wall and also extensive inducible ischemia involving most of the remaining viable myocardium sparing only the basal septum and the adjacent basal part of the anterior wall. PET, positron emission tomography.

it is based on sympathetic stimulation. Release of norepinephrine from stimulated sympathetic neurons activates α-adrenoceptors on the endothelium that mediate the release of nitric oxide. In the presence of an intact endothelium, this leads to a 30% to 65% increase in myocardial blood flow (MBF) compared to baseline levels. α-Adrenergic stimulation of vascular smooth muscle cells that causes vasoconstriction is normally counteracted; however, if endothelial integrity is impaired, it prevails over the endothelium-derived vasodilatation. CPT is probably the most appropriate test for early detection of endothelial dysfunction in individuals with risk factors for coronary atherosclerosis, as impairment of the endothelial health precedes abnormalities in smooth muscle cell vasodilator function, but requires extensive procedural standardization.[2,51,53]

Imaging Protocols and Image Interpretation

Two sets of images are acquired: at rest and following a stress test. In contemporary general purpose scanners that combine PET with CT, PET MPI is accomplished by obtaining a CT scan first for AC followed by perfusion imaging. A scout image or a topogram to determine the precise location of the heart in the thorax and to position the patient correctly is required, and afterward, a low-dose CT scan is performed covering the heart region. This is usually a nongated, fast (<1 minute), low-resolution scan that is obtained during tidal expiration, breath hold, or shallow breathing. Upon termination of this scan, a resting injection of radiotracer is given and resting images are acquired. After completion of the resting images, pharmacologic stress is performed (as for SPECT imaging), during which a second tracer injection is given. A second transmission scan is then acquired for AC. Both rest and stress images can be combined with ECG gating, thus allowing also assessment of global and regional LV function. With ^{82}Rb, total imaging time is less than 30 minutes, while with ^{13}N-ammonia, this takes longer due to the tracer's longer half-life. The injected activity with ^{82}Rb is 1,500 to 2,500 MBq at rest and the same dose at stress. For ^{13}N-ammonia, the options are either to use a lower activity for rest (370 MBq) and a higher activity for the stress (1,100 MBq) resulting in a faster termination of the study or to inject the same dose (370 MBq) for both studies, but to wait for ^{13}N to sufficiently decay to background levels before the second dose is administered to the patient.[2,51,53]

Myocardial perfusion and hence tracer distribution is uniform in normal myocardium. It should be noted though that with ^{13}N-ammonia, in normal volunteers, there is a mild heterogeneity in the lateral wall of the LV compared with the other segments. As in SPECT MPI, a reversible perfusion defect indicates myocardial ischemia whilst a fixed defect, myocardial infarction. In addition to regional myocardial uptake, other features of the images are important. Of particular significance is LV dilatation in stress images that is less marked on the resting ones since this implies extensive inducible ischemia and is associated with an adverse prognosis. Enlargement of ventricles seen on both the rest and stress studies indicates ventricular dysfunction. The increased right ventricular (RV) uptake is an indicator of pulmonary hypertension with or without RV hypertrophy. In patients with depressed LV systolic function or chronic pulmonary disease or even in smokers, there might be an increase in the uptake of ^{13}N-ammonia or ^{82}Rb in the lungs. To optimize the contrast between myocardial and background activity, it is better in such cases to increase the time between injection and image acquisition. Attention should be paid also to extracardiac findings in the mediastinum or the lungs observed in the CT scan. These findings might have a clinical importance, as they might be associated with malignancy or an inflammatory process.

As in SPECT MPI, the perfusion defects are characterized qualitatively as mild, moderate, and severe, but also semiquantitatively by obtaining measurements (scores) of segmental perfusion according to the standard of 17 segments (see above).

Quantification

In human studies, PET is the gold standard for quantifying myocardial perfusion in absolute terms (mL/min/g) both at rest and stress and also the assessment of coronary vasodilator reserve (CFR). This is because PET has a high sensitivity and temporal resolution, which allow fast dynamic imaging of tracer kinetics and extensively validated algorithms for accurate correction of photon attenuation. Global and regional myocardial perfusion is measured by compartmental (usually one or two tissue compartments) tracer kinetic models, which are then combined with appropriate corrections for physical decay of the radioisotope, partial volume-related underestimation of the true myocardial tissue concentrations, and spillover of radioactivity between the left ventricular blood pool and the myocardium. ^{15}O-water is the ideal tracer for quantification as it diffuses freely across plasma membranes and exhibits a linear relationship between uptake and flow at high flow rates. However, other PET radiopharmaceuticals are quite satisfactory for quantification as well.[51,53] ^{82}Rb compares reasonably well with ^{13}N-ammonia or ^{15}O-water in absolute measurements of myocardial perfusion, and it is therefore an attractive option for hospitals without easy access to a cyclotron.

Clinical Applications of Radionuclide Myocardial Perfusion Imaging

The Role of SPECT MPI in the Diagnosis of CAD

The hallmark of stable CAD is the predictable central chest pain provoked by exertion and relieved by rest. This is caused by obstructive atherosclerosis that results in reduction of myocardial perfusion (and thus ischemia) upon exhaustion of CFR. The need for and the appropriate choice of further investigation of chest pain should be decided on the basis of the pretest likelihood of significant CAD, which can be estimated by different predictive nomograms. Amongst them, the Diamond and Forrester predictive table integrates three clinical variables (quality of chest pain, gender, and age) to provide an estimation of the likelihood of angiographically significant coronary disease.[55] This approach can be refined by incorporating other powerful predictors, such as serum cholesterol levels, systolic blood pressure, and diabetes.[56] Most predictors of pretest likelihood are able to distinguish those at low and high likelihood of CAD but leave many to be classified as intermediate. According to Bayes' theorem,[57] these patients have the most to gain from further investigation, as a positive or negative result allows reclassification of intermediate pretest likelihood to either high or low posttest likelihood, respectively. A positive or negative result can revise the intermediate value to high or low, respectively, while a positive test in patients with low probability of CAD (<15%) is likely to be a false positive, and thus, further investigation would only increase the cost, exposing the patient to unnecessary procedures and risks. On the other hand, most patients with high pretest probability of disease (>85%) do not require further noninvasive investigation for diagnostic purposes, but functional imaging can be performed for risk stratification and management decisions. Exercise electrocardiography (ExECG) remains the test of first choice in many centers, especially in the United States, because it is widely available, is easy to perform, and does not involve radiation exposure. Noninvasive CT coronary angiography is performed in patients unable to exercise or when a stress test is contraindicated, but in some centers, it is a first-line investigation in patients with low to intermediate likelihood of CAD, because it can be carried out quickly and easily and has a high negative predictive value (NPV) (up to 98%).[58] It should be pointed out that while the latter provides information on the morphology of the lumen of the coronary vessels and whether there is stenosis, a stress test enables assessment of hemodynamic response, ECG changes, symptoms, and exercise tolerance during stress, which probably match (or in several instances exceed) the usual level of a patient's activity. Meta-analyses indicate that the average sensitivity and specificity of ExECG are 68% and 77%, respectively.[59] ExECG is of limited value if the patient cannot exercise adequately or has an abnormal resting ECG that precludes ST-segment assessment on exercise (preexcitation, left ventricular hypertrophy, and changes due to the use of digoxin). In these patients, but also in those with a nondiagnostic ExECG result, stress/rest MPI is ideally suited for use in the diagnosis of stable CAD due to its ability to assess directly myocardial perfusion and its alterations during exercise or pharmacologic stress. Normal myocardial perfusion after stress indicates the absence of functionally significant CAD and is associated with a low risk (<1%; see below) of future coronary events.[60]

It should be noted that normal stress perfusion is *not* synonymous with the absence of CAD, as coronary atherosclerosis need not necessarily cause stenosis of sufficient severity to result in impairment of CFR. In the presence of abnormal perfusion, the site, depth, and extent of the demonstrated ischemia provide diagnostic information and can guide subsequent management. On a recent meta-analysis, sensitivity and specificity were 85% to 90% and 70% to 75%, respectively, for the detection of angiographically significant CAD.[61] It is important to recognize that conventional coronary angiography (ICA) is an anatomical rather than a functional technique and that a "significant" stenosis on ICA may be associated with normal CFR. In clinical practice therefore, and unless ICA is combined with functional indexes of the coronary status (e.g., intracoronary Doppler velocity wire flow reserve or coronary pressure wire measurements), the techniques should be seen as providing complementary rather than necessarily equivalent information.

The sensitivity and specificity of SPECT MPI can be improved using ECG gated[62] and AC. ECG gated allows quantitation of global and regional ventricular function that, aside from providing important prognostic information, aids in the distinction of artifacts from true perfusion defects, thus improving specificity and normalcy. Fixed defects in the anterior and inferior walls, commonly due to breast and diaphragmatic attenuation artifacts in women and men, respectively, may be mistaken for myocardial infarction, but myocardial motion and thickening in these areas are normal on gated images. Similarly, the use of AC to recover counts in these areas further improves the recognition of attenuation artifacts and hence diagnostic accuracy. A common cause of suboptimal specificity of SPECT MPI reported in earlier studies is posttest referral bias. In other words, when the reference standard (in this case ICA) is not performed in all patients and referral to angiography is more likely when SPECT MPI is reported as abnormal, then the results are affected by posttest referral bias and specificity appears falsely low. Normalcy, the number of patients at low likelihood of coronary disease with normal SPECT MPI, is a better index for assessing the performance of the test for excluding disease, and this was found to be consistently high (around 90%) irrespective of tracer or method of stress.[61]

SPECT MPI in Risk Stratification and Management of Patients

Risk Assessment in Patients with Suspected or Confirmed CAD

The risk of future cardiac events, such as myocardial infarction or death, is a significant determinant of treatment type. A number of factors, such as extent of anatomic disease, total ischemic burden, degree of LV dysfunction, threshold of angina, presence of comorbidities such as severe peripheral vascular disease or diabetes, and uncontrolled CAD risk factors, contribute to the annual risk of cardiac events, which may be classified as low (<1%), intermediate (1% to 3%), or high (>3%).[63] Numerous studies have confirmed the excellent prognostic power of SPECT MPI and its important role in risk stratification and patients' management.[64–66] In addition, SPECT MPI provides incremental information over and above that obtained by clinical or stress ECG data. Several large studies reporting prognostic analyses of MPI in cohorts using exercise, vasodilator, or both types of stress in various clinical settings have documented the incremental value of MPI.[67–69] The incremental value of SPECT MPI can be increased further for assessing the probability of death due to cardiovascular causes by incorporating information on LVEF and LV end-systolic volume derived from the gated data.

A normal SPECT MPI is associated with a 0.7% annual risk of MI and cardiac death, which is similar to the general population.[70] This has important clinical implications because a normal study obviates the need for invasive investigation or revascularization. It should be noted, however, that the value 0.7% per year represents an average annual event rate and a normal perfusion study should always be interpreted in the context of the individual patient. For instance, patients with normal myocardial perfusion but significant ST segment depression during adenosine stress are at increased risk for nonfatal myocardial infarction, (7.6% compared to 0.5% in patients without such findings, during a mean follow-up period of 29 +/– 12 months).[71] In addition, higher heart rate at rest and a blunted heart rate increase during adenosine infusion have also been found to be predictors of severe future events. Specific groups, such as the elderly, those with diabetes, or those with known CAD, have an annual event rate somewhat higher (1.4% to 1.8% per year) despite normal SPECT MPI.[65] In general, the "warranty period" of a normal SPECT MPI in this setting is around 2 years, after which repeat scanning may be necessary to redefine prognosis.

An abnormal scan confers around a sevenfold increase in annual cardiac events compared to a normal study.[72] The probability of a cardiovascular event increases in parallel with increasing depth and extent of reversibility of inducible ischemia, which are markers of the stenosis severity and the amount of myocardium subtended by the stenosed vessels, respectively. Those with only mild inducible ischemia have an annual event rate of around 3%, which rises to 7% in those with severe ischemia. The presence of corollary markers of severe 3-vessel disease, such as transient left ventricular dilatation[73] or increased lung uptake of ^{201}Tl,[74] increases the event rate still further (Table 23.4).

TABLE
23.4 High-Risk Imaging Variables

- Multiple myocardial perfusion defects
- Extensive reversibility of a perfusion defect
- Transient left ventricular dilation
- Multiple regional wall motion or wall thickening abnormalities
- Left ventricular ejection fraction <35%
- Increased end-diastolic and/or end-systolic volume in ECG-gated SPECT
- Increased lung tracer uptake
- LV dyssynchrony assessed by phase analysis

Patients with mildly abnormal SPECT MPI are generally at low risk of cardiac death; therefore, if they are not limited by their symptoms, these patients might be candidates for aggressive medical therapy/risk factor modification. However, this is not the case in patients with significant comorbidities (e.g., advanced age, prior CAD, diabetes mellitus, atrial fibrillation, pharmacologic stress, etc).[68] The decision, therefore, whether or not to catheterize a patient with a mildly abnormal perfusion scan becomes a function of the underlying patient condition.

In the current era, SPECT MPI is used increasingly to test the effectiveness of different management strategies both on a clinical basis and cost-effectiveness basis. The largest and most representative study included 13, 969 patients who were investigated with SPECT MPI and followed up over 8 years.[75] The results showed that patients without extensive scar but significant (at least 10%) ischemic myocardium were likely to realize a survival benefit from early revascularization. In contrast, patients with minimal ischemia fared better on medical therapy without early revascularization. These findings agree with those from the SPECT MPI substudy of the Clinical Outcomes Using Revascularization and Aggressive Drug Evaluation trial, which included 314 patients with known CAD.[76] Patients who were randomized to receive percutaneous coronary intervention (PCI) in addition to optimal medical therapy (OMT) had a greater reduction in inducible ischemia than did those randomized to receive OMT alone. Reduction in ischemia was associated with improvement in angina frequency and stability, and this was more pronounced in patients with baseline moderate-to-severe ischemia.

In view of the large body of evidence on the diagnostic and prognostic value of SPECT MPI, a number of guidelines recommend its use in a wide range of clinical scenarios. Both European and American guidelines recommend SPECT MPI in patients with an intermediate likelihood of disease.[77–79] All guidelines emphasize the accuracy of vasodilator stress with SPECT MPI in patients with LBBB, paced rhythm, resting ST segment depression greater than 1 mm, or preexcitation. When CAD is already known, SPECT MPI is recommended for symptomatic patients to assess the severity of ischemic burden, and in the presence of significant ischemia, coronary angiography is recommended. When the latter has already taken place and an assessment of the functional significance of a coronary stenosis is required, SPECT MPI is also indicated.

The Role of SPECT MPI in the Assessment of Special Populations

Asymptomatic Patients

The role of SPECT MPI in the assessment of *asymptomatic patients* with risk factors but absence of known CAD has been the focus of numerous studies recently. Although more precise risk stratification is achieved following SPECT MPI in subjects with an intermediate (6% to 20% risk for MI or death over 10 years) or high (>20% over 10 years) Framingham Risk Score (FRS), there are no outcome data from randomized trials evaluating the clinical impact and cost-effectiveness of imaging-based treatment. According to the recommendations of European and American professional societies, SPECT MPI is indicated for assessment of asymptomatic subjects with a family history of premature CAD as well as in patients with diabetes and increased coronary calcium score (CAC) score.[80,81] A debatable point is the indication of SPECT MPI in subjects with intermediate FRS and elevated CAC score. The 2010 ACC/AHA Guideline for Assessment of Cardiovascular Risk in Asymptomatic Adults recommends the use of SPECT MPI in this group (in moderate-risk patients according to the FRS and CAC score >400 or in high risk and CAC score 100 to 400), while the position statement of the Working Group on Nuclear Cardiology and Cardiac CT of the ESC advocates against this approach favoring aggressive medical management.[80,81] The value of SPECT MPI in medical conditions that portend a similar cardiovascular risk to established CAD has also been studied. This spectrum includes peripheral vascular disease, abdominal aortic aneurysm, and erectile dysfunction. Novel data suggest that patients with any of these conditions may benefit from SPECT MPI, but at present, there is no sufficient level of evidence to make concrete recommendations.[82]

A special group of patients for which the existing data suggest that the SPECT MPI has an excellent diagnostic accuracy and independent prognostic value is that of subjects with chronic kidney disease (CKD). Greater extent of inducible perfusion abnormalities and greater degrees of renal dysfunction are associated with higher risks of cardiac complications. What is yet to be ascertained is whether coronary revascularization improves outcomes in such patients with CKD and abnormal findings on SPECT MPI.[82] Finally, SPECT MPI can be useful for follow-up assessment at 2-year or longer intervals in asymptomatic patients with known stable disease and prior evidence of silent ischemia or who are at an increased risk for a coronary event and (a) are unable to exercise to an adequate workload, (b) have an *uninterpretable ECG, or (c) have a history of* incomplete coronary revascularization.

Preoperative Evaluation of Patients Who Are to Undergo Noncardiac Surgery

For assessment of patients who are scheduled to undergo noncardiac surgery, the ACC/AHA guidelines recommend limited use of SPECT MPI. In all patients, the assessment begins by determining the Revised Cardiac Risk Index (RCRI), which is formed on the presence or absence of six factors, each of which receives a point. These factors are high-risk surgery, history of ischemia, congestive HF, stroke, preoperative treatment with insulin, and high preoperative serum creatinine levels (>2 mg/dL). SPECT MPI is suitable for preoperative evaluation of asymptomatic patients scheduled to undergo intermediate-risk surgery and have an RCRI score ≥1 *and* low (<4 METs) or uncertain functional capacity and for those with RCRI score ≥ 1 *or* low functional capacity scheduled for high-risk surgery.[83]

Investigation of Women with Chest Pain

In female patients, the different hormonal substrate compared to men results in higher incidence of atherosclerosis with diffuse vascular abnormalities and lower rate of stenotic lesions, but different composition of atherosclerotic plaque with more fibrous tissue.[84] Overall, in female patients, ExECG shows moderate accuracy for detecting CAD. In contrast, SPECT MPI is equally accurate for male and female patients.[85] In combination with dynamic or pharmacologic stress, SPECT MPI is a very reliable noninvasive imaging technique for evaluation of women with intermediate to high pretest likelihood of CAD.[86–89] In the most recent meta-analysis (26 studies, 1,148 women), the sensitivity and specificity values of SPECT MPI were 84.2% and 78.7%, respectively.[90] The diagnostic accuracy of SPECT MPI in women may be affected by breast attenuation, the small size of LV cavity, and the high prevalence of single-vessel disease; however, use of ECG gating or AC can improve specificity. In terms of risk assessment, SPECT MPI is equally robust in women as it is in men, and in both populations, prognosis is refined when factors such as diabetes, metabolic syndrome, or peripheral vascular disease are considered along with the scan result.[86–92] The pretest likelihood is an important factor for the choice of the appropriate stress test when investigating women with chest pain. In the recent results from the "what is the optimal method for ischemia evaluation in women" (women) randomized study comprising 824 female patients and comparing ExECC with stress SPECT MPI, there were no significant differences in terms of major cardiovascular events in women with normal results (0.4% for ExECG vs. 1.2% for SPECT MPI).[93] These findings suggest that for lower-risk patients with good functional capacity and not known CAD, ExECG should be the initial test to assess whether myocardial ischemia is present or not.

Investigation of Patients with Diabetes Mellitus

Several studies have investigated the diagnostic and prognostic value of SPECT MPI demonstrating that overall, the high diagnostic value of SPECT MPI and its ability to prognosticate accurately are maintained in patients with diabetes.[94,95] More recently, however, the multicenter study Detection of Ischemia in Asymptomatic Diabetics, which included 1,123 asymptomatic patients with type II diabetes, showed significantly lower rate of cardiovascular events than it was expected to during a follow-up period of 4.8 years. Mortality rates did not differ significantly in patients who underwent SPECT MPI and those who were not (2.7% vs. 3.0%), while similar rates were reported for revascularization (5.5% vs. 7.8%) in the two groups. The positive predictive value (PPV) of moderate and severe perfusion defects was only 12%. According to this study, routine use of SPECT MPI in the above group of patients is not justified either on clinical or cost-effectiveness grounds.[96] Considering that in asymptomatic patients with diabetes, CAC score is a useful parameter for risk assessment, an alternative strategy is to apply sequential risk stratification based on careful assessment of risk factors, followed by CAC score measurement, and then SPECT MPI for individuals with a score >400.[80,97,98] In addition, SPECT MPI is recommended in asymptomatic diabetic patients with autonomic neuropathy, or when other evidence of vascular disease, such as peripheral arterial disease (e.g., carotid, renal, femoral), is present or when there is an abnormal ECG. For symptomatic patients, SPECT MPI is recommended for those with mild angina and normal ECG and in patients with multiple risk factors and atypical chest pain.[99] It should always be born in mind that this is a challenging group for management decisions and a referral of an individual patient to SPECT MPI should be carefully examined, taking into consideration also the existing data on the value of different therapeutic strategies. Interestingly, the main Bypass Angioplasty Revascularization Investigation 2 Diabetes study did not reveal any survival advantage after revascularization compared with medical therapy, which is different from the results of a previous randomized study by Sorajja et al., suggesting that coronary artery bypass graft (CABG) improves survival even in asymptomatic patients, if there are high-risk features in SPECT MPI.[100,101]

Postrevascularization

Several studies performed before the introduction of drug-eluting stents, investigating the value of routine SPECT MPI in patients post-PCI at different time intervals, have shown that SPECT provides useful information on restenosis, disease progression, and additional risk stratification in this patient population. In the current era, where the majority of patients undergo PCI with drug-eluting stents and the rate of restenosis is significantly lower compared to bare metal stents and angioplasty, there is no direct evidence to support routine use of SPECT MPI after the intervention.[82,102,103] Current guidelines recommend SPECT MPI in patients presenting with symptoms suggestive of underlying ischemia. Based on published guidelines and appropriate use criteria, regarding asymptomatic patients who have undergone PCI, SPECT MPI is recommended in patients with high risk-features, such as decreased LV function, multivessel disease, or proximal LAD disease, or when there is history of sudden cardiac death, diabetes mellitus, employment in a hazardous occupations, or incomplete revascularization.[104] If the aforementioned features are not present, SPECT MPI is not recommended earlier than 2 years from the date of the intervention. The physician who reads the SPECT MPI scans should be very careful when interpreting such studies soon after PCI as reversible perfusion abnormalities can occur after intervention in the absence of restenosis and are attributable to microvascular disturbances or endothelial damage. Reduced response to vasodilator stress can last from 7 days to 3 months.[105]

Regarding patients with CABG, studies on those with recurrent symptoms have shown that SPECT MPI is useful in detecting ischemia due to unrevascularized myocardial segments or early graft failure. A strategy of routine testing 1 year after bypass found that the overall event rate was low and that routine perfusion imaging early after bypass did not add any important prognostic information.[102,103] Several studies have demonstrated the independent and incremental predictive value of SPECT MPI for future coronary events in asymptomatic patients more than 5 years after CABG; however, recent data suggest that repeat revascularization in asymptomatic patients provides no survival benefit even if inducible ischemia is present. SPECT MPI has a good diagnostic accuracy for demonstrating graft occlusion or stenosis post-CABG with sensitivity and specificity values of 81% and 79%, respectively.[106,107] A normal result excludes significant restenosis or worsening of underlying CAD, with good prognosis. According to international guidelines, patients with normal SPECT MPI or small perfusion defects after revascularization if respond well to conservative treatment usually do not require further investigation. In contrast, symptomatic patients with large reversible perfusion defects should be directed to coronary angiography.[106]

The Role of PET Perfusion Imaging in the Evaluation of Patients with Suspected or Known CAD

PET has higher spatial resolution and an improved contrast as compared to SPECT. This allows a more conspicuous identification of regional differences in radiotracer uptake during stress, thus increasing the sensitivity for detecting flow-limiting CAD. In addition, PET affords a more robust AC than does SPECT.[108,109] Such properties make PET a superior modality compared to SPECT, particularly for cases where image quality can be degraded with SPECT, as it occurs in obese patients or in women where a breast attenuation artifact can lead to a false-positive result. In a recent meta-analysis (total of 23 studies), which focused on the diagnostic accuracy for detecting CAD, PET had sensitivity and specificity of 90% and 88%, respectively. For SPECT, the corresponding values of both the sensitivity and specificity were 85%.[110]

PET has also been used for risk stratification, and its overall prognostic value over and above clinical and angiographic evaluation has been demonstrated in several studies that included large series of patients. Total cardiac events (hard events, revascularization, and hospitalization) and in particular cardiac mortality are uncommon when the scan result is normal, with 3-year event rates of 1.7% and 1%, respectively.[111,112] Event rates increase with SSS, which is the strongest predictor of total cardiac events. In the study by Yoshinaga et al.,[113] the annual cardiac event rate was 0.4% for normal, 2.3% for mildly abnormal, and 7% for moderately and severely abnormal PET scans. An abnormal vasodilator LVEF reserve (stress minus rest LVEF) is not only a marker of extensive anatomic obstructive CAD (providing higher sensitivity than do the perfusion data alone) (79% vs. 50%) but also an independent and incremental marker for patients' outcomes. In line with previous studies from the SPECT literature, the direct relationship between the scan result and event rate was confirmed, and in addition, the annualized rates of coronary events (2.1% vs. 5.3%, $p < 0.001$) and all-cause death (4.3% vs. 9.2%, $p < 0.001$) were higher in patients with an LVEF reserve <0% compared with those with an LVEF reserve ≥0%[114,115].

Absolute quantification of myocardial perfusion (mL/min/g) that is currently performed only in specialized centers has also been used for diagnosis and prognosis assessment. Quantification enables calculation of CFR, the ratio of myocardial perfusion during pharmacologically induced vasodilatation to resting perfusion. Quantitative assessment of the hyperemic response to stress and CFR can enhance further the sensitivity of myocardial perfusion PET, particularly for detection of multivessel disease or balanced ischemia that cannot be appreciated by assessment of relative perfusion.[116] Recent data demonstrate that absolute quantification may be more accurate than CFR, because the latter is a ratio, and therefore, factors that influence either the numerator or the denominator may affect its calculation. The optimal threshold values of hyperemic myocardial perfusion and CFR are dependent on PET tracer and methodology used for quantification. In a recent study with ^{13}N-ammonia, a threshold of <1.85 mL/min/g has provided a diagnostic accuracy of 90% for detecting a >50% angiographic stenosis, while in a different study with ^{15}O-water, a higher threshold of 2.5 mL/min/g provided the highest diagnostic accuracy. Similar differences for cutoff values exist for CFR. Quantification, however, may lead to a reduced specificity as causes other than epicardial disease, such as microvascular dysfunction, can also affect myocardial perfusion and CFR. Therefore, interpretation of reduced values should be made with caution taking into consideration the clinical setting and the presence of factors that may affect the microcirculation. On the other hand, if coronary anatomy is known, quantification provides accurate information on the functional significance of a coronary lesion that can be utilized for management decisions. Recent studies of centers with great experience in PET have shown that the quantification increases the diagnostic accuracy, enhancing the sensitivity of the method, to 96%, without loss of specificity, and further improves the detection of multivessel disease.[116,117]

In patients with CAD, both the hyperemic response and CFR are inversely and nonlinearly related to stenosis severity.[118,119] Regarding prognosis, as shown in multiple studies, including the largest and most recent to date, that of Murthy et al. comprising 2,783 patients who underwent PET study with ^{82}Rb, the overall reduction in CFR is associated with poor prognosis, providing information over and above that obtained by semiquantitative analysis alone.[120–122] This allows a more accurate risk stratification of patients investigated for CAD, particularly those with moderate or no ischemia based on qualitative assessment. Perfusion quantification in combination with pharmacologic stress using vasodilators or CPT may also be helpful for detection of early stages of atherosclerosis or microvascular dysfunction and prognosis assessment of individuals with risk factors for CAD, as well as for monitoring of therapeutic strategies.[123,124]

Comparison of SPECT and PET with Other Imaging Techniques

There are alternative techniques for the noninvasive assessment of myocardial perfusion, and these include echocardiography and cardiac magnetic resonance (CMR). Perfusion imaging by CT is also feasible following similar principles to first-pass gadolinium chelate CMR and is currently under investigation.[125] Stress echo with the use of exercise or dobutamine identifies the presence of flow-limiting coronary stenosis in the form of ischemia-induced regional wall motion abnormality with a sensitivity of 89% for exercise and 72% for dobutamine stress.[126] An important advance is the addition of real-time perfusion, which improves the sensitivity to 98% for exercise and 85% for dobutamine echocardiography. This is a procedure without the use of ionizing radiation that can be performed with standard, widely available equipment. There are however some limitations yet to overcome. The procedure remains highly operator dependent, and there is a considerable learning curve for both image acquisition and interpretation. As for conventional transthoracic echocardiography (TTE), the diagnostic yield depends greatly on image quality.

Perfusion CMR is another alternative to PET or SPECT for perfusion imaging with reported sensitivity and specificity values of 84% to 91% and 58% to 94%, respectively. CMR provides detailed information on cardiac morphology and structure including tissue characterization and is currently regarded as the reference method for assessment of ventricular function. While CMR does not involve ionizing radiation, the gadolinium chelate–based contrast agents are not without risk, and this is greater in patients with significantly impaired renal function.[127] Although new and MRI compatible devices have been engineered, at present, CMR cannot be carried out in most patients with implanted pacemakers and ICDs. Compared to PET, the most recent meta-analysis that focuses on diagnostic accuracy for detecting CAD and includes also comparisons with SPECT has demonstrated that CMR has superior sensitivity compared to SPECT MPI but lags behind PET both in specificity and overall diagnostic accuracy.[128] Constant improvements in CMR technology such as blood oxygen level dependent or whole-heart coverage with dynamic 3D-CMR perfusion imaging that utilizes undersampling in k-space and time (k-t) allow performance of perfusion quantification; however, the correlation of measurements between CMR and PET (reference method) is weak.[129,130]

Cost-Effectiveness of SPECT and PET Myocardial Perfusion Studies

The application of SPECT MPI allows a cost advantageous risk stratification of patients as compared with other noninvasive imaging methods, but also with coronary angiography. The Economics of Noninvasive Diagnosis (END) study showed that when stable chest pain patients undergo a diagnostic strategy based on direct catheterization have higher diagnostic costs and greater rates of intervention and follow-up costs, compared to strategy according to which patients with stable angina undergo initial SPECT MPI and then selective angiography.[131] The results of the Economics of Myocardial Perfusion Imaging in Europe also showed that strategies that used SPECT MPI for diagnostic and management decisions were cheaper but equally effective compared to strategies that are not using SPECT MPI. This was true both in terms of cost per patient up to the final diagnosis and the final outcome of each patient after 2 years.[132] Regarding cost-effectiveness of PET in the diagnosis and management of CAD, there are limited studies. Patterson et al.[133] have compared cost-effectiveness and cost utility of exercise ECG, SPECT, PET, and coronary angiography to diagnose obstructive CAD. Effectiveness was defined as the number of patients with diagnosed CAD and utility as the number of quality-adjusted life years extended by therapy after the diagnosis.[134] They observed that in patients with a pretest likelihood of CAD less than 70%, PET is the most cost-effective test, with the lower cost per utility. This was due to its superior diagnostic accuracy and avoidance of false-positive and false-negative studies. On the contrary, when the pretest likelihood of CAD is above 70%, coronary angiography is the most cost effective approach. More recently, Merhige et al. have studied the frequency of diagnostic arteriography, revascularization, costs, and 1-year clinical outcomes of 102 patients with an intermediate probability of CAD who have undergone PET and compared costs, procedure rates, and outcomes both with an internal and an additional external group studied with SPECT MPI and matched for CAD probability. They have confirmed the results by Patterson et al. demonstrating that PET with ^{82}Rb in patients with intermediate pretest likelihood of CAD results in more than 50% reduction in invasive coronary arteriography and CABG rates and a 30% cost savings, with no significant difference in cardiac death or MI at 1-year follow-up compared with SPECT.[135] The issue of cost-effectiveness of different noninvasive imaging strategies is explored currently by ongoing and better designed studies such as SPARC (Study of Myocardial Perfusion and Coronary Anatomy Imaging Roles in Coronary Artery Disease) and EVINCI (Evaluation of INtegrated Cardiac Imaging for the Detection, Characterization and Monitoring of Ischemic Heart Disease), the results of which are expected with a great interest by the medical community.[136,137]

Hybrid imaging and Atherosclerotic Coronary Disease

Combined assessment of coronary anatomy and function is an attractive option that is feasible with the new PET/CT and SPECT/CT systems. Recent data suggest that combined evaluation of myocardial perfusion by SPECT MPI and CAC may achieve a higher sensitivity for detecting CAD than does perfusion assessment alone. This approach is more clinically relevant in the presence of a normal SPECT MPI scan, where a high (>400) CAC score is associated with an increased cardiac event rate (3% per year). Furthermore, the addition of CAC score defines more precisely the warranty period of a normal SPECT MPI study with a shorter "event-free" period in subjects with normal perfusion but a high CAC score. Moreover, combined SPECT MPI and coronary computed tomography angiogram (CTA) using fusion software has an incremental value over SPECT MPI alone, mainly by allowing a more accurate assignment of perfusion defects to the involved vessels, thus improving diagnostic accuracy on per vessel analysis and detection of multivessel disease. Other studies have shown that hybrid SPECT/CTA imaging shows excellent diagnostic accuracy in stenoses of ≥50% in the coronary vessels compared with SPECT MPI and allows better risk stratification for patients with known or suspected CAD for future cardiovascular events. It has also been shown that SPECT/CTA can guide more accurately the management of CAD patients.[138,139]

Regarding the combination of PET and angiographic data from CT, the largest of these studies has included 107 patients with chest pain and intermediate likelihood of CAD. The study compares hybrid ^{15}O-water PET and CTA versus CTA or PET alone for detecting hemodynamically significant CAD using quantitative coronary angiography along with fractional flow reserve measurements for lesions of intermediate severity.[140] Although both PET and CTA alone demonstrated high (97%) NPV, CTA was suboptimal in assessing the severity of stenosis (PPV 76%) and PET could not separate microvascular disease from epicardial stenoses (PPV 77%) in all patients. The combined use of PET-CTA improved significantly diagnostic accuracy to 98%. Sensitivity, specificity, PPV, and NPV were 93%, 99%, 96%, and 99%, respectively. Combining CAC with PET imaging is also feasible. In a recent study, Schenker et al.[141] have assessed patients with an intermediate pretest likelihood of CAD and demonstrated that the annualized event rate in patients with normal PET MPI and no CAC was substantially lower than among those with a CAC score ≥1,000 (2.6% vs. 12.3%). Likewise, the annualized event rate in patients with ischemia on PET and no CAC was also lower than among those with a CAC score ≥1,000 (8.2% vs. 22.1%). More recently, the same group has assessed 901 consecutive patients undergoing ^{82}Rb PET and CAC scan. All patients had a normal PET scan by qualitative assessment. They found that among symptomatic patients without obstructive CAD, although both the severity of coronary calcium deposits and the presence of coronary vascular dysfunction were associated with increased risk of adverse cardiac events, after adjustment for clinical risk, only coronary vascular dysfunction (assessed by CFR) improved risk assessment. These results suggest that direct measures of coronary vascular function, reflecting disease activity in the coronary circulation, may improve phenotypic characterization of atherosclerosis and result in enhanced risk stratification and prediction of cardiovascular events among symptomatic patients.[142]

Future studies are needed to assess the impact of PET/CTA or SPECT/CTA imaging on clinical outcomes and to investigate the cost-effectiveness of a hybrid approach. Until the results of such studies become available, a logical approach is to perform anatomical or functional imaging sequentially, selecting cardiac CT or PET (or SPECT) according to the pretest probability of disease. In patients with a rather low likelihood of CAD, CTA would be appropriate because of its high NPV, while PET (or SPECT) should be performed first in patients with a higher probability of disease. The decision to perform a second study should be made on an individual basis and must balance risks and benefits. Total radiation burden is an issue, if a patient is to undergo a combined examination; however, improvements in CT image acquisition (e.g., prospective ECG-triggered sequential scanning), along with the possibility to omit the resting perfusion study if the stress scan is normal, may achieve considerable reduction in radiation exposure.[143]

Recently, the combination of PET imaging with MRI with its excellent soft tissue contrast is a very appealing possibility for investigating several cardiovascular diseases. The main differences of PET/MRI compared with PET/CT are the reduction of radiation dose, the improvement of soft tissue resolution, but limited means of imaging the coronaries and extended examination times. From a technical point of view, the challenge of hybrid PET/MRI is that the conventional design of PET scanners uses photomultiplier tubes (PMTs), which are used to detect the positron annihilation photons. PMTs are very sensitive to even weak magnetic fields and cannot be used in integrated PET/MRI.[144] After overcoming those technical obstacles, however, PET/MRI appears now to be a very promising modality for improved tissue characterization and also atherosclerotic plaque imaging. For the latter, it can combine the high sensitivity of PET to demonstrate accumulation of a specific agent with MRI's high-resolution depiction of the morphology of plaques. With respect to tissue characterization in the assessment of myocardial viability/hibernation, PET/MRI may also be an ideal technique because it allows a detailed delineation of the amount of viable tissue simultaneously with the amount of myocardial scarring and its transmural distribution (see below and elsewhere in this book). In addition, hybrid PET/MRI may prove a valuable tool for assessing novel therapeutic strategies such as cell and gene therapies by allowing localization of the gene expression or the cell engraftment area at high spatial resolution together with morphologic and functional description of the target myocardium.[145]

Diagnosis and Management of Patients with Acute Chest Pain and Acute Coronary Syndrome

SPECT MPI is a very sensitive test for detection of acute myocardial infarction. SPECT MPI is especially useful in those patients with an intermediate likelihood of CAD and chest pain in the absence of diagnostic ECG changes.[146,147] Abnormal resting SPECT MPI in this setting has a high sensitivity for acute infarction particularly if it is associated with regional wall motion abnormalities on gated imaging. Normal resting SPECT MPI excludes acute infarction and suggests that either ExECG or stress SPECT MPI should be the next diagnostic step. If tracer injection occurs during chest pain, normal SPECT MPI rules out an ACS and allows the patient to be discharged. SPECT MPI is therefore especially useful in the stratification of patients with symptoms suggestive of ACS but without ECG changes to either admission or discharge. In those with definitive acute cardiac ischemia on ECG, SPECT MPI has no impact on the clinical decision making. In those without definitive ischemia, acute resting SPECT MPI may reduce unnecessary admissions by up to 20% with a mean cost saving per patient of $4258, irrespective of gender, age, or risk factors for CAD.[148]

SPECT MPI has been used in patients with acute myocardial infarction to assess the extent of the myocardium at risk as well as the effect of intracoronary thrombolysis or intervention.[149] The most appropriate radiotracers are MIBI or tetrofosmin, administered before reperfusion. Due to the nonsignificant redistribution, imaging can be performed later, when the patient is stable, because the obtained image represents the perfusion conditions that existed in the myocardium before reperfusion. Reinjection of radiotracer and then imaging takes place a few days later, and the difference between the two images allows accurate assessment of the salvaged myocardium.[150]

The prognosis of patients with acute MI depends on several factors, and therefore, it is particularly important to identify those patients who are at risk to suffer a second MI or die. In the acute phase, important clinical markers of high risk are history of prior myocardial infarction especially in the anterior wall, advanced age, Killip class >I, increased serum creatinine, recurrence of angina, hypotension, HF, AV block, and serious arrhythmias. Therefore, patients with one or more of the above characteristics should be referred for coronary angiography and PCI if it is possible. Stratification of patients can also occur after reperfusion therapy, and at this stage, it is important to identify patients at high risk for future events (such as myocardial infarction or death), to ensure timely intervention in order to avoid them. The assessment of the extent of myocardial infarction and function of LV at rest, which are important prognostic factors, is usually done by echocardiography, but also with nuclear techniques, which are accurate enough to estimate the above parameters. A number of studies have shown that there is a close relationship between the size of the perfusion defect (as assessed with SPECT MPI at rest with MIBI/tetrofosmin or ^{201}Tl) corresponding to myocardial fibrosis and measurements that have traditionally been used in clinical practice to assess infarct size, including EF, end-systolic volumes, regional wall motion, and enzymes.

Whether further investigation will follow immediately before or after hospital discharge depends on the available means and whether PCI has been successful. When PCI is performed in patients with acute ST elevation MI (STEMI), it is usually not necessary to perform a stress test for risk stratification. However, for patients with multivessel disease, or in those for whom a further revascularization procedure is considered, a stress test is indicated for assessment of myocardial ischemia. In the group of patients with severe impairment of ventricular function, SPECT MPI at rest is recommended for viability assessment in the infarct area and also for prediction of recovery of LV function postrevascularization. Additionally, in post-STEMI stable patients who have not undergone coronary angiography, early SPECT MPI (2 to 4 days after acute MI) can be performed safely for assessment of myocardial ischemia, which contributes to risk stratification and management decisions.[151,152] The risk of future events is related to the infarct location (an anterior infarct usually has worse prognosis than does an inferior one), its extent (this is related to the number of fixed deficits), the presence or not of LV remodeling, and the severity of myocardial ischemia. European and American guidelines also support the use of SPECT MPI for detection of ischemia in patients with non–ST segment myocardial infarction who are not candidates for early intervention.[153] The most recent study underpinning the contribution of SPECT MPI in ACS is the adenosine MIBI SPECT Post-Infarction Evaluation (INSPIRE) study, which showed that SPECT MPI can identify a lower-risk population that is best managed with OMT alone and separate also higher-risk patients for whom revascularization would be beneficial.[154] Moreover, new data suggest that infarct size and LV volumes by SPECT MPI can predict with reasonable accuracy LV remodeling following acute STEMI treated with primary PCI.[155]

SPECT and PET Perfusion Imaging in Heart Failure

Approximately 23 million people worldwide suffer from HF, 5.8 from them in the United States.[156,157] There are multiple causes of HF: CAD is the underlying etiology of approximately two-thirds of cases of systolic HF, although hypertension and diabetes are probable contributing factors in many cases. There are many other causes of systolic HF, which include previous viral infection (recognized or unrecognized), alcohol abuse, chemotherapy (e.g., doxorubicin or trastuzumab), and "idiopathic" dilated cardiomyopathy (DCM). Regardless of etiology of HF, a number of neurohormonal, immunologic, and biochemical alterations may be common in these patients and reflected in a series of biomarkers, which are detected in the circulation and support the diagnosis and prognosis of the disease course, in parallel with the clinical evaluation and imaging techniques.[158] These changes include (a) activation of molecular mechanisms, (b) structural changes in the heart and other organs such as the kidneys and lungs, and (c) systemic changes such as chronic inflammation.

Investigation of Etiology of Heart Failure

In addition to objective evidence of a structural or functional abnormality of the heart, HF can be diagnosed by the presence of typical symptoms and signs such as dyspnea, cough, anorexia, nausea, lower extremity edema, etc. Common investigations in this setting include laboratory tests (natriuretic peptides, troponins) and noninvasive imaging. TTE is the recommended test for evaluation of systolic and diastolic dysfunction and is considered mandatory in patients with suspected HF. Radionuclide and CMR imaging are also used, particularly the latter in subjects with inadequate echocardiographic images or where the echocardiographic findings are inconclusive or incomplete. Current guidelines recommend myocardial perfusion/ischemia imaging (echocardiography, CMR, SPECT, or PET) in patients thought to have CAD and who are considered suitable for coronary revascularization, to determine whether there is inducible myocardial ischemia or viable myocardium.[159,160]

Radionuclide imaging plays a pivotal role in the identification of myocardial ischemia as underlying cause of HF as its treatment may improve symptoms, ventricular function, and, importantly, long-term outcome. The latter is related to the severity of the ischemic burden as well as to the degree of LV dysfunction. These parameters can be measured accurately by radionuclide imaging techniques using either single-photon or positron-emitting radiotracers.[161] The most recent study in this field, the Imaging HF study, has confirmed findings from previous studies demonstrating that in hospitalized patients with newly diagnosed HF, SPECT imaging has a high NPV for excluding CAD (close to 100%), but its PPV is around 50%.[26,161] This is because significant myocardial fibrosis and impaired CFR during hyperemic stress may all occur in the absence of epicardial coronary obstruction with resultant abnormalities that can mimic significant CAD on SPECT MPI.

Specific Issues on Radionuclide Imaging of the Ischemic HF

Assessment of Perfusion and Myocardial Viability

The term viable myocardium means "alive" myocardium without special reference to the metabolic state of perfusion and function. Often, the terms "viable" and "hibernating" myocardium are used as synonyms, ignoring the fact that the definition of viability is wide and covers different pathophysiologic entities, one of which is the "hibernating" myocardium. Cardiac radionuclide imaging and PET in particular have been used extensively in this setting and contributed significantly to our understanding of the underlying pathophysiology. Two pathophysiologic phenomena have been described: stunning and hibernation. Stunning refers to the phenomenon of regional contractile impairment, usually as a result of an ischemic insult, which persists for hours or weeks even after restoration of CBF. Recovery of myocardial function is spontaneous provided that myocardial perfusion remains normal. Hibernation, in its original definition, refers to dysfunctional myocardium that is in a state of metabolic downregulation in response to reduced perfusion. However, resting flow in hibernating myocardial segments may not be decreased to the extent that would account for the degree of cardiac dysfunction. In most cases, there is impairment of CFR, with reduction of resting perfusion seen in only the most advanced cases. Hibernation, therefore, probably represents a spectrum with chronic repetitive stunning showing normal or near normal resting perfusion and impaired CFR at one end and reduced resting perfusion at the other. Recovery of function in hibernating myocardium requires coronary revascularization, which in turn restores an adequate CFR. Although the exact underlying phenomena in hibernation remain to a significant degree unclear, alteration of structural proteins and metabolism, disorganization of the cytoskeleton, loss of myofilaments, glycogen vacuoles, and sarcomeric instability may all result from impairment of regional perfusion and lead to myocardial dysfunction.[162,163]

SPECT is a well-established and widely available technique. ^{201}Tl is not only a perfusion agent but also a tracer of myocardial viability due to the reliance of tracer uptake on both myocardial blood flow and sarcolemmal integrity. It has therefore been used widely for identifying myocardial hibernation. Various imaging criteria have been proposed for the identification of viable myocardium. The most commonly used is the ratio of the radiotracer uptake in the relevant region to the uptake seen in the best perfused region of the myocardium (maximum tracer uptake), which shows directly proportional relationship with the amount of viable myocardium and inversely proportional with the amount of fibrotic tissue. A common threshold for defining clinically significant viability is $\geq$50% of maximal myocardial uptake, although the best threshold may be higher.[164,165] This criterion is highly specific, especially if there is coexisting ischemia at rest. As thallium redistribution may be slow or incomplete in regions of reduced perfusion, the usual stress/redistribution protocol can underestimate myocardial viability and additional steps may be required. These include late redistribution imaging at 8 to 72 hours after stress injection, reinjection of tracer at rest after redistribution imaging, and a resting injection on a separate day with both early (20 minutes) and delayed imaging (4 hours).

MIBI and tetrofosmin have also been used for detection of viable and hibernating myocardium. In theory, these tracers may underestimate viability in areas with reduced resting perfusion because they do not redistribute and cannot thus allow independent distinction of perfusion and viability. Some studies have therefore found ^{201}Tl SPECT MPI to be a more sensitive test for the assessment of viability.[166] However, the use of sublingual nitrates improves resting perfusion and thus the detection of myocardial viability using technetium tracers. An important advantage of using MIBI or tetrofosmin SPECT is the ability to perform ECG gating and thus assess ventricular function. Comparative studies between MRI and ECG-gated SPECT have shown good agreement for myocardial wall motion and thickening where myocardial tracer uptake is present.[167] Since detection of hibernation requires knowledge of viability, perfusion, and function, ECG-gated SPECT is ideally suited for the assessment of patients with HF by providing information on all these parameters in a single study.

Radiolabeled fatty acids for SPECT imaging have also been used to detect myocardial hibernation. Fatty acids serve as the primary source of energy for the myocardium. During periods of ischemia, however, stores are quickly exhausted and myocardial metabolism switches to glucose. This switch may persist for several hours, even after restoration of normal myocardial perfusion. Myocardial metabolism may be imaged through the use of radiolabeled fatty acid (FFA) analogues, of which the most widely studied is ß-methyl-p-[123I]-iodophenylpentadecanoic acid (BMIPP). This tracer is taken up by metabolically active myocardium but not by myocytes that have switched to glucose as their primary energy source. In patients with chronic CAD, myocardial segments demonstrating inducible ischemia may have larger resting BMIPP defects compared to resting ^{201}Tl images, suggesting that the metabolic abnormality may be more severe than would be expected from the defect in perfusion.[168] Uptake within areas of infarcted myocardium is similar for both BMIPP and ^{201}Tl. In patients with chronic CAD and depressed LV function, the presence and extent of discordant BMIPP uptake compared to both ^{201}Tl- and ^{99m}Tc-labeled agents is a reasonable predictor of functional recovery after revascularization.[166,169]

The use of PET is related to its ability to assess accurately alterations of myocardial metabolism that occur following myocardial ischemia. Uptake of glucose by the myocardium is increased with mild-to-moderate ischemia and hypoxia but decreased with very severe ischemia. Conversely under ischemic conditions, the extraction, uptake, and oxidation of FFA are reduced.[170] PET has been considered for many years as the "gold standard" for assessment of myocardial hibernation using ^{18}F-FDG. ^{18}F-FDG competes with glucose for transport into the cell and phosphorylation by the hexokinase reaction to ^{18}F-FDG-6-phosphate, but it is not further metabolized and it is trapped in the myocyte.

The usual dose of ^{18}F-FDG is 370 MBq, and imaging is performed 40 to 90 minutes after intravenous injection. In order to maximize myocardial uptake and overcome tracer inhomogeneity that is observed after fasting conditions,[171] ^{18}F-FDG is normally given after an oral glucose load (some centers also use nicotinic acid derivatives), and in patients with glucose intolerance or diabetes, it is also important to combine tracer injection with glucose and insulin infusion: the "euglycemic hyperinsulinemic clamp."[172] Qualitative assessment of the relative distribution of the radiotracer in the LV is the usual approach, but absolute quantification of glucose metabolic rates is also feasible, and this is accomplished by dynamic imaging that begins immediately during the injection of the radiotracer. Exogenous glucose utilization can be measured from the rate of supply and incorporation of ^{18}F-FDG into the myocardium, correcting for the different rates of transport and phosphorylation of glucose and ^{18}F-FDG. Current guidelines propose ^{18}F-FDG studies to be combined with assessment of myocardial perfusion (Fig. 23-9).[173] ^{13}N-Ammonia/^{18}F-FDG PET and ^{82}Rb/^{18}F-FDG PET are common combinations for detection of hibernation in clinical practice. Alternatively, SPECT with MIBI or tetrofosmin can be used instead of ^{13}N-ammonia or ^{82}Rb in centers with no access to PET perfusion tracers. ^{18}F-FDG PET studies can be combined with ECG gating, thus obtaining also information on regional and global function as well as assessing ventricular synchronization by phase analysis.

Studies based on assessment of ^{13}N-ammonia and ^{82}Rb uptake only (without using ^{18}F-FDG) have also been used for predicting functional recovery of dysfunctional myocardium. ^{15}O-water has also been proposed as another option since the fraction of tissue that can exchange water (water-perfusable tissue fraction, WPTF) can be measured and potentially used as a marker of myocardial viability.

Dysfunctional myocardial segments with higher ^{18}F-FDG uptake compared to that of ^{13}N-ammonia or ^{82}Rb (mismatch between and perfusion and metabolism) represent hibernating

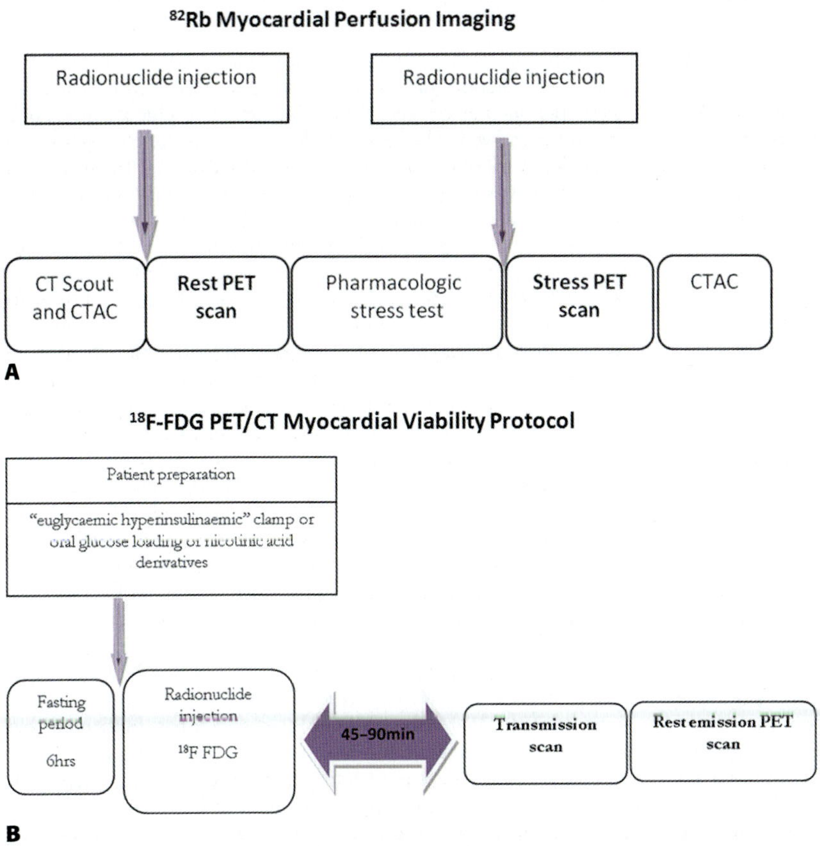

Figure 23-9. A: ^{82}Rb myocardial perfusion imaging protocol. **B:** ^{18}F-FDG PET/CT protocol for myocardial viability. (^{82}Rb, rubidium 82; CT, computed tomography; PET, positron emission tomography; CTAC, computed tomography attenuation correction; ^{18}F-FDG PET/CT, ^{18}F-fluorodeoxyglucose positron emission tomography/computed tomography.)

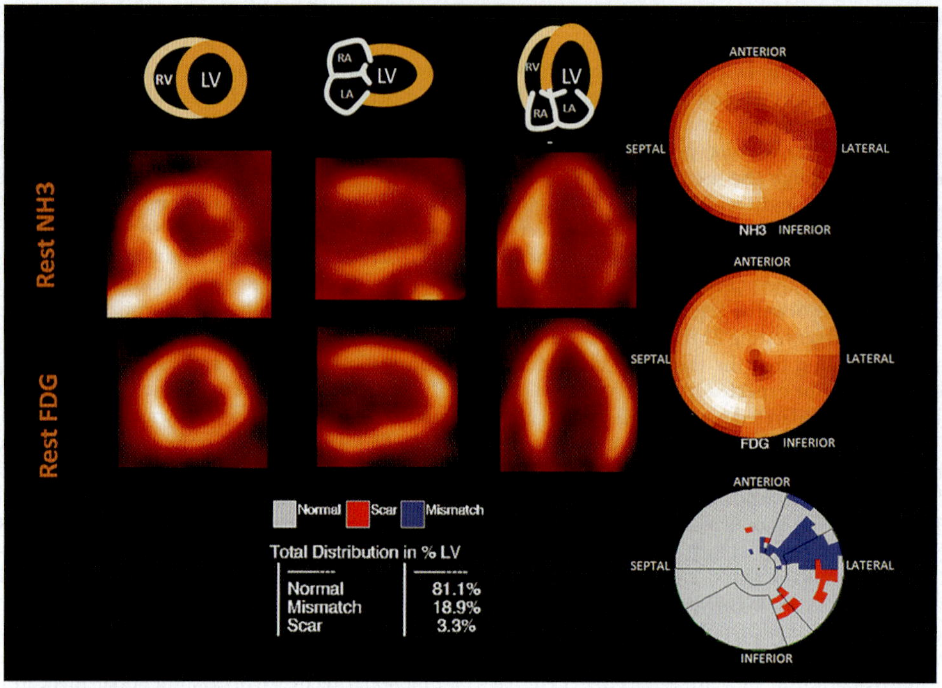

Figure 23-10. **Resting ^{13}N-ammonia and ^{18}F-FDG tomographic images and polar maps of a 68-year-old male with known CAD, previous myocardial infarctions, impaired LV function, and multiple previous PCIs.** He underwent a PET study for assessment of myocardial viability. Combined assessment of the resting ^{13}N-ammonia and the ^{18}F-FDG images shows a large mismatch between perfusion and metabolism (19% of the total myocardial mass) in the anterolateral region compatible with hibernating myocardium. There is an area with minor match inferolaterally (indicative of very limited myocardial damage involving only 3.1% of the total myocardial mass) but otherwise well-preserved perfusion and viability in the LV myocardium. (^{18}F-FDG: ^{18}F-fluorodeoxyglucose, CAD: coronary artery disease, LV: left ventricle, PCI: percutaneous coronary intervention, PET: positron emission tomography, RV: right ventricle, RA: right atrium, LA: left atrium). (From Anagnostopoulos C, Georgakopoulos A, Pianou N, et al. Assessment of Myocardial Perfusion and Viability by Positron Emission Tomography. *Int J Cardiol* 2013;167(5):1737–1749.)

myocardium, while reduction on both perfusion and metabolism suggests the presence of scarring (Fig. 23-10). In cases of myocardial stunning, perfusion is normal or almost normal while ^{18}F-FDG uptake is variable. Indeed, this may be even reduced compared to perfusion (reverse mismatch). This pattern has been observed in situations of repetitive stunning, following revascularization early post-MI when the myocardium is stunned, in patients with LBBB, and in some patients with diabetes.

Diagnostic Performance of Noninvasive Imaging Modalities for Detection of Viability and Hibernation

Several techniques have been developed for assessment of myocardial viability and hibernation. These include PET, SPECT, and also stress echo and CMR. Each technique uses different physiologic processes to image myocardial viability and can delineate irreversibly scarred from dysfunctional but viable myocardium with varying sensitivity and specificity. Myocardial perfusion, cell membrane integrity, mitochondrial function, glucose utilization, and contractile reserve may all be assessed, and their presence or absence relates to the severity of ultrastructural damage at the myocyte level. The accuracy for predicting improvement in regional or global function postrevascularization has been tested in numerous studies. Despite their limitations, which include variations in the definition of viability/hibernation and only rare evaluation of graft patency at the time of postrevascularization assessment, these studies consistently show that radionuclide techniques are most sensitive for prediction of functional recovery, whereas techniques challenging contractile reserve such as CMR and dobutamine stress echocardiography (DSE) are more specific.[174,175] This discrepancy may be related to different levels of ultrastructural cell damage in dysfunctional myocardium. The inotropic response during dobutamine stimulation may no longer be intact while more basic characteristics such as cell membrane integrity and glucose utilization are still preserved. The relatively low specificity of the techniques of nuclear cardiology, however, is not a disadvantage because other factors, such as the improvement of symptoms and prognosis after revascularization are more important than is the exact prediction of improvement of regional wall systolic function. Reperfusion of the hibernating myocardium stabilizes the myocardial blood flow conditions by eliminating repetitive episodes of ischemia and protects the myocardium from remodeling, apoptosis, and cell death even when it does not lead to an improvement of LV function. In a recent meta-analysis by Schinkel et al.[176] (24 studies from 1980 to 2007, 756 patients), the sensitivity and specificity values of PET were 92% and 63%, respectively. The corresponding values of DSE and dobutamine CMR for predicting recovery of regional function postrevascularization were 80% and 78% versus 74% and 82%, respectively. For ^{201}Tl SPECT and MIBI SPECT, these values were 87% and 54% and 83% and 65%, respectively. For contrast-enhanced CMR, the corresponding values in the same meta-analysis were 84% and 63%, respectively. Regarding improvement of global LV function, the study by Schinkel et al. demonstrated a higher sensitivity for radionuclide imaging (SPECT or PET) but comparable specificity for all imaging tests. A different meta-analysis that included more recent studies (performed between 1998 and 2006), focusing on patients with LV dysfunction (LVEF $<$ 45%), has confirmed that PET was more sensitive but less specific compared to nonnuclear techniques.[177] A consistent finding of all the aforementioned studies is that a meaningful improvement in LVEF postrevascularization can only be expected when a significant amount of chronically stunned/hibernating involving approximately 20% for PET or 25% for SPECT of the LV mass is present. Beyond the time of LV function assessment postrevascularization, it has also been shown that in patients with ischemic LV dysfunction and a mixture of viable and nonviable tissue, the extent of scar tissue should also be taken into account in order to accurately predict functional recovery after revascularization.[178] In addition, remodeling and enlargement of the left ventricle should also be considered. Remodeling of the left ventricle resulting in an enlarged end-systolic volume may prevent global recovery, even in patients with substantial viability.

Assessment of Prognosis and Contribution to Patients' Management

A major goal of viability studies is to identify patients with low LVEF who are at the highest clinical risk and in whom revascularization may offer the greatest survival benefit. Several mostly retrospective studies have shown that ^{18}F-FDG PET is a valuable tool for risk stratification of patients with LV dysfunction and viable myocardium by revealing significantly worse outcomes for those not undergoing timely revascularization.[179–181] In contrast, there was no apparent benefit from revascularization over medical therapy in the absence of demonstrated myocardial viability. A recent meta-analysis has shown that the annualized mortality rates in patients with viable myocardium assessed by ^{18}F-FDG PET in relation to treatment were 4% for patients undergoing revascularization and 17% for those on medical treatment. Compared to ^{18}F-FDG PET, the corresponding values for dobutamine echocardiography were 3% and 12%, while for SPECT ^{201}Tl and SPECT ^{99m}Tc, these were 4% and 7% versus 3% and 9%, respectively.[182]

In the first prospective randomized controlled trial, Siebelink et al.[181] compared MIBI SPECT to $^{13}NH_3$/^{18}F-FDG PET in 103 patients. They found no significant difference in outcomes; however, only approximately 30% of patients had severe LV dysfunction, and in addition, there were long delays to revascularization, which may limit the benefit of viability imaging and therefore may have affected the study's ability to detect differences. More recently, a multicenter randomized controlled trial, the PET and Recovery Following Revascularization (PARR-2), has been conducted to assess whether the use of ^{18}F-FDG PET in clinical decision making can lead to better clinical outcome compared with standard care where PET was not available. The study population included patients with an LVEF $\leq$ 35% who were being considered for revascularization, transplantation, or HF workup. The primary outcome was a composite of cardiac death, myocardial infarction, or cardiac repeat hospital stay at 1 year. In the PET arm, extent and severity of scar and mismatch were incorporated together with clinical parameters in a previously derived model for prediction of LV recovery postrevascularization.[183] This trial did not demonstrate statistically significant differences between the two groups; however, in a post hoc analysis focusing on adherence to PET recommendations, there was a significant decrease in the hazard ratio for the primary outcome compared with standard care for revascularized patients with a mismatch size of at least 7%.[184] This was even lower than the cutoff value of 25.8% (CI = 16.6% to 35.0%), which was found, in a recent meta-analysis of seven mostly retrospective PET studies, to be the optimal threshold above which a survival benefit was achieved by revascularization in comparison to medical therapy. Compared to PET, the same meta-analysis has shown that the corresponding values were 35.9% (95% CI: 31.6% to 40.3%) for stress echo using contractile reserve or ischemic responses and 38.7% (95% CI: 27.7% to 49.7%) for SPECT using ^{201} Tl or MIBI. PARR-2 and its substudies[184–187] provide good evidence for using ^{18}F-FDG PET to identify high-risk patients who may benefit from revascularization; however, further randomized trials incorporating viability imaging as part of the workup for management of ischemic HF are still required to assess the value of imaging in this setting. The Alternative Imaging Modalities in Ischemic Heart Failure is one such trial that is currently underway and is expected to address the issue around the role of cardiac imaging in management decisions and to ascertain which methods are most suitable for which types of patients (for instance, patients with severely dilated hearts and LVEF < 25%).[188] Its results are eagerly awaited by the scientific community particularly after the recent publication of the substudy of the Surgical Treatment for Ischemic Heart Failure trial.[189] According to this, the presence of viable myocardium was associated with an increased probability of survival but viability assessment failed to identity patients with a survival benefit from surgical revascularization as compared with medical therapy alone. These results need to be interpreted with caution bearing in mind some important limitations of the study. First of all, the definition of viability as predictor of functional recovery after revascularization included myocardial segments that were alive but not necessarily dysfunctional, hence defying the concept of hibernation, which refers to viable but severely dysfunctional myocardium. Second, information on viability (assessed either by SPECT or stress echo) was available in 50% of randomized patients only, and test performance was subject to test availability and clinical judgment. Finally, the patient population was different from that reported in prior observational studies and in PARR-2 in that the recruited individuals had less comorbid disease, including frequently having single-vessel disease, low incidence of renal dysfunction, and lower rates of significant HF, as well as only 19% of them were considered not to have viable myocardium.

Prediction of Improvement of Symptoms, Exercise Capacity, and Quality of Life

Issues such as New York Heart Association (NYHA) class of symptoms, exercise capacity, and quality of life are also important; however, the related studies are rather limited. Di Carli et al.[190] have demonstrated the usefulness of ^{18}F-FDG PET to predict improvement of HF symptoms and exercise capacity. These findings were confirmed by Marwick et al.[191] and Haas et al.,[192] respectively, with the latter group showing, in addition, that patients selected for revascularization based on ^{18}F-FDG PET presented fewer perioperative complications and better short-term outcome compared to those who underwent revascularization without prior viability assessment. Similar results were reported by Gunning et al.[193] using SPECT. More recently, Shukla et al.[194] demonstrated that patients whose treatment is directed by ^{18}F-FDG PET imaging have a better quality of life versus those with standard care. Improvement of quality is likely related to the fact that ^{18}F-FDG PET offers a better treatment selection in patients who need or not revascularization.

Recommendations for Viability/Hibernation Assessment by Noninvasive Imaging

The role of viability imaging in patients with ischemic HF is discussed in various international guidelines. Current ACC/AHA and also ESC guidelines on HF recommend (class IIa, level of evidence: B) viability assessment in patients with known CAD who present with HF symptoms but no angina.[195,196] In addition, the consensus statement of Canadian Cardiovascular Society on HF supports performance of viability testing prior to revascularization.[197] ACC/AHA guidelines on revascularization recommend CABG (class IIa, level of evidence: B) to improve survival for patients with CAD and mild-to-moderate LV systolic dysfunction (EF 35% to 50%) "when viability is present in the territory of intended revascularization." Regarding patients with severe LV systolic dysfunction (EF < 35%), the guidelines state that "CABG might be considered with the primary or sole intent of improving survival whether or not viable myocardium is present" (class IIb, level of evidence: B). ESC guidelines on revascularization for patients with ischemic LV dysfunction and HF state that "revascularization in the absence of myocardial viability study is not recommended."[198]

The aforementioned documents do not make concrete recommendations on which test to perform in clinical practice. Typically, the choice will usually depend upon availability, local expertise, cost, and on whether the clinical question requires a sensitive or a specific technique for predicting recovery of segmental function.[199] In many centers with multimodality imaging facilities, performance of SPECT MPI and stress echocardiography are often first-line examinations. In this case, imaging in the form of PET or MRI can be reserved for patients with a body habitus that could affect image quality with SPECT MPI or stress echocardiography, or for patients with severe LV remodeling and reduction of LVEF, or for situations when clinical suspicion of viability/hibernation remains after other imaging techniques have proved negative. When there is coexistent valvular regurgitation, MRI is conceivably the technique of choice, but in situations such as presence of pacemakers, defibrillators, renal insufficiency, and claustrophobia, its use is restricted.

Radionuclide Imaging and Cardiac Resynchronization Therapy

Current guidelines recommend CRT to reduce morbidity and mortality in (NYHA III or IV) patients who are symptomatic despite OMT with LV EF ≤35% and prolonged QRS interval (≥120 milliseconds).[199,200] In this population, delayed electrical activation and impaired excitation–contraction coupling result in a dispersion of regional mechanical activation. This results in dyssynchronous contraction both within the LV (intraventricular dyssynchrony) and between the left and right ventricles (interventricular dyssynchrony). These phenomena are associated with presystolic mitral valve regurgitation, decreased LV diastolic filling time, reduced LV contractility, and occasionally with septal wall dyskinesia. Biventricular pacing results in resynchronization of ventricular contraction, which may optimize LV filling, reduce functional mitral regurgitation, and reduce or even reverse LV remodeling. These effects may thus improve LV function and hence reduce the symptoms of HF and also improve exercise capacity. Current data suggest that around one-third of patients who meet the criteria for CRT fail to respond symptomatically. As the insertion of CRT devices, whether or not combined with implantable cardiac defibrillator, is costly and not without risk, considerable effort has been expended on the noninvasive prediction of patients who stand to benefit.

Noninvasive imaging approaches have been extensively used for the prediction of the response to CRT therapy as well as of long-term outcome including the most recent techniques such as real-time 3D echocardiography and MRI. Amongst other noninvasive techniques, interest is focused currently on phase analysis of equilibrium RNV and ECG-gated SPECT or PET. ECG-gated MPI SPECT permits assessment of perfusion, viability, scar tissue, and LV dyssynchrony from a single study, so that this technique may provide a one-stop shop for predicting CRT response.[201] In patients with HF (NYHA classes III–IV), QRS duration greater than 120 milliseconds, and LV EF <35%, a phase histogram bandwidth of greater than 72.5 degrees has a sensitivity of 83% and a specificity of 81% for predicting response (improvement by one functional class) to CRT at 6 months. For phase SD, a cutoff value of 19.6 degrees yielded similar sensitivity and specificity.[54] Dyssynchrony assessment by ECG-gated MPI SPECT or PET can also be useful for risk stratification in a broad spectrum of patients including those of LV dysfunction of ischemic etiology, providing incremental information beyond that obtained by established imaging-derived predictors.[202]

Monitoring Regenerative Cell Therapy with PET and SPECT

Regenerative cell therapy using embryonic stem cells, bone marrow–derived stem cells, and endothelial progenitor cells is being investigated for HF. Such therapy, delivered by intracoronary, intramyocardial, or systemic venous injection, requires monitoring of the homing, engraftment, and survival of the injected cells. In addition to providing information on these aspects, radionuclide techniques have the advantage of being able to assess myocardial remodeling as well as imaging different aspects of the myocardial microenvironment in which the cells are engrafted such as regional myocardial perfusion and viability. Global and regional function can also be measured and along with changes of perfusion and viability can be used as measures of outcome in regenerative therapy.[203,204] The majority of preclinical studies thus far have shown that engraftment of various cell types into ischemic or infarcted myocardium can lead in reduced infarct size, reversible ventricular remodeling, and improved left ventricular systolic function.[205]

SPECT and PET Perfusion Imaging in Other Cardiac Diseases

Coronary Disease of Nonatherosclerotic Etiology

MPI with SPECT or PET is also performed in patients with angina or pain, which resembles angina without substrate of atherosclerotic disease in order to assess the presence or not of underlying ischemia. A variety of conditions such as congenital coronary anomalies (see below), arteritis, emboli, thrombi, metabolic disorders (e.g., Hunter and Hurler diseases), intimal proliferation (e.g., irradiation therapy, transplantation), and external compression or Kawasaki disease may compromise the coronary lumen. A special group of patients discussed in this chapter includes individuals with angina or angina-like pain but angiographically unobstructed coronary arteries and no evidence of coronary artery spasm. These are labeled as "syndrome X" patients or patients with a "sensitive heart syndrome."[204] PET studies have demonstrated reduced CFR in approximately two-thirds of patients, while with SPECT, transient abnormalities of myocardial perfusion were found in up to 60% of "syndrome X" patients, suggesting that vascular dysfunction is common in this population.[206–208]

In *Kawasaki disease*, the relationship between visually assessed coronary artery lesions on angiography and CFR has been shown to be variable. A study focusing on the functional significance of coronary aneurysms in patients with *Kawasaki disease* has demonstrated that CFR was reduced in aneurysms of moderate to large size only.[209] Both exercise and vasodilator stress test have been utilized in this setting, and they were shown to be safe and effective.[210,211] The diagnostic accuracy of SPECT in the detection of flow-limiting coronary stenosis in Kawasaki disease has been investigated by Fukuda et al. In this study, a sensitivity of 90% and specificity of 100% for angiographic coronary stenosis ≥75% were demonstrated with dipyridamole–tetrofosmin SPECT.[209] Serial monitoring of patients with nuclear imaging techniques may be useful to predict late progression in coronary stenosis and assist decision making for angiography.[212,213] Furthermore, scintigraphic evaluation permits not only functional assessment of the demonstrated coronary aneurysms[214] but also documentation of changes with therapy.[215] Some studies have showed a poor agreement between SPECT and coronary angiography, but this can be explained by the fact that the former assesses perfusion while the latter provides anatomical information.[216,217] This distinction is also supported by evidence from dynamic PET studies. Such studies have demonstrated that adenosine-induced absolute hyperemic coronary flow and CFR remain depressed in patients with previous Kawasaki disease even in the absence of angiographic coronary stenosis.[218] Furthermore, a study in children with diagnosed Kawasaki disease showed that PET is the most sensitive method for detection of regional ischemia, when there are symptoms or signs of ischemia, even if there is no indication of coronary vascular stenosis by ultrasound or coronary angiography.[219]

There are also data on the prognostic value of nuclear imaging techniques in patients with Kawasaki disease. In a prospective study of 90 patients, followed up for a mean of 8.8 years, the presence of ^{201}Tl redistribution on SPECT imaging was found to be the most significant independent predictor ($\chi^2 = 54.4$, $p < 0.0001$) and the best multivariate independent predictor (relative risk 57.8) of future cardiac events. Patients with no redistribution (in other words, no ischemia) on ^{201}Tl imaging had a low late cardiac event rate of 1.6% ± 1.6%. This powerful prognostic value of SPECT imaging makes a strong case for its use in the management of all patients with Kawasaki disease.[220]

Cardiomyopathies

According to a recent *AHA Scientific Statement on* Cardiomyopathies, these are define as "a heterogeneous group of diseases of the myocardium associated with mechanical and/or electrical dysfunction that usually (but not invariably) exhibit inappropriate ventricular hypertrophy or dilatation and are due to a variety of causes that frequently are genetic. Cardiomyopathies either are confined to the heart or are part of generalized systemic disorders, often leading to cardiovascular death or progressive heart failure–related disability."[221] The role of radionuclide imaging in the various cardiomyopathies is diverse.[222] Regarding perfusion assessment, SPECT and PET are often used to assess the presence or absence of CAD but also to assess prognosis, even if CAD is not present based on myocardial perfusion patterns.

In patients with HCM, PET offers the unique ability to quantify MBF in the absence of epicardial CAD.[223] A blunted response to vasodilators has been demonstrated in patients with HCM, and in addition, it was found that impaired vasodilatory response can be a remodeling predictor as well as a powerful prognostic factor of future events including progressive HF, ventricular tachyarrhythmias, and death, which are directly linked to the severity of microvasculature dysfunction. Patients with HCM and chest pain might have functionally significant epicardial CAD, which can be assessed by SPECT MPI. Defects, both reversible and fixed, have been reported in 10% to 100% of patients suggesting myocardial ischemia or fibrosis even in the absence of significant epicardial coronary artery stenosis (Fig. 23-11). These abnormalities may reflect impaired CFR or decreased sympathetic neural function in hypertrophied areas. In HCM, stress SPECT MPI provides important prognostic information by identifying patients at increased risk of cardiovascular death, with a significantly lower survival at 10 years for those with an abnormal study compared to patients with a normal SPECT result (67% vs. 89% $p < 0.04$).[224] A common SPECT MPI finding in HCM patients is that of relatively increased counts at the septum compared to the lateral wall, but such "hot spots" can occur in other walls too. This could be related to LV hypertrophy and/or increased regional blood flow at rest. In the posttreatment setting (after alcohol septal reduction therapy), SPECT MPI has also been utilized and it was found that fixed septal perfusion defects are present involving the basal septum in all patients and the midseptum in 38% of patients.

Dilated cardiomyopathy is a major cause of HF at younger ages. While 35% to 50% of cases of DCM may be hereditary, myocarditis can explain up to 10% of cases of idiopathic DCM. Myocardial perfusion defects can be seen in DCM (Fig. 23-12). As mentioned earlier, this is because significant myocardial fibrosis and impaired CFR may occur in the absence of epicardial coronary obstruction

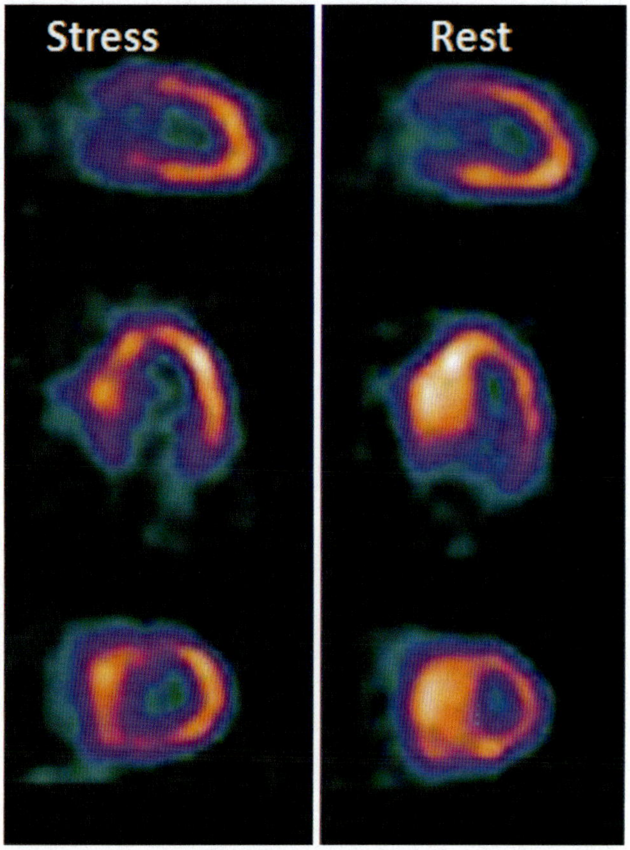

Figure 23-11. **Example of hypertrophic cardiomyopathy.** Stress and rest images from a 21-year-old male patient. There is an inducible perfusion abnormality of the severely hypertrophied septum.

resulting in perfusion abnormalities that can mimic significant CAD on MPI. Usually, patients with underlying CAD as a cause for LV dysfunction have more extensive and severe defects, which lie within a typical coronary distribution; those with nonischemic LV dysfunction tend to have smaller, milder defects, which do not correspond to any particular coronary territory. However, even in nonischemic LV dysfunction, larger and more extensive inducible abnormalities are associated with increased mortality.[225–227]

Cardiac involvement can be detected at postmortem in 20% to 30% of patients with *sarcoidosis* but is clinically evident in only 5%. Detection of this subclinical involvement is a major challenge as most clinically important cases present with heart block, tachyarrhythmias, ventricular dysfunction, and even sudden death. Sarcoid granulomas usually involve the myocardium with rare focal extensions into the pericardium and endocardium causing inflammation and healing by fibrosis. MPI with ^{201}Tl has been used in patients with suspected cardiac sarcoidosis in conjunction with ^{67}Ga imaging. Perfusion defects on thallium SPECT MPI correspond to the areas of fibrogranulomatous replacement, whereas gallium uptake represents active inflammation and infiltration by sarcoid granulomas and is thus a marker of disease activity. ^{67}Ga uptake often disappears after treatment with steroids indicating the inflammatory component of active sarcoid granulomas.[228] PET assessment using ^{18}FDG may also be useful, with focal uptake within cardiac granulomas a potentially characteristic feature of sarcoidosis. ^{18}FDG PET may be used in conjunction with $^{13}NH_3$ perfusion[229] imaging or gadolinium-enhanced CMR to improve the sensitivity of the detection of sarcoidosis. Radionuclide imaging

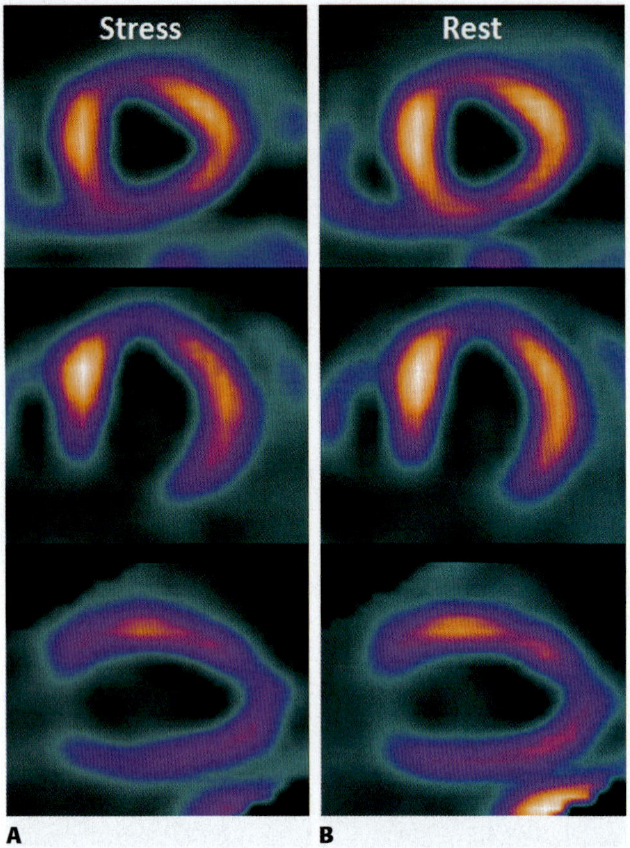

Figure 23-12. Example of dilated cardiomyopathy of nonischemic etiology. Stress and rest images from a 37-year-old male patient. **A:** Inhomogeneous radiotracer uptake in the apical region and inferior wall as well as higher uptake in the septum compared to the lateral wall instead of the usual reverse order. **B:** There is no significant change after reinjection of the radiotracer.

can therefore be used to monitor disease activity and assess the efficacy of treatment.

Congenital Heart Disease

Assessment of cardiac anatomy in patients with congenital heart disease is performed by ECHO and CMR. Occasionally, imaging with noninvasive techniques is supplemented by CT, although its use is limited in the pediatric population. Assessment of physiology is accomplished by CMR as well as radionuclide imaging. The latter has an important role in selected patients particularly in the investigation of individuals at increased risk of myocardial ischemia. The most common applications of SPECT and PET in patients with biventricular circulation are those related to the investigation of congenital anomalies of the coronary arteries as in (a) abnormal origin or course of coronary artery from the aorta or pulmonary trunk, (b) unusual coronary epicardial course, (c) severe stenosis or atresia of orifice of the coronary artery, (d) coronary artery fistulas, and (e) myocardial bridging. The abnormal origin of a coronary artery from the aorta does not necessarily mean impaired perfusion unless is accompanied by anatomic or functional stenosis of the coronary artery. In adult patients operated because of left coronary artery arising from the pulmonary artery (ALCAPA), myocardial ischemia can be due to problematic grafts or stenosis of the reimplanted coronary arteries, and it can be manifested as ischemic mitral regurgitation. In patients with unusual epicardial course of coronary arteries, ischemia can occur at stress due to compression of the lumen of the coronary artery, which is located between the trunk of the dilated large vessels. Coronary orifices located in the tubular part of the aorta may also be associated with decreased coronary perfusion.[230] Myocardial bridging, which is another cause of ischemia, occurs when a segment of an epicardial coronary artery courses below the epicardial surface, which leads to compression of the artery during ventricular contraction. The most frequent site is the middle portion of the left anterior descending coronary artery. The endomyocardial section of the coronary artery is often free of atherosclerotic changes, although there can be atheromatous plaques without significant stenosis proximal of the myocardial bridge.[231] Finally, coronary artery fistulas, which most commonly occur between a coronary artery and a large vessel or endocardial cavity (right atrium, right ventricle, coronary sinus, pulmonary artery), may be responsible for the presence of myocardial ischemia and perfusion deficits in the region distal to the fistula (steal phenomenon).

Another group where assessment of myocardial perfusion is important is that of patients with a previous switch operation of the large vessels. The procedure was first described by Jatene in 1975 although started to gain widespread acceptance in the early 1980s.[232] The prevalence of coronary abnormalities can be as high as 29%, if the patients are symptomatic, but they can also occur, although far less frequently (up to 7%), in asymptomatic individuals. Several mechanisms of lesions of coronary arteries after surgical anatomical correction have been reported. Delayed obstruction is usually secondary to fibrocellular intimal thickening or to thrombus formation. The stenosis of the coronary arteries can also be due to scar formation that surrounds the proximal portion of the reimplanted vessels. Tsuda et al[233] reported mortality rate up to 10% in the series of their patients as a result of these interventions in the coronary vessels. The usual cause of death was subendocardium infarction resulting from stenosis of the coronary vessels.

Patients with coarctation of the aorta (CoA) are at risk of developing premature atherosclerosis and CAD. This may be due to known defects in the composition of tunica media in patients with CoA, leading to increased stiffness of the vessel (aortic wall stiffness), but also in persistent hypertension proximal of stenosis, which remains even after successful surgical correction in childhood.

Technical Considerations: Stress Techniques, Image Acquisition, and Interpretation

In patients with congenital defects, dynamic exercise is the stress method of choice for SPECT imaging, typically on a treadmill or bicycle ergometer. This is the most physiologic form of stress and provides additional useful information such as exercise capacity and hemodynamic changes. However, sudden death is associated with some congenital anomalies, especially during exercise—this has been particularly documented for anomalous origin of the left main coronary artery from the right aortic sinus and anomalous origin of the right coronary artery from the left aortic sinus (as the vessel can be compressed between the great vessels secondary to an exercise-induced rise in cardiac output).[234] While there is potentially legitimate concern with exercising such patients, there has been no reported mortality in the literature.[235,236] These patients may be safely exercised if stress is terminated at the onset of symptoms consistent with ischemia. With PET studies, pharmacologic stress with vasodilators has been used to induce coronary hyperaemia.[237,238]

Dextrocardia, if present, should be noted as the acquisition protocol should be changed to start at 45-degree right posterior oblique and end at 45-degree left anterior oblique (instead of the usual 45-degree RAO to 45-degree LPO rotation). Even in the absence of dextrocardia, many patients with congenital heart disease have a rotated heart, and the arc of acquisition may be changed accordingly to allow optimal myocardial counts registration.

The interpretation of myocardial perfusion images is in principle no different from that of patients without congenital defects. Indeed, image interpretation in patients with simple congenital defects, such as isolated congenital coronary anomaly or a small septal defect, is relatively straightforward. However, image interpretation in patients with complex congenital defects who have gross distortion of cardiac anatomy may be extremely difficult. This is partly related to the limited resolution of the gamma camera and difficulties in axis and slice selection and stress–rest comparison (particularly if transient perfusion abnormalities are also present), but is also related to the unpredictable effect of surgery and underlying myocardial disease on regional tracer uptake.

SPECT and PET Findings in Specific Types of Congenital Heart Disease

Early studies have demonstrated that planar resting thallium imaging can be used to diagnose myocardial infarction in patients with anomalous origin of the left coronary artery and single-trunk anomalous origin of both coronary arteries from the pulmonary artery.[239–241] Early studies with exercise thallium imaging in patients with muscle bridging have failed to demonstrate associated ischemia in these patients.[242] More recent studies with intravascular ultrasound, however, have shown that bridged segments show a marked reduction in luminal area throughout ventricular systole that persists into diastole. Studies have also shown that coronary flow velocities are increased and flow reserve is reduced in arteries in which bridging is present.[243] Several case reports have highlighted the possible association between bridging and ischemia and/or infarction.[244]

Perfusion studies are also helpful in patients with congenitally corrected transposition of the great arteries. These patients often present in adulthood with symptoms of HF or more rarely of angina.[245] Many of these patients develop progressive systemic RV dysfunction. A postulated mechanism is myocardial ischemia and/or infarction secondary to an imbalance in oxygen supply and demand as a result of ventricular hypertrophy.[246] Both reversible and fixed perfusion abnormalities have been demonstrated on SPECT imaging in such patients, lending support to this hypothesis.[247,248] Furthermore, adenosine-induced hyperemic coronary flow and CFR have been shown to be attenuated in these patients using dynamic PET with ^{13}N-ammonia. A similar situation arises in patients with simple transposition of the great arteries (TGAs) following treatment with switch procedure. Long-term follow-up studies with SPECT have shown a high incidence of reversible and fixed perfusion defects in such patients. The extent of myocardial perfusion abnormalities has been found to correlate well with the impairment in ventricular function.[249] For patients with TGA treated with an arterial switch operation, there is also evidence from SPECT that late perfusion abnormalities are present. Dynamic PET studies have also demonstrated that CFR is significantly reduced in these patients, even in the absence of symptoms. A postulated mechanism is coronary obstruction, secondary to coronary mobilization and reimplantation, which is an integral part of the arterial switch operation.[250,251]

Assessment of Myocardial Perfusion in Patients with Diseases of the Connective Tissue

Patients with connective tissue diseases compared to healthy population show two to five times more frequently diseases of the cardiovascular system, which reduce the life expectancy by 5 to 10 years. Diseases of the cardiovascular system can appear during or after diagnosis. Most commonly are observed in rheumatoid arthritis and in systemic lupus erythematosus (SLE).[252] The events are different per disease and affect different structures of the heart and may even cause death. The impaired function of the endothelium and the existence of low-grade inflammation have a major role in the development of atherosclerosis in these patients. A higher CAC score has been documented in the above patients compared with the healthy population of similar age. SPECT MPI reveals perfusion defects in 28% of female patients with SLE and nonstenosed coronary vessels. Especially for asymptomatic patients with SLE, it has been found that both SPECT and PET imaging can show impaired myocardial perfusion. Furthermore, PET can reveal endothelial dysfunction through quantitative measurements.[253–256] Similarly, perfusion defects were found in patients with advanced systemic sclerosis, which have been attributed to microcirculation impairment.

Myocardial Perfusion for Assessment of Complications Post–Heart Transplantation

Despite advances in the management of HF and the application of ventricular implantable devices, cardiac transplantation still offers the best survival probability for patients with end-stage HF. Early detection of graft rejection and adequate immunosuppressive therapy remain fundamental targets after heart transplantation. Intravascular ultrasound is the imaging method with the highest sensitivity for the diagnosis of vasculopathy after cardiac transplant. However, SPECT MPI with ^{201}Tl or ECG-gated MIBI shows excellent NPV for identifying vasculopathy in the graft, thus acting as a "gatekeeper" to coronary catheterization, which can then be reserved only for patients with perfusion abnormalities.[257]

Conclusions

The increasing number of available imaging modalities has made the investigation of myocardial perfusion feasible by a range of different techniques. In the field of radionuclide imaging, technologic developments, such as new γ camera detectors along with AC improvements, enhance diagnostic accuracy, while analysis of left ventricular phase from ECG gating studies for detecting dyssynchrony increases the derived information from a single perfusion study. In PET imaging, the broader availability of scanners as well as standardization of dynamic studies have enhanced the technique's potential in terms of both diagnostic and risk stratification capabilities. Radionuclide MPI plays a pivotal role in the diagnosis and management of patients investigated for CAD. The clinical value and cost-effectiveness, particularly for SPECT MPI, have been recognized in numerous international guidelines, which recommend SPECT or PET in various clinical scenarios both in the acute and chronic settings. Radionuclide perfusion imaging has also been used in other entities such as the cardiomyopathies and the congenital heart diseases with important diagnostic and prognostic contribution.

REFERENCES

1. **Erlandsson K, Kacperski K, van Gramberg D, et al.** Performance evaluation of D-SPECT: a novel SPECT system for nuclear cardiology. *Phys Med Biol* 2009;54(9):2635–2649.
2. **Al-Mallah MH, Sitek A, Moore SC, et al.** Assessment of myocardial perfusion and function with PET and PET/CT. *J Nucl Cardiol* 2010;17(3):498–513.
3. **Marban E, Koretsune Y, Corretti M, et al.** Calcium and its role in myocardial cell injury during ischemia and reperfusion. *Circulation* 1989;80(6 suppl):IV17–IV22.
4. **Ishizaka H, Kuo L.** Acidosis-induced coronary arteriolar dilation is mediated by ATP-sensitive potassium channels in vascular smooth muscle. *Circ Res* 1996;78:50–57.
5. **Leong-Poi H, Rim SJ, Le DE, et al.** Perfusion versus function: the ischemic cascade in demand ischemia. *Circulation* 2002;105:987–992.
6. **Gould KL, Lipscomb K.** Effects of coronary stenoses on coronary flow reserve and resistance. *Am J Cardiol* 1974;34:48–55.
7. **Hesse B, Tagil K, Cuocolo A, et al.** EANM/ESC procedural guidelines for myocardial perfusion imaging in nuclear cardiology. *Eur J Nucl Med Mol Imaging* 2005;32(7):855–897.

8. **Goldhaber SZ, Newell JB, Ingwall JS, et al.** Effects of reduced coronary flow on thallium-201 accumulation and release in an in vitro rat heart preparation. *Am J Cardiol* 1983;51:891–896.
9. **Grunwald AM, Watson DD, Holzgrefe HH Jr, et al.** Myocardial thallium-201 kinetics in normal and ischaemic myocardium. *Circulation* 1981;64:610–618.
10. **Weich H, Strauss HW, Pitt B.** The extraction of thallium-201 by the myocardium. *Circulation* 1977;56(2):188–191.
11. **Administration of Radioactive Substances Advisory Committee.** Notes for Guidance on the Clinical Administration of Radiopharmaceuticals and Use of Sealed Radioactive Sources. March 2006, Revised 2006, 2007 (twice), 2011 and 2014.
12. **Li QS, Solot G, Frank TL, et al.** Myocardial redistribution of technetium-99m-methoxyisobutylisonitrile (SESTAMIBI). *J Nucl Med* 1990;31(6):1069–1076.
13. **Jain D, Wackers FJ, Mattera J, et al.** Biokinetics of technetium-99m-tetrofosmin: myocardial perfusion imaging agent: implications for a one-day imaging protocol. *J Nucl Med* 1993;34(8):1254–1259.
14. **Anagnostopoulos C, Harbinson M, Kelion A, et al.** Procedure guidelines for radionuclide myocardial perfusion imaging. *Heart* 2004; 90(suppl 1):i1–i10.
15. **Ranhosky A, Kempthorne-Rawson J.** The safety of intravenous dipyridamole thallium myocardial perfusion imaging. Intravenous Dipyridamole Thallium Imaging Study Group. *Circulation* 1990;81:1205–1209.
16. **Verani MS, Mahmarian JJ, Hixson JB, et al.** Diagnosis of coronary artery disease by controlled coronary vasodilation with adenosine and thallium-201 scintigraphy in patients unable to exercise. *Circulation* 1990;82:80–87.
17. **Iskandrian AE, Bateman TM, Belardinelli L, et al.; ADVANCE MPI Investigators.** Adenosine versus regadenoson comparative evaluation in myocardial perfusion imaging: results of the ADVANCE phase 3 multicenter international trials. *J Nucl Cardiol* 2007;14:645–658.
18. **Cerqueira MD, Nguyen P, Staehr P et al.; ADVANCE-MPI Trial Investigators.** Effects of age, gender, obesity, and diabetes on the efficacy and safety of the selective A_{2a} agonist regadenoson versus adenosine in myocardial perfusion imaging: integrated ADVANCE-MPI trial results. *J Am Coll Cardiol Img* 2008;1:307–316.
19. **Leaker BR, O'Connor B , Hansel TT, et al.** Safety of regadenoson, an adenosine A_{2A} receptor agonist for myocardial perfusion imaging, in mild asthma and moderate asthma patients: a randomized, double-blind, placebo-controlled trial. *J Nucl Cardiol* 2008;15:329–336.
20. **Thomas GS, Tammelin BR, Schiffman GL, et al.** Safety of regadenoson, a selective adenosine A_{2A}agonist, in patients with chronic obstructive pulmonary disease: a randomized, double-blind, placebo-controlled trial (RegCOPD trial). *J Nucl Cardiol* 2008;15:319–328.
21. **Iskandrian AE.** State of the art of pharmacological stress imaging. In: Zaret BL, Beller GA, eds. *Nuclear Cardiology, state of the art and future direction*, 2nd ed. St Louis, MO: Mosby; 1999:19:312.
22. **Dilsizian V, Rocco TP, Freedman NM, et al.** Enhanced detection of ischemic but viable myocardium by the reinjection of thallium after stress-redistribution imaging. *N Engl J Med* 1990;323(3):141–146.
23. **Henzlova MJ, Cerqueira MD, Hansen CL, et al.** ASNC Imaging guidelines for nuclear cardiology procedures. Stress protocols and tracers. *J Nucl Med* 2009; doi: 10.1007/s12350-009-9062-4.
24. **Heo J, Kegel J, Iskandrian AS, et al.** Comparison of same-day protocols using technetium-99m-sestamibi myocardial imaging. *J Nucl Med* 1992;33(2):186–191.
25. **Ben-Haim S, Kacperski A, Hain S, et al.** Simultaneous dual-radionuclide myocardial imaging with a solid state dedicated cardiac camera. *Eur J Nucl Med Mol Imaging* 2010;37:1710–1721.
26. **Hesse B, Lindhardt TB, Acampa W, et al.** EANM/ESC guidelines for radionuclide imaging of cardiac function. *Eur J Nucl Med Mol Imaging* 2008;35:851–885.
27. **Marcassa C, Campini R, Zoccarato O, et al.** Wide beam reconstruction for half-dose or half-time cardiac gated SPECT acquisitions: optimization of resources and reduction in radiation exposure. *Eur J Nucl Med Mol Imaging* 2011;38:499–508.
28. **Valenta I, Treyer V, Husmann L, et al.** New reconstruction algorithm allows shortened acquisition time for myocardial perfusion SPECT. *Eur J Nucl Med Mol Imaging* 2010;37:750–757.
29. **Bateman TM, Heller GV, McGhie AI, et al.** Multicenter investigation comparing a highly efficient half-time stress-only attenuation correction approach against standard rest-stress Tc-99m SPECT imaging. *J Nucl Cardiol* 2009;16:726–735.
30. **Sharir T, Ben-Haim S, Merzon K, et al.** High-speed Myocardial Perfusion Imaging. Initial comparison with conventional dual detector anger camera imaging. *JACC Cardiovasc Imaging* 2008;1:156–163.
31. **Sharir T, Slomka PJ, Hayes SW, et al.** Multicenter Trial of High-Speed Versus Conventional Single-Photon Emission Computed Tomography Imaging. Quantitative results of myocardial perfusion and left ventricular function. *J Am Coll Cardiol* 2010;55:1965–1974.
32. **Bocher M, Blevis IM, Tuskerman L, et al.** A fast cardiac gamma camera with dynamic SPECT capabilities: design, system validation and future potential. *Eur J Nucl Med Mol Imaging* 2010;37:1887–1902.
33. **Esteves FP, Raggi P, Folks RD, et al.** Novel solid-state-detector dedicated cardiac camera for fast myocardial perfusion imaging: multicentre comparison with standard dual detector cameras. *J Nucl Cardiol* 2009;16:927–934.
34. **Duvall WL, Croft LB, Ginsberg ES, et al.** Reduced isotope dose and imaging time with a high-efficiency CZT SPECT camera. *J Nucl Cardiol* 2011;18:847–857.
35. **Hamad EA, Travin MI.** The complementary roles of radionuclide myocardial perfusion imaging and cardiac computed tomography. *Semin Roentgenol* 2012;47:228–239.
36. **Heller GV, Links J, Bateman TM, et al.** American Society of Nuclear Cardiology and Society of Nuclear Medicine joint position statement: attenuation correction of myocardial perfusion SPECT scintigraphy. *J Nucl Cardiol* 2004;11:229–230.
37. **Sharma P, Patel C, Karunanithi S, et al.** Comparative accuracy of CT attenuation-corrected and non-attenuation—corrected SPECT myocardial perfusion imaging. *Clin Nucl Med* 2012;37:332–338.
38. **Weiss AT, Berman DS, Lew AS, et al.** Transient ischemic dilatation of the left ventricle on stress thallium-201 scintigraphy: a marker of severe and extensive coronary artery disease. *J Am Coll Cardiol* 1987;9(4): 752–759.
39. **Xu Y, Arsanjani R, Clond M, et al.** Transient ischemic dilation for coronary artery disease in quantitative analysis of same-day sestamibi myocardial perfusion SPECT. *J Nucl Cardiol* 2012;19(3):465–473.
40. **Petretta M, Acampa W, Daniele S, et al.** Transient ischemic dilation in SPECT myocardial perfusion imaging for prediction of severe coronary artery disease in diabetic patients. *J Nucl Cardiol* 2013;20:45–52.
41. **Arrighi JA, Soufer R.** Reverse redistribution: is it clinically relevant or a washout? *J Nucl Cardiol* 1998;5:195–201.
42. **Moralidis E, Spyridonidis T, Arsos G, et al.** Identification of advanced coronary artery disease with exercise myocardial perfusion imaging: the clinical value of a novel approach for assessing lung thallium-201 uptake. *Eur J Nucl Med Mol Imaging* 2007;34:573–583.
43. **Bacher-Stier C, Sharir T, Kavanagh P, et al.** Post exercise lung uptake of 99m-Tc-sestamibi determined by a new automatic technique: validation and application in detection of severe and extensive coronary artery disease and reduced left ventricular ejection fraction. *J Nucl Med* 2000;41(7):1190–1197.
44. **Leslie WD, Tully SA, Yogendran MS, et al.** Prognostic value of lung sestamibi uptake in myocardial perfusion imaging of patients with known or suspected coronary artery disease. *J Am Coll Cardiol* 2005;45(10):1676–1682.
45. **Mahmarian JJ, Boyce TM, Goldberg RK, et al.** Quantitative exercise thallium-201 single photon emission computed tomography for the enhanced diagnosis of ischemic heart disease. *J Am Coll Cardiol* 1990;15(2):318–329.
46. **Tilkemeier PL, Cooke CD, Ficaro EP, et al.** American Society of Nuclear Cardiology information statement: standardized reporting matrix for radionuclide myocardial perfusion imaging. *J Nucl Cardiol* 2006;13(6):e157–e171.
47. **Berman DS, Kiat H, Friedman JD, et al.** Separate acquisition rest thallium-201/stress technetium- 99m sestamibi dual-isotope myocardial perfusion single-photon emission computed tomography: a clinical validation study. *J Am Coll Cardiol* 1993;22(5):1455–1464.
48. **Slomka P, Xu Y, Berman D, et al.** Quantitative analysis of perfusion studies: strengths and pitfalls. *J Nucl Cardiol* 2012;19(2):338–346.
49. **Mohamed A, Gnanasegaran G, Buscombe JR, et al.** *Integrating cardiology for nuclear physicians.* Berlin, Germany: Springer; 2009:4–20.
50. **Gaemperli O, Bengel FM, Kaufmann PA.** Cardiac hybrid imaging. *Eur Heart J* 2011;32(17):2100–2108.
51. **Boogers MM, Van Kriekinge SD, Henneman MM, et al.** Quantitative gated SPECT-derived phase analysis on gated myocardial perfusion SPECT defects left ventricular dyssynchrony and predicts response to cardiac resynchronization therapy. *J Nucl Med* 2009;50:718–725.

52. **Di Carli MF, Dorbala S, Meserve J, et al.** Clinical myocardial Perfusion PET/CT. *J Nucl Med* 2007;48(5):783–793.
53. **Anagnostopoulos C, Georgakopoulos A, Pianou N, et al.** Assessment of myocardial perfusion and viability by positron emission tomography. *Int J Cardiol* 2013;167(5):1737–1749.
54. **Maddahi J, Czernin J, Lazewatsky J, et al.** Phase I, first-in-human study of BMS747158, a Novel 18 F-labeled tracer for myocardial perfusion PET: dosimetry, biodistribution, safety, and imaging characteristics after a single injection at rest. *J Nucl Med* 2011;52(9):1490–1498.
55. **Diamond GA, Forrester JS.** Analysis of probability as an aid in the clinical diagnosis of coronary-artery disease. *N Engl J Med* 1979; 300(24):1350–1358.
56. **Wilson PW, D'Agostino RB, Levy D, et al.** Prediction of coronary heart disease using risk factor categories. *Circulation* 1998;97(18): 1837–1847.
57. **Goodman SN.** Toward evidence-based medical statistics. 2: the Bayes factor. *Ann Intern Med* 1999;130(12):1005–1013.
58. **Chong FY, Soon K, Brown F, et al.** Negative coronary CT angiography for chest pain assessment predicts low event rate in 5 years. *J Med Imaging Radiat Oncol* 2012;56(1):55–57.
59. **Gibbons RJ, Balady GJ, Bricker JT, et al.** ACC/AHA 2002 guideline update for exercise testing: summary article. A report of the American College of Cardiology/American Heart Association Task Force on Practice Guidelines (Committee to Update the 1997 Exercise Testing Guidelines). *J Am Coll Cardiol* 2002;40(8):1531–1540.
60. **Hachamovitch R, Berman DS, Shaw LJ, et al.** Incremental prognostic value of myocardial perfusion single photon emission computed tomography for the prediction of cardiac death: differential stratification for risk of cardiac death and myocardial infarction. *Circulation* 1998;97(6):535–543.
61. **Loong CY, Anagnostopoulos C.** The diagnosis of coronary artery disease by radionuclide myocardial perfusion imaging. *Heart* 2004; V.90(suppl 5):V2–V9.
62. **Smanio PE, Watson DD, Segalla DL, et al.** Value of gating of technetium-99m sestamibi single-photon emission computed tomographic imaging. *J Am Coll Cardiol* 1997;30(7):1687–1692.
63. **Gibbons RJ, Abrams J, Chatterjee K, et al.** ACC/AHA 2002 guideline update for the management of patients with chronic stable angina—summary article: a report of the American College of Cardiology/American Heart Association Task Force on Practice Guidelines (Committee on the Management of Patients With Chronic Stable Angina). *Circulation* 2003;107(1):149–158.
64. **Berman D, Hachamovitch R, Shaw L, et al.** Roles of nuclear cardiology, cardiac computed tomography, and cardiac magnetic resonance: noninvasive risk stratification and a conceptual framework for the selection of noninvasive imaging tests in patients with known or suspected coronary artery disease. *J Nucl Med* 2006;47:1107–1118.
65. **Hachamovitch R, Hayes S, Friedman JD, et al.** Determinants of risk and its temporal variation in patients with normal stress myocardial perfusion scans: what is the warranty period of a normal scan? *J Am Coll Cardiol* 2003;41:1329–1340.
66. **Underwood SR, Anagnostopoulos C, Cerqueiera M, et al.** Myocardial perfusion scintigraphy: the evidence. *Eur J Nucl Med Mol Imaging* 2004;31(2):262–291.
67. **Berman D, Hachamovitch R, Shaw L, et al.** Roles of nuclear cardiology, cardiac computed tomography, and cardiac magnetic resonance: assessment of patients with suspected coronary artery disease. *J Nucl Med* 2006;47:74–82.
68. **Clark AN, Beller GA.** The present role of nuclear cardiology in clinical practice. *Q J Nucl Med Mol Imaging* 2005;49:43–58.
69. **Hendel R, Berman D, Di Carli M, et al.** ACCF/ASNC/ACR/AHA/ASE/SCCT/SCMR/SNM 2009 appropriate use criteria for cardiac radionuclide imaging: a report of the American College of Cardiology Foundation Appropriate Use Criteria Task Force, the American Society of Nuclear Cardiology, the American College of Radiology, the American Heart Association, the American Society of Echocardiography, the Society of Cardiovascular Computed Tomography, the Society for Cardiovascular Magnetic Resonance, and the Society of Nuclear Medicine: endorsed by the American College Of Emergency Physicians. *Circulation* 2009; 119:561–587.
70. **Klocke FJ, Baird MG, Lorell BH, et al.** ACC/AHA/ASNC guidelines for the clinical use of cardiac radionuclide imaging—executive summary: a report of the American College of Cardiology/American Heart Association Task Force on Practice Guidelines (ACC/AHA/ASNC Committee to Revise the 1995 Guidelines for the Clinical Use of Cardiac Radionuclide Imaging). *Circulation* 2003;108(11): 1404–1418.
71. **Abbott BG, Afshar M, Berger AK, et al.** Prognostic significance of ischemic electrocardiographic changes during adenosine infusion in patients with normal myocardial perfusion imaging. *J Nucl Cardiol* 2003;10(1):9–16.
72. **Marcassa C, Bax JJ, Bengel F, et al.** Clinical value, cost-effectiveness, and safety of myocardial perfusion scintigraphy: a position statement. *Eur Heart J* 2008;29(4):557–563.
73. **Bidov A, Bax JJ, Hayes SW, et al.** Transient ischemic dilation ratio of the left ventricle is a significant predictor of future cardiac events in patients with otherwise normal myocardial perfusion SPECT. *J Am Coll Cardiol* 2003;42(10):1818–1825.
74. **Gill JB, Ruddy TD, Newell JB, et al.** Prognostic importance of thallium uptake by the lungs during exercise in coronary artery disease. *N Engl J Med* 1987;317(24):1486–1489.
75. **Hachamovitch R, Rozanski A, Shaw LJ, et al.** Impact of ischaemia and scar on the therapeutic benefit derived from myocardial revascularization vs. medical therapy among patients undergoing stress-rest myocardial perfusion scintigraphy. *Eur Heart J* 2011;32:1012–1024.
76. **Shaw LJ, Berman DS, Maron DJ, et al.** Optimal medical therapy with or without percutaneous coronary intervention to reduce ischemic burden: results from the Clinical Outcomes Utilizing Revascularization and Aggressive Drug Evaluation (COURAGE) trial nuclear substudy. *Circulation* 2008;117:1283–1291.
77. **Gibbons RJ, Abrams J, Chatterjee K, et al.** American College of Cardiology; American Heart Association Task Force on Practice Guidelines. Committee on the Management of Patients with Chronic Stable Angina ACC/AHA 2002 guideline update for the management of patients with chronic stable angina: summary article. *Circulation* 2003;107:149–158.
78. **Fox K, Garcia MA, Ardissino D, et al.** Guidelines on the management of stable angina pectoris: executive summary. *Eur Heart J* 2006;27: 1341–1381.
79. **Hendel RC, Berman DS, Di Carli MF, et al.** ACCF/ASNC/ACR/AHA/ASE/SCCT/SCMR/SNM 2009 appropriate use criteria for cardiac radionuclide imaging. *J Am Coll Cardiol* 2009;53:2201–2229.
80. **Greenland P, Alpert JS, Beller GA, et al. American College of Cardiology Foundation/American Heart Association Task Force on Practice Guidelines.** 2010 ACCF/AHA guideline for assessment of cardiovascular risk in asymptomatic adults. *Circulation* 2010;122:e584–e636.
81. **Perrone-Filardi P, Achenbach S, Möhlenkamp S, et al.** Cardiac computed tomography and myocardial perfusion scintigraphy for risk stratification in asymptomatic individuals without known cardiovascular disease. *Eur Heart J* 2011;32(16):1986–1993.
82. **Hendel RC, Abbott BG, Bateman TM, et al.** The role of radionuclide myocardial perfusion imaging for asymptomatic individuals. *J Nucl Cardiol* 2011;18:3–15.
83. **Fleisher LA, Beckman JA, Brown KA, et al.** 2009 ACCF/AHA focused update on perioperative beta blockade incorporated into the ACC/AHA 2007 guidelines on perioperative cardiovascular evaluation and care for noncardiac surgery. *Circulation* 2009;120:169–276.
84. **Mautner SL, Lin F, Mautner GC, et al.** Comparison in women versus men of composition of atherosclerotic plaques in native coronary arteries and saphenous veins used as aorto-coronary conduits. *J Am Coll Cardiol* 1993;21:1312–1318.
85. **Cerqueira MD.** Diagnostic testing strategies for coronary artery disease: specific issues related to gender. *Am J Cardiol* 1995;75:52D–60D.
86. **Hachamovitch R, Berman DS, Kiat H, et al.** Effective risk stratification using exercise myocardial perfusion SPECT in women: gender-related differences in prognostic nuclear testing. *J Am Coll Cardiol* 1996;28:34–44.
87. **Marwick TH, Swaw LJ, Laurere MS, et al.** The noninvasive prediction of cardiac mortality in man and women with known or suspected coronary artery disease. *Am J Med* 1999;106:172–178.
88. **Swah LJ, Hachamovitch R, Redberg RF.** Current evidence on diagnostic testing in women with suspected coronary artery disease: choosing the appropriate test. *Cardiol Rev* 2000;8:65–74.
89. **Chen G, Redberg RF.** Noninvasive diagnostic testing of coronary artery disease in women. *Cardiol Rev* 2000;8(6):354–360
90. **Iskandar A, Limone B, Parker MW.** Gender differences in the diagnostic accuracy of SPECT myocardial perfusion imaging: a bivariate meta-analysis. *J Nucl Cardiol* 2013;20(1):53–63.

91. **Pianou N, Georgakopoulos A, Anagnostopoulos CD.** Positron emission tomography for risk assessment in women investigated for coronary artery disease. *Cardiology* 2011;118:164–167.
92. **Cerci MS, Cerci JJ, Cerci RJ, et al.** Myocardial Perfusion Imaging is a strong predictor of death in women. *JACC Cardiovasc Imaging* 2011; 4(8)880–888.
93. **Shaw LJ, Mieres JH, Hendel RH, et al.** Comparative effectiveness of exercise electrocardiography with or without myocardial perfusion single photon emission computed tomography in women with suspected coronary artery disease: results from the What Is the Optimal Method for Ischemia Evaluation in Women (WOMEN) trial. *Circulation* 2011;124(11):1239–1249.
94. **Berman DS, Kang X, Hayes SW, et al.** Adenosine myocardial perfusion single-photon emission computed tomography in women compared with men. Impact of diabetes mellitus on incremental prognostic value and effect on patient management. *J Am Coll Cardiol* 2003;41(7):1125–1133.
95. **Kang X, Berman DS, Lewin H, et al.** Comparative ability of myocardial perfusion single-photon emission computed tomography to detect coronary artery disease in patients with and without diabetes mellitus. *Am Heart J* 1999;137(5):949–957.
96. **Young LH, Wackers FJ, Chyun DA, et al.** Cardiac outcomes after screening for asymptomatic coronary artery disease in patients with type 2 diabetes: the DIAD study: a randomized controlled trial. *JAMA* 2009;301(15):1547–1555.
97. **Agarwal S, Morgan T, Herrington DM, et al.** Coronary calcium score and prediction of all-cause mortality in diabetes: the diabetes heart study. *Diabetes Care* 2011;34(5):1219–1224.
98. **Anand DV, Lim E, Hopkins D, et al.** Risk stratification in uncomplicated type 2 diabetes: prospective evaluation of the combined use of coronary artery calcium imaging and selective myocardial perfusion scintigraphy. *Eur Heart J* 2006;27(6):713–721.
99. **Bax JJ, Young LH, Frye RL, et al.** Screening for coronary artery disease in patients with diabetes. *Diabetes Care.* 2007;30(10):2729–2736.
100. **BARI 2D Study Group; Frye RL, August P, Brooks MM et al.** A randomized trial of therapies for type 2 diabetes and coronary artery disease. *N Engl J Med* 2009;360(24):2503–2515.
101. **Sorajja P, Chareonthaitawee P, Rajagopalan N, et al.** Improved survival in asymptomatic diabetic patients with high-risk SPECT imaging treated with coronary artery bypass grafting. *Circulation* 2005;112 (9 suppl):I311–I316.
102. **Shaw LJ, Weintraub WS, Maron DJ, et al.** Baseline stress myocardial perfusion imaging results and outcomes in patients with stable ischemic heart disease randomized to optimal medical therapy with or without percutaneous coronary intervention. *Am Heart J* 2012; 164(2):243–250.
103. **Abreu A.** Can myocardial perfusion scintigraphy predict the future for patients after percutaneous coronary intervention? *Rev Port Cardiol* 2002;21(12):1405–1410.
104. **Underwood SR, Anagnostopoulos C, Cerqueira M.** Myocardial perfusion scintigraphy: the evidence. *Eur J Nucl Med Mol Imaging* 2004;31(2):261–291.
105. **Elhendy A, van Domburg RT, Bax JJ, et al.** Dobutamine-atro-pine stress myocardial perfusion SPECT imaging in the diagnosis of graft stenosis after coronary artery bypass grafting. *J Nucl Cardiol* 1998; 5:533–537.
106. **Hendel RC, Abbott BG.** Bateman TM myocardial perfusion imaging after coronary revascularization: a clinical appraisal. *Eur J Nucl Med Mol Imaging* 2013;40(8):1275–1282.
107. **Bourque JM, Beller GA.** Stress myocardial perfusion imaging for assessing prognosis: an update. *JACC Cardiovasc Imaging* 2011;4(12): 1305–1319.
108. **Gould KL, Johnson NP, Bateman TM, et al.** Anatomic versus physiologic assessment of coronary artery disease. Role of coronary flow reserve, fractional flow reserve, and positron emission tomography imaging in revascularization decision-making. *J Am Coll Cardiol* 2013; 62(18):1639–1653.
109. **Parker MW, Iskandar A, Limone B, et al.** Diagnostic accuracy of cardiac positron emission tomography versus single photon emission computed tomography for coronary artery disease: a bivariate meta-analysis. *Circ Cardiovasc Imaging* 2012;5(6):700–707.
110. **Mc Ardle BA, Dowsley TF, Dekemp RA, et al.** Does Rubidium-82 PET have superior accuracy to SPECT perfusion imaging for the diagnosis of obstructive coronary disease? A systematic review and meta-analysis. *J Am Coll Cardiol* 2012;60(18):1828–1837.
111. **Marwick TH, Shan K, Patel S, et al.** Incremental value of Rubidium-82 Positron Emission Tomography for prognostic assessment of known or suspected coronary artery disease. *Am J Cardiol* 1997;80: 865–870.
112. **Chow BJ, Wong JW, Yoshinaga K, et al.** Prognostic significance of dipyridamole-induced ST depression in patients with normal ^{82}Rb PET Myocardial Perfusion Imaging. *J Nucl Med* 2005;46:1095–1101.
113. **Yoshinaga K., Chow BJ, Williams K, et al.** What is the prognostic value of myocardial perfusion imaging using Rubidium-82 positron emission tomography? *J Am Coll Cardiol* 2006;48(5):1029–1039.
114. **Dorbala S, Vangala D, SaMPIon U, et al.** Value of left ventricular ejection fraction reserve in evaluating the magnitude of myocardium at risk and the extent of angiographic coronary artery disease: a ^{82}Rb PET/CT study. *J Nucl Med* 2007;3:349–358.
115. **Dorbala S, Hachamovitch R, Curillova Z, et al.** Incremental prognostic value of gated Rb-82 positron emission tomography myocardial perfusion imaging over clinical variables and rest LVEF. *JACC Cardiovasc Imaging* 2009;2(7):846–854.
116. **Hajjiri MM, Leavitt MB, Zheng H, et al.** Comparison of positron emission tomography measurement of adenosine stimulated absolute myocardial blood flow versus relative myocardial tracer content for physiological assessment of coronary artery stenosis severity and location. *JACC Cardiovasc Imaging* 2009;2(6):751–758.
117. **Nesterov SV, Han C, Maki M, et al.** Myocardial perfusion quantitation with ^{15}O-labelled water PET: high reproducibility of the new cardiac analysis software (CARIMAS™). *Eur J Nucl Med Mol Imaging* 2009;36:1594–1602.
118. **Uren NG, Melin JA, De Bruyne B, et al.** Relation between myocardial blood flow and the severity of coronary artery stenosis. *N Engl J Med* 1994;330(25):1782–1788.
119. **Di Carli M, Czernin J, Hoh CK, et al.** Relation among stenosis severity, myocardial blood flow, and flow reserve in patients with coronary artery disease. *Circulation* 1995;91(7):1944–1951.
120. **Murthy VL, Naya M, Foster CR, et al.** Improved cardiac risk assessment with non invasive measures of coronary flow reserve. *Circulation* 2011;124(20):2215–2224.
121. **Herzog BA, Husmann L, Valenta I, et al.** Long-term prognostic value of 13N-ammonia myocardial perfusion positron emission tomography added value of coronary flow reserve. *J Am Coll Cardiol* 2009;54(2):150–156.
122. **Ziadi MC, Dekemp RA, Williams KA, et al.** Impaired myocardial flow reserve on rubidium-82 positron emission tomography imaging predicts adverse outcomes in patients assessed for myocardial ischemia. *J Am Coll Cardiol* 2011;58(7):740–748.
123. **Camici PG, Crea F.** Coronary microvascular dysfunction. *N Engl J Med* 2007;356:830–840.
124. **Wielepp P, Baller D, Gleichmann U, et al.** Beneficial effects of atorvastatin on myocardial regions with initially low vasodilatory capacity at various stages of coronary artery disease. *Eur J Nucl Med Mol Imaging* 2005;32:1371–1377.
125. **Williams MC, Reid JH, McKillop G, et al.** Cardiac and coronary CT comprehensive imaging approach in the assessment of coronary heart disease. *Heart* 2011;97:1198–1205.
126. **Dodla S, Xie F, Smith M, et al.** Real-time perfusion echocardiography during treadmill exercise and dobutamine stress testing. *Heart* 2010;96:220–225.
127. **Goulle JP, Cattaneo A, Saussereau E, et al.** MRI gadolinium-based contrast agents. Radiologists beware! *Ann Pharm Fr* 2009;67(5):335–339.
128. **Jaarsma C, Leiner T, Bekkers S, et al.** Diagnostic performance of non-invasive myocardial perfusion imaging using single-photon emission computed tomography, cardiac magnetic resonance, and positron emission tomography imaging for the detection of obstructive coronary artery disease. *J Am Coll Cardiol* 2012;59:1719–1728.
129. **Bernhardt P, Manzke R, Bornstedt A, et al.** Blood oxygen- level dependent magnetic resonance imaging using T2-prepared steady-state free-precession imaging in comparison to contrast–enhanced myocardial perfusion imaging. *Int J Cardiol* 2011;147:416–419.
130. **Gebker R, Jahnke C, Manka R, et al.** High spatial resolution myocardial perfusion imaging during high dose dobutamine/atropine stress magnetic resonance using k-t SENSE. *Int J Cardiol* 2012;158: 411–416.

131. **Shaw LJ, Hachamovitch R, Berman DS, et al.** The economic consequences of available diagnostic and prognostic strategies for the evaluation of stable angina patients: an observational assessment of the value of precatheterization ischemia. Economics of Noninvasive Diagnosis (END) Multicenter Study Group. *J Am Coll Cardiol* 1999; 33(3):661–669.
132. **Brindis RG, Douglas PS, Hendel RC, et al.** ACCF/ASNC appropriateness criteria for single-photon emission computed tomography myocardial perfusion imaging (SPECT MPI): a report of the American College of Cardiology Foundation Quality Strategic Directions Committee Appropriateness Criteria Working Group and the American Society of Nuclear Cardiology endorsed by the American Heart Association. *J Am Coll Cardiol* 2005;46(8):1587–1605.
133. **Patterson RE, Eisner RL, Horowitz SF.** Comparison of cost-effectiveness and utility of exercise ECG, single photon computed tomography, positron emission tomography, and coronary angiography for diagnosis of coronary artery disease. *Circulation* 1995;91(1):54–65.
134. **Löthgren M, Zethraeus N.** Definition, interpretation and calculation of costeffectiveness acceptability curves. *Health Econ* 2000;9(7): 623–630.
135. **Merhige ME, Breen WJ, Shelton V, et al.** Impact of myocardial perfusion imaging with PET and (82) Rb on downstream invasive procedure utilization, costs, and outcomes in coronary disease management. *J Nucl Med* 2007;48(7):1069–1076.
136. **Hachamovitch R, Nutter B, Hlatky MA, et al.** Patient management after noninvasive cardiac imaging results from SPARC (Study of myocardial perfusion and coronary anatomy imaging roles in coronary artery disease). *J Am Coll Cardiol* 2012;59(5):462–474.
137. **Gaemperli, O, Husmann L, Schepis T, et al.** Coronary CT angiography and myocardial perfusion imaging to detect flow-limiting stenoses: a potential gatekeeper for coronary revascularization? *Eur Heart J* 2009; 30:2921–2929.
138. **Pazhenkottil AP, Nkoulou RN, Ghadri JR, et al.** Prognostic value of cardiac hybrid imaging integrating single-photon emission computed tomography with coronary computed tomography angiography. *Eur Heart J* 2011;32:1465–1471.
139. **Kajander S, Joutsiniemi E, Saraste M, et al.** Cardiac positron emission tomography/computed tomography imaging accurately detects anatomically and functionally significant coronary artery disease. *Circulation* 2010;122(6):603–613.
140. **Esteves FP, Khan A, Corrreia LC, et al.** Absent coronary artery calcium excludes inducible myocardial ischemia on computed tomography/ positron emission tomography. *Int J Cardiol* 2011;147(3):424–427.
141. **Schenker MP, Dorbala S, Hong EC, et al.** Interrelation of coronary calcification, myocardial ischemia, and outcomes in patients with intermediate likelihood of coronary artery disease: a combined positron emission tomography computed tomography study. *Circulation* 2008; 117(13):1693–1700.
142. **Hausleiter J, Meyer T, Hermann F, et al.** Estimated radiation dose associated with cardiac CT angiography. *JAMA* 2009;301(5):500–507.
143. **Pichler BJ, Wehrl HF, Judenhofer MS.** Latest advances in molecular imaging instrumentation. *J Nucl Med* 2008;49 (suppl 2):5S–23S.
144. **Nekolla SG, Martinez-Moeller A, Saraste A.** PET and MRI in cardiac imaging: from validation studies to integrated applications. *Eur J Nucl Med Mol Imaging* 2009;36(suppl 1):S121–S130.
145. **Kontos MC, Jesse RL, Schmidt KL, et al.** Value of acute rest sestamibi perfusion imaging for evaluation of patients admitted to the emergency department with chest pain. *J Am Coll Cardiol* 1997;30:976–982.
146. **Heller GV, Stowers SA, Hendel RC, et al.** Clinical value of acute rest technetium-99m tetrofosmin tomography myocardial perfusion imaging in patients with acute chest pain and nondiagnostic electrocardiograms. *J Am Coll Cardiol 1998*;31:1011–1017.
147. **Kapetanopoulos A, Heller GV, Selker HP, et al.** Acute resting myocardial perfusion imaging in patients with diabetes mellitus: results from the Emergency Room Assessment of Sestamibi for Evaluation of Chest Pain (ERASE Chest Pain) trial. *J Nucl Cardiol* 2004; 11:570–577.
148. **van Der Werf F, Ardissino D, Betriou A, et al.** Management of acute myocardial infarction in patients presenting with ST-segment elevation. *Eur Heart J* 2003;24:28–66.
149. **Anagnostopoulos C, Underwood R.** Myocardial perfusion scintigraphy: the evidence. *Heart* 2004;90(suppl V):v1–v40.
150. **Antman EM, Anbe DT, Armstrong PW, et al.** ACC/AHA guidelines for the management of patients with ST-elevation myocardial infarction; A report of the American College of Cardiology/American Heart Association Task Force on Practice Guidelines (Committee to Revise the 1999 Guidelines for the Management of patients with acute myocardial infarction). *J Am Coll Cardiol* 2004;44:E1–E211.
151. **Brown KA, Heller GV, Landin RS, et al.** Early dipyridamole (99m) Tc-sestamibi single photon emission computed tomographic imaging 2 to 4 days after acute myocardial infarction predicts in-hospital and postdischarge cardiac events: comparison with submaximal exercise imaging. *Circulation* 1999;100:2060–2066.
152. **Travin MI, Dessouki A, Cameron T, et al.** Use of exercise technetium-99m sestamibi SPECT imaging to detect residual ischaemia and for risk stratification after acute myocardial infarction. *Am J Cardiol* 1995;75:665–669.
153. **Wright RS, Anderson JL, Adams CD, et al.** ACCF/AHA focused update incorporated into the ACC/AHA 2007 guidelines for the management of patients with unstable angina/non-ST-elevation myocardial infarction: a report of the American College of Cardiology Foundation/American Heart Association Task Force on Practice Guidelines Developed in Collaboration with the American Academy of Family Physicians, Society for Cardiovascular Angiography and Interventions, and the Society of Thoracic Surgeons. *J Am Coll Cardiol* 2011;57:e215–e367.
154. **Mahmarian JJ, Shaw LJ, Olszewski GH, et al.** Adenosine sestamibi SPECT post-infarction evaluation (INSPIRE) trial: a randomized, prospective multicenter trial evaluating the role of adenosine Tc-99m sestamibi SPECT for assessing risk and therapeutic outcomes in survivors of acute myocardial infarction. *J Nucl Cardiol* 2004 ;11(4):458–469.
155. **Zellweger MJ, Tabacek G, Zutter AW, et al.** Evidence for left ventricular remodeling after percutaneous coronary intervention: effect of percutaneous coronary intervention on left ventricular ejection fraction and volumes. *Int J Cardiol* 2004;96(2):197–201.
156. **Roger VL.** The heart failure epidemic. *Int J Environ Res Public Health* 2010;7:1807.
157. **Braunwald E.** The management of heart failure: the past, the present, and the future. *Circ Heart Fail* 2008;1(1):58–62.
158. **European Society of Cardiology.** Recommendations for guidelines production. *ESC/Task Force Instructions.* 2010;1–14.
159. **Hunt SA, Abraham WT, Chin MH, et al.** Focused update incorporated into the ACC/AHA 2005 guidelines for the diagnosis and management of heart failure in adults: a report of the American College of Cardiology Foundation/American Heart Association Task Force on Practice Guidelines Developed in Collaboration with the International Society for Heart and Lung Transplantation. *J Am Coll Cardiol* 2009;53:e1–e90.
160. **Soman P, Lahiri A, Mieres J, et al.** Etiology and pathophysiology of new-onset heart failure: evaluation by myocardial perfusion imaging. *J Nucl Cardiol* 2009;16(1):82–91.
161. **Atchley AE, Kitzman DW, Whellan DJ.** Myocardial perfusion, function, and dyssynchrony in patients with heart failure: baseline results from the single-photon emission computed tomography imaging ancillary study of the Heart Failure and A Controlled Trial Investigating Outcomes of Exercise TraiNing (HF-ACTION) Trial. *Am Heart J* 2009;158(4 suppl):S53–S63.
162. **Anagnostopoulos C, Neill J, Reyes E, et al.** Myocardial perfusion scintigraphy: technical innovations and evolving clinical applications. *Heart* 2012;98(5):353–359.
163. **Stirrup J, Wechalekar K, Maenhout A, et al.** Radionuclide imaging in ischaemic heart failure. *Br Med Bull* 2009;92:43–59.
164. **Kayden DS, Sigal S, Sonfer R, et al.** Thallium-201 for assessment of myocardial viability: quantitative comparison of 24 hour redistribution imaging with reinjection at rest. *J Am Coll Cardiol* 1991;18:1480–1486.
165. **Gunning MG, Anagnostopoulos C, Knight CJ, et al.** Identification of hibernating myocardium. A comparison of TI-201, Tc-99m tetrofosmin and dobutamine cine magnetic resonance imaging. *Circulation* 1998;98:1869–1874.
166. **Hambye AS, Dobbeleir AA, Vervaet AM, et al.** BMIPP imaging to improve the value of sestamibi scintigraphy for predicting functional outcome in severe chronic ischemic left ventricular dysfunction. *J Nucl Med* 1999;40(9):1468–1476.
167. **Anagnostopoulos C, Gunning MG, Pennell DJ, et al.** Regional myocardial motion and thickening assessed by ECG-Gated ^{99m}Tc-MIBI emission tomography and by magnetic resonance imaging. *Eur J Nucl Med* 1996;23:909–916. The reference is included in the Year Book of Nuclear Medicine 1998.

168. **Taki J, Nakajima K, Matsunari I, et al.** Impairment of regional fatty acid uptake in relation to wall motion and thallium-201 uptake in ischaemic but viable myocardium: assessment with iodine-123-labelled beta-methyl-branched fatty acid. *Eur J Nucl Med* 1995;22(12): 1385–1392.
169. **Taki J, Nakajima K, Matsunari I, et al.** Assessment of improvement of myocardial fatty acid uptake and function after revascularization using iodine-123-BMIPP. *J Nucl Med* 1997; 38(10):1503–1510.
170. **Slart RH, Bax JJ, Van Veldhuisen DJ, et al.** Imaging techniques in nuclear cardiology for the assessment of myocardial viability. *Int J Cardiovasc Imaging* 2006;22(1):63–80.
171. **Inglese E, Leva L, Matheoud R, et al.** Spatial and temporal heterogeneity of regional myocardial uptake in patients without heart disease under fasting conditions on repeated whole-body 18F-FDG PET/CT. *J Nucl Med* 2007;48(10):1662–1669.
172. **Dilsizian V, Bacharach SL, Beanlands RS, et al.** ASNC Imaging Guidelines for Nuclear Cardiology Procedures. ASNC imaging guidelines for nuclear cardiology procedures. PET myocardial perfusion and metabolism clinical imaging. *J Nucl Cardiol* 2009.
173. **Kitsiou AN, Bacharach SL, Bartlett ML, et al.** 13N-ammonia myocardial blood flow and uptake: relation to functional outcome of asynergic regions after revascularization. *J Am Coll Cardiol* 1999;33(3):678–686.
174. **Lida H, Ruotsalainen U, Mäki M, et al.** F-18 fluorodeoxyglucose uptake and water-perfusable tissue fraction in assessment of myocardial viability. *Ann Nucl Med* 2012;26(8):644–655.
175. **Schinkel AF, Bax JJ, Delgado V, et al.** Clinical relevance of hibernating myocardium in ischemic left ventricular dysfunction. *Am J Med* 2010;123 (11):978–986.
176. **Schinkel AF, Bax JJ, Poldermans D, et al.** Hibernating myocardium: diagnosis and patient outcomes. *Curr Probl Cardiol* 2007;32(7):375–410.
177. **Bengel FM, Higuchi T, Javadi MS, et al.** Cardiac positron emission tomography. *J Am Coll Cardiol* 2009;54(1):1–15.
178. **Landoni C, Lucignani G, Paolini G, et al.** Assessment of GABG -related risk in patients with CAD and LVD. Contribution of PET with [18F] FDG to the assessment of myocardial viability. *J Cardiovasc Surg* 1999;40:363–372.
179. **Eitzman D, al-Aouar Z, Kanter HL, et al.** Clinical outcome of patients with advanced coronary artery disease after viability studies with positron emission tomography. *J Am Coll Cardiol* 1992;20(3):559–565.
180. **Rohatgi R, Epstein S, Henriquez J, et al.** Utility of positron emission tomography in predicting cardiac events and survival in patients with coronary artery disease and severe left ventricular dysfunction. *Am J Cardiol* 2001;87(9):1096–1099.
181. **Siebelink HM, Blanksma PK, Crijns HJ, et al.** No difference in cardiac event free survival between positron emission tomography–guided and single-photon emission computed tomography-guided patient management: a prospective, randomized comparison of patients with suspicion of jeopardized myocardium. *J Am Coll Cardiol* 2001;37(1):81–88.
182. **Camici PG, Prasad SK, Rimoldi OE.** Stunning hibernation and assessment of myocardial viability. *Circulation* 2008;117(1):103–114.
183. **Beanlands RS, Nichol G, Huszti E, et al.** F-18-fluorodeoxyglucose positron emission tomography imaging-assisted management of patients with severe left ventricular dysfunction and suspected coronary disease: a randomized controlled trial (PARR-2). *J Am Coll Cardiol* 2007;50(20):2002–2012.
184. **D' Egidio G, Nichol G, Williams KA, et al.** Increasing benefit from revascularization is associated with increasing amounts of myocardial hibernation: a substudy of the PARR-2 trial. *JACC Cardiovasc Imaging* 2009;2(9):1060–1068.
185. **Inaba Y, Chen JA, Bergmann SR.** Quantity of viable myocardium required to improve survival with revascularization in patients with ischemic cardiomyopathy: a meta-analysis. *J Nucl Cardiol* 2010; 17(4):646–654.
186. **Abraham A, Nichol G, Williams KA, et al.** 18-F-FDG PET imaging of myocardial viability in an experienced center with access to 18 F-FDG and integration with clinical management teams: the Ottawa-Five substudy of the PARR 2 trial. *J Nucl Med* 2010;51(4):567–574.
187. **Bourge RC, Abraham WT, Adamson PB, et al.** Randomized controlled trial of an implantable continuous hemodynamic monitor in patients with advanced heart failure: the COMPASS-HF study. *J Am Coll Cardiol* 2008;51(11):1073–1079.
188. **Meara O, Mielniczuk E, Wells LM, et al.** Alternative Imaging modalities in ischemic Heart Failure (AIMI-HF) IMAGE HF Project I-A: study protocol for a randomized controlled trial. *Trials* 2013;14:218.
189. **Bonow RO, Maurer G, Lee KL, et al.** Myocardial viability and survival in ischemic left ventricular dysfunction. *N Engl J Med* 2011; 364(17):1617–1625.
190. **Di Carli MF, Davidson M, Little R, et al.** Value of metabolic imaging with positron emission tomography for evaluating prognosis in patients with coronary artery disease and left ventricular dysfunction. *Am J Cardiol* 1994;73(8):527–533.
191. **Marwick TH, Nemec JJ, Lanfont A, et al.** Prediction by postexercise fluoro-18 deoxyglucose positron emission tomography of improvement in exercise capacity after revascularization. *Am J Cardiol* 1992; 69(9):854–859.
192. **Haas F, Haehnel CJ, Picker W, et al.** Preoperative positron emission topographic viability assessment and perioperative and postoperative risk in patients with advanced ischemic heart disease. *J Am Coll Cardiol* 1997;30:1693–1700.
193. **Gunning MG, Chua TP, Harrington D, et al.** Hibernating myocardium: clinical and functional response to revascularisation. *Eur J Cardiothorac Surg* 1997(6):1105–1112.
194. **Shukla T, Nichol G, Wells G, et al.** Does FDG PET–assisted management of patients with left ventricular dysfunction improve quality of life? A substudy of the PARR-2 trial. *Can J Cardiol.* 2012;28(1):54–61.
195. **Bonow RO, Ganiats TG, Beam CT, et al.** ACCF/AHA/AMA-PCPI 2011 performance measures for adults with heart failure: a report of the American College of Cardiology Foundation/American Heart Association Task Force on performance measures and the American Medical Association–Physician consortium for performance improvement. *Circulation* 2012;125(19):2382–2401.
196. **Jessup M, Abraham WT, Casey DE, et al.** 2009 focused update: ACCF/AHA guidelines for the diagnosis and management of heart failure in adults: a report of the American College of Cardiology Foundation/American Heart Association Task Force on practice guidelines: developed in collaboration with the International Society for Heart and Lung Transplantation. *Circulation* 2009;119(14):1977–2016.
197. **Howlett JG, McKelvie RS, Costigan J, et al.** The 2010 Canadian Cardiovascular Society guidelines for the diagnosis and management of heart failure update: heart failure in ethnic minority populations, heart failure and pregnancy, disease management, and quality improvement/assurance programs. *Can J Cardiol* 2010;26(4):185–202.
198. **Dickstein K, Cohen-Solal A, Filippatos G, et al.** ESC guidelines for the diagnosis and treatment of acute and chronic heart failure 2008: the Task Force for the diagnosis and treatment of acute and chronic heart failure 2008 of the European Society of Cardiology. Developed in collaboration with the Heart Failure Association of the ESC (HFA) and endorsed by the European Society of Intensive Care Medicine (ESICM). *Eur J Heart Fail* 2008;10:933–989.
199. **Underwood SR, Bax JJ, vom Dahl J, et al.** Imaging techniques for the assessment of myocardial hibernation Report of a study group of the European Society of Cardiology. *Eur Heart J* 2004;25(10):815–836.
200. **Henneman MM, van der Wall EE, Ypenburg C, et al.** Nuclear imaging in cardiac resynchronization therapy. *J Nucl Med* 2007; 48(12):2001–2010.
201. **Chen J, Boogers MJ, Bax JJ, et al.** The use of nuclear imaging for cardiac resynchronization therapy. *Curr Cardiol Rep* 2010;12(2):185–191.
202. **Al Jaroudi W, Alraies MC, Hachamovittch R, et al.** Association of left ventricular mechanical dyssynchrony with survival benefit from revascularization: a study of gated positron emission tomography in patients with ischemic LV dysfunction and narrow QRS. *Eur J Nucl Med Mol Imaging* 2012;39(10):1581–1591.
203. **Penicka M, Lang O, Widimsky P, et al.** One-day kinetics of myocardial engraftment after intracoronary injection of bone marrow mononuclear cells in patients with acute and chronic myocardial infarction. *Heart* 2007;93:837–841.
204. **Chen IY, Wu JC.** Cardiovascular molecular imaging. Focus on clinical translation. *Circulation* 2011;123:425–443.
205. **Lanza GA.** Cardiac syndrome X: a critical overview and future perspectives. *Heart* 2007;93(2):159–166.
206. **Ong P, Athanasiadis A, Mahrholdt H, et al.** Increased coronary vasoconstrictor response to acetylcholine in women with chest pain and normal coronary arteriograms (cardiac syndrome X). *Clin Res Cardiol* 2012;101(8):673–681.

207. **Graf S, Khorsand A, Gwechenberger M, et al.** Typical chest pain and normal coronary angiogram: cardiac risk factor analysis versus PET for detection of microvascular disease. *J Nucl Med* 2007;48(2):175–181.
208. **Demir H, Kahraman G, Isgoren S, et al.** Evaluation of post-stress left ventricular dysfunction and its relationship with perfusion abnormalities using gated SPECT in patients with cardiac syndrome X. *Nucl Med Commun* 2008;29(3):208–214.
209. **Prabhu AS, Singh TP, Morrow WR, et al.** Safety and efficacy of intravenous adenosine for pharmacologic stress testing in children with aortic valve disease or Kawasaki disease. *Am J Cardiol* 1999;83(2):284–286.
210. **Fukuda T, Ishibashi M, Yokoyama T, et al.** Myocardial ischemia in Kawasaki disease: evaluation with dipyridamole stress technetium 99m tetrofosmin scintigraphy. *J Nucl Cardiol* 2002;9(6):632–637.
211. **Jan SL, Hwang B, Fu YC, et al.** Comparison of 201Tl SPET and treadmill exercise testing in patients with Kawasaki disease. *Nucl Med Commun* 2000;21(5):431–435.
212. **Kondo C, Nakanishi T, Sonobe T, et al.** Scintigraphic monitoring of coronary artery occlusion due to Kawasaki disease. *Am J Cardiol* 1993;71(8):681–685.
213. **Hijazi ZM, Udelson JE, Snapper H, et al.** Physiologic significance of chronic coronary aneurysms in patients with Kawasaki disease. *J Am Coll Cardiol* 1994;24(7):1633–1638.
214. **Nienaber CA, Spielmann RP, Hausdorf G.** Dipyridamole-thallium-201 tomography documenting improved myocardial perfusion with therapy in Kawasaki disease. *Am Heart J* 1988;116(6 Pt 1):1575–1579.
215. **Fukazawa M, Fukushige J, Takeuchi T, et al.** Discordance between thallium-201 scintigraphy and coronary angiography in patients with Kawasaki disease: myocardial ischemia with normal coronary angiogram. *Pediatr Cardiol* 1993;14(2):67–74.
216. **Fu YC, Kao CH, Hwang B, et al.** Discordance between dipyridamole stress Tc-99m sestamibi SPECT and coronary angiography in patients with Kawasaki disease. *J Nucl Cardiol* 2002;9(1):41–46.
217. **Muzik O, Paridon SM, Singh TP, et al.** Quantification of myocardial blood flow and flow reserve in children with a history of Kawasaki disease and normal coronary arteries using positron emission tomography. *J Am Coll Cardiol* 1996;28(3):757–762.
218. **Ohmochi Y, Onouchi Z, Oda Y, et al.** Assessment of effects of intravenous dipyridamole on regional myocardial perfusion in children with Kawasaki disease without angiographic evidence of coronary stenosis using positron emission tomography and H2(15)O. *Coron Artery Dis* 1995;6(7):555–559.
219. **Hwang B, Liu RS, Chu LS, et al.** Positron emission tomography for the assessment of myocardial viability in Kawasaki disease using different therapies. *Nucl Med Commun* 2000;21(7):631–636.
220. **Miyagawa M, Mochizuki T, Murase K, et al.** Prognostic value of dipyridamole-thallium myocardial scintigraphy in patients with Kawasaki disease. *Circulation* 1998;98(10):990–996.
221. **Maron BJ, Towbin JA, Thiene G, et al.** Contemporary definitions and classification of the cardiomyopathies: an American Heart Association Scientific Statement from the Council on Clinical Cardiology, Heart Failure and Transplantation Committee; Quality of Care and Outcomes Research and Functional Genomics and Translational Biology Interdisciplinary Working Groups; and Council on Epidemiology and Prevention. *Circulation* 2006;113(14):1807–1816.
222. **Thiene G, Corrado D, Basso C.** Revisiting definition and classification of cardiomyopathies in the era of molecular medicine. *Eur Heart J* 2008;29:144–146.
223. **Morton G, Chiribiri A, Ishida M, et al.** Quantification of absolute myocardial perfusion in patients with coronary artery disease: comparison between cardiovascular magnetic resonance and positron emission tomography. *J Am Coll Cardiol* 2012;60:1546–1555.
224. **Sorajja P, Chareonthaitawee P, Ommen SR, et al.** Prognostic utility of single-photon emission computed tomography in adult patients with hypertrophic cardiomyopathy. *Am Heart J* 2006;151(2):426–435.
225. **O'Neill JO, McCarthy PM, Brunken RC, et al.** PET abnormalities in patients with nonischemic cardiomyopathy. *J Card Fail* 2004;10(3):244–249.
226. **Sobajima M, Nozawa T, Suzuki T, et al.** Impact of myocardial perfusion abnormality on prognosis in patients with non-ischemic dilated cardiomyopathy. *J Cardiol* 2010;56(3):280–286.
227. **Fank W, Zhang J, He ZX.** Myocardial ischemia in patients with dilated cardiomyopathy. *Nucl Med Commun* 2010;31(11):981–984.
228. **Okayama K, Kurata C, Tawaraha K, et al.** Diagnostic and prognostic value of myocardial scintigraphy with thallium-201 and gallium-67 in cardiac sarcoidosis. *Chest* 1995;107:330–334.
229. **Ohira H, Tsujino I, Yoshinaga K.** 18F-Fluoro-2-deoxyglucose positron emission tomography in cardiac sarcoidosis. *Eur J Nucl Med Mol Imaging* 2011;38:1773–1778.
230. **Polacek P, Kralove H.** Relation of myocardial bridges and loops on the coronary arteries to coronary occlusions. *Am Heart J* 1961;61:44–52.
231. **Mohlenkamp S, Hort W, Ge J, et al.** Update on myocardial bridging. *Circulation* 2002;106(20):2616–2622.
232. **Jatene AD, Fontes VF, Paulista PP, et al.** Anatomic correction of transposition of the great vessels. *J Thorac Cardiovasc Surg* 1976;72(3):364–370.
233. **Tsuda E, Imakita M, Yagihara T, et al.** Late death after arterial switch operation for transposition of the great arteries. *Am Heart J* 1992;124:1551–1557.
234. **Taylor AJ, Rogan KM, Virmani R.** Sudden cardiac death associated with isolated congenital coronary artery anomalies. *J Am Coll Cardiol* 1992;20(3):640–647.
235. **Rajfer SI, Oetgen WJ, Weeks KD, et al.** Thallium-201 scintigraphy after surgical repair of hemodynamically significant primary coronary artery anomalies. *Chest* 1982;81(6):687–692.
236. **Hauser M, Bengel FM, Hager A, et al.** Impaired myocardial blood flow and coronary flow reserve of the anatomical right systemic ventricle in patients with congenitally corrected transposition of the great arteries. *Heart* 2003;89(10):1231–1235.
237. **Bengel FM, Hauser M, Duvernoy CS, et al.** Myocardial blood flow and coronary flow reserve late after anatomical correction of transposition of the great arteries. *J Am Coll Cardiol* 1998;32(7):1955–1961.
238. **Moodie DS, Cook SA, Gill CC, et al.** Thallium-201 myocardial imaging in young adults with anomalous left coronary artery arising from the pulmonary artery. *J Nucl Med* 1980;21(11):1076–1079.
239. **Gutgesell HP, Pinsky WW, DePuey EG.** Thallium-201 myocardial perfusion imaging in infants and children. Value in distinguishing anomalous left coronary artery from congestive cardiomyopathy. *Circulation* 1980;61(3):596–599.
240. **Goldblatt E, Adams AP, Ross IK, et al.** Single-trunk anomalous origin of both coronary arteries from the pulmonary artery. Diagnosis and surgical management. *J Thorac Cardiovasc Surg* 1984;87(1):59–65.
241. **Voss H, Kupper W, Hanrath P, et al.** Clinical correlations, lactate extraction, coronary venous bloodflow and Thallium-201 myocardial imaging in patients with isolated left anterior descending muscle bridges: normal variant or obstruction? (author's transl). *Z Kardiol* 1980;69(5):347–352.
242. **Klues HG, Schwarz ER, vom Dahl J, et al.** Disturbed intracoronary hemodynamics in myocardial bridging: early normalization by intracoronary stent placement. *Circulation* 1997;96(9):2905–2913.
243. **Agirbasli M, Martin GS, Stout JB, et al.** Myocardial bridge as a cause of thrombus formation and myocardial infarction in a young athlete. *Clin Cardiol* 1997;20(12):1032–1036.
244. **Roul G, Sens P, Germain P, et al.** Myocardial bridging as a cause of acute transient left heart dysfunction. *Chest* 1999;116(2):574–580.
245. **Connelly MS, Liu PP, Williams WG, et al.** Congenitally corrected transposition of the great arteries in the adult: functional status and complications. *J Am Coll Cardiol* 1996;27(5):1238–1243.
246. **Bajwa N, Bianco JA, Stone CK.** Thallium myocardial scintigraphy in congenitally-corrected transposition of the great arteries. *J Nucl Med* 1991;32(8):1611–1613.
247. **Hornung TS, Bernard EJ, Celermajer DS, et al.** Right ventricular dysfunction in congenitally corrected transposition of the great arteries. *Am J Cardiol* 1999;84(9):1116–1119.
248. **Lubiszewska B, Gosiewska E, Hoffman P, et al.** Myocardial perfusion and function of the systemic right ventricle in patients after atrial switch procedure for complete transposition: long-term follow-up. *J Am Coll Cardiol* 2000;36(4):1365–1370.
249. **Weindling SN, Wernovsky G, Colan SD, et al.** Myocardial perfusion, function and exercise tolerance after the arterial switch operation. *J Am Coll Cardiol* 1994;23(2):424–433.
250. **Yates RW, Marsden PK, Badawi RD, et al.** Evaluation of myocardial perfusion using positron emission tomography in infants following a neonatal switch operation. *Pediatr Cardiol* 2000;21:111–118.

251. **Hayes AM, Baker EJ, Kakadeker A, et al.** Influence of anatomic correction for transposition of the great arteries on myocardial perfusion: radionuclide imaging with technetium-99m 2-methoxy isobutyl isonitrile. *J Am Coll Cardiol* 1994;24(3):769–777.
252. **Owlia MB, Mostafavi Pour Manshadi SM, Naderi N.** Cardiac manifestations of rheumatological conditions: a narrative review *ISRN Rheumatol* 2012;2012:463620. doi: 10.5402/2012/463620.
253. **Hürlimann D, Enseleit F, Ruschitzka F.** Rheumatoid arthritis, inflammation, and atherosclerosis. *Herz* 2004;29(8):760–768.
254. **Kao AH, Wasko MC, Krishnaswami S, et al.** C-reactive protein and coronary artery calcium in asymptomatic women with systemic lupus erythematosus or rheumatoid arthritis. *Am J Cardiol* 2008; 102(6):755–760.
255. **Baharfard N, Shiroodi MK, Fotoohi F, et al.** Myocardial perfusion imaging using a technetium-99m sestamibi in asymptomatic and low risk for coronary artery disease patients diagnosed systemic lupus erythematosus. *Perfusion* 2011;26(2):151–157.
256. **Alexanderson E, Ochoa JM, Calleja R, et al.** Endothelial dysfunction in systemic lupus erythematosus: evaluation with ^{13}N-Ammonia PET. *J Nucl Med* 2010;51:1927–1931.
257. **Schmauss D, Weis M.** Cardiac allograft vasculopathy: recent developments. *Circulation* 2008;117:2131–2141.

CHAPTER

24 Myocardial Perfusion Imaging with Contrast Echocardiography

Kevin Wei, MD

Introduction

Echocardiography plays an important role in the management of patients, especially in its ability to evaluate left ventricular (LV) global and regional function. Its portability, lack of ionizing radiation, and relatively low cost make it the initial test of choice in many clinical situations. Its clinical utility, however, may be impacted by image quality. It has been estimated that between 10% and 15% of routine echocardiograms, and up to 25% to 30% of studies performed in intensive care units, have incomplete resolution of the endocardial border.[1,2] Left ventricular opacification (LVO) with microbubble ultrasound contrast agents (UCAs) have been shown in numerous studies to enhance delineation of the endocardial border, which improves both the qualitative and quantitative assessment of LV function, and decreases inter- and intraobserver variability.[3–7] LVO has also been shown to improve delineation of intracardiac pathology especially at the LV apex—such as aneurysms and pseudoaneurysms, masses, thrombi, hypertrophic cardiomyopathy, and isolated noncompaction.[1] UCAs also enhance delineation of systemic Doppler signals, like pulmonary venous inflows or aortic outflow signals.[8]

Many may not realize, however, that the imaging methods that are used for LVO today were all developed with an alternate goal in mind—namely, to assess myocardial perfusion with UCAs. Since coronary artery disease (CAD) continues to remain the leading cause of morbidity and mortality worldwide, myocardial perfusion imaging (MPI) with UCAs has wide applications and clinical benefit. However, MPI with UCAs is still an off-label application, because to date, no UCA has yet gained approval from the Federal Drug Administration for an MPI indication.

This chapter will discuss various ultrasound imaging methods that have been developed for qualitative and quantitative assessment of MPI. Furthermore, aspects of the coronary microcirculation that form the basis for MPI with myocardial contrast echocardiography (MCE) will be discussed, as well as the clinical applications that have been studied.

Principles of Quantitative MCE

Properties of Microbubble Tracers

There are currently two commercially available microbubble UCAs in the United States—Optison (GE Healthcare) and Definity (Lantheus Medical Imaging). The mean diameter of the microbubbles is less than 5 μm, allowing them to pass unimpeded through the capillary beds of tissues, and the gas contained within the microbubbles is a high molecular weight gas (perfluoropropane) that has low diffusibility and solubility, so the size of the microbubbles remains stable after their administration into the circulation.

The microbubbles used as tracers during MCE have a number of properties that make them ideal for measuring microcirculatory flow. They approximate the size of red blood cells (RBCs) and can pass unimpeded through the coronary microcirculation.[9] The microbubbles are hemodynamically inert and, therefore, do not influence coronary or systemic flow. The microbubbles have also been shown to have the same intravascular rheology as RBCs and can therefore be used to track the transit of RBCs through tissue.[10,11]

Backscatter signals from microbubbles (see below) are processed into pixels of brightness or acoustic intensity (AI) in the ultrasound system. In order to quantitate the microbubble backscatter signal, the relationship between microbubble concentration and AI must be known. Figure 24-1 shows that at low concentration of microbubbles, the relationship between AI and microbubble concentration is linear (Fig. 24-1, inset).[12] As microbubble concentration increases, the AI saturates and the relation between the two variables plateaus. At even higher microbubble concentrations, AI actually decreases due to attenuation of ultrasound by the microbubbles. For quantitative MPI, it is essential to ensure that the microbubble concentration is maintained within the linear range so that the AI remains directly proportional to microbubble concentration. Since it is impractical to derive the microbubble concentration versus AI relation for each patient prior to a perfusion study, a simple way of ensuring that saturation has not been reached within the myocardium is to keep myocardial enhancement visually less bright than the LV cavity.

The Generation and Detection of Microbubble Ultrasound Signal

Ultrasound can be described as a wavefront of alternating positive and negative pressure fluctuations that occur at a frequency above the audible range for humans (>20 KHz). The gas-containing microbubbles are four to five times more compressible than water or tissue. Since microbubbles are compressible and are generally smaller than the wavelength of ultrasound used during clinical

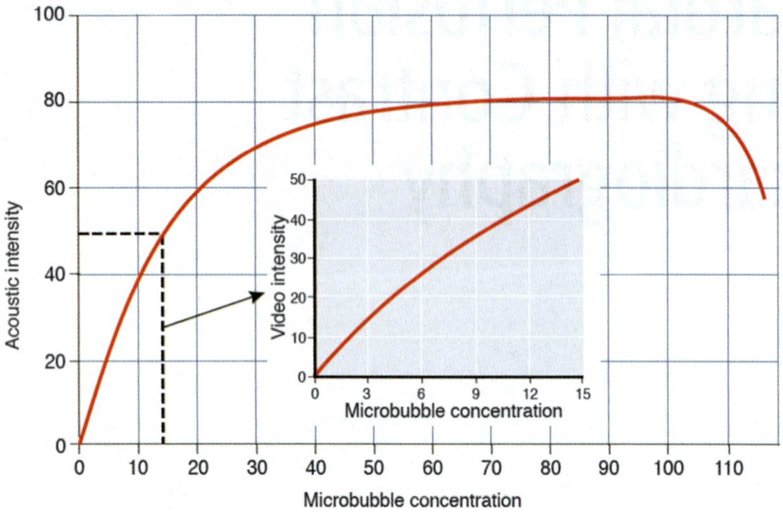

Figure 24-1. **Relation between microbubble concentration and backscatter acoustic intensity.** The relation is linear only at low concentrations of microbubbles (**inset**). (From Skyba DM, Jayaweera AR, Goodman NC, et al. Quantification of myocardial perfusion with myocardial contrast echocardiography during left atrial injection of contrast: implications for venous injection. *Circulation* 1994;90:1513–1521.)

imaging, they undergo volumetric oscillation in the acoustic field since they are compressed during the pressure peaks and expand during the low pressure phases of ultrasound (Fig. 24-2A).[13,14] Radial oscillations of microbubbles generate backscatter that result in bright signals in ultrasound images. Myocardial tissue, however, also produces strong ultrasound backscatter. For MPI, in order to detect the microbubbles within the tissue, the system must differentiate microbubble backscatter signals from those of tissue (which is considered "noise" during MCE).

An unique property of the oscillating microbubbles is the nonlinear microbubble behavior. Microbubbles have an ideal resonant frequency at which radial oscillation is particularly efficient and exaggerated. The ideal resonant frequency for a microbubble is inversely related to the square of its radius and is also influenced by the viscoelastic and compressive properties of the shell and gas.[15,16] By serendipity, for the size and shell properties of currently available microbubble UCAs, the resonant frequency is in the range of those used for echocardiographic imaging in adults. Furthermore, when the acoustic pressure of the insonating beam is sufficiently high, the oscillation of the microbubbles becomes nonlinear, so the alternate compression and expansion of the microbubbles are unequal or asymmetric (Fig. 24-2B).[17–19]

The asymmetric acoustic signals from nonlinear microbubble behavior can be shown to consist of fundamental and harmonic frequencies using fast Fourier transform.[19] An example of harmonics is illustrated by the frequency–amplitude histogram received from a microbubble contrast agent in Figure 24-2C. A very strong signal is returned at the frequency that was transmitted (the fundamental frequency or f_o). A second peak is produced by the microbubbles at twice the fundamental frequency, termed the second harmonic signal ($2f_o$). Tissue produces lower amplitude signals at the second harmonic compared to UCAs and come from gradual distortion of the acoustic pulse as it propagates from the near to the far-field through the tissue.[20] Filtering all but the harmonic signals (so-called harmonic imaging) enhances the signal-to-noise ratio during contrast imaging, thereby improving contrast detection compared to fundamental imaging for MPI with MCE.[19]

The degree of nonlinear oscillation is related to the power of the transmitted ultrasound. Exaggerated microbubble oscillation at high powers leads to microbubble destruction from abrupt fragmentation of the microbubbles, which can occur with only a single pulse of ultrasound. Although intense harmonic backscatter signals can be derived from UCAs as they burst with high-power ultrasound, continual destruction of microbubbles prevents effective contrast enhancement of tissue. Ultrasound systems commonly display the acoustic power in terms of the mechanical index (MI), which is directly proportional to the acoustic pressure (peak negative pressure in MPa) and is inversely proportional to the square root of the frequency. An MI greater than 0.5 usually results in rapid microbubble destruction during imaging. In order to assess myocardial perfusion using high MI imaging methods, the frame rate of imaging must therefore be dramatically reduced to allow microbubbles to populate myocardial capillaries in between destructive pulses. Typically, ultrasound transmission will be triggered using the electrocardiogram, so it was termed "intermittent" imaging. The method initially developed to quantify flow with MCE utilized this type of intermittent high MI imaging (see below).

After intermittent harmonic imaging, the next generation of imaging methods developed to further enhance signal-to-noise ratio for MPI with MCE utilized algorithms that incorporated various receive filters or Doppler processing. As shown in Figure 24-3, amplitude of microbubble backscatter signals (red line at "a") are of equal intensity to tissue signals (blue line at "b") at the fundamental frequency (f_o), so the signal-to-noise ratio of fundamental imaging is poor and is inadequate for MPI. With second harmonic imaging (transmit at f_o with receive only at $2f_o$), improvement in the signal-to-noise ratio ("c" vs. "d") is achieved, but strong tissue clutter ("d") is still present. With the development of broaderband transducers, further improvement in the signal-to-noise ratio ("e" vs. "f") has been accomplished with ultraharmonic imaging (transmit at f_o with receive only at $5/2f_o$), which takes advantage of low tissue noise ("f") at the ultraharmonic while microbubble destruction produces strong microbubble signals ("e"). Harmonic and ultraharmonic imaging use B-mode processing techniques to suppress tissue noise, but Doppler processing can also be used. With the latter, received signals from tissue show little spectral decorrelation compared to the transmitted signal, which can then be suppressed by an appropriate wall filter. Conversely, microbubble destruction produces received signals that are markedly different from those transmitted—consequently, only the power spectrum of microbubbles is displayed (this was called power harmonic Doppler imaging).

The use of high MI imaging modes discussed above mandated the use of low frame rates which removed the ability to simultaneously assess myocardial perfusion and wall motion, and also made imaging cumbersome and slow. Therefore, MPI methods using a low MI were sought. When the MI of ultrasound is reduced to very low levels (approximately 0.1), and the frequency of ultrasound approximates the resonant frequency of the microbubble,

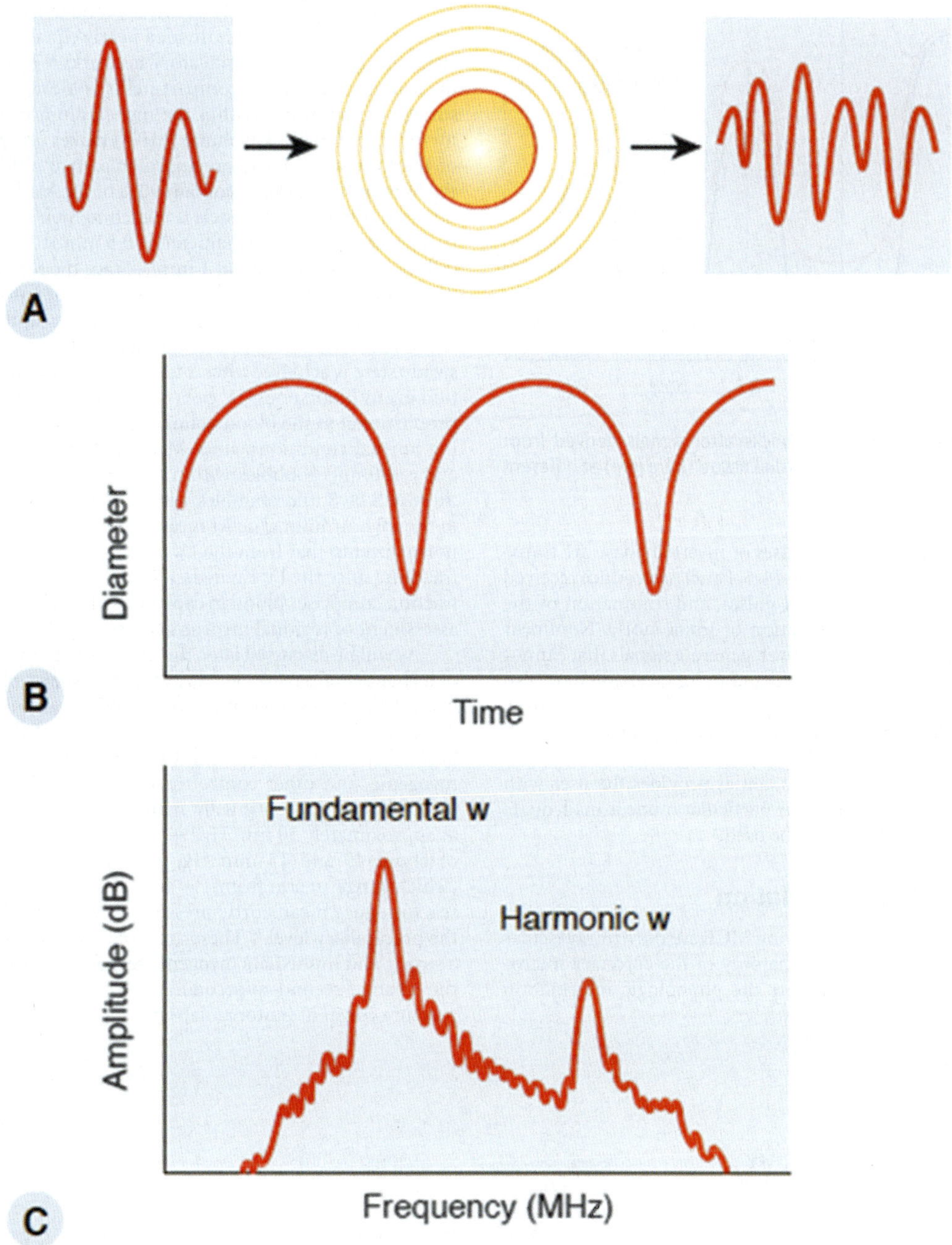

Figure 24-2. Panel A: Sound waves cause compressible microbubbles to oscillate, resulting in the production of ultrasound backscatter signals. **Panel B:** Graph depicting changes in microbubble diameter over time when it is oscillating at its resonant frequency. The alternate expansion and compression phases of the microbubble are unequal (nonlinear). **Panel C:** The acoustic spectrum arising from nonlinear oscillation of the microbubble contains fundamental and harmonic frequencies.

nonlinear microbubble oscillation (and harmonic signals) can still be induced without the microbubbles being destroyed. Tissue, on the other hand, responds "linearly" to low MI ultrasound, which means that tissue backscatter contains very low amplitude harmonic signals, making the separation of nonlinear microbubble signals from that of the myocardium possible. Tissue clutter can also be suppressed using multipulse schemes (the transmission of multiple ultrasound pulses sequentially along the same line), where the amplitude (power modulation) or phase (pulse inversion) of sequential pulses are altered. With power modulation (Fig. 24-4), pulses at half-height ("A") and full-height amplitude ("B") are transmitted sequentially. The received signals from a linear scatterer such as tissue (Fig. 24-4, Panel A) are identical to the transmitted pulses. Subsequently, the received echoes from the half-height transmitted pulses are scaled and subtracted from the full-height signal, which results in effective removal of tissue clutter. On the other hand, nonlinear scatterers such as microbubbles (Panel B) produce received signals that are different from the transmitted pulses (especially from the full-height pulse), resulting in residual microbubble signal even after subtraction. With pulse

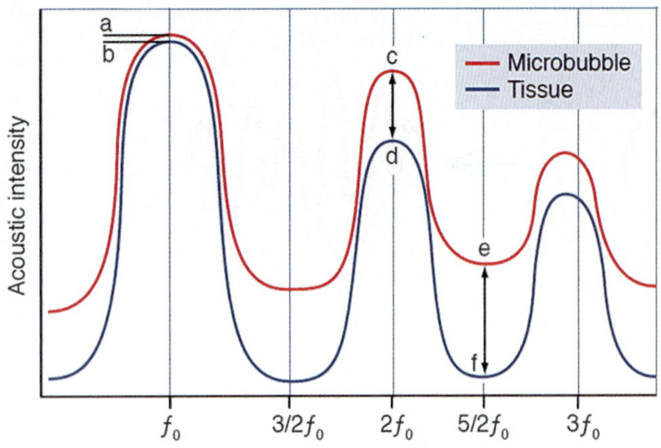

Figure 24-3. Schematic showing backscatter signals derived from microbubbles (*red line*) and myocardial tissue (*blue line*) at different frequencies. See text for details.

inversion (Fig. 24-5), sequential pulses of inverted phase are transmitted. Again, linear scatterers (Fig. 24-5, Panel A) produce received signals identical to the transmitted pulses, and summation of the received signals results in cancellation of tissue noise. Nonlinear scatterers (Fig. 24-5, Panel B), however, generate signals that cannot be summed. Both power modulation and pulse inversion have also been combined into a single modality (contrast pulse sequencing), where alternate ultrasound pulses have differing amplitude as well as phase.

The wide array of imaging modalities provides the user with great range and flexibility, and if any particular mode is inadequate for a patient, a different one could be used.

The Coronary Microcirculation

Because the microbubbles used during MCE are pure intravascular tracers, an understanding of the anatomy of the coronary microcirculation is required to appreciate the physiologic information represented by MCE images.

There is approximately 45 mL of blood in the adult human coronary circulation, which is divided nearly equally between the arterial, venous, and microcirculatory networks.[21] Most of the blood in the arterial and venous compartments is located on the epicardial surface of the heart. Within the myocardium itself, microcirculatory myocardial blood volume (MBV) makes up approximately 8% of the LV mass.[22] There are approximately 8 million capillaries in the human heart, which contain 90% of the MBV.[22] The velocity of blood in the coronary vessels is related to their size. At the capillary level (mean length and diameter of 0.5 mm × 7 μm), the mean red cell velocity at rest is about 1 mm/s. Since the red cells traverse capillaries in single file, it has been estimated that 1 mL of blood would take approximately 1 year to traverse a single capillary![23]

When microbubbles are administered as a constant infusion, steady state is achieved after 2 to 3 minutes, where their concentration in any blood pool (LV cavity, myocardium, etc.) is constant and proportional to the blood volume fraction of that pool. Thus, during normal conditions, since MBV represents 8% of LV mass, for every 100 microbubbles within a sample volume in the LV cavity, there will be 8 microbubbles within a similar sized sample volume in the myocardium. The AI measured from the myocardium, when normalized to that from the LV cavity, provides a measure of MBV fraction (since the LV cavity is 100% blood). Because 90% of MBV fraction comprises blood in capillaries, the MCE image provides an assessment of regional myocardial capillary density.

As will be discussed later, the microcirculation not only consists of a channel of passive networks that transports blood through the myocardium, but also an active site of blood flow control as well as metabolic activity. Indeed, the regulation of flow through these networks is complicated and depends on a number of metabolic, myogenic, and other control mechanisms.[24] The capillary hydrostatic pressure is continually maintained within the myocardium at approximately 30 mm Hg, with pre- and postcapillary pressures of about 45 and 15 mm Hg, respectively.[25] Coronary arterioles (which range in size from 150 to 300 μm) act as a resistance vessels to reduce mean aortic pressure (approximately 90 mm Hg) to the precapillary level.[26] These arterioles have smooth muscles with a strong and immediate myogenic response, so arteriolar resistance can change second-to-second in order to keep the precapillary pressure constant (autoregulation).[27]

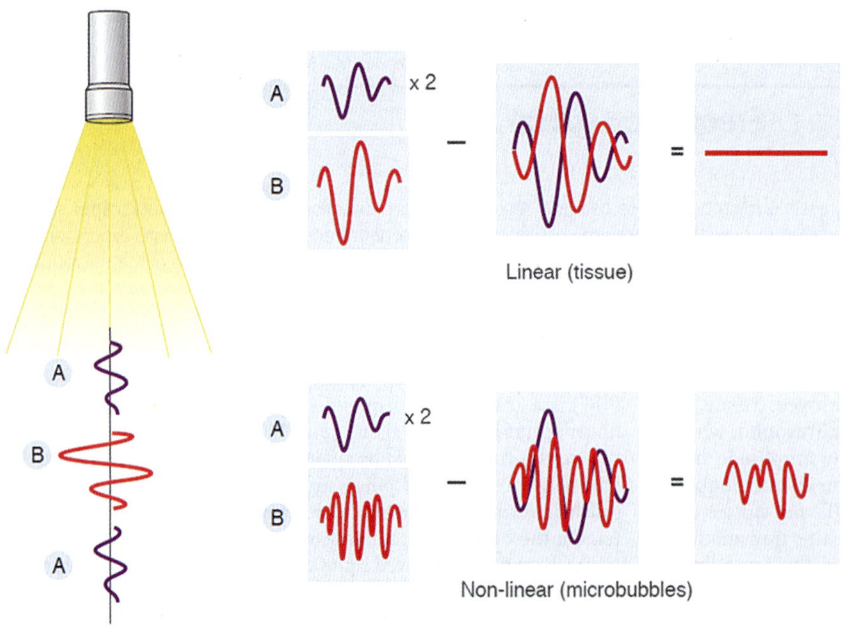

Figure 24-4. Schematic demonstrating power modulation imaging. Along each line of ultrasound, pulses of different amplitude (*A* and *B*) are sequentially transmitted. The backscatter signal derived from the half-height amplitude pulses are summed, and then subtracted from the full-height amplitude pulse. See text for details.

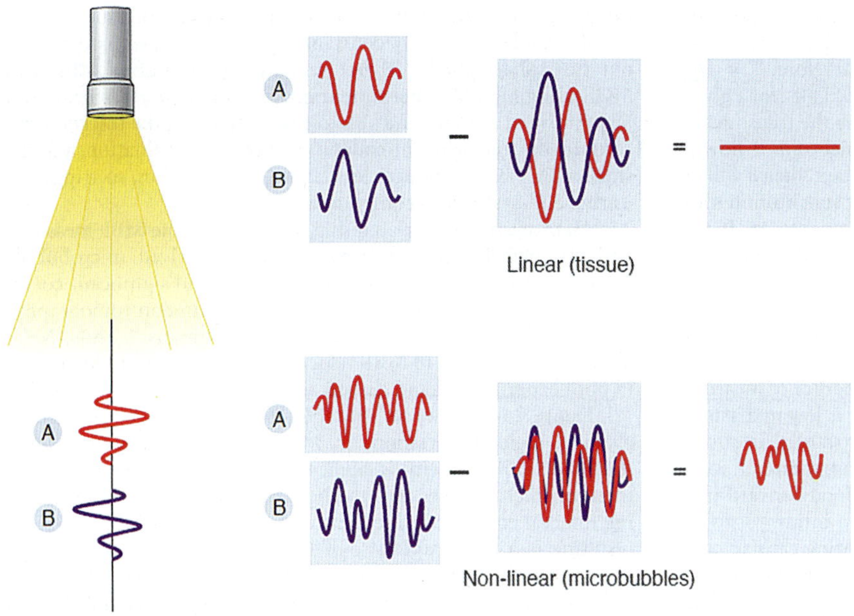

Figure 24-5. Schematic demonstrating pulse inversion imaging. Along each line of ultrasound, sequential pulses of inverted phase are transmitted. The backscatter signals received from tissue and microbubbles are then subtracted from each other. See text for details.

Quantification of Myocardial Blood Flow with MCE

At steady state, the inflow and outflow of microbubbles in any microcirculatory unit is constant, and is dependent only on the flow rate of microbubbles (which is identical to RBCs) through those vessels. The method for quantification of myocardial blood flow (MBF) with MCE is based on measuring the rate of microbubble transit through the myocardial capillary bed,[28] which occurs at a velocity of approximately 1 mm/s at rest, as discussed above.

Microbubbles within the myocardium can be destroyed with high-energy ultrasound, and rapidly eliminated from the myocardium.[29] By triggering the transmission of ultrasound to 1 point in the cardiac cycle, new microbubbles are allowed to replenish the microcirculation between destructive pulses of ultrasound, so each image provides a snapshot of the degree of replenishment of the microcirculation in a particular time interval. By making the time interval between destructive pulses longer and longer, more microbubble replenishment can occur and the degree of contrast enhancement increases.

To understand this concept mathematically, assume that all microbubbles within an ultrasound field are destroyed by a single ultrasound pulse and that the elevation (thickness) of the ultrasound beam E is uniform (Fig. 24-6). If new microbubbles enter this field with a flat profile at a velocity v, then the distance (d) they will travel within the beam elevation as the pulsing interval is prolonged (t_1 to t_4, Fig. 24-6B through E) will be given by the equation $E = vt$. Thus, as the time interval between consecutive destructive ultrasound pulses is increased, more time is allowed for microbubble replenishment, which is dependent on the velocity of the microbubbles. As pulsing interval lengthens, the rise in microbubble concentration is displayed as a corresponding rise in myocardial AI, provided that the relationship between AI and microbubble concentration remains linear (as discussed above). As shown in Figure 24-6F, when the pulsing interval exceeds T, AI will remain constant. This plateau phase will reflect the effective microbubble concentration within the myocardial microcirculation. At any given concentration of microbubbles, the AI at the plateau phase will be proportional to the sum of the cross-sectional area of microvessels (a) within the beam thickness.

The model predicts a sharp demarcation between the upslope and plateau phases of the pulsing interval–AI relation. In reality, however, neither the beam elevation nor the degree of microbubble destruction are expected to be entirely uniform. The profile of the microbubbles is also not expected to be entirely flat. The actual relationship between AI and pulsing interval is therefore more likely to be curvilinear (Fig. 24-6F) and can be described by the exponential function: $y = A(1 - e^{-\beta t})$, where y is AI at a pulsing interval of t, A is the plateau AI, and β is the rate constant that determines the rate of rise of AI.

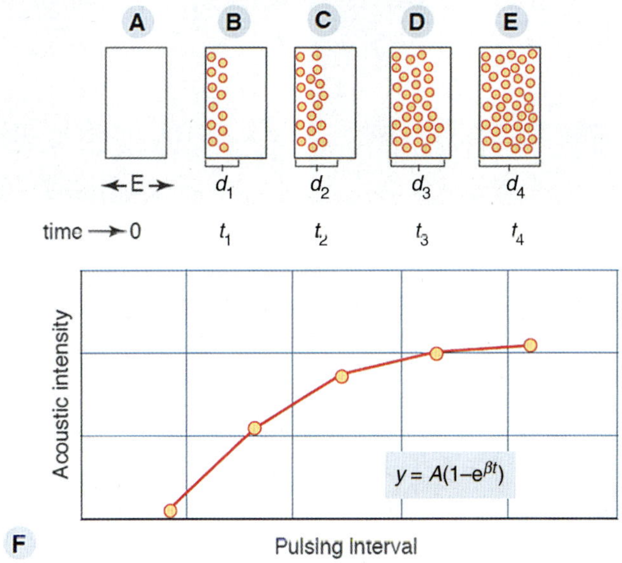

Figure 24-6. **The elevation dimension (E or thickness) of the ultrasound beam is represented as a rectangle (Panels A to E).** At steady state during a continuous infusion of microbubbles, high MI ultrasound is used to destroy all the microbubbles in the elevation (**Panel A**). As the time interval (t) between successive destructive pulses is prolonged (t_1–t_4), the degree of microbubble replenishment into the ultrasound elevation increases (d_1–d_4) and produces greater AI backscatter. The pulsing interval to AI relation (**Panel F**) can be fitted to an exponential function. See text for details.

Because the slope of the tangent to the curve is given by $dv/dt = A\beta E^{-\beta t}$, the slope at the origin ($t = 0$) is $A\beta$. As shown in Figure 24-6F, this slope is also equal to A/T. Therefore, $T = 1/\beta$. Eliminating T between equations results in: $v = E\beta$. Thus, for a given beam elevation (thickness at a given distance from the transducer), the mean velocity of microbubbles is proportional to β. If flow, f, occurs through an area, a, then: $f = av$. If E is constant, then a will be proportional to A. Therefore, with rearrangement substitution for v we get: $f \propto A\beta E$. When E is constant, f is proportional to $A\beta$. If E is known, then v can be expressed in cm/s. Similarly, if the microvascular cross-sectional area is known, then A can be expressed in cm^2. The product of A and v will then represent f in mL/s.[28]

Does it matter whether imaging is performed in diastole or systole during intermittent imaging? After all, it is known that flow in epicardial coronary arteries and veins is phasic in nature. Myocardial vessels fill with blood when myocardial elastance is low in diastole. In systole, the high elastance compresses intramyocardial arterioles which empty out retrogradely.[30] Likewise, intramyocardial veins are compressed during systole, which propels blood forward into the coronary sinus.[31] Although phasic changes in intramyocardial arteriolar dimensions have been documented during cardiac contraction, what happens to capillary dimensions during this period? We have shown that because arterioles and venules are larger than capillaries, they are compressed in systole prior to capillaries, causing an increase in their resistances that would result in functional isolation of the capillaries (i.e., no flow occurs through the capillaries during systole, but only during diastole).[32] Capillary pressure thus increases concurrently with intramyocardial pressure during systole, resulting in fairly constant capillary dimensions throughout the cardiac cycle.[32,33] Therefore, for quantification of MBF with MCE using high MI intermittent imaging methods, triggering can be performed at either end-diastole or systole, but the thicker myocardium during systole provides more tissue for evaluation, and the smaller LV cavity produces less far-field attenuation, so triggering during end-systole is recommended.

An excellent linear relationship between absolute MBF measured with radiolabeled microspheres and MCE-derived microbubble velocity has been found in animal studies,[28] and significant correlations have been found between positron emission tomography-derived MBF and MCE-derived MBF in humans.[34] Thus, MCE allows quantification of MBF velocity (β), MBV (A), and MBF ($A\beta$) in both experimental and clinical settings.

Figure 24-7 shows an example of how MCE can be used to evaluate regional variations in MBF velocity. In regions where the blood flow velocity is high, there will be greater replenishment of microbubbles into the beam elevation at any given pulsing interval compared to regions with a lower blood flow velocity, resulting in a more rapid rise of AI.[28] Panels A to D show images obtained with the pulsing intervals triggered to every 1, 3, 5, and 8 cardiac cycles (corresponding to intervals of approximately 100, 300, 500, and 800 milliseconds at a heart rate of 60 bpm, respectively). Regions of interest have been drawn over the septum and apex to generate theoretical pulsing interval versus AI curves (Panel E) using off-line image analysis software. At the shortest pulsing

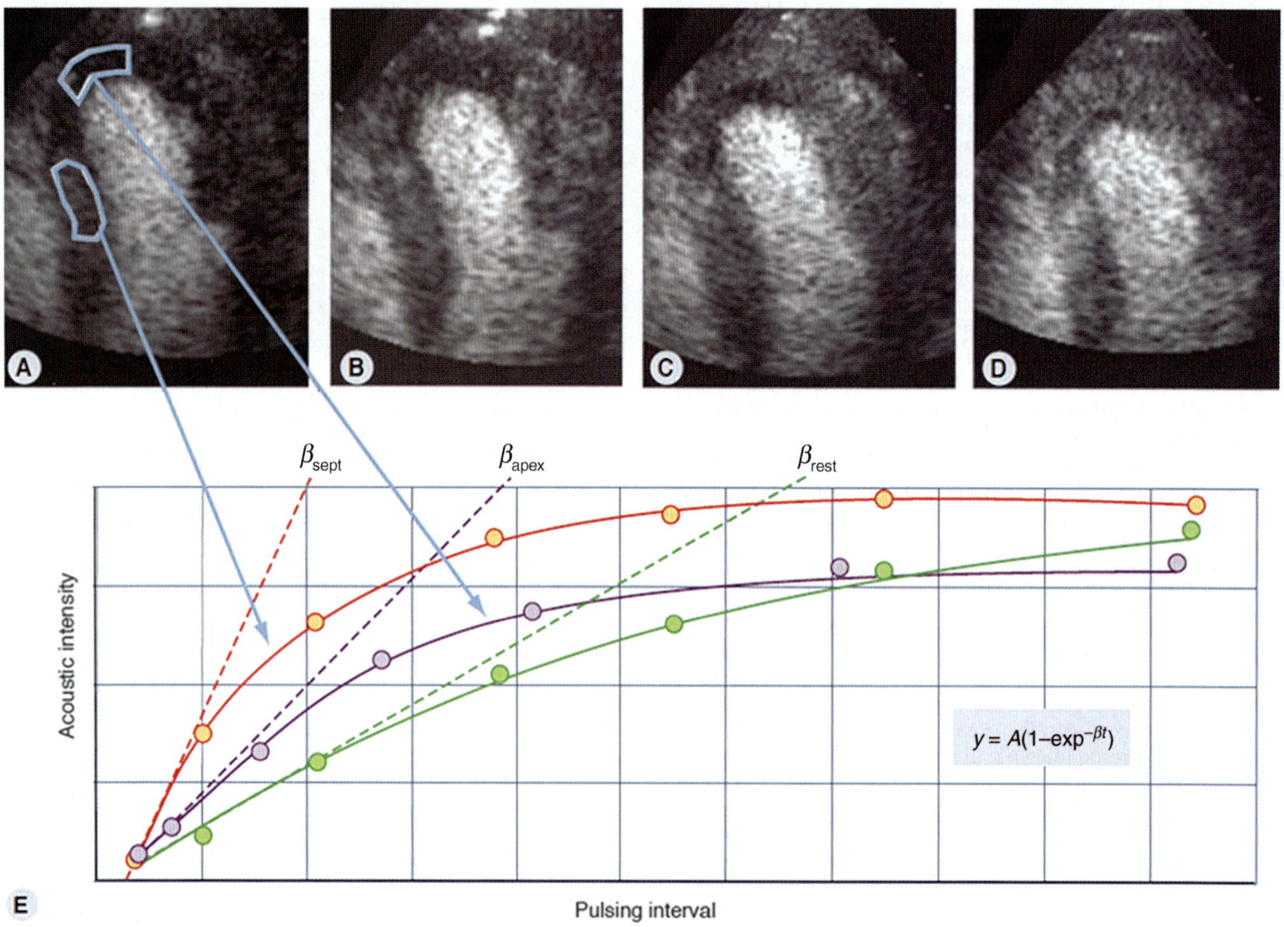

Figure 24-7. Contrast-enhanced images from the apical four-chamber view at four different pulsing intervals (**Panels A to D**). Pulsing interval versus AI plots derived from regions of interest drawn in the septum (*orange*) and apex (*purple*) are showing in **Panel E**. See text for details.

interval (Panel A), contrast cannot be seen in any myocardial segment, indicating that the pulsing interval was too short to allow replenishment of measurable amounts of microbubbles into the myocardium. At longer pulsing intervals (Panels B to D), contrast enhancement increases in both beds as more time is available for microbubble replenishment into the microcirculation. The higher flow velocity in the septum results in a greater degree of microbubble replenishment than the apex at any pulsing interval. Thus, the rate of rise of AI from the pulsing interval versus AI curves (Panel E) is higher for the septum (orange line) compared to the apex (purple line).

When the pulsing interval is long enough for the entire ultrasound beam elevation to be completely replenished with microbubbles, further increases in pulsing interval do not result in further increases in tissue AI, and the pulsing interval versus AI relation plateaus. As stated earlier, as long as the relation between microbubbles and AI is linear, the steady-state myocardial AI represents myocardial (or capillary) blood volume.[24] Since the normal blood flow velocity within the capillaries is very low (approximately 1 mm/s), and the ultrasound beam elevation measures approximately 5 mm in thickness, more than 5 seconds are required between pulses of ultrasound to allow complete replenishment for estimation of capillary blood volume at rest.

The pulsing interval versus myocardial AI relation (Fig. 24-7, Panel E) can be fitted to an exponential function: $y = A(1 - e^{-\beta t})$, where y is AI at a PI of t, A is the plateau AI representing MBV, and β represents the mean microbubble velocity. MBF velocity of the septum (β_{sept}) derived from a function fitted to the data points would be found to be greater than β_{apex}.[24]

Venous Administration of Microbubbles: Bolus or Continuous Infusion

The method described above for assessment of MBF using MCE mandates the use of continuous infusions of microbubbles to achieve "steady-state" concentrations of microbubbles in the circulation. There are other advantages for using continuous infusions. The rate of the infusion can be titrated to attain optimal myocardial opacification and yet avoid significant attenuation. With a bolus injection, high microbubble concentrations at some points during imaging will impede the ability to assess all myocardial segments due to far-field shadowing. Furthermore, excessive concentrations of microbubbles may exceed the linear portion of the relationship between AI and microbubble concentration. Thirdly, a continuous infusion allows time for the acquisition of multiple views, whereas multiple boluses will be required to accomplish the same. A continuous infusion also allows a single operator to perform the entire study alone, without necessitating the presence of a second person to administer the bolus injections.

On the other hand, bolus injections can be performed rapidly. This is especially relevant in the setting of exercise or ionotropic stress, where the time available for image acquisition is limited. With foresight and experience, however, an infusion could be started at an appropriate rate prior to the end of exercise or peak dobutamine stress, so that steady state will already be achieved when it is time to image. A much lower volume of agent is administered with each bolus, so a single vial of the agent is almost always adequate to image every segment even in technically difficult patients where multiple off-axis views are required. A bolus produces higher instantaneous concentrations of microbubbles in the circulation, which is advantageous for low MI techniques that produce smaller backscatter signals from microbubbles.

Overall, our bias is toward the use of continuous infusions because obtaining steady-state concentrations is essential for accurate assessment of the quantitative parameters discussed above, and for reducing attenuation artifacts.

High versus Low Mechanical Index MCE Methods for Quantification of MBF Velocity

More recently, a number of low MI "real-time" MCE techniques have been developed. These techniques produce nonlinear oscillations of microbubbles without destroying them. With low MI imaging, a "flash" impulse consisting of one or several high-power ultrasound frames destroys the microbubbles within the beam elevation, and microbubble replenishment into the microcirculation can then be assessed with continuous imaging at a relatively high frame rate (>15 Hz).[35,36] Apart from the ability to visualize both perfusion and myocardial function simultaneously, the main advantage of these techniques for evaluation of MBF is the rapidity with which the entire microbubble replenishment curve can be acquired (15 s compared to >5 min for intermittent imaging techniques).

With real-time imaging, frames throughout the cardiac cycle are acquired after each flash impulse. In contradistinction to intermittent high MI techniques where imaging can be triggered to either systolic or diastolic frames, however, replenishment curves with low MI techniques must be fitted to only end-systolic frames. This is because in diastole, large intramyocardial vessels rapidly replenish with microbubbles due to their high flow velocity (Fig. 24-8, Panel A).[37] Fitting a replenishment curve to sequential end-diastolic frames results in overestimation of MBF velocity by 41%.[37] Fitting the exponential function to all frames (including diastolic and systolic) within the cardiac cycle will overestimate MBF velocity by 24%.[37] The use of end-systolic frames is accurate compared to radiolabeled microspheres ($r = 0.53, p = 0.04$).[37]

Since only end-systolic frames should be used for quantification of MBF velocity even with a low MI MCE imaging method, some ultrasound systems allow only end-systolic frames to be digitally acquired while imaging is performed in real time. The sonographer can therefore follow an image on the monitor in real time, but a digital cine-loop of only systolic frames from each cardiac cycle will be acquired, and can subsequently be used for quantification. Most off-line MCE analysis software allows the user to select only the end-systolic frames for use prior to drawing a region of interest. Another method of acquiring only end-systolic frames is achieved by triggering during low MI imaging—so called tissue replenishment imaging. After the flash impulse, low MI imaging is performed at each sequential end-systole over the desired number of cardiac cycles, which are then used to assess microbubble replenishment kinetics.

Despite assessment of only end-systolic frames with both high and low MI imaging techniques, differences in the quantitative parameters are still obtained using the two modalities. The ability of the two modalities to assess the physiologic significance of coronary stenoses have been compared to ^{99m}Tc-sestamibi **single photon emission computed tomography** (SPECT) in patients.[38]

Intermittent ultraharmonic imaging (high MI) and power modulation Angio (low MI) were performed during continuous infusions of Optison at rest and after dipyridamole stress in 39 patients. ^{99m}Tc-sestamibi SPECT was performed simultaneously. MBF velocity and MBF velocity reserve (hyperemic/resting MBF velocity) were quantified from pulsing interval versus AI curves. MBF velocity derived from both MCE methods increased significantly after dipyridamole in normal patients compared to those with either reversible or fixed defects on SPECT. Consequently, MBF velocity reserve was significantly greater in patients with normal perfusion using both techniques. Receiver–operator characteristic curves obtained for MBF velocity reserve provided a sensitivity 82% versus 64% for low MI imaging for detection of defects compared to SPECT. The absolute value of β was also significantly lower during low compared to high MI imaging.

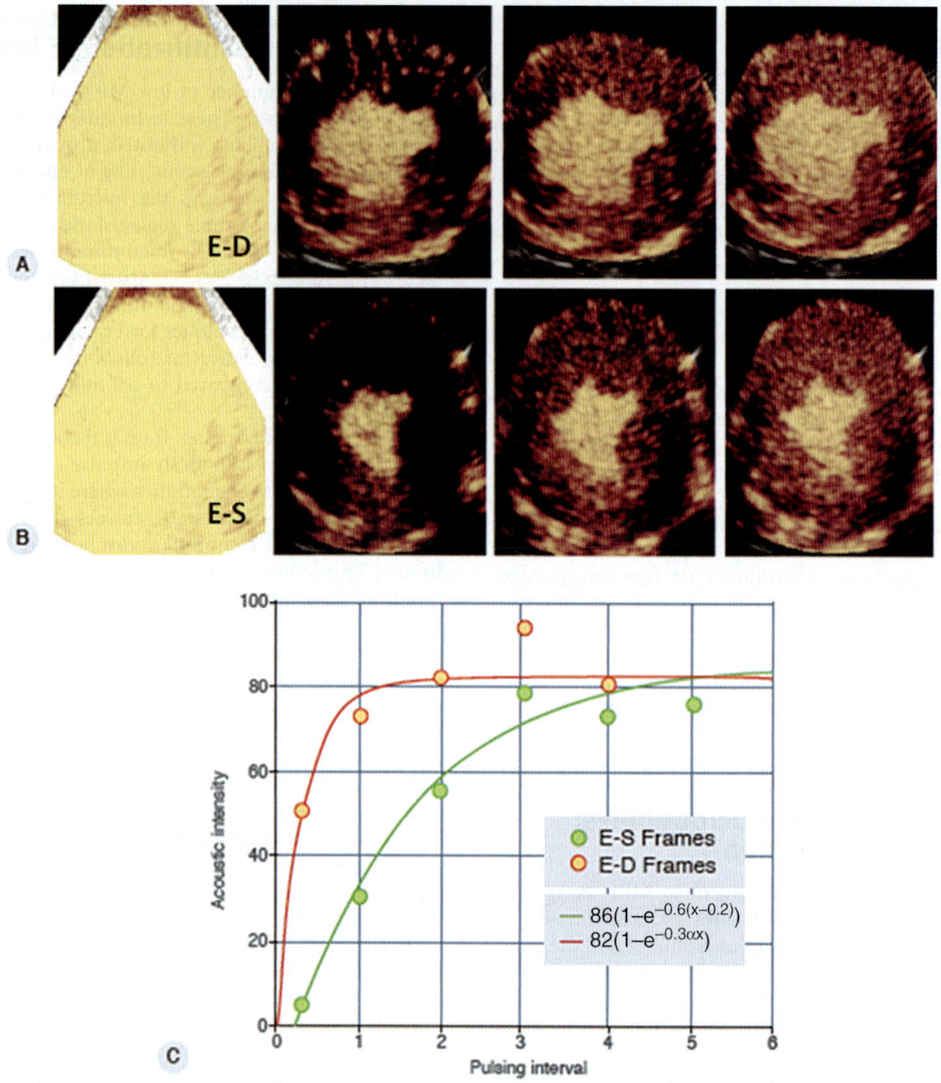

Figure 24-8. Panel A: Sequential end-diastolic frames acquired after "flash destruction" of microbubbles. In the first end-diastolic frame, linear signals are seen from microbubbles within large intramyocardial arteries. **Panel B:** Sequential end-systolic frames acquired after "flash destruction of microbubbles." **Panel C:** The pulsing interval versus acoustic intensity plots derived from end-diastolic (E-S, *orange circles*) and end-systolic frames (E-D, *green circles*). See text for details.

There are several potential reasons for differences in absolute β between the two types of imaging techniques, as well as for the lower sensitivity of quantitative parameters derived from the low MI technique. Excessive destruction of microbubbles in the LV cavity from multiple flash frames could result in distortion of the myocardial input function and prolongation of the output function. Microbubble destruction may also occur due to high frame rates despite the low MI. Most importantly, however, the variability probably occurs from differences in dynamic range, incorrect curve fitting, and noise between the two techniques.

Nonetheless, due to the relatively ease of image acquisition for real-time low MI techniques compared to high MI-triggered techniques, and the rapidity with which an entire replenishment curve can be derived, the low MI techniques have by-and-large eclipsed the high MI techniques. Although there may be differences in the absolute β between the two types of imaging techniques, regional differences in the rate of replenishment of microbubbles remains valid with low MI techniques.

Stress-Induced Perfusion Defects

So far, this chapter has focused mainly on differences in the rate of replenishment of microbubbles and demonstrated how that parameter can be used to distinguish differences in MBF velocity between perfusion beds. Let us now examine the plateau phase of the pulsing interval versus AI relationship, that is, myocardial or capillary blood volume.

While resting epicardial coronary blood flow remains normal despite the presence of a severe luminal stenosis (up to 85%), flow during maximal hyperemia is reduced when the luminal diameter stenosis severity exceeds 50%.[39] It has always been assumed that during maximal hyperemia, the resistance vessels are maximally dilated and the decrease in hyperemic flow is due to resistance offered by the epicardial coronary stenosis. Since they do not have smooth muscle, capillaries have always been thought to be passive conductors of flow.

With MCE, it has been realized that capillary blood volume actually decreases during hyperemia in the presence of a stenosis, and that this decrease is proportional to stenosis severity.[40,41] It is actually the decrease in capillary blood volume that results in perfusion defects on MCE. Since the length of each capillary remains constant, and they cannot dilate or constrict in the absence of smooth muscle, the only way capillary volume can decrease is through the derecruitment of capillary units during hyperemia.

If one examines the distribution of pressures across the coronary circulation, the mean aortic pressure is approximately 90 mm Hg, which is reduced to a precapillary pressure of 45 mm Hg resistance arterioles. There is a further 30 mm Hg drop of pressure across the capillary bed. Each individual capillary is very small and offers high resistance, but since there are so many capillaries in each tissue bed and they are arranged in parallel, the total capillary resistance is relatively small. The drop across the venous bed is only 15 mm Hg since these are high-capacitance vessels, but nevertheless they have some smooth muscle. Thus, at rest, approximately 60% of total myocardial vascular resistance is offered by the arterioles, 25% by the capillaries, and 15% by the venules.[41]

When hyperemia is induced in the normal coronary circulation, smooth muscle vasodilation results in dilatation of the arterioles and venules with no change in the size of capillaries. The total myocardial vascular resistance can decreases by 68% during hyperemia compared to at rest, with arterial and venular resistances decreasing by 86% and 98%, respectively. Capillary resistance now accounts for 75% of the total myocardial vascular resistance. Thus, capillaries offer the most resistance to MBF during hyperemia and limit the maximal increase in hyperemic MBF.[41] Because they are laid in parallel, a greater number of capillaries allows a higher hyperemic MBF and vice versa. Conditions that are associated with capillary loss, such as myocardial infarction, are associated with reduced MBF reserve even in the absence of an epicardial coronary stenosis.

In the presence of a noncritical stenosis during hyperemia, capillary resistance increases due to capillary derecruitment. This likely occurs in an effort to prevent changes in capillary hydrostatic pressure.

It has been shown that the decrease in capillary blood volume distal to a stenosis during hyperemia is proportional to stenosis severity.[40,42,43] Therefore, more severe stenoses will be associated with "darker" perfusion defects. Figure 24-9 shows background-subtracted, color-coded short-axis images from an experimental study. All images were obtained during hyperemia, at baseline (Panel A), in the presence of a mild stenosis (trans-stenotic pressure gradient of 14 mm Hg; Panel B), and a moderate stenosis (transstenotic pressure gradient of 22 mm Hg; Panel C) of the left anterior descending coronary artery. The degree of capillary derecruitment, and thus the severity of the perfusion defect becomes greater with increasing levels of stenosis. The corresponding time–intensity curves from the normal and stenosed beds also shows progressive decreases in the peak AI obtained from the stenosed bed with greater stenoses. The ratio of myocardial AI between the stenosed and normal beds during hyperemia was shown to correlate very well with microsphere-derived MBF ratios between the two beds ($r = 0.81$, $p < 0.001$).[40]

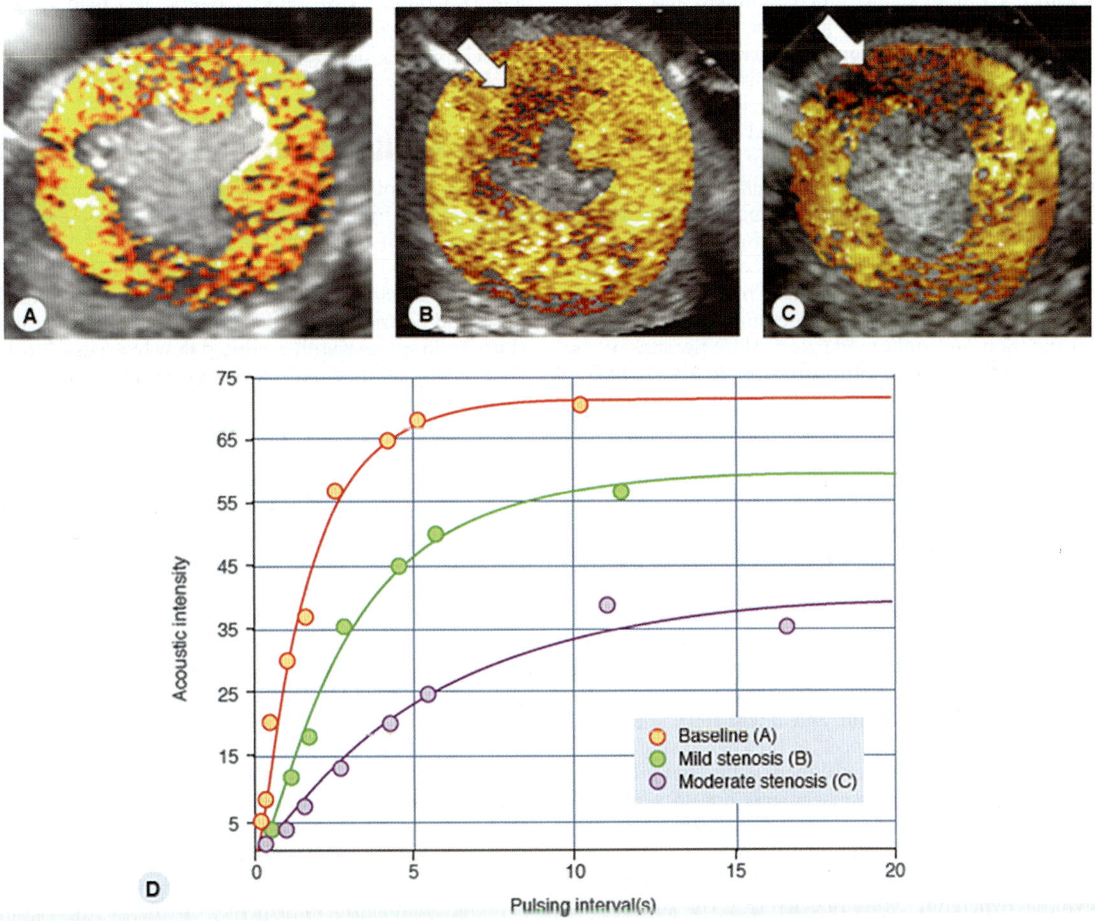

Figure 24-9. Offline background-subtracted color-coded short-axis images from an experimental study during hyperemia. The images were obtained at baseline (**Panel A**), and in the presence of a mild (**Panel B**) or moderate (**Panel C**) left anterior descending (LAD) coronary artery stenosis. The corresponding pulsing interval versus acoustic intensity curves from the LAD bed (*white arrows*) are shown (**Panel D**). See text for details.

As discussed above, capillary resistance also determines how much hyperemic flow will increase in a stenosed bed during hyperemia. This means that with more severe stenoses during hyperemia, there is more capillary derecruitment and larger increases in myocardial vascular resistance, which attenuates the increase in hyperemic flow distal to a stenosis.[41] Since the degree of capillary derecruitment determines both the severity of a perfusion defect and how much hyperemic flow is attenuated, these two parameters are physiologically coupled.

Thus, for the detection of CAD with MCE, both regional differences in hyperemic MBF velocity (β), and volume (A) are useful parameters. MBF velocity reserve on MCE may be a more robust and accurate method to detect CAD than relative MBV in the clinical setting for several reasons. Firstly, the assessment of regional plateau AI is complicated by heterogeneity of acoustic power in different sections of the ultrasound beam, artifacts, and regional differences in ultrasound attenuation—all of which may cause spurious decreases in AI. The limited dynamic range of some imaging modalities may also narrow the linear range and decrease the sensitivity for detection of mild defects. On the other hand, the assessment of MBF velocity is relatively independent of microbubble concentration, and appreciation of the relative change in AI at different pulsing intervals can often be achieved despite the factors mentioned above.

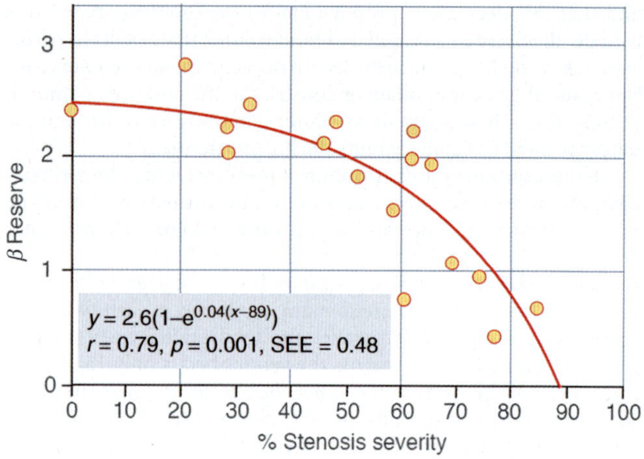

Figure 24-10. Relation between percent stenosis severity and MCE-derived flow velocity (β) reserve. See text for details. (From Wei K, Ragosta M, Thorpe J, et al. Noninvasive quantification of coronary blood flow reserve in humans using myocardial contrast echocardiography. *Circulation* 2001;103:2560–2565.)

Quantification of Coronary Stenosis Severity with MCE

In patients with CAD, both capillary derecruitment and a lesser increase in hyperemic MBF velocity form the basis for stenosis detection using continuous infusions of microbubbles. During hyperemia, the normal myocardium replenishes rapidly after microbubble destruction (1 to 1.5 s), while in regions subserved by a stenotic artery, the rate of filling is slower and depends upon the severity of stenosis. The rate of replenishment of microbubbles and perfusion defects in a stenosed bed are particularly evident in the endocardium, and, in milder stenoses, may be localized only within the endocardium.[43,44] The good spatial resolution of echocardiography and its ability to resolve subendocardial abnormalities may be one reason that MCE has been shown to be more sensitive than SPECT for the detection of coronary stenoses in patients with normal regional function and only moderate CAD.[45] Because of its poorer spatial resolution (cm vs. mm) compared to MCE, SPECT cannot detect defects located only in the endocardium. MCE may also superior in identifying multivessel CAD because each myocardial segment at stress is compared to its own resting state, while on SPECT the comparison is across segments, so that left main or "balanced" multivessel CAD can be missed.

MCE can noninvasively quantify the physiologic significance of stenoses in patients by determining MBF reserve.[46] These experiments were performed in the cardiac catheterization laboratory where coronary blood flow velocity was measured using a Doppler flow wire simultaneously with MCE measurements. The images in Figure 24-7 were actually obtained during hyperemia induced with 140 μg/kg/min of adenosine. The apex replenishes more slowly with microbubbles compared to the septum and anterolateral segments, producing an obvious "perfusion defect" at the apex at short pulsing intervals. The slower rate of replenishment at the apex is caused by a lower hyperemic MBF in those segments due to a midleft anterior descending coronary artery stenosis. The slower replenishment is evident by examining the pulsing interval versus AI curves (Fig. 24-7E) from regions of interest drawn at the apex and septum. By dividing hyperemic MBF velocity (β_{apex} or β_{sept}) from β obtained at rest, absolute MBF velocity reserve can be calculated. β_{apex} divided by β_{sept} will determine relative MBF velocity reserve. Figure 24-10 shows the relation between percent luminal diameter narrowing derived using quantitative coronary angiography (QCA) versus MCE-derived absolute MBF velocity reserve. The relation closely resembles that described by Gould and Lipscomb.[39] MBF velocity reserve less than 1.5 indicates the presence of greater than 70% epicardial stenosis.[46]

The discussion above demonstrates how MCE can be used to qualitatively or quantitatively evaluate CAD.

Vasodilator versus Inotropic Stress

In CAD without collateral development or infarction, inducible abnormalities in wall thickening during inotropic stress are related to the degree of endocardial MBF reserve.[47]

Figure 24-11 shows the wall thickening responses to different doses of dobutamine in three groups of animals: group I had no stenoses and normal endocardial flow reserve of greater than 3; group II had mild stenoses with a reduced flow reserve of 2 to 3; and group III animals had moderate stenoses with a flow reserve of less than 2. All three groups of animals had normal wall thickening at rest. As the dobutamine dose was increased from 5 to 10, 20, 30, and 40 μg/kg/min, wall thickening progressively increased in group I animals. In group II, abnormal endocardial flow reserve resulted in supply–demand mismatch at a dobutamine dose higher than 25 μg/kg/min, resulting in abnormal wall thickening and a classic biphasic response. Group III animals developed ischemia and wall thickening abnormalities beginning at only 20 μg/kg/min of dobutamine, and the severity of the wall thickening abnormalities were more severe than group II animals. These data demonstrate that the individual response of each segment to dobutamine was influenced by the endocardial MBF reserve in that segment.

Inotropic agents induce regional decreases in MBV distal to a noncritical stenosis just like vasodilators.[48] Compared to intracoronary adenosine, a similar degree of capillary derecruitment occurred with intracoronary dobutamine.[48] Regional myocardial perfusion defects during dobutamine stress are no different than those induced by vasodilators, and allow the detection of CAD with good agreement compared to quantitative angiography.

The attenuation of hyperemic MBF in the stenosed bed is also similar with intracoronary dobutamine and adenosine.[48] The reduction in endocardial flow reserve in the presence of a stenosis is also manifested as slow microbubble replenishment in the subendocardium compared using MCE during dobutamine stress.[49]

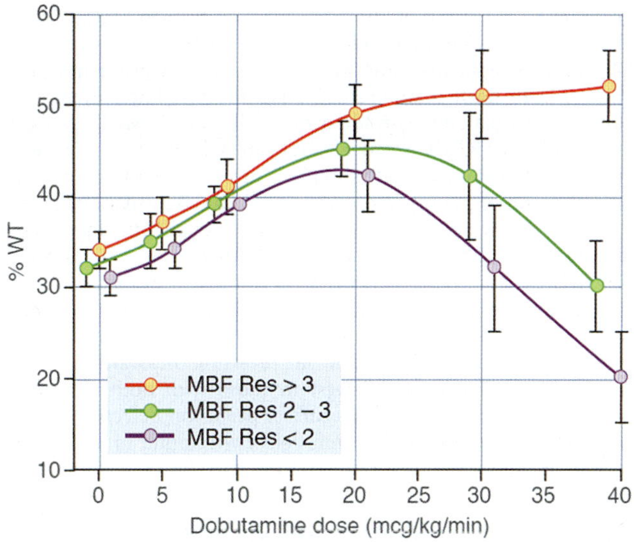

Figure 24-11. **Relation between dobutamine dose and % wall thickening in myocardial segments with endocardial MBF reserve >3 (*orange*), 2 to 3 (*green*), and <2 (*purple*).** (Redrawn from Bin JP, Wei K, Pelberg RA, et al. Relation between regional function and coronary blood flow reserve in multivessel coronary artery stenosis. *Am J Physiol* 2000;279:H3058–H3064.)

Thus, perfusion imaging with MCE may be a useful adjunct to the wall thickening information obtainable from dobutamine stress echocardiography (DSE). The ischemic cascade predicts that since perfusion abnormalities develop prior to the onset of ischemia and wall thickening abnormalities, and perfusion defects using MCE were detected in animal studies before the development of significant wall thickening abnormalities.[49] The spatial extent of perfusion defects is larger than that of abnormal wall thickening during stress, so the addition of perfusion may enhance the sensitivity of DSE.[50]

Thus, abnormal MBF velocity reserve and regional perfusion defects can be used to detect CAD during inotropic stress using MCE. Inducible perfusion defects may be a useful parameter when coupled with abnormal wall thickening to increase sensitivity for detection of milder stenoses or single-vessel CAD.

Clinical Detection of CAD with MCE

Based on the principles outlined above, a large number of clinical studies have now been performed to evaluate the ability of MCE to detect CAD in patients. These trials have utilized high[38,45,46,51–54] and low MI[35,36,38,55–58] imaging modalities, coupled with exercise,[36,55] or pharmacologic stress with either vasodilators[46,51–54,56–58] or inotropes.[35,55] All of these studies performed only visual "qualitative" assessments of MCE data. Overall good concordance was found between MCE and SPECT or quantitative coronary angiography when the latter two were used as the gold standard. When all three modalities were performed, the sensitivity of MCE was equivalent or higher than SPECT, with equivalent or slightly lower specificity compared to SPECT.[56–58] A summary of the results from representative studies are shown in Table 24.1 for patient-by-patient analyses.

Apart from the diagnosis of CAD, MCE is comparable to SPECT in terms of localizing perfusion defects in territory-by-territory analyses or segment-by-segment analyses. MCE can also accurately classify defects into those that are fixed or reversible. Greater discrepancies between MCE and SPECT have been found in the right coronary and left circumflex artery territories, where attenuation of basal segments on MCE results in false-positive perfusion defects or prevents analysis.[53,54] Off-axis views that diminish rib shadowing or that position the segment of interest in the middle of the imaging

TABLE **24.1** **Detection of CAD with MCE**

Study	Year	No. of Patients	MCE Mode	Stress Method	Gold Standard	Sensitivity	Specificity	Concordance	Kappa
Kaul et al.	1997	30	High MI	DP	SPECT			86%	0.71
Porter et al.	1997	28	High MI	DP	SPECT	92%	84%	84%	—
Heinle et al.	2000	123	High MI	Ad	SPECT	—	—	81%	0.60
Cwajg et al.	2000	45	Low MI	Ex./Db	Angio	—	—	80%	0.61
Shimoni et al.	2001	100	Low MI	Ex.	SPECT	—	—	76%	0.50
Shimoni et al.	2001	44	Low MI	Ex.	Angio	75%	100%	—	0.67
Porter et al.	2001	117	Low MI	Db	DSE	—	—	91%	0.70
Porter et al.	2001	40	Low MI	Db	Angio	—	—	83%	0.65
Oraby et al.	2001	27	High MI	DP	SPECT	—	—	82%	0.49
Haluska et al.	2001	49	High MI	DP	SPECT	83%	55%	—	—
Wei et al.	2003	43	High MI	DP	SPECT	96%	63%	84%	0.63
Jeetley et al.	2006	123	Low MI	DP	Angio	84%	56%	—	—
Porter et al.	2011	100	Low MI	Reg	Angio	80%	74%	—	—
Senior et al.	2013	628	Low MI	DP	Angio	75%	52%	—	—

Key: MI, mechanical index; DP, dipyridamole; Ad, adenosine; Ex, exercise; Db, dobutamine; SPECT, single photon emission computed tomography; Angio, angiography; Reg, regadenoson.

sector (where acoustic power is higher) may help to minimize this limitation. The presence of bright tissue backscatter, especially from thin fibrotic segments, may lead to false-negative studies due to an inability to visually distinguish tissue noise from myocardial perfusion. In these circumstances, quantitative methods that use offline background subtraction or color-coding algorithms may be of significant benefit. The presence of subtle microbubble replenishment in segments that are hypoperfused or collateral dependent, or areas that are affected by attenuation, may also be difficult to determine visually, but incremental changes in AI at different pulsing intervals is an extremely useful finding that helps distinguish viable from infarcted segments.

A method that qualitatively determines regional differences in MBF velocity (a visual assessment of the rate of microbubble replenishment between rest and stress stages) has also been shown to be a robust method for detection of CAD in patients.[45] Since normal resting capillary blood flow velocity is approximately 1 mm/s, complete myocardial replenishment of the microcirculation within the ultrasound beam elevation should be seen in 4 to 5 seconds (or at a pulsing interval of approximately 4 beats for high MI-triggered imaging) at rest. Since MBF velocity normally increases four to five times at peak hyperemia, complete replenishment would be expected in only 1 or 2 seconds (one to two cardiac cycles for triggered imaging) during stress. The lack of significant myocardial opacification by 5 seconds at rest would signify the presence of a resting perfusion defect, and delayed replenishment after 2 seconds during hyperemia would identify segments with abnormal flow reserve. Good concordance was found using this approach for the detection of normal segments, and for classification of perfusion defects as reversible and fixed compared to SPECT.[45]

Clinical studies have also been done to evaluate the incremental benefit of adding perfusion imaging to wall thickening for the detection of CAD. This has been performed using either vasodilator[59,60] or inotropic[61] stress. In Moir et al., the sensitivity for detection of stenoses greater than 50% in severity increased from 74% for wall thickening alone to 91% after perfusion imaging was added ($p = 0.02$). There was a nonsignificant reduction in specificity from 81% to 70%. The benefit persisted even after patients who failed to achieve target heart rate and technically challenging cases were excluded. The extent of CAD that was diagnosed also increased significantly after perfusion imaging was incorporated, and more patients with multivessel disease were recognized although the difference was not statistically significant (79% vs. 58%, $p = 0.09$).[59] The results were similar in Elhendy et al.,[61] where the sensitivity for detection of stenoses greater than 50% in severity increased from 71% to 91% after perfusion imaging was added during DSE. The improvement in sensitivity was particularly impressive at intermediate levels of stress, where sensitivity increased from 20% for wall thickening to 84% for myocardial perfusion.[61] In this study, however, specificity was significantly lower for perfusion (51%) compared to wall motion (74%, $p = 0.01$), but overall accuracy was still higher for perfusion. Again, the detection of multivessel disease was superior for perfusion imaging compared to wall motion alone (44% vs. 18%, $p = 0.001$).

The presence of normal resting wall motion can be used as a surrogate for normal resting perfusion, so a resting perfusion study can be omitted for these patients. Inducible perfusion defects during stress in these patients allows accurate classification of defects as "reversible" compared to rest/stress sestamibi SPECT. In patients with abnormal resting wall motion, however, a resting MCE study still has to be performed to distinguish stunned from infarcted segments. By taking advantage of both the excellent spatial and temporal characteristics of echocardiography, the time and cost of stress testing for patients may be reduced.

The prognostic utility of stress MCE has been evaluated in retrospective[62–64] and more recently prospective studies.[65,66] In Porter et al.,[65] a group of 2014 intermediate-to-high pretest probability patients were randomly assigned to undergo conventional DSE or DSE with real-time MCE (RTMCE) perfusion imaging. Patients with normal studies had a significantly lower event rate compared to patients with abnormal DSE and RTMCE. Patients with abnormal RTMCE had a significantly lower event-free survival (events included death, nonfatal myocardial infarction, and revascularization) compared to patients with abnormal DSE, over a median follow-up of 2.6 years. In Gaibazzi et al.,[66] the incremental benefit of adding MPI to high-dose dipyridamole stress MCE was evaluated in 1,252 patients with known or suspected CAD. The 2-year event-free survival was best in patients with normal wall motion and myocardial perfusion (97.9%), intermediate in those with normal wall motion but reversible myocardial perfusion defects (91.9%), and lowest in those with both abnormal wall motion and reversible myocardial perfusion defects (67.4%). A reversible myocardial perfusion defect was found to add incremental predictive value over wall motion and clinical factors.

Assessment of Myocardial Viability

Both morbidity and mortality from myocardial infarction are significantly affected by infarct size, which can be characterized by its endocardial length and transmural extent. Experimental studies in dogs have shown that the time course of cell death begins approximately 30 to 40 minutes after acute coronary occlusion, and occurs initially in the subendocardium where ischemia is most severe.[67] Necrosis extends toward the subepicardium over time, and becomes transmural after 6 hours.[68] Reperfusion within 2 hours can result in functional recovery of the ischemic tissue. This forms the basis for achieving early reperfusion of the infarct-related artery to salvage viable myocardium within the infarct bed.

Evaluation of Collateral Flow in AMI with MCE

Another determinant of infarct size, however, is the adequacy of collateral flow within the risk area.[69–71] Even though collaterals may not be present de novo in normal subjects, patients with chronic CAD develop abundant collaterals to ischemic territories.[71] The presence of adequate collateral-derived blood flow maintains myocardial viability and spares tissue from necrosis despite persistent coronary occlusion in patients with recent myocardial infarction.[72]

MCE can be used to determine the amount of collateral blood flow within the risk area before the infarct-related artery is reperfused.[73–75] Because collateral-derived flow has a lower MBF velocity than normal antegrade flow, enough time has to be given during imaging for microbubbles to replenish into the risk area after their destruction.[74] The presence of myocardial opacification identifies regions where MBF exceeds approximately 20% of normal resting levels, which is adequate to maintain myocardial viability.

Figure 24-12 shows short-axis images obtained in the presence of an occlusion of the left circumflex coronary artery in two different animals during a continuous intravenous (IV) infusion of microbubbles using high MI intermittent imaging. Both MCE images (Panels A and C) were obtained at long pulsing intervals (9.2 and 16.2 seconds, respectively, between pulses of ultrasound). Despite the long pulsing interval, a hypoperfused zone is seen in the left circumflex perfusion bed (1 to 5 o'clock) compared to the normal myocardial perfusion in the left anterior descending perfusion bed (7 to 1 o'clock). There is attenuation from LV cavity contrast from 5 to 7 o'clock. The hypoperfused zone at this pulsing interval represents the risk area because there is insufficient MBF to maintain viability. However, both the length and transmural extent of the hypoperfused zone is obviously very different between Panels A and C (denoted by the white arrows). The presence of

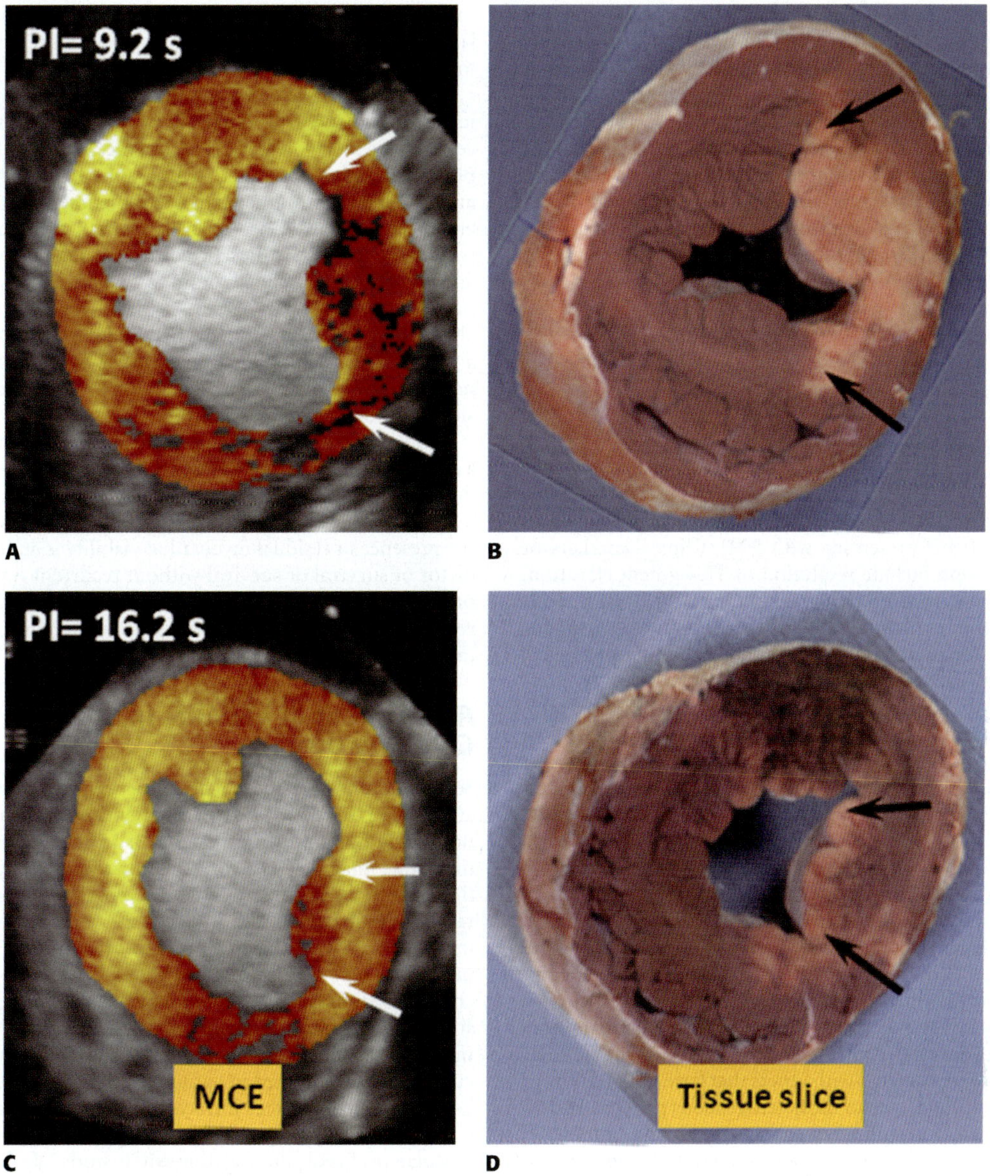

Figure 24-12. Offline background-subtracted and color-coded short-axis images from two different animals during occlusion of the left circumflex coronary artery (**Panels A and C**), and corresponding 2,3,5-triphenyltetrazolium chloride stained tissue slices from the same animals postmortem (**Panels B and D**). See text for details. (From Coggins MP, Sklenar J, Le E, et al. Noninvasive prediction of ultimate infarct size at the time of acute coronary occlusion based on the extent and magnitude of collateral-derived myocardial blood flow. *Circulation* 2001;104:2471–2477.)

perfusion denotes collateral-derived MBF and the spatial distribution of perfusion within the risk area identifies tissue that may be spared from necrosis despite persistent coronary occlusion. The 2,3, 5-triphenyltetrazolium chloride stained tissue slices in Panels B and D show the extent of myocellular necrosis (unstained area denoted by the black arrows) after a 6-hour occlusion. In Panel C, the animal had good collateral blood flow to the entire left circumflex perfusion bed except for the tip of the posteromedial papillary muscle, which was the only area that became infracted (Panel D). On the other hand, the animal with poor collateral blood flow (Panel A) sustained a large transmural infarct (Panel B).

The example above illustrates how collateral flow can prevent myocellular necrosis despite prolonged occlusion of the epicardial coronary artery, and how the extent of necrosis can be predicted by MCE. MCE is superior to wall motion in this regard—although the circumferential extent of abnormal wall thickening correlates well with the size of the initial risk area on MCE, it overestimates the eventual infarct size. During acute occlusion, the entire risk area is akinetic, including regions that receive collateral flow. The extent and severity of the wall thickening abnormality remains constant for the entire duration of coronary occlusion. Thus, collateral flow within the risk area may be adequate to maintain viability, but is insufficient to allow wall thickening. Assessments of wall thickening alone therefore provide only limited information in patients presenting with acute myocardial infarction (AMI). It cannot predict eventual infarct size, as wall thickening remains severely abnormal even in the presence of adequate collateral flow that can maintain viability. MCE therefore has the potential to provide important adjunctive information that may impact on the management of patients presenting with AMI in future.

The protective effect of collateral flow has been shown in patients with chronic total occlusion.[76] In this study, 64 patients with a chronic total occlusion greater than 2 weeks in duration underwent MCE with direct intracoronary injections of microbubbles. Patients were then revascularized percutaneously. Those with good contrast enhancement of the risk area (well collateralized) were shown to have a significant improvement in wall motion score index by 1 month after revascularization, with further improvement at 6 months. Patients without good enhancement of the risk area only developed some improvement in wall thickening at 6 months after revascularization, and had significantly less improvement compared to those with good collateralization. Likewise, LV ejection fraction increased significantly more in patients with good collaterals compared to the other group of patients after revascularization.[76]

Assessment of the Success of Reperfusion with MCE

Early reperfusion of the infarct-related artery is the primary goal of therapy for patients presenting with AMI. Clinical markers of successful reperfusion include resolution of ST-segment elevation, alleviation of angina, and ventricular arrhythmias such as an accelerated idioventricular rhythm. None of these parameters are sensitive or specific for successful reperfusion. The ability of clinical markers to identify successful thrombolysis was previously compared to patency of the infarct-related artery at 90 minutes after therapy.[77] None of the clinical markers, either independently or in combination, adequately predicted failure of thrombolytic therapy to open the infarct-related artery.[77] A method that can easily and rapidly define tissue reperfusion would therefore be useful. Apart from assessing the success of therapy, identifying patients with unsuccessful thrombolysis may be beneficial, as they may require further interventions such as rescue angioplasty.[78,79]

After blood flow is restored to an occluded bed, myocardial contrast enhancement should be seen in regions with successful reperfusion. Blood flow within the reperfused bed is heterogeneous, and exhibits dynamic fluctuations over time.[80] Regions of significant myocellular injury (necrosis) have microvascular disruption, and show no myocardial contrast enhancement or "no reflow." These regions may be admixed with others that have normal flow or even reactive hyperemia. Due to the heterogeneous patterns of flow in the reperfused myocardium, the spatial extent of the "no reflow" zone on MCE may underestimate the true infarct size determined using other methods, such as 2,3,5-triphenyltetrazolium chloride staining.[80,81] In order not to overestimate the extent of myocardial salvage after reperfusion, resting MCE studies to evaluate infarct size should be performed after reactive hyperemia has abated, or about 24 hours after reperfusion.[82,83] Alternatively, almost all regions that have sustained some injury will exhibit impaired flow reserve, so MCE defect sizes determined after administration of vasodilators or inotropes correspond closely to the area of infarction—even early after reperfusion.[80,81]

It is now recognized that simple recanalization of the infarct-related artery is inadequate to ensure a good outcome. Despite patency of the infarct-related artery, there may be reduced microvascular flow due to small vessel spasm, plugging from thrombi, inflammatory cells, or debri. MCE, which provides an assessment of microvascular perfusion, can be used to assess the status of the microcirculation.

Clinical studies have evaluated the relationship between antegrade epicardial flow using the Thrombolysis in Myocardial Infarction (TIMI) study group grading system and the adequacy of microvascular perfusion on MCE. Patients with TIMI grades 1 and 2 flow have a higher incidence of microvascular injury or "no-reflow" on MCE, than those with TIMI grade 3 flow.[84,85] Even in patients with TIMI grade 3 flow, however, 16% had microvascular no-reflow on MCE,[84] and other studies have found even higher incidences.[86]

The extent of no-reflow on MCE has been shown to have significant consequences. Studies done with intravenously administered contrast agents show good concordance between MCE and single photon emission computed tomography for detection of viability, and dysfunctional segments that demonstrated myocardial contrast enhancement had better recovery of wall motion than segments with no-reflow.[87] The presence of reflow defined by MCE 24 hours after reperfusion has been found to be associated with higher coronary flow reserve than patients with no-reflow, and these authors also found that these segments had better improvement in regional and global ventricular function at follow-up.[88] Patients with low- or no-reflow had poor recovery of LV function, greater infarct expansion, remodeling, and LV dilation.[89–91]

Moreover, patients with poor microvascular reperfusion have a significantly higher incidence of cardiac events including cardiac death, nonfatal myocardial infarction, and congestive heart failure over a 1-year follow-up period.[92] The ability of MCE to determine the presence of residual myocardial viability is an independent predictor of survival or survival without recurrent AMI,[93] because the presence of microvascular perfusion is the major determinant of reverse LV remodeling, and reverse LV remodeling is an important predictor of event-free survival.[94]

Assessment of Viability in Chronic Coronary Disease

Several noninvasive approaches have been developed for the evaluation of myocardial viability in patients with chronic LV dysfunction, including perfusion imaging (such as nuclear scintigraphy), metabolic imaging (positron emission tomography), and the functional assessment of contractile reserve (dobutamine echocardiography). Similar to its use in AMI, the presence of microvascular integrity and viability are denoted by myocardial contrast enhancement on MCE. Determining the extent of viability in patients with chronic CAD and LV dysfunction helps to define optimal treatment strategies and patient prognosis. Irrespective of the method used, many studies have now shown that the greatest benefit from revascularization is obtained in patients with significant viability.[95–97]

Studies using direct intracoronary injections of microbubbles during MCE have shown that the spatial distribution of microvascular perfusion on a resting MCE study can be used to determine the presence of myocardial viability.[98] Higher contrast scores (denoting greater contrast enhancement) were associated with better improvement in LV function 1 month after revascularization, and was found on multiple regression analysis to be a better predictor than baseline wall motion, or final percent stenosis of the vessel supplying the dysfunctional segments.[98]

We have unpublished data using IV infusions of microbubbles to identify viability in patients with chronic ischemic LV dysfunction (ejection fraction <40%). We hypothesized that the presence of microvascular integrity would identify patients who would benefit from revascularization. We enrolled 90 patients and performed 2D echocardiographic studies at baseline, as well as 3, 6, and 12 months after enrollment. End-diastolic and systolic volumes and LV ejection fraction were measured. Patients were divided into four groups based on the presence or absence of viability on MCE, as well as whether or not they underwent revascularization. Patients with viability who underwent revascularization had significant decreases in volumes and a significant $30 \pm 30\%$ improvement in LV ejection fraction, whereas those parameters remained unchanged or deteriorated over the follow-up period in all other groups.

MCE using direct intracoronary injections of microbubbles has also been compared to nuclear scintigraphy and dobutamine echocardiography for predicting recovery of resting function after revascularization.[99] Similar to thallium uptake, normalized peak contrast intensity of dysfunctional segments that recovered function was significantly higher than segments that did not improve after revascularization. Both perfusion modalities were found to have similar sensitivity, but a lower specificity compared to dobutamine echocardiography. Other studies have confirmed the excellent sensitivity of MCE, and also found a lower specificity for predicting recovery of function after revascularization.[100,101] It was noted that a combined assessment of perfusion and contractile reserve provided the most optimum sensitivity and specificity.[100]

The disparity in sensitivity and specificity between techniques that evaluate perfusion and contractile reserve is due to the use of "recovery of resting function after revascularization" as the gold standard for viability. Because the subendocardium is responsible for most of the resting LV wall thickening, a subendocardial infarction that involves only 30% of the transmural thickness of the wall will result in akinesis of the affected segments.[102,103] Although the majority of the transmural extent of the myocardium is viable, revascularization of these segments will not result in recovery of resting wall thickening. Even though the mid- and epicardial regions may contribute little to resting function, viability in those areas are of great importance. These segments can be recruited during inotropic stimulation, and can contribute to increases in wall thickening during exercise.[104] The viable epicardial segments that overly regions of necrosis may also act as a buffer to prevent infarct expansion and remodeling and have been shown to help preserve LV volumes and geometry.[105] Even in the absence of improvement in global LV ejection fraction, revascularization of ischemic (and therefore viable) myocardium has been found to decrease angina, increase functional capacity, and allow similar survival as patients who have an improvement in LV function.[106]

Apart from trying to determine which patients may have improvement in resting LV function after revascularization, a more important goal in the assessment of myocardial viability may be to distinguish tissue that is alive from that which is necrotic, and to determine its potential for long-term maintenance of viability.

Diagnostic and Prognostic Utility of MCE for Patients with Suspected Acute Coronary Syndromes

Even after a brief coronary occlusion (5 to 15 minutes), regional systolic function is severely reduced.[107] These functional changes occur briskly and are evident for hours after the initial insult, despite reperfusion, and may take up to 48 hours to normalize.[107–111] The duration and severity of systolic dysfunction directly relates to the duration of ischemic insult, the severity of the insult, and the adequacy of reperfusion.[108–112] In order to have high sensitivity, it is of utmost importance to clearly visualize each myocardial segment, so the use of contrast agents for LV endocardial border delineation is critical for this application of echocardiography. Furthermore, as noted below, MPI using MCE can provide incremental prognostic utility.

Several studies have evaluated MCE in the evaluation of patients presenting with CP but no ST elevation in the emergency department. A multicenter, prospective study compared MCE and SPECT to diagnose AMI and risk stratify 203 patients for the development of "hard" cardiovascular endpoints (AMI, urgent revascularization or death) within 48 hours.[111] MCE was found to be equivalent to SPECT in diagnosing AMI but was inferior with respect to predicting other adverse cardiac events. Both MCE and SPECT added significant additional information (17% and 23.5%, respectively) for diagnosis and short-term prognosis over routine clinical methods (ECG, history, and risk factors). This study demonstrated for the first time the incremental value of MCE in the diagnosis and short-term prognosis of AMI. The assessment of myocardial perfusion played a dominant role in the value of MCE. Surprisingly, the evaluation of regional function was less powerful. The use of bolus administration of the microbubble contrast agent could have resulted in far-field attenuation and affected the assessment of regional function. Additionally, UA was not included as an endpoint that may have underestimated the diagnostic and prognostic capabilities of MCE in this study.

Both wall motion and perfusion with MCE were used to evaluate 100 patients with "first time chest pain" to demonstrate the ability of MCE to detect acute coronary syndromes (unstable angina, non-ST elevation MI) compared to traditional clinical tests.[112] Those with ST elevation, known CAD or previous myocardial infarction were excluded. Contrast agents were administered as a slow bolus, and MCE was performed using low MI real-time imaging. Thirty-seven patients were diagnosed with an ACS. An abnormal MCE exam was the most powerful predictor of an ACS (89% sensitivity, 93% specificity, $p < 0.001$). Myocardial perfusion was superior to wall motion analysis for detecting an ACS. In 21 patients, MCE was performed before the initial troponin data were available, and 95/98 underwent MCE before follow-up troponins were performed—so MCE can identify high-risk patients more quickly than the use of serum cardiac markers. In two patients with abnormal troponin values, MCE was found to be normal but identified the presence of pericardial effusions. Subsequent angiography was also normal and these individuals were diagnosed with perimyocarditis—demonstrating the excellent negative predictive value of MCE.

The use of MCE was further strengthened the findings in a prospective study of 114 patients presenting to the emergency room with "suspected cardiac chest pain."[113] The main study endpoint was the diagnosis of an ACS. Patients who had Q waves on ECG or a history of myocardial infarction were excluded. All patients underwent MCE and coronary angiography in addition to ECG and serologic testing. Microbubbles were administered using a more contemporary "continuous infusion" method. An ACS was diagnosed in 87 patients. Myocardial perfusion defects demonstrated 77% sensitivity for the detection of ACS compared to 28% and 34%, respectively, with ECG and troponin while maintaining similar specificity (89% to 96%). Abnormal myocardial perfusion was the only independent variable for diagnosing an ACS (odds ratio 87, $p < 0.001$). Regional function was not as powerful as perfusion for predicting an ACS but was more sensitive than ST changes or troponin alone (65% compared to 33% and 54%, respectively). This study similarly found incremental benefit for MCE over ECG and cardiac biomarkers in the setting of suspected cardiac CP.

The largest study to date evaluating MCE in patients with CP included 1,017 patients presenting to the ED who were greater than 30 years of age, with CP lasting at least 30 minutes occurring within the previous 12 hours. Primary endpoints included all cause mortality and acute MI. Secondary endpoints included revascularization or unstable angina (typical chest pain, dynamic ECG changes, and/or mild troponin elevation). Late prognostic utility was also evaluated and patients were followed for up to 2 years. MCE was performed with a continuous infusion of microbubbles and images were interpreted separately for regional function and myocardial perfusion by experienced clinicians blinded to all clinical information. In contradistinction to the last few studies presented, patients with a prior MI were not excluded from enrollment.

The short- and long-term prognostic significance of MCE on primary and secondary cardiovascular endpoints in the study from Rinkevich et al.[114] Total short-term events (48 h) were noted in 16% of patients, 9% of whom had AMI. Patients with abnormal regional function were sixfold more likely to have an early event compared to those with normal function. Patients with abnormal perfusion were 2.5-fold more likely to have an adverse event, but those with both abnormal regional function and myocardial perfusion were 14.3-fold ($p < 0.001$) more likely to have events—demonstrating the incremental benefit of combined wall thickening and perfusion data over regional function alone in these patients. Similar findings were noted over late follow-up where patients with abnormal regional function had a fivefold increased incidence of an adverse event compared those with normal function, and the patients with both abnormal perfusion and function were at the highest risk of adverse events (10-fold increase).

In clinical practice, it is important not only to diagnose an ACS but to risk stratify patients appropriately for decisions regarding triage and management. A commonly used clinical tool is the TIMI risk score.[115] However, because there is an inherent delay in obtaining serum cardiac biomarker data, a full TIMI risk score cannot be derived in patients at the time of a patient's presentation to the ED. MCE may therefore provide better risk stratification early in the assessment of chest pain patients than even a composite risk score. This hypothesis was evaluated by Tong et al.[116] Normal regional function and perfusion on MCE were used to identify a low-risk population (adverse event rate of 0.4%) and was found to have a better negative predictive value than the TIMI score without troponins (2% adverse event rate in patients with a modified TIMI score of 0 to 1). As shown in Figure 24-13, even when patients are considered low risk by clinical criteria, MCE can further subdivide those patients into low, intermediate, and high risk groups based on their regional function and myocardial perfusion findings. The same holds true for patients who are clinically intermediate risk.

Although the ability of MCE to detect a patient with an ongoing ACS or AMI is excellent, regional function and myocardial perfusion abnormalities may resolve in patients with only transient ischemia, especially if there is a significant delay between the ischemic episode and imaging. The effect of the timing of MCE and patient presentation were evaluated in a study where the patients were divided into four quartiles (0, 1, 4, and 12 h) based on their last episode of CP.[117] The negative predictive value of MCE was found to remain extremely high (94% for the development of any cardiac event) even up to 12 hours after chest pain had resolved.[117] Thus, even in

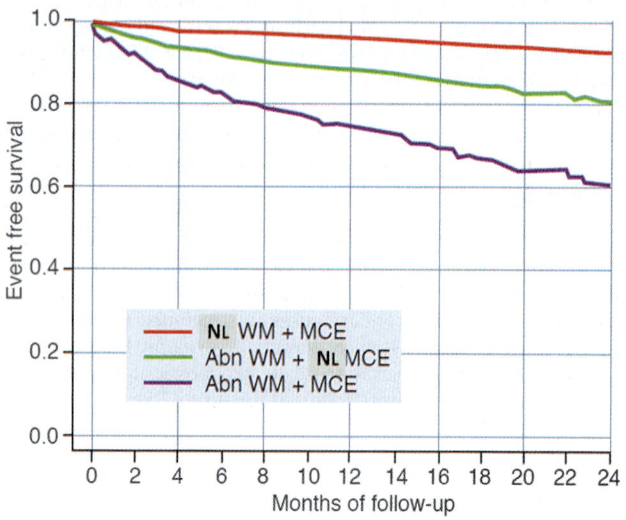

Figure 24-13. Long-term event-free survival in low-risk patients presenting with chest pain to the emergency department. Patients with normal wall motion and perfusion (NL WM + MCE) had the best outcome, while those with both abnormal wall motion and perfusion (Abn WM + MCE) had the worst. Patients with abnormal wall motion but normal perfusion (Abn WM + NL MCE) had intermediate outcome.

the setting of spontaneous reperfusion and restoration of normal antegrade flow, the presence of myocardial stunning in patients who have suffered significant ischemia persists for many hours.

The cost associated with the performance of echocardiography (especially if contrast is used for every case) is substantial. It has been shown, though, that by reducing the number of unnecessary admissions to hospital and other downstream costs for low-risk patients that MCE is cost-efficient, and can even reduce the costs of managing patients with undifferentiated CP by as much as $900 per patient.[118]

Some advantages of MCE over other potential modalities are its cost, its speed, and its transportability. It is smaller and portable, compared to SPECT, CMR, and CT. Echo is also relatively cheap compared to these other methods. No image processing is required. Limitations would include operator-dependent image quality, lack of quantitative variables for evaluation, and inadequate acoustic windows in some patients despite using contrast.

Summary

UCAs can be used to help define the LV endocardial border and assess myocardial perfusion, which provides multiple benefits for echocardiography.

In order to use MCE as a clinical tool, it is important to have a working knowledge of the imaging protocols, and also understand the complex coronary physiology that allows the user to interpret the information provided by perfusion imaging. In this chapter, we have attempted to provide insights into the microbubble contrast agents, the specific imaging methods employed, and coronary anatomy/physiology relevant to MCE.

Clinical studies have clearly established the role of LVO in routine practice, and perfusion imaging provides significant incremental diagnostic and prognostic information in many scenarios, but its role is still evolving.

REFERENCES

1. **Mulvagh SL, Rakowski H, Vannan MA, et al.** American Society of Echocardiography Consensus Statement on the Clinical Applications of Ultrasonic Contrast Agents in Echocardiography. *J Am Soc Echocardiogr* 2008;21:1179–1201.
2. **Senior R, Dwivedi G, Hayat S, et al.** Clinical benefits of contrast-enhanced echocardiography during rest and stress examinations. *Eur J Echocardiogr* 2006;6(suppl 2):S6–S13.
3. **Cohen JL, Cheirif J, Segar DS, et al.** Improved left ventricular endocardial border delineation and opacification with OPTISON (FS069), a new echocardiographic contrast agent: results of a phase III multicenter trial. *J Am Coll Cardiol* 1998;32(3):746–752.
4. **Hundley WG, Kizilbash AM, Afridi I, et al.** Effect of contrast enhancement of transthoracic echocardiographic assessment of left ventricular regional wall motion. *Am J Cardiol* 1999;84:1365–1369.
5. **Kitzman DW, Goldman ME, Gillam LD, et al.** Efficacy and safety of the novel ultrasound contrast agent perflutren (definity) in patients with suboptimal baseline left ventricular echocardiographic images. *Am J Cardiol* 2000;86(6):669–674.
6. **Lang RM, Mor-Avi V, Zoghbi WA, et al.** The role of contrast enhancement in echocardiographic assessment of left ventricular function. *Am J Cardiol* 2002;90:28J–34J.
7. **Nanda NC, Kitzman DW, Dittrich HC, et al.** Imagent improves endocardial delineation, inter-reader agreement, and the accuracy of segmental wall motion assessment. *Echocardiography* 2003;20:151–161.
8. **Terasawa A, Miyatake K, Nakatani S, et al.** Enhancement of Doppler flow signals in the left heart chambers by intravenous injection of sonicated albumin. *J Am Coll Cardiol* 1993;21(3):737–742.
9. **Keller MW, Segal SS, Kaul S, et al.** The behaviour of sonicated albumin microbubbles in the microcirculation: a basis for their use during myocardial contrast echocardiography. *Circ Res* 1989;65:458–466.

10. **Jayaweera AR, Edwards N, Glasheen WP, et al.** In vivo myocardial kinetics of air-filled albumin microbubbles during myocardial contrast echocardiography: comparison with radiolabeled red blood cells. *Circ Res* 1994;74:1157–1165.
11. **Skyba DM, Camarano G, Goodman NC, et al.** Hemodynamic characteristics, myocardial kinetics, and microvascular rheology of FS-069, a second generation echocardiographic contrast agent capable of producing myocardial opacification from a venous injection. *J Am Coll Cardiol* 1996;28:1292–1300.
12. **Skyba DM, Jayaweera AR, Goodman NC, et al.** Quantification of myocardial perfusion with myocardial contrast echocardiography during left atrial injection of contrast: implications for venous injection. *Circulation* 1994;90:1513–1521.
13. **de Jong N, Frinking PJ, Bouakaz A, et al.** Optical imaging of contrast agent microbubbles in an ultrasound field with a 100-MHx camera. *Ultrasound Med Biol* 2000;26:487–492.
14. **Dayton PA, Morgan KE, Klibanov AL, et al.** Optical and acoustical observations of the effects of ultrasound on contrast agents. *IEEE Trans Ultrason Ferroelectr Freq Control* 1999;46:220–232.
15. **DeJong N, Hoff L, Skotland T, et al.** Absorption and scatter of encapsulated gas filled microspheres: theoretical considerations and some measurements. *Ultrasonics* 1992;30:95–103.
16. **Hoff L, Sontum PC, Hoff B.** Acoustic properties of shell-encapsulated, gas-filled ultrasound contrast agents. *Proc IEEE Ultrason Symp* 1996;2: 1441–1444.
17. **DeJong N, Cornet R, Lancee CT.** Higher harmonics of vibrating gas filled microspheres. *Ultrasonics* 1994;32:455–459.
18. **Miller DL.** Ultrasonic detection of resonant cavitation bubbles in a flow tube by their second harmonic emission. *Ultrasonics* 1981;19:217–224.
19. **Burns PN, Powers JE, Simpson DH, et al.** Harmonic imaging: principles and preliminary results. *Clin Radiol* 1996;51(suppl):50–55.
20. **Thomas JD, Rubin DN.** Tissue harmonic imaging: why does it work? *J Am Soc Echocardiogr* 1998;11:803–808.
21. **Kassab GS, Lin DH, Fung YB.** Topology and dimensions of pig coronary capillary network. *Am J Physiol* 1994;267:H319–H325.
22. **Kassab GS, Lin DH, Fung YB.** Morphometry of pig coronary venous system. *Am J Physiol* 1994;267:H2100–H2113.
23. **Kaul S, Jayaweera AR.** Coronary and myocardial blood volumes: noninvasive tools to assess the coronary microcirculation? *Circulation* 1997; 96:719–724.
24. **Johnson PC.** Autoregulation of blood flow. *Circ Res* 1986;59:483–495.
25. **Jarhult J, Mellander S.** Autoregulation of capillary hydrostatic pressure in skeletal muscle during regional arterial hypo- and hypertension. *Acta Physiol Scand* 1974;91:32–41.
26. **Chilian WM, Layne SM, Klausner ED, et al.** Redistribution of coronary microvascular resistance produced by dipyridamole. *Am J Physiol* 1989;256;H383–H390.
27. **Canty JM Jr.** Coronary pressure-function and steady-state pressure-flow relations during autoregulation in the unanesthetized dog. *Circ Res* 1988;63:821–836.
28. **Wei K, Jayaweera AR, Firoozan S, et al.** Quantification of myocardial blood flow with ultrasound-induced destruction of microbubbles administered as a constant infusion. *Circulation* 1998;97:473–483.
29. **Pelberg RA, Wei K, Kamiyama N, et al.** Advantages of 'Flash Echocardiography'—a new technique for assessing myocardial perfusion. *J Am Soc Echocardiogr* 1999;12:85–93.
30. **Chilian WM, Marcus ML.** Phasic coronary blood flow velocity in intramural and epicardial coronary arteries. *Circ Res* 1982;50:772–781.
31. **Kajiya F, Tsujioka K, Goto M, et al.** Evaluation of phasic blood flow velocity in the great cardiac vein by a laser Doppler method. *Heart Vessels* 1985;1:16–23.
32. **Wei K, Le E, Bin JP, et al.** Non-invasive detection of coronary artery stenosis at rest without recourse to exercise or pharmacologic stress. *Circulation* 2002;105:218–223.
33. **Toyota E, Fujimoto K, Ogasawara Y, et al.** Dynamic changes in three-dimensional architecture and vascular volume of transmural coronary microvasculature between diastolic- and systolic-arrested rat hearts. *Circulation* 2002;105:621–626.
34. **Ay T, London V, d'Hondt A-M, et al.** Quantification of coronary flow reserve with myocardial contrast echocardiography in humans: comparison with positron emission tomography. *Circulation* 2001;104 (suppl II):II-589; (abstract).
35. **Porter TR, Xie F, Silver M, et al.** Real-time perfusion imaging with low mechanical index pulse inversion Doppler imaging. *J Am Coll Cardiol* 2001;37:748–753.
36. **Shimoni S, Zoghbi WA, Xie F, et al.** Real-time assessment of myocardial perfusion and wall motion during bicycle and treadmill exercise echocardiography: comparison with single photon emission computed tomography. *J Am Coll Cardiol* 2001;37:741–747.
37. **Leong-Poi H, Le E, Rim SJ, et al.** Quantification of myocardial perfusion and determination of coronary stenosis severity during hyperemia using real-time myocardial contrast echocardiography. *J Am Soc Echocardiogr* 2001;14:1173–1182.
38. **Dawson D, Rinkevich D, Belcik T, et al.** Measurement of myocardial blood flow velocity reserve with myocardial contrast echocardiography in patients with suspected coronary artery disease: comparison with quantitative gated ^{99m}Tc sestamibi SPECT. *J Am Soc Echocardiogr* 2003;16:1171–1177.
39. **Gould KL, Lipscomb K.** Effects of coronary stenoses on coronary flow reserve and resistance. *Am J Cardiol* 1974;34:48–55.
40. **Wei K, Jayaweera AR, Firoozan S, et al.** Basis for detection of stenosis using venous administration of microbubbles during myocardial contrast echocardiography: bolus or continuous infusion? *J Am Coll Cardiol* 1998;32:252–260.
41. **Jayaweera AR, Wei K, Bin JP, et al.** Role of capillaries in determining coronary blood flow reserve. *Am J Physiol* 1999;227:H2363–H2372.
42. **Ismail S, Jayaweera AR, Goodman NC, et al.** Detection of coronary stenoses and quantification of the degree and spatial extent of blood flow mismatch during coronary hyperemia with myocardial contrast echocardiography. *Circulation* 1995;91:821–830.
43. **Firschke C, Lindner JR, Wei K, et al.** Myocardial perfusion imaging in the setting of coronary artery stenosis and acute myocardial infarction using venous injection of a second-generation echocardiographic contrast agent. *Circulation* 1997;96:959–967.
44. **Linka AZ, Sklenar J, Wei K, et al.** Spatial distribution of microbubble velocity and concentration within the myocardium: insights into the transmural distribution of myocardial blood flow and volume. *Circulation* 1998;98:1912–1920.
45. **Wei K, Crouse L, Weiss J, et al.** Dipyridamole stress myocardial contrast echocardiography compared to ^{99m}Tc-sestamibi single photon emission computed tomography for detection of coronary artery disease: PB127 multicenter phase 2 trial results. *Am J Cardiol* 2003;91:1293–1298.
46. **Wei K, Ragosta M, Thorpe J, et al.** Noninvasive quantification of coronary blood flow reserve in humans using myocardial contrast echocardiography. *Circulation* 2001;103:2560–2565.
47. **Bin JP, Wei K, Pelberg RA, et al.** Relation between regional function and coronary blood flow reserve in multivessel coronary artery stenosis. *Am J Physiol* 2000;279:H3058–H3064.
48. **Bin J-P, Le E, Jayaweera AR, et al.** Direct effects of dobutamine on the coronary microcirculation: comparison with adenosine using myocardial contrast echocardiography. *J Am Soc Echocardiogr* 2003;16: 871–879.
49. **Leong-Poi H, Rim SJ, Le DE, et al.** Perfusion versus function: the ischemic cascade in demand ischemia: implications of single-vessel versus multivessel stenosis. *Circulation* 2002;105(8):987–992.
50. **Leong-Poi H, Coggins MP, Sklenar J, et al.** Role of collateral blood flow in the apparent disparity between the extent of abnormal wall thickening and perfusion defect size during acute myocardial infarction and demand ischemia. *J Am Coll Cardiol* 2005;45:565–572.
51. **Kaul S, Senior R, Dittrich H, et al.** Detection of coronary artery disease with myocardial contrast echocardiography: comparison with ^{99m}Tc-sestamibi single-photon emission computed tomography. *Circulation* 1997;96:785–792.
52. **Porter TR, Li S, Kricsfeld D, et al.** Detection of myocardial perfusion in multiple echocardiographic windows with one intravenous injection of microbubbles using transient response second harmonic imaging. *J Am Coll Cardiol* 1997;29:791–799.
53. **Heinle SK, Noblin J, Goree-Best P, et al.** Assessment of myocardial perfusion by harmonic power Doppler imaging at rest and during adenosine stress. Comparison with ^{99m}Tc-Sestamibi SPECT Imaging. *Circulation* 2000;102:55–60.
54. **Oraby MA, Hays J, Maklady FA, et al.** Assessment of myocardial perfusion during pharmacologic contrast stress echocardiography. *Am J Cardiol* 2002;89:640–644.

55. **Cwajg J, Feng X, O'Leary E, et al.** Detection of angiographically significant coronary artery disease with accelerated intermittent imaging after intravenous administration of ultrasound contrast material. *Am Heart J* 2000;139:675–683.
56. **Jeetley P, Hickman M, Kamp O, et al.** Myocardial contrast echocardiography for the detection of coronary artery stenosis. A prospective multicenter study in comparison with single-photon emission computed tomography. *J Am Coll Cardiol* 2006:141–145.
57. **Porter TR, Adolphson M, High RR, et al.** Rapid detection of coronary artery stenoses with real-time perfusion echocardiography during regadenoson stress. *Circ Cardiovasc Imaging* 2011;4:628–635.
58. **Senior R, Moreo A, Gaibazzi N, et al.** Comparison of sulfur hexafluoride microbubble (SonoVue)-enhanced contrast echocardiography with gated single-photon emission computed tomography for detection of significant coronary artery disease. A large European multicenter study. *J Am Coll Cardiol* 2013;62:1353–1361.
59. **Moir S, Haluska BA, Jenkins C, et al.** Incremental benefit of myocardial contrast to combined dipyridamole-exercise stress echocardiography for the assessment of coronary artery disease. *Circulation* 2004;110:1108–1113.
60. **Gabazzi N, Rigo F, Squeri A, et al.** Incremental value of contrast myocardial perfusion to detect intermediate versus severe coronary artery stenosis during stress echocardiography. *Cardiovasc Ultrasound* 2010;8:16–24.
61. **Elhendy A, O'Leary EL, Xie F, McGrain AC, et al.** Comparative accuracy of real-time myocardial contrast perfusion imaging and wall motion analysis during dobutamine stress echocardiography for the diagnosis of coronary artery disease. *J Am Coll Cardiol* 2004;44:2185–2191.
62. **Dawson D, Kaul S, Peters D, et al.** Prognostic value of dipyridamole stress myocardial contrast echocardiography: comparison with single photon emission computed tomography. *J Am Soc Echocardiogr* 2009;22:954–960.
63. **Miszalski-Jamka T, Kuntz-Hehner S, Schmidt H, et al.** Myocardial contrast echocardiography enhances long-term prognostic value of supine bicycle stress two-dimensional echocardiography. *J Am Soc Echocardiogr* 2009;22:1179–1201.
64. **Tsutsui JM, Xie F, Cloutier D, et al.** Real-time dobutamine stress myocardial perfusion echocardiography predicts outcome in the elderly. *Eur Heart J* 2008;29:377–385.
65. **Porter TR, Smith LM, Wu J, et al.** Patient outcome following 2 different stress imaging approaches. *J Am Coll Cardiol* 2013;61:2446–2455.
66. **Gaibazzi N, Reverberi C, Lorenzoni V, et al.** Prognostic value of high-dose dipyridamole stress myocardial contrast perfusion echocardiography. *Circulation* 2012;126:1217–1224.
67. **Kloner RA, Rude RE, Carlson N, et al.** Ultrastructural evidence of microvascular damage and myocardial cell injury after coronary artery occlusion: which one comes first? Circulation 1980;62:945–952.
68. **Reimer KA, Jennings RB.** The "wavefront phenomenon" of myocardial ischemic cell death. II. Transmural progression of necrosis within the framework of ischemic bed size (myocardium at risk) and collateral flow. *Lab Invest* 1979;40:633–644.
69. **Kaul S, Pandian NG, Guerrero L, et al.** Effects of selectively altering collateral driving pressure on regional perfusion and function in occluded coronary bed in the dog. *Circ Res* 1987;61:77–85.
70. **Piek J, Becker AE.** Collateral blood supply to the myocardium at risk in human myocardial infarction: a quantitative postmortem assessment. *J Am Coll Cardiol* 1988;11:1290–1296.
71. **Levin DC.** Pathways and functional significance of the coronary collateral circulation. *Circulation* 1974;50:831–837.
72. **Schaper WR, Frenzel H, Hort W.** Experimental coronary artery occlusion 1: measurement of infarct size. *Basic Res Cardiol* 1979;74:46–53.
73. **Sabia PJ, Powers ER, Jayaweera AR, et al.** Functional significance of collateral blood flow in patients with recent acute myocardial infarction: a study using myocardial contrast echocardiography. *Circulation* 1992;85:2080–2089.
74. **Coggins MP, Sklenar J, Le E, et al.** Noninvasive prediction of ultimate infarct size at the time of acute coronary occlusion based on the extent and magnitude of collateral-derived myocardial blood flow. *Circulation* 2001;104:2471–2477.
75. **Lafitte S, Higashiyama A, Masugata H, et al.** Contrast echocardiography can assess risk area and infarct size during coronary occlusion and reperfusion: experimental validation. *J Am Coll Cardiol* 2002;39:1546–1554.
76. **Jin J, Huang L, Wang H, et al.** Value of myocardial regional perfusion on long-term function in collateral-dependent myocardium. *South Med J* 2008;101:894–899.
77. **Califf RM, O'Neill W, Stacks RS, et al.** Failure of simple clinical measurements to predict perfusion status after intravenous thrombolysis. *Ann Intern Med* 1988;108:658–662.
78. **Belenkie I, Traboulsi M, Hall C, et al.** Rescue angioplasty during myocardial infarction has a beneficial effect on mortality: a tenable hypothesis. *Can J Cardiol* 1992;8:357–362.
79. **Ellis SG, da Silva ER, Heyndrickx G, et al.** Randomized comparison of rescue angioplasty with conservative management of patients with early failure of thrombolysis for acute anterior myocardial infarction. *Circulation* 1994;90:2280–2284.
80. **Villanueva FS, Glasheen WP, Sklenar J, et al.** Characterization of spatial patterns of flow within the reperfused myocardium by myocardial contrast echocardiography. Implications in determining extent of myocardial salvage. *Circulation* 1993;88:2562–2569.
81. **Sklenar J, Ismail S, Villanueva FS, et al.** Dobutamine echocardiography for determining the extent of myocardial salvage after reperfusion. An experimental evaluation. *Circulation* 1994;90:1502–1512.
82. **Kamp O, Lepper W, Vanoverschelde JL, et al.** Serial evaluation of perfusion defects in patients with a first acute myocardial infarction referred for primary PTCA using myocardial contrast echocardiography. *Eur Heart J* 2001;22:1485–1495.
83. **Main ML, Magalski A, Chee NK, et al.** Full-motion pulse inversion power Doppler contrast echocardiography differentiates stunning from necrosis and predicts recovery of left ventricular function after acute myocardial infarction. *J Am Coll Cardiol* 2001;38:1390–1394.
84. **Ito H, Okamura A, Iwakura K, et al.** Myocardial perfusion patterns related to thrombolysis in myocardial infarction perfusion grades after coronary angioplasty in patients with acute anterior wall myocardial infarction. *Circulation* 1996;93:1993–1999.
85. **Iwakura K, Ito H, Takiuchi S, et al.** Alternation in the coronary blood flow velocity pattern in patients with no reflow and reperfused acute myocardial infarction. *Circulation* 1996;94:1269–1275.
86. **Porter TR, Li S, Oster R, et al.** The clinical implications of no reflow demonstrated with intravenous perfluorocarbon containing microbubbles following restoration of thrombolysis in myocardial infarction (TIMI) 3 flow in patients with acute myocardial infarction. *Am J Cardiol* 1998;82:1173–1177.
87. **Rocchi G, Kasprzak JD, Galema TW, et al.** Usefulness of power Doppler contrast echocardiography to identify reperfusion after acute myocardial infarction. *Am J Cardiol* 2001;87:278–282.
88. **Lepper W, Hoffmann R, Kamp O, et al.** Assessment of myocardial reperfusion by intravenous myocardial contrast echocardiography and coronary flow reserve after primary percutaneous transluminal coronary angiography in patients with acute myocardial infarction. *Circulation* 2000;101:2368–2374.
89. **Ujino K, Hillis GS, Mulvagh SL, et al.** Usefulness of real-time intravenous myocardial contrast echocardiography in predicting left ventricular dilation after successfully reperfused acute myocardial infarction. *Am J Cardiol* 2005;96:17–21.
90. **Galiuto L, Gabrielli FA, Lombardo A, et al.** Reversible microvascular dysfunction coupled with persistent myocardial dysfunction: implications for post-infarct left ventricular remodeling. *Heart* 2007;93:565–571.
91. **Galiuto L, Garramone B, Scara A, et al.** The extent of microvascular damage during myocardial contrast echocardiography is superior to other known indexes of post-infarct reperfusion in predicting left ventricular remodeling. Results of the multicenter AMICI study. *J Am Coll Cardiol* 2008;51:552–559.
92. **Ito H, Maruyama A, Iwakura K, et al.** Clinical implications of the 'no reflow' phenomenon. A predictor of complications and left ventricular remodeling in reperfused anterior wall myocardial infarction. *Circulation* 1996;93:223–228.
93. **Dwivedi G, Janardhanan R, Hayat SA, et al.** Prognostic value of myocardial viability detected by myocardial contrast echocardiography early after acute myocardial infarction. *J Am Coll Cardiol* 2007;50:327–334.
94. **Funaro S, La Torre G, Madonna M, et al.** Incidence, determinants, and prognostic value of reverse left ventricular remodeling after primary percutaneous coronary intervention: results of the acute myocardial infarction contrast imaging (AMICI) multicenter study. *Eur Heart J* 2009;30:566–575.

95. **Pagley PR, Beller GA, Watson DD, et al.** Improved outcome after coronary bypass surgery in patients with ischemic cardiomyopathy and residual myocardial viability. *Circulation* 1997;96:793–800.
96. **Senior R, Kaul S, Lahiri A.** Myocardial viability on echocardiography predicts long-term survival after revascularization in patients with congestive heart failure. *J Am Coll Cardiol* 1999;33:1848–1854.
97. **Afridi I, Grayburn PA, Panza JA, et al.** Myocardial viability during dobutamine echocardiography predicts survival in patients with coronary artery disease and severe left ventricular dysfunction. *J Am Coll Cardiol* 1998;32:921–926.
98. **Camarano G, Ragosta M, Gimple LW, et al.** Identification of viable myocardium with contrast echocardiography in patients with poor left ventricular systolic function caused by recent or remote myocardial infarction. *Am J Cardiol* 1995,75:215–219.
99. **Nagueh SF, Vaduganathan P, Ali N, et al.** Identification of hibernating myocardium: comparative accuracy of myocardial contrast echocardiography, rest-redistribution thallium-201 tomography and dobutamine echocardiography. *J Am Coll Cardiol* 1997;29:985–993.
100. **Meza MF, Ramee S, Collins T, et al.** Knowledge of perfusion and contractile reserve improves the predictive value of recovery of regional myocardial function postrevascularization. A study using the combination of myocardial contrast echocardiography and dobutamine echocardiography. *Circulation* 1997;96:3459–3465.
101. **deFilippi CR, Willett DL, Irani WN, et al.** Comparison of myocardial contrast echocardiography and low-dose dobutamine stress echocardiography in predicting recovery of resting left ventricular function after coronary revascularization in chronic ischemic heart disease. *Circulation* 1995;92:2863–2868.
102. **Myers JH, Stirling MC, Choy M, et al.** Direct measurement of inner and outer wall thickening dynamics with epicardial echocardiography. *Circulation* 1986;74:164–172.
103. **Weintraub WS, Hattori S, Agarwal JB, et al.** The relationship between myocardial blood flow and contraction by myocardial layer in the canine left ventricle during ischemia. *Circ Res* 1981;48:430–438.
104. **Afridi I, Qureshi U, Kopelen HA, et al.** Serial changes in responses of hibernating myocardium to inotropic stimulation after revascularization. A dobutamine echocardiographic study. *J Am Coll Cardiol* 1997;30:1233–1240.
105. **Senior R, Lahiri A, Kaul S.** Effect of revascularization on left ventricular remodeling in patients with heart failure from severe chronic ischemic left ventricular dysfunction. *Am J Cardiol* 2001;88(6): 624–629.
106. **Samady H, Elefteriades JA, Abbott BG, et al.** Failure to improve left ventricular function after coronary revascularization for ischemic cardiomyopathy is not associated with worse outcome. *Circulation* 1999; 100:1298–1304.
107. **Heyndrickx GR, Baig H, Nellens P, et al.** Depression of regional blood flow and wall thickening after brief coronary occlusions. *Am J Physiol* 1978;234:H653–H659.
108. **Kloner RA, Jennings RB.** Consequences of brief ischemia: stunning, preconditioning, and their clinical implications: part 1. *Circulation* 2001;104:2981–2989.
109. **Nixon JV, Brown CN, Smitherman TC.** Identification of transient and persistent segmental wall motion abnormalities in patients with unstable angina by two-dimensional echocardiography. *Circulation* 1982;65:1497–1503.
110. **Ito H, Tomooka T, Sakai N, et al.** Time course of functional improvement in stunned myocardium in risk area in patients with reperfused anterior infarction. *Circulation* 1993;87:355–362.
111. **Kaul S, Senior R, Firschke C, et al.** Incremental value of cardiac imaging in patients presenting to the emergency department with chest pain and without ST-segment elevation: a multicenter study. *Am Heart J* 2004;148:129–136.
112. **Korosoglou G, Labadze N, Hansen A, et al.** Usefulness of real-time myocardial perfusion imaging in the evaluation of patients with first time chest pain. *Am J Cardiol* 2004;94:1225–1231.
113. **Kang DH, Kang SJ, Song JM, et al.** Efficacy of myocardial contrast echocardiography in the diagnosis and risk stratification of acute coronary syndrome. *Am J Cardiol* 2005;96:1498–1502.
114. **Rinkevich D, Kaul S, Wang XQ, et al.** Regional left ventricular perfusion and function in patients presenting to the emergency department with chest pain and no ST-segment elevation. *Eur Heart J* 2005;26:1606–1611.
115. **Antman E, Cohen M, Bernink PJL, et al.** The TIMI risk score for unstable angina/non-ST elevation MI. A method for prognostication and therapeutic decision making. *JAMA* 2000;284:835–842.
116. **Tong KL, Kaul S, Wang XQ, et al.** Myocardial contrast echocardiography versus thrombolysis in myocardial Infarction score in patients presenting to the emergency department with chest pain and a nondiagnostic electrocardiogram. *J Am Coll Cardiol* 2005;46:920–927.
117. **Kalvaitis S, Kaul S, Tong KL, et al.** Effect of time delay on the diagnostic use of contrast echocardiography in patients presenting to the emergency department with chest pain and no S-T segment elevation. *J Am Soc Echocardiogr* 2006;19:1488–1493.
118. **Wyrick JJ, Kalvaitis S, McConnell J, et al.** Cost efficiency of myocardial contrast echocardiography in patients presenting to the emergency department with chest pain of suspected cardiac origin and a nondiagnostic electrocardiogram. *Am J Cardiol* 2008;102:649–652.

CHAPTER

25 Pulmonary Perfusion Imaging with MR

Sebastian Ley, MD

Introduction

The main task of the lung is establishing a highly effective gas exchange. For this purpose, ventilation and perfusion of the lung need to match on a local level. Many conditions, including pulmonary embolism, pulmonary hypertension (PH), chronic obstructive disease, and tumors, alter pulmonary perfusion. Furthermore, pulmonary perfusion changes after surgical lung resection and during physiologic processes, such as change of body position or during physical activity. Therefore, assessment of the pulmonary perfusion is of physiologic and clinical importance. For studying such a large heterogeneous moving organ in detail, techniques providing good to excellent spatial resolution are required. One of these techniques is magnetic resonance imaging (MRI). For more than 20 years, MRI has been available as a technique for assessment of pulmonary perfusion.[1] Given the tremendous technical developments of the recent years regarding hardware and new sequences, MR-based perfusion imaging became broadly available. Two principal techniques are established: arterial spin-labeling and contrast-enhanced perfusion.[2] These two techniques are presented theoretically and within the clinical context.

Non–Contrast-Enhanced Pulmonary Perfusion

Technique

MR offers the possibility to mark a specific part of spins magnetically by selective radiofrequency (RF) excitation, leading to a specific magnetization to a selected fraction of blood. This technique is called arterial spin labeling (ASL) and requires no intravenous application of contrast material and is therefore considered to be completely noninvasive.[3]

In principle, two ECG-gated images of a selected slice (one slice location) are taken 5 to 8 seconds apart during a single apnea.[4] Images are acquired in diastole using a pulse sequence. To visualize pulmonary perfusion, the first image is preceded by a slice-selective inversion/saturation RF preparation overlaid on the imaged slice, the effect of which is to minimize the available MR signal in the imaged slice. The preceding saturation pulse is followed by the pulse sequence after one cardiac ejection to bring in unsaturated blood, resulting in a bright-blood image. For the second image, the process is repeated, except that this time the tagging preparation is spatially nonselective, so that blood flowing into the imaged slice has also been subject to the signal minimization (dark-blood image). Subtraction of the dark-blood image from the bright-blood image eliminates signal from any static elements in both images, leaving an image of blood delivered to the slice in one systolic ejection period.[5] Most important is that on the subtraction image, the signal from a volume element (voxel) is proportional to the amount of pulmonary arterial blood delivered during the previous heart cycle.[3,6–12] In principle, ASL preparation can be combined with many fast data recording techniques. True fast imaging with steady precession (true FISP) sequences in particular has been found to be ideally suited for assessment of pulmonary perfusion.

Specific types of ASL techniques that allow for quantification of regional pulmonary perfusion during a single breath hold are called "flow-sensitive alternating inversion recovery" (FAIR) and "flow-sensitive alternating inversion recovery with an extra radiofrequency (RF) pulse" (FAIRER).[13,14] The potential sources of artifacts are cardiac and respiratory motion. Cardiac motion and pulsatile flow of the descending aorta can generate smearing and flow artifacts, respectively. Spatial variation between the control images can lead to ghosting of the blood vessels, and spatial movement between the control and tag images causes the appearance of the adjacent dark–bright pairs of the blood vessels.

A closely related technique, called the T1 method, has also been used to measure pulmonary perfusion (Fig. 25-1).[15,16] Methodologically, this technique is similar to the ASL techniques. It differs primarily in how the experiment is conceptualized—as the delivery of a bolus of tagged spins or as an apparent alteration of the longitudinal relaxation time. Perfusion-weighted images are acquired in a single shot by completely saturating the static background tissue before image acquisition. The decrease of the lung T1 values in the same slice position from the global to the selective experiment is statistically significant and results from the wash-in effect of the noninverted blood water ^{1}H spins outside the imaging slice. Because the perfusion-weighted image is acquired in a single shot, artifacts arising from patient motion or different respiratory levels can be avoided. Furthermore, only very short acquisition times (≤5 seconds per slice) are required for the perfusion-weighted image, facilitating rapid and comfortable examinations. This is especially important for lung imaging, as some patients are not able to hold their breath for more than a few seconds.

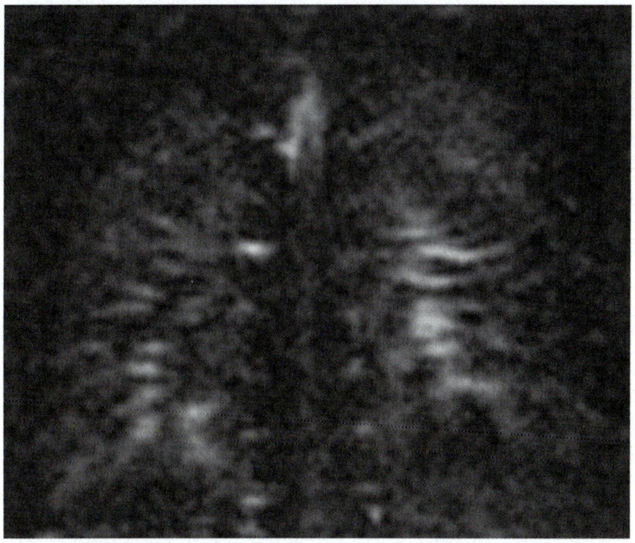

Figure 25-1. Arterial spin-labeling (ASL) image in a healthy volunteer (coronal orientation). The spatial resolution is 3.9 × 3.9 × 10 mm. The major drawback of this technique is low signal-to-noise ratio making a detailed evaluation difficult.

Lately, a technique called Fourier decomposition (FD) has been proposed for non–contrast-enhanced functional lung MRI.[17] This method was implemented on a standard 1.5-T whole-body MR system with an optimized two-dimensional (2-D) balanced steady-state free precession (bSSFP) sequence to produce time-resolved data stacks. Application of image registration combined with Fourier analysis of the data along the temporal dimension allowed for spectral separation of the signal changes caused by lung parenchyma contraction and blood flow.[18]

The non–contrast-enhanced sequences have the advantage that measurements can be made repeatedly over very short time periods (seconds). The absence of contrast also means that the measurements can be repeated indefinitely as it has not to be cleared out from the blood before reimaging is possible (also, the absolute number of measurements is limited by the total amount of contrast material that can be applied in 1 day). There are some limitations of these techniques: (a) more difficulty in implementation compared with dynamic contrast-enhanced imaging, (b) requirement of a regular cardiac cycle, (c) requirement of single-slice technique and five to eight slices to cover the whole lung, and (d) the limited voxel resolution (i.e., 5 × 5 × 30 mm^3).[14]

Quantification

ASL-based techniques allow for calculation of relative pulmonary blood flow (rPBF) in mL/100 g/min.[13,19,20] For conversion of rPBF into PBF, the lung density is required, which is usually assumed to be constant with 0.33 g/mL (at functional residual capacity).[21] However, this might not be the case in lung diseases like fibrosis or emphysema. Normal values are reported to be in the range of 5.5 mL/g/min.

Using a rapid IR Snapshot FLASH technique, a spin-labeling method within the imaging slice was used in combination with a simple two-compartment lung tissue model. The measured pulmonary perfusion rates of the healthy lung parenchyma were on the order of 400 to 600 mL/100 g/min, depending on the subject investigated and the actual slice position in the lung.[22]

In healthy volunteers ($n = 6$), a quantitative comparison between non–contrast-enhanced and contrast-enhanced techniques was performed.[23] Two coronal slices (middle and dorsal part of the lung) were assessed, and maps of rPBF were calculated—no absolute perfusion measures were calculated. By placing 10 regions of interest in each lung, a right-to-left perfusion ratio analysis was performed. For the dorsal slice, the differences between both techniques were not statistically different. The middle position however showed a 16% to 43% underestimation of FAIR-derived rPBF in the right lung. This was explained by tracer saturation for the right lung as the right pulmonary artery is in the plane of both pulses needed for tagging and readout. In an internal control, this difference was not present if slices were acquired in a sagittal orientation.

The Fourier decomposition method was tested qualitatively against gadolinium-enhanced MR perfusion in patients with cystic fibrosis showing a good intrareader agreement between both techniques.[24] However, it was shown that the image quality of Fourier decomposition technique was significantly inferior to that of gadolinium-enhanced MR perfusion in patients with non–small cell cancer.[25]

Application

Based on the strength and limitations noted above, the clinical application so far has been limited. However, the strength of the techniques lies in the ability to study physiologic aspects of the lung perfusion on a regional level.[26–29] Important for all perfusion studies is to notice that the signal-to-noise ratio (SNR) of ASL images is low, particularly in the anterior portions of the lung. Therefore, positioning the patient so that the area of interest is down, gravity may increase SNR and improve visibility of perfusion defects. Also, signal intensity and subsequently perfusion increase during examination on end-expiratory breath hold compared to end-inspiratory breath hold.[30,31]

Normal aging is associated with a decline in pulmonary function and efficiency of gas exchange. The effect of aging on spatial heterogeneity of pulmonary perfusion was studied on 56 healthy, nonsmoking volunteers with an age range of 21 to 76 years.[32] Relative dispersion increased significantly with increasing age by 0.1 per decade until age 50 to 59 years, and a significant positive relationship between relative dispersion and age was found. No regional lung density measurements were performed. Therefore, it was not possible to investigate if the age-related parenchymal changes were the cause for this phenomenon. In an early study, Keilholz et al.[33] demonstrated the ability of ASL to depict the gravity-dependent perfusion effects. Healthy volunteers were placed inside the scanner on their right and left lateral side, and coronal images were acquired within a 10-s breath hold using a FAIRER HASTE sequence. In both positions, an increase in the intensity of the dependent lung was found (229% for left lateral, 40% for right lateral). No change was seen along an isogravitational plane. These results were confirmed for volunteers lying on their back.[16]

In six rabbits, a pulmonary emboli model was introduced using a balloon catheter, which was placed in the left pulmonary artery.[34] After occlusion of the left pulmonary artery, a set of FAIRER images followed by a contrast-enhanced angiography was performed. The huge perfusion defect (whole left lung) was depicted by both imaging techniques. It has to be noted again that 8 seconds were required for a single slice of ASL, while the 3-D acquisition of the contrast-enhanced perfusion needed 30 seconds. A similar experiment was done in five rabbits where ASL perfusion and ventilation images using hyperpolarized helium-3 were assessed.[35] After occlusion of the pulmonary artery by a balloon catheter, the ventilation was unchanged and the ASL perfusion images demonstrated the large perfusion defect.

In patients susceptible to high-altitude pulmonary edema (HAPE), it was possible to demonstrate the uneven hypoxic pulmonary vasoconstriction compared to nonsusceptible patients by assessing the relative dispersion of blood flow.[36]

Future Developments

Up to now, only few reports exist on the clinical application of non–contrast-enhanced perfusion techniques. Due to the lengthy acquisition times and relatively low signal increase, the clinical usage will be limited in the future. The main application will be in exploration of physiologic processes were the possibility of unrestricted measurements outweighs the prolonged acquisition time.[3] It may be the imaging technique of choice for pregnant women to rule out pulmonary emboli. However, in this stetting, other native imaging techniques, like steady-state free precession sequences, also showed a good clinical potential.[37] In patients with severely impaired kidney function, application of contrast media should be avoided to reduce the risk of nephrogenic systemic fibrosis (NSF). As this patient population increases, the demand of non–contrast-enhanced techniques for visualization of pulmonary perfusion increases. Thus, this patient population could benefit from future developments within this area.

Contrast-Enhanced MR Perfusion

Technique

Contrast-enhanced lung perfusion is realized by rapid imaging of the first pass of contrast material through the lungs after intravenous bolus injection. To visualize the peak enhancement of the lungs, the temporal resolution of contrast-enhanced MRI of lung perfusion has to be below the transit time of a contrast bolus through the lungs being in the range of 3 to 4 seconds.[38]

Especially with older machines, 2-D approaches are quite commonly used as they can be acquired in a timely fashion such as 0.3 second for each slice. As a drawback, they lack sufficient spatial resolution and anatomic coverage to characterize most of the perfusion defects or inhomogeneities. For clinical usage, a reasonable spatial resolution and anatomic coverage are required to allow for visualization of perfusion changes on a segmental level. Thus, nowadays 3-D techniques are most frequently used. Even if the temporal resolution is not sufficient for quantification of pulmonary perfusion, a visual analysis can be performed in any case allowing to visualization of the perfusion distribution and defects. Most frequently, a 3-D gradient echo pulse sequence (FLASH) with a short TE and TR with a resulting temporal resolution of 1.0 to 1.5 seconds for each 3-D data set is used, dependent on the used slice thickness of 10 mm down to 5 mm.[39,40] Improvements in k-space sampling techniques such as the use of parallel imaging techniques allow for increased spatial resolution without reduction of temporal resolution.[41] A second strategy is to use echo sharing (time-resolved echo-shared angiographic technique [TREAT], time-resolved imaging of contrast kinetics [TRICKS]), where the low-frequency k-space data are updated more often than are the high-frequency k-space data, which are interpolated between consecutive time frames, thus leading to an effective shortening of the total acquisition time. Image quality of both techniques was assessed in nine patients.[42] Using the same temporal resolution, the voxel size was decreased by 24% in the TREAT data sets compared to the standard perfusion technique (both techniques used parallel imaging with an acceleration factor of 2). For central and peripheral vascular perception, the TREAT perfusion was rated significantly superior to the standard technique. Basic evaluation of MR perfusion was performed qualitatively in comparison to perfusion scintigraphy. Intermodality comparison showed a good agreement (kappa = 0.74) in 14 patients with various diseases (chronic obstructive pulmonary disease [COPD], lung cancer, …).[43] Rapid acquisition of multiple images during bolus contrast administration is essential to pulmonary perfusion imaging. A direct comparison between different k-space acquisition techniques was performed recently.[44] Three k-space acquisition techniques were compared for image quality and SNR: (a) generalized autocalibrating partial parallel acquisition (GRAPPA) with an internal acquisition of reference lines, (b) GRAPPA with a single "external" acquisition of reference lines before the measurement, and (c) a combination of GRAPPA with an internal acquisition of reference lines and view sharing. All examinations were performed in 10 healthy volunteers (5-mL gadobutrol with an injection speed of 2.5 mL/s) with a constant voxel size: 3.9 × 3.9 × 5 mm^3. At 1.5 T, view sharing resulted in the best image quality and SNR. Furthermore, the temporal resolution was the shortest with 1.07 seconds. k-t BLAST (broad-use linear speed-up technique) is a method employed to reduce scan time using undersampling of data in k-t space.[41] With this technique, faster images with an acceleration factor of 5 are achieved with acceptable error.

Contrast Media

So far, most of the studies used 0.1-mmol Gd-DTPA/kg body weight for visualization of pulmonary perfusion. Different amounts of contrast media (0.05 mmol/kg body weight and 0.1 mmol/kg body weight), contrast media concentrations (0.5 mmol/L and 1 mmol/L), and injection protocols (2.5 mL/s and 5 mL/s) were compared in 10 healthy volunteers.[45] By analyzing the SNR, no difference was found between the different contrast media concentrations giving the same injection speed. For both contrast agents, a dose of 0.1 mmol/kg body weight was superior to the half-dose protocol. In combination with a rapid injection (5 mL/s), the highest SNR in all vascular segments were achieved. Regarding the contrast media injection speed, a small bolus profile and fast attenuation of the lung parenchyma are optimal. It was found that with increased speed, the mean transit time (MTT) for the pulmonary arteries decreased significantly.[46] However, this decrease was not linear: a fourfold increase in injection rate leads to a twofold decrease in MTT. In the same study, it was found that the cardiac function parameters had no significant influence on the bolus profile. Overall, an injection speed of 3 mL/s was recommended for pulmonary perfusion.[47] A summary of frequently used contrast media injection regimens are provided in Table 25.1.

Basic postprocessing for improvement of visualization of perfusion is done by subtraction of the data set with the highest signal intensity from a baseline data set (Fig. 25-2). In most cases, this allows for a rapid analysis of the clinical situation of the patient. However, for any detailed analysis, therapy monitoring, or presurgical estimation of the regional pulmonary function, a quantitative analysis is important.

Quantification

Quantification of pulmonary perfusion is based on the indicator dilution theory where the maximum of signal intensity and the temporal course of the signal change are used. For quantification, an arterial input function (AIF) has to be defined by placing a region of interest (ROI) in the main pulmonary artery. The tissue response function of the lung parenchyma can be either determined by multiple single small ROIs or, better, for the whole lung. The placement of ROIs usually is done manually with known inter- and intraobserver variabilities during (repeated) evaluations. This has significant implications on the quantification results derived from this technique. Recently, a technique for automatic lung segmentation was published overcoming this above-mentioned shortcomings.[56]

Assuming a linear relation between the signal and the concentration of contrast agent, signal intensity–time curves are converted to concentration–time curves.[57] Hypothesizing a negligible amount of extravasating contrast agent during the first pass of the bolus in the lungs, the principles of the indicator dilution theory[58] were applicable. The central volume theorem states the relationship between the perfusion parameters regional pulmonary blood

TABLE

25.1 Summary of Used Contrast Media Injection Protocols and Spatial Resolution of Perfusion-Weighted MR

Injection Speed (mL/s)	Dose	Spatial Resolution (mm³)	Reference
2.5	5-mL gadobutrol	3.9 × 3.9 × 5	44
5	5-mL Magnevist	1.9 × 1.8 × 10	48
3	0.05 mmol/kg BW Magnevist	3.9 × 3.9 × 6.3	49
4	0.125 mmol/kg BW Magnevist	2.9 × 1.6 × 10	50
5	5-mL Omniscan	1.9 × 1.8 × 12	51
5	0.1 mmol/kg BW Magnevist	3.5 × 1.9 × 4	52
5	0.1 mmol/kg BW Magnevist	1.9 × 3.8 × 3.6	53
5	0.1 mmol/kg BW Multihance	1.9 × 3.8 × 4	54
3–5	3- to 5-mL Magnevist	1.9 × 1.8 × 10	39
5	0.1 mmol/kg BW Omniscan	1.9 × 3.6 × 4	55

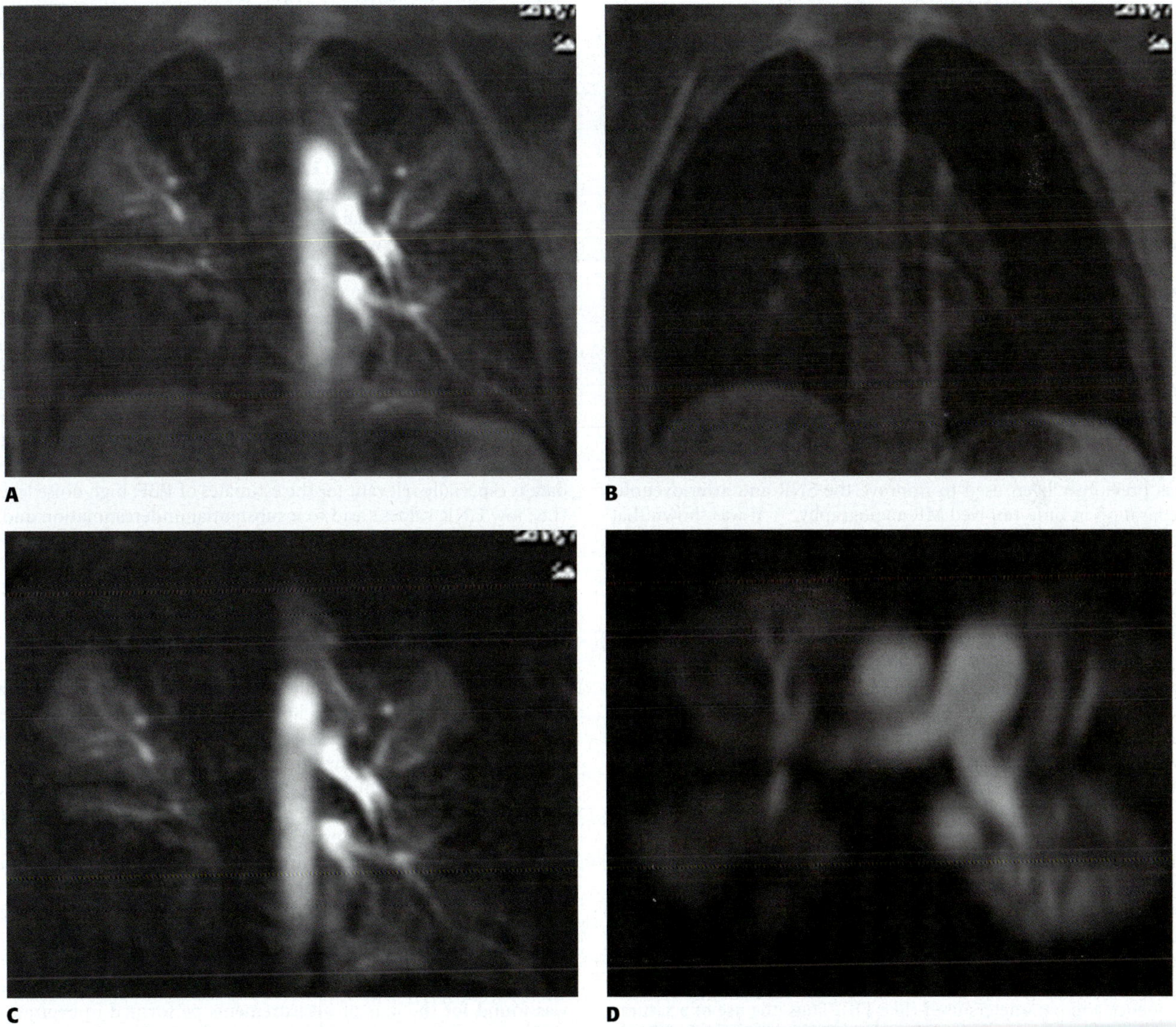

Figure 25-2. Concept of subtraction of perfusion images in a patient with acute pulmonary embolism. **(A)** represents the data set with the maximum contrast enhancement. **(B)** is an early data set without contrast media. Subtraction of both data sets **(C)** results in an image with suppressed background and therefore enhanced perfusion. The 3-D nature of the data sets allow for reformation in any plane, like axial **(D)**. The contrast-enhanced lung areas are nicely visible in contrast to the nonenhanced areas due to the perfusion defects. Typically, for acute pulmonary embolism, the defects are wedge shaped with the broad basis in the periphery.

flow (PBF mL/100 mL lung tissue/min), regional pulmonary blood volume (PBV) (PBV mL/100 mL lung tissue), and the mean transit time (MTT, s):

$$MTT = \frac{PBV}{PBF}$$

Regional PBV can be calculated by normalizing the area under the tissue concentration–time curve to the integral of the arterial input function (AIF):

$$PBV = \frac{\int C(t)dt}{\int AIF(t)dt}$$

In consideration of the finite length of the bolus and its dispersion during its way to the tissue volume, the relationship between the AIF and the tissue concentration–time curve is described by the convolution of the AIF and a residue function R(t):

$$C(t) = PBF \int AIF(\tau) \bullet R(t-\tau)d\tau$$

where R(t) is the amount of contrast agent remaining in the tissue at time t. PBF is therefore the initial height of R(t 0) and the maximum of R(t) in case of a delay between the AIF(t) and C(t) and can be assessed by deconvolving AIF(t) and C(t). The deconvolution of the last equation is performed using singular value decomposition,[59] a model-independent nonparametric deconvolution analysis with the potentiality of reducing the noise contribution by applying a suitable threshold to a singular value matrix. This method has shown reliable results for first-pass bolus tracking in clinical studies.[60]

Inclusion of the central pulmonary arteries leads to a systematic overestimation of pulmonary perfusion. Therefore, the use of small ROIs in the lung periphery can be beneficial. However, if the spatial distribution of the underlying lung disease is unknown, or if lung perfusion quantification is required for an entire lung (e.g., to assess side differences of lung perfusion), a measurement of a limited lung sample in a small ROI will only reflect a poor estimate of lung perfusion. One study used a cross-correlation analysis (CCA) of perfusion data sets for suppression of central pulmonary vessels.[61] CCA has previously been used to improve the SNR and arteriovenous separation in time-resolved MR angiography.[62,63] It was shown that it is feasible to identify vessels with a similar signal intensity–time curve as a reference vessel using CCA. For this purpose, reference ROIs have to be drawn in the pulmonary artery and pulmonary vein. The approach was evaluated in seven healthy volunteers. The quantification of PBV and PBF resulted in an average reduction of 25% for PBV and 15% for PBF compared with the segmentations without vessel exclusion. A comparison of the manual exclusion of vessel structures and the CCA revealed an average reduction of 13% for the PBV and 8% for PBF. The reduction by applying the CCA was significant ($p \leq 0.001$) compared with the results with manual and without blood vessel exclusion for all calculated parameters.

Basically, during quantitative perfusion evaluation, the signal intensity–time curves are converted into concentration–time curves. Therefore, a linear relationship between signal intensity and concentration is mandatory. This is especially important for the AIF where all contrast media pass by in a compact bolus.[64] A linear relationship, however, is only seen for a small range of concentrations of 3, 4, or 5 mmol/L as seen in in vitro experiments.[65–67] The linearity between signal and concentration is dependent on the sequence and parameters used (like TE). Thus, the use of a saturation recovery–prepared FLASH sequence was proposed,[67] which is often used in myocardial perfusion imaging, to improve the linearity of the measurements and thus the contrast-to-noise ratio (CNR) at higher doses. Applied to volunteers, the usage of 0.057 mmol/kg body weight was feasible,[67] while in an animal experiment, it was found that already 0.05 mmol Gd-DTPA/kg body weight resulted in in vivo concentrations outside the linearity range.[66] However, comparing the quantitative measures of the 0.05 mmol/kg body weight, the values were too high compared to results from PET where PBF was found to be 121 mL/min/100 mL[68] and PBV 17 to 20 mL/100 mL.[69] In a prospective trial, different injection protocols and contrast media concentrations were investigated and compared to quantitative analysis of perfusion SPECT.[48] The amount of the MR contrast bolus was fixed with 5 mL and an injection speed of 5 mL/s, followed by a 20-mL saline flush. This approach ensured similar bolus widths in all applications. It was found that for patients weighting less than 70 kg, a concentration of 0.3 mmol/mL showed the highest accordance to SPECT and 0.5 mmol/mL for patients weighing more than 70 kg. However, this study used 10-mm-thick slice partitions. Therefore, the small amount of 5 mL of contrast media resulted in an appropriate contrast-to-noise ratio.

Another solution for this complex problem was the usage of a dual-bolus approach.[65] In this experiment, the AIF is determined by a low-volume application of contrast media (i.e., 0.01 mmol/kg body weight) to achieve a linear relationship between contrast agent concentration and signal intensity in the large pulmonary vessels. This is followed by boluses with higher doses to obtain sufficient CNR in lung tissue. This may allow absolute quantification as well as the visual analysis of perfusion in lung tissue, which is often not possible when a single low dose is used for absolute perfusion quantification. The drawback of this approach is the small and therefore short bolus (i.e., 1.5 mL) for the AIF, which requires an extremely high temporal resolution of the perfusion sequence to assess the peak signal. The combination of a small prebolus (0.01 mmol/kg bodyweight) with a main bolus of 0.04 mmol/kg bodyweight resulted in perfusion parameters best comparable with literature data. A combination of the prebolus with a main bolus of 0.08 mmol/kg body weight resulted in an underestimation of PBV.[65]

For perfusion imaging of the lung, the optimal combination of temporal resolution and contrast-to-noise ratio is essential. This complex interaction was studied using a Monte Carlo simulation and volunteer examinations.[70] It was found that a temporal resolution of approximately 2 seconds has to be achieved for correct application of the deconvolution algorithm. The influence of noise in the data is especially relevant for the estimates of PBF: high noise levels (i.e., low CNR values) lead to a substantial underestimation and a significant loss of accuracy in the PBF estimates. It was concluded that the assessment of PBF might benefit from less aggressive acceleration, for example, by a lower acceleration factor of 2. The CNR can be notably increased if larger voxel sizes are employed; the voxel size should thus be chosen as large as clinically acceptable.

Repeatability of quantitative perfusion measurements was tested in two patient groups and one large volunteer study. In one study, 10 patients with bronchoalveolar carcinoma were scanned twice within 3 days in inspiratory breath hold.[48] Evaluation was performed by manually placing three regions of interest in the data set. An excellent agreement between both measurements was found, without any significant difference. Ten patients with pulmonary hypertension were rescanned 3 weeks after the initial scan.[71] 3-D perfusion data sets were acquired in inspiratory breath hold and evaluation comprised the whole lung. No significant difference was found for PBF, PBV, and MTT. Fourteen volunteers were examined twice after 24 hours in inspiratory and expiratory breath hold.[49] Evaluation was done comprising quantitative whole lung evaluation and was performed by two observers. No significant difference was found for the pair of measurements performed in expiration and evaluated by the same observer. The inspiratory data sets however showed significant differences for PBF. Significant differences were found in inspiration and expiration for the interobserver variability. These three studies demonstrate the significant influence of the observer on the quantitative results. Therefore, for a broad usage of the technique, an automatic segmentation approach assisting evaluation should be developed. Especially in data sets with pathologically changed perfusion (i.e., peripheral perfusion defects), automatic segmentation algorithms will be difficult to be implemented. An initial study used morphologic HASTE images for segmentation of the lung borders.[72] These contours were applied to the perfusion data sets after image registration of the HASTE and perfusion images. This reduced the time needed for evaluation of the perfusion data sets to approximately 10 minutes. However, this technique was only applied to data sets of healthy volunteers, and no reproducibility experiments were performed.

So far, MR perfusion of the lung parenchyma has been performed at 1.5 T. Given the benefits of higher field strengths (like 3 T), a higher SNR can be expected, which should be beneficial regarding quantification or which allow an increase in spatial resolution.

An example of first-pass pulmonary perfusion MR technique using coronal 3-D spoiled gradient echo imaging with TRICKS at 1.5 T includes TR/TE/flip angle, 2.5/0.8/30 degrees; parallel imaging acceleration factor, 2; matrix 256 × 128; field of view (FOV), 480 mm; slice thickness, 10 mm reconstructed at 5-mm intervals (i.e., 50% slice overlap) using zero-fill interpolation; 28 to 44 coronal slices (depending on the size of thorax); scan time, 60 seconds; and temporal resolution of rate of 1.2 to 1.8 seconds. A bolus of 0.1 mmol/kg bodyweight Gd-DTPA followed by a saline flush of 20 mL is injected at 5 mL/s. The AIF for absolute quantification of pulmonary perfusion is derived from a first-pass contrast bolus injection with an ROI in the right ventricle on a short-axis slice. After injection of 0.05 mmol/kg contrast at 5 mL/s, an ECG-gated multiphase inversion recovery fast gradient echo sequence is acquired (three to five slices): TR/TE, 6.4/1.3 milliseconds; flip angle, 25 degrees; inversion time, 176 milliseconds; slice thickness/gap, 8/5 mm; number of slices, 3; and phases reconstructed per slice, 40. Pulmonary perfusion is then calculated using signal intensity–time curves of the lung parenchyma (TRICKS sequence) and the right ventricular AIF.

Different models are proposed for absolute quantification of pulmonary parenchymal perfusion. However, these techniques are challenging and time consuming and requires specific imaging and contrast protocols as well as dedicated postprocessing software. In contrast, semiquantitative measures can be calculated quickly and reliably from signal intensity–time curves of the lung parenchyma and do not require a specific MRI protocol and dedicated deconvolution software. Hueper et al.[73] have shown a good correlation between quantitative (e.g., MTT, PBV) and semiquantitative (e.g., time to peak, upslope, maximum signal) parameters of the regional lung perfusion in both normal and COPD patients.

Measurement of total or regional pulmonary parenchymal perfusion by MRI can demonstrate the physiologic distribution of lung perfusion in healthy lungs. Mean values for total lung perfusion in normal individuals are PBF of 122 ± 25 mL/min/100 mL, PBV of 10 ± 4 mL/100 mL, and MTT of 4.7 ± 1.7 seconds.[39] These values are much lower (almost half) in COPD. PBF values in the posterior normal lung (148 ± 17 mL/min/100 mL lung) are higher than in the anterior (97.6 ± 13.7 mL/100 mL lung) lung, but mean MTT is shorter in the posterior than in the anterior lung parenchyma.[39]

Application

In clinical routine, contrast-enhanced perfusion can be easily applied for visual assessment of disease characteristics. For a qualitative approach, the discussion of temporal resolution and contrast media dose is obsolete, and it can be performed at any MR scanner. Perfusion defects due to vascular obstruction show a typical wedge shape including the lung periphery (Fig. 25-2).[74] In 41 patients with acute PE, the agreement of MR perfusion with SPECT perfusion for perfusion defects down to the subsegmental level was assessed.[74] MR perfusion showed a very high agreement with SPECT (0.98 for kappa value per examination and 0.98, 0.83, and 0.69 for lobar, segmental, and subsegmental perfusion defects, respectively). By a quantitative segmental perfusion analysis in patients with acute pulmonary embolism, it was possible to determine the obstruction index.[51] This perfusion-based index showed a higher correlation with clinical severity and also was a significant predictor of outcome. This initial report brings MR perfusion in the pole position for being discussed as new modality of choice for PE assessment. Furthermore, this radiation-free technique is optimally suited for follow-up studies and treatment monitoring.[75] Visual evaluation is also sufficient to differentiate between different causes of pulmonary hypertension (PH) like pulmonary arterial hypertension (PAH) and chronic thromboembolic PH (CTEPH).[52] Perfusion was diffusely reduced in PAH, and focal defects occurred in CTEPH (Fig. 25-3). In 45 patients with moderate-to-severe COPD, perfusion was matched to parenchymal alterations demonstrated by multidetector-row computed tomography (MDCT).[53] A high agreement on a lobar level was found between parenchymal destruction and reduction of perfusion in patients with severe emphysema (kappa of 0.8). In patients with cystic fibrosis, the functional score, based on the visual evaluation of the perfusion defects, showed an acceptable intra- and interreader agreement (concordance correlation coefficient 0.89 and 0.8, respectively) (Fig. 25-4).[76]

Semiquantitative analysis of 3-D perfusion data sets in eight healthy volunteers allowed for calculation of the left-to-right perfusion ratio (ratio 0.9), which was confirmed by phase-contrast flow measurements.[77] Furthermore, a shorter transit time and higher peak signal were found in the dorsal lung regions. Quantitative evaluation of perfusion was compared to perfusion scintigraphy for assessment of left-to-right perfusion ratios in 23 patients with various lung diseases.[54] The MR estimations of left-to-right perfusion ratios correlated significantly with those of perfusion scintigraphy scans ($p < 0.01$). The MR ratios computed from PBF showed the highest accuracy, followed by those from peak concentration and PBV.

One important clinical field for perfusion assessment is estimation of postsurgical lung function, for example, after lung cancer

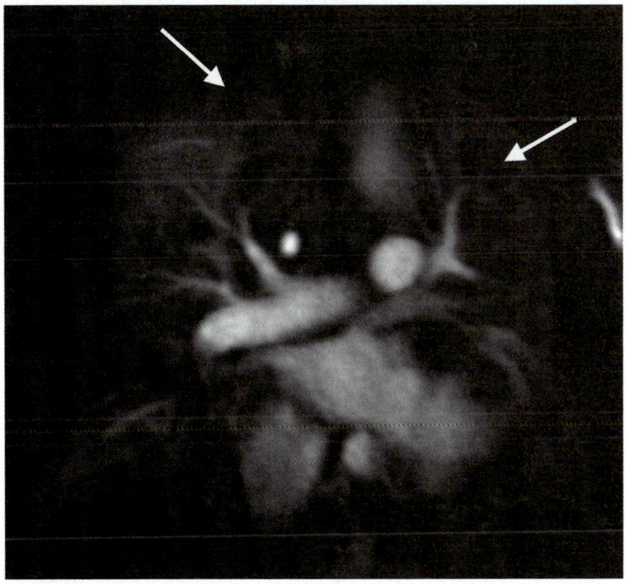

Figure 25-3. A patient with primary pulmonary hypertension is shown. Note the overall well-preserved perfusion of the lung parenchyma. There are small perfusion defects visible (two examples highlighted by the *arrows*); the distribution and localization is typical for pulmonary hypertension.

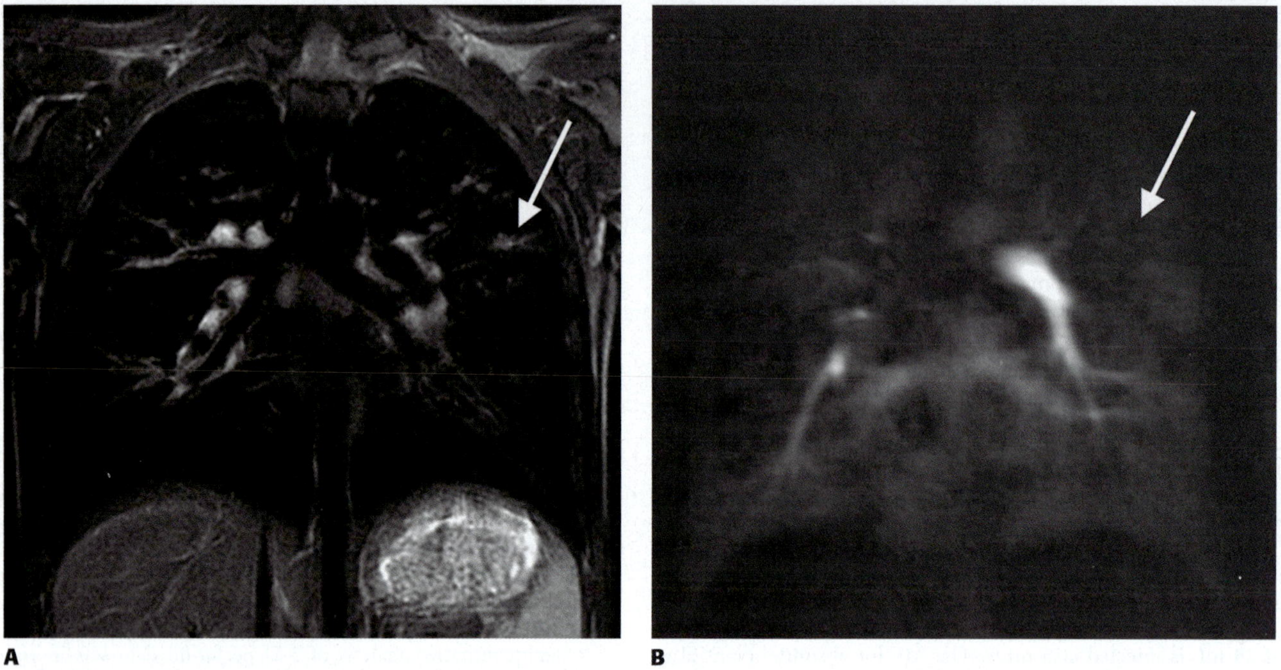

Figure 25-4. A 16-year-old patient with cystic fibrosis is shown. **(A)** is a coronal T2 TSE image with respiratory gating and **(B)** is a subtraction of the perfusion data set. MR is one of the few modalities allowing studying the functional impact of morphologic changes. In this example, it can be seen that especially mucus plugging (*arrow*) and bronchiectasis lead to perfusion defects.

resection. So far, perfusion scintigraphy is routinely used for this purpose. In 60 patients with lung cancer, regional blood flow was assessed by scintigraphy and MR.[39] MR outperformed scintigraphy for assessment of postoperative FEV 1 ($r = 0.93$ and $r = 0.89$, respectively). Therefore, it was concluded that perfusion MR is a feasible alternative to pulmonary perfusion scintigraphy for predicting postoperative lung function in patients with lung cancer.

Quantitative evaluation of different physiologic effects was performed in nine healthy volunteers.[78] Examinations were performed in inspiratory and expiratory breath holds. A significantly higher perfusion was observed at expiratory breath hold. Also, a higher PBF was observed for the right lung. However, no ventrodorsal perfusion gradient was observed, which was explained by the inclusion of central pulmonary vessels in the evaluation. After application of a vasodilative agent (inhalation of 100% oxygen), a significant increase and redistribution of the pulmonary perfusion was found in 10 healthy volunteers.[79] Therefore, MR perfusion seems to be suited for estimation of therapy response in patients with PH after administration of vasodilative drugs.

In a group of 13 COPD patients, the pulmonary perfusion was found to be heterogeneously altered—PBF and PBV were significantly reduced and MTT prolonged.[80]

Despite the pure quantification, another aspect of perfusion, although harder to establish, is the degree of homogeneity. In patients susceptible to high-altitude pulmonary edema (HAPE-S), the perfusion inhomogeneity was compared between HAPE-resistant volunteers and HAPE-S patients after 2 hours of hypoxia (being equivalent to an altitude of 4,500 m).[55] Parameters indicating perfusion inhomogeneity increased during hypoxia in both populations, particularly in HAPE-S subjects where they increased significantly for almost all evaluations. These results were in accordance with those obtained by ASL technique.[36] Therefore, this kind of analysis, although not yet broadly used, may be important for future applications in diseases with peripheral vasoconstriction like pulmonary hypertension. So far, only conventional perfusion parameters are assessed in patients with pulmonary hypertension. Compared to healthy, age-matched volunteers, perfusion parameters are different in patients with pulmonary hypertension, with reduced PBF and PBV and increased MTT.[81,82] Only the MTT showed a moderate linear relationship with MPAP ($r = 0.54$ and $r = 0.56$, respectively). Therefore, a severity assessment for pulmonary hypertension is currently not possible. It remains to be determined if perfusion MR might have a role for follow-up after treatment.[71]

Solitary Pulmonary Nodules

Solitary pulmonary nodules are one of the most common findings on imaging studies. Noninvasive differentiation of malignant from benign nodules is not always easy, and relying on morphologic characteristics can be misleading. Arterial supply to normal lung is provided by the pulmonary and bronchial arterial branches. However, the contribution of the bronchial system to this dual blood supply is only 3%.[50] The major outflow of the pulmonary intravascular space is through the pulmonary veins into the left atrium, whereas venous drainage by the bronchial veins into the azygos system is minor.[83] The rate of contrast material inflow into the interstitial space depends on the blood flow and permeability of the vessels, whereas the rate of contrast washout from the interstitial space depends on amount of the lymphatic vessels and the capillary backflow. The volumes of the intravascular and interstitial spaces in the normal lung are approximately equal, so that transport of contrast medium produces a uniform background blush throughout the entire lung.

In general, primary lung cancer is mainly supplied by bronchial arteries with various degrees of contribution from the pulmonary circulation depending on the type of tumor histology.[84] However, in metastatic lung lesions, the contribution of the pulmonary circulation is generally higher than that in primary tumors of the lung. In tumors, contrast outflow may be delayed because of the lack of pulmonary venous drainage and that it is mainly performed by the bronchial veins. Washout from the interstitial space of malignant or benign nodules is also markedly reduced due to the lack of lymphatic outflow. As a result, contrast drainage in tumors can be delayed compared with normal lung tissue. Furthermore, the volume of microcirculation increases in tumors compared with those in normal lung, which further contributes to retention of contrast medium.

Overexpression of vascular endothelial growth factor is the major factor for angiogenesis and increased vascular permeability in malignant nodules and tumors.[85,86] As a result of increased vascular permeability and paucity of lymphatic vessels in tumors, the interstitial pressure increases and the size of interstitial (extravascular) space may reach up to three to five times larger than that of normal tissue, which leads to compression of vessels inside the tumor.[50] Consequently, in spite of a high global blood flow, various parts of the tumor may become hypoperfused and hypoxic. Development of arteriovenous shunts in some tumors can also contribute to focal ischemic zones within the tumors.[87]

Dynamic contrast-enhanced CT and MR and FDG PET have been extensively used to differentiate malignant from benign tumors.[87–92] The blood supply and metabolism of malignant neoplasms are different from those of chronic infection and benign neoplasms according to biologic and histopathologic findings.[50]

Initial changes in signal intensity–time curve during the first pass of contrast in DCE MRI correlates with the blood flow, the relative blood volume, the capillary surface area, and the capillary permeability. These components are generally increased in most malignant nodules compared with benign tumors. However, distinguishing active infection from a malignant neoplasm by using perfusion characteristics can be extremely difficult especially in those that they coexist.[88] Increased blood flow and capillary permeability are observed in both conditions, and the maximum relative enhancement ratio and slope of enhancement are significantly higher than are those for the benign nodules.[88]

Fluorodeoxyglucose uptake at PET has been used to diagnose malignant tumors in several ways. For visual analysis, a cutoff standard uptake value of 2.5 is frequently used.[89,93] However, this value can range widely depending on blood glucose concentration, time to imaging after injection, and lesion size.[84,89] The tissue contrast resolution of MRI is generally superior to CT, and, therefore, MRI may better characterize internal composition of the nodules. For perfusion studies, both MR and CT will provide valuable information.

In a recent meta-analysis, no significant differences we found for the sensitivity, specificity, and area under the ROC curve for four imaging modalities: dynamic CT, dynamic MR imaging, FDG PET, and 99mTc-depreotide SPECT.[93] In another study, it was shown that the specificity and accuracy of the slope of the enhancement ratio of dynamic MR were significantly higher than were those of dynamic CT indices and SUV(max).[94] It is suggested that in routine clinical practice dynamic MRI may be used as a substitute for CT and FDG PET or PET/CT to determine whether further intervention and treatment are indicated rather than as the primary modality to differentiate pulmonary malignant nodules from other nodules.[84,94] In another study by Zou et al., MR time–signal intensity curves were obtained at the first, second, and fourth minutes after contrast injections in different pulmonary nodules and classified into three groups.[88] In malignant nodules, enhancement increased in the early phase (peak enhancement seen within 120 seconds) and a decrease or plateau occurred in the following phase (Fig. 25-5). In active inflammation, there was no peak enhancement and enhancement increased with time steadily. In benign nodules, no significant increase over baseline was present. It was shown that with enhancement ratio 65% or less at the fourth minute, malignant nodules were differentiated from active inflammatory lesions with high sensitivity (93%) and high specificity (100%).[88]

Perfusion MRI has also been used to study the effect of chemotherapy drugs on lung cancer perfusion. Chang et al. investigated

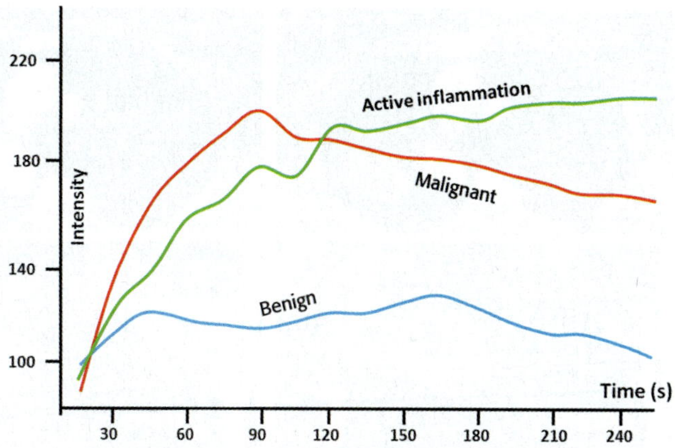

Figure 25-5. Time–signal intensity curve types for malignant, benign, and active inflammatory lesions. (From Zou Y, Zhang M, Wang Q, et al. Quantitative investigation of solitary pulmonary nodules: dynamic contrast-enhanced MRI and histopathologic analysis. *AJR Am J Roentgenol* 2008;191(1):252–259. doi: 10.2214/AJR.07.2284.)

patients with advanced non–small cell lung cancer (NSCLC) patients treated with antiangiogenic agent (bevacizumab) combined with gemcitabine and cisplatin.[95] In this DCE MRI study, four contiguous sagittal slices (6-mm slice thickness, 20% interslice gap) for measuring the targeted tumor and one axial slice for measuring AIF of the aorta were obtained with a temporal resolution of 1 second using a saturation recovery–prepared turbo FLASH (repetition time/echo time/inversion time = 200/1.1/100 milliseconds flip angle =18 degrees). Dynamic images were obtained for 100 seconds. Responders showed a significant decrease of mean of the K^{trans} and k_{ep} histograms (Fig. 25-6).

Different software programs are used to analyze data obtained from DCE MR images. Volume, MTT, time to peak (TTP), and maximum enhancement (Emax) can easily be calculated from time–signal intensity curves. More recently, attention has been given to the investigation of pharmacokinetic parameters.[95,96] These parameters, also derived from the dynamic data, include transendothelial transfer constant (K^{trans}, min^{-1}), rate constant (k_{ep}, min^{-1}), interstitial (extravascular extracellular space) volume fraction ($0 < v_p < 1$, dimensionless), and plasma volume fraction ($0 < v_p < 1$, dimensionless).

The product PS (permeability/surface area densities of the plasma/interstitial interface) is often denoted K^{trans}. K^{trans} depends on the balance between capillary permeability and blood flow. In a high-permeability situation, the transfer constant K^{trans} is equal to the blood plasma flow per unit volume of tissue.[96] The characteristic rate of transfer of contrast tracer to and from plasma and the interstitial space is given by k_{ep}, which is equal to the ratio K^{trans}/v_e. Therefore, it is dependent on both endothelial permeability and the interstitial volume fraction. From all perfusion parameters, kep is shown the most significant index in differentiating malignant from benign nodules.[96] Most benign nodules show $k_{ep} < 1.0$ min^{-1}, and more than two-thirds of malignant nodules show $k_{ep} > 1.0$ min^{-1}.[96]

Summary

Non–contrast-enhanced techniques for assessment of pulmonary perfusion are an important tool for understanding of lung physiology. Given the low spatial resolution and limited SNR ratio, a broad clinical application appears to be difficult. Contrast-enhanced perfusion techniques are broadly available and are easily and quickly performed, even in critical ill patients. Perfusion MR has shown good agreement with perfusion scintigraphy and SPECT. Therefore, this technique is ready to be used in a broader clinical area.

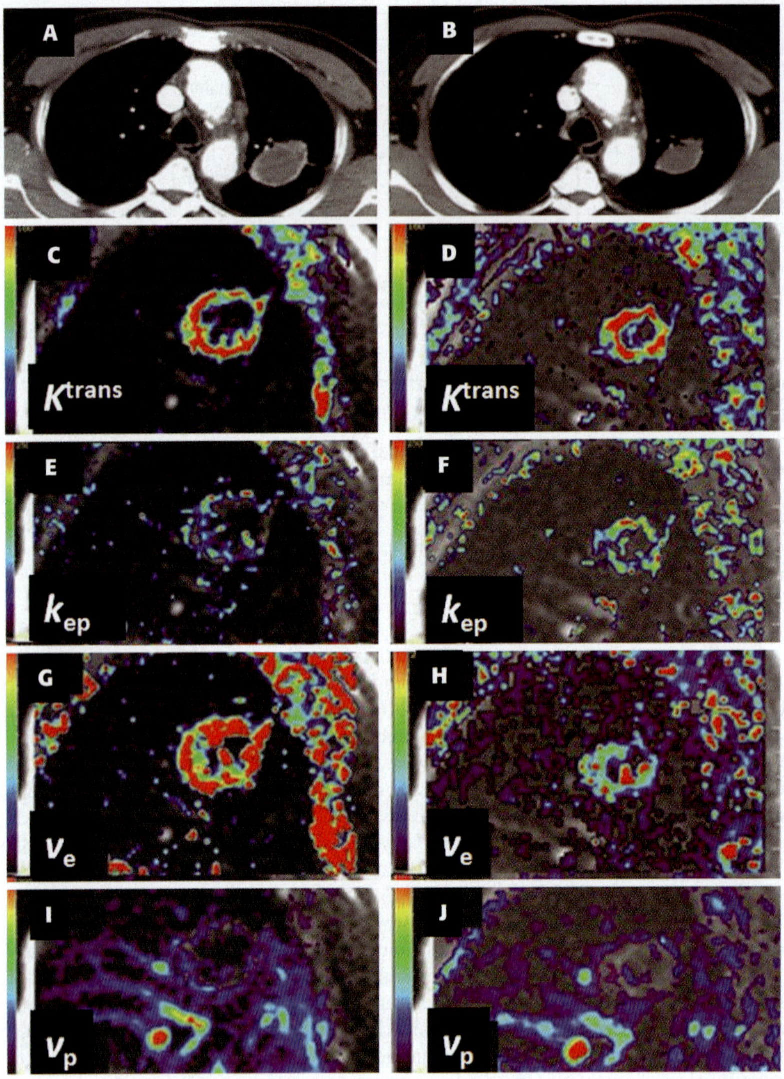

Figure 25-6. A 68-year-old male with lung adenocarcinoma at the left upper lobe **(A)** before and **(B)** after three courses of bevacizumab combined with gemcitabine and cisplatin in axial contrast-enhanced CT. There was decreased tumor size of about 25.9% of the largest transverse dimension, categorized as stationary disease. Images of color MR K^{trans}, k_{ep}, v_e, and v_p mapping before **(C,E,G,I)** and after **(D,F,H,J)** chemotherapy shows decreased values of K^{trans}, v_e, and v_p after treatment. The value of k_{ep} mapping was increased. (From Chang YC, Yu CJ, Chen CM, et al. Dynamic contrast-enhanced MRI in advanced nonsmall-cell lung cancer patients treated with first-line bevacizumab, gemcitabine, and cisplatin. *J Magn Reson Imaging* 2012;36(2): 387–396. doi: 10.1002/jmri.23660., with permission.)

REFERENCES

1. **Berthezène Y, Vexler V, Clément O, et al.** Contrast-enhanced MR imaging of the lung: assessment of ventilation and perfusion. *Radiology* 1992;183:667–672.
2. **Attenberger UI, Ingrisch M, Busing K, et al.** Magnetic resonance imaging of pulmonary perfusion. Technical requirements and diagnostic impact. *Radiologe* 2009;49:739–747.
3. **Hopkins SR, Prisk GK.** Lung perfusion measured using magnetic resonance imaging: new tools for physiological insights into the pulmonary circulation. *J Magn Reson Imaging* 2010;32:1287–1301.
4. **Mai VM, Berr SS.** MR perfusion imaging of pulmonary parenchyma using pulsed arterial spin labeling techniques: FAIRER and FAIR. *J Magn Reson Imaging* 1999;9:483–487.
5. **Miller GW, Mugler JP III, Sa RC, et al.** Advances in functional and structural imaging of the human lung using proton MRI. *NMR Biomed* 2014;27(12):1542–1556.
6. **Hatabu H, Tadamura E, Prasad PV, et al.** Noninvasive pulmonary perfusion imaging by STAR-HASTE sequence. *Magn Reson Med* 2000;44:808–812.
7. **Roberts DA, Gefter WB, Hirsch JA, et al.** Pulmonary perfusion: respiratory-triggered three-dimensional MR imaging with arterial spin tagging—preliminary results in healthy volunteers. *Radiology* 1999;212: 890–895.
8. **Lipson DA, Roberts DA, Hansen-Flaschen J, et al.** Pulmonary ventilation and perfusion scanning using hyperpolarized helium-3 MRI and arterial spin tagging in healthy normal subjects and in pulmonary embolism and orthotopic lung transplant patients. *Magn Reson Med* 2002;47:1073–1076.
9. **Rizi RR, Lipson DA, Dimitrov IE, et al.** Operating characteristics of hyperpolarized 3He and arterial spin tagging in MR imaging of ventilation and perfusion in healthy subjects. *Acad Radiol* 2003;10:502–508.
10. **Suga K, Ogasawara N, Okada M, et al.** Regional lung functional impairment in acute airway obstruction and pulmonary embolic dog models assessed with gadolinium-based aerosol ventilation and perfusion magnetic resonance imaging. *Invest Radiol* 2002;37:281–291.
11. **Ogasawara N, Suga K, Kawakami Y, et al.** Assessment of regional lung function impairment in airway obstruction and pulmonary embolic dogs with combined noncontrast electrocardiogram-gated perfusion and gadolinium diethylenetriaminepentaacetic acid aerosol magnetic resonance images. *J Magn Reson Imaging* 2004;20:46–55.
12. **Martirosian P, Boss A, Fenchel M, et al.** Quantitative lung perfusion mapping at 0.2 T using FAIR True-FISP MRI. *Magn Reson Med* 2006;55: 1065–1074.
13. **Bolar DS, Levin DL, Hopkins SR, et al.** Quantification of regional pulmonary blood flow using ASL-FAIRER. *Magn Reson Med* 2006;55: 1308–1317.
14. **Martirosian P, Boss A, Schraml C, et al.** Magnetic resonance perfusion imaging without contrast media. *Eur J Nucl Med Mol Imaging* 2010;37(suppl 1):S52–S64. doi: 10.1007/s00259-010-1456-7 (online first).
15. **Pracht ED, Fischer A, Arnold JF, et al.** Single-shot quantitative perfusion imaging of the human lung. *Magn Reson Med* 2006;56:1347–1351.
16. **Fischer A, Pracht ED, Arnold JF, et al.** Assessment of pulmonary perfusion in a single shot using SEEPAGE. *J Magn Reson Imaging* 2008; 27:63–70.

17. **Bauman G, Puderbach M, Deimling M, et al.** Non-contrast-enhanced perfusion and ventilation assessment of the human lung by means of Fourier decomposition in proton MRI. *Magn Reson Med* 2009;62:656–664.
18. **Lederlin M, Bauman G, Eichinger M, et al.** Functional MRI using Fourier decomposition of lung signal: reproducibility of ventilation- and perfusion-weighted imaging in healthy volunteers. *Eur J Radiol* 2013;82:1015–1022.
19. **Buxton RB, Frank LR, Wong EC, et al.** A general kinetic model for quantitative perfusion imaging with arterial spin labeling. *Magn Reson Med* 1998;40:383–396.
20. **Mai VM, Chen Q, Edelman RR.** Absolute quantification of pulmonary perfusion rates using flow-sensitive alternating inversion recovery with an extra radio frequency pulse (FAIRER). Proceedings of the 8th Annual Meeting of ISMRM,171; 01-07 April; 2000, Denver, CO.
21. **Brudin LH, Rhodes CG, Valind SO, et al.** Regional lung density and blood volume in nonsmoking and smoking subjects measured by PET. *J Appl Physiol* 1987;63:1324–1334.
22. **Wang T, Schultz G, Hebestreit H, et al.** Quantitative perfusion mapping of the human lung using 1H spin labeling. *J Magn Reson Imaging* 2003;18:260–265.
23. **Lin YR, Wu MT, Huang TY, et al.** Comparison of arterial spin labeling and first-pass dynamic contrast-enhanced MR imaging in the assessment of pulmonary perfusion in humans: the inflow spin-tracer saturation effect. *Magn Reson Med* 2004;52:1291–1301.
24. **Bauman G, Puderbach M, Heimann T, et al.** Validation of Fourier decomposition MRI with dynamic contrast-enhanced MRI using visual and automated scoring of pulmonary perfusion in young cystic fibrosis patients. *Eur J Radiol* 2013;82:2371–2377.
25. **Sommer G, Bauman G, Koenigkam-Santos M, et al.** Non-contrast-enhanced preoperative assessment of lung perfusion in patients with non-small-cell lung cancer using Fourier decomposition magnetic resonance imaging. *Eur J Radiol* 2013;82:e879–e887.
26. **Mai VM, Hagspiel KD, Christopher JM, et al.** Perfusion imaging of the human lung using flow-sensitive alternating inversion recovery with an extra radiofrequency pulse (FAIRER). *Magn Reson Imaging* 1999;17:355–361.
27. **Hopkins SR, Henderson AC, Levin DL, et al.** Vertical gradients in regional lung density and perfusion in the supine human lung: the Slinky effect. *J Appl Physiol* 2007;103:240–248.
28. **Henderson AC, Prisk GK, Levin DL, et al.** Characterizing pulmonary blood flow distribution measured using arterial spin labeling. *NMR Biomed* 2009;22:1025–1035.
29. **Hopkins SR, Levin DL, Emami K, et al.** Advances in magnetic resonance imaging of lung physiology. *J Appl Physiol* 2007;102: 1244–1254.
30. **Mai VM, Chen Q, Bankier AA, et al.** Effect of lung inflation on arterial spin labeling signal in MR perfusion imaging of human lung. *J Magn Reson Imaging* 2001;13:954–959.
31. **Fan L, Liu SY, Xiao XS, et al.** Demonstration of pulmonary perfusion heterogeneity induced by gravity and lung inflation using arterial spin labeling. *Eur J Radiol* 2010;73:249–254.
32. **Levin DL, Buxton RB, Spiess JP, et al.** Effects of age on pulmonary perfusion heterogeneity measured by magnetic resonance imaging. *J Appl Physiol* 2007;102:2064–2070.
33. **Keilholz SD, Knight-Scott J, Christopher JM, et al.** Gravity-dependent perfusion of the lung demonstrated with the FAIRER arterial spin tagging method. *Magn Reson Imaging* 2001;19:929–935.
34. **Keilholz SD, Mai VM, Berr SS, et al.** Comparison of first-pass Gd-DOTA and FAIRER MR perfusion imaging in a rabbit model of pulmonary embolism. *J Magn Reson Imaging* 2002;16:168–171.
35. **Altes TA, Mai VM, Munger TM, et al.** Pulmonary embolism: comprehensive evaluation with MR ventilation and perfusion scanning with hyperpolarized helium-3, arterial spin tagging, and contrast-enhanced MRA. *J Vasc Interv Radiol* 2005;16:999–1005.
36. **Hopkins SR, Garg J, Bolar DS, et al.** Pulmonary blood flow heterogeneity during hypoxia and high-altitude pulmonary edema. *Am J Respir Crit Care Med* 2005;171:83–87.
37. **Kluge A, Muller C, Hansel J, et al.** Real-time MR with TrueFISP for the detection of acute pulmonary embolism: initial clinical experience. *Eur Radiol* 2004;14:709–718.
38. **Fishman AP.** Dynamic of the pulmonary circulation. In: *Handbook of physiology*. Washington D.C.: American Physiological Society; 1963;1708. Section 2: Circulation.
39. **Ohno Y, Hatabu H, Higashino T, et al.** Dynamic perfusion MRI versus perfusion scintigraphy: prediction of postoperative lung function in patients with lung cancer. *AJR Am J Roentgenol* 2004;182:73–78.
40. **Fink C, Ley S, Kroeker R, et al.** Time-resolved contrast-enhanced three-dimensional magnetic resonance angiography of the chest: combination of parallel imaging with view sharing (TREAT). *Invest Radiol* 2005;40:40–48.
41. **Hsu JS, Tsai SY, Wu MT, et al.** Fast dynamic contrast-enhanced lung MR imaging using k-t BLAST: a spatiotemporal perspective. *Magn Reson Med* 2012;67(3):786–792.
42. **Fink C, Puderbach M, Ley S, et al.** Time-resolved echo-shared parallel MRA of the lung: observer preference study of image quality in comparison with non-echo-shared sequences. *Eur Radiol* 2005;15:2070–2074.
43. **Fink C, Bock M, Puderbach M, et al.** Partially parallel three-dimensional magnetic resonance imaging for the assessment of lung perfusion—initial results. *Invest Radiol* 2003;38:482–488.
44. **Attenberger UI, Ingrisch M, Dietrich O, et al.** Time-resolved 3D pulmonary perfusion MRI: comparison of different k-space acquisition strategies at 1.5 and 3 T. *Invest Radiol* 2009;44:525–531.
45. **Fink C, Bock M, Kiessling F, et al.** Time-resolved contrast-enhanced three-dimensional pulmonary MR-angiography: 1.0 M gadobutrol vs. 0.5 M gadopentetate dimeglumine. *J Magn Reson Imaging* 2005;19: 202–208.
46. **Kreitner KF, Kunz RP, Weschler C, et al.** Analysis of first-pass bolus geometry in contrast-enhanced MRA of thoracic vessels. *Fortschr Röntgenstr* 2005;177:646–654.
47. **Fink C, Risse F, Semmler W, et al.** MRI of pulmonary perfusion. *Radiologe* 2006;46:290–299.
48. **Ohno Y, Murase K, Higashino T, et al.** Assessment of bolus injection protocol with appropriate concentration for quantitative assessment of pulmonary perfusion by dynamic contrast-enhanced MR imaging. *J Magn Reson Imaging* 2007;25:55–65.
49. **Ley-Zaporozhan J, Molinari F, Risse F, et al.** Repeatability and reproducibility of quantitative whole-lung perfusion MRI. *J Thorac Imaging* 2011;26:230–239.
50. **Ohno Y, Nishio M, Koyama H, et al.** Dynamic contrast-enhanced CT and MRI for pulmonary nodule assessment. *AJR Am J Roentgenol* 2014;202(3):515–529. doi: 10.2214/AJR.13.11888.
51. **Ohno Y, Koyama H, Matsumoto K, et al.** Dynamic MR perfusion imaging: capability for quantitative assessment of disease extent and prediction of outcome for patients with acute pulmonary thromboembolism. *J Magn Reson Imaging* 2010;31:1081–1090.
52. **Ley S, Fink C, Zaporozhan J, et al.** Value of high spatial and high temporal resolution magnetic resonance angiography for differentiation between idiopathic and thromboembolic pulmonary hypertension: initial results. *Eur Radiol* 2005;15:2256–2263.
53. **Ley-Zaporozhan J, Ley S, Eberhardt R, et al.** Assessment of the relationship between lung parenchymal destruction and impaired pulmonary perfusion on a lobar level in patients with emphysema. *Eur J Radiol* 2007;63:76–83.
54. **Molinari F, Fink C, Risse F, et al.** Assessment of differential pulmonary blood flow using perfusion magnetic resonance imaging: comparison with radionuclide perfusion scintigraphy. *Invest Radiol* 2006;41:624–630.
55. **Dehnert C, Risse F, Ley S, et al.** Magnetic Resonance Imaging of Uneven Pulmonary Perfusion in Hypoxia in Humans. *Am J Respir Crit Care Med* 2006;174:1132–1138.
56. **Kohlmann P, Strehlow J, Jobst B, et al.** Automatic lung segmentation method for MRI-based lung perfusion studies of patients with chronic obstructive pulmonary disease. *Int J Comput Assist Radiol Surg* 2014. [Epub ahead of print July 3, 2014].
57. **Risse F, Fink C, Ley S, et al.** Perfusion quantification of the whole lung using singular value decomposition with optimized threshold. *Proc Intl Soc Mag Med* 2004;11:2611.
58. **Meier P, Zierler KL.** On the theory of the indicator-dilution method for measurement of blood flow and volume. *J Appl Physiol* 1954;6:731–744.
59. **Ostergaard L, Weisskoff RM, Chesler DA, et al.** High resolution measurement of cerebral blood flow using intravascular tracer bolus passages. Part I: Mathematical approach and statistical analysis. *Magn Reson Med* 1996;36:715–725.
60. **Ostergaard L, Sorensen AG, Kwong KK, et al.** High resolution measurement of cerebral blood flow using intravascular tracer bolus passages. Part II: Experimental comparison and preliminary results. *Magn Reson Med* 1996;36:726–736.

61. **Risse F, Kuder TA, Kauczor HU, et al.** Suppression of pulmonary vasculature in lung perfusion MRI using correlation analysis. *Eur Radiol* 2009;19:2569–2575.
62. **Bock M, Schoenberg SO, Floemer F, et al.** Separation of arteries and veins in 3D MR angiography using correlation analysis. *Magn Reson Med* 2000;43:481–487.
63. **Santini F, Patil S, Meckel S, et al.** Double-reference cross-correlation algorithm for separation of the arteries and veins from 3D MRA time series. *J Magn Reson Imaging* 2008;28:646–654.
64. **Kostler H, Ritter C, Lipp M, et al.** Prebolus quantitative MR heart perfusion imaging. *Magn Reson Med* 2004;52:296–299.
65. **Risse F, Semmler W, Kauczor HU, et al.** Dual-bolus approach to quantitative measurement of pulmonary perfusion by contrast-enhanced MRI. *J Magn Reson Imaging* 2006;24:1284–1290.
66. **Puderbach M, Risse F, Biederer J, et al.** In vivo Gd-DTPA concentration for MR lung perfusion measurements: assessment with computed tomography in a porcine model. *Eur Radiol* 2008;18:2102–2107.
67. **Nikolaou K, Schoenberg SO, Brix G, et al.** Quantification of pulmonary blood flow and volume in healthy volunteers by dynamic contrast-enhanced magnetic resonance imaging using a parallel imaging technique. *Invest Radiol* 2004;39:537–545.
68. **Schuster DP, Kaplan JD, Gauvain K, et al.** Measurement of regional pulmonary blood flow with PET. *J Nucl Med* 1995;36:371–377.
69. **Brudin LH, Valind SO, Rhodes CG, et al.** Regional lung hematocrit in humans using positron emission tomography. *J Appl Physiol* 1986;60:1155–1163.
70. **Ingrisch M, Dietrich O, Attenberger UI, et al.** Quantitative pulmonary perfusion magnetic resonance imaging: influence of temporal resolution and signal-to-noise ratio. *Invest Radiol* 2010;45:7–14.
71. **Ley S, Gruenig E, Risse F, et al.** *Treatment monitoring in patients with pulmonary arterial hypertension (PAH) using quantitative 3D MR pulmonary perfusion. ECRB-818* 2008.
72. **Bottger T, Grunewald K, Schobinger M, et al.** Implementation and evaluation of a new workflow for registration and segmentation of pulmonary MRI data for regional lung perfusion assessment. *Phys Med Biol* 2007;52:1261–1275.
73. **Hueper K, Parikh MA, Prince MR, et al.** Quantitative and semiquantitative measures of regional pulmonary microvascular perfusion by magnetic resonance imaging and their relationships to global lung perfusion and lung diffusing capacity: the multiethnic study of atherosclerosis chronic obstructive pulmonary disease study. *Invest Radiol* 2013;48(4):223–230.
74. **Kluge A, Gerriets T, Stolz E, et al.** Pulmonary perfusion in acute pulmonary embolism: agreement of MRI and SPECT for lobar, segmental and subsegmental perfusion defects. *Acta Radiol* 2006;47:933–940.
75. **Fink C, Ley S, Schoenberg SO, et al.** Magnetic resonance imaging of acute pulmonary embolism. *Eur Radiol* 2007;17:2546–2553.
76. **Eichinger M, Optazaite DE, Kopp-Schneider A, et al.** Morphologic and functional scoring of cystic fibrosis lung disease using MRI. *Eur J Radiol* 2012;81:1321–1329.
77. **Ley S, Fink C, Puderbach M, et al.** Contrast-enhanced 3D MR perfusion of the lung: application of parallel imaging technique in healthy subjects. *Fortschr Röntgenstr* 2004;176:330–334.
78. **Fink C, Ley S, Risse F, et al.** Effect of inspiratory and expiratory breathhold on pulmonary perfusion: assessment by pulmonary perfusion magnetic resonance imaging. *Invest Radiol* 2005;40:72–79.
79. **Ley S, Puderbach M, Risse F, et al.** Impact of oxygen inhalation on the pulmonary circulation: assessment by magnetic resonance (MR)-perfusion and MR-flow measurements. *Invest Radiol* 2007;42:283–290.
80. **Ohno Y, Hatabu H, Murase K, et al.** Quantitative assessment of regional pulmonary perfusion in the entire lung using three-dimensional ultrafast dynamic contrast-enhanced magnetic resonance imaging: preliminary experience in 40 subjects. *J Magn Reson Imaging* 2004;20:353–365.
81. **Ohno Y, Hatabu H, Murase K, et al.** Primary pulmonary hypertension: 3D dynamic perfusion MRI for quantitative analysis of regional pulmonary perfusion. *AJR Am J Roentgenol* 2007;188:48–56.
82. **Ley S, Mereles D, Risse F, et al.** Quantitative 3D pulmonary MR-perfusion in patients with pulmonary arterial hypertension: correlation with invasive pressure measurements. *Eur J Radiol* 2007;61:251–255.
83. **Littleton JT, Durizch ML, Moeller G, et al.** Pulmonary masses: contrast enhancement. *Radiology* 1990;177:861–871.
84. **Ohno Y, Hatabu H, Takenaka D, et al.** Solitary pulmonary nodules: potential role of dynamic MR imaging in management initial experience. *Radiology* 2002;224(2):503–511.
85. **Dvorak HF, Brown LF, Detmar M, et al.** Vascular permeability factor/vascular endothelial growth factor, microvascular hyperpermeability, and angiogenesis. *Am J Pathol* 1995;146:1029–1039.
86. **Han H, Silverman JF, Santucci TS, et al.** Vascular endothelial growth factor expression in stage I non-small cell lung cancer correlates with neoangiogenesis and a poor prognosis. *Ann Surg Oncol* 2001;8:72–79.
87. **Delorme S, Knopp MV.** Non-invasive vascular imaging: assessing tumour vascularity. *Eur Radiol* 1998;8:517–527.
88. **Zou Y, Zhang M, Wang Q, et al.** Quantitative investigation of solitary pulmonary nodules: dynamic contrast-enhanced MRI and histopathologic analysis. *AJR Am J Roentgenol* 2008;191(1):252–259. doi: 10.2214/AJR.07.2284.
89. **Gupta NC, Frank AR, Dewan NA, et al.** Solitary pulmonary nodules: detection of malignancy with PET with 2-[F-18]-fluoro-2-deoxy-D-glucose. *Radiology* 1992;184:441–444.
90. **Satoh S, Nakaminato S, Kihara A, et al.** Evaluation of indeterminate pulmonary nodules with dynamic MR imaging. *Magn Reson Med Sci* 2013;12(1):31–38.
91. **Kono R, Fujimoto K, Terasaki H, et al.** Dynamic MRI of solitary pulmonary nodules: comparison of enhancement patterns of malignant and benign small peripheral lung lesions. *AJR Am J Roentgenol* 2007;188:26–36.
92. **Ohno Y, Koyama H, Matsumoto K, et al.** Differentiation of malignant and benign pulmonary nodules with quantitative first-pass 320-detector row perfusion CT versus FDG PET/CT. *Radiology* 2011; 258:599–609.
93. **Cronin P, Dwamena BA, Kelly AM, et al.** Solitary pulmonary nodules: meta-analytic comparison of cross-sectional imaging modalities for diagnosis of malignancy. *Radiology* 2008;246(3):772–782. doi: 10.1148/radiol.2463062148.
94. **Ohno Y, Koyama H, Takenaka D, et al.** Dynamic MRI, dynamic multidetector-row computed tomography (MDCT), and coregistered 2-[fluorine-18]-fluoro-2-deoxy-D-glucose-positron emission tomography (FDG-PET)/CT: comparative study of capability for management of pulmonary nodules. *J Magn Reson Imaging* 2008;27:1284–1295.
95. **Chang YC, Yu CJ, Chen CM, et al.** Dynamic contrast-enhanced MRI in advanced nonsmall-cell lung cancer patients treated with first-line bevacizumab, gemcitabine, and cisplatin. *J Magn Reson Imaging* 2012;36(2):387–396. doi: 10.1002/jmri.23660.
96. **Mamata H, Tokuda J, Gill RR, et al.** Clinical application of pharmacokinetic analysis as a biomarker of solitary pulmonary nodules: dynamic contrast-enhanced MR imaging. *Magn Reson Med* 2012;68(5): 1614–1622. doi: 10.1002/mrm.24150.

CHAPTER

26 Pulmonary Perfusion Imaging with CT

Sonja Sudarski, MD and Thomas Henzler, MD

Introduction

Multiple approaches to assess pulmonary perfusion by means of CT have emerged over the past decades. In the year 2000, Schoepf et al.[1] used dynamic multisection electron beam CT for the assessment of pulmonary blood flow (BF). However, the technique was limited to a *z*-axis coverage of 7.6 cm and required a long patient breath hold. Moreover, the technique used in this feasibility study was associated with a substantial amount of ionizing radiation limiting its clinical acceptance. Major basic research on the feasibility of multidetector CT pulmonary perfusion imaging has been performed by the group of Wildberger[2–5]: in 2001, perfusion-derived color maps of the density of lung parenchyma in single-energy CT pulmonary angiography (CT-PA) of patients with suspected pulmonary embolism (PE) were generated.[3] A later animal study by the same group used a subtraction technique to compare density values of whole-thorax multidetector CT scans before and after intravenous contrast injection in a single breath hold; however, this technique was again limited by the breath-hold length and the additional radiation dose the patient was exposed to.[2] Moreover, one has to acknowledge that the term perfusion was misleading in these studies since only one contrast phase during the first pass of contrast material was imaged by CT. Thus, the term first-pass perfusion seems to be more appropriate also within the context of today's dual-energy CT (DE-CT).

To date, the probably most important step towards the broad introduction of first-pass pulmonary perfusion imaging into clinical routine was the advent of DE-CT: the principle of DE-CT was initially introduced in the late 1970s and allows for the differentiation of materials based on their x-ray attenuation at different tube voltages. DE-CT has been investigated for a variety of organ systems. At that time point, with regard to thoracic imaging, limited temporal resolution and respiratory misregistration were the main reasons wherefore DE-CT did not enter clinical routine at that time. Different vendors reintroduced DE-CT in the second half of 2000 using different technical approaches like the dual-source CT (DS-CT) technology, single-source rapid kV switching, or a dual-layer approach to separate different x-ray spectra.[6–9]

Since then, pulmonary DE-CT imaging has been intensively studied[10–15]: DE-derived iodine maps allow the visualization of parenchymal iodine distribution, which can be considered as a surrogate for pulmonary first-pass perfusion.

Ventilation and Perfusion of the Lung

To properly interpret perfusion imaging, the interaction of ventilation and perfusion has to be considered in the first place: In the presence of hypoxia without presence of hypercapnia, blood flow will be directed to lung segments and alveoli with a higher oxygen concentration. Therefore, pulmonary arteries will constrict in the presence of low oxygen blood levels. This physiologic phenomenon of hypoxic pulmonary vasoconstriction is generally known as the Euler-Liljestrand mechanism.[16] Although the process might seem paradoxical at first impression, the redistribution of blood flow to higher-ventilated areas of the lung increases the area involved in gaseous exchange and consequently improves the ventilation–perfusion ratio and arterial oxygenation as a last consequence. This compensation mechanism can be observed in patients with chronic obstructive pulmonary disease and heart failure or as well in healthy individuals at altitude.

Due to patient's supine position during a CT scan, lung perfusion images have to be seen in the light of an abolished craniocaudal perfusion gradient in an upright thorax and a gravity-dependent gradient in ventrodorsal direction instead.

Furthermore, morphologic alterations of small pulmonary vessels have to be considered, as larger cross-sectional areas have been shown to influence pulmonary perfusion.[17]

DE-CT-PA is consequently able to provide both morphologic and functional information for an accurate assessment of lung physiology, that is, vascular morphology, regional perfusion, and ventilation.

DE-CT Techniques

Various approaches for acquiring multiple energy data of an anatomic area of interest have been developed by different vendors. Dual-source technique, single-source rapid kV switching technique, and dual-layer technique are the most common and promising ones with regard to pulmonary imaging: while DS-CT and double-layer technology derive their information from one set of data acquired at identical time points, in fast kilovoltage-switching technique, there is a delay of a few milliseconds between the acquisitions. In DS-DE-CT, two x-ray tubes and two corresponding detectors at different kilovoltages and tube currents are simultaneously run.[6] The single-source CT-derived double-layer detectors conduct compartmentalization of detected x-ray photons into energy bins.[18]

In another single-source DE-CT approach, the rapid kV switching technique, the tube voltage alternates between a high voltage and a low voltage, and for every projection, data are acquired twice. The rotation speed has to be therefore reduced in order to account for the acquisition of these additional projections and the rise and fall times of the voltage modulation. Therefore, the gantry rotation time usually must be at least 0.5 seconds.[9,18]

Most evidence on DE-CT pulmonary perfusion imaging was gained with the DS-CT technique so far. The DS-DE-CT technique allows differentiation, separation, and quantification of tissue or material with high atomic numbers such as iodine and xenon. The two x-ray tubes and two corresponding detectors are positioned 90 degrees apart from each other in the gantry. Initially, a combination of 80/140 kVp was used for dual-energy scanning. Then, 100 kVp was suggested as an alternative to 80 kVp for dual-energy scanning of thicker body regions and/or larger adults in order to improve image quality by means of noise reduction. Because of the low-attenuation profile of the thoracic region, using 80 kVp is usually sufficient for DE-CT of the chest. In order to compensate for the lower photon output of the low-kilovoltage tube, the reference tube current has to be increased. Nevertheless, this technical approach has been proven to be the best with regard to radiation dose efficiency. In second-generation DS-CT scanner systems, a better separation of x-ray spectra could be achieved by application of a tin filter to the 140-kVp tube, resulting in less photon starvation of low-spectrum photons within the patient and consequently in further noise reduction and dose savings. In third-generation DS-CT scanner systems, both tubes are equipped with tin filters, although in DE-CT mode, only the high-kVp tube is run with the tin filter, at this case with 150 kVp. Three-material decomposition is used for both perfusion and ventilation CT, in which iodine or xenon, respectively, is decomposed from body tissue and air by calculating volume fractions of the three materials for each voxel.

DE-CT thereby is able to provide both anatomic and functional information in a variety of pulmonary diseases by means a contrast-enhanced chest scan using only a single contrast material application (Fig. 26-1): furthermore, in the course of image postprocessing, virtual nonenhanced DE-CT–derived images can be created as well, which are then used to characterize pulmonary nodules, which abolishes the need to acquire additional true nonenhanced CT data.

Principle of Dynamic Contrast-enhanced CT

Besides DE-CT–derived iodine maps, with the advent of newer scanner generations and continuously lower radiation doses required for CT examinations, 4-D time-resolved dynamic contrast-enhanced CT (DCE-CT) has been proposed as a new single-energy method to visualize pulmonary perfusion. However, due to additional radiation exposure, DCE-CT has been mainly investigated for different tumor entities in order to quantify tumor perfusion over time so far[19–30]: tumor angiogenesis leads to an increase of regional blood flow and blood volume. Newly developed antiangiogenic therapies—so-called targeted therapies—are aiming at activation of molecular antiangiogenic pathways with the overall goal to reduce tumor nourishment. Consequently, imaging modalities used in the diagnostic workup of such patients for the purpose of staging, restaging, and follow-up examinations have to keep up with the innovations in oncology: with the acquisition of CT angiographic data of multiple repetitive CT scans with only one bolus of iodinated contrast material given and subsequent summation of the gathered information resulting in time–density curves, functional information is added to mere morphometric information. Assessment of contrast enhancement of lung cancer tissue, tumor perfusion, and perfusion changes in the course of therapy by means of dynamic perfusion computed tomography (dPCT) in patients with lung cancer therefore seems to be a promising new approach with regard to evaluation of response to therapy.[31,32] Until recently, the biggest drawback of dPCT was the fact that time–density curves could only be acquired for selected transverse sections within the tumors but not for the whole tumor volume, limiting its representative value for response to therapy, especially in large tumor masses.[33] Reproducibility of dPCT values was further reduced due to tumor motion during the breathing cycle and differing transverse tumor sections evaluated in different intraindividual examinations as a possible consequence.[34] These limitations have been overcome by dPCT of whole tumor volumes with sufficient motion correction, subsequently referred to as dynamic volume perfusion CT (dVPCT).[35–37] DCE-CT–derived dPCT or dVPCT is thereby able to provide quantitative data of blood flow, blood volume, permeability, and the mean transit time of iodinated contrast material through the whole tumor.[38–44]

Despite robust results regarding visualization of vasculature and promising results regarding visualization of tissue perfusion, to date, the technique of dVPCT is not routinely used, as ideal time points of perfusion imaging are not yet standardized and multiple shuttle protocols are existing with varying scan time points from every 1.5 seconds up to every 6 seconds with introduction of third-generation DS-CT. This chapter will focus on the DE-CT technique, as indications are broader and more evidence as well as established and robust protocols do already exist.

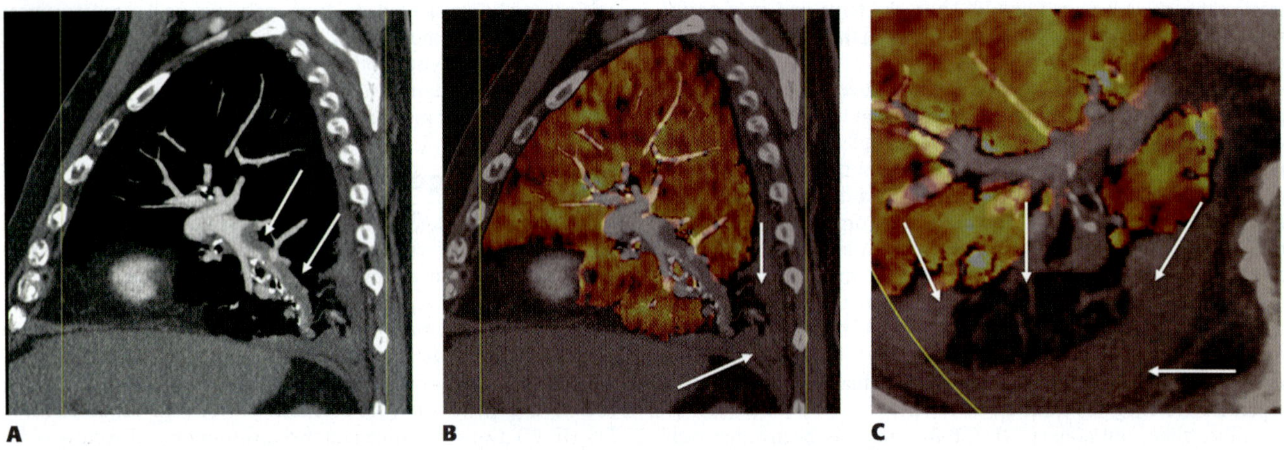

A B C

Figure 26-1. **Contrast-enhanced dual-energy CT pulmonary angiography of a 76-year-old patient with pulmonary embolism of the right lower lobe.** Sagittal gray-scale images **(A)** depict large embolic mass (*white arrows*) within the right lower lobe artery. The color-coded sagittal **(B)** and axial **(C)** iodine DE perfusion maps show in this case the complete lack of first-pass perfusion of the affected lung parenchyma. The resultant large perfusion defect (*white arrows*) indicates a total obstruction with subsequent consolidation due to PE and is rather contradictive of acute pulmonary embolism.

Clinical Applications

Pulmonary perfusion imaging plays an important role in the diagnostic workup of PE, thoracic malignancies, vascular disorders, and parenchymal diseases.[8,45]

Pulmonary Embolism

Acute PE

CT-PA is the reference standard for the diagnosis of acute PE and has replaced catheter pulmonary angiography and ventilation–perfusion scintigraphy as the first-line imaging method.[46,47] Suspected pulmonary embolism is the most common indication of lung perfusion by means of DE-CT in both children and adults.[15,48–52] Aside from visualizing pulmonary blood pool deficits for diagnosing PE, DE-CT can be used for monitoring success of PE treatment.[53]

Chronic PE

DE-CT-PA can also allow diagnosis of chronic PE and chronic thromboembolic pulmonary hypertension. DE-CT has also been found to aid in the differentiation of ground-glass attenuation of vascular origin in chronic PE patients (by means of the high iodine content within the areas of ground-glass attenuation) from ground-glass attenuation secondary to bronchioloalveolar diseases.[54] Also, image series generated from lower x-ray energies have been reported to be useful for an improved visualization of the systemic collateral supply in chronic PE, originating from bronchial and nonbronchial (i.e., chest wall, abdomen) systemic arteries.[55]

Emphysema

Chronic obstructive pulmonary disease is defined as airway obstruction due to irreversible parenchymal destruction. Assessment of emphysema severity has gained increasing importance with regard to treatment planning for lung volume reduction surgery. DE-CT can be performed for emphysema quantification and regional perfusion evaluation using virtual unenhanced series and iodine maps simultaneously.[56]

Functional Resectability

DE-CT pulmonary perfusion imaging can also be used to determine functional resectability not only in patients with emphysema but also in patients with malignancies prior to surgical lobectomy. Preoperative exact quantification of FEV1 to calculate postsurgical FEV1 is necessary in these patients. DE-CT can help to determine the exact percentage a distinct segment owns in overall ventilation.[57–59]

Lung Cancer

The feasibility of DCE-CT to characterize pulmonary nodules has been proven by a prospective, multicenter trial evaluating DCE-CT for the classification of benign and malignant pulmonary nodules.[60] In solitary pulmonary nodules (SPNs) with a diameter greater than 10 mm, CT perfusion could significantly reduce the number of SPNs, diagnosed as undetermined at morphologic CT, thereby skipping the need for follow-up CT examinations, additional FDG-PET studies, biopsy, or even surgery.[61]

DCE-CT may be furthermore used for the assessment of tumor response to targeted therapy or radiotherapy. Good intraobserver agreement has been reported for lung cancer DCE-CT measurements, encouraging its use for tumor characterization and therapy response monitoring.[62] Moreover, whole tumor DCE-CT may allow advanced subclassification of different lung cancer entities.[35]

Excursion: Angioinvasive Aspergillosis

Another rare indication for DCE-CT is diagnosis of suspected angioinvasive aspergillosis as a severe and life-threatening complication in immunosuppressed patients (Fig. 26-2). DCE-CT can help to accurately identify vessel interruption caused by angioinvasive aspergillosis that has been reported as a relatively specific sign of disease.[63]

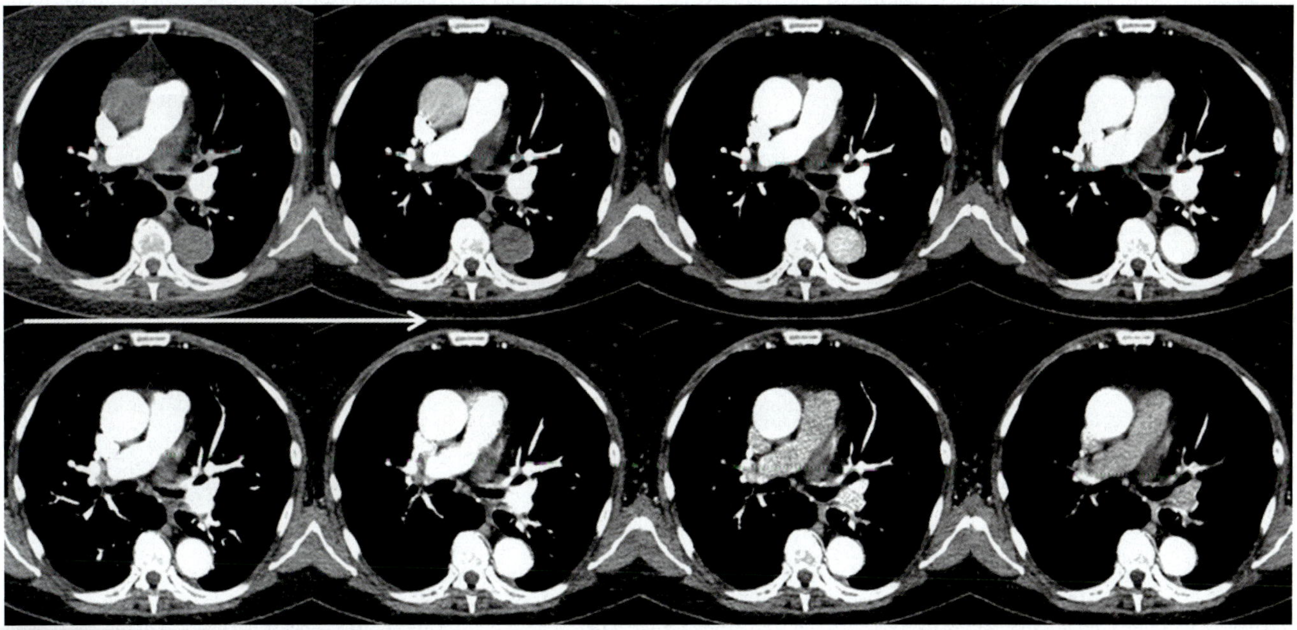

Figure 26-2. Dynamic contrast-enhanced CT performed at 70-kV tube voltage on a third-generation dual-source CT system in a 71-year-old patient with suspected angioinvasive pulmonary aspergillosis. The images demonstrate the dynamic inflow of the contrast material through the pulmonary arteries, pulmonary veins, and aorta. The dose-length product (DLP) of the scan was 800, which is comparable to a standard biphasic chest CT at 120-kV tube voltage.

DE-CT Protocols

Adults

Various image acquisition protocols for DS-DE-CT image acquisition have been proposed in the literature; however, currently, only few protocols are available for single-source DE-CT techniques.[8] The scanning protocols aim at evaluating both the pulmonary arteries and lung perfusion from a single contrast-enhanced CT examination.[64] To evaluate both the pulmonary arteries and lung perfusion, the scanning delay should be slightly longer (e.g., 4 to 7 seconds) than that for regular CT-PA examinations to allow the contrast material to distribute in the lung parenchyma.[8,64] Dual-energy lung perfusion CT should be obtained at peak lung parenchymal enhancement in order to avoid underestimation of regional lung perfusion.[8]

With regard to this, it should be always kept in mind that, in contrast to DCE-CT, the DE-CT-PA–derived perfusion map merely reflects iodine distribution in the lung parenchyma at a given single time point.

Thoracic DE-CT scans should be acquired in the caudocranial direction so that the saline chaser bolus reaches the upper chest by the time this area is acquired to avoid streak artifacts from highly concentrated contrast material in the subclavian vein or superior vena cava.[64,65] Patients should be instructed to hold their breath at a shallow inspiratory level during scan acquisition to avoid excessive influx of unenhanced blood from the inferior vena cava from the Valsalva maneuver associated with deep inspiration.[66]

With regard to contrast material doses, high iodine concentration and high iodine delivery rate have been shown to provide the best image quality of both CT-PA and perfusion map images of the lung through high attenuation within the pulmonary arteries and minimization of beam-hardening artifacts.

Nance et al.[67] reported that a contrast material protocol using a high iodine concentration and a high injection delivery rate for contrast material delivery (iomeprol 400 at 4 mL/s, corresponding to an injection delivery rate of 1.6 g I/s) resulted in the best image quality of both CT-PA images and perfusion map images of the lung by virtue of high attenuation in the pulmonary arteries and minimization of beam-hardening artifacts compared with protocols comprising a lower concentration or lower delivery rate. Despite controversial reports about increased artifacts on iodine perfusion maps when using highly concentrated iodinated contrast material combined with high flow rates, consensus exists about improved diagnostic image quality and the highest target-tract attenuation with these DE-CT-PA protocols.[68]

Concerning the determination of an optimal scan delay after application of contrast material, test bolus and bolus tracking were determined to provide equal image quality and diagnostic accuracy in patients with suspected PE, while use of a fixed delay is not recommended.[49,69] Regarding the number of phases acquired in contrast-enhanced chest scans, a triphasic contrast medium injection protocol (50 mL of undiluted contrast medium in the first phase, followed by a constant volume of 30 mL of a 70% to 30% NaCl–contrast medium mixture and 50 mL of pure NaCl in the third phase) has been shown to avoid streak artifacts from high-attenuation contrast material in the superior vena cava.[70]

Children

Shorter scan time may be beneficial not only with regard to motion artifact reduction and shortening of breath hold in children: a combination of faster scan speed (gantry rotation time, 0.28 s; pitch, 0.55 to 0.7) and greater longitudinal coverage (64 × 2 [z flying focal spot] × 0.6 mm) likely results in improved image quality of dual-energy thoracic CT in children by creating a uniform longitudinal distribution of contrast agent in the lung parenchyma.[48,71,72]

Technical Limitations

An obvious drawback has been the limited field of view, being dependent on the smaller detector array. In first-generation dual-source DE-CT, the high-kVp detector (corresponding to tube A) provides a field of view of 50 cm, while the other detector array (corresponding to tube B) is limited to field of view of 26 cm. Peripheral parts of the lungs were not completely covered by the 80-kVp B detector in 85% of patients using these scanner systems.[13] However, in second-generation dual-source CT systems, this problem has been addressed and the field of view for tube B (in this case the low-kVp tube) had been extended from 33 second-generation to 35 cm in third-generation dual-source CT scanner systems (Fig. 26-3).

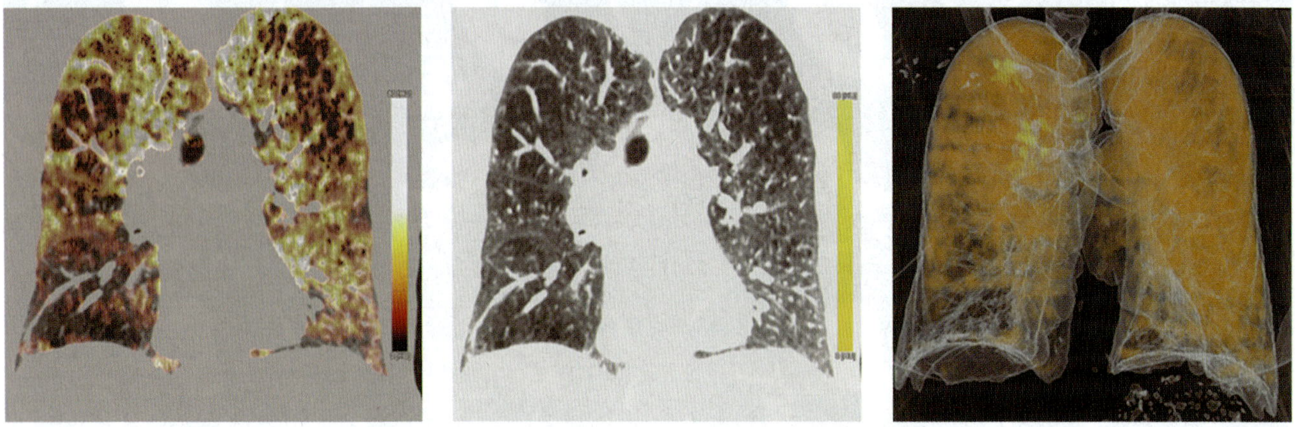

A B C

Figure 26-3. Contrast-enhanced dual-energy CT of an 84-year-old patient with inhomogeneous pulmonary emphysema. Coronal color-coded iodine distribution map **(A)** shows diffuse perfusion defects of the most affected areas within the left upper lobe and right lower lobe, in analogy to the gray-scale coronal multiplanar reformation displayed in lung window setting **(B)**. The 3-D reconstruction **(C)** shows full coverage of the chest even in this emphysema patient, which became feasible by enlarging the angle between the two fan beams of second- and third-generation dual-source CT resulting in a field of view of 33 and 35 cm, respectively, (compared to 26 cm in first-generation dual-source CT systems). This allows iodine distribution imaging of both lungs without exclusion of distal lung parenchyma.

Image Evaluation

Lung parenchymal iodine distribution reflecting regional lung perfusion obtained from dual-energy CT scanning can be assessed qualitatively,[11] semiquantitatively,[73] or quantitatively.[14,71]

The minimum and maximum CT numbers (−1,024 HU and −500 HU, respectively) are defined to include only the lung parenchyma in contrast agent map. This default range generally works well in older children and adults. However, the maximum value needs to be increased appropriately (e.g., −200 to −300 HU) in young children because normal lung density is higher in young children.[48] Such adjustment of the maximum value is also necessary for evaluating ground-glass opacities in the lung parenchyma.[48,71,72]

In order to calculate iodine distribution within the lung parenchyma on the basis of DS-DE-CT-PA, the postprocessing software application aims at selective extraction of iodine. The following material decomposition parameters for iodine mapping within the lung parenchyma are recommended: −1,000 HU for air at 80 kVp, −1,000 HU for air at 140 kVp, 60 HU for soft tissue at 80 kVp, and 54 HU for soft tissue at 140 kVp; these parameters should not be changed for patient examinations.[74] Other ranges recommend to use are −960 HU as lower margin and −200 to −300 HU as upper margin.[8] The "range" refers to the number of adjacent voxels used for interpolation during the calculation of the three-material decomposition, with small values yielding higher spatial resolution and large values improving detection of small contrast differences.[75]

For evaluation of iodine perfusion maps, color coding using 16-bit gray-scale or "hot metal" 16-bit color coding (default setting) is applied, with different optional color scales: the software enables a multiplanar view of the lung parenchyma and allows the user to define a mixing ratio between a non–color-coded 120-kV–equivalent dataset (0%) and the pure color map (100%).[64] The mixing ratio can be varied freely between 0% and 100%.

Qualitative

Physiologic pulmonary perfusion maps show homogeneous perfusion with symmetric as well as so-called dependent lung iodine distribution: dependent lung perfusion at DE-CT refers to a relatively lower blood pool content in the ventral regions and a relatively higher blood pool content in the dorsal regions with the patient in the supine position.[76]

Lung perfusion may be generally decreased in some lung diseases, for example, hypoxic pulmonary vasoconstriction present in chronic obstructive airway disease with parenchymal destruction. Usefulness of minimum-intensity projection images (MinIP) has been reported to identify these hypoattenuating lung lesions.[77] Expiratory CT including cine-CT[78] and dual-energy ventilation CT[79] can also be used for that purpose.

As a simple but effective means to differentiate between pathologies, the shape of perfusion defects may be used[11]: perfusion defects typically observed in patients with acute PE include peripherally located, wedge-shaped defects and are often found in a segmental or lobar distribution.[80] All other perfusion defects, such as patchy or band-like defects without segmental distribution or complete loss of color coding (indicating a lack of air-containing voxels due to consolidation [Fig. 26-1]), are ordinarily considered inconsistent with acute PE.[64]

Iodine distribution images may also assist in detecting small PEs that are not evident with conventional CT-PA.[13,15] The idea is that the observed pulmonary perfusion defects corresponded to segments of prior embolism with in the meantime reperfused segmental vessels and residual peripheral thrombosed vessels that were too small to visualize on CT-PA.

With regard to evaluation of chronic PE by means of DE-CT, the following characteristic patterns should be mentioned: first of all, a typical perfusion pattern occurring in chronic PE is a mosaic-like blood pool distribution, which can be clearly differentiated from the localized, wedge-shaped appearance of acute PE. When present, these findings are highly suggestive of redistribution of blood flow, although they are not specific for chronic PE.[81] DE-CT was also proposed to aid in the differentiation of ground-glass attenuation of vascular origin in PE patients (by means of the high iodine content within the areas of ground-glass attenuation) from ground-glass attenuation secondary to bronchioloalveolar diseases.[54] Secondly, DE-CT can show the relationship between the severity of pulmonary arterial obstruction and a perfusion impairment, the latter being influenced by the degree to which the systemic collateral vascular supply has developed: the most severe pulmonary arterial features of chronic thromboembolic pulmonary hypertension were observed to be seen with a significantly higher frequency in segments with blood pool defects than in segments with normal perfusion.[82] Thirdly, in chronic PE, DE-CT can correlate blood pool defects with embolus-containing pulmonary arteries. The three following perfusion patterns can be distinguished in chronic PE: matched defects, defined as occluded pulmonary arteries and negligible residual blood flow; mismatched defects, occluded artery and visible residual blood flow; and normal lung regions, unobstructed pulmonary arteries with visible normal or increased flow.[83] Areas of mismatch with maintained blood supply despite of occluded pulmonary arteries can be interpreted a result of a collateral systemic supply. Lastly, chronic PE can lead to the development of calcifications within partially or completely occlusive chronic clots and within pulmonary artery walls when chronic PE is complicated by long-standing or severe pulmonary hypertension.[81] Generation of virtual unenhanced images can help with the diagnosis, which poses another major advantage of acquisition of DE-CT data in this pathology.

Quantitative

It has been shown that in patients with acute PE, the extent of DE-CT-PA–derived perfusion defect volume (PDvol) correlates with the risk to experience adverse clinical outcome.[73,84,85] Perfusion defect volume can be also used as a surrogate marker for right heart strain, which is known to be predictive for 30-day mortality[53,73]: patients with right heart strain have significantly higher perfusion defect volumes than do patients without right heart strain. Furthermore, a good correlation between the RV diameter–LV diameter ratio with a proposed DE-CT lung perfusion score or with the number of pulmonary segments with perfusion defects could be demonstrated.[64,86] Readmission and death due to PE occurred only in patients with a relative perfusion defect size of more than 5% of the total lung volume, whereas no such event was recorded for patients with less than 5% affected lung volume.[64,86] The median survival time is observed to be significantly lower in patients with more than 5% blood pool deficits with an increased relative hazard ratio for death compared with patients with less than 5% lung volume affected and the control group without PE.[80] Thus, DE-CT-based quantification of pulmonary blood pool deficits may serve as an additional means for risk stratification and outcome prediction in patients with acute PE.

Regarding emphysema, automated quantification of lung perfused blood volume (PBV) in DE-CT-PA for assessment of the severity and regional distribution of pulmonary hypoperfusion has been proposed as a promising method[87]: in patients with pulmonary emphysema, automated quantification of pulmonary PBV in DE-CT-PA correlated with the lung function parameters residual volume, forced expiratory volume in 1 second, and diffusing lung capacity for carbon monoxide. The authors concluded that automated quantification of pulmonary PBV can be used for a quick, reader-independent estimation of global and regional pulmonary perfusion.[87]

Other very recent work in emphysema patients investigated the feasibility of simultaneous assessment of emphysema quantification performed on the DE-CT-derived virtual noncontrast (VNC) images and regional perfusion evaluation by means of iodine maps in emphysema patients: moderate correlations between quantitative parameters on VNC images and pulmonary function tests patients underwent as well were found.[56] Furthermore, moderate correlations between the severity of parenchymal destruction, as determined from VNC images, and perfusion status, as determined from iodine maps, were seen.

Exact quantification of global and/or regional perfusion is also an important instrument with regard to the clinical application of DE-CT in assessment of pulmonary functional resectability: preoperative exact quantification of FEV1 to calculate postsurgical FEV1 is necessary in these patients. Normally, expected postoperative calculation of FEV1 is done under the rather rough assumption of every lobe participating equally in ventilation assessed with conventional lung function assessment, and according to the number of resected segments, the reduced FEV1 is estimated. DE-CT maps may help to determine the exact percentage a distinct segment owns in overall ventilation as well as in perfusion.[57–59]

Regarding usefulness and application indications of pulmonary perfusion imaging in lung cancer patients, DE-CT, on the one hand, has been observed to be of use for the characterization of pulmonary nodules[60]: DE-CT-measured iodinated contrast enhancement correctly classified 45 of 49 nodules into benign or malignant tumors. DCE-CT, on the other hand, has been recently shown to add to the characterization of SPNs as well: valid in SPNs with a diameter greater than 10 mm, CT perfusion could reduce the number of SPNs, diagnosed as undetermined at morphologic CT, thereby skipping the need for follow-up CT examinations, additional FDG-PET studies, biopsy, or even surgery.[61]

With regard to the assessment of tumor response to targeted therapies as well as radiotherapy, recent work by Henzler et al.,[88] which has reviewed functional CT imaging techniques for the assessment of angiogenesis in lung cancer, has also elaborated on applications of DCE-CT in lung cancer patients: tumor blood flow assessed in patients with advanced NSCLC correlated with the response to antiangiogenic and anti-EGFR targeted therapy (i.e., sorafenib and erlotinib)[89]: DCE-CT was performed at baseline as well as 3 and 6 weeks after the initiation of treatment, and tumor perfusion was lower in responders than in nonresponders at week 3 and 6. Patients with a large decrease of blood flow at week 6 tended to have a longer progression-free survival. A similar study in patients with advanced lung adenocarcinoma suggests performing DCE-CT at day 40 and 90 after initiation of conventional and antiangiogenic chemotherapy[90]: in this study, BF, BV, and permeability values were higher in responding patients than in the other patients, with significant differences for BF, BV, and permeability at second follow-up. The time to peak contrast enhancement was higher in nonresponding patients than in treatment responders.

With regard to tumor response to radiotherapy, microvascular damage has been determined as one of the key mechanisms.[91] It has been demonstrated that fractionated radiotherapy increases both the tumor vascular blood volume and the permeability of NSCLC with greater vascular changes being reported at the tumor rim compared with the center.[92] Also, NSCLC with higher pretherapeutic perfusion values, as measured by DCE-CT, has been observed to show higher sensitivity to radiochemotherapy than do tumors with initially lower perfusion values.[31] Moreover, the resultant DCE-CT measurements have shown predictive value for early tumor response and overall survival among patients with NSCLC.

Despite these promising results, DCE-CT has not yet been established as a standard procedure in clinical routine since the applicability of this technique was limited in the past because data acquisition was restricted to single or few slides throughout a tumor. However, with currently available state-of-the-art CT systems, whole tumor coverage with an acceptable radiation dose using low tube voltage settings became feasible (see Fig. 26-4)[35,38,90,92] and good intraobserver agreement for lung cancer DCE-CT measurements has been demonstrated, encouraging its use for tumor characterization and therapy response monitoring.[62]

Artifacts

In the analysis of DE-CT-derived perfusion maps, one should be familiar with sources of pitfalls to avoid misdiagnoses: streaks and beam-hardening effects resulting from ribs, metal, and especially high-concentration contrast material in the superior vena cava or right cardiac chambers are probably the most common artifacts in iodine perfusion maps.[64] All these kinds of artifacts must be considered when an unexpected abnormal blood pool pattern is detected. In the case of contrast material inflow artifacts, the resulting pseudoperfusion defects may appear band-like and are most commonly located in the upper lung lobes. These artifacts were found to be present in up to 97% of iodine maps of patients[67] and have the potential to at worst obscure true perfusion defects or lead to false-positive reports. As a means to reduce streak artifacts from undiluted contrast agent, caudocranial scan direction has been reported.[71]

Diaphragmatic or cardiac motion may as well cause artificial decreases in the pulmonary blood pool adjacent to the diaphragm or cardiac chambers[64]: in this setting, the perfusion defect appears mostly crescent shaped and blurring. Additionally, double lines adjacent to the diaphragm or heart border can be seen when viewing the data in lung or mediastinal window settings.[64] Breath-holding techniques can reduce diaphragmatic motion artifacts. Normal physiologic, gravity-dependent variations in the pulmonary blood pool should also be recognized. Functional reconstructions should be viewed alongside the anatomic CT reconstructions for recognition of pulmonary abnormalities and diseases like emphysema (see Fig. 26-3), tumors invading or compressing the pulmonary arteries, pulmonary consolidation, vasculitis, or vascular anomalies, all of which will result in blood pool defects or unphysiologic blood flow patterns.[64] Also, the considerable reduction in the pulmonary capillary bed often seen in elderly patients or patients with emphysema can cause diffuse decreases in the pulmonary blood pool.[76]

Knowledge of occurrence of all the aforementioned artifacts should prevent everyone from solely using iodine perfusion maps to assess pulmonary perfusion disorders and to instead always correlate findings to morphologic CT-PA images.

Discussion

Correlation to Other Imaging Modalities

Diagnostic accuracy of dual-energy lung perfusion CT was initially proven in multiple animal studies.[2,93–96] In the literature, DE-CT pulmonary perfusion imaging has shown especially good correlation when compared to nuclear medicine–based imaging modalities used for pulmonary perfusion and ventilation assessment at that time including primarily perfusion scintigraphy, single photon emission computed tomography (SPECT) and SPECT/CT. For DE-CT-PA, sensitivities/specificities of 100% and 100% of for the diagnosis of acute pulmonary perfusion deficits were reported when compared to SPECT/CT and a per-segment sensitivity/specificity of 83%/99% with a negative predictive value of 93% for DE-CT when compared to pulmonary scintigraphy.[12,13,57,97–103]

Time-resolved contrast-enhanced MR angiography and phase contrast MRI have been also proposed as valuable modalities to visualize pulmonary perfusion, and mostly positive results were reported regarding correlation of CT-derived lung perfusion

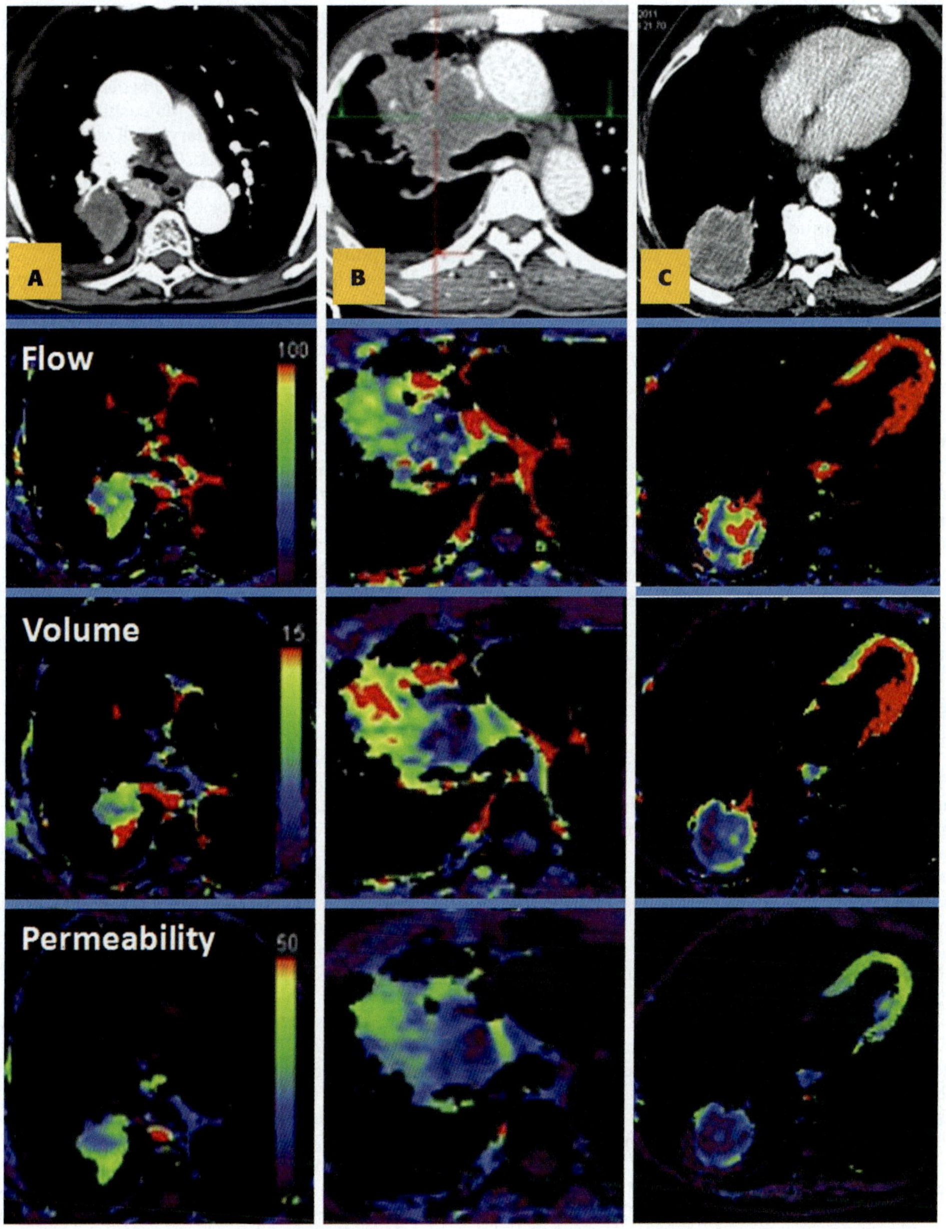

Figure 26-4. Dynamic volume perfusion CT study. **A:** A 78-year-old man with T3, N2, M1a adenocarcinoma of the right upper lobe (*first column*). **B:** A 61-year-old man with small cell lung cancer of the right upper lobe (*second column*). **C:** A 76-year-old man with a T3, N2, M0 squamous cell carcinoma of the right lower lobe (*third column*). The upper row shows standard 80-kV images during a midarterial phase; the second row demonstrates color-coded images representing tumor blood flow (mL/100 mL/min). The third row shows color-coded images representing tumor blood volume (mL/100 mL), and the fourth row demonstrates color-coded images representing tumor permeability (mL/100 mL/min). (With kind permission of T. Henzler, MD.)

imaging with functional MRI perfusion imaging.[71,104–108] In contrast to that, a recent study found moderate visual but not statistically significant correlation between DE-CT iodine maps and perfusion parameter maps of DCE-MRI.[109] However, the study cohort was small, and the time span between MRI and CT was supposed to account in part for this mismatch.

Radiation Dose

Conventional CT-PA reference dose value set in the "European Guidelines on Quality Criteria for Multi-Slice Computed Tomography" is 650 mGy*cm.[110] In the literature, the average reported dose of a conventional CT-PA is around 900 mGy × cm.[8] Previously uttered concerns about an increase in radiation exposure due to the use of DE-CT-based pulmonary angiography have been revealed as unfounded.

Regarding dual-source DE-CT-PA, dose-length products (DLP) of around 150 to 380 mGy*cm have been reported with various tube current settings, and DE-CT-PA therefore results in a radiation dose between a 100-kV and a 120-kV single-source PA scan.[15,74,110–112]

One also has to bear in mind that the use of DE-CT for diagnostic workup of patients might obviate additional examinations where radiation is applied, due to additional functional information beyond morphology gained, finally resulting in an intraindividual radiation dose reduction for the patient.

In contrast to dose-neutral perfusion imaging with DE-CT, DCE-CT examinations are associated with an additional radiation exposure and therefore up to now mostly used in cancer patients. Yet, with the advent of newer CT scanner generations, and especially the technical possibility to perform time-resolved CT angiographies at 70-kV tube voltage in most of the body regions, the promising technique will probably become more widely adopted.

Conclusions

DE-CT-derived iodine perfusion imaging has already found its way into clinical routine as it can be easily implemented into clinical postprocessing workflow along with standard reconstructions and as the generation of DE-CT-derived iodine perfusion maps does not imply additional radiation exposure. Functional information and morphologic information can be simultaneously obtained with this method. However, lung perfusion in CT imaging of pulmonary diseases is not meant to replace conventional morphologic pulmonary CT angiographic data, but is intended to add diagnostic and prognostic value and always has to be evaluated in conjunction. DCE-CT pulmonary perfusion imaging on the other hand is an emerging technique, which requires future research with regard to standardization of protocols and interpretation of quantitative results in order to gain broad clinical relevance.

REFERENCES

1. **Schoepf UJ, Bruening R, Konschitzky H, et al.** Pulmonary embolism: comprehensive diagnosis by using electron-beam CT for detection of emboli and assessment of pulmonary blood flow. *Radiology* 2000;217:693–700.
2. **Wildberger JE, Klotz E, Ditt H, et al.** Multislice computed tomography perfusion imaging for visualization of acute pulmonary embolism: animal experience. *Eur Radiol* 2005;15:1378–1386.
3. **Wildberger JE, Niethammer MU, Klotz E, et al.** Multi-slice CT for visualization of pulmonary embolism using perfusion weighted color maps. *Rofo* 2001;173:289–294.
4. **Wildberger JE, Klotz E, Ditt H, et al.** Multi-slice CT for visualization of acute pulmonary embolism: single breath-hold subtraction technique. *Rofo* 2005;177:17–23.
5. **Wildberger JE, Schoepf UJ, Mahnken AH, et al.** Approaches to CT perfusion imaging in pulmonary embolism. *Semin Roentgenol* 2005;40:64–73.
6. **Johnson TR, Krauss B, Sedlmair M, et al.** Material differentiation by dual energy CT: initial experience. *Eur Radiol* 2007;17:1510–1517.
7. **Flohr TG, McCollough CH, Bruder H, et al.** First performance evaluation of a dual-source CT (dsct) system. *Eur Radiol* 2006;16:256–268.
8. **Lu GM, Zhao Y, Zhang LJ, et al.** Dual-energy CT of the lung. *AJR Am J Roentgenol* 2012;199:S40–S53.
9. **Johnson TRC.** Dual-energy CT: general principles. *AJR Am J Roentgenol* 2012;199:S3–S8.
10. **Thieme SF, Johnson TR, Reiser MF, et al.** Dual-energy lung perfusion computed tomography: a novel pulmonary functional imaging method. *Semin Ultrasound CT MR* 2010;31:301–308.
11. **Thieme SF, Johnson TR, Lee C, et al.** Dual-energy CT for the assessment of contrast material distribution in the pulmonary parenchyma. *AJR Am J Roentgenol* 2009;193:144–149.
12. **Thieme SF, Graute V, Nikolaou K, et al.** Dual energy CT lung perfusion imaging—correlation with SPECT/CT. *Eur J Radiol* 2012;81:360–365.
13. **Thieme SF, Becker CR, Hacker M, et al.** Dual energy CT for the assessment of lung perfusion—correlation to scintigraphy. *Eur J Radiol* 2008;68:369–374.
14. **Fink C, Johnson TR, Michaely HJ, et al.** Dual-energy CT angiography of the lung in patients with suspected pulmonary embolism: initial results. *Rofo* 2008;180:879–883.
15. **Pontana F, Faivre JB, Remy-Jardin M, et al.** Lung perfusion with dual-energy multidetector-row CT (MDCT): feasibility for the evaluation of acute pulmonary embolism in 117 consecutive patients. *Acad Radiol* 2008;15:1494–1504.
16. **Euler USv, Liljestrand G.** Observations on the pulmonary arterial blood pressure in the cat. *Acta Physiol Scand* 1946;12:301–320.
17. **Matsuoka S, Yamashiro T, Matsushita S, et al.** Relationship between quantitative ct of pulmonary small vessels and pulmonary perfusion. *AJR Am J Roentgenol* 2014;202:719–724.
18. **Johnson T, Fink C, Schoenberg SO, et al.** eds. *Dual energy CT in clinical practice. Medical radiology*. Berlin, Heidelberg: Springer-Verlag; 2011.
19. **Afaq A, Akin O.** Imaging assessment of tumor response: past, present and future. *Future Oncol* 2011;7:669–677.
20. **Bellomi M, Petralia G, Sonzogni A, et al.** CT perfusion for the monitoring of neoadjuvant chemotherapy and radiation therapy in rectal carcinoma: initial experience. *Radiology* 2007;244:486–493.
21. **Bellomi M, Viotti S, Preda L, et al.** Perfusion CT in solid body-tumours. Part II: Clinical applications and future development. *Radiol Med* 2010;115:858–874.
22. **Bisdas S, Rumboldt Z, Wagenblast J, et al.** Response and progression-free survival in oropharynx squamous cell carcinoma assessed by pretreatment perfusion CT: comparison with tumor volume measurements. *AJNR Am J Neuroradiol* 2009;30:793–799.
23. **Choi H.** Critical issues in response evaluation on computed tomography: lessons from the gastrointestinal stromal tumor model. *Curr Oncol Rep* 2005;7:307–311.
24. **d'Assignies G, Couvelard A, Bahrami S, et al.** Pancreatic endocrine tumors: tumor blood flow assessed with perfusion CT reflects angiogenesis and correlates with prognostic factors. *Radiology* 2009;250:407–416.
25. **Faivre S, Zappa M, Vilgrain V, et al.** Changes in tumor density in patients with advanced hepatocellular carcinoma treated with sunitinib. *Clin Cancer Res* 2011;17:4504–4512.
26. **Fournier LS, Oudard S, Thiam R, et al.** Metastatic renal carcinoma: evaluation of antiangiogenic therapy with dynamic contrast-enhanced CT. *Radiology* 2010;256:511–518.
27. **Frampas E, Lassau N, Zappa M, et al.** Advanced hepatocellular carcinoma: early evaluation of response to targeted therapy and prognostic value of perfusion CT and dynamic contrast enhanced-ultrasound. Preliminary results. *Eur J Radiol* 2013;82:e205–e211.
28. **Gandhi D, Chepeha DB, Miller T, et al.** Correlation between initial and early follow-up CT perfusion parameters with endoscopic tumor response in patients with advanced squamous cell carcinomas of the oropharynx treated with organ-preservation therapy. *AJNR Am J Neuroradiol* 2006;27:101–106.
29. **Coche E.** Assessment of lung tumor response by perfusion CT. *JBR-BTR* 2013;96:172–174.
30. **Tacelli N, Santangelo T, Scherpereel A, et al.** Perfusion CT allows prediction of therapy response in non-small cell lung cancer treated with conventional and anti-angiogenic chemotherapy. *Eur Radiol* 2013;23:2127–2136.
31. **Wang J, Wu N, Cham MD, et al.** Tumor response in patients with advanced non-small cell lung cancer: perfusion CT evaluation of chemotherapy and radiation therapy. *AJR Am J Roentgenol* 2009;193:1090–1096.
32. **Ng Q-S, Goh V, Fichte H, et al.** Lung cancer perfusion at multi–detector row CT: reproducibility of whole tumor quantitative measurements. *Radiology* 2006;239:547–553.
33. **Ng CS, Chandler AG, Wei W, et al.** Reproducibility of perfusion parameters obtained from perfusion ct in lung tumors. *AJR Am J Roentgenol* 2011;197:113–121.
34. **Ng QS, Goh V, Klotz E, et al.** Quantitative assessment of lung cancer perfusion using mdct: does measurement reproducibility improve with greater tumor volume coverage? *AJR Am J Roentgenol* 2006;187:1079–1084.
35. **Shi J, Schmid-Bindert G, Fink C, et al.** Dynamic volume perfusion CT in patients with lung cancer: baseline perfusion characteristics of different histological subtypes. *Eur J Radiol* 2013;82:e894–e900.
36. **Sun YS, Zhang XY, Cui Y, et al.** Spectral CT imaging as a new quantitative tool? Assessment of perfusion defects of pulmonary parenchyma in patients with lung cancer. *Chin J Cancer Res* 2013;25:722–728.
37. **Zhang G, Dilling TJ, Stevens CW, et al.** Functional lung imaging in thoracic cancer radiotherapy. *Cancer Control* 2008;15:112–119.
38. **Li Y, Yang ZG, Chen TW, et al.** Whole tumour perfusion of peripheral lung carcinoma: evaluation with first-pass CT perfusion imaging at 64-detector row CT. *Clin Radiol* 2008;63:629–635.

39. **Swensen SJ.** Functional CT: lung nodule evaluation. *Radiographics* 2000;20:1178–1181.
40. **Swensen SJ, Brown LR, Colby TV, et al.** Pulmonary nodules: CT evaluation of enhancement with iodinated contrast material. *Radiology* 1995;194:393–398.
41. **Swensen SJ, Morin RL, Schueler BA, et al.** Solitary pulmonary nodule: CT evaluation of enhancement with iodinated contrast material—a preliminary report. *Radiology* 1992;182:343–347.
42. **Swensen SJ, Viggiano RW, Midthun DE, et al.** Lung nodule enhancement at CT: multicenter study. *Radiology* 2000;214:73–80.
43. **Yamashita K, Matsunobe S, Tsuda T, et al.** Solitary pulmonary nodule: preliminary study of evaluation with incremental dynamic CT. *Radiology* 1995;194:399–405.
44. **Zhang M, Kono M.** Solitary pulmonary nodules: evaluation of blood flow patterns with dynamic CT. *Radiology* 1997;205:471–478.
45. **Remy-Jardin M, Faivre JB, Pontana F, et al.** Thoracic applications of dual energy. *Semin Respir Crit Care Med* 2014;35:64–73.
46. **Remy-Jardin M, Pistolesi M, Goodman LR, et al.** Management of suspected acute pulmonary embolism in the era of CT angiography: a statement from the fleischner society. *Radiology* 2007;245:315–329.
47. **Torbicki A, Perrier A, Konstantinides S, et al.** Guidelines on the diagnosis and management of acute pulmonary embolism: the task force for the diagnosis and management of acute pulmonary embolism of the european society of cardiology (esc). *Eur Heart J* 2008;29:2276–2315.
48. **Goo HW.** Dual-energy lung perfusion and ventilation CT in children. *Pediatr Radiol* 2013;43:298–307.
49. **Geyer LL, Scherr M, Korner M, et al.** Imaging of acute pulmonary embolism using a dual energy CT system with rapid kvp switching: Initial results. *Eur J Radiol* 2012;81:3711–3718.
50. **Henzler T, Barraza JM Jr, Nance JW Jr, et al.** CT imaging of acute pulmonary embolism. *J Cardiovasc Comput Tomogr* 2011;5:3–11.
51. **Hong YJ, Kim JY, Choe KO, et al.** Different perfusion pattern between acute and chronic pulmonary thromboembolism: evaluation with two-phase dual-energy perfusion CT. *AJR Am J Roentgenol* 2013;200:812–817.
52. **Kim BH, Seo JB, Chae EJ, et al.** Analysis of perfusion defects by causes other than acute pulmonary thromboembolism on contrast-enhanced dual-energy CT in consecutive 537 patients. *Eur J Radiol* 2012;81:e647–e652.
53. **Zhang LJ, Yang GF, Zhao YE, et al.** Detection of pulmonary embolism using dual-energy computed tomography and correlation with cardiovascular measurements: a preliminary study. *Acta Radiol* 2009;50:892–901.
54. **Pontana F, Remy-Jardin M, Duhamel A, et al.** Lung perfusion with dual-energy multi-detector row ct: can it help recognize ground glass opacities of vascular origin? *Acad Radiol* 2010;17:587–594.
55. **Remy-Jardin M, Abbott G.** Modern diagnosis in the evaluation of pulmonary vascular disease. In: Hodler J, von Schulthess GK, Zollikofer CL, eds. *Diseases of the heart and chest, including breast 2011–2014.* Milan, Italy: Springer; 2011:55–59.
56. **Lee CW, Seo JB, Lee Y, et al.** A pilot trial on pulmonary emphysema quantification and perfusion mapping in a single-step using contrast-enhanced dual-energy computed tomography. *Invest Radiol* 2012;47:92–97.
57. **Chae EJ, Kim N, Seo JB, et al.** Prediction of postoperative lung function in patients undergoing lung resection: dual-energy perfusion computed tomography versus perfusion scintigraphy. *Invest Radiol* 2013;48:622–627.
58. **Nagayama H, Sueyoshi E, Hayashida T, et al.** Quantification of lung perfusion blood volume (lung pbv) by dual-energy CT in pulmonary embolism before and after treatment: preliminary results. *Clin Imaging* 2013;37:493–497.
59. **Yanagita H, Honda N, Nakayama M, et al.** Prediction of postoperative pulmonary function: preliminary comparison of single-breath dual-energy xenon CT with three conventional methods. *Jpn J Radiol* 2013;31:377–385.
60. **Chae EJ, Song JW, Krauss B, et al.** Dual-energy computed tomography characterization of solitary pulmonary nodules. *J Thorac Imaging* 2010;25:301–310.
61. **Mazzei MA, Cioffi Squitieri N, Guerrini S, et al.** Quantitative CT perfusion measurements in characterization of solitary pulmonary nodules: new insights and limitations. *Recenti Prog Med* 2013;104: 430–437.
62. **Sauter AW, Merkle A, Schulze M, et al.** Intraobserver and interobserver agreement of volume perfusion CT (VPCT) measurements in patients with lung lesions. *Eur J Radiol* 2012;81(10):2853–2859.
63. **Stanzani M, Battista G, Sassi C, et al.** Computed tomographic pulmonary angiography for diagnosis of invasive mold diseases in patients with hematological malignancies. *Clin Infect Dis* 2012;54:610–616.
64. **Zhao Y, Zhang LJ, Lu GM, et al.** Dual source, dual energy computed tomography in pulmonary embolism. In: Çobanoğlu U, ed. *Pulmonary embolism*; 2012.
65. **Apfaltrer P, Hanna EL, Henzler T, et al.** CT imaging of pulmonary embolism: current status. *Curr Cardiovasc Imaging Rep* 2011;4:476–484.
66. **Krissak R, Fink C.** Lung perfusion. In: Johnson T, et al., eds. *Dual energy CT in clinical practice.* Berlin, Heidelberg: Springer; 2011:83–90.
67. **Nance JW Jr, Henzler T, Meyer M, et al.** Optimization of contrast material delivery for dual-energy computed tomography pulmonary angiography in patients with suspected pulmonary embolism. *Invest Radiol* 2012;47:78–84.
68. **Hansmann J, Fink C, Jost G, et al.** Impact of iodine delivery rate with varying flow rates on image quality in dual-energy CT of patients with suspected pulmonary embolism. *Acad Radiol* 2013;20:962–971.
69. **Henzler T, Meyer M, Reichert M, et al.** Dual-energy CT angiography of the lungs: comparison of test bolus and bolus tracking techniques for the determination of scan delay. *Eur J Radiol* 2012;81:132–138.
70. **Kerl JM, Bauer RW, Renker M, et al.** Triphasic contrast injection improves evaluation of dual energy lung perfusion in pulmonary CT angiography. *Eur J Radiol* 2011;80:e483–e487.
71. **Goo HW.** Initial experience of dual-energy lung perfusion CT using a dual-source CT system in children. *Pediatr Radiol* 2010;40:1536–1544.
72. **Goo HW.** Current trends in cardiac CT in children. *Acta Radiol* 2013;54:1055–1062.
73. **Chae EJ, Seo JB, Jang YM, et al.** Dual-energy CT for assessment of the severity of acute pulmonary embolism: pulmonary perfusion defect score compared with CT angiographic obstruction score and right ventricular/left ventricular diameter ratio. *AJR Am J Roentgenol* 2010;194:604–610.
74. **Kang MJ, Park CM, Lee CH, et al.** Dual-energy CT: clinical applications in various pulmonary diseases. *Radiographics* 2010;30:685–698.
75. **Hagspiel KD, Flors L, Housseini AM, et al.** Pulmonary blood volume imaging with dual-energy computed tomography: spectrum of findings. *Clin Radiol* 2012;67:69–77.
76. **Lu GM, Wu SY, Yeh BM, et al.** Dual-energy computed tomography in pulmonary embolism. *Br J Radiol* 2010;83:707–718.
77. **Ferda J, Ferdova E, Mirka H, et al.** Pulmonary imaging using dual-energy CT, a role of the assessment of iodine and air distribution. *Eur J Radiol* 2011;77:287–293.
78. **Goo HW, Kim HJ.** Detection of air trapping on inspiratory and expiratory phase images obtained by 0.3-second cine CT in the lungs of free-breathing young children. *AJR Am J Roentgenol* 2006;187:1019–1023.
79. **Thieme SF, Hoegl S, Nikolaou K, et al.** Pulmonary ventilation and perfusion imaging with dual-energy CT. *Eur Radiol* 2010;20:2882–2889.
80. **Bauer RW, Kerl JM, Weber E, et al.** Lung perfusion analysis with dual energy CT in patients with suspected pulmonary embolism—influence of window settings on the diagnosis of underlying pathologies of perfusion defects. *Eur J Radiol* 2011;80:e476–e482.
81. **Boroto K, Remy-Jardin M, Flohr T, et al.** Thoracic applications of dual-source ct technology. *Eur J Radiol* 2008;68:375–384.
82. **Renard B, Remy-Jardin M, Santangelo T, et al.** Dual-energy CT angiography of chronic thromboembolic disease: can it help recognize links between the severity of pulmonary arterial obstruction and perfusion defects? *Eur J Radiol* 2011;79:467–472.
83. **Hoey ET, Mirsadraee S, Pepke-Zaba J, et al.** Dual-energy CT angiography for assessment of regional pulmonary perfusion in patients with chronic thromboembolic pulmonary hypertension: initial experience. *AJR Am J Roentgenol* 2011;196:524–532.
84. **Apfaltrer P, Bachmann V, Meyer M, et al.** Prognostic value of perfusion defect volume at dual energy cta in patients with pulmonary embolism: correlation with cta obstruction scores, CT parameters of right ventricular dysfunction and adverse clinical outcome. *Eur J Radiol* 2012;81:3592–3597.
85. **Miura S, Ohno Y, Kimura H, et al.** Quantitative lung perfused blood volume imaging on dual-energy CT: capability for quantitative assessment of disease severity in patients with acute pulmonary thromboembolism. *Acta Radiol* 2014. [Epub ahead of print February 24, 2014].

86. **Kim WY, Ahn S, Lee CW.** Risk stratification of submassive pulmonary embolism: the role of chest computed tomography as an alternative to echocardiography. In: Çobanoğlu U, ed. *Pulmonary embolism*. 2012.
87. **Meinel FG, Graef A, Thieme SF, et al.** Assessing pulmonary perfusion in emphysema: automated quantification of perfused blood volume in dual-energy ctpa. *Invest Radiol* 2013;48:79–85.
88. **Henzler T, Shi J, Jafarov H, et al.** Functional CT imaging techniques for the assessment of angiogenesis in lung cancer. *Transl Lung Cancer Res* 2012;1:78–83.
89. **Lind JS, Meijerink MR, Dingemans AM, et al.** Dynamic contrast-enhanced CT in patients treated with sorafenib and erlotinib for non-small cell lung cancer: a new method of monitoring treatment? *Eur Radiol* 2010;20:2890–2898.
90. **Fraioli F, Anzidei M, Zaccagna F, et al.** Whole-tumor perfusion CT in patients with advanced lung adenocarcinoma treated with conventional and antiangiogenetic chemotherapy: initial experience. *Radiology* 2011;259:574–582.
91. **Garcia-Barros M, Paris F, Cordon-Cardo C, et al.** Tumor response to radiotherapy regulated by endothelial cell apoptosis. *Science* 2003;300:1155–1159.
92. **Ng Q-S, Goh V, Milner J, et al.** Acute tumor vascular effects following fractionated radiotherapy in human lung cancer: in vivo whole tumor assessment using volumetric perfusion computed tomography. *Int J Radiat Oncol Biol Phys* 2007;67:417–424.
93. **Chai X, Zhang LJ, Yeh BM, et al.** Acute and subacute dual energy CT findings of pulmonary embolism in rabbits: correlation with histopathology. *Br J Radiol* 2012;85:613–622.
94. **Zhang LJ, Zhao YE, Wu SY, et al.** Pulmonary embolism detection with dual-energy CT: experimental study of dual-source ct in rabbits. *Radiology* 2009;252:61–70.
95. **Chung MJ, Goo JM, Im JG, et al.** CT perfusion image of the lung: value in the detection of pulmonary embolism in a porcine model. *Invest Radiol* 2004;39:633–640.
96. **Screaton NJ, Coxson HO, Kalloger SE, et al.** Detection of lung perfusion abnormalities using computed tomography in a porcine model of pulmonary embolism. *J Thorac Imaging* 2003;18:14–20.
97. **Suga K, Yasuhiko K, Iwanaga H, et al.** Relation between lung perfusion defects and intravascular clots in acute pulmonary thromboembolism: assessment with breath-hold spect-ct pulmonary angiography fusion images. *Eur J Radiol* 2008;67:472–480.
98. **Yang GF, Yang X, Zhang LJ, et al.** Pulmonary enhancement imaging with dual energy CT for the detection of pulmonary embolism in a rabbit model: comparison to perfusion planar scintigraphy, spect and SPECT-CT modalities. *Acad Radiol* 2011;18:605–614.
99. **Bury B.** Scintigraphy or multidetector CT angiography for suspected pulmonary embolism? *J Nucl Med* 2008;49:864; author reply 864.
100. **Larcos G, Chi KK, Shiell A, et al.** Suspected acute pulmonary emboli: cost-effectiveness of chest helical computed tomography versus a standard diagnostic algorithm incorporating ventilation-perfusion scintigraphy. *Aust N Z J Med* 2000;30:195–201.
101. **Nyman U.** Routine use of a v/q spect/low-dose CT hybrid system to diagnose pulmonary embolism seems premature. *J Nucl Med* 2010;51:1329–1330; author reply 1330.
102. **Rossi A, Attina D, Borgonovi A, et al.** Evaluation of mosaic pattern areas in hrct with min-ip reconstructions in patients with pulmonary hypertension: could this evaluation replace lung perfusion scintigraphy? *Eur J Radiol* 2012;81:e1–e6.
103. **Suga K, Kawakami Y, Iwanaga H, et al.** Comprehensive assessment of lung CT attenuation alteration at perfusion defects of acute pulmonary thromboembolism with breath-hold SPECT-CT fusion images. *J Comput Assist Tomogr* 2006;30:83–91.
104. **Fink C, Henzler T, Shirinova A, et al.** Thoracic magnetic resonance imaging: pulmonary thromboembolism. *J Thorac Imaging* 2013;28:171–177.
105. **Henzler T, Schmid-Bindert G, Schoenberg SO, et al.** Diffusion and perfusion mri of the lung and mediastinum. *Eur J Radiol* 2010;76: 329–336.
106. **Kjorstad A, Corteville DM, Fischer A, et al.** Quantitative lung perfusion evaluation using Fourier decomposition perfusion mri. *Magn Reson Med* 2014;72(2):558–562.
107. **Zhang LJ, Lu L, Bi J, et al.** Detection of pulmonary embolism comparison between dual energy CT and MR angiography in a rabbit model. *Acad Radiol* 2010;17:1550–1559.
108. **Zhang Q, Shi B, Liu Z, et al.** Preliminary study of CT in combination with MRI perfusion imaging to assess hemodynamic changes during angiogenesis in a rabbit model of lung cancer. *Onco Targets Ther* 2013;6:685–692.
109. **Hansmann J, Apfaltrer P, Zoellner FG, et al.** Correlation analysis of dual-energy CT iodine maps with quantitative pulmonary perfusion MRI. *World J Radiol* 2013;5:202–207.
110. **Bongartz GS, Jurik AG, Leonardi M.** *European guidelines on quality criteria for multislice computed tomography*. Luxembourg, Germany; 2004.
111. **Schenzle JC, Sommer WH, Neumaier K, et al.** Dual energy CT of the chest: how about the dose? *Invest Radiol* 2010;45:347–353.
112. **De Zordo T, von Lutterotti K, Dejaco C, et al.** Comparison of image quality and radiation dose of different pulmonary cta protocols on a 128-slice CT: high-pitch dual source CT, dual energy CT and conventional spiral CT. *Eur Radiol* 2012;22:279–286.

CHAPTER

27 Liver Perfusion Imaging with MR

Maxime Ronot, MD, PhD, Benjamin Leporq, PhD,
Simon A. Lambert, PhD, Jean-Luc Daire, PhD,
Bernard E. Van Beers, MD, PhD, and Valérie Vilgrain, MD, PhD

Introduction

The liver is a large, highly vascularized, subcutaneous solid organ that is easily accessible with various imaging techniques, including magnetic resonance imaging (MRI). Perfusion imaging provides information about tissue microcirculation or the movement of water and solutes at levels far below the spatial resolution of imaging techniques. Thus, perfusion imaging is not the dynamic qualitative analysis commonly obtained with tissue enhancement, but a quantitative extraction of physiologic perfusion parameters of the liver. MR perfusion imaging of the liver is based on the same principles as those used in other organs: the injection of a gadolinium chelate contrast medium (called a tracer) and acquisition by rapid temporal sampling of signal-intensity/time curves that provide information on variations in tracer concentrations over time. The physiologic parameters are extracted from these curves by adjusting them to mathematical perfusion models. Because of certain features of the liver, perfusion imaging is more challenging than in other organs. Indeed, the liver is a large, mobile organ that deforms with respiratory movements and has a dual vascular supply through the hepatic artery and the portal vein. In addition, the sinusoidal capillaries are fenestrated in the normal liver so the tracer readily diffuses from them.

Liver perfusion imaging is based on the hypothesis that local or diffuse pathologic processes result in measurable changes in perfusion parameters. Information is obtained about the presence or progression of these pathologic processes by quantifying these changes. Perfusion imaging is indicated in the liver for two main conditions: (a) Malignant liver tumors, in particular hepatocellular carcinoma (HCC) and liver metastases; and (b) the investigation of chronic liver diseases. Imaging already plays an important role in these two fields because imaging techniques (mainly CT and MRI) provide highly accurate qualitative data for the detection and characterization of liver lesions, treatment assessment, and patient follow-up. Therefore, the benefits of perfusion imaging must be evaluated not to replace existing techniques but as a complementary tool to adapt patient management or provide an earlier and more reproducible evaluation.

This chapter describes the bases and limitations of the different MR perfusion imaging techniques of the liver and discusses the clinical indications for liver perfusion studies.

The Vascular Physiology of the Liver

The liver has a dual blood supply and receives approximately 25% of its blood from the hepatic artery and the remaining 75% from the portal vein. There is no hepatic capillary network per se. It is replaced by fenestrated sinusoids. These two afferent vascular systems communicate through transsinusoidal and transvasal communications as well as the peribiliary plexuses. One of the fundamental adaptive mechanisms involved in vascular abnormalities of the liver is the presence of an arterioportal balance called the "hepatic buffer response" characterized by a compensatory increase in arterial blood supply when portal supply decreases, although the reverse does not occur.[1]

MR Imaging Techniques

In 1999, Scharf et al.[2] found a significant correlation between MRI and thermal dilution probe flow measurements in pigs using 1.0 T T1-weighted (T1W) sequences. Many MRI techniques can be used for analysis of the microcirculation, including arterial spin labeling (ASL)[3] in which the circulating blood is magnetically labeled, and the more recent combination of ASL with diffusion.[4] In blood oxygen level dependency (BOLD) imaging,[5] the ratio of oxygenated hemoglobin and paramagnetic deoxygenated hemoglobin can be used to obtain an indirect analysis of the oxygen supply in tissue. The two latter techniques are not used in the liver and will not be discussed.

The most common approach is a kinetic analysis following injection of a bolus of contrast material through tissue. When negative enhancement is evaluated (signal drop due to the effects induced by the first-pass of a bolus of concentrated contrast agent in T2/T2*-weighted MRI sequences), the technique is called dynamic susceptibility contrast-MRI (DSC-MRI). Although this was one of the first techniques to be investigated, today it is essentially indicated in brain perfusion analysis. Indeed, strictly speaking, DSC-MRI is not used to investigate capillary leakage, and its analysis theoretically implies the presence of an intact blood–organ barrier, impermeable to contrast agents. Thus, it is not used in the liver and will not be discussed in this chapter. The evaluation of positive enhancement (T1 effect of the contrast agent) is called "dynamic contrast-enhanced-imaging" or DCE imaging. This is the most common technique used in the liver, and the rest of the chapter describes it in detail. Besides conventional DCE sequences, sequences that measure molecular diffusion (diffusion-weighted MRI) are also influenced by microperfusion. This notion, which is called the IVIM model (intravoxel incoherent motion), was initially developed by Le Bihan et al.[6] to quantitatively measure the microscopic movements that contribute to the diffusion MR signal. In biologic tissue, these movements are mainly due to the molecular diffusion of water and the microcirculation of blood in the capillary network (perfusion). Le Bihan et al. developed the notion that water circulating in randomly oriented capillaries (at a voxel level) imitates random motion ("pseudodiffusion"). This attenuates the diffusion MRI signal, which depends upon the speed of the circulating blood and the vascular architecture. Like true molecular diffusion, the effect of pseudodiffusion on signal attenuation depends on the *b* value. The amount of signal attenuation that occurs from pseudodiffusion, however, is greater than molecular diffusion in tissue, and, as a result, the relative contribution to the diffusion-weighted signal is only significant at very low *b* values, theoretically allowing diffusion and microperfusion components to be separated.

Dynamic Contrast-Enhanced MR Imaging

Contrast-enhanced MRI corresponds to the acquisition of images of the liver during the arterial, portal venous, and delayed phases following a bolus injection of a gadolinium chelate (0.2 mmol/kg followed by 20 mL saline flush at 3 mL/s). When a hepatocyte-specific contrast agent such as gadoxetic acid (Gd-EOB-DTPA) is used, a hepatobiliary phase (20 minutes) is added to the dynamic phase to assess intracellular retention of the contrast agent. To perform DCE-MRI, sequences can be accelerated (or time resolved) to obtain multiple dynamic scans.[7] DCE-MRI is usually performed with diffusible agents. High temporal resolution is needed because the concentration changes rapidly in the arterial vessels during the first pass and correct sampling of the concentration versus time curves is essential. A temporal resolution less than 3 seconds is usually recommended, but a resolution of 1 second may be needed to visualize aortic peak enhancement. It is difficult to obtain this time resolution with whole-liver 3D MRI. Moreover, the relationship between signal intensity and tracer concentrations is not linear with MRI, unlike CT scan, in which the tracer concentration curve over time is proportional to changes in attenuation measured in Hounsfield units. A common DCE-MRI protocol is coronal 3D T1W fast gradient echo such as FLASH (TR = 2.7 milliseconds, TE = 0.9 millisecond, flip angle = 18 degrees, partition thickness = 8 mm, temporal resolution = 2 seconds for a 10 slice slab). A total of 180 consecutive measurements will be obtained. Precontrast images are obtained with two different flip angles (4 and 18 degrees) to analyze T1 values. The contrast will be injected after completion of first noncontrast measurement. In 3D acquisition, the first and the last couple slices will be excluded from analysis to remove wrap artifacts.

Nonlinear Relationship between Signal Intensity and Tracer Concentration

The nonlinearity of signal intensity and tracer concentrations can be seen when looking at the pulse sequence used for DCE-MRI. Indeed, these sequences are very sensitive to signal saturation and flow resulting in nonlinearity. Gadolinium concentration can be calculated from differences in T1 relaxation time before and after contrast. Precontrast T1 can be calculated from two or more sets of precontrast images using different flip angles, and postcontrast T1 values can be obtained from postcontrast and precontrast series with different flip angles.

Signal Saturation

Traditionally, the pulse sequences used were based on a spoiled gradient echo scheme with a short echo time (<1 millisecond) to decrease the T2* effect and a short repetition time (<4 to 5 milliseconds) to keep a suitable temporal resolution. The sequence dynamic is poor in this case, and depends upon the flip angle that significantly influences the linearity between T1 (thus concentration) and signal intensity (Fig. 27-1). The signal for long T1 structures—such as the liver—can be maintained with a small flip angle (<10 degrees) before enhancement, while the signal saturates during the enhancement peak of short T1 structures, such as the aorta.

Indeed, during these sequences the spins receive repeated RF pulses and there is not enough repetition time for longitudinal recovery of magnetization. As a result, spin magnetic moments are likely to be in the spin down direction and enter in a saturated state inducing signal saturation. This effect is emphasized by a large flip angle, by a short repetition time, and by the number of impulses. For conventional cartesian acquisitions, the *k*-space profile order is linear and the central lines are acquired halfway through the acquisition, after a significant number of repetitions (depending on the spatial resolution). Since this part of the *k*-space encodes for contrast, the saturation effect is predominant and may artificially erase contrast enhancement. This is very important to consider for quantitative perfusion imaging. A centric low-to-high profile may also be used (Fig. 27-2). This allows central lines of the *k*-space to be read first, limiting saturation as well as providing a better signal-to-noise ratio. A reverse linear profile is also an alternative with partial Fourier imaging in the phase direction.

Sensitivity to Flow

It is also very important to understand that the pulse sequences used for DCE-MRI are highly flow sensitive and influenced by a flow-related enhancement effect and entry slice phenomena. During the flow-related enhancement effect, the RF pulse selectively excites a volume while the rephasing gradient is applied to the entire body. Therefore, a flowing spin receiving an excitation pulse will be rephased regardless of its position. A stationary spin receives repeated RF pulses that tend to saturate, so flowing spin appears to have a higher signal. This phenomenon is emphasized by short

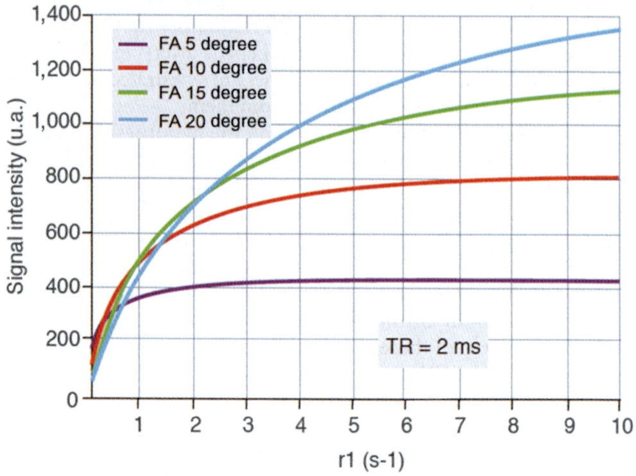

Figure 27-1. Simulation representing the signal intensity according to the longitudinal relaxation rate (1/T1) for different flip angles and with an ultrashort repetition time (2 milliseconds). These simulations illustrate the nonlinearity of the sequence according to r1 and the strong effect of flip angle on the dynamic. With small flip angles, dynamic is poor and saturation appears for short T1 structures.

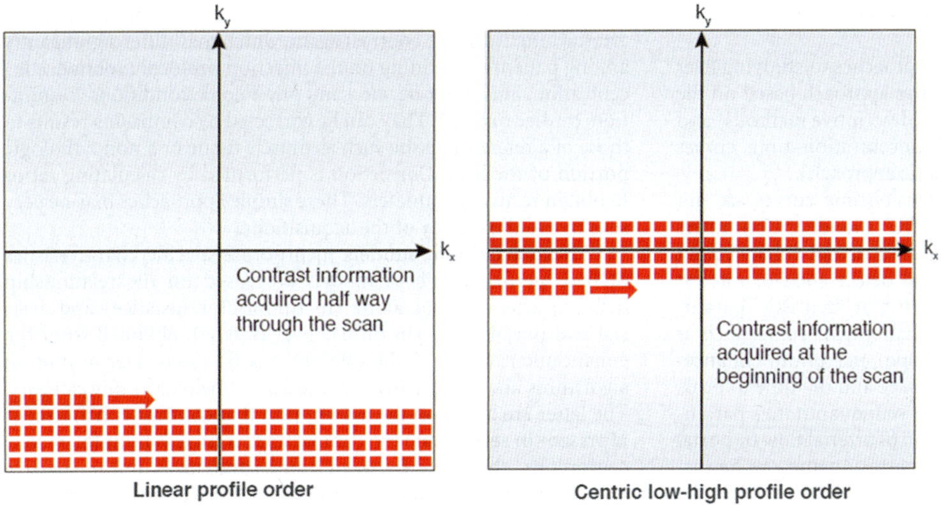

Figure 27-2. Scheme illustrating two *k*-space filling according to a linear profile order and to a centric low-high profile order.

repetition times and short echo times as well as when the thickness of slice increases; thus it is predominant in DCE-MRI.

During the slice entry effect, the magnetic moments of spins receiving repeated RF pulses are usually oriented in the spin-down direction since the repetition time is not long enough for longitudinal recovery of magnetization in the tissue where the spin resides. Spins that have not received repeated RF pulses are called "fresh" since their magnetic moment is mainly orientated in the spin-up direction. Thus, flowing spins, perpendicular to the slice, enter it "fresh" because they have not received repeated RF pulses, and they produce a higher signal than do stationary spins in the slice. This effect increases with velocity and countercurrent flows and is therefore very strong in large vessels such as the abdominal aorta and the main portal trunk.

The Nonlinear Relationship between Signal Intensity and Concentration

The relationship between the signal and tracer concentrations need not necessarily be linear but must be clear. One simple solution to prevent the above-mentioned effects would be "spatial presaturation," which delivers a selective 90-degree pulse to a volume outside the field of view (FOV) or the use of a nonselective preparation pulse in the sequence.

Several strategies have been suggested to manage the nonlinear relationship between signal intensity and gadolinium agent concentrations. First, precalibration can be performed by preparing scans with different tracer concentrations.[8,9] Although the results of this method are accurate, it is complicated to perform in clinical practice and may decrease reproducibility. Autocalibration is another alternative. This involves computing a T1 precontrast map with a multiple flip angle acquisition corresponding to a dynamic acquisition flip angle in order to derive the T1 postinjection. Finally, plasma concentrations can be determined based on knowledge of tracer r_1 relaxivity. Indeed, although the longitudinal relaxation rate and the signal intensity do not vary linearly, the relationship between r_1 and the contrast agent concentration is linear based on:

$$R1_{post} - R1_{pre} = r_1 \times C \tag{1}$$

where $R1_{post}$ is the postcontrast longitudinal relaxation rate, $R1_{pre}$ is the precontrast longitudinal relaxation rate, r_1 is the longitudinal relaxivity of the contrast agent, and C is its concentration. This equation assumes that the relaxivity of the contrast agent is the same in blood and tissue, and that exchanges of water between intravascular, extravascular, and intracellular spaces are fast.[8]

However, this method is sensitive to the nonuniformity of the transmitted B_1 field as well as to the nonlinearity of the RF transmission chain that affects small flip angles in particular, especially with 2D acquisitions. This can be corrected using a B_1 map. Moreover, these measurements should be obtained from 3D images because of the imperfect slice selection profile of 2D images. Finally, a simple linear relationship between signal intensity and contrast agent concentrations is often assumed. In this case, low contrast agent concentrations (0.025 mmol/kg) and/or lower injection rates should be used to avoid saturation of signal enhancement at high concentrations. The pulse sequence setting should also be carefully performed to minimize the nonlinearity effect. While most groups use conventional gadolinium chelates, recent studies have reported the use of specific hepatobiliary contrast agents with similar results.[10]

The Technical Challenges of Liver Perfusion Analysis

Pandharipande et al.[11] published a list of requirements for an ideal liver perfusion analysis:

- Accurate quantification of overall or regional arterial and portal perfusion to assess focal or diffuse abnormalities
- High spatial resolution to examine small lesions
- High temporal resolution to correctly identify the kinetic properties of tracers, which may differ within tissue lesions
- Accurate quantitative analysis by measuring concentrations of reliable tracers
- Robust modeling of the physiology of liver perfusion
- "Whole-liver" imaging
- Compatibility with morphologic imaging modalities so that complementary perfusion studies can be performed with more conventional studies

This list highlights the difficulties of studying the liver. Besides the well-known limitations of MRI—such as accessibility and cost—liver perfusion imaging involves several specific challenges and limitations that result in significant variability of results, in particular, the difficulty of accurately modeling liver perfusion and the size and mobility of this organ.

Liver Perfusion Modeling

Perfusion analysis relies entirely on the analysis of tracer concentration–time curves whose shape depends on tissue perfusion parameters, the characteristics of the tracer bolus (volume, injection rate), and the patient's cardiovascular parameters (cardiac output, ejection fraction).

There are two main mathematical approaches to studying liver perfusion (Fig. 27-3): The semiquantitative approach based on the shape of the signal intensity/time curves (descriptive methods) and the quantitative approach based on concentration–time curves using a perfusion model (pharmacokinetic approach).

Descriptive methods of signal intensity/time curves are not based on any physiologic hypothesis (free models). Computers can be used to automate shape recognition of the enhancement process to create enhancement maps and detect areas of interest (e.g., hypervascular areas). Several descriptive or "heuristic" parameters can be analyzed from the tissue enhancement curve, such as the slope of enhancement (maximum slope), maximum enhancement (peak height) expressed in a percentage and the time to peak. Hepatic perfusion index (HPI) is another semiquantitative parameter that describes the relative contribution of arterial flow or portal flow to the total (arterial + portal) liver perfusion and can be easily calculated using different imaging techniques. HPI reflects the amount of arterial supply to the tumor or liver and its calculation does not require AIF or modeling. The time to peak in the splenic enhancement curve is used to distinguish between the arterial and portal venous phases of the liver. For perfusion analysis, the radiologist will place ROIs in the aorta, main portal vein, normal liver parenchyma, lesion, and the spleen. Liver arterial or venous perfusion will be estimated by the maximum slope in the liver enhancement curve before or after the splenic peak, respectively, divided by the peak aortic enhancement.

It should be noted that descriptive parameters may be affected by the instability of curves due to liver and vessel displacement. The area under the curve (AUC), that is, the integral under the enhancement curve, is a common parameter, because it is less affected by noise and does not require a mathematical model.[12] Finally, raw semiquantitative evaluation does not take into account the intra-arterial kinetics of the contrast agent, which may differ significantly among patients depending on the injection protocol (volume, concentration, injection rate, etc.) and physiologic conditions (respiration, cardiac output). They can be corrected by comparing results to those of a reference tissue such as muscle tissue or a nonpathologic portion of the liver. Correction is performed by calculating ratios to obtain relative parameters. These simple approaches may be very sensitive to the quality of the acquisitions.

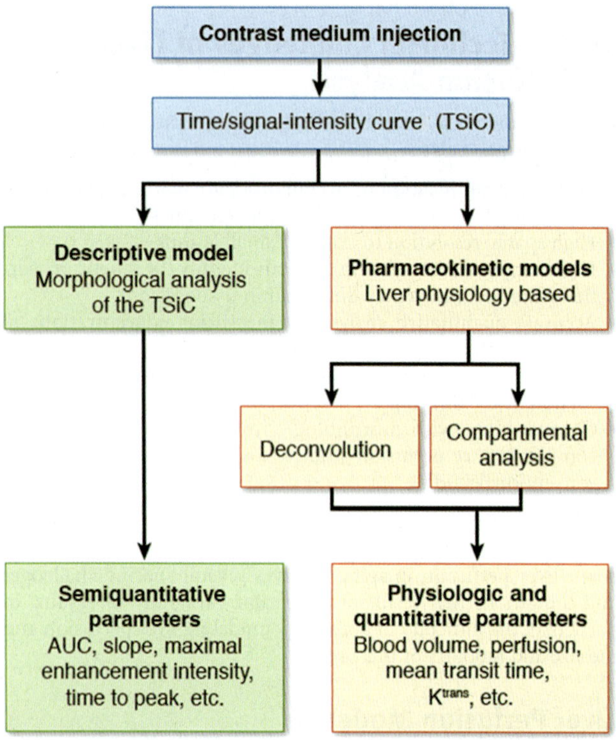

Figure 27-3. Schematic representation of the different models used in liver perfusion imaging analysis. (AUC, area under the curve.)

Pharmacokinetic models incorporate specific characteristics of liver perfusion. These models are based on the relationship between arterial input alone (in tumors for instance) and arterial and portal input (in diffuse liver disease), obtained from the enhancement curve of the afferent blood vessels. Deconvolution algorithms and compartmental models[13,14] belong to this category. The latter are based on the assumption that contrast enhancement is present in several hepatic compartments mixed in uniform concentrations, that flow between compartments is linear (passive exchange only) and that the parameters describing compartments do not vary during data acquisition. The parameters being studied are then extracted, depending on the models, which vary in the number of compartments and afferent blood vessels. Normal liver tissue can be considered a single compartment since there is free passage of contrast between the sinusoid (intravascular compartment) and the space of Disse (extravascular component). Therefore, in normal liver tissue, parameters related to extravasation of contrast into the interstitial space (such as permeability–surface area product) are not measurable. In contrast, in cirrhosis, the sinusoids become capillary-like and increased deposition of collagen in the space of Disse separates the intravascular from the extravascular space and contrast kinetics in the interstitial space become measurable.[13]

The T1 relaxation rate (i.e., tracer concentration) versus time curves can be analyzed with a dual-input model in the liver because it has two vascular inputs. The dual-input, single-compartmental model validated by Materne et al.[8] is often used. The arterial, portal venous, and total liver blood transfer constants K_{1a}, K_{1p}, and K_{1t}, respectively (mL/min/100 mL) can be assessed with this model as well as the distribution volume (DV) (%) and the mean transit time (MTT) (s) ($1/k_2$).

K_1 represents total perfusion and permeability as follows:

$$K_1 = F \times E \tag{2}$$

where F is the perfusion and E is the extraction fraction, varying between 0 and 1. When permeability is high as in the normal liver—which has fenestrated sinusoids—the extraction fraction equals 1 and K_1 represents perfusion. If permeability is low, K_1 represents PS, the permeability–surface area product.[15] To measure vascular input, an ROI is placed in the portal vein and the abdominal aorta to be used as a surrogate for hepatic arterial blood supply. For dual-input one-compartment models, it is mandatory to include two delays (arterial and portal) in the model to take into account the temporal offset between central compartment input and measured input from arterial and portal ROIs.[9] Nevertheless, the addition of two fitting parameters in the model increases the degree of freedom involving local minima problems. Thus, some groups have proposed to fix the delays manually. While arterial delay can be simply estimated from a curve analysis, manual estimation of portal delay is tricky. To address this issue, some groups have assumed the equality between portal and arterial delays. This approach has two main limitations. First, since delays spatially vary (depending on the ROI location), this approach is restricted to small ROI analysis and unsuited for mapping. Secondly, the assumption of equality between arterial and portal delays is very approximate since the delays are dependent on the blood flows. An alternative could be to include both delays in the model and to use an advanced optimization procedures such as multistart approaches for the fitting procedure. Classically, the modeling is achieved using solvers based on a nonlinear least square fit. These methods are prone to local minima problems mainly linked at the choice of starting values. Multistart methods, by repeating the fitting procedure with pseudorandom starting values reinitialized each time, uncorrelate the fitting procedure from the choice of starting values, and reduce local minima problem. The main limitation of these approaches is the computing time increase due to repetition of fitting procedure.

In contrast to the liver parenchyma, primary and secondary tumors of the liver, except very early stage, have only arterial but no portal venous input.[16] Therefore, the perfusion of hepatic tumors can be analyzed with single-input rather than dual-input models. There are several single-input models available to assess tumors. The most frequently used models include a simple single-compartmental model, known as the Tofts (or Kety) model in which K^{trans} (=K_1) and the extravascular extracellular volume ($v_e = v_d$) are assessed; the extended Tofts (or extended Kety) model (which takes into account the contribution of the tracer in the vascular space), in which K^{trans}, v_e, and plasma volume (v_p) are assessed; and the St. Lawrence and Lee model, which is a distributed-parameter model with four free parameters: tissue plasma flow (F), the extraction fraction (E), the extravascular extracellular volume (v_e), and the mean capillary transit time (MTT). The capillary permeability–surface area product (PS) and the plasma volume (v_p) can be derived from these parameters.[17] Although a consensus conference has been published,[18] there is still no consensus about the best model. The distributed St. Lawrence and Lee model is more physiologic with a separate calculation for perfusion and permeability, but is less precise than are the compartmental models due to the interdependency of the free parameters and their sensitivity to initial values. The problem of the uniqueness of the solutions may be even more complex when a dual-input distributed model is used, as recently proposed.[19] Thus, the extended Tofts model may be a good compromise to estimate perfusion parameters in tumors because neither data interpolation nor supervised fitting is required.[18]

The transfer constant K^{trans} and the extravascular extracellular volume v_e are the recommended primary and secondary end points, respectively, of perfusion measurements.[18] Both variables should be obtained, although the reproducibility of v_e is better than that of K^{trans} (repeatability coefficient of 30% for v_e vs. 100% for K^{trans}), and it can be used to assess vascular permeability by determining the volume accessible to contrast agents with different molecular wei ghts.[17,20,21] However, the data obtained are not independent from the model or the software package used for analysis. This has been clearly demonstrated with CT perfusion studies.[22]

The Liver Is a Mobile Organ

Radiographic studies using fixed landmarks, radioscopy, and even CT[23] have shown that the liver is an organ that moves considerably during breathing, shifting approximately 20 mm along its craniocaudal axis, 10 mm along its anteroposterior axis, and 5 mm laterally.

Due to long acquisition times (2 to 3 minutes) and because regular sampling is preferable for quantitative perfusion imaging, free-breathing acquisitions are highly recommended. Thus, to prevent pixel scale mismatches and to obtain diagnostic information from quantitative pharmacokinetic data analysis, correct registration of the different images/time points is essential.

In a noncoregistered data set of 2D + t images, respiratory motion may introduce "temporal noise" in both input and tissue functions, reducing the robustness of perfusion modeling. This effect is especially marked in portal input function because of portal trunk orientation in relation to the main motion (craniocaudal). To reduce this effect, coronal rather than axial views may be acquired. Another possibility is to include a registration-based motion correction method in the postprocessing chain.

Several registration-based methods correct respiratory motion and are classified according to the search space used (rigid, elastic, and optical flow). Rigid search spaces are based on matrix algebra, in which a single matrix characterizes the transformation of the entire image or volume. Typical operations include translation, rotation, isotropic or anisotropic scaling, bi- or trilinear transformation, and quadratics. Elastic search spaces allow the transformation parameters to exhibit spatial dependence. These parameters are often defined by certain key points only and interpolated on a region-by-region basis. Optical flow is a result of a continuous functional optimization scheme, in which independent displacement is computed for each point in the image, with constraints arising from a priori regularization.

These methods can be also classified according to the reference image feature, including methods based on a geometric approach or an iconic approach. Geometric approaches use landmarks or geometric primitives (curves or surfaces) chosen manually by the user or semiautomatically by segmentation algorithms (snake, mathematical morphology operators, and level set). Similarity functions used to quantify the transformation matrix are based on distance (euclidian norm, iterative closest point, head and hat algorithm). Iconic approaches use the entire pixel, and the similarity functions are based on pixel intensity or on information theory such as minimization of the sum of squared intensity difference, correlations, minimization of the variance of intensity ratio, minimization of joint entropy, or maximization of mutual information.

Quantitative perfusion imaging is limited by the "semiautomatic" aspect of geometric approaches in relation to the number of co-registered sequences (normally between 100 and 200 dynamics, depending on the temporal resolution). Moreover, landmark locations are user dependent and could reduce reproducibility. Nevertheless, these approaches seem to be more accurate than are fully automatic iconic approaches in this context. Indeed, similarity functions used by iconic methods assume that the differences in intensity between images are only due to gaussian noise, while geometric approaches are based on anatomical information providing high level and more discriminative information. However, data are often oversimplified by landmarks and geometric primitives.

In conclusion, the "ideal method" to correct respiratory motion artifacts in quantitative perfusion imaging of the liver is still a challenge. If we assume that liver displacement induced by respiratory motion does not deform liver volume, rigid registration based motion correction by the geometric approach seems to be the most accurate existing approach.

The Liver Is a Large Organ

Time-resolved sequences are necessary to accurately sample tracer kinetics for quantitative perfusion. High spatial resolution and/or extensive coverage are also important, but both decrease maximum temporal resolution. Thus, imaging of dynamic processes usually involves a compromise between temporal resolution, spatial resolution, and spatial coverage. As a result, spatial resolution and exploratory volume are often reduced to obtain satisfactory temporal resolution, which can create a problem for small lesions or diffuse diseases with locoregional variations.

Partial k-space updating methods can also be used. The 4D sequences will probably help resolve this issue. These sequences combine a keyhole acquisition and an optimized k-space filling. Keyhole acquisition is based on the assumption that dynamic information is band limited in k-space. The keyhole methods repeatedly update data in the center of k-space more frequently than in other parts of k-space. For each dynamic, only a central elliptical cylinder of the k-space (low frequencies including dynamic information) is refreshed with a random readout. Dynamic sequences are followed or preceded by the readout of the periphery of k-space (high frequencies including static information). This technique drastically decreases the acquisition time of dynamic. These acquisitions may be combined with parallel and partial Fourier imaging to decrease the dynamic acquisition time further. In this way, it is possible to use the time gained to add slices and cover the entire liver, with adequate spatial and temporal resolution. The k-space filling scheme used in these sequences also reduces motion sensitivity, which is an important issue for free-breathing perfusion imaging.

The Reproducibility Issue

Variability of the results depending on the model or the software, the patient's breathing, and perfusion analysis limited to a portion of the liver, results in significant intra- and interpatient variability. For instance, Ng et al.[24] have shown that the intrapatient coefficients of variation of K^{trans} and the initial AUC for liver lesions were 8.9% and 9.9%. In that study, a 20% reduction of a parameter value due to the treatment resulted, in a given patient, in confidence estimates changes ranging from 71% to 87%. Finally, reproducibility of the perfusion parameters of the IVIM model has also been shown to be poor, limiting their use in routine clinical practice.[25,26] Thus, reproducibility should be assessed before beginning clinical trials with perfusion MRI of the liver.

Clinical Applications

The two main clinical applications of liver perfusion imaging are liver oncology and chronic liver diseases. Imaging is important in both cases for the noninvasive detection and characterization of solid focal liver lesions, treatment evaluation, and patient follow-up. Because of its limitations especially in relation to spatial resolution and because of the difficulty of this technique and the learning curve, the goal is not to compare perfusion imaging with conventional imaging techniques such as ultrasound, computed tomography, MRI, or positron tomography emission. It is more interesting to determine the potential benefits of adding perfusion imaging to the conventional imaging protocol, and its influence on patient management and access to earlier or more accurate disease assessment.

Liver Oncology

A combination of conventional imaging techniques has been shown to be highly accurate in detecting and characterizing lesions. Thus, indications for DCE-MRI are limited and it is not performed in routine clinical practice. Imaging is also needed to evaluate antitumoral locoregional or systemic treatments. The Response Evaluation Criteria in Solid Tumors (RECIST) guidelines were recently approved as a standard method to evaluate tumor response in patients in clinical trials and are considered to be a surrogate endpoint to predict survival in patients with solid tumors.[27,28] Other imaging criteria have been evaluated in the liver and other organs to assess the efficacy of treatment on tumor vascularization based on changes in contrast-enhanced images.[29–31] These morphologic criteria are obtained several weeks after the initiation of treatment to identify responders and nonresponders. Thus, nonresponders who could benefit from an early change in treatment are assessed later, which could influence outcome. Functional techniques such as perfusion imaging could discriminate responders from nonresponders earlier because they record microscopic phenomenon and might even predict patient response before treatment begins.

Detection and Characterization of Focal Liver Lesions

Most studies have focused on DCE-MRI in HCC and liver metastases. Alicioglu et al.[32] showed differences between liver hemangiomas, HCC, and metastases using semiquantitative descriptive models and the best parameter was the AUC. The pattern of tissue signal intensity–time curve may help to differentiate tumors. Hypervascular tumors usually have a larger vascular space relative to the interstitial space and demonstrate rapid arterial enhancement followed by washout. In contrast, a hypovascular tumor with a larger interstitial space relative to the vascular space (e.g., colorectal metastasis) shows progressive enhancement from arterial to portal and to equilibrium phases. Recently, Yoon et al. and Penner et al.[33,34] published their experience with the IVIM model and showed that pseudodiffusion and the vascular fraction were significantly higher in hypervascular than in hypovascular focal liver lesions, although these parameters did not seem to improve the characterization of focal liver lesions with MRI.[35] DCE-MRI can improve the detection of hypervascular tumors, especially HCC, which show transient enhancement during the arterial phase.[36]

However, most studies in HCC have evaluated the characterization of lesions to assess tissue differentiation and distinguish dysplastic nodules and HCC. Arterial hepatic blood flow and the arterial fraction were found to be higher, while the DV and portal venous hepatic blood flow were significantly lower in HCC compared to the liver parenchyma.[37] Similar results have been found with perfusion CT,[38,39] suggesting that perfusion techniques can provide quantitative information about tumor-related angiogenesis in patients with cirrhosis and HCC. Another study identified a correlation between IVIM model perfusion parameters and hypervascularity,[40] although reproducibility of these results was poor.[25] Perfusion parameters (evaluated by perfusion CT) were correlated with tumor differentiation; well-differentiated HCC had significantly higher perfusion values than did other grades.[41]

The presence of overt liver metastases results in hemodynamic changes including an increase in arterial perfusion and a decrease in portal perfusion. This was first shown on scintigraphy and CT scan[42–44] and has been confirmed in MRI.[45] However, these changes are of limited use because the tumors were already visible with morphologic imaging techniques. Studies showing similar results in occult liver metastases (with either Doppler or perfusion CT)[46–48] are of more interest, although results have not been confirmed in humans. A multicenter French institutional CT study including approximately 400 patients until 2012 has evaluated whether liver perfusion parameters are significantly different in patients with colon cancer who develop liver metastases than in those who do not.

Assessing Response to Treatment

Locoregional Therapies

Perfusion studies of locoregional treatment of liver tumors, especially HCC do not provide additional information during percutaneous ablation (using radiofrequency or microwave) because the tumor response and recurrence criteria are well described and robust.[49,50] In a study of perfusion CT by Meijerink et al.,[51] blood volume was shown to be useful for detecting recurrence in contact with ablation zones, but similar results were not reported with MRI.

Numerous studies have been published about transarterial chemoembolization using either perfusion CT or MRI. Treatment involves the selective intra-arterial injection of different chemotherapy molecules, either mixed with iodized oil—the conventional approach—or with loaded drug delivery beads. The arterial supply in the tumor is interrupted in both techniques either by injection of embolic agents during conventional treatment or due to the embolic effect of the loaded particles. Thus, significant modifications in tumoral and peritumoral perfusion parameters can be expected following chemoembolization. Choi et al. prospectively evaluated the feasibility of perfusion CT to follow-up hepatic artery chemoembolization in rabbits and showed early changes in perfusion (at 1 week) in treated compared to untreated areas. They concluded that perfusion CT could help assess the rapid response to treatment and detect early tumor recurrence.[52] There are very few studies in humans. Ippolito et al.[53] obtained perfusion parameters in tumor residues following transarterial chemoembolization, and found differences between completely and incompletely treated tumors similar to those of Choi et al. in animals.

Results from a rabbit model have validated the use of DCE-MRI to quantify tumor perfusion after several sequences of embolization.[54] A group from Chicago has also reported significant changes in perfusion during embolization using a descriptive semiquantitative approach.[55–57] As expected, they found a significant decrease in the AUC of time–intensity curves of tumors following treatment. Similar results were reported by Taouli et al.,[37] who showed a higher arterial fraction and lower portal venous hepatic blood flow value in untreated HCCs than in those treated with transarterial chemoembolization. These studies may suggest that perfusion imaging provide information equivalent to conventional techniques based on the morphologic modifications induced by treatment, and therefore, may be of limited in this setting. The use of perfusion imaging to show early changes related to tumoral necrosis or to predict good or poor responders, might be a more interesting indication for this technique. Recently, Braren et al.[58] showed that the extravascular extracellular volume fraction $v_{(e)}$ assessed by DCE-MRI 1 day after an embolization procedure in a rodent model was promising for the prediction of tumor necrosis. Michielsen et al.[59] showed that pretreatment perfusion parameters before transarterial chemoembolization were predictive of progression-free survival, independent of tumor size and number of lesions.[59]

Selective internal radiation therapy (SIRT) is a locoregional technique that has been found to be of interest in malignant liver tumors.[60] Radioactive microspheres are injected into the arteries that feed the tumors. Like other intra-arterial procedures, SIRT is usually performed in unresectable tumors and in patients with diffuse, infiltrating, and/or multifocal disease. Unlike transarterial chemoembolization, it is difficult to assess tumor response because most changes occur 3 to 6 months after treatment. Morsbach et al.[61] recently published preliminary results with perfusion CT in a series of colorectal liver metastases treated with SIRT. The authors showed that a significant difference in arterial perfusion was found in pretreatment CT perfusion between responders and nonresponders and that 1-year survival was significantly higher in patients with a high pretreatment arterial perfusion. There are no published data on the use of DCE-MRI.

Systemic Chemotherapy and Targeted Therapies

Systematic treatment of liver metastases, especially colorectal, is based on cytotoxic agents that can be associated with targeted therapy. In contrast, the only systemic treatment that has been shown to benefit overall survival in advanced HCC is targeted therapy (sorafenib). This explains the differences in imaging criteria for tumoral response, because cytotoxic agents can cause tumor shrinkage, while targeted therapies are known to result in sustained tumor stabilization and reduce tumor vascularization provoking tumor necrosis. Thus, the determination of changes in perfusion following targeted therapy could be of major interest (Figs. 27-4 and 27-5). Although DCE-MRI is rarely used in oncologic trials for the moment, certain studies have included this functional technique in their study design together with conventional tumoral evaluation criteria such as RECIST.

Hsu et al.[62] performed DCE-MRI before treatment and after 14 days of treatment in a phase II study evaluating "sorafenib" combined with metronomic tegafur/uracil as first-line therapy for advanced HCC.[62] They selected the most contrast-enhanced region of the tumor and measured the volume transfer constant, K^{trans}. The baseline K^{trans} was significantly higher in patients in whom the disease was controlled than in those with progressive disease, and it significantly decreased after treatment. A vascular response, defined as a ≥40% decrease in K^{trans} after treatment, was associated with improved Progression free survival (PFS) and Overall survival (OS). Another study evaluating "sunitinib" in the treatment of advanced HCC found a significant decrease in K^{trans} in all patients, and a greater decrease in patients with controlled disease than in those with progressive disease.[63]

Most published studies evaluating liver metastases have focused on colorectal metastases treated with targeted therapies in combination with conventional cytotoxic agents, and similar results have been reported with K^{trans} and other perfusion parameters. Coenegrachts et al.[64] showed that the baseline K_{ep} was significantly higher in responders than in nonresponders and that responders had a significant decrease in K_{ep} after 6 weeks of treatment. De Bruyne et al.[65] showed an improvement in progression-free survival in patients with a greater than 40% reduction in K^{trans}. These results were supported by those from Hirashima et al.[66] in lesions treated with bevacizumab and FOLFIRI showing that a variation in both K^{trans} and K_{ep} as early as 1 week after treatment could help predict response to chemotherapy. There are very few studies on other liver metastases, such as neuroendocrine tumors, but existing results are consistent with those observed in colorectal liver metastases.[67]

Chronic Liver Disease

The development and progression of liver fibrosis to cirrhosis is associated with microarchitectural vascular changes and modified perfusion: sinusoids gradually convert into continuous nonfenestrated capillaries with an organized basal membrane containing laminin, an increase in vascular resistance and a decrease in portal perfusion, partly compensated by an increase in arterial perfusion (buffer response) and later by an overall decrease in global perfusion.

The first studies evaluating chronic liver diseases with perfusion CT were published in the 1990s. Miles et al. and Blomley et al.[68,69] described the buffer response, and Van Beers et al.[70] reported an increase in the arterial fraction and MTT in a group of patients with cirrhosis compared to a control group using a compartmental model.[70] They also confirmed the decrease in total liver blood flow in patients with cirrhosis compared to controls. The increase in MTT was attributed to the reduced mobility of low molecular weight tracer molecules in the space of Disse in fibrotic livers, since mobility was preserved and the distribution of volumes was unchanged. We recently showed that perfusion CT could identify the early stages of fibrosis.[71]

There are fewer DCE-MRI studies in chronic liver diseases. Studies in animal models[8,72,73] have confirmed previous results. In patients with cirrhosis, Annet et al. and Baxter et al.[74,75] described a reduction in portal perfusion and an increase in both arterial perfusion and MTT. Perfusion changes were also observed at intermediate stages of liver fibrosis,[74,76] but were more marked in cirrhosis, where they were correlated with the degree of liver dysfunction and portal hypertension.[74] Although it must be

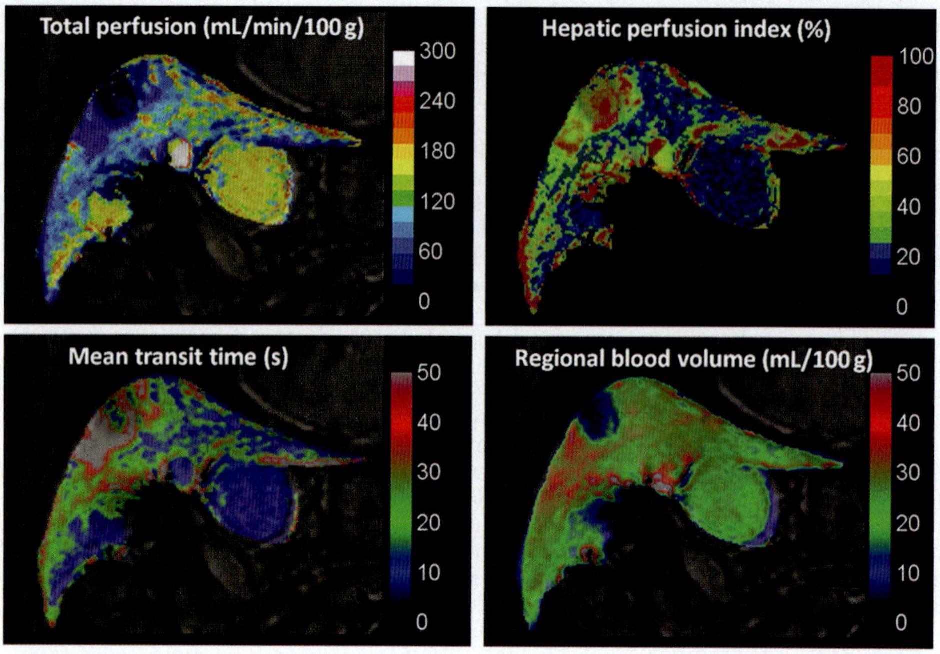

A

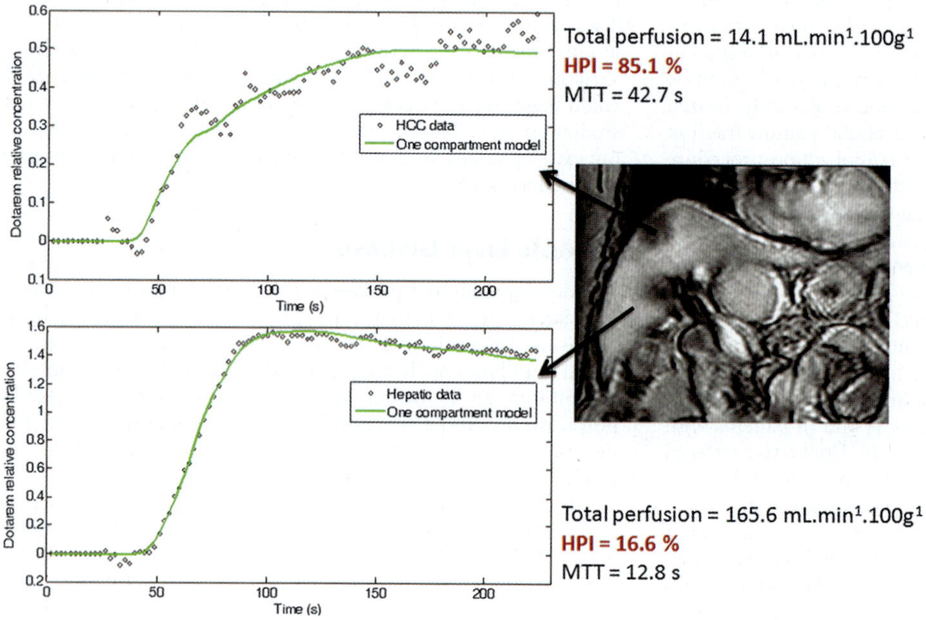

B

Figure 27-4. A: Example of perfusion parametric maps (arterial, portal and total perfusion, hepatic perfusion index, mean transit time, and regional blood volume) obtained from a patient with hepatocarcinoma 7 days after the initiation of sorafenib treatment. These maps were computed from images acquired with a 3D FLASH acquisition with 2.0 seconds temporal resolution. Gd-DOTA was used as a tracer. Perfusion parameters were extracted using a nonlinear least square fit on a dual-input one-compartment model including two delays (arterial and portal). **B:** The lesion was located in the dome of the liver. Comparison between the lesion **(upper part)** and the surrounding liver **(lower part)**. The lesion showed a significant total perfusion decrease, with significant hepatic perfusion index (HPI) and mean transit time (MTT) increase consistent with a tumoral response to the treatment.

confirmed, this suggests that DCE-MRI could be useful in assessing the different stages of fibrosis and the severity of cirrhosis (Fig. 27-6).

Another approach to evaluate the microvascular disorders in patients with chronic liver disease is the IVIM model. One experimental study showed that rats with liver fibrosis had reduced in vivo ADC (apparent diffusion coefficient) values compared to controls, although this difference disappeared ex vivo.[14] A study published by Luciani et al.[77] in patients with cirrhosis confirmed the decrease in ADC in the former compared to controls, and showed that the restriction in diffusion was largely due to changes in microperfusion and to a lesser extent to a reduction in pure hepatic diffusion. These results were confirmed by Yoon et al.[78] in patients with chronic liver disease, and by Chow et al. and Zhang et al.[79,80] in rodents. More recently, several teams have investigated the IVIM model for the assessment of steatohepatitis with contradictory results. A study by Lee et al. did not show any significant correlation between the hepatic fat fraction and IVIM-assessed perfusion parameters,[81] while Guiu et al.[82] found a reduction in "pseudodiffusion" reflecting decreased parenchymal perfusion in steatosis. Finally, in a study in rabbits by Joo et al.,[83] the perfusion fraction was found to be significantly lower in rabbits with nonalcoholic fatty liver disease (NAFLD) than in controls with a progressive decrease in this fraction as the severity of NAFLD increased. IVIM parameters are probably affected by liver steatosis, but further studies are needed to confirm these results.

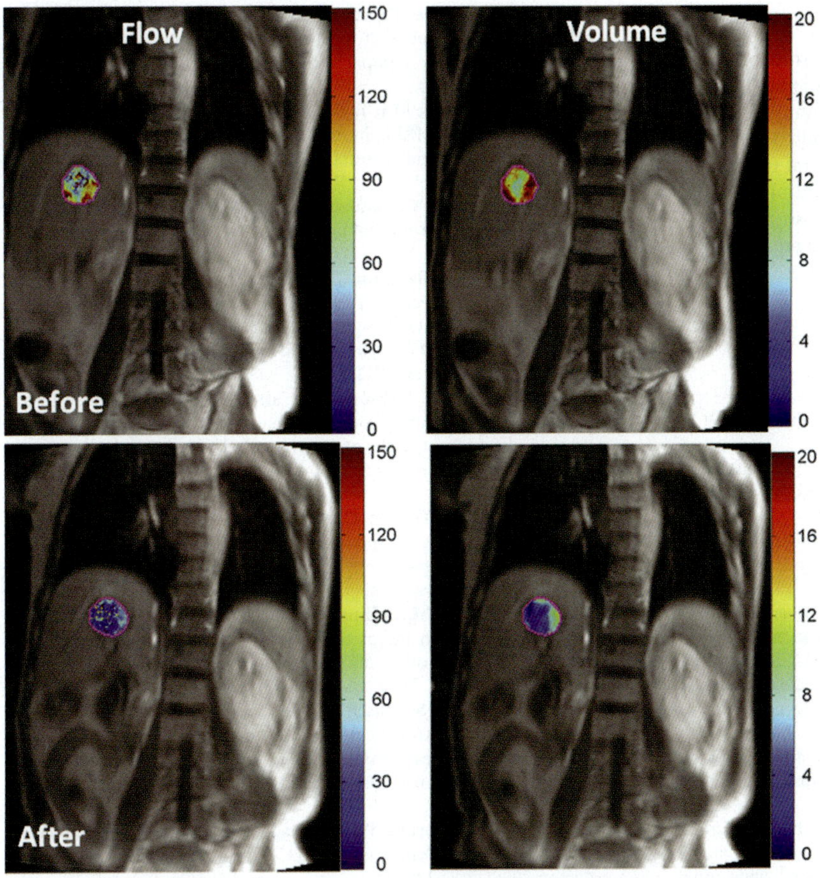

Figure 27-5. Decrease in flow (mL/min/100 mL) and percentage of intravascular space volume (mL/100 mL) evaluated by dual-input distributed parameter model in a 59-year-old man with HCC after therapy with antiangiogenic therapy (a combination of sorafenib and selumetinib). The decrease after therapy can be appreciated by a change in color from the red spectrum toward the blue spectrum. (From Thng CH, Koh TS, Collins DJ, et al. Perfusion imaging in liver MRI. *Magn Reson Imaging Clin N Am* 2014;22(3):417–432., with permission.)

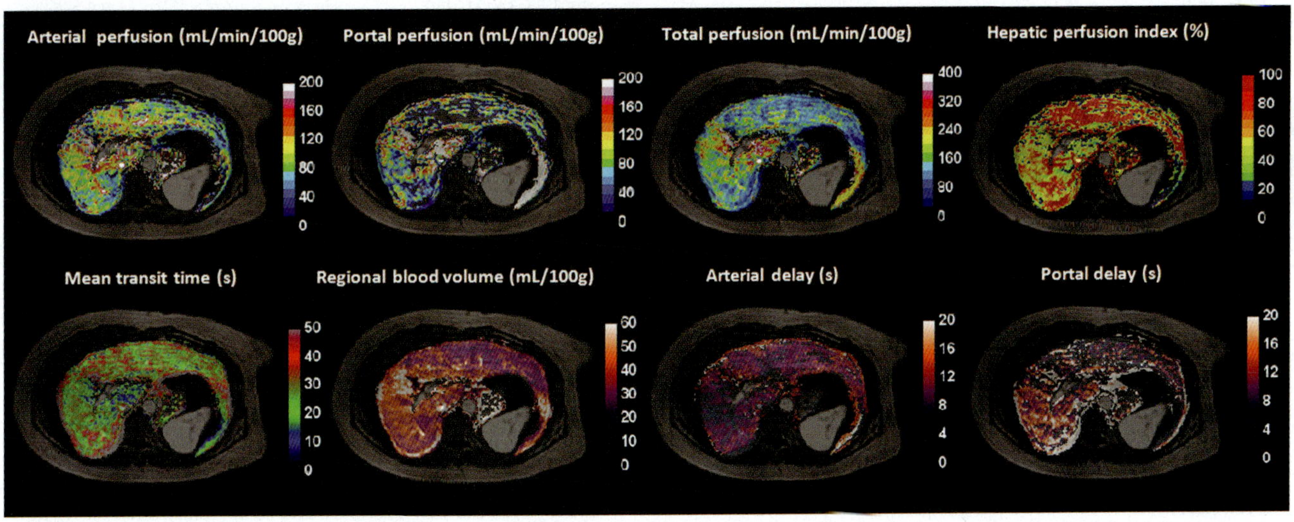

Figure 27-6. Example of perfusion parametric maps (arterial, portal, and total perfusion, hepatic perfusion index, mean transit time, and regional blood volume) obtained from a patient with cirrhosis. These maps were computed from images acquired with a 4D keyhole acquisition with 1.7 seconds temporal resolution. Gd-DOTA was used as a tracer. Perfusion parameters were extracted using a nonlinear least square fit on a dual-input one-compartment model including to delays (arterial and portal). These maps well illustrate the adaptive response in the liver aiming to counterbalance the portal perfusion drop by increasing arterial perfusion in order to keep the total perfusion. This explains the significant rise in the hepatic perfusion index. Mean transit time increased illustrating the restriction of the low molecular weight tracer molecules in the Disse due to collagen deposition in liver cirrhosis. Mean perfusion parameters values were—arterial, portal, and total perfusion: 72, 54, and 126 mL/min/100 g, respectively; hepatic perfusion index: 57.1%; mean transit time: 27.2 seconds; and regional blood volume: 57.1 mL/100 g.

Conclusions

Perfusion imaging is not part of the routine MRI protocol in the liver. For the moment, this technique is usually performed in clinical and experimental research. Results are encouraging, showing the potential use of this technique in liver tumors and chronic liver diseases mainly for the early evaluation of antitumoral treatments and the staging of fibrosis. However, like other quantitative tools, acquisition, mathematical algorithms, and postprocessing of DCE–MRI must be standardized to increase clinical use and reproducibility. Indeed, large multicenter studies are necessary before perfusion parameters can be considered reliable biomarkers.

REFERENCES

1. **Itai Y, Matsui O.** Blood flow and liver imaging. *Radiology* 1997;202(2):306–314.
2. **Scharf J, Zapletal C, Hess T, et al.** Assessment of hepatic perfusion in pigs by pharmacokinetic analysis of dynamic MR images. *J Magn Reson Imaging* 1999;9(4):568–572.
3. **Katada Y, Shukuya T, Kawashima M, et al.** A comparative study between arterial spin labeling and CT perfusion methods on hepatic portal venous flow. *Jpn J Radiol* 2012;30(10):863–869.
4. **St. Lawrence KS, Owen D, Wang DJ.** A two-stage approach for measuring vascular water exchange and arterial transit time by diffusion-weighted perfusion MRI. *Magn Reson Med* 2012;67(5):1275–1284.
5. **Gillis P, Peto S, Moiny F, et al.** Proton transverse nuclear magnetic relaxation in oxidized blood: a numerical approach. *Magn Reson Med* 1995;33(1):93–100.
6. **Le Bihan D, Breton E, Lallemand D, et al.** MR imaging of intravoxel incoherent motions: application to diffusion and perfusion in neurologic disorders. *Radiology* 1986;161(2):401–407.
7. **Beck GM, De Becker J, Jones AC, et al.** Contrast-enhanced timing robust acquisition order with a preparation of the longitudinal signal component (CENTRA plus) for 3D contrast-enhanced abdominal imaging. *J Magn Reson Imaging* 2008;27(6):1461–1467.
8. **Materne R, Smith AM, Peeters F, et al.** Assessment of hepatic perfusion parameters with dynamic MRI. *Magn Reson Med* 2002;47(1):135–142.
9. **Leporq B, Dumortier J, Pilleul F, et al.** 3D-liver perfusion MRI with the MS-325 blood pool agent: a noninvasive protocol to asses liver fibrosis. *J Magn Reson Imaging* 2012;35(6):1380–1387.
10. **Sourbron S, Sommer WH, Reiser MF, et al.** Combined quantification of liver perfusion and function with dynamic gadoxetic acid-enhanced MR imaging. *Radiology* 2012;263(3):874–883.
11. **Pandharipande PV, Krinsky GA, Rusinek H, et al.** Perfusion imaging of the liver: current challenges and future goals. *Radiology* 2005;234(3):661–673.
12. **Roberts C, Issa B, Stone A, et al.** Comparative study into the robustness of compartmental modeling and model-free analysis in DCE-MRI studies. *J Magn Reson Imaging* 2006;23(4):554–563.
13. **Thng CH, Koh TS, Collins DJ, et al.** Perfusion imaging in liver MRI. *Magn Reson Imaging Clin N Am* 2014;22(3):417–432.
14. **Annet L, Peeters F, Abarca-Quinones J, et al.** Assessment of diffusion-weighted MR imaging in liver fibrosis. *J Magn Reson Imaging* 2007;25(1):122–128.
15. **Tofts PS, Brix G, Buckley DL, et al.** Estimating kinetic parameters from dynamic contrast-enhanced T(1)-weighted MRI of a diffusable tracer: standardized quantities and symbols. *J Magn Reson Imaging* 1999;10(3):223–232.
16. **Liu Y, Matsui O.** Changes of intratumoral microvessels and blood perfusion during establishment of hepatic metastases in mice. *Radiology* 2007;243(2):386–395.
17. **Michoux N, Huwart L, Abarca-Quinones J, et al.** Transvascular and interstitial transport in rat hepatocellular carcinomas: dynamic contrast-enhanced MRI assessment with low- and high-molecular weight agents. *J Magn Reson Imaging* 2008;28(4):906–914.
18. **Leach MO, Brindle KM, Evelhoch JL, et al.** Assessment of antiangiogenic and antivascular therapeutics using MRI: recommendations for appropriate methodology for clinical trials. *Br J Radiol* 2003;76 (Spec No. 1):S87–S91.
19. **Koh TS, Thng CH, Lee PS, et al.** Hepatic metastases: in vivo assessment of perfusion parameters at dynamic contrast-enhanced MR imaging with dual-input two-compartment tracer kinetics model. *Radiology* 2008;249(1):307–320.
20. **Galbraith SM, Lodge MA, Taylor NJ, et al.** Reproducibility of dynamic contrast-enhanced MRI in human muscle and tumours: comparison of quantitative and semi-quantitative analysis. *NMR Biomed* 2002;15(2):132–142.
21. **Padhani AR, Hayes C, Landau S, et al.** Reproducibility of quantitative dynamic MRI of normal human tissues. *NMR Biomed* 2002;15(2):143–153.
22. **Goh V, Halligan S, Bartram CI.** Quantitative tumor perfusion assessment with multidetector CT: are measurements from two commercial software packages interchangeable? *Radiology* 2007;242(3):777–782.
23. **Langen KM, Jones DT.** Organ motion and its management. *Int J Radiat Oncol Biol Phys* 2001;50(1):265–278.
24. **Ng CS, Raunig DL, Jackson EF, et al.** Reproducibility of perfusion parameters in dynamic contrast-enhanced MRI of lung and liver tumors: effect on estimates of patient sample size in clinical trials and on individual patient responses. *AJR Am J Roentgenol* 2010;194(2):W134–W140.
25. **Kakite S, Dyvorne H, Besa C, et al.** Hepatocellular carcinoma: short-term reproducibility of apparent diffusion coefficient and intravoxel incoherent motion parameters at 3.0 T [Epub ahead of print January 10, 2014]. *J Magn Reson Imaging.*
26. **Andreou A, Koh DM, Collins DJ, et al.** Measurement reproducibility of perfusion fraction and pseudodiffusion coefficient derived by intravoxel incoherent motion diffusion-weighted MR imaging in normal liver and metastases. *Eur Radiol* 2013;23(2):428–434.
27. **Therasse P, Arbuck SG, Eisenhauer EA, et al.** New guidelines to evaluate the response to treatment in solid tumors. European Organization for Research and Treatment of Cancer, National Cancer Institute of the United States, National Cancer Institute of Canada. *J Natl Cancer Inst* 2000;92(3):205–216.
28. **Eisenhauer EA, Therasse P, Bogaerts J, et al.** New response evaluation criteria in solid tumours: revised RECIST guideline (version 1.1). *Eur J Cancer* 2009;45(2):228–247.
29. **Bruix J, Sherman M, Llovet JM, et al.** Clinical management of hepatocellular carcinoma. Conclusions of the Barcelona-2000 EASL conference. European Association for the Study of the Liver. *J Hepatol* 2001;35(3):421–430.
30. **Lencioni R, Llovet JM.** Modified RECIST (mRECIST) assessment for hepatocellular carcinoma. *Semin Liver Dis* 2010;30(1):52–60.
31. **Choi H, Charnsangavej C, Faria SC, et al.** Correlation of computed tomography and positron emission tomography in patients with metastatic gastrointestinal stromal tumor treated at a single institution with imatinib mesylate: proposal of new computed tomography response criteria. *J Clin Oncol* 2007;25(13):1753–1759.
32. **Alicioglu B, Guler O, Bulakbasi N, et al.** Utility of semiquantitative parameters to differentiate benign and malignant focal hepatic lesions. *Clin Imaging* 2013;37(4):692–696.
33. **Yoon JH, Lee JM, Yu MH, et al.** Evaluation of hepatic focal lesions using diffusion-weighted MR imaging: comparison of apparent diffusion coefficient and intravoxel incoherent motion-derived parameters. *J Magn Reson Imaging* 2014;39(2):276–285.
34. **Penner AH, Sprinkart AM, Kukuk GM, et al.** Intravoxel incoherent motion model-based liver lesion characterisation from three b-value diffusion-weighted MRI. *Eur Radiol* 2013;23(10):2773–2783.
35. **Doblas S, Wagner M, Leitao HS, et al.** Determination of malignancy and characterization of hepatic tumor type with diffusion-weighted magnetic resonance imaging: comparison of apparent diffusion coefficient and intravoxel incoherent motion-derived measurements. *Invest Radiol* 2013;48(10):722–728.
36. **Takahashi N, Yoshioka H, Yamaguchi M, et al.** Accelerated dynamic MR imaging with a parallel imaging technique for hypervascular hepatocellular carcinomas: usefulness of a test bolus in examination and subtraction imaging. *J Magn Reson Imaging* 2003;18(1):80–89.
37. **Taouli B, Johnson RS, Hajdu CH, et al.** Hepatocellular carcinoma: perfusion quantification with dynamic contrast-enhanced MRI. *AJR Am J Roentgenol* 2013;201(4):795–800.
38. **Ippolito D, Sironi S, Pozzi M, et al.** Perfusion computed tomographic assessment of early hepatocellular carcinoma in cirrhotic liver disease: initial observations. *J Comput Assist Tomogr* 2008;32(6):855–858.

39. **Ippolito D, Sironi S, Pozzi M, et al.** Hepatocellular carcinoma in cirrhotic liver disease: functional computed tomography with perfusion imaging in the assessment of tumor vascularization. *Acad Radiol* 2008;15(7):919–927.
40. **Woo S, Lee JM, Yoon JH, et al.** Intravoxel incoherent motion diffusion-weighted MR imaging of hepatocellular carcinoma: correlation with enhancement degree and histologic grade. *Radiology* 2014;270(3):758–767.
41. **Sahani DV, Holalkere N-S, Mueller PR, et al.** Advanced hepatocellular carcinoma: CT perfusion of liver and tumor tissue—initial experience. *Radiology* 2007;243(3):736–743.
42. **Miles KA, Kelley BB.** Altered perfusion adjacent to hepatic metastases. *Clin Radiol* 1997;52(2):162–163.
43. **Leggett DA, Kelley BB, Bunce IH, et al.** Colorectal cancer: diagnostic potential of CT measurements of hepatic perfusion and implications for contrast enhancement protocols. *Radiology* 1997;205(3):716–720.
44. **Meijerink MR, van Waesberghe JH, van der Weide L, et al.** Total-liver-volume perfusion CT using 3-D image fusion to improve detection and characterization of liver metastases. *Eur Radiol* 2008;18(10):2345–2354.
45. **Totman JJ, O'Gorman RL, Kane PA, et al.** Comparison of the hepatic perfusion index measured with gadolinium-enhanced volumetric MRI in controls and in patients with colorectal cancer. *Br J Radiol* 2005;78(926):105–109.
46. **Leen E, Angerson WG, Cooke TG, et al.** Prognostic power of Doppler perfusion index in colorectal cancer. Correlation with survival. *Ann Surg* 1996;223(2):199–203.
47. **Tsushima Y, Blomley MJ, Yokoyama H, et al.** Does the presence of distant and local malignancy alter parenchymal perfusion in apparently disease-free areas of the liver? *Dig Dis Sci* 2001;46(10):2113–2119.
48. **Cuenod C, Leconte I, Siauve N, et al.** Early changes in liver perfusion caused by occult metastases in rats: detection with quantitative CT. *Radiology* 2001;218(2):556–561.
49. **Chopra S, Dodd GD III, Chintapalli KN, et al.** Tumor recurrence after radiofrequency thermal ablation of hepatic tumors: spectrum of findings on dual-phase contrast-enhanced CT. *AJR Am J Roentgenol* 2001;177(2):381–387.
50. **Forner A, Ayuso C, Varela M, et al.** Evaluation of tumor response after locoregional therapies in hepatocellular carcinoma: are response evaluation criteria in solid tumors reliable? *Cancer* 2009;115(3):616–623.
51. **Meijerink MR, van Waesberghe JH, van der Weide L, et al.** Early detection of local RFA site recurrence using total liver volume perfusion CT initial experience. *Acad Radiol* 2009;16(10):1215–1222.
52. **Choi SH, Chung JW, Kim HC, et al.** The role of perfusion CT as a follow-up modality after transcatheter arterial chemoembolization: an experimental study in a rabbit model. *Invest Radiol* 2010;45(7):427–436.
53. **Ippolito D, Bonaffini P-A, Ratti L, et al.** Hepatocellular carcinoma treated with transarterial chemoembolization: dynamic perfusion-CT in the assessment of residual tumor. *World J Gastroenterol* 2010;16(47):5993–6000.
54. **Wang D, Bangash AK, Rhee TK, et al.** Liver tumors: monitoring embolization in rabbits with VX2 tumors—transcatheter intraarterial first-pass perfusion MR imaging. *Radiology* 2007;245(1):130–139.
55. **Larson AC, Wang D, Atassi B, et al.** Transcatheter intraarterial perfusion: MR monitoring of chemoembolization for hepatocellular carcinoma—feasibility of initial clinical translation. *Radiology* 2008;246(3):964–971.
56. **Gaba RC, Wang D, Lewandowski RJ, et al.** Four-dimensional transcatheter intraarterial perfusion MR imaging for monitoring chemoembolization of hepatocellular carcinoma: preliminary results. *J Vasc Interv Radiol* 2008;19(11):1589–1595.
57. **Wang D, Jin B, Lewandowski RJ, et al.** Quantitative 4D transcatheter intraarterial perfusion MRI for monitoring chemoembolization of hepatocellular carcinoma. *J Magn Reson Imaging* 2010;31(5):1106–1116.
58. **Braren R, Altomonte J, Settles M, et al.** Validation of preclinical multiparametric imaging for prediction of necrosis in hepatocellular carcinoma after embolization. *J Hepatol* 2011;55(5):1034–1040.
59. **Michielsen K, De Keyzer F, Verslype C, et al.** Pretreatment DCE-MRI for prediction of PFS in patients with inoperable HCC treated with TACE. *Cancer Imaging* 2011;11(Spec No A):S114.
60. **Memon K, Lewandowski RJ, Kulik L, et al.** Radioembolization for primary and metastatic liver cancer. *Semin Radiat Oncol* 2011;21(4):294–302.
61. **Morsbach F, Pfammatter T, Reiner CS, et al.** Computed tomographic perfusion imaging for the prediction of response and survival to transarterial radioembolization of liver metastases. *Invest Radiol* 2013;48(11):787–794.
62. **Hsu C-Y, Shen Y-C, Yu C-W, et al.** Dynamic contrast-enhanced magnetic resonance imaging biomarkers predict survival and response in hepatocellular carcinoma patients treated with sorafenib and metronomic tegafur/uracil. *J Hepatol* 2011;55(4):858–865.
63. **Zhu AX, Sahani DV, Duda DG, et al.** Efficacy, safety, and potential biomarkers of sunitinib monotherapy in advanced hepatocellular carcinoma: a phase II study. *J Clin Oncol* 2009;27(18):3027–3035.
64. **Coenegrachts K, Bols A, Haspeslagh M, et al.** Prediction and monitoring of treatment effect using T1-weighted dynamic contrast-enhanced magnetic resonance imaging in colorectal liver metastases: potential of whole tumour ROI and selective ROI analysis. *Eur J Radiol* 2012;81(12):3870–3876.
65. **De Bruyne S, Van Damme N, Smeets P, et al.** Value of DCE-MRI and FDG-PET/CT in the prediction of response to preoperative chemotherapy with bevacizumab for colorectal liver metastases. *Br J Cancer* 2012;106(12):1926–1933.
66. **Hirashima Y, Yamada Y, Tateishi U, et al.** Pharmacokinetic parameters from 3-Tesla DCE-MRI as surrogate biomarkers of antitumor effects of bevacizumab plus FOLFIRI in colorectal cancer with liver metastasis. *Int J Cancer* 2012;130(10):2359–2365.
67. **Miyazaki K, Orton MR, Davidson RL, et al.** Neuroendocrine tumor liver metastases: use of dynamic contrast-enhanced MR imaging to monitor and predict radiolabeled octreotide therapy response. *Radiology* 2012;263(1):139–148.
68. **Miles KA, Hayball MP, Dixon AK.** Functional images of hepatic perfusion obtained with dynamic CT. *Radiology* 1993;188(2):405–411.
69. **Blomley MJ, Coulden R, Dawson P, et al.** Liver perfusion studied with ultrafast CT. *J Comput Assist Tomogr* 1995;19(3):424–433.
70. **Van Beers BE, Leconte I, Materne R, et al.** Hepatic perfusion parameters in chronic liver disease: dynamic CT measurements correlated with disease severity. *AJR Am J Roentgenol* 2001;176(3):667–673.
71. **Ronot M, Asselah T, Paradis V, et al.** Liver fibrosis in chronic hepatitis C virus infection: differentiating minimal from intermediate fibrosis with perfusion CT. *Radiology* 2010;256(1):135–142.
72. **Van Beers BE, Materne R, Annet L, et al.** Capillarization of the sinusoids in liver fibrosis: noninvasive assessment with contrast-enhanced MRI in the rabbit. *Magn Reson Med* 2003;49(4):692–699.
73. **Zhou L, Chen TW, Zhang XM, et al.** Liver dynamic contrast-enhanced MRI for staging liver fibrosis in a piglet model. *J Magn Reson Imaging* 2014;39(4):872–878.
74. **Annet L, Materne R, Danse E, et al.** Hepatic flow parameters measured with MR imaging and Doppler US: correlations with degree of cirrhosis and portal hypertension. *Radiology* 2003;229(2):409–414.
75. **Baxter S, Wang ZJ, Joe BN, et al.** Timing bolus dynamic contrast-enhanced (DCE) MRI assessment of hepatic perfusion: initial experience. *J Magn Reson Imaging* 2009;29(6):1317–1322.
76. **Hagiwara M, Rusinek H, Lee VS, et al.** Advanced liver fibrosis: diagnosis with 3D whole-liver perfusion MR imaging—initial experience. *Radiology* 2008;246(3):926–934.
77. **Luciani A, Vignaud A, Cavet M, et al.** Liver cirrhosis: intravoxel incoherent motion MR imaging—pilot study. *Radiology* 2008;249(3):891–899.
78. **Yoon JH, Lee JM, Baek JH, et al.** Evaluation of hepatic fibrosis using intravoxel incoherent motion in diffusion-weighted liver MRI. *J Comput Assist Tomogr* 2014;38(1):110–116.
79. **Chow AM, Gao DS, Fan SJ, et al.** Liver fibrosis: an intravoxel incoherent motion (IVIM) study. *J Magn Reson Imaging* 2012;36(1):159–167.
80. **Zhang Y, Jin N, Deng J, et al.** Intra-voxel incoherent motion MRI in rodent model of diethylnitrosamine-induced liver fibrosis. *Magn Reson Imaging* 2013;31(6):1017–1021.
81. **Lee JT, Liau J, Murphy P, et al.** Cross-sectional investigation of correlation between hepatic steatosis and IVIM perfusion on MR imaging. *Magn Reson Imaging* 2012;30(4):572–578.
82. **Guiu B, Petit JM, Capitan V, et al.** Intravoxel incoherent motion diffusion-weighted imaging in nonalcoholic fatty liver disease: a 3.0-T MR study. *Radiology* 2012;265(1):96–103.
83. **Joo I, Lee JM, Yoon JH, et al.** Nonalcoholic fatty liver disease: intravoxel incoherent motion diffusion-weighted MR imaging-an experimental study in a rabbit model. *Radiology* 2014;270(1):131–140.

CHAPTER

28 Liver Perfusion Imaging with CT

Marco Rengo, MD, PhD, Marco Maria Maceroni, MD, and Andrea Laghi, MD

Introduction

Advances in therapeutic options for primitive or metastatic liver malignancies raised the demands on diagnostic and surveillance tests. Existing imaging modalities provide limited assessment beyond morphologic and structural criteria; perfusion imaging, conversely, has potential to improve this shortcoming. Earlier detection of liver malignancies or cirrhosis may be possible on the basis of hepatic disease–related changes in blood flow (BF). The advent of multidetector CT (MDCT), thanks to its high temporal and spatial resolution, is a noninvasive and robust imaging modality for the evaluation and quantification of tissue perfusion.

Functional imaging is becoming increasingly important in both research and clinical diagnostic radiology. Perfusion computed tomography (pCT) is a readily available tool that allows an objective measurement of tissue perfusion through the mathematical analysis of CT data. pCT analysis has been validated against the current standard of reference and has been proven to be reproducible.[1,2] Several papers stating a correlation between perfusion parameters and histologic results of angiogenesis, such as microvessel density, validate the use of pCT as an in vivo biomarker of angiogenesis.

A robust acquisition technique, an accurate data analysis, and an adequate interpretation of results are essential to make pCT a valid diagnostic and prognostic tool into clinical context.

Background

The process of tumor neoangiogenesis plays a central role in the growth and spread of tumors, and it is currently a leading theme in oncology. Expanding tumors become hypoxic, and tumor cells express transcription factors, which induce the release of proangiogenic growth factors such as vascular endothelial growth factors (VEGF) and transforming growth factor that promote the formation of new capillaries by recruiting, activating, and stimulating endothelial cells. The newly grown vessels are immature and differ from normal capillaries. They are tortuous, irregular, and leaky (especially to macromolecules), and they are independent of the normal mechanisms of regulation of the capillary BF. Evaluation of neoangiogenesis can be used as a prognostic marker to evaluate the aggressiveness of tumor and as a potential predictive marker of antiangiogenic treatment response.

The assumption of angiogenesis process as a prognostic feature in the growth and metastatic spread of several tumors[3] encouraged finding new drugs targeting tumor vascularization.[4,5]

For this reasons, monitoring vessel pattern changes is currently a fundamental concern in oncology. Microvascular density has been considered as a gold standard method to take count of angiogenesis or aggressiveness of many cancers.[6,7] Unfortunately, microvascular density indexes require invasive tissue sampling, and therefore, it is unfeasible for monitoring response to antiangiogenic drugs; furthermore, it is also limited by random sampling errors and limited reproducibility, and thus, it is not feasible in routine clinical practice.[8] It has become a challenging goal for radiologists to assess noninvasively the physiology of the tumor microcirculation, in addition to conventional morphology. Angiogenesis is now extensively studied by dynamic contrast-enhanced (DCE) magnetic resonance imaging (MRI)[9–11] and MDCT.[12–14] Over the last few years, substantial gains have been made with pCT imaging, and the role of CT has been investigated to assess angiogenesis in the malignant lesions of the lung, colon–rectum, liver, esophagus, and pancreas.[15–21] Because the resulting pCT parameters are dependent on the kinetic model and the software employed in analysis, efforts to further improve the reproducibility and to understand the relationship with cancer angiogenesis are currently justified.

CT Perfusion

Although a range of other imaging modalities ensure tissue perfusion analysis, CT is particularly suitable in everyday clinical practice due to its widespread availability and reproducibility. Another advantage of pCT is the linear relation between iodine concentration and tissue attenuation modifications, which makes mathematic modeling relatively simpler against MR imaging. Furthermore, the increasing availability of commercial software for pCT makes this technique easily incorporated into existing CT protocols. Until a few years ago, the main limitation was related to reduced anatomic coverage of the first-generation scanners and the low speed of acquisition and processing of images. With the advent of MDCT, decrease in the gantry rotation time (about 0.4 seconds), and the capability to cover major volumes at each rotation of the tube, this limit falls inexorably.[2,22] Further, the development of MDCT systems has motivated growing interest to a volume-based examination. The principles, on which pCT studies are based, continue to reside in continuous acquisition of a serial high temporal resolution images at stationary table (imposed by the geometry of the scanner) following rapid intravenous injection of iodinated contrast media and in assessing attenuation differences of tissue over time that indirectly reflects tissue vascularity and vascular physiology. The neoangiogenesis is a biologic phenomenon of extreme importance in growth and distant spread of the tumor. The liver pCT study represents a noninvasive tool able to provide useful information regarding the vascular network modifications; it allows an in vivo assessment of BF, blood volume (BV), the mean transit time (MTT), permeability–surface (PS) area product, arterial liver perfusion (ALP), portal liver perfusion (PLP), hepatic perfusion index (HPI), and indexes of tumor angiogenic modifications and liver function reserve. These tissue perfusion parameters reflect physiologic angiogenic markers and may be visually assessed by using colored functional maps created in pCT analysis.[22] The key point in performing liver pCT is to resolve hepatic dual vasculature. Arterial and portal venous supply of the liver parenchyma enhancement may be distinctly resolved using the beginning of dominant portal venous perfusion, highlighted by peak splenic enhancement (Fig. 28-1). PLP and ALP values are computed by normalizing the slopes of the attenuation rise in arterial and portal venous phases of liver enhancement, respectively, to peak aortic enhancement. HPI is calculated by dividing the derived arterial perfusion by the sum of portal and arterial perfusion values.[2,22] The average time required for blood to cross the vascular network from the arterial inlet to venous outlet is defined as MTT. Further, the PS area product for circulating molecules reflects the speed of transfer of a contrast agent from the intravascular to the extravascular/extracellular compartment.

pCT is used in oncology because it is believed that it can serve as an indicator of the angiogenic events in solid tumors. By definition, angiogenesis is the formation of new blood vessels from preexisting vessels; theoretically, the pCT is capable of measuring the BV inside of the newly formed microvessels, because it gives a numerical value to the parameter of BV, expressed in mL/100 g tissue. The newly formed vessels also have an altered wall and therefore are abnormally permeable, and the pCT is able to provide an estimate of the capillary permeability through the calculation of the PS. For these reasons, the pCT would theoretically be able to quantify the phenomenon of angiogenesis in solid tumors: compared to other potential angiogenic biomarkers as the measurement of MVD, circulating levels of the VEGF, or circulating endothelial cells, it presents undeniable advantages of being noninvasive, inexpensive, and widely available.

Perfusion CT Technique

The perfusion is by definition the transport of blood to unit of volume of tissue in the unit of time. In theory, pCT is a tool able to quantify (through the usage of mathematical models) in an objective manner (by the use of dedicated software) "real" tissue perfusion, as it only assesses the attenuation differences produced by the arrival of contrast agent (and therefore blood) to the tissues. The pCT is based on two technical requirements. The first is the acquisition of dynamic CT scans of the volume of interest before, during, and after the intravenous administration of iodinated contrast media, in order to study the variations of the attenuation over time. The density measured by CT in a voxel-by-voxel analysis (i.e., x-ray attenuation expressed in Hounsfield unit [HU]) is directly

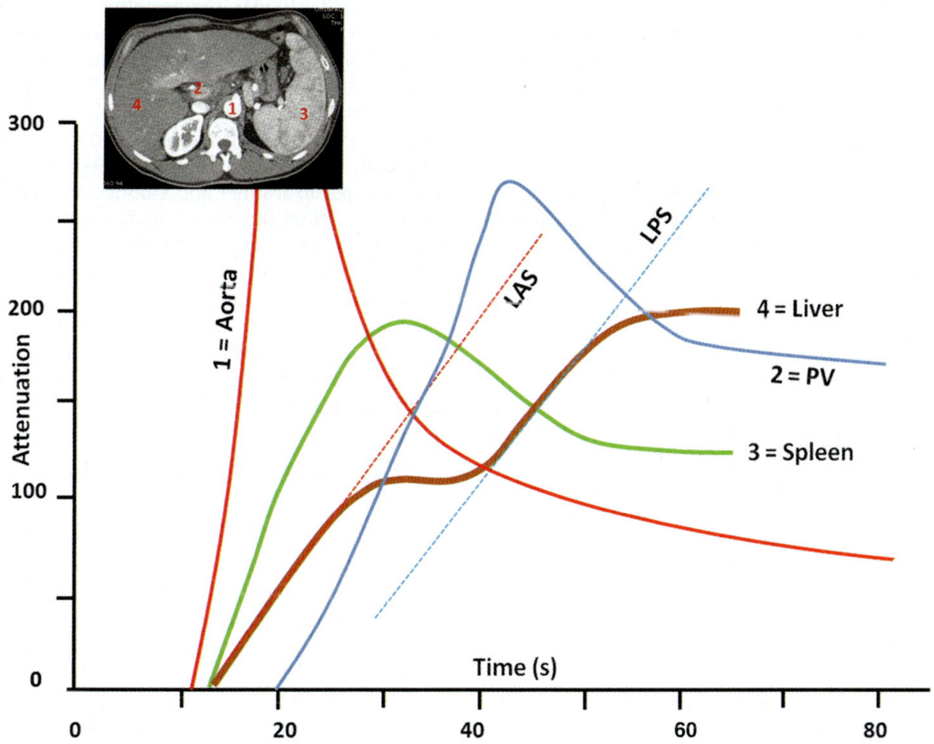

Figure 28-1. Schematic diagram showing dual liver supply and time–attenuation curves for the abdominal aorta (1 = *red*), portal vein (2 = *blue*), spleen (3 = *green*), and normal liver (4 = *brown*). The peak splenic attenuation (3) is used to separate the arterial phase from the portal venous phase. The liver arterial perfusion maximal slope (LAS) and the liver portal perfusion maximal slope (LPS) are obtained as shown by *red* and *blue* dotted lines. To calculate hepatic arterial and portal perfusions, the maximal slope in each phase is divided by the peak aortic (1) and portal (2) enhancement. PV, portal vein

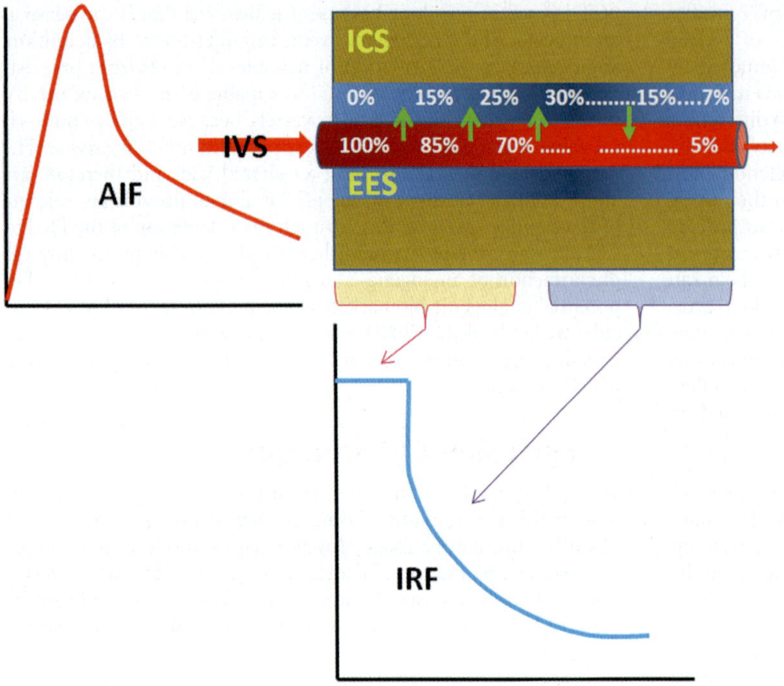

Figure 28-2. **Simplified two-compartment model of the capillary intravascular interstitial tissue exchange system.** In this system, the injected contrast (impulse) that is transported from the intravascular space (IVS) into the interstitial space (extravascular–extracellular space or EES) will in part renter the IVS and soon is washed off from both spaces. Mathematical kinetics of the tracer transport in the tissue is known as impulse retention (residue) function or IRF. As shown in this diagram, the recorded attenuation values for the early flat plateau of the IRF remains highest because the sum of contrast concentration in both IVS and EES adds up to 100%. Soon with entrance of contrast into the venules, its concentration in the system drops. This decay in attenuation reflects the first-pass extraction of contrast in this two-compartment model and in overall depends on the capillary PS area product. Intracellular space (ICS) does not participate in the exchange. AIF, arterial input function. (From Thng CH, Koh TS, Collins D, et al. Perfusion imaging in liver MRI. *Magn Reson Imaging Clin N Am* 2014;22(3):417–432.)

proportional to the amount of contrast agent in the tissue; the contrast medium (CM) present in the volume of tissue is due to the presence of contrast agent in the vessels and in the interstitium (extravascular/extracellular space), by passive diffusion. The second requirement is the selection of an arterial input. The placement of a region of interest (ROI) on an artery (arterial input) allows to obtain an attenuation/time curve, expressed in HU/s, which is compared to that related to the tissue analysis obtained through the placement of an ROI (Fig. 28-1). This comparison allows one to distinguish the amount of contrast agent inside the vessels (vascular compartment) from that in the interstitium (extravascular compartment). The ensuing attenuation modifications over time are analyzed by using one of the known kinetic models (Appendix) to calculate perfusion parameters that reflect the functional status of the vascular system.[23]

Perfusion CT Protocols

The primary objective of hepatic perfusion imaging is to increase the detection of liver disease. Distinct pCT protocols have been developed, depending on the target organ, kinetic model, CT scan configuration, and clinical objective. A typical pCT examination takes place by performing a baseline acquisition without contrast enhancement, followed by a sequential high temporal resolution acquisition after intravenous injection of CM. The baseline-unenhanced CT acquisition serves as a localizer to select the ROI to be included in the dynamic series. According to the scanner configuration, a 2-cm coverage area (for a 4- or 16-row CT scanner) or a 4-cm coverage area (for a 64-row CT scanner) can be selected for dynamic scanning. Larger z-axis coverage (8 to 16 cm) is now achievable with the introduction of newer scanners with 128 to 320 rows of detectors.[24] Depending on the bicompartmental kinetic of contrast media (intra- and extravascular components), two sets of physiologic data have to be quantified for contrast enhancement on CT. The intravascular phase assesses tissue perfusion (i.e., BF per unit volume or mass of tissue and relative BV, parameters usually increased in malignancies in relation to the high MVD found in neoplastic tissue). In this phase, the enhancement is mainly attributable to the distribution of contrast within the intravascular space, and it usually lasts approximately 40 to 60 seconds from the time of contrast arrival (first pass). The extravascular phase, conversely, can be used to exploit the abnormally leaky vessels to circulating molecules (contrast material) in malignant tissue, reflecting the increased vascular permeability due to immature basement membrane. In this second phase, tissue enhancement results from contrast distribution between the intra- and extravascular compartments (delayed phase) (Fig. 28-2). The two most common analytic methods to estimate tissue perfusion from the dynamic CT data are compartmental analysis and deconvolution analysis.[12,21,24,25] The analytic methods used and the acquisition protocols vary from scanner to scanner and among commercial vendors. General Electric works on the deconvolution approach and allows calculation of parametric maps of BF, BV, MTT, and PS. The Philips pCT software works on the slope method to calculate the perfusion maps and to estimate the tissue peak enhancement, time to peak enhancement, and MTT. Siemens perfusion software similarly exploits the slope method to calculate perfusion and also to estimate the BV and time to peak enhancement. In Table 28.1 is reported a glossary of terms commonly used in CT perfusion.

Contrast Media Administration

The shape of the bolus of CM is a key point for pCT. An optimal perfusion analysis is adequately performed by injecting a 40 to 70 mL at a rate ranging from to 3.5 to 10 mL/s.[12,21,24,25] According to the linear relation between tissue enhancement and iodine concentration, it is preferable to use a higher concentration of CM (>370 mgI/mL). For compartmental analysis the use of a short and rapid bolus is recomended (40 to 50 mL administered with an injection rate between 5 and 10 mL/s) to obtain perfusion parameters, because this kinetic model requires that peak arterial iodine concentration come early the maximal increase in tissue enhancement. By using deconvolution kinetic model, lower injection rates may be used though higher rates may still be advisable by maximizing tissue enhancement and to improve the signal-to-noise ratio (50 to 70 mL administered with an injection rate between 4 and 6 mL/s). Depending on the linear relation between iodine concentration and

TABLE 28.1 Glossary of Terms Commonly Used in Perfusion CT

Perfusion Parameters	Definition	Units
BF	Flow rate through vascular bed in tissue region	mL/100 g/min
BV	Volume of flowing blood within a vascular bed in tissue region	mL/100 g
ALP	The slope of the attenuation increase in arterial phases of liver enhancement normalized to peak aortic enhancement	mL/min/100 mL
PLP	The slope of the attenuation increase in portal venous phases of liver enhancement normalized to peak aortic enhancement	mL/min/100 mL
HPI	Calculated by dividing the arterial perfusion by the sum of portal and arterial perfusion values	%
MTT	Average time to pass from the arterial inlet to venous outlet	Seconds
PS	Total flux from plasma to interstitial space	mL/100 g/min
TTP	Time from arrival of the contrast in major arterial vessels to the peak enhancement	Seconds
PEI	Maximum attenuation tissue increase after contrast injection	HU

BF, blood flow; BV, blood volume; ALP, arterial liver perfusion; PLP, portal liver perfusion; HPI, hepatic arterial index; MTT, mean transit time; PS, permeability surface product; TTP, time to peak; PEI, peak enhancement index.

tissue enhancement, a higher concentration of CM (370 mg/mL or greater) is recommended; however, regardless iodine concentration, it is important to maintain an iodine injection rate of 2 g/s.[21]

Acquisition Parameters

Volume of Interest

The standard protocol needs to acquire a preliminary CT images without contrast material (thickness of 2.5 to 5 mm) for locating the tumor and select the volume on which to perform the perfusion scans. This volume is limited by the detector configuration used (e.g., 20 mm for the 16-slice CT scanners and 40 mm for the 64 layers), if first-pass study is needed, because it requires scanning at high temporal resolution (0.5 to 1 seconds using a defined protocol for perfusion analysis with the "deconvolution" kinetic model and 3 to 5 seconds using a defined protocol for perfusion analysis with the model kinetic unicompartmental or bicompartmental), possible only with the stationary table. Increased coverage along the z-axis is possible if we decide to study only the interstitial phase, because they are sufficient scans with low temporal resolution (10 to 20 seconds). If the tumor had a volume greater than that perfusion scans may include, it is preferable to identify the section with the maximum viewable area of the tumor and place it on the center of the volume used for the perfusion study.

Perfusion Scans

The perfusion scans performed during the first pass (up to 45 to 60 seconds from the start of the administration of contrast media) require a high temporal resolution (at least 1 second to the protocols defined for the analysis of perfusion with the "deconvolution" kinetic model and 3 to 5 seconds to those defined for the analysis of perfusion with the mono- or bicompartmental kinetic model).[12,25] The precise time interval depends on the cardiac output and BV of the patient. During this phase, the CM is primarily intravascular, and perfusion indexes, which can be calculated following an acquisition "cine mode" for such a protracted period, are only the BF and the BV.

Over time, the amount of CM that diffuses in extravascular space increases. Once the equilibrium is reached, the percentage of CM moving from the intravascular to the extravascular space is balanced by the percentage of CM that moves within the vascular system from the interstitium. In solid tumors, the greatest amount of CM moves within the vascular space in a couple of minutes. For this reason, the measurement of the PS requires scanned images to a maximum of 2 minutes. Since the variations of the enhancement in this phase (after the first pass) are less rapid, the images can be obtained at a frequency less than that required for a study of the first pass.[26] For assessing permeability measurements, the perfusion scans performed during interstitial phase after the study of the first pass according to the deconvolution kinetic model must be performed with temporal resolution of 10 seconds and have a duration of no more than 2 minutes after the beginning of the administration of contrast material, to apply the adiabatic approximation of St. Lawrence and Lee. The perfusion scans performed during interstitial phase after the study of the first pass according to the mono- or bicompartmental kinetic model must be performed with temporal resolution of between 10 and 20 seconds and have a duration of between 2 and 10 minutes after the start of the administration of contrast material. A second delayed phase ranging from 2 to 10 minutes is supplemented after the first-pass study, according to the parameters that need to be assessed.[27] The serial high-frequency acquisitions (cine mode), required for a study of the first pass, may be limited by the volume of tissue to be investigated. This limit does not affect the delayed phase as the attenuation variations over time are so slow as to allow serial acquisitions at very low frequency (every 10 to 20 seconds), allowing for larger volume coverage.[26]

Acquisition Parameters

For dose savings purpose, recommended values are relatively low tube voltage (80 to 100 kVp) and tube current (120 to 200 mA) for perfusion scans, as most recently published studies reported for most body investigations.[25,27] The radiation burden associated with pCT is dependent on the number of images acquired and the tube current (mAs) and tube voltage (kVp) used. By acquiring a greater number of images (high temporal resolution), more time points on the time–attenuation curve are available, and hence, higher-quality perfusion measurements may be provided. Likewise, a higher tube current results in less image noise and, therefore, a more reliable evaluation of tissue enhancement. Further, increasing slice thickness can also reduce image noise but at the expense of spatial resolution.

The judicious selection of these parameters must also be customized according to the kinetic model used and the body part scanned, to keep the radiation exposure acceptable. By using deconvolution model–based protocols, Miles et al. recommended setting a tube current ranging from 50 to 100 mAs, because this kinetic model is less sensitive to image noise and therefore tolerates lower tube current and allows a higher temporal resolution. Contrariwise, a compartmental model–based protocol requires a tube current of 100 to 250 mAs because it is more sensitive to image noise; depending on three images (baseline and immediately before and after maximal parenchymal enhancement images), the presence of noise in one of the acquisitions may determine a miscalculation of perfusion parameters.[23] A study by Lee et al. showed that perfusion scans performed with 80 kV allow a dose reduction of 30% compared to those with 120 kV, with a loss in the signal-to-noise ratio only dell 11%. Finally, a slice thickness not less than 5 mm, which ensures a balance between the needs of spatial resolution and signal-to-noise ratio in the perfusion scans, is recommended and almost universally used in published studies.

Practical Issues

Respiratory motion is the most important cause of image misregistration during the liver dynamic acquisition, leading to errors in the estimation of perfusion values. Therefore, to minimize motion artifacts is the main goal by using approaches such as breath holding or quiet breathing. Miles states that higher quality perfusion images can be obtained using quiet breathing, but the patient must be exhorted to avoid to take a deep breath during the rapid CM bolus administration. Breath holding is not recommended because of the first-pass longer acquisition time (45 to 60 seconds) and the tendency to exhale during images acquisition, leading to motion artifacts. Beam-hardening artifacts secondary to metallic stents and surgical implants can negatively affect the perfusion measurements. Finally, avoiding excessive tumor necrosis areas or areas near metallic stents, clips, or surgical implants is crucial to perform accurate perfusion analysis.

Perfusion Indexes

BF, expressed in mL/100 g tissue/min, is calculated using the kinetic model of the "deconvolution." It represents the BF through the vascular network of the tumor. It includes flow in the arteries, arterioles, capillaries, venules, and veins. In addition, it also includes the flow at the level of arteriovenous shunts, which are much more present in neoplastic tissues compared to healthy ones.

BV, expressed in mL/100 g tissue, is calculated using the kinetic model of the "deconvolution." It measures the volume of blood "flows" in the examined tissue. It therefore includes the volume of blood present in the vessels arteries, arterioles, capillaries, venules, and veins. The amount of "stagnant" blood is not included in the measurement of BV.

MTT, expressed in seconds, is calculated with the "deconvolution" kinetic model. It represents the average time it takes for the blood to cross the microvascular structures from the arterial to venous end. If the BF is high, the MTT will be low.

PS, expressed in mL/100 g tissue/min, is calculated using the adiabatic approximation of the St. Lawrence and Lee. It measures the product between the permeability and the total surface of the capillary endothelium in a unit mass of tumor (normally 100 g). The PS can then be interpreted as the unidirectional flow of contrast material from the vascular to the extravascular (the interstitium) compartment.

Perfusion values measured with pCT significantly higher than the healthy tissue of the same organ were observed in hepatocellular carcinomas (HCCs), tumors of the rectum, lung, and upper digestive tract. A higher value of BF (or perfusion, in agreement with the kinetic model used) in the tumor tissue compared to healthy one could be the expression of a large number of arteriovenous shunts that, being a compartment with low resistance, lead to an increase in the microvascular flow. With increasing BF, the MTT of the blood in the microvessels of the analyzed volume decreases. A higher value of BV in the tumor compared to healthy tissue could be expression of the increase in the tumor microvascular network due to the formation of new vessels, in relation to the angiogenic process. Finally, a larger value of permeability (PS) in the tumor compared to healthy tissue may reflect the increased permeability of the endothelium of newly formed vessels compared to that of normal microvessels.

Image Analysis

The calculation of perfusion parameters is obtained by the use of dedicated software. These software are semiautomatic applications that require the intervention of the operator in the ROI positioning and the optimization of the process, but they play automatically mathematical analysis of the data.

Arterial Input Selection

The ROI for arterial input should be positioned on an artery whitin the scan volume. Theoretically, this is the ideal condition for a reliable analysis of CT perfusion, as the arterial input is specific for each patient and for each examination made by the same patient at different times. However, the selection of the arterial input may introduce a source of variability. It is an actual issue, for example, if the positioning of the ROI on an ipsilateral versus contralateral artery in relation to the site of the tumor may be a source of variations in the measurements of perfusion, because of the anatomical diversity between the right and left side. Another current issue is the selection of the artery: large caliber to avoid artifacts from tortuosity of the flow or small caliber because directly tributary of the tumor. It is advisable to select as arterial input an artery of adequate caliber (>4 to 5 mm) and well imaged in the perfusion scans but not necessarily a tributary of the tumor. In addition, many studies with pCT in various body regions have successfully used as arterial input the aorta or arteries not directly tributary of the tumor.[26] The selection of the arterial input, finally, must avoid motion and partial volume artifacts, which could severely affect the reliability of the analysis of pCT.

ROI Positioning

This step consists in manually draw an ROI along the margins of the tumor so that the software accurately quantify the perfusion values. During ROI positioning, special attention should be taken not to include the great vessels, air, or surrounding fatty tissue. It is important that the ROI is positioned at the inner margins of the tumor in all the images of perfusion scans; for this purpose, accurate evaluation of all the images must be done, preferably in cine-loop mode, and make sure that the ROI does not come out the margins of the tumor.

Clinical Interpretation

Qualitative Analysis

It consists in the analysis of the color-coded maps, which are generated automatically by the software for each perfusion parameter. They assign a color to each pixel of a CT, which represents the numeric value of the perfusion parameter calculated for that pixel; the color scale is chosen by the radiologist, in order to maximize the differences between the areas with different perfusion. The qualitative analysis of color-coded maps allows a panoramic view of the perfusion inside the whole volume scanned, reflecting the different perfusion areas of the tumor and making easy the identification of possible angiogenic spots (theoretically, more perfused areas) or of possible areas of necrosis or hypoxia (theoretically, the less perfused areas).[26] Finally, most of the commercially available software allows to overlay the map color to the native CT images; this overlap can help when the identification of tumor margins is difficult, as, for example, in the presence of a complex anatomy or after chemotherapy or radiotherapy.

Quantitative Analysis

It consists in the interpretation of the numerical values of perfusion computed by the software in the ROI positioned on the tumor. Perfusion parameters represent the average of the numerical values of perfusion for each voxel included in ROI drawn on the tumor. This method of quantification has, on the one side, the advantages of providing an estimate of the overall perfusion of the selected tumor volume and to ensure a high repeatability between different observers but, from the other side, has the defect to mask the differences in perfusion inside the tumor (i.e., the heterogeneity of its perfusion), as these are lost in the calculation of the average between the values of the single voxels. The assessment of the heterogeneity of tumor perfusion can be performed in a subjective manner, when the operator assesses visually the heterogeneity of colors generated on the color-coded maps, or in an objective manner, through the graphical representation of the distribution in the classes of the perfusion values of each voxel (histograms): theoretically, a tumor with high perfusion heterogeneity presents a number of colors and classes wider compared to a tumor with homogeneous perfusion.[26,28] However, in the literature, there are no studies that have used the method of graphs and histograms to assess the heterogeneity of tumor perfusion performed by using pCT.

Clinical Applications

The functional imaging is gaining an increasing role in both research and clinical work in diagnostic imaging. pCT imaging ensures qualitative and quantitative evaluation of liver perfusion. pCT imaging more reliably detects perfusion abnormalities than accurately does conventional CT.[29] Functional evaluation of normal and pathologic tissues perfusion is obtained by using quantitative or semiquantitative parameters that provide valuable information for diagnosis.

Perfusion Imaging in Cirrhosis

Cirrhosis is characterized by progressive disruption of the normal liver anatomy and physiology, leading to regional and global hemodynamic changes. Actually, liver biopsy is the gold standard for diagnosis. The current imaging modalities (US, MRI, and CT) provide morphologic assessment of liver disease and are commonly used for the diagnosis of liver cirrhosis. The arrangement of normal sinusoidal architecture results in an increase in sinusoidal BF resistance and portal venous flow decrease. As a result, BF begins to bypass the hepatic parenchyma by means of portosystemic shunts. Conversely, this modification in portal venous flow is balanced by an increase in hepatic arterial flow that acts as reserve for liver function and oxygenation, process known as arterial buffer response. More accurate information about diffuse liver diseases is obtained by the evaluation of hemodynamic alterations by using cross-sectional imaging.[30] According to the described physiologic adjustments of liver vascular network, the perfusion parameters result in a decrease in the portal fraction (PLP) and in an increase in arterial fraction (ALP) of hepatic perfusion. In cirrhotic liver parenchyma, the ALP determined by quantitative color-coded map significantly correlates with the severity of cirrhosis.[31]

Perfusion Imaging in HCC Detection

Liver cancer incidence has risen greatly in the last years, and up to 90% of liver cancers are HCCs. During the evolution from dysplastic nodule to HCC, the process of capillarization (formation of nontriadal arteries) explains the modifications in hemodynamic components of tumor areas that reflect the HCC dynamic behavior.[29] Classically, HCC receives its blood supply primarily by the hepatic artery that reflects its typical vascular pattern in dynamic acquisitions, consisting in high attenuation relative to the liver parenchyma during the early arterial phase.[32] Liver pCT imaging ensures quantitative resolution and assessment of the portal venous and arterial components of hepatic BF, making diagnosis of HCC more reliable. The perfusion parameters of HCC show great differences compared to the nontumor liver parenchyma. According to literature,[20,33] the typical hemodynamic characteristics of HCC are an increase of BF, BV, and ALP and a decrease of PLP (Fig. 28-3). Hence, pCT imaging can quantitatively assess the blood supply and its distribution in liver cancer, providing useful parameter for assessing angiogenesis of liver cancer. pCT may also investigate the therapeutic effectiveness of interventional procedures by providing quantitative functional parameters related to residual arterial structures in viable tumors.[33] Furthermore, it can positively affect the management of patients with HCC, as it could potentially measured changes in angiogenic parameters after target therapies. In this regard, Zhu et al.[34] have found significant reduction in BF, BV, and PS and an increase in MTT within HCC tissues after therapy with agents targeted to tumor vasculature.

Perfusion Imaging in Metastatic Disease

Metastatic disease begins with extravasation of tumoral cells within hepatic parenchyma. Neoangiogenesis plays an important role in tumor growth. Similar in the hepatocarcinogenesis, capillarization process occurs in the peritumoral region, resulting in nontriadal arteries formation to sustain neoplastic cells growth and ensuing increase in BF and BV (Fig. 28-4). Increased values of HPI and ALP and decrease PLP, also, can suggest the presence of hepatic metastases, reflecting the vascular changes related to the process of neoangiogenesis.[32] Early diagnosis of liver metastatic disease is of value for staging, prognosis, and treatment. Leggett et al. proved increased ALP in colorectal metastases. Further, in this study, PLP presented decreased values in three patients with metastatic progressive disease.[35] These results suggested the diagnosis of disease progression when metastatic lesions showed decreased PLP values. In another study by Cuenod et al. were reported decrease PLP and increase MTT values in rats with subclinical hepatic metastases. The modifications in PLP and MTT were related to a higher intrahepatic resistance owing to capillarization process. The authors also hypothesized that there was an increase in ALP secondary to a hepatic arterial buffer response in patients with occult micrometastatic disease.[14] As stated in the literature, pCT also provide useful prognostic data, showing reduction in BF, BV, and PS values in solid tumors[36,37] in response to antiangiogenic drugs (Fig. 28-5).

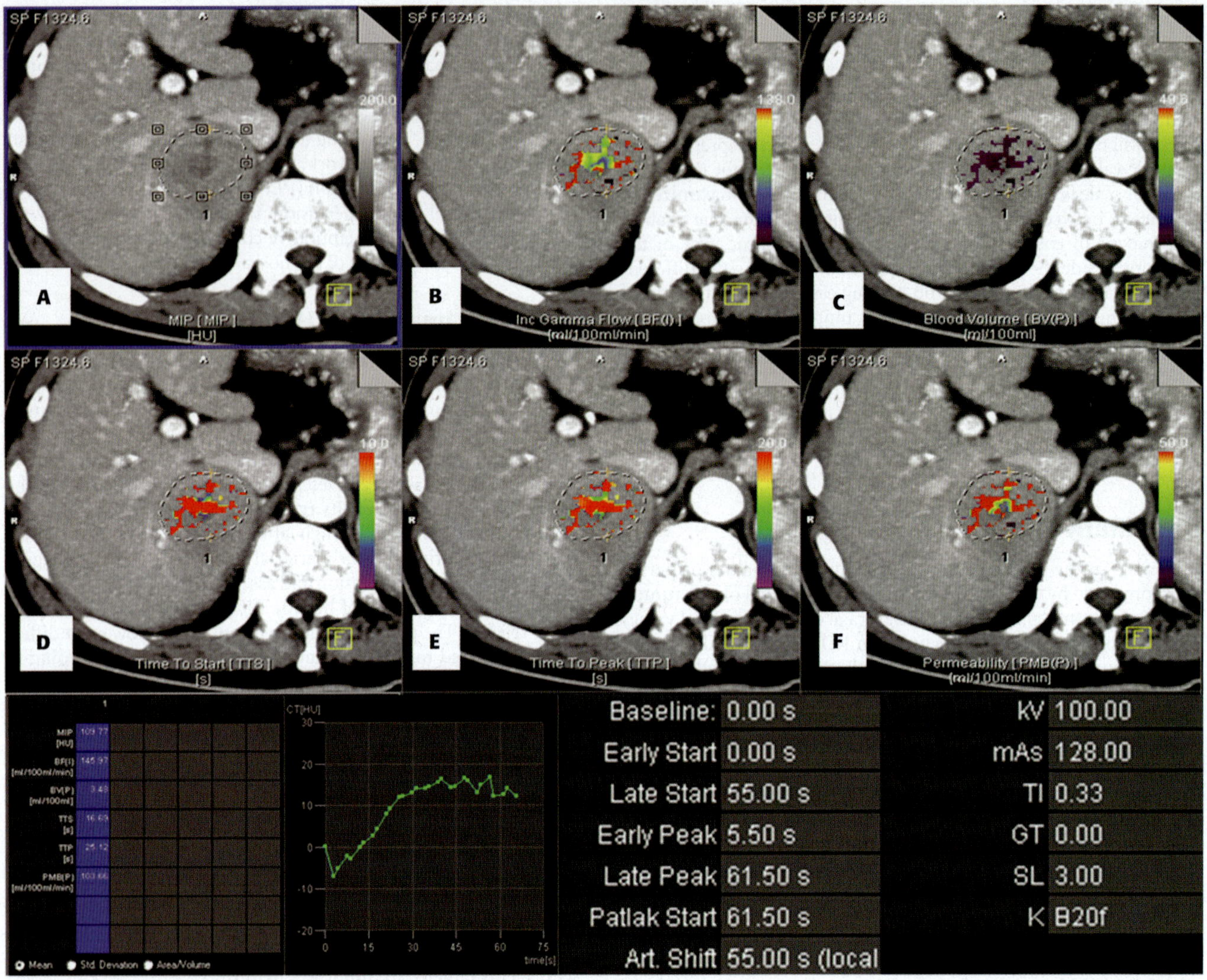

Figure 28-3. Axial CT images **(A)** and pCT maps (B–F) of a 65-year-old man with HCC in the right lobe of the liver. The functional map shows the increase in blood flow (BF) **(B)** and blood volume (BV) **(C)** as the result in hemodynamic changes owing to hepatocarcinogenesis. **D**, time to start; **E**, time to peak; **F**, permeability. Time–attenuation curve and perfusion parameter values are shown in the lower row.

Perfusion Imaging in Cholangiocarcinoma

Cholangiocarcinoma is the second liver malignant tumor arising from the biliary tract. Cross-sectional imaging cannot always provide diagnosis of intrahepatic cholangiocarcinoma in a straightforward manner. Delayed enhancement is the radiologic key findings along with segmentary biliary dilatation owing to obstruction.[38] Functional pCT imaging can aim to investigate tumor vascularity in cholangiocarcinoma.[12,36] Increased values of BF, BV, ALP, and HPI, and decreased values of PLP are usually found in cholangiocarcinoma. Finally, pCT can also be used in treatment response monitoring, particularly in antiangiogenic drugs or novel targeted therapies, by demonstrating modifications in tumor vascularization before and after treatment.

Perfusion Imaging in Postinterventional Procedure

Patients affected by HCC cannot undergo surgery because of their severe hepatic dysfunction and/or advanced liver disease; transarterial chemoembolization (TACE) has been proved to increase the survival rate. Other interventional procedure, such as percutaneous ethanol injection and radiofrequency tumor ablation, may be selected according to clinical setting. Postprocedural peripheral enhancement at DCE cross-sectional imaging may be suggestive of incomplete tumor ablation. This scenario may be complicated by marginal reactive hyperemia, an inflammatory response after treatment; however, it is usually well resolve from pathologic tissue on the basis of its regular shape and enhancement characteristics at dynamic imaging[39]; further, this finding generally resolves within 1 to 4 months. Perfusion imaging of HCC can be used as an in vivo marker for therapeutic response to therapy. Contrariwise to RECIST criteria based on tumor size evaluation, tumor response may be better depicted by considering hemodynamic modifications in tumor area.[38] BF and BV along with ALP, total liver perfusion, and HPI show significant reduction after a month course of TACE (Fig. 28-6). Persistent increase of BV, BV, and ALP following chemoembolization is suggestive for residual or recurrent tumor (Fig. 28-7).[40]

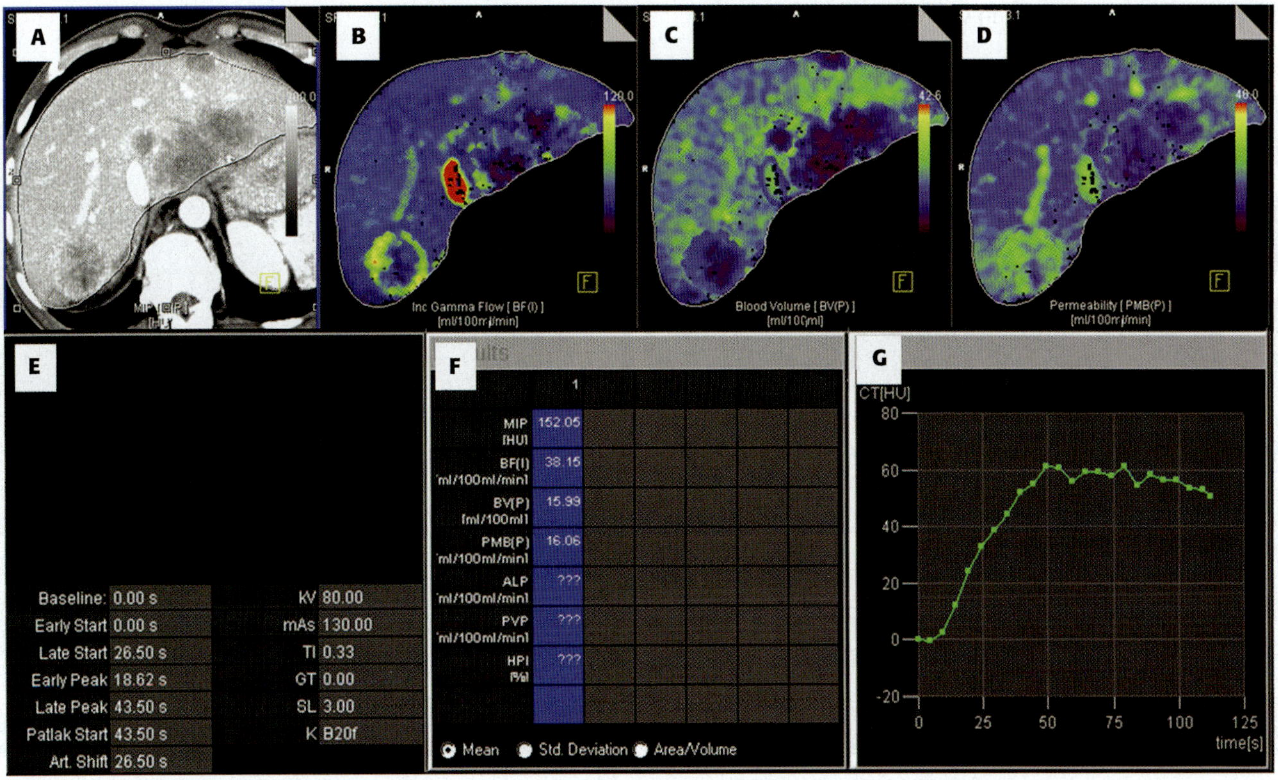

Figure 28-4. Axial images (A) and pCT maps (B–G) of a 70-year-old woman with liver metastasis. The perfusion images show increased blood flow (BF) **(B)** and blood volume (BV) **(C)** compared with normal liver parenchyma. Perfusion parameter values **(E and F)** and time–attenuation curve **(G)** are shown in the lower row.

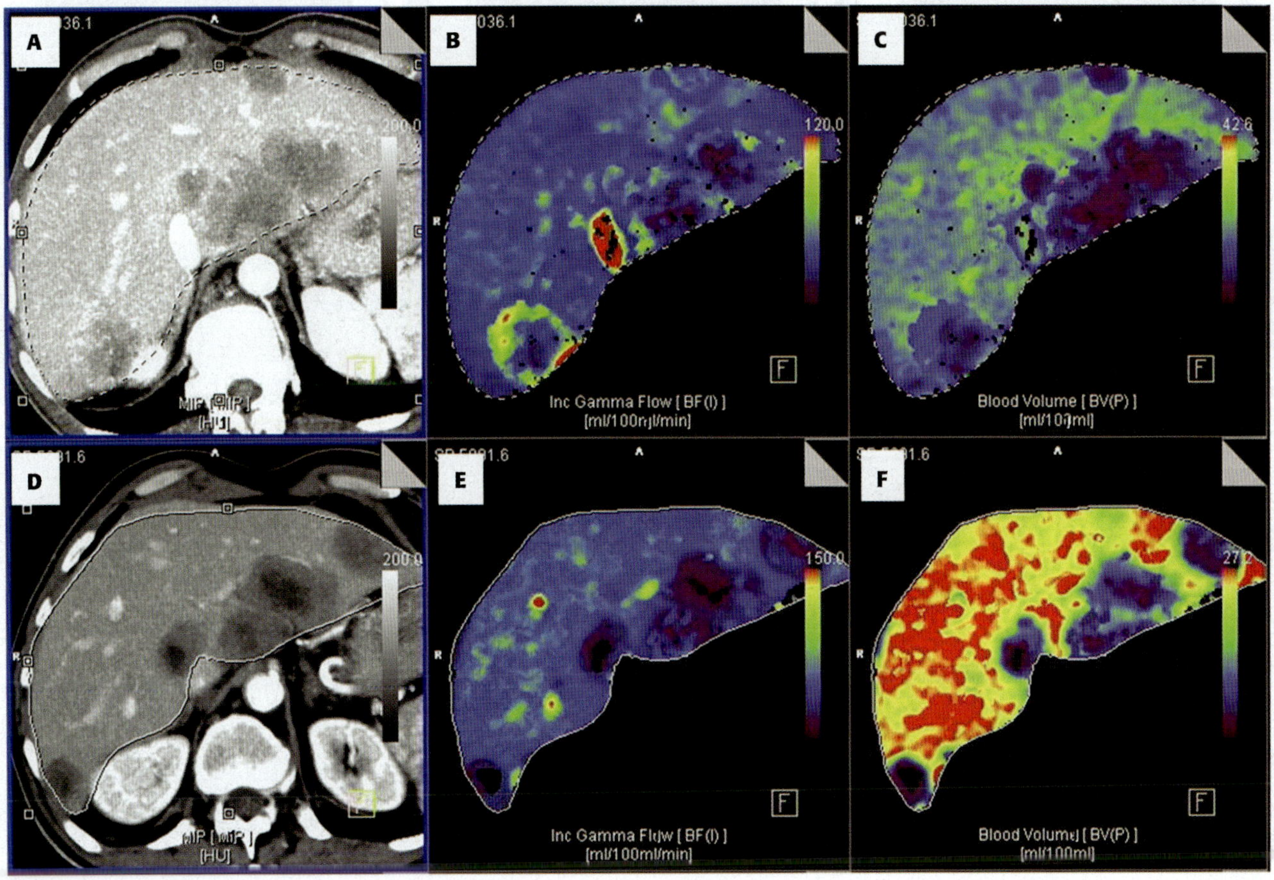

Figure 28-5. Axial CT images (A and D) and pCT maps (B, C, E, and F) of a 70-year-old man with multiple colorectal cancer metastasis, pre- **(A–C)** and postantiangiogenic therapy **(D–F)**. The functional maps show a significant decrease in blood flow (BF) **(E)** and blood volume (BV) **(F)** as the result of therapies with agents targeted to tumor vasculature.

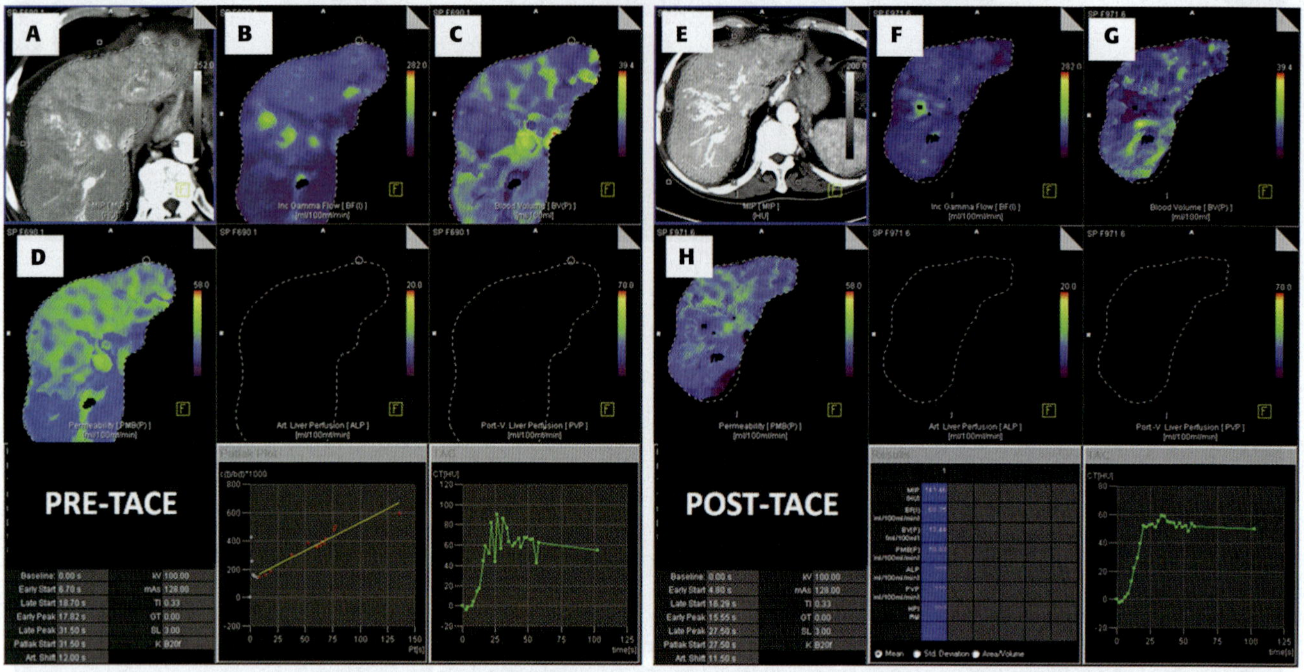

Figure 28-6. Axial CT images (A and E) and pCT maps of multifocal HCC following before (B–D) and after transarterial chemoembolization (TACE) (F–H). The functional map shows a decrease in blood flow (BF) **(B** vs. **F)** and blood volume (BV) **(C** vs. **G)** values, resulting in tumor response to TACE.

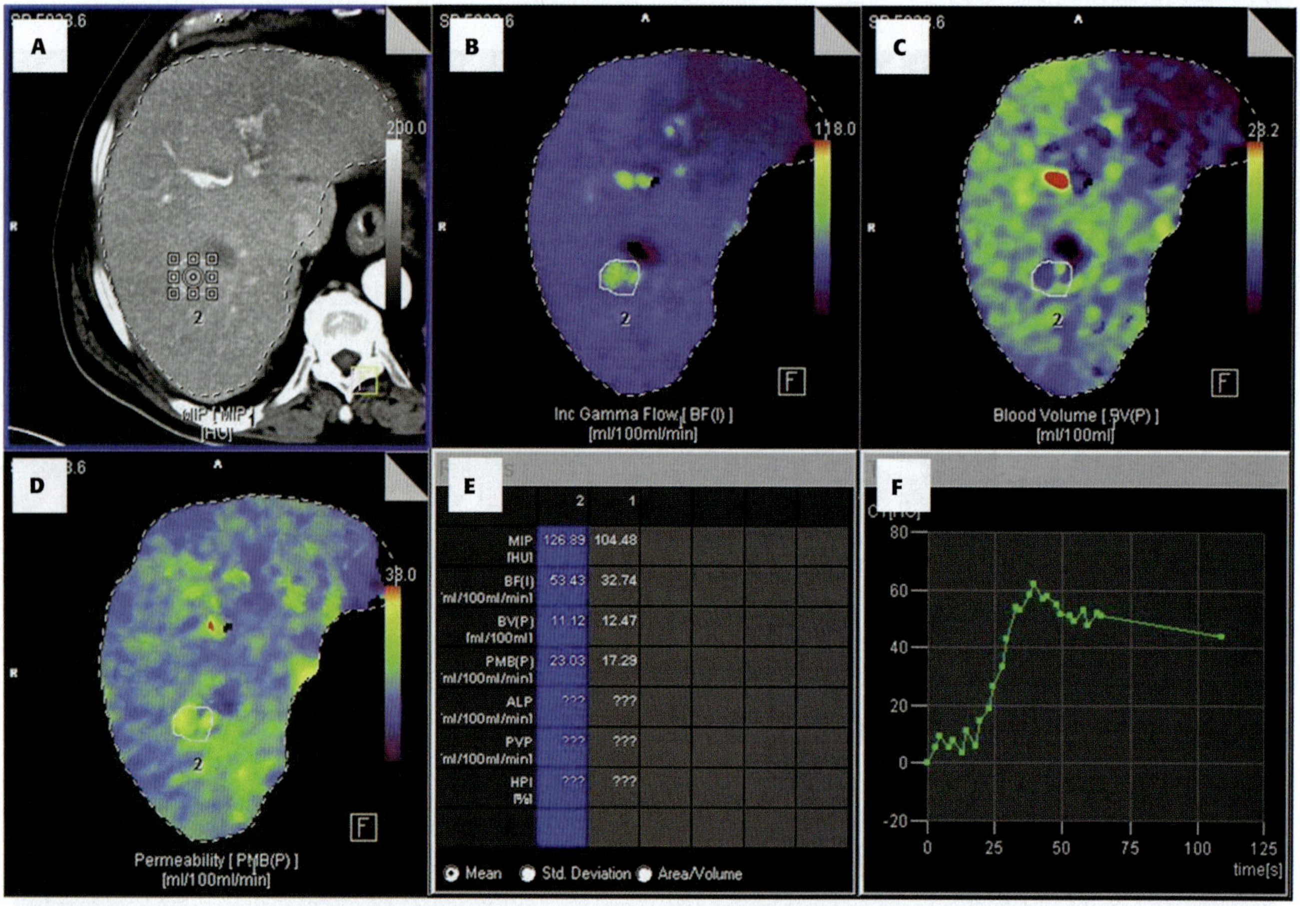

Figure 28-7. Axial CT images (A) and pCT maps (B–D) of a 70-year-old man with HCC in the right lobe of the liver following TACE. The functional map shows an increase in blood flow (BF) **(B)** and blood volume (BV) **(C)** in the peritumoral area suggesting HCC recurrence after transarterial chemoembolization. Perfusion parameter values **(E)** and time–attenuation curve **(F)** are shown in the lower row.

Limitations

The greatest drawback of pCT is radiation burden. The radiation dose to which patients are exposed is high, especially because the pCT is often performed in the same session of the conventional CT examination. Exposure to a high radiation dose is one of the main factors that limit the wide applications of pCT, which in oncology should only be performed inside of research protocols approved by the ethics committee. Therefore, dose reduction strategies such as tube current or voltage modulation, scanning parameters customization, helical pitch, automatic exposure control, and image filters should be used during the CT examination. Image quality is strongly related to radiation dose. Images obtained with low kVp contain a high degree of noise, which is relieved by increasing the mAs. Iterative reconstruction algorithms provide a comparable image quality compared to the usual filtered back-projection algorithm, with a significant saving of dose delivered to the patient depending on the algorithm used.

Although there are encouraging preliminary results on the reproducibility of the pCT, as well as on the determination of intra- and inter-observer in the analysis of the data, more experience in different organs and with more advanced pCT techniques is needed to confirm the reliability of this method. Finally, there is a lack of multicentric studies on pCT, which are necessary to finally validate the technique.

Appendix

The bicompartmental kinetic model (or Patlak) differentiates the vascular compartment and the extravascular/extracellular (interstitium) compartment, and it quantifies the compartmental exchanges. It provides an estimate of the volume of blood inside the microvessels (BV) and the extraction fraction, also known as constant of transit (Ktrans), which is the sum of the flow inside of the microvessels and capillary permeability.

The single-compartment kinetic model (or the slope method) allows the calculation of perfusion with perfusion scans of short duration. The perfusion can be calculated as the ratio between the maximum slope of the curve density/time of the tissue and the peak density reached by the artery selected as arterial input. The main advantage of this method is to allow the calculation of the perfusion with scans of short duration, because the density/time curve of the tissue reaches its maximum slope much before its peak density. The scans of short duration are defined to include only the first pass of the CM in the volume in the analysis (first pass), to prevent the recirculation of the blood can interfere with the quantification of perfusion; they also offer the advantage of being able to be made with breath-hold acquisition in critical districts, limiting the possibility of motion artifacts. However, this kinetic model is by nature very sensitive to noise present in the acquired images, as they are analyzed in a discontinuous way. Furthermore, the perfusion is calculated using only four images: the baseline, that in the moment of the peak density of the artery, and the two subsequent, that show the greatest differences of density in the tissues: The presence of noise in one of these images may affect the quantification of perfusion.

The "deconvolution" kinetic model applies a mathematical operation of deconvolution to compare the attenuation/time curves obtained from the input from the arterial and tissue analysis, in order to obtain a theoretical curve of concentration (of contrast agent in the tissue under analysis)/time, said impulse residue function (IRF)[41] (Fig. 28-2). Using the first part of the curve of concentration of the contrast agent in the tissue is applicable to the assumption that the contrast agent is only in the vascular compartment; thus, it is possible to calculate the BF, BV, and the MTT inside of the microvessels according to the "central volume principle" BF = BV/MTT. In fact, the contrast agent is only distributed in the vascular parenchyma in the healthy brain (where the blood–brain barrier prevents passage into the extravascular/extracellular compartment), in the testis, and in the retina; in all other organs, the contrast agent diffuses through the capillaries into the interstitium. However, most of the contrast agent lately diffuses into the interstitium, and the proportion that will spread during its first pass is small (first pass); therefore, it can be assumed that the contrast agent is theoretically only in the vascular compartment also in all other parenchyma, if only early scans are used for the analysis of perfusion (within 45 to 60 seconds from the start of the administration of contrast material), with a maximum error of 15%. Using the last part of the curve, through adiabatic approximation of St. Lawrence and Lee, it is possible to quantify the passage of contrast material into the interstitial compartment, including also the analysis of pCT scans carried out after the first pass (interstitial phase). The calculation of the PS takes place according to the following equation: $PS = -BF [\ln (1 - E)]$, where E represents the fraction of contrast agent that diffuses into the interstitium of the vascular space (extraction fraction).

REFERENCES

1. **Gillard JH, Antoun NM, Burnet NG, et al.** Reproducibility of quantitative CT perfusion imaging. *Br J Radiol* 2001;74:552–555.
2. **Miles KA, Hayball MP, Dixon AK.** Functional images of hepatic perfusion obtained with dynamic CT. *Radiology* 1993;188:405–411.
3. **Kai L, Wang J, Ivanovic M, et al.** Targeting prostate cancer angiogenesis through metastasis-associated protein 1 (MTA1). *Prostate* 2011;71(3):268–280.
4. **Aragon-Ching JB, Dahut WL.** VEGF inhibitors and prostate cancer therapy. *Curr Mol Pharmacol* 2009;2(2):161–168.
5. **Kluetz PG, Figg WD, Dahut WL.** Angiogenesis inhibitors in the treatment of prostate cancer. *Expert Opin Pharmacother* 2010;11(2) 233–247.
6. **Bunsiripaiboon P, Sornmayura P, Wilasrusmee C, et al.** The prognostic significance of microvessel density in intrahepatic cholangiocarcinoma. *J Med Assoc Thai* 2010;93(1):66–72.
7. **Erbersdobler A, Isbarn H, Dix K, et al.** Prognostic value of microvessel density in prostate cancer: a tissue microarray study. *World J Urol* 2010;28(6):687–692.
8. **Cuenod CA, Fournier L, Balvay D, et al.** Tumor angiogenesis: pathophysiology and implications for contrast-enhanced MRI and CT assessment. *Abdom Imaging* 2006;31(2):188–193.
9. **Brasch R, Turetschek K.** MRI characterization of tumors and grading angiogenesis using macromolecular contrast media: status report. *Eur J Radiol* 2000;34:148–155.
10. **Griebel J, Mayr NA, de Vries A, et al.** Assessment of tumor microcirculation: a new role of dynamic contrast MR imaging. *J Magn Reson Imaging* 1997;7:111–119.
11. **Neeman M.** Preclinical MRI experience in imaging angiogenesis. *Cancer Metastasis Rev* 2000;19:39–43.
12. **Miles KA.** Functional computed tomography in oncology. *Eur J Cancer* 2002;38(16):2079–2084.
13. **Lee TY, Purdie TG, Stewart E.** CT imaging of angiogenesis. *Q J Nucl Med* 2003;47:171–187.
14. **Cuenod C, Leconte I, Siauve N, et al.** Early changes in liver perfusion caused by occult metastases in rats: detection with quantitative CT. *Radiology* 2001;218:556–561.
15. **Chen TW, Yang ZG, Wang QL, et al.** Whole tumour quantitative measurement of first-pass perfusion of oesophageal squamous cell carcinoma using 64-row multidetector computed tomography: correlation with microvessel density. *Eur J Radiol* 2011;79(2):218–223.
16. **Jiang NC, Han P, Zhou CK, et al.** Dynamic enhancement patterns of solitary pulmonary nodules at multi-detector row CT and correlation with vascular endothelial growth factor and microvessel density. *Ai Zheng* 2009;28(2):164–169.
17. **Feng ST, Sun CH, Li ZP, et al.** Evaluation of angiogenesis in colorectal carcinoma with multidetector-row CT multislice perfusion imaging. *Eur J Radiol* 2009;75:191–196.

18. **Faggioni L, Neri E, Bartolozzi C.** CT perfusion of head and neck tumors: how we do it. *AJR Am J Roentgenol* 2010;194:62–69.
19. **Ng CS, Wang X, Faria SC, et al.** Perfusion CT in patients with metastatic renal cell carcinoma treated with interferon. *AJR Am J Roentgenol* 2010;194:166–171.
20. **Yang HF, Du Y, Ni JX, et al.** Perfusion computed tomography evaluation of angiogenesis in liver cancer. *Eur Radiol* 2010;20:1424–1430.
21. **Miles KA, Griffiths MR.** Perfusion CT: a worthwhile enhancement? *Br J Radiol* 2003;76:220–231.
22. **Miles KA, Hayball M, Dixon AK.** Colour perfusion imaging: a new application of computed tomography. *Lancet* 1991;337:643–645.
23. **Kambadakone AR, Sahani DV.** Body perfusion CT: technique, clinical applications, and advances. *Radiol Clin North Am* 2009;47(1):161–178. doi: 10.1016/j.rcl.2008.11.003. Review. PubMed PMID: 19195541.
24. **Miles KA.** Tumour angiogenesis and its relation to contrast enhancement on computed tomography: a review. *Eur J Radiol* 1999;30(3):198–205.
25. **Miles KA.** Perfusion CT for the assessment of tumour vascularity: which protocol? *Br J Radiol* 2003;76 (Spec No 1):S36–S42.
26. **Petralia G, Preda L, D'Andrea G, et al.** CT perfusion in solid-body tumours. Part I: technical issues. *Radiol Med* 2010;115(6):843–857. doi: 10.1007/s11547-010-0519-y. English, Italian. PubMed PMID: 20177989.
27. **Miles KA, Charnsangavej C, Lee FT, et al.** Application of CT in the investigation of angiogenesis in oncology. *Acad Radiol* 2000;7(10):840–850.
28. **Goh V, Halligan S, Bartram CI.** Quantitative tumor perfusion assessment with multidetector CT: are measurements from two commercial software packages interchangeable? *Radiology* 2007;242(3):777–782. PubMed PMID: 17325066.
29. **Ogul H, Kantarci M, Genc B, et al.** Perfusion CT imaging of the liver: review of clinical applications. *Diagn Interv Radiol* 2014;20:379–389. doi: 10.5152/dir.13396. PubMed PMID: 24834487.
30. **Chen ML, Zeng QY, Huo JW, et al.** Assessment of the hepatic microvascular changes in liver cirrhosis by perfusion computed tomography. *World J Gastroenterol* 2009;15(28):3532–3537. PubMed PMID: 19630110; PubMed Central PMCID: PMC2715981.
31. **Hashimoto K, Murakami T, Dono K, et al.** Assessment of the severity of liver disease and fibrotic change: the usefulness of hepatic CT perfusion imaging. *Oncol Rep* 2006;16(4):677–683. PubMed PMID: 16969479.
32. **Pandharipande PV, Krinsky GA, Rusinek H, et al.** Perfusion imaging of the liver: current challenges and future goals. *Radiology* 2005;234(3):661–673.
33. **Ippolito D, Capraro C, Casiraghi A, et al.** Quantitative assessment of tumour associated neovascularisation in patients with liver cirrhosis and hepatocellular carcinoma: role of dynamic-CT perfusion imaging. *Eur Radiol* 2012;22(4):803–811. doi: 10.1007/s00330-011-2307-z. PubMed PMID: 22086560.
34. **Zhu AX, Holalkere NS, Muzikansky A, et al.** Early antiangiogenic activity of bevacizumab evaluated by computed tomography perfusion scan in patients with advanced hepatocellular carcinoma. *Oncologist* 2008;13(2):120–125. doi: 10.1634/theoncologist.2007-0174. PubMed PMID: 18305056.
35. **Leggett DA, Kelley BB, Bunce IH, et al.** Colorectal cancer: diagnostic potential of CT measurements of hepatic perfusion and implications for contrast enhancement protocols. *Radiology* 1997;205(3):716–720. PubMed PMID: 9393526.
36. **Jain RK.** Normalization of tumor vasculature: an emerging concept in antiangiogenic therapy. *Science* 2005;307:58–62.
37. **Hinnen P, Eskens FA.** Vascular disrupting agents in clinical development. *Br J Cancer* 2007;96:1159–1165.
38. **Sainani NI, Catalano OA, Holalkere NS, et al.** Cholangiocarcinoma: current and novel imaging techniques. *Radiographics* 2008;28(5):1263–1287. doi: 10.1148/rg.285075183. Review. PubMed PMID: 18794305.
39. **Bartolozzi C, Crocetti L, Cioni D, et al.** Assessment of therapeutic effect of liver tumor ablation procedures. *Hepatogastroenterology* 2001;48:352–358.
40. **Yang L, Zhang XM, Zhou XP, et al.** Correlation between tumor perfusion and lipiodol deposition in hepatocellular carcinoma after transarterial chemoembolization. *J Vasc Interv Radiol* 2010;21:1841–1846.
41. **Thng CH, Koh TS, Collins D, et al.** Perfusion imaging in liver MRI. *Magn Reson Imaging Clin N Am* 2014;22(3):417–432.

CHAPTER

29 Renal Perfusion Imaging with MRI

Byron Gaing, MD, Henry Rusinek, PhD, and Hersh Chandarana, MD

Introduction

Evaluation of renal function with noninvasive methods has become an important topic in medicine both in clinical practice and in research. Subtle changes in renal function occur before anatomic changes are manifested, and early detection of functional impairment can allow for earlier, more effective treatment. The most widely used indicator of renal function is based on estimated glomerular filtration rate (GFR), calculated from patient serum creatinine (SCR) and corrected for age, gender, and race. The most often used estimate, known as Modification of Diet in Renal Disease formula,[1,2] is as follows:

$$\mathrm{GFR}\left(\text{in mL/min/1.73 m}^2\right) = 186 \times \mathrm{SCR}^{-1.154} \times \mathrm{age}^{-0.203} \quad (1)$$

$$\left[\begin{array}{l}\text{Correction factors for special populations:}\\ \times 0.742\left(\text{if female}\right); \times 1.212\left(\text{if African American}\right)\end{array}\right]. \quad (2)$$

A different equation is used for children.[3]

However, SCR-based GFR estimates are of limited accuracy in certain patient populations,[4,5] especially those that do not fit into the demographics that were used to define the equations. SCR is insensitive to early renal dysfunction; thus, abnormalities in SCR are often discovered late when irreversible renal damage may have already taken place. Furthermore, SCR-based equations provide estimated GFR for total kidney function rather than for single-kidney function. Determination of single-kidney function is important for many clinical applications including renal artery stenosis (RAS), preoperative evaluation for partial nephrectomy, and determination of split renal function in cases of obstructive uropathy.

Other techniques such as inulin clearance and technetium 99m–based renal scintigraphy have been used to estimate single-kidney renal function. These methods, however, are time consuming and not practical for routine clinical use.[6] Furthermore, nuclear studies that provide single kidney functional information are limited by poor spatial resolution and thus do not provide detailed morphologic information. Dynamic computed tomography (CT) perfusion techniques provide superior spatial resolution and direct correlation between iodine quantification and attenuation values. However, this is associated with significant radiation exposure as well as nephrotoxicity of iodinated contrast agents, particularly in a subset of patients with chronic kidney disease (CKD).[7]

Magnetic resonance (MR) imaging has a proven track record for anatomic imaging of the kidneys. The role of MR is expanding to include functional assessment of the kidneys (Table 29.1). Techniques such as dynamic contrast-enhanced (DCE) MRI, diffusion-weighted imaging (DWI), blood oxygenation level–dependent MRI, and arterial spin labeling (ASL) have potential to noninvasively assess multiple aspects of renal function. MR renography (MRR) is an emerging technique that can monitor the transit of gadolinium-containing tracers through the renal cortex, medulla, and collecting system. Widely available low molecular weight gadolinium chelate are filtered but not secreted or reabsorbed by the tubules. The pharmacokinetics of gadolinium chelates is similar to conventional tracers like inulin or iodinated contrast agents. Thus, analyzing enhancement of renal tissue over time allows measurement of single-kidney parameters that are clinically relevant such as GFR. MRR has a number of important advantages over other imaging techniques in noninvasive measurement of renal function:

1. Superior anatomic depiction and resolution is advantageous over nuclear imaging.
2. No ionizing radiation or iodinated contrast material is utilized.
3. It requires only a small dose of gadolinium-based contrast agent and is safe for most patients except those with severely impaired renal function.
4. It can be easily incorporated into routine clinical MRI protocols.[8] For example, at our institution, the addition of MRR has been successfully implemented into preoperative imaging of renal masses, adding only about 10 minutes of additional scan time.

The first part of this chapter briefly reviews the anatomy and physiology of the kidney. We then discuss the details of MRR technique and technical aspects of the image analysis pipeline. Finally, we survey clinical applications of MRR in evaluating renal disease.

Anatomy and Physiology of the Kidney

The primary function of the kidney is to maintain homeostasis through filtering and secreting metabolites from blood for excretion as urine, while at the same time reabsorbing water and essential electrolytes. The kidney also plays several secondary endocrine

TABLE 29.1 **Functional MRI Techniques and the Physiologic Processes They Measure**

Physiologic Process	MRI Technique
Perfusion	ASL, DCE, DWI (IVIM)
Glomerular filtration	DCE
Interstitial diffusion	DWI
Tissue oxygenation	BOLD
Sodium concentration	Sodium imaging

ASL, arterial spin labeling; DCE, dynamic contrast enhanced; DWI, diffusion-weighted imaging; IVIM, intravoxel incoherent motion; BOLD, blood oxygen level dependent.

functions, including regulating systemic blood pressure through secretion of renin. The kidneys receive approximately 20% of cardiac output. There is differential perfusion in the kidney with the cortex receiving approximately 400 to 500 mL/min/100 g and the medulla receiving 100 to 150 mL/min/100 g as measured by CT perfusion.[9,10]

The kidney can be divided into two main anatomic regions: the renal cortex and renal medulla (Fig. 29-1). The cortex is situated peripherally, whereas the medulla is located more centrally and is organized into conical aggregates of tissue called pyramids. Each pyramid converges into its apex, referred to as the renal papilla. Fluids and electrolytes flow through the renal cortex and medulla through the renal papilla and are excreted as urine into the calyces of the collecting system. Multiple renal calyces converge in the renal pelvis at the renal hilum and flow into the ureter, which finally drains urine from each kidney into the urinary bladder. Aside from containing the renal pelvis, the renal hilum is the point of entry and exit of the renal artery and vein.

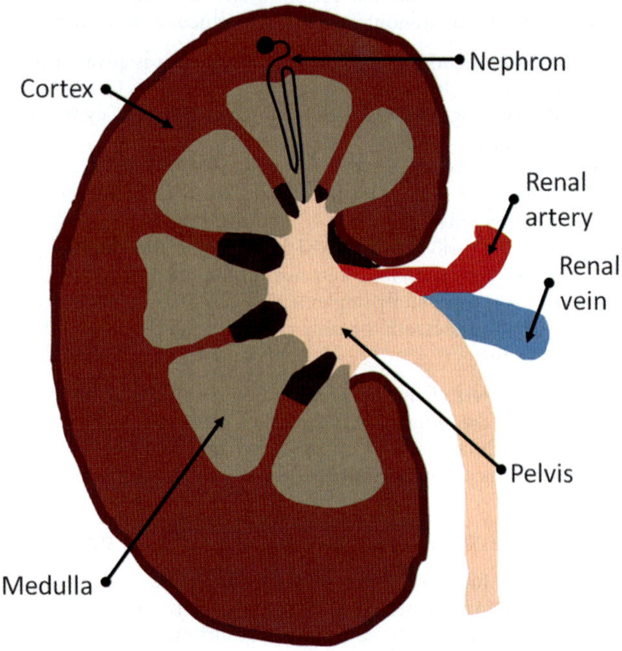

Figure 29-1. Macroscopic depiction of the kidney in coronal section.

Nephron

The kidney contains about 1 million nephrons, which are the functional units of the kidney. The main components of the nephron are the corpuscle, where plasma is initially filtered, and the tubules, where essential electrolytes are reabsorbed and other wastes are secreted. The renal corpuscle consists of an outer layer called the Bowman capsule and an inner component called the glomerulus. The glomerulus is made of bundles of capillary loops that enter the nephron via afferent arterioles. Blood is filtered at the level of the glomerulus and exits via the efferent arteriole. Filtered plasma enters the proximal tubule via the Bowman space and capsule. This process of filtration removes about 20% of the incoming renal plasma flow. The total GFR is typically 120 mL/min (60 mL/min per kidney); however, urine is produced at a rate of only 1 mL/min due to massive reabsorption of filtered contents carried out by the properly functioning kidney.

Tubules

The renal tubules carry out the reabsorption and secretion functions of the kidney. The tubules carry the filtrate from the Bowman capsule to the renal medulla where the final filtrate is excreted as urine. The tubules consist of a proximal convoluting tubule (PT), loop of Henle (LH), and distal convoluting tubule (DT). As filtrate flows through the tubules, the varying osmolarity differences either drive solutes into the filtrate or cause them to be reabsorbed back into the systemic circulation via the peritubular capillary network and vasa recta. The final renal filtrate passes from the DT to the collecting duct, which empties into the collecting system as urine.

Water and Sodium Reabsorption

The bulk of electrolyte and water exchanges that occur in the nephron are via hydrostatic and oncotic forces, with the remainder being an active process by way of energy driven ion transporters. The PT is the site of a majority of the sodium (Na) reabsorption (approximately 65%). This is accomplished through a Na/H transporter. Water follows Na via osmotic forces out of the PT, which is highly permeable to water due to abundance of aquaporin water channels. Water continues to be absorbed as the filtrate makes its way through the descending LH. The ascending limb of the LH contains abundant Na-K-2Cl active transporters, which result in an additional 25% of Na being absorbed. The ascending limb and DT are impermeable to water. About 5% of Na is absorbed in the DT via a Na/Cl transporter. These transporters are driven by the Na/K pump, which utilizes energy in the form of ATP. As previously mentioned, the renal medulla receives a small fraction of total renal blood flow (RBF). When considered along with the abundance of energy-consuming active sodium transport that occurs in the medulla, this setting creates an environment of hypoxia (oxygen pressure PO_2 is only 10 to 20 mm Hg in the medulla vs. 50 to 60 mm Hg in the cortex).[11,12] In the collecting ducts, water absorption is controlled by antidiuretic hormone, which allows added fine-tuning of water and salt homeostasis depending on the subject's hydration status. The role of each component of the nephron in salt and water homeostasis is summarized in Table 29.2.

Renal Autoregulation

The renin–angiotensin feedback loop allows the kidney to maintain RBF and GFR despite variations in systemic blood pressure. In states of relative renal hypoperfusion such as shock or dehydration, decreased pressure on the renal arterial side leads to decreased glomerular filtration. The result is decreased renal tubular Na concentration, which is readily detected by chemoreceptors called

TABLE 29.2 **The Role of Each Nephron Component in Salt and Water Homeostasis**

Component	Function
Corpuscle (Bowman capsule + glomerulus)	Initial filtration of plasma
Proximal tubule	Active reabsorption of sodium Water reabsorption by osmosis
Descending limb loop of Henle	Water reabsorption by osmosis
Ascending limb loop of Henle	Active reabsorption of sodium
Distal tubule	Active reabsorption of sodium
Collecting duct	Water reabsorption under the influence of ADH

ADH, antidiuretic hormone.

macula densa. These receptors stimulate the renin and angiotensin cascade, whose final action is to constrict the efferent arteriole thus maintaining GFR. Angiotensin-converting enzyme (ACE) inhibitors are a class of drugs that counteract this pathway and are useful in unmasking the compensatory effects of the renin–angiotensin system in cases of renovascular hypertension.

MR Renography Technique

MRI allows distinct visualization of the renal cortex, medulla, and collecting system allowing for accurate segmentation. MRR requires that we capture the time course of cortical and medullary kidney signal intensity after contrast agent injection. Development of advanced mathematical models of kidney function has allowed us to determine various measures of renal function noninvasively. Most of these models require that we also acquire the dynamic signal in the arterial blood (arterial input function [AIF]). It must be emphasized that there is no consensus regarding the optimal model or protocol for performing MRR. The following section attempts to give the reader a broad overview of the technique rather than focusing on any specific protocol.

Technical Factors

One advantage of MRR is that it can be added to any conventional abdominal MRI protocol. Either two-dimensional (2D) or three-dimensional (3D) interpolated spoiled gradient-echo acquisitions are performed in the axial or coronal plane for perfusion-weighted imaging (PWI). The optimal sequence should have sufficiently high temporal resolution (<5 seconds) and volumetric coverage for accurate characterization of renal parenchymal enhancement. Currently available MR units can achieve these standards using a combination of high-powered gradients, parallel imaging, and view-sharing techniques.

Perfusion imaging can be performed on either 1.5 or 3.0 T units. We routinely use a coronal 3D-spoiled T1-weighted gradient-echo sequence, sometimes with a view-sharing undersampling method called time-resolved angiography with stochastic trajectories (TWIST). This allows acquisition of data at sufficiently high spatial and temporal resolution but at the expense of lower signal-to-noise ratio (SNR).[13,14] In our opinion, a 3D acquisition method, while more complex to analyze, is preferable to a 2D acquisition to allow whole-organ coverage and account for regional organ perfusion differences. Because the entire volume is acquired, the radiologist or technologist is not required to manually select the appropriate coverage area, minimizing operator dependency. 2D technique may suffice in certain situations where the disease process affects the entire kidney homogenously and no regional differences are expected. 2D acquisition also allows acquisition at a higher temporal resolution at the expense of decreased volumetric coverage. Temporal blurring due to view sharing between time points may occur with the TWIST technique and is a concern with this type of 3D acquisition (Fig. 29-2). The imaging field of view should cover both the abdominal aorta and the kidneys. This poses a problem in 2D technique, requiring one to set up an interleaving coronal protocol,[15] with one coronal section through the abdominal aorta to measure the AIF and another coronal section through the long axis of both kidneys. Coronal acquisition minimizes through-plane inflow-related artifacts.[16] Parallel imaging factors of 2 to 3 are used

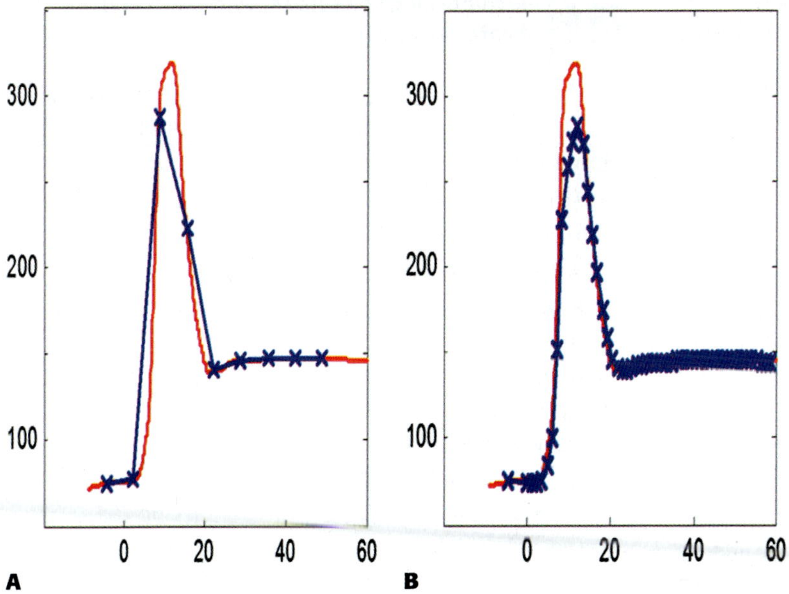

Figure 29-2. TWIST-sampled aortic SI curves (*blue line and markers*) compared with the true ideal aortic curves (*red line*) during the initial minute. TWIST method splits the frequency domain k < kmax into two separate subregions, A and B. Region A consist of lower spatial frequency samples, k < kc. Region B consists of higher frequency k >= kc samples. Region B is further divided into N polar wedges. Sampling of entire region A is interleaved with sampling of successive wedges from region B. pA = kc/kmax, pB = 1/N. **A:** Moderate undersampling (pA = 0.5, pB = 0.5) results in lower temporal resolution. **B:** High undersampling (pA = 0.1, pB = 0.1) leads to high temporal resolution. Note, however, that even with high temporal resolution, the aortic peak is underestimated because of data sharing with adjacent images where aortic signal is lower.

TABLE 29.3 **Example of a Clinical Renal MR Protocol with Inclusion of MR Renography**

MR Protocol with Incorporation of MRR
Transverse breath-hold T1-weighted in- and opposed-phase GRE
Transverse and coronal breath-hold T2-weighted half-Fourier single-shot turbo spin echo (HASTE)
Transverse 3D fat-suppressed T1-weighted interpolated spoiled GRE (VIBE) prior to contrast administration
Low-dose MRR: coronal 3D T1-weighted GRE FLASH initiated 5 s after administration of 4 mL of contrast at 2 mL/s
▪ 10 measures at 3-s temporal resolution over a 30-s breath-hold
▪ 18 measures at 3-s temporal resolution over a series of 15-s breath-holds
▪ 7 measures every 30 s
▪ 7 measures every 60 s
High-resolution anatomic imaging: coronal breath-hold 3D T1-weighted GRE FLASH prior to and three times following injection of the remainder of the standard weight–based dose of gadolinium-DTPA contrast at 2 mL/s

GRE, gradient recalled echo; FLASH, fast low-angle shot.

to accelerate image acquisition times. To obtain renal signal intensities at baseline, three to five volume acquisitions are performed before contrast administration.

It has been shown that gadolinium concentrations on the order of 0.02 mmol/kg (approximately 4 mL) in healthy individuals and 0.025 mmol/kg (approximately 5 mL) in patients with renal insufficiency allow measurement of GFR with greatest precision.[17] High concentrations of gadolinium should be avoided to minimize T2* effects and loss of signal. For a typical examination, approximately 4 mL of extracellular contrast agent (gadopentetate dimeglumine, Bayer HealthCare) is administered at a rate of 2 mL/s via power injector followed by a 20 mL saline flush. Imaging begins immediately after contrast administration. With current scanner technology, continuous 3D frames of 30 to 40 3D interpolated (15 to 20 noninterpolated) sections can be acquired every 3 to 5 seconds. With the 2D approach, the temporal resolution can be 1 second per frame or faster. Images can be obtained in multiple breath-holds or in free-breathing. Both of these acquisition schemes would require coregistration of dynamic data sets. We routinely acquire dynamic data during multiple breath-holds at end expiration to minimize misregistration artifacts. This is followed by 4 to 5 seconds of shallow respiration between breath-holds. Oxygen is administered to facilitate breath-holding.[18] Total acquisition time ranges from about 3 to 10 minutes. A summary of the MRR protocol and technical parameters we have used at our institution is provided in Tables 29.3 and 29.4.

Postprocessing Techniques

Image analysis is considered to be the main challenge limiting widespread clinical use of MRR. The basic data output of a perfusion sequence is a signal intensity over time curve. Various postprocessing techniques have been used to analyze these data including semiquantitative and quantitative methods, the choice of which depends on the particular clinical application.

Semiquantitative analysis has been used in many other clinical applications such as oncologic imaging and breast MRI.[19,20] These have the advantage of relative ease of image analysis without the need for a pharmacokinetic mathematical model to convert signal intensity to gadolinium contrast concentration as with quantitative methods. Common parameters that are used include initial upslope or maximal slope, time to peak, maximum signal intensity, initial area under the curve, and washout. The disadvantages of semiquantitative analysis are in the variability in measurements and difficulties in interpreting the results. Poor reliability stems from a variety of factors such as technical imprecision associated with defining bolus arrival time, image noise, observer bias, and patient-specific factors such as cardiac output. This can limit reproducibility between different scanners and between patients. Also the output parameters are indirect surrogates for true physiologic measures, and the exact biophysiologic correlate for these parameters is unclear.

Quantitative analysis involves converting signal intensity data into clinically useful metrics such as GFR, renal plasma flow, and split renal function. This process can be divided into three basic steps: (a) image registration and segmentation, (b) conversion of MR signal to gadolinium concentration versus time curves, and (c) applying a tracer kinetic model to derive clinically relevant metrics such as GFR. Each of these steps has its own challenges and is discussed.

TABLE 29.4 **Technical Parameters for Perfusion and Anatomic Imaging Sequences**

	Low-Dose MRR	High-Resolution FLASH
Plane	Coronal	Coronal
TR/TE (ms)	2.8/1.0	3.1/1.2
Flip angle (degrees)	12	25
Slice thickness (mm)	2.5	1.2
Bandwidth (Hz/voxel)	650	650
Voxel size (mm)	2.2 × 1.4 × 2.5	1.5 × 0.9 × 1.2
Parallel imaging factor (GRAPPA)	3	2
Slices per measure	40	88
Acquisition time (per volume)	3–5 s	10–20 s

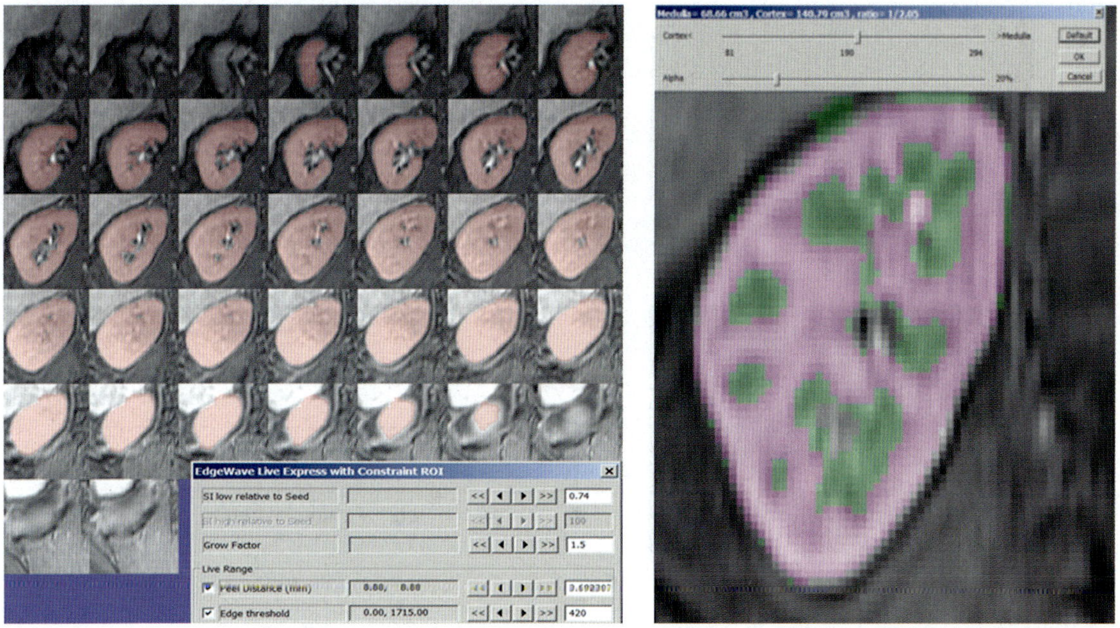

A **B**

Figure 29-3. Three-dimensional segmentation of the right kidney from high-resolution postcontrast VIBE perfusion sequence (**A**). Cortex–medulla segmentation (**B**).

Image Registration and Segmentation

Manual regions of interest (ROIs) are created circumscribing the kidney and aorta at the level of the renal arteries. Additionally, separate ROIs can be drawn to only include the renal cortex or medulla for further segmentation[21] (Fig. 29-3). This step partially accounts for patient respiratory motion and can be used to generate renal parenchymal volume. Over the course of the 3- to 5-minute acquisition, there is considerable patient motion in the imaging field, mostly from respiration. Newer techniques have been developed for automated motion and registration correction.[22,23] Additionally, imaging in the coronal plane limits the majority of motion secondary to respiration within the in-plane direction, which facilitates the use of automated coregistration software.

Conversion of MR Signal to Gadolinium Concentration

Modeling RBF and function requires obtaining an accurate measure of the enhancement or time–intensity curve of the feeding vessel (in this case the aorta), otherwise known as the AIF. This poses several challenges as arterial signal on MRI suffers from various artifacts including inflow effect, spin dephasing, partial volume effect, and pulsation artifact. Coronal imaging helps minimize AIF inflow artifact (Fig. 29-4). Flow variations along the course of the abdominal aorta result in a heterogeneous distribution of the AIF depending on the portion of the aorta being measured. Additionally, the size of the ROI drawn to capture the aortic signal also influences the AIF.[24,25] Early attempts at overcoming these issues relied on surrogate markers for arterial input, such as the signal in renal cortex.[26,27] However, these methods did not provide information on RBF.

A simple population-based approach averaged the AIF on healthy volunteers and applied this value to the study of subsequent patients. However, application to a diverse patient population with varying comorbidities was limited. It is known that cardiac output affects significantly the shape of the AIF, thus this attribute of the control group from which the average is obtained needs to match the study group.[28,29]

More sophisticated methods to directly measure the AIF while compensating for flow artifacts were subsequently explored in the MRR literature. One technique involved using a double bolus to compensate for potential distortion of the first-pass AIF at low temporal resolution. Precisely timed dual-injection protocol is designed to reduce the impact of temporal undersampling on the initial AIF bolus passage. The hypothesis is that missampling of one peak could be compensated by the properly sampled second peak, improving the overall accuracy and reproducibility of the measurement.[30]

A method based on indicator dilution theory incorporated the patient's cardiac output, injected dose of contrast, and area under the first-pass AIF curve to accurately depict the AIF of each individual patient.[31] The patient's cardiac output can be measured during the same MR perfusion scan by simply acquiring an additional cardiac phase-contrast sequence.

MRI signal intensities are converted into gadolinium concentration curves over time. Unlike glomerular tracers used for CT (iodine) and scintigraphy (^{99m}Tc-DTPA or ^{51}Cr-EDTA), which show a linear relationship between attenuation and contrast agent concentration, gadolinium-based contrast agents have a nonlinear relationship between measured signal intensity and gadolinium concentration. The complex relationships between concentration and the effect on T_1, T_2, and T_2* weighting all factor into the observed signal intensity.[32] With MRI, the signal intensities in most sequences are based on weighted T_1 and T_2 values. As such, the aortic and renal signal intensity values must be first converted into T_1 values in order to measure gadolinium concentration. The additivity of relaxivity allows one to derive gadolinium concentration curves from the T_1 values based on the following formula:

$$[\mathrm{Gd}] = \left(1/\mathrm{T}_1 - 1/\mathrm{T}_1 0\right)/\mathrm{R}_1, \tag{3}$$

where [Gd] is gadolinium concentration, R_1 is the relaxivity of gadolinium, and $T_1 0$ is the measured unenhanced T_1 value for the ROI (aorta, renal cortex, or medulla).[33] The formula requires that for each tissue and each time point, the measured variable signal

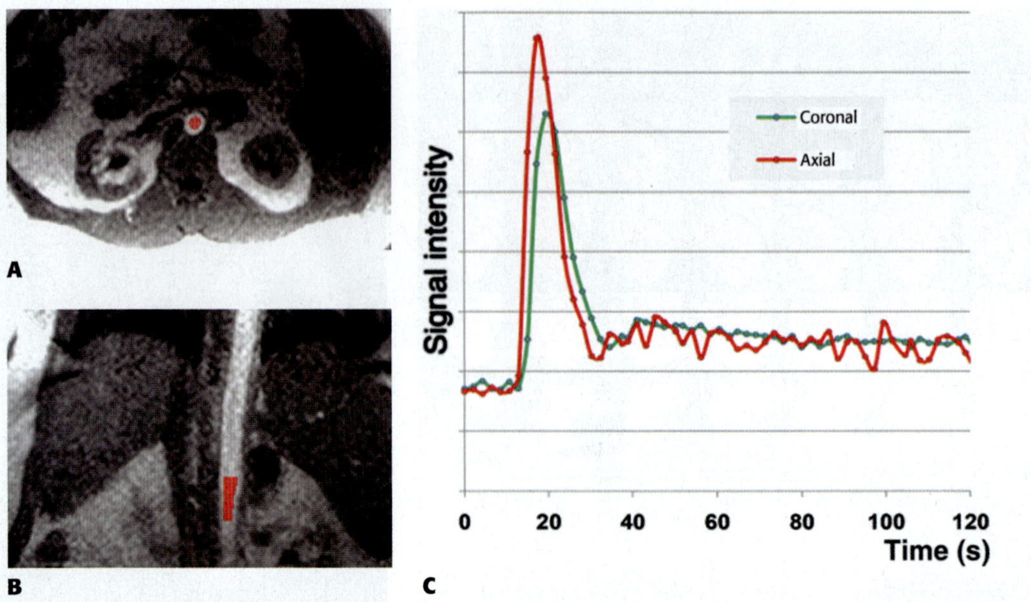

Figure 29-4. Variability in aortic input function. A: Dynamic axial acquisition showing an ROI in *red*; **B:** interleaved coronal acquisition for the same dynamic exam, with an ROI in *red* at approximately the same level; **C:** Signal intensity versus time curves sampled from these two regions shows different shapes, most likely due to larger inflow effect for axial acquisition. Coronal acquisition is preferred.

intensity SI(t) be converted to a corresponding T_1 value $T_1(t)$. A recent study[34] discusses advantages and disadvantages of two different approaches for implementing such a conversion appropriate for a given acquisition sequence: (a) linear approximation and (b) nonlinear approach. To date, the most widely accepted tissue-specific relaxivities for Gd-DTPA measured using a 1.5-T system are R_1 of 1.1 to 1.2/s/mM for the renal cortex and 1.3 to 1.6/s/mM for the renal medulla,[35,36] whereas the relaxivity of plasma is 4 to 5/s/mM. The precontrast T_1 value (T_10) of various tissues can be obtained with techniques that have been described, which include the variable flip angle method and inversion recovery method.[37–39]

Quantitative Tracer Kinetic Modeling

A tracer kinetic model is finally applied to the derived gadolinium concentration curves to yield perfusion parameters for one or both kidneys. These models rely on accurate segmentation of the kidneys, particularly for complex three-compartment modeling where missegmentation of the cortex and medulla could result in partial volume effect that lowers the accuracy of GFR estimates.[21,40] Several such models have been described in the literature.[41–43] At this time, there is no consensus regarding the optimal model to be used. This may ultimately depend on the clinical question being answered or the biomarker being measured.

The simplest method to describe the transit of contrast through the kidney is the two-compartment model restricted to vascular and tubular compartments only[43] as described in the Rutland-Patlak plot. However, the major limitation of this model is that it does not account for transit of gadolinium-based contrast out of the tubular compartment. Further work led to refinement of this model by allowing a time delay from when the contrast bolus from the aorta reached the intrarenal vasculature. Additionally, contrast exit from the tubular compartment was described using an exponential decay function.[41] The promising results of this animal model were successfully applied to healthy human volunteers to measure renal perfusion and GFR.[44] However, a follow-up comparison study on human subjects showed that this technique tended to overestimate single-kidney GFR although there was a better overall fit to the experimental data compared to the Rutland-Patlak approach.[42] Yet another approach models the vascular and tubular transit as a parallel, two-pathway model.[45]

The ability to better segment the renal cortex and medulla led to more elaborate modeling using three compartments. In our practice, we have used a three-compartment corticomedullary tracer kinetic model to obtain single-kidney GFR normalized to the patient's total body surface area[31,33,46] (Fig. 29-5). The added benefit of using three-compartment models is to allow functional assessment of the renal tubules.

The advances in MR imaging technique as well as refinements in postprocessing and mathematical modeling described above have allowed practical application of MRR to various disease processes affecting the kidney as will be discussed in the next section.

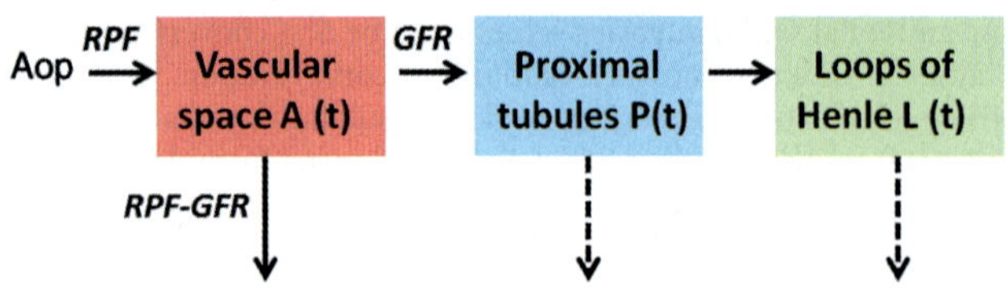

Figure 29-5. Multicompartmental corticomedullary tracer kinetic model. Vascular, tubular, and loop of Henle compartments are modeled as shown. RPF and GFR can be extracted knowing the Aop. Aop, aortic input function; RPF, renal plasma flow; GFR, glomerular filtration rate.

Clinical Applications

Preoperative Planning for Nephron-Sparing Surgery

With advances in surgical techniques, nephron-sparing procedures are being performed with increasing frequency.[47] Minimally invasive procedures such as laparoscopic and robotic partial nephrectomy have been shown to have equal oncologic outcomes compared to open approaches with decrease in adverse measures such as pain, shorter length of hospital stay, and better cosmetic outcome.[48–50] However, compared to open procedures, the minimally invasive techniques subject the kidney to warm ischemia times. There is concern for ischemic injury to the kidney secondary to renal artery clamping during the procedure.[51,52] It has been shown that even with nephron-sparing procedures, CKD develops in up to 50% of patients postoperatively.[53] In addition to loss of nephrons, the ischemic injury to the renal parenchyma during the procedure may contribute to future loss of renal function. Thus, it is important to assess and monitor patient renal function both before and after partial nephrectomy.

Historically, this type of assessment has been limited by the inability to measure the individual kidney response to ischemic insult during surgery. Existing techniques measuring global GFR are confounded due to inability to account for the compensatory effect of the contralateral kidney. With the advent of MRR, measurement of single-kidney function has become a clinical reality, particularly in the perioperative period (Fig. 29-6). MRR can be used not only to study the reversibility of renal function loss in the postoperative kidney but also to measure the compensatory increase in GFR of the contralateral kidney. The same techniques can be used to calculate renal parenchymal volume loss or gain, as these factors may ultimately contribute to subsequent renal function.[8] MRR can be easily performed as an adjunct to standard renal MRI with only a small increase in scan time. The low doses of gadolinium used for perfusion do not interfere with the subsequent routine DCE imaging.[15] If MRR can predict the development of CKD in post–partial nephrectomy patients, it will help in the selection of appropriate patients for partial nephrectomy and develop risk stratification schemes to allow appropriate renal protective procedures during the operation. This may influence the surgeon on the surgical approach (open vs. minimally invasive) as cold ischemia during open procedures can be used to protect the at-risk kidney.

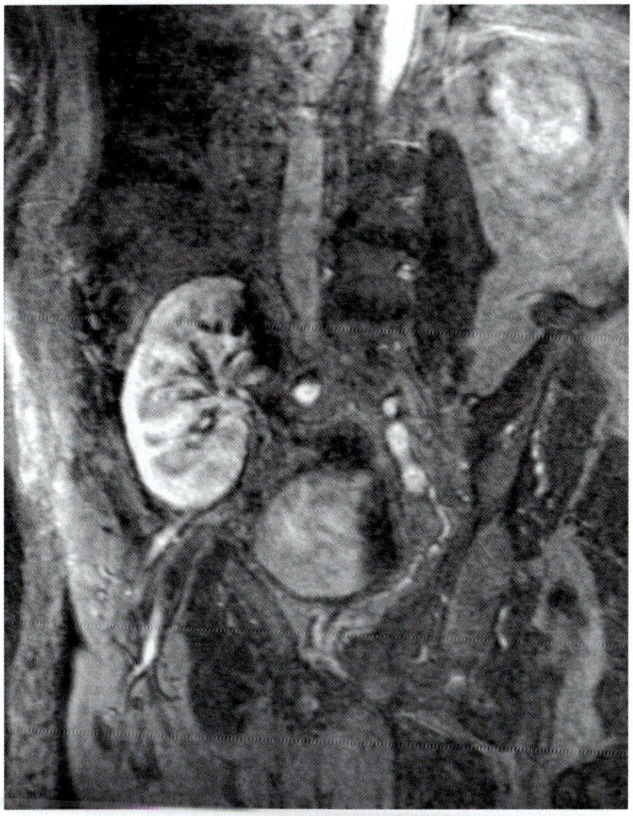

Figure 29-6. Coronal oblique view of a right iliac fossa renal transplant. MRR is useful for measuring single-kidney GFR in the perioperative period.

Renal Mass Characterization

Renal MRI is being increasingly used in clinical practice for characterization of incidentally detected renal masses.[54–56] Although the main reason for further imaging workup remains differentiation between benign and malignant masses, advances in MRI techniques, specifically DWI and perfusion weighted imaging (PWI), may also allow noninvasive assessment of tumor aggressiveness by predicting tumor grade and subtype. MRI can also serve as a powerful tool to guide clinical management of renal cell carcinoma (RCC) by assisting with surgical planning and assessment of treatment response to targeted chemotherapy.

It has been well-established that the papillary subtype of RCC enhances more homogeneously and to a lesser degree compared to the clear cell subtype.[57–60] Although it is possible with routine clinical sequences to differentiate between these two subtypes based on the degree and homogeneity of enhancement on corticomedullary phase imaging,[61] there is a need for quantitative imaging biomarkers as a more direct and less subjective way to characterize renal lesions.

PWI techniques in the kidney are showing promise in the differentiation of renal tumor subtypes, especially between benign and malignant lesions, which is sometimes not possible with conventional imaging. For example, Notohamiprodjo et al. showed distinct perfusion patterns for clear cell RCC versus papillary RCC using high temporal resolution PWI and a two-compartment-exchange model that simultaneously provided perfusion and permeability data.[62] A more recent study suggests that benign oncocytoma and chromophobe RCC, despite showing similar degree of enhancement on routine morphologic evaluation have significant differences in perfusion metrics including gadolinium exchange constant (K^{trans}) obtained with a generalized kinetic model.[63] Although these initial observations are promising, the small number of patients in these studies, as well as lack of a standardized imaging technique, and cumbersome post processing currently limits widespread adoption of these advances in daily practice. Further clinical evaluation with larger patient cohorts and different histologic subtypes should be performed to better appraise the diagnostic value of PWI in the differentiation of renal tumor subtypes.

Another clinically useful application for renal PWI is monitoring tumor response to targeted molecular therapies in patients with metastatic renal cancer. The limitations of commonly used size criteria (e.g., RECIST) for monitoring treatment response to new targeted therapies are becoming clear,[64–66] given that the biologic efficacy of these newer agents do not necessarily result in tumor size regression. Antiangiogenic drugs are now routinely used to treat metastatic RCC[67–70]; thus, new imaging biomarkers are needed to monitor their efficacy. Both qualitative and quantitative changes in PWI have been demonstrated in response to antiangiogenic drug therapy.[71,72] Quantitative parameters such as K^{trans} (gadolinium exchange constant) are shown to change early in response to targeted therapy. In one study, a high baseline K^{trans} between blood and tumor interstitium was associated with better treatment response to sorafenib as well as longer disease-free survival.[73]

Renovascular Hypertension

RAS, although an uncommon cause of hypertension, is nevertheless an important diagnosis as it is potentially treatable using catheter-directed techniques. The most common etiologies include atherosclerosis and fibromuscular dysplasia. Evaluation of RAS as a cause of systemic hypertension is confounded by the fact that many patients with renovascular hypertension also have atherosclerotic calcification without significant narrowing and/or underlying essential hypertension; thus, it is of utmost importance to identify patients with clinically significant RAS who might benefit from revascularization.

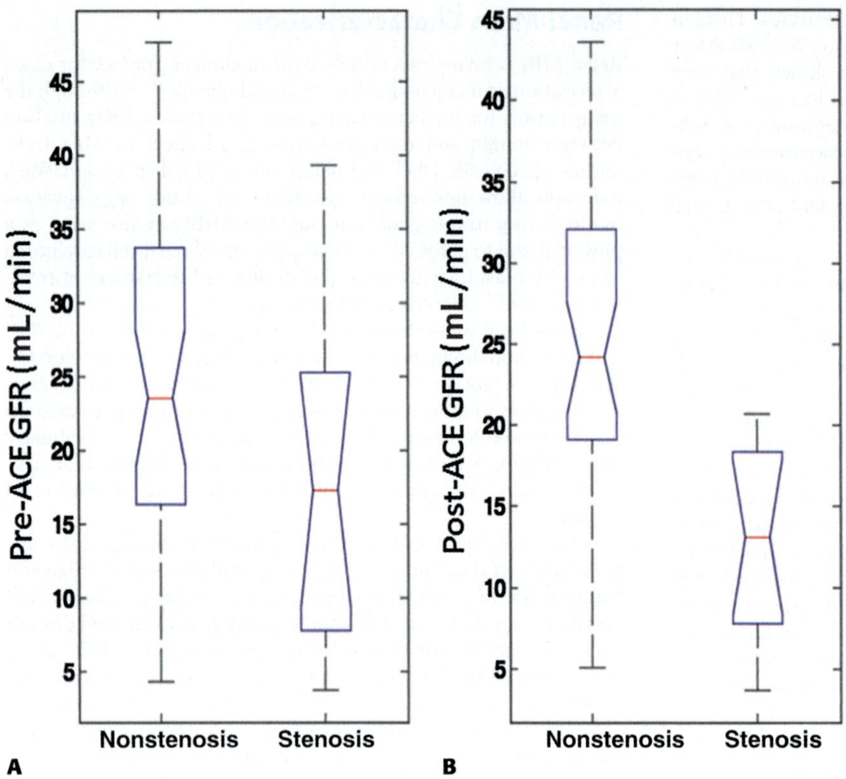

Figure 29-7. Box and whiskers plots before **(A)** and after **(B)** ACE-I administration. In hemodynamically significant renal artery stenosis, the GFR drops after administration of ACE-I compared to the normal renal artery. ACE-I, angiotensin-converting enzyme inhibitor; GFR, glomerular filtration rate.

Traditionally, nuclear renography with Captopril challenge has been used for this diagnosis.[74] However, a dual-injection MRR exam performed before and after angiotensin-converting enzyme inhibitor (ACE-I) challenge offers reliable and reproducible measures of GFR with acceptable precision and accuracy.[75–77] A significant decrease in single-kidney GFR on the affected side after administration of ACE-I indicates the presence of clinically significant RAS (Fig. 29-7). Other MR perfusion parameters that have been useful in evaluation of RAS include mean transit time, maximum upslope, and time-to-peak signal intensity.[78] These can be calculated from first-pass tracer kinetics.

Functional Urinary Obstruction

A common clinical question encountered when dealing with a hydronephrotic kidney is whether the collecting system is merely dilated without functional obstruction or whether true obstruction exists. Functional renal obstruction is an important clinical diagnosis, as long-standing obstruction can lead to renal atrophy and irreversible loss of function. The most commonly used methods for differentiating these two entities relied heavily on nuclear renography by way of diuretic challenge to assess obstruction, split renal function, and organ damage. However, scintigraphy is limited by lack of anatomic detail in the projection images as well as the need for depth correction and background subtraction.

MRR can assess renal morphology, crossing vessels, and function in a single imaging session. Dynamic contrast enhancement can be used to assess renal parenchymal loss by measuring differential renal function (DRF), which is analogous to nuclear split renal function.[79] Several methods have been proposed for assessing DRF. In order of increasing complexity, these include measurements based on renal parenchymal volume,[80] area under the tubular phase of signal versus time curve,[81] Rutland-Patlak plot,[82] or advanced models measuring MR-GFR of each kidney.[83,84]

For assessment of renal functional obstruction, renal transit time (RTT), defined as the interval between appearance of the tracer in the kidney and subsequently in the collecting system, has been shown to be elevated in obstructed kidneys.[85] With accurate segmentation of the renal cortex, medulla, and collecting system, it is possible to generate time–intensity curves showing both uptake of contrast and washout within the various segments allowing analysis of RTT.[86] Although statistically significant differences in RTT between normal, equivocal, and obstructed kidneys were demonstrated,[87] there was some overlap in the range of values, and further investigation is needed. Quoted reference ranges are listed in Table 29.5.

It has been suggested that various MRR parameters can be used to identify ureteropelvic junction (UPJ) obstructions that would

TABLE **29.5** **Reference Values for Determining Functional Urinary Obstruction by MR Renography**

Renal Transit Time (s)	Diagnosis
<245	Normal kidney
245–490	Equivocal: close follow-up needed to ensure stability of renal function
>490	Obstructed kidney

Adapted from Grattan-Smith JD, Jones RA. MR urography: technique and results for the evaluation of urinary obstruction in the pediatric population. *Magn Reson Imaging Clin N Am* 2008;16(4):643–660, viii–ix.

benefit from surgery. For example, delay in the corticomedullary crossover point as measured on signal intensity–time curves has been correlated with increased intratubular pressure from clinically significant UPJ obstruction in pediatric patients.[80] Obstructed kidneys also showed reduced ability to concentrate gadolinium contrast as manifested by decreased peak amplitude of concentration. Our group has recently shown that renal pelvic uptake rate, defined as the rate of increase in signal intensity in the renal pelvis, in mechanically obstructed kidneys was significantly lower compared to functionally obstructed kidneys[83] (Fig. 29-8).

In summary, MRR is well suited to evaluate urinary obstruction given its ability to assess both morphologic and functional changes in one comprehensive examination with superb spatial and temporal resolution.

Renal Transplant Complications

Differentiating acute graft rejection (AR) from acute tubular necrosis (ATN) in the early posttransplant period (1 to 2 weeks) remains an important clinical challenge. Whereas ATN is self-limiting, AR requires immediate treatment to prevent graft loss. Clinically, these two entities are difficult to differentiate, and percutaneous biopsy is often necessary. Nonspecific findings of graft dysfunction can be attributed to several causes in addition to AR and ATN including renal artery or vein thrombosis, cyclosporine toxicity, perinephric collections, ureteric obstruction, or arteriovenous fistula related to renal biopsy. Although ultrasound remains the primary diagnostic tool for evaluation of posttransplant complications, particularly those with morphologic or anatomic manifestations (hydronephrosis, perinephric collections), MRR may be a useful adjunct tool as investigated by various researchers.

Initial studies using semiquantitative analysis of MR enhancement curves showed that AR manifests as decreased cortical and medullary enhancement, whereas ATN predominantly affects medullary enhancement.[88] Similarly, AR is associated with a larger reduction in cortical and medullary perfusion as compared to ATN.[89] However, in that study, ATN could not be differentiated from normal kidneys based on perfusion parameters alone. Additionally, MRR with semiquantitative analysis shows promise in differentiating AR and cyclosporine toxicity.[90] As ATN essentially represents ischemic injury to the tubules resulting in reduced blood flow, decreased GFR, and tubular dysfunction, it was postulated that ATN might affect tubular transit time. Using a quantitative three-compartment model, it was shown that mean transit time showed significant differences between AR and ATN compared to normal functioning transplants.[91]

Other MR Perfusion Techniques

Arterial Spin Labeling

Initially developed for cerebral perfusion quantification, ASL has increasingly been investigated for abdominal applications including renal perfusion. Magnetically labeled protons within blood serve to provide an endogenous contrast agent, as such no exogenous contrast agent is necessary.[92] In a commonly described technique,

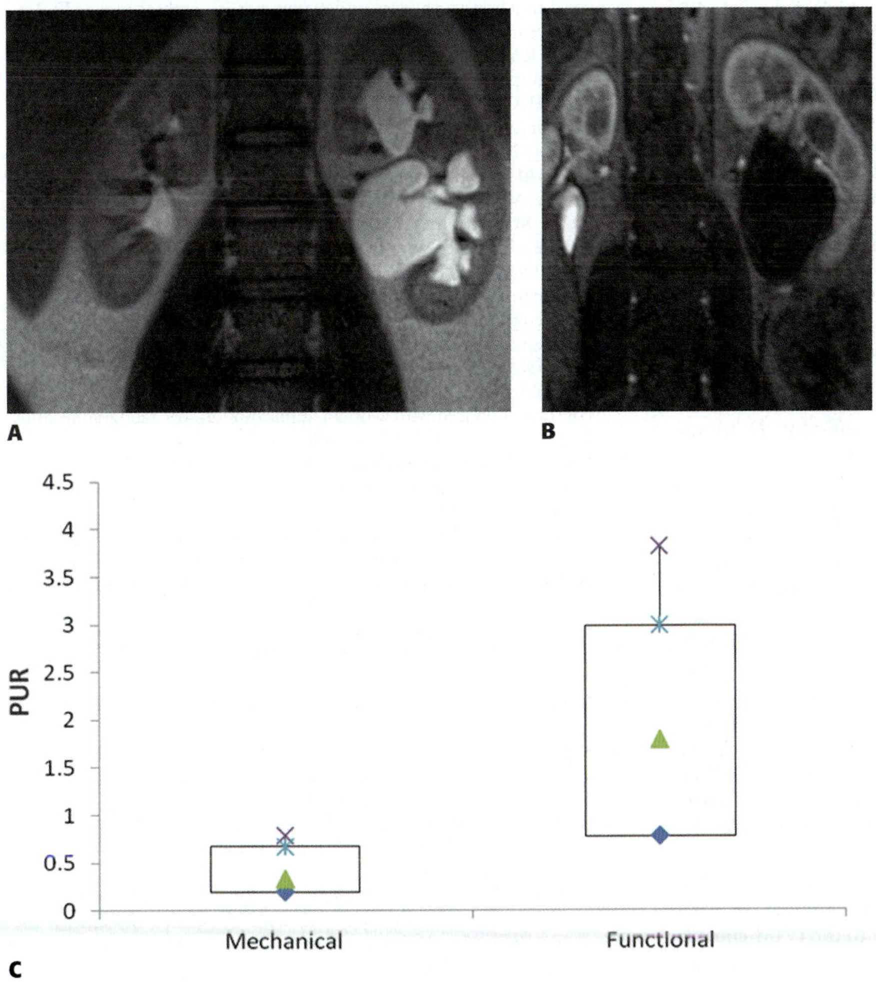

Figure 29-8. Differentiation of functional versus mechanical UPJ obstruction. **A:** Coronal HASTE and **B:** high-resolution coronal FLASH sequences through the kidneys for anatomic assessment show left hydronephrosis secondary to UPJ obstruction. However, determination of functional versus mechanical obstruction cannot be made on anatomic images alone. **C:** MRR-derived renal PUR in our study showed significantly lower values in mechanical obstruction. HASTE, half-Fourier single-shot turbo spin echo; FLASH, fast low-angle shot; MRR, MR renography; PUR, pelvic uptake rate.

the first step is to label the blood protons, usually using a FAIR (flow-sensitive alternating inversion recovery) sequence. Then, imaging is performed with a True-FISP (true fast imaging with steady-state precession) sequence. Tissue perfusion is related to the difference between the section-selective and nonselective inversion recovery sequence.[93,94] A handful of studies have applied ASL to perfusion imaging in the human and animal kidney with renal transplants,[95,96] RAS,[97] as well as contrast-induced nephropathy and acute kidney injury in animal models.[98,99]

Several challenges of ASL technique limit its widespread use. Low intrinsic SNR of this technique requires high-field strength magnets (3 T) and multiple averages. The labeled spins decay rather quickly (within a few seconds) so imaging must be performed rapidly. Generating clinically useful images requires subtraction of the unlabeled data set from the labeled data thus introducing misregistration if there is any patient motion. Dual navigator gating may partially compensate for misregistration; however, further work is needed to achieve reliable results.[100]

Diffusion-Weighted Imaging and Intravoxel Incoherent Motion

DWI is a technique that allows qualitative and quantitative assessment of random (Brownian) motion of water molecules within tissues. The difference in motility of protons in water between different tissues generates tissue contrast. The signal from DW-MRI captures the properties of tissue cellularity, integrity of cell membranes, T2-relaxation time, and microcapillary perfusion.[101–103] The key measure is the apparent diffusion coefficient (ADC). Calculation of the ADC requires two or more acquisitions with different diffusion weightings (known as *b* values). A low ADC corresponds to restricted diffusion.

However, several studies have highlighted the limitations of using the monoexponential fit (or ADC) in interpreting diffusion data in lesions,[104,105] as well as in the renal parenchyma.[106,107] Thus, the intravoxel incoherent motion (IVIM) model that performs biexponential fitting of the diffusion signal has been described as follows:

$$S(b) = S_0\left(f_p \exp(-bD_P) + (1 - f_P)\exp(-bD_t)\right) \quad (4)$$

Where $S(b)$ is the signal intensity at a given b value, and S_0 is the signal intensity before application of the diffusion gradient. f_p represents the volume fraction of the vascular compartment with its corresponding diffusion coefficient, D_p (pseudodiffusivity). The remaining volume fraction $(1 - f_p)$ represents the tissue compartment with its corresponding diffusion coefficient, D_t (tissue diffusivity).

The IVIM model shows promise for generating both perfusion and diffusion information by biexponential fitting of the diffusion data without the use of exogenous contrast agents.[108,109] With this technique, true diffusion effect can be separated from tissue perfusion by performing DWI with *b* values in both the low range (0 to 200 s/mm) and high range (>200 s/mm).

Currently, this is a rapidly expanding area of research in DWI, and applications are being developed to assess tumor response to treatment, tumor subtype differentiation, and various nononcologic applications using IVIM parameters.[104,110,111] However, several limitations of this technique require further investigation. The source data for DWI needs to be optimized for respiratory motion. Slight inaccuracies in DWI data lead to greater error propagation in calculating IVIM parameters such as f_p and D_p compared to the error involved in calculation of ADC. In addition to blood flow from microcapillary perfusion, theoretical contributions to the IVIM effect stemming from tubular flow can confound IVIM analysis. The relative contribution of tubular flow to the IVIM effect is not yet elucidated. More accurate measurement of pure perfusion based on DWI techniques requires further separation of these components that may contribute to fast diffusion.

In conclusion, MRR imaging with high spatial and temporal resolution provides a method to accurately measure renal perfusion and function. These techniques are being increasingly utilized in the clinical realm to answer relevant clinical questions.

REFERENCES

1. **Levey AS, Bosch JP, Lewis JB, et al.** A more accurate method to estimate glomerular filtration rate from serum creatinine: a new prediction equation. Modification of Diet in Renal Disease Study Group. *Ann Intern Med* 1999;130(6):461–470.
2. **Levey AS, Stevens LA, Schmid CH, et al.** A new equation to estimate glomerular filtration rate. *Ann Intern Med* 2009;150(9):604–612.
3. **Schwartz GJ, Work DF.** Measurement and estimation of GFR in children and adolescents. *Clin J Am Soc Nephrol* 2009;4(11):1832–1843.
4. **Poggio ED, Nef PC, Wang X, et al.** Performance of the Cockcroft-Gault and modification of diet in renal disease equations in estimating GFR in ill hospitalized patients. *Am J Kidney Dis* 2005;46(2):242–252.
5. **Poggio ED, Wang X, Greene T, et al.** Performance of the modification of diet in renal disease and Cockcroft-Gault equations in the estimation of GFR in health and in chronic kidney disease. *J Am Soc Nephrol* 2005;16(2):459–466.
6. **Gates GF.** Split renal function testing using Tc-99m DTPA. A rapid technique for determining differential glomerular filtration. *Clin Nucl Med* 1983;8(9):400–407.
7. **Lemoine S, Papillard M, Belloi A, et al.** Renal perfusion: noninvasive measurement with multidetector CT versus fluorescent microspheres in a pig model. *Radiology* 2011;260(2):414–420.
8. **Kang SK, Huang WC, Lee VS, et al.** MR renographic measurement of renal function in patients undergoing partial nephrectomy. *AJR Am J Roentgenol* 2013;200(6):1204–1209.
9. **Miles KA.** Measurement of tissue perfusion by dynamic computed tomography. *Br J Radiol* 1991;64(761):409–412.
10. **Zhao H, Gong J, Wang Y, et al.** Renal hemodynamic changes with aging: a preliminary study using CT perfusion in the healthy elderly. *Clin Imaging* 2010;34(4):247–250.
11. **Brezis M, Rosen S.** Hypoxia of the renal medulla—its implications for disease. *N Engl J Med* 1995;332(10):647–655.
12. **Evans RG, Gardiner BS, Smith DW, et al.** Intrarenal oxygenation: unique challenges and the biophysical basis of homeostasis. *Am J Physiol Renal Physiol* 2008;295(5):F1259–F1270.
13. **Herrmann KH, Baltzer PA, Dietzel M, et al.** Resolving arterial phase and temporal enhancement characteristics in DCE MRM at high spatial resolution with TWIST acquisition. *J Magn Reson Imaging* 2011;34(4):973–982.
14. **Song T, Laine AF, Chen Q, et al.** Optimal k-space sampling for dynamic contrast-enhanced MRI with an application to MR renography. *Magn Reson Med* 2009;61(5):1242–1248.
15. **Vivier PH, Storey P, Rusinek H, et al.** Kidney function: glomerular filtration rate measurement with MR renography in patients with cirrhosis. *Radiology* 2011;259(2):462–470.
16. **Ivancevic MK, Zimine I, Foxall D, et al.** Inflow effect in first-pass cardiac and renal MRI. *J Magn Reson Imaging* 2003;18(3):372–376.
17. **Rusinek H, Lee VS, Johnson G.** Optimal dose of Gd-DTPA in dynamic MR studies. *Magn Reson Med* 2001;46(2):312–316.
18. **Hagiwara M, Rusinek H, Lee VS, et al.** Advanced liver fibrosis: diagnosis with 3D whole-liver perfusion MR imaging—initial experience. *Radiology* 2008;246(3):926–934.
19. **Evelhoch JL.** Key factors in the acquisition of contrast kinetic data for oncology. *J Magn Reson Imaging* 1999;10(3):254–259.
20. **Kuhl CK, Mielcareck P, Klaschik S, et al.** Dynamic breast MR imaging: are signal intensity time course data useful for differential diagnosis of enhancing lesions? *Radiology* 1999;211(1):101–110.
21. **Rusinek H, Boykov Y, Kaur M, et al.** Performance of an automated segmentation algorithm for 3D MR renography. *Magn Reson Med* 2007;57(6):1159–1167.
22. **de Senneville BD, Mendichovszky IA, Roujol S, et al.** Improvement of MRI-functional measurement with automatic movement correction in native and transplanted kidneys. *J Magn Reson Imaging* 2008;28(4):970–978.

23. **Giele EL, de Priester JA, Blom JA, et al.** Movement correction of the kidney in dynamic MRI scans using FFT phase difference movement detection. *J Magn Reson Imaging* 2001;14(6):741–749.
24. **Cutajar M, Mendichovszky IA, Tofts PS, et al.** The importance of AIF ROI selection in DCE-MRI renography: reproducibility and variability of renal perfusion and filtration. *Eur J Radiol* 2010;74(3):e154–e160.
25. **Mendichovszky IA, Cutajar M, Gordon I.** Reproducibility of the aortic input function (AIF) derived from dynamic contrast-enhanced magnetic resonance imaging (DCE-MRI) of the kidneys in a volunteer study. *Eur J Radiol* 2009;71(3):576–581.
26. **Baumann D, Rudin M.** Quantitative assessment of rat kidney function by measuring the clearance of the contrast agent Gd(DOTA) using dynamic MRI. *Magn Reson Imaging* 2000;18(5):587–595.
27. **Bokacheva L, Rusinek H, Zhang JL, et al.** Assessment of renal function with dynamic contrast-enhanced MR imaging. *Magn Reson Imaging Clin N Am* 2008;16(4):597–611, viii.
28. **Parker GJ, Roberts C, Macdonald A, et al.** Experimentally-derived functional form for a population-averaged high-temporal-resolution arterial input function for dynamic contrast-enhanced MRI. *Magn Reson Med* 2006;56(5):993–1000.
29. **Wang Y, Huang W, Panicek DM, et al.** Feasibility of using limited-population-based arterial input function for pharmacokinetic modeling of osteosarcoma dynamic contrast-enhanced MRI data. *Magn Reson Med* 2008;59(5):1183–1189.
30. **Roberts C, Buckley DL, Parker GJ.** Comparison of errors associated with single- and multi-bolus injection protocols in low-temporal-resolution dynamic contrast-enhanced tracer kinetic analysis. *Magn Reson Med* 2006;56(3):611–619.
31. **Bokacheva L, Rusinek H, Zhang JL, et al.** Estimates of glomerular filtration rate from MR renography and tracer kinetic models. *J Magn Reson Imaging* 2009;29(2):371–382.
32. **Grenier N, Cornelis F, Le Bras Y, et al.** Perfusion imaging in renal diseases. *Diagn Interv Imaging* 2013;94(12):1313–1322.
33. **Bokacheva L, Rusinek H, Chen Q, et al.** Quantitative determination of Gd-DTPA concentration in T1-weighted MR renography studies. *Magn Reson Med* 2007;57(6):1012–1018.
34. **Aronhime S, Calcagno C, Jajamovich GH, et al.** DCE-MRI of the liver: effect of linear and nonlinear conversions on hepatic perfusion quantification and reproducibility. *J Magn Reson Imaging* 2014;40(1):90–98.
35. **Shuter B, Tofts PS, Wang SC, et al.** The relaxivity of Gd-EOB-DTPA and Gd-DTPA in liver and kidney of the Wistar rat. *Magn Reson Imaging* 1996;14(3):243–253.
36. **Morkenborg J, Taagehoj JF, Vaever PN, et al.** In vivo measurement of T1 and T2 relaxivity in the kidney cortex of the pig—based on a two-compartment steady-state model. *Magn Reson Imaging* 1998;16(8): 933–942.
37. **Bokacheva L, Huang AJ, Chen Q, et al.** Single breath-hold T1 measurement using low flip angle TrueFISP. *Magn Reson Med* 2006; 55(5):1186–1190.
38. **Fram EK, Herfkens RJ, Johnson GA, et al.** Rapid calculation of T1 using variable flip angle gradient refocused imaging. *Magn Reson Imaging* 1987;5(3):201–208.
39. **Scheffler K, Hennig J.** T(1) quantification with inversion recovery TrueFISP. *Magn Reson Med* 2001;45(4):720–723.
40. **Li S, Zollner FG, Merrem AD, et al.** Wavelet-based segmentation of renal compartments in DCE-MRI of human kidney: initial results in patients and healthy volunteers. *Comput Med Imaging Graph* 2012;36(2):108–118.
41. **Annet L, Hermoye L, Peeters F, et al.** Glomerular filtration rate: assessment with dynamic contrast-enhanced MRI and a cortical-compartment model in the rabbit kidney. *J Magn Reson Imaging* 2004;20(5):843–849.
42. **Buckley DL, Shurrab AE, Cheung CM, et al.** Measurement of single kidney function using dynamic contrast-enhanced MRI: comparison of two models in human subjects. *J Magn Reson Imaging* 2006;24(5):1117–1123.
43. **Hackstein N, Heckrodt J, Rau WS.** Measurement of single-kidney glomerular filtration rate using a contrast-enhanced dynamic gradient-echo sequence and the Rutland-Patlak plot technique. *J Magn Reson Imaging* 2003;18(6):714–725.
44. **Sourbron SP, Michaely HJ, Reiser MF, et al.** MRI-measurement of perfusion and glomerular filtration in the human kidney with a separable compartment model. *Invest Radiol* 2008;43(1):40–48.
45. **Koh TS, Zhang JL, Ong CK, et al.** A biphasic parameter estimation method for quantitative analysis of dynamic renal scintigraphic data. *Phys Med Biol* 2006;51(11):2857–2870.
46. **Lee VS, Rusinek H, Bokacheva L, et al.** Renal function measurements from MR renography and a simplified multicompartmental model. *Am J Physiol Renal Physiol* 2007;292(5):F1548–F1559.
47. **Uzzo RG, Novick AC.** Nephron sparing surgery for renal tumors: indications, techniques and outcomes. *J Urol* 2001;166(1):6–18.
48. **Dash A, Vickers AJ, Schachter LR, et al.** Comparison of outcomes in elective partial vs radical nephrectomy for clear cell renal cell carcinoma of 4-7 cm. *BJU Int* 2006;97(5):939–945.
49. **Park H, Byun SS, Kim HH, et al.** Comparison of laparoscopic and open partial nephrectomies in t1a renal cell carcinoma: a Korean multicenter experience. *Korean J Urol* 2010;51(7):467–471.
50. **Gill IS, Kavoussi LR, Lane BR, et al.** Comparison of 1,800 laparoscopic and open partial nephrectomies for single renal tumors. *J Urol* 2007;178(1):41–46.
51. **Ojo AO, Wolfe RA, Held PJ, et al.** Delayed graft function: risk factors and implications for renal allograft survival. *Transplantation* 1997;63(7):968–974.
52. **Thompson RH, Lane BR, Lohse CM, et al.** Renal function after partial nephrectomy: effect of warm ischemia relative to quantity and quality of preserved kidney. *Urology* 2012;79(2):356–360.
53. **Huang WC, Levey AS, Serio AM, et al.** Chronic kidney disease after nephrectomy in patients with renal cortical tumours: a retrospective cohort study. *Lancet Oncol* 2006;7(9):735–740.
54. **Kang SK, Chandarana H.** Contemporary imaging of the renal mass. *Urol Clin North Am* 2012;39(2):161–170, vi.
55. **Allen BC, Tirman P, Jennings Clingan M, et al.** Characterizing solid renal neoplasms with MRI in adults. *Abdom Imaging* 2014;39(2): 358–387.
56. **Gilet AG, Kang SK, Kim D, et al.** Advanced renal mass imaging: diffusion and perfusion MRI. *Curr Urol Rep* 2012;13(1):93–98.
57. **Chandarana H, Rosenkrantz AB, Mussi TC, et al.** Histogram analysis of whole-lesion enhancement in differentiating clear cell from papillary subtype of renal cell cancer. *Radiology* 2012;265(3):790–798.
58. **Egbert ND, Caoili EM, Cohan RH, et al.** Differentiation of papillary renal cell carcinoma subtypes on CT and MRI. *AJR Am J Roentgenol* 2013;201(2):347–355.
59. **Pedrosa I, Alsop DC, Rofsky NM.** Magnetic resonance imaging as a biomarker in renal cell carcinoma. *Cancer* 2009;115(10 suppl): 2334–2345.
60. **Young JR, Margolis D, Sauk S, et al.** Clear cell renal cell carcinoma: discrimination from other renal cell carcinoma subtypes and oncocytoma at multiphasic multidetector CT. *Radiology* 2013;267(2):444–453.
61. **Sun MR, Ngo L, Genega EM, et al.** Renal cell carcinoma: dynamic contrast-enhanced MR imaging for differentiation of tumor subtypes—correlation with pathologic findings. *Radiology* 2009;250(3):793–802.
62. **Notohamiprodjo M, Sourbron S, Staehler M, et al.** Measuring perfusion and permeability in renal cell carcinoma with dynamic contrast-enhanced MRI: a pilot study. *J Magn Reson Imaging* 2010; 31(2):490–501.
63. **Chandarana H, Amarosa A, Huang WC, et al.** High temporal resolution 3D gadolinium-enhanced dynamic MR imaging of renal tumors with pharmacokinetic modeling: preliminary observations. *J Magn Reson Imaging* 2013;38(4):802–808.
64. **Ratain MJ, Eckhardt SG.** Phase II studies of modern drugs directed against new targets: if you are fazed, too, then resist RECIST. *J Clin Oncol* 2004;22(22):4442–4445.
65. **Rosner GL, Stadler W, Ratain MJ.** Randomized discontinuation design: application to cytostatic antineoplastic agents. *J Clin Oncol* 2002;20(22):4478–4484.
66. **Teng FF, Meng X, Sun XD, et al.** New strategy for monitoring targeted therapy: molecular imaging. *Int J Nanomedicine* 2013;8:3703–3713.
67. **Albiges L, Choueiri T, Escudier B, et al.** A systematic review of sequencing and combinations of systemic therapy in metastatic renal cancer. *Eur Urol* 2014;671:100–110.
68. **Escudier B, Michaelson MD, Motzer RJ, et al.** Axitinib versus sorafenib in advanced renal cell carcinoma: subanalyses by prior therapy from a randomised phase III trial. *Br J Cancer* 2014;11012:2821–2828.
69. **Lee-Ying R, Lester R, Heng DY.** Current management and future perspectives of metastatic renal cell carcinoma. *Int J Urol* 2014; 219:847–855.

70. **Philips GK, Atkins MB.** New agents and new targets for renal cell carcinoma. *Am Soc Clin Oncol Educ Book* 2014;34:e222–e227.
71. **Hillman GG, Singh-Gupta V, Al-Bashir AK, et al.** Dynamic contrast-enhanced magnetic resonance imaging of sunitinib-induced vascular changes to schedule chemotherapy in renal cell carcinoma xenograft tumors. *Transl Oncol* 2010;3(5):293–306.
72. **Galbraith SM, Maxwell RJ, Lodge MA, et al.** Combretastatin A4 phosphate has tumor antivascular activity in rat and man as demonstrated by dynamic magnetic resonance imaging. *J Clin Oncol* 2003;21(15):2831–2842.
73. **Flaherty KT, Rosen MA, Heitjan DF, et al.** Pilot study of DCE-MRI to predict progression-free survival with sorafenib therapy in renal cell carcinoma. *Cancer Biol Ther* 2008;7(4):496–501.
74. **Taylor A, Nally J, Aurell M, et al.** Consensus report on ACE inhibitor renography for detecting renovascular hypertension. Radionuclides in Nephrourology Group. Consensus Group on ACEI Renography. *J Nucl Med* 1996;37(11):1876–1882.
75. **Grenier N, Trillaud H, Combe C, et al.** Diagnosis of renovascular hypertension: feasibility of captopril-sensitized dynamic MR imaging and comparison with captopril scintigraphy. *AJR Am J Roentgenol* 1996;166(4):835–843.
76. **Lee VS, Rusinek H, Johnson G, et al.** MR renography with low-dose gadopentetate dimeglumine: feasibility. *Radiology* 2001;221(2):371–379.
77. **Zhang JL, Rusinek H, Bokacheva L, et al.** Angiotensin-converting enzyme inhibitor-enhanced MR renography: repeated measures of GFR and RPF in hypertensive patients. *Am J Physiol Renal Physiol* 2009;296(4):F884–F891.
78. **Michaely HJ, Schoenberg SO, Oesingmann N, et al.** Renal artery stenosis: functional assessment with dynamic MR perfusion measurements—feasibility study. *Radiology* 2006;238(2):586–596.
79. **Grattan-Smith JD, Perez-Bayfield MR, Jones RA, et al.** MR imaging of kidneys: functional evaluation using F-15 perfusion imaging. *Pediatr Radiol* 2003;33(5):293–304.
80. **McDaniel BB, Jones RA, Scherz H, et al.** Dynamic contrast-enhanced MR urography in the evaluation of pediatric hydronephrosis: Part 2, anatomic and functional assessment of ureteropelvic junction obstruction. *AJR Am J Roentgenol* 2005;185(6):1608–1614.
81. **Rohrschneider WK, Haufe S, Wiesel M, et al.** Functional and morphologic evaluation of congenital urinary tract dilatation by using combined static-dynamic MR urography: findings in kidneys with a single collecting system. *Radiology* 2002;224(3):683–694.
82. **Grattan-Smith JD, Little SB, Jones RA.** MR urography evaluation of obstructive uropathy. *Pediatr Radiol* 2008;38 suppl 1:S49–S69.
83. **Krepkin K, Won E, Ramaswamy K, et al.** Dynamic contrast-enhanced MR renography for renal function evaluation in ureteropelvic junction obstruction: feasibility study. *AJR Am J Roentgenol* 2014;202(4): 778–783.
84. **Lee VS, Rusinek H, Noz ME, et al.** Dynamic three-dimensional MR renography for the measurement of single kidney function: initial experience. *Radiology* 2003;227(1):289–294.
85. **Jones RA, Perez-Brayfield MR, Kirsch AJ, et al.** Renal transit time with MR urography in children. *Radiology* 2004;233(1):41–50.
86. **Jones RA, Easley K, Little SB, et al.** Dynamic contrast-enhanced MR urography in the evaluation of pediatric hydronephrosis: part 1, functional assessment. *AJR Am J Roentgenol* 2005;185(6):1598–1607.
87. **Grattan-Smith JD, Jones RA.** MR urography: technique and results for the evaluation of urinary obstruction in the pediatric population. *Magn Reson Imaging Clin N Am* 2008;16(4):643–660, viii–ix.
88. **Szolar DH, Preidler K, Ebner F, et al.** Functional magnetic resonance imaging of human renal allografts during the post-transplant period: preliminary observations. *Magn Reson Imaging* 1997;15(7):727–735.
89. **Wentland AL, Sadowski EA, Djamali A, et al.** Quantitative MR measures of intrarenal perfusion in the assessment of transplanted kidneys: initial experience. *Acad Radiol* 2009;16(9):1077–1085.
90. **Agildere AM, Tarhan NC, Bozdagi G, et al.** Correlation of quantitative dynamic magnetic resonance imaging findings with pathology results in renal transplants: a preliminary report. *Transplant Proc* 1999;31(8):3312–3316.
91. **Yamamoto A, Zhang JL, Rusinek H, et al.** Quantitative evaluation of acute renal transplant dysfunction with low-dose three-dimensional MR renography. *Radiology* 2011;260(3):781–789.
92. **Martirosian P, Boss A, Schraml C, et al.** Magnetic resonance perfusion imaging without contrast media. *Eur J Nucl Med Mol Imaging* 2010;37 (suppl 1):S52–S64.
93. **Kim SG.** Quantification of relative cerebral blood flow change by flow-sensitive alternating inversion recovery (FAIR) technique: application to functional mapping. *Magn Reson Med* 1995;34(3):293–301.
94. **Kwong KK, Chesler DA, Weisskoff RM, et al.** MR perfusion studies with T1-weighted echo planar imaging. *Magn Reson Med* 1995;34(6):878–887.
95. **Lanzman RS, Wittsack HJ, Martirosian P, et al.** Quantification of renal allograft perfusion using arterial spin labeling MRI: initial results. *Eur Radiol* 2010;20(6):1485–1491.
96. **Wang JJ, Hendrich KS, Jackson EK, et al.** Perfusion quantitation in transplanted rat kidney by MRI with arterial spin labeling. *Kidney Int* 1998;53(6):1783–1791.
97. **Fenchel M, Martirosian P, Langanke J, et al.** Perfusion MR imaging with FAIR true FISP spin labeling in patients with and without renal artery stenosis: initial experience. *Radiology* 2006;238(3):1013–1021.
98. **Hueper K, Gutberlet M, Rong S, et al.** Acute kidney injury: arterial spin labeling to monitor renal perfusion impairment in mice-comparison with histopathologic results and renal function. *Radiology* 2014;270(1):117–124.
99. **Liu YP, Song R, Liang C, et al.** Arterial spin labeling blood flow magnetic resonance imaging for evaluation of renal injury. *Am J Physiol Renal Physiol* 2012;303(4):F551–F558.
100. **Song R, Loeffler RB, Hillenbrand CM.** Improved renal perfusion measurement with a dual navigator-gated Q2TIPS fair technique. *Magn Reson Med* 2010;64(5):1352–1359.
101. **Koh DM, Collins DJ.** Diffusion-weighted MRI in the body: applications and challenges in oncology. *AJR Am J Roentgenol* 2007; 188(6):1622–1635.
102. **Le Bihan D, Breton E, Lallemand D, et al.** Separation of diffusion and perfusion in intravoxel incoherent motion MR imaging. *Radiology* 1988;168(2):497–505.
103. **Taouli B, Koh DM.** Diffusion-weighted MR imaging of the liver. *Radiology* 2010;254(1):47–66.
104. **Luciani A, Vignaud A, Cavet M, et al.** Liver cirrhosis: intravoxel incoherent motion MR imaging—pilot study. *Radiology* 2008;249(3):891–899.
105. **Patel J, Sigmund EE, Rusinek H, et al.** Diagnosis of cirrhosis with intravoxel incoherent motion diffusion MRI and dynamic contrast-enhanced MRI alone and in combination: preliminary experience. *J Magn Reson Imaging* 2010;31(3):589–600.
106. **Wittsack HJ, Lanzman RS, Mathys C, et al.** Statistical evaluation of diffusion-weighted imaging of the human kidney. *Magn Reson Med* 2010;64(2):616–622.
107. **Zhang JL, Sigmund EE, Chandarana H, et al.** Variability of renal apparent diffusion coefficients: limitations of the monoexponential model for diffusion quantification. *Radiology* 2010;254(3):783–792.
108. **Chandarana H, Lee VS, Hecht E, et al.** Comparison of biexponential and monoexponential model of diffusion weighted imaging in evaluation of renal lesions: preliminary experience. *Invest Radiol* 2011;46(5):285–291.
109. **Koh DM, Collins DJ, Orton MR.** Intravoxel incoherent motion in body diffusion-weighted MRI: reality and challenges. *AJR Am J Roentgenol* 2011;196(6):1351–1361.
110. **Kang KM, Lee JM, Yoon JH, et al.** Intravoxel incoherent motion diffusion-weighted MR imaging for characterization of focal pancreatic lesions. *Radiology* 2014;270(2):444–453.
111. **Chandarana H, Kang SK, Wong S, et al.** Diffusion-weighted intravoxel incoherent motion imaging of renal tumors with histopathologic correlation. *Invest Radiol* 2012;47(12):688–696.

CHAPTER

30 Renal Perfusion Imaging with CT and PET

Sandrine Lemoine, MD, PhD and Laurent Juillard, MD, PhD

Rationale

Perfusion and renal blood flow (RBF) are key determinant of renal function, altered in most kidney diseases. The ability to quantify accurately intrarenal blood flow would contribute substantially to our understanding of a variety of renal disease mechanisms. Nevertheless, this measurement is difficult to obtain noninvasively and in a manner applicable to humans. Indeed, in clinical practice, RBF can be estimated indirectly by the clearance of the para-aminohippuric acid (PAH), corrected for hematocrit and possibly PAH extraction. These corrections impair the accuracy of RBF measurement and make it unsuitable in cases of chronic renal failure. Moreover, PAH clearance provides only a two-kidney measurement of RBF and cannot be evaluated within periods of less than 30 minutes. These limitations have stimulated research for a method that would allow a direct measurement of RBF, with the ability to record regional perfusion, at least a single-kidney evaluation.

Functional imaging methods address these goals by measuring quantitatively and noninvasively renal perfusion and RBF, potentially with addition of a morphologic analysis. Moreover, some modalities such as multidetector computer tomography (MDCT) and position electron tomography (PET) can also measure either glomerular filtration rate (GFR) or oxidative metabolism. The choice of the initial imaging method depends on patient's characteristics, local availability, and expertise.

Renal Perfusion

The total RBF corresponds to about 20% of cardiac output (about 1 L/min) for about 1% of the total body weight. Renal perfusion is maximal in the cortex (420 mL/min/100 g) and minimal in the papilla (50 mL/min/100 g). In comparison, perfusion of the heart is approximately 84 mL/min/100 g and perfusion of the liver is 58 mL/min/100 g in dogs.[1] Indeed, the distribution of perfusion is very heterogeneous even within the renal parenchyma.[2,3] The renal cortex receives the most RBF. In the renal medulla, blood flow accounts only for 1% to 2% of the total RBF. An essential function of the renal medulla is to regulate the concentration of the urine, requiring the maintenance of a corticopapillary gradient (from about 50 mOsm/kg in the superficial cortex, up to 1,200 mOsm/kg in the deepest medulla). Approximately only 20% of the plasma in the arteriolar capillary is filtered, and only a small amount of urine is formed from this high blood flow. Then, it is important to note that this high blood flow greatly exceeds the metabolic needs of the kidney, but it is mandatory for an efficient regulation of renal function.

Kidneys have also the highest basal oxidative metabolism, representing 10% of the basal body metabolism.[4] This very high oxidative metabolism is mainly due to sodium reabsorption, and changes in renal oxidative metabolism correlate closely with changes in sodium reabsorption. It is, therefore, most likely that renal oxidative metabolism could be changed significantly in chronic renal diseases, such as ischemic nephropathy.

In this review, we will describe the measure of RBF and perfusion with computer tomography and PET scan.

Multidetector Computed Tomography and Electron Beam Computer Tomography

Method Description

MDCT is the latest evolution of the computer tomography technology and is a powerful modality allowing the measurement of RBF, perfusion, and GFR. CT allows a fast acquisition of renal images, with isolation of vascular and tissue peak concentration of the CM after intravenous (IV) injection.

The principle of CT imaging is based on the attenuation of x-rays by tissue structures (measured in Hounsfield units). The relationship between the attenuation measured in renal tissue and the concentration of iodinated CM is strictly linear, allowing a robust and quantitative modeling. Similar to inulin, iodine is eliminated by glomerular filtration. They are not reabsorbed nor are secreted by the tubules and thus can be used as a tracer for GFR measurement. The density observed in the renal parenchyma corresponds to the sum of the density of the parenchyma before injection, and the iodine density accumulated in the renal vessels and tubules.[5]

Electron beam computer tomography (EBCT) has been used since the 1980s in the United States. In this scanner, there is no rotation of the acquisition ring. The electron source, located at a distance behind the acquisition ring, produces an electron beam which is deflected electromagnetically toward the eight rows of x-ray emitters underneath the patient. The spatial resolution of EBCT is lower than a standard CT scanner but remains acceptable for renal functional

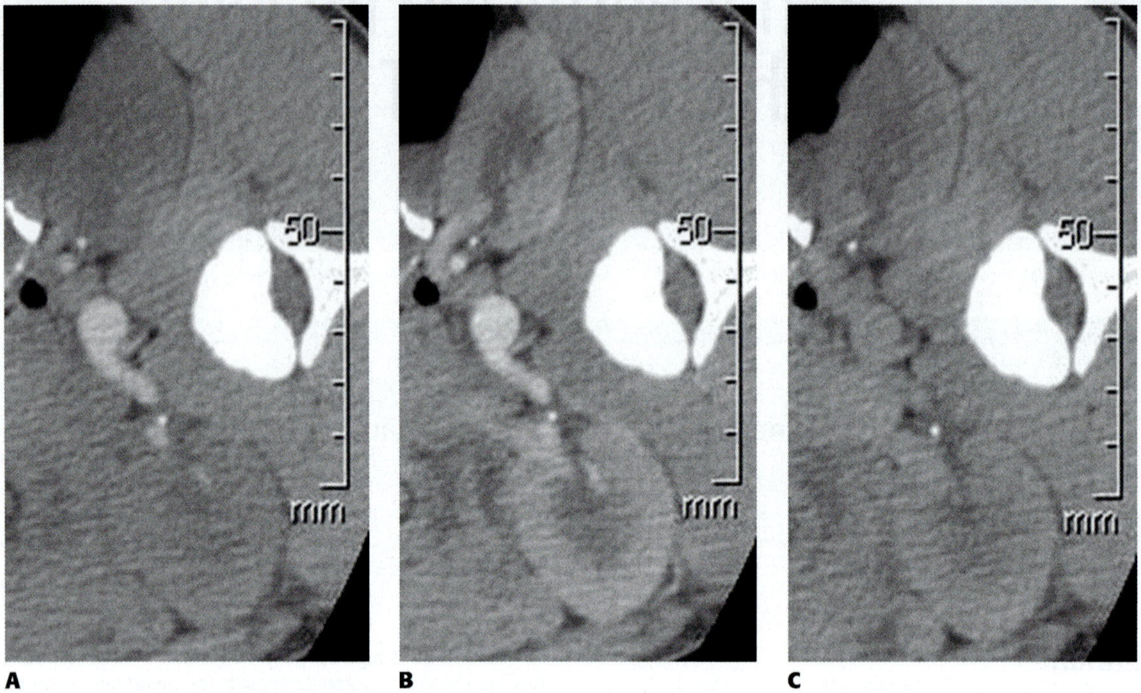

Figure 30-1. Dynamic multidetector CT images in a pig model. **A:** Maximum aortic density enhancement. **B:** Cortical and **(C)** medullary phases. Top of image = pig's left side and right of image = pig's ventral side.

imaging. The temporal resolution is fast enough (<100 milliseconds), thanks to the absence of limitation forced by the mechanical rotation of the detector ring. These two features allow the extraction of renal perfusion and DFG using gamma variate modeling.

Modeling

The repeated acquisition of images at the same level of a cross section after the iodinated CM bolus permits to obtain a kinetic of the vascular and tissue density as a function of time. Following the vascular phase, the contrast appears first in the cortex and the amount of cortical enhancement corresponds to the glomerular filtration of CM into the proximal tubule. A second enhancement is observed when the CM transits within the distal tubules (Fig. 30-1). Time density curves are obtained after manual drawing of regions of interest (ROI) corresponding to the aorta and renal cortices on each cross section. To obtain reliable and accurate kinetics, the temporal resolution of the scanner must be high, especially during the vascular transit of the CM, in order to monitor the rapid changes in density. Moreover, to prevent any errors related to respiratory movements, it is essential to acquire simultaneously several cross section images at contiguous levels of the kidney. The *Gamma Variate* modeling[6] (Fig. 30-2) and the *Rutland-Patlak Method*[7] are the two validated methods for extracting renal parameters from the density kinetic. Only the Gamma variate modeling allows measuring perfusion.

Gamma Variate Modeling

The most commonly applied analytic models for perfusion analysis based on dynamic CT data include compartment models and deconvolution methods.

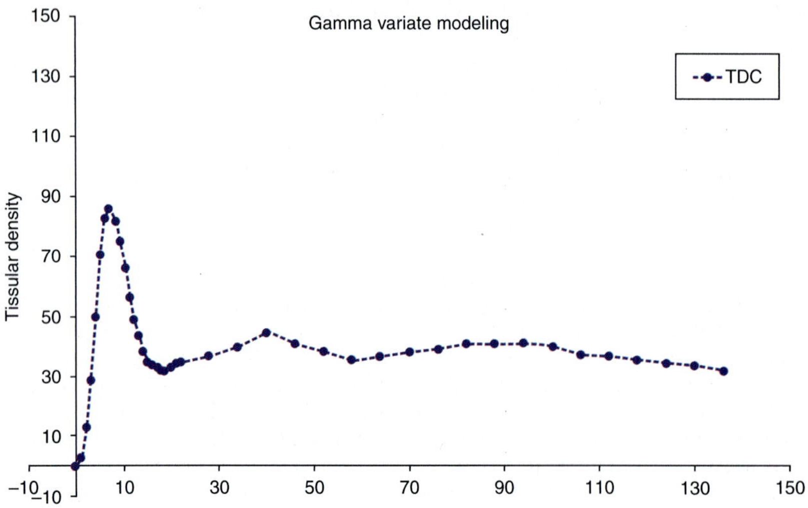

Figure 30-2. Time density curve (TDC) obtained from a region of interest in the left cortex.

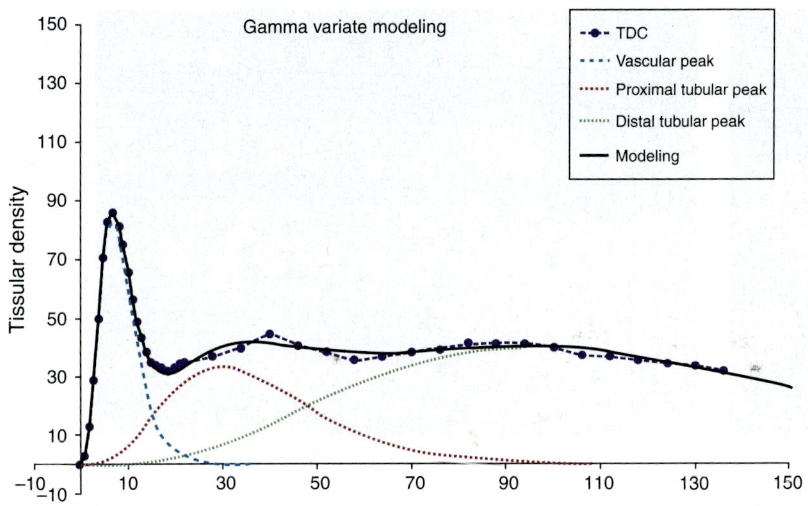

Figure 30-3. **Gamma variate modeling.** TDC from Figure 30-2 in gray, gamma variate modeling in black line from corresponding time density curve. The TDC is broken down in to three peaks: vascular (*dotted black line*), proximal tubular (*dotted gray line*), and distal tubular (*little gray dotted line*) peaks.

The *Gamma Variate Method* allows to measure the most functional parameters (perfusion, RBF, and GFR). This method was developed by Krier et al.[8] The initial formula of gamma variate was $[C(t) = c \times t^a \times \exp(-t/b)]$ that permits to describe the kinetic of a vascular peak of iodinated CM.[9] An extend formula of gamma variate permits to measure perfusion and glomerular filtration. $[C(t) = c \times t^a \times [\exp(-t/b) + d \times \exp(-t/h) + i \times t^j \times \exp(-t/k)]$, where $C(t)$ corresponds to the concentration of iodinated CM in function of time, where a, b, and c describe the vascular transit of iodinated CM, d and h are the accumulation and the transit in the proximal tubule and i, j, and k in the distal tubule (Fig. 30-3). This model required a high-rate of CM injection (i.e., 15 mL/s) to obtain a bolus as short as possible because it used the maximum slope model in a single-compartment model that neglects venous outflow. This high rate injection is impossible to deliver using a peripheral catheter because of the small diameter of the peripheral vein; therefore, a central venous catheter was mandatory, the method remained invasive and cannot be used easily in routine clinical practice. Lemoine et al. validated the measurement of renal perfusion with MDCT using a low-rate injection of CM (i.e., 3 mL/s) with gamma variate extended modeling validated with a reference method using fluorescent microspheres (MS) that permits to use this technique in clinical practice.[10] Kandel et al. showed that the duration of CM bolus injection does not influence perfusion measurement substantially in pigs. They recommended to use the same scheme of duration of bolus injection for longitudinal perfusion measurements in a same patient.[11]

Kidney Applications

The *Gamma Variate* method has been used in experimental and clinical practice for evaluation renal function in ischemic nephropathy, renal obstruction, and renal carcinoma.

Experimental Practice

Bentley et al. showed that the renal tissue perfusion is more dependent on the microvascular distribution volume than the vascular transit time in dogs.[12] They showed that the cortical perfusion was significantly decreases when RBF was significantly reduced, whereas the medulla perfusion remain unchanged. Lerman et al. demonstrated that, in case of a unilateral chronic renal ischemia, there was a hypertrophy of the contralateral kidney and an increase of RBF.[13] Krier et al. showed that in a model of renal artery stenosis in pigs the RBF was reduced significantly and proportional to the degree of the renal artery stenosis (RAS).[8] Other studies show that the RAS leads to a redistribution of the intrarenal blood flow.[14]

With the EBCT, the microvasculature was also studied by quantifying the regional perfusion before and after injection of vasodilators in pigs with atherosclerotic RAS showing that the coexistence of an early hypercholesterolemia and hypoperfusion was associated with a greater renal functional and structural impairment, especially in the tubular and glomerular systems, compared with each condition alone.[15,16] The same author showed also that the renal perfusion increased significantly after blocking oxidative stress.[17]

Other studies have examined the impact of an acute ureteral obstruction. After ureteral obstruction, Pelaez et al. observed a reduction of the cortical perfusion without medullary perfusion modification with a maintenance of the GFR during the first 30 minutes.[18] Itano et al. showed that there was a decrease in cortical blood flow during severe chronic obstruction, whereas GFR and proximal tubular function were preserved.[19]

Human Renal Disease

Lerman et al studied regional renal perfusion in patients with high blood pressure due to essential hypertension and RAS either due to atherosclerosis or due to fibrodysplasia.[20] Global and cortical perfusion was lower in patients with RAS due to atherosclerosis than in patients with RAS due to dysplasia or patients with essential hypertension. As mentioned before, CT allowed measuring regional perfusion in the cortex and medulla. This study showed that medullary perfusion was identical in all groups.

Helck et al. used CT to distinguish acute tubular necrosis and acute rejection in kidney allografts.[21] The RBF measurements were significantly lower ($p = 0.001$) in allografts undergoing acute rejection compared with those with acute tubular necrosis. No significant difference ($p = 0.71$) was observed regarding creatinine level. The mean amount of CM injected was limited to 34.5 ± 5.1 mL. Renal perfusion has also been measured by MDCT in renal tumor. In a preliminary prospective study, the renal carcinoma perfusion determined with MDCT could help predict a biologic response to antiangiogenic drugs.[22]

Advantages and Limitations

For transferring this method to clinical practice, radiation exposure would be a concerning issue. However, Liu et al. reported a postprocessing with a HYPR-LR algorithm of images acquired with one-tenth of the typical radiation dose (80 kV, 16 mAs). She showed that MDCT perfusion measurements were unchanged with this acquisition processing. Indeed, this finding is critical and needs to be applied systematically in MDCT perfusion measurements for reducing radiation exposure to patients significantly.

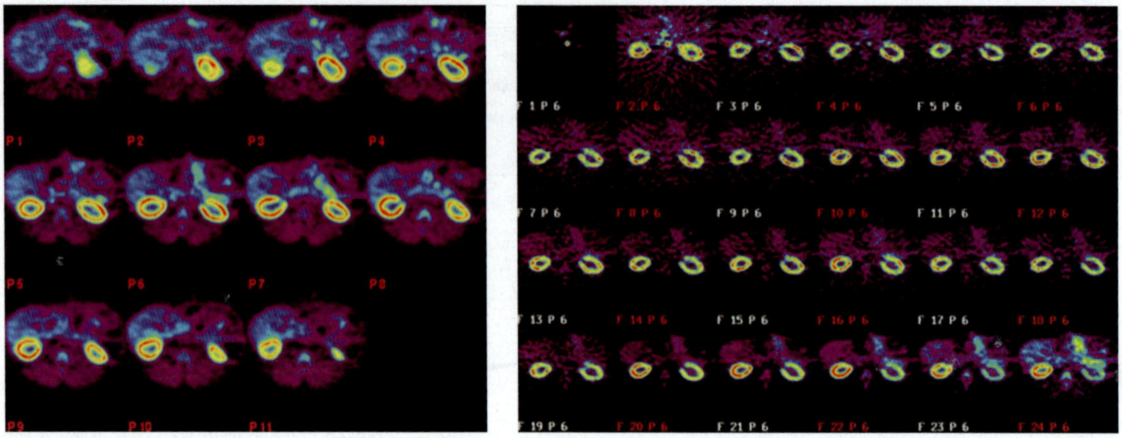

A B

Figure 30-4. Static **(A)** and dynamic **(B)** images with ^{11}C-acetate injection. (From Juillard L, Lemoine S, Janier MF, et al. Validation of renal oxidative metabolism measurement by positron-emission tomography. *Hypertension* 2007;50(1):242–247.)

Another potential limitation of this technique in clinical practice is the increased risk of a CM induced nephropathy in patients with preexisting chronic kidney disease (CKD). In this setting, patients should be selected with caution and the use of low osmolality CM is preferred. Effective prevention of CM nephropathy can be performed by hydration but with an unknown risk of modifying RBF or GFR.

Positron Electron Tomography

Principles

PET is a nuclear imaging technique that uses physiologic labeled tracers, such as water or acetate. The disintegrated isotopes emit a positron, an antiparticle of the electron. The encounter between electron and positron (annihilation) produces two gamma photons of 511 keV emitted in the same direction, but in opposite sides. A computerized system generated static and dynamic images representing, pixel by pixel, the absolute concentration of the tracer (Fig. 30-4). PET is a tool used routinely in humans for measuring myocardial or cerebral blood flow, but its widespread use in nephrology is not yet established.

Modeling

PET can measure different parameters such as RBF or oxidative metabolism. For renal RBF, PET methods have been described for imaging and quantification of renal perfusion using cyclotron-produced ^{15}O-water and ^{13}N-ammonia. These two tracers are different: ^{15}O-water can diffuse freely between blood and tissue and $^{13}NH_3$ accumulates in the renal tissue. For oxidative metabolism, the tracer validated is carbon 11–labeled acetate.

For each isotope used, a mathematical modeling is required to obtain the quantitation of the renal functional parameters. As previously described with MDCT, ROIs are drawn on renal cortex using summed images from them time activity curve is created (Fig. 30-5).

Perfusion and Renal Blood Flow

RBF can be measured with ^{13}N with the Patlak modeling or a bicompartmental model. Nitzsche et al.[23] showed that the Patlak method, as previously described, can be used only if the kinetic data are recorded from 40 to 90 seconds after the injection of the tracer. Indeed, the assumption of unidirectional transport model needed for Patlak method is available only early after tracer accumulation in renal cortex. The authors concluded that,

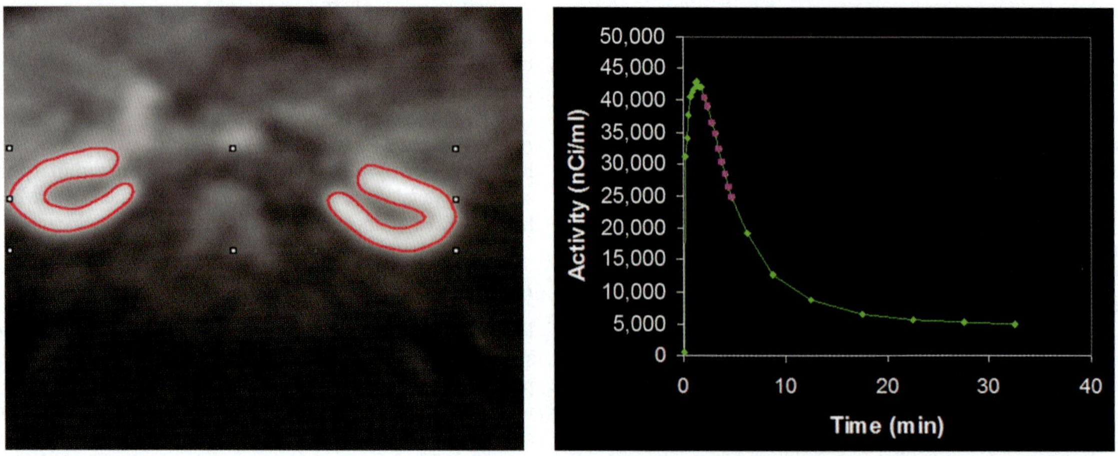

A B

Figure 30-5. Renal ROI **(A)** and time activity curve **(B)**.

in animals or in humans, the comparisons between the two mathematical models with ^{15}O-labeled water as reference method was good ($r = 0.86$ and $r = 0.91$ for the bicompartmental and the Patlak models, respectively).

$H_2{}^{15}O$ is a diffusible tracer, neither extracted nor metabolized like $^{13}NH_3$ and is more accurate for high flow as in the kidney. First, PET with $H_2{}^{15}O$ was used with the Kety-Smith model on the observation of renal monoexponential clearance of radioactive water injected in renal arteries.[24] Then, Juillard et al.[25] validated experimentally the measurement of renal cortical flow with $H_2{}^{15}O$ with the reference method of radiolabeled MSs under a large range of RBF (baseline, with dopamine infusion and angiotensin II infusion). A monocompartmental model was used as previously described in the heart and the correlation between labeled MSs and RBF was excellent ($r = 0.93$, $p < 0.001$). Moreover, the PET imaging method provides absolute value of RBF and allows fast repeated measurements of this parameter.

$H_2{}^{15}O$ appears to be more suitable because of its shorter half-life (2 vs. 11 minutes) that allows measurements at shorter time intervals (15 vs. 60 minutes).

Oxidative Metabolism

Oxidative metabolism before the development of the PET needed invasive techniques to be measured. The PET scan allowed measuring oxidative metabolism noninvasively to be used in clinical practice, using carbon 11–labeled acetate (^{11}C-acetate). Acetate is extracted from the blood after carbon 11–labeled acetate IV injection. Then, acetate is metabolized rapidly and transformed in acetyl-CoA. It can either be oxidized in the Krebs cycle in the mitochondria where the consumption of acetyl-CoA-^{11}C lead to the formation of $^{11}CO_2$ and H_2O (catabolic pathways) or be involved in the anabolic pathway. The pathway used depends on the type of cell. In tumor cells, it is the anabolic pathway that is predominant. In myocardial tissue, it has been showed that the acetate is mainly metabolized in the Krebs cycle, depending on the intensity of oxidative metabolism.[26] Using this principle, acetate turnover measurement by PET has been extensively used in cardiology to evaluate heart viability. Like the heart, the kidney is an organ with a very high oxidative metabolism, because of the important energy required to reabsorb sodium by active transport. Shreve et al showed first that the renal acetate turnover measured by PET was changed markedly in human renal diseases.[27] Shreve et al showed the safety of ^{11}C-acetate in human patients and showed also that ^{11}C-acetate is not excreted by the kidney and will not accumulate in diseases that decrease renal function. In preclinical study, ^{11}C-acetate was validated with the invasive reference method of oxygen metabolism measurement. Juillard et al showed that oxidative metabolism was better correlated with the monoexponential fit ($r = 0.82$) than with the biexponential fit ($r = 0.72$).[28] This study demonstrates that PET using ^{11}C-acetate measures quantitatively renal oxidative metabolism and correlates with the amounts of filtrated and reabsorbed sodium, which are the physiologic processes that affect renal oxygen consumption primarily (Fig. 30-6).

Kidney Applications

Juillard et al. conducted a study to test whether PET imaging with ^{15}O-labeled water could detect the variations of RBF induced by angiotensin-converting enzyme inhibitor (ACEI) in patients with CKD and hypertension. The whole RBF was measured by PAH clearance as the reference method.[29] As expected, the mean baseline RBF (measured by the two methods) was decreased because of the CKD and the administration of ACEI leaded to a decrease of mean blood pressure, ACE activity and filtration fraction. However, only the PET-measured RBF showed a detectable increase after ACEI injection, whereas there were no significant changes with PAH-measured RBF. Furthermore, a good correlation was observed between the values of RBF obtained by the two methods ($r = 0.81$; $p < 0.001$).

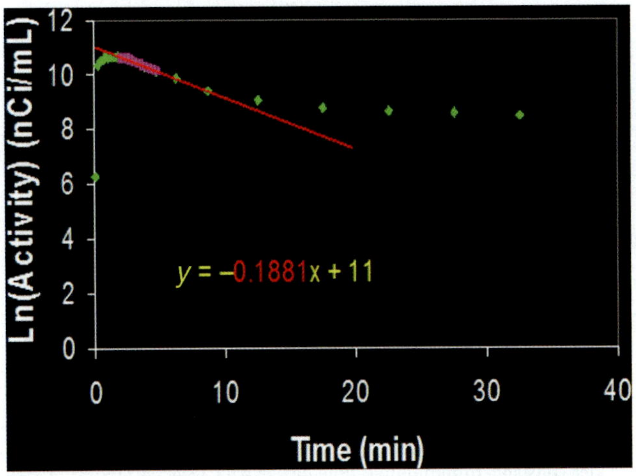

Figure 30-6. Monocompartment fit with ^{11}C-acetate injection.

Alpert and colleagues also tested the validity of the measurement of RBF by PET imaging in patients with or without CKD.[30] The reference method used was also the RBF measured by PAH clearance. No dynamic measurements were made in this study. The measurements obtained by the two methods were strongly correlated ($r^2 = 0.78$). Moreover, the investigators showed that taking benefic for 7 days did not change the measurements obtained by PET imaging (whereas diminishing notably the PAH-measured RBF both in healthy volunteers and in CKD patients). Therefore, they concluded that the PET-measured RBF with ^{15}O-labeled water is reliable and reproducible and could be used in patients with nephropathy and tubular injury. Koivuviita et al. showed a negative correlation between the degree of RAS and the cortical renal perfusion at baseline. However, dilatation of RAS did not improve the renal perfusion.[31]

The results of these studies demonstrated the feasibility and reliability of the measurement of RBF by PET imaging. Several tracers and mathematical modeling are suitable to get measurement of RBF.

Advantages and Limitations

One limitation of this technique is the use of radioactive tracers with a very short radioactive half life (2 minutes for $H_2{}^{15}O$, 11 minutes for $^{13}NH_3$, and 20 minutes for acetate), which requires close access to the imager and a cyclotron to produce the isotope; therefore, it is only limited to some experimental centers. PET imaging device is expensive equipment which diffusion needs to be implemented presently. However, the possibilities of noninvasive and reliable quantitation of RBF and oxygen consumption with PET imaging should lead to its increased use, both in basic and clinical research and in clinical practice. It is now possible to couple PET and MDCT to improve the quality and numbers of functional parameters.

Conclusions

Functional imaging could evaluate physiologic parameters that permits better therapeutic decisions. Different imaging methods are available. PET and MDCT were described in this chapter. Other methods include, MRI or BOLD MRI, and contrast Doppler. These techniques allow measuring intrarenal perfusion patterns and function in animals and patients, and may provide insights into the effects of chronic unilateral or bilateral renovascular disease on both the hypoperfused and intact kidneys. This methodology may thereby prove to be very useful in the evaluation of renal disease in general, and the renovascular hypertensive patients in particular.

REFERENCES

1. **Clausen G, Hope A, Kirkebø A, et al.** Distribution of blood flow in the dog kidney. I. Saturation rates for inert diffusible tracers, ^{125}I-iodoantipyrine and titrated water, versus uptake of microspheres under control conditions. *Acta Physiol Scand* 1979;107(1):69–81.
2. **Chade AR.** Renovascular disease, microcirculation, and the progression of renal injury: Role of angiogenesis. *Am J Physiol Regul Integr Comp Physiol* 2011;300:R783–R790.
3. **Stein JH, Fadem SZ.** The renal circulation. *JAMA* 1978;239(13): 1308–1312.
4. **Munger KA, et al.** The renal circulations and glomerular ultrafiltration. In: Taal MW, et al., eds. *Brenner and Rector's the kidney*. 9th ed. Philadelphia, PA: Elsevier; 2012:Chapter 3.
5. **Lerman LO, Rodriguez-Porcel M, Romero JC.** The development of x-ray imaging to study renal function. *Kidney Int* 1999;55(2):400–416.
6. **Thompson HK, Starmer CF, Whalen RE, et al.** Indicator transit time considered as a gamma variate. *Circ Res* 1964;14:502–515.
7. **Patlak CS, Blasberg RG.** Graphical evaluation of blood-to-brain transfer constants from multiple-time uptake data. Generalizations. *J Cereb Blood Flow Metab* 1985;5(4):584–590.
8. **Krier JD, Ritman EL, Bajzer Z, et al.** Noninvasive measurement of concurrent single-kidney perfusion, glomerular filtration, and tubular function. *Am J Renal Physiol* 2001;281(4):F630–F638.
9. **Krier JD, Ritman EL, Bajzer Z, et al.** Noninvasive measurement of concurrent single-kidney perfusion, glomerular filtration, and tubular function. *Am J Physiol Renal Physiol* 2001;281(4):F630–F638.
10. **Lemoine S, Papillard M, Belloi A, et al.** Renal perfusion: noninvasive measurement with multidetector CT versus fluorescent microspheres in a pig model. *Radiology* 2011;260(2):414–420.
11. **Kandel SM, Meyer H, Boehnert M, et al.** How influential is the duration of contrast material bolus injection in perfusion CT? Evaluation in a Swine model. *Radiology* 2014;270(1):125–130.
12. **Bentley MD, Lerman LO, Hoffman EA, et al.** Measurement of renal perfusion and blood flow with fast computed tomography. *Circ Res* 1994;74(5):945–951.
13. **Lerman LO, Schwartz RS, Grande JP, et al.** Noninvasive evaluation of a novel swine model of renal artery stenosis. *J Am Soc Nephrol* 1999; 10(7):455–465.
14. **Romero JC, Lerman LO.** Novel noninvasive techniques for studying renal function in man. *Semin Nephrol* 2000;20(5):456–462.
15. **Chade AR, Rodriguez-Porcel M, Grande JP, et al.** Distinct renal injury in early atherosclerosis and renovascular disease. *Circulation* 2002;106(9):1165–1171.
16. **Feldstein A, Krier JD, Sarafov MH, et al.** In vivo renal vascular and tubular function in experimental hypercholesterolemia. *Hypertension* 1999;34(4 Pt 2):859–864.
17. **Chade AR, Krier JD, Rodriguez-Porcel M, et al.** Comparison of acute and chronic antioxidant interventions in experimental renovascular disease. *Am J Physiol Renal Physiol* 2004;286(6):F1079–F1086.
18. **Pelaez LI, Juncos LA, Stulak JM, et al.** Non-invasive evaluation of bilateral renal regional blood flow and tubular dynamics during acute unilateral ureteral obstruction. *Nephrol Dial Transpl* 2005;20(1): 83–88.
19. **Itano NB, Sherrill LE, Lerman LO, et al.** Electron beam computerized tomography assessment of in vivo single kidney glomerular filtration rate and tubular dynamics during chronic partial unilateral ureteral obstruction in the pig. *J Urol* 2001;166(6):2530–2535.
20. **Lerman LO, Taler SJ, Textor SC, et al.** Computed tomography-derived intrarenal blood flow in renovascular and essential hypertension. *Kidney Int* 1996;49(3):846–854.
21. **Helck A, Wessely M, Notohamiprodjo M, et al.** CT perfusion technique for assessment of early kidney allograft dysfunction: preliminary results. *Eur Radiol* 2013;23(9):2475–2481.
22. **Fournier LS, Oudard S, Thiam R, et al.** Metastatic renal carcinoma: evaluation of antiangiogenic therapy with dynamic contrast-enhanced CT. *Radiology* 2010;256(2):511–518.
23. **Nitzsche EU, Choi Y, Killion D, et al.** Quantification and parametric imaging of renal cortical blood flow in vivo based on Patlak graphical analysis. *Kidney Int* 1993;44(5):985–996.
24. **Inaba T, Yamashita M, Kawase Y, et al.** Quantitative measurement of renal plasma flow by positron emission tomography with oxygen-15 water. *Tohoku J Exp Med* 1989;159(4):283–289.
25. **Juillard L, Janier MF, Fouque D, et al.** Renal blood flow measurement by positron emission tomography using ^{15}O-labeled water. *Kidney Int* 2000;57(6):2511–2518.
26. **Randle PJ, England PJ, Denton RM.** Control of the tricarboxylate cycle and its interactions with glycolysis during acetate utilization in rat heart. *Biochem J* 1970;117(4):677–695.
27. **Shreve P, Chiao PC, Humes HD.** Carbon-11-acetate PET imaging in renal disease. *J Nucl Med* 1995;36(9):1595–1601.
28. **Juillard L, Lemoine S, Janier MF, et al.** Validation of renal oxidative metabolism measurement by positron-emission tomography. *Hypertension* 2007;50(1):242–247.
29. **Juillard L, Janier MF, Fouque D, et al.** Dynamic renal blood flow measurement by positron emission tomography in patients with CRF. *Am J Kidney Dis* 2002;40(5):947–954.
30. **Alpert NMN, Rabito CAC, Correia DJAD, et al.** Mapping of local renal blood flow with PET and H(2)(15)O. *J Nucl Med* 2002;43(4): 470–475.
31. **Koivuviita N, Liukko K, Kudomi N, et al.** The effect of revascularization of renal artery stenosis on renal perfusion in patients with atherosclerotic renovascular disease. *Nephrol Dial Transpl* 2012;27(10): 3843–3848.

CHAPTER

31 Prostate Perfusion Imaging with MR

Jurgen J. Fütterer, MD, PhD

Introduction

Prostate cancer is the second most frequently diagnosed malignancy and the sixth leading cause of cancer-related death mortality in males worldwide.[1] The widespread use of prostate-specific antigen (PSA) as a screening test for prostate cancer resulted in earlier detection of high-grade prostate cancer at a curative stage. A major concern related to prostate cancer screening and early detection is overdiagnosis and overtreatment of indolent disease. Strategies to reduce overdiagnosis are necessary, as are strategies to differentiate indolent from aggressive tumors.[2,3] The prevalence of prostate cancer increases with age; 40% of men in the sixth decade of life and up to 60% aged 80 years or older have histologic evidence of prostate cancer.[4]

The conventional diagnostic pathway in men with elevated serum PSA levels and/or abnormal digital rectal examination consists of a random "blind" systematic transrectal ultrasound (TRUS)-guided prostate biopsy. The clinical stage is identified using clinical variables (digital rectal examination, PSA, and Gleason score) and is expressed in the TNM staging classification. The Gleason score is a histopathologic score that correlates with prostate cancer prognosis. In order to determine the treatment that optimally suits the individual patient, it is necessary to evaluate all patient and clinical characteristics.

Due to its high soft tissue contrast, high resolution, and ability to simultaneously image functional parameters, magnetic resonance (MR) imaging provides the best visualization of the prostate compared to other available imaging methods. The following functional MR imaging techniques are applied in the prostate: (a) diffusion-weighted MR imaging (DWI); (b) dynamic contrast-enhanced MRI (DCE-MRI); and (c) MR spectroscopy imaging.[5–12] This multiparametric MR imaging approach has resulted in accurate prostate cancer detection and localization.[12,13] Multiparametric prostate MR imaging plays an important role in the detection, localization, staging, image-guided targeted prostate biopsy, and the assessment of posttreatment changes in prostate cancer.

The microvascular network formed by the capillaries supplies the tissues and permits their function. It provides a considerable surface area for exchanges between blood and tissues.[14] All pathologic conditions cause changes in the microcirculation. These changes can be used as imaging biomarkers for the diagnosis of lesions. This book chapter focuses on the role MR imaging and dynamic contrast-enhanced MR imaging (i.e., perfusion MR imaging) of the prostate.

Prostate Cancer Pathophysiology

Prostate cancer is a multifactorial disease. Age and a positive family history of prostate cancer are the main risk factors. Other factors are the type of diet, lifestyle-related factors, and certain genetic defects.[15] There is also a distinct geographical and racial difference in prostate cancer incidence with higher rates in Western countries and among Black men, as compared to Asian countries and White men, respectively.

The primary function of the prostate gland is to produce prostatic fluid and to lubricate the sperm produced in the testes during ejaculation.[16,17] In healthy prostatic epithelial cells, the enzyme aconitase is inhibited by high levels of zinc present in the cells. This, in turn, blocks the oxidation of citrate in the Krebs cycle, thus accumulating citrate in the prostatic lumina.[18]

The earliest determinable pathologic changes in characteristics of the healthy prostatic cells are atrophic and inflammatory changes. A cascade of these and other factors may lead to the histopathologically defined precursor of high-grade prostatic intraepithelial neoplasia. It is the only accepted facultative precursor lesion for acinar prostate cancer. While high-grade prostatic intraepithelial neoplasia shows many similarities to prostate cancer, it is most probably not a precursor of every prostate cancer variant. However, the detection of high-grade prostatic intraepithelial neoplasia in needle biopsies is a significant risk factor for the subsequent diagnosis of invasive prostate cancer.[19]

Prostate Anatomy

The prostate gland is a complex organ composed of different zones that have different embryologic origin and different functional activities. It is a small gland and situated directly caudal to the bladder. The prostate gland envelops the prostatic urethra and the ejaculatory ducts. The seminal vesicles are paired grape-like pouches filled with fluid that are located caudolateral to the corresponding deferent duct between the bladder and rectum. The prostate is divided into apex and base (directed upward to the inferior border of the bladder). The neurovascular bundle courses bilaterally along the posterolateral aspect of the prostate and is a preferential pathway of tumor spread.

The prostate is anatomically divided on the basis of embryologic origins into three zones that are eccentrically located around the urethra: the innermost transition zone, the central zone, and the outermost peripheral zone. Knowledge of the zonal anatomy of the prostate is very useful considering that many prostatic diseases have

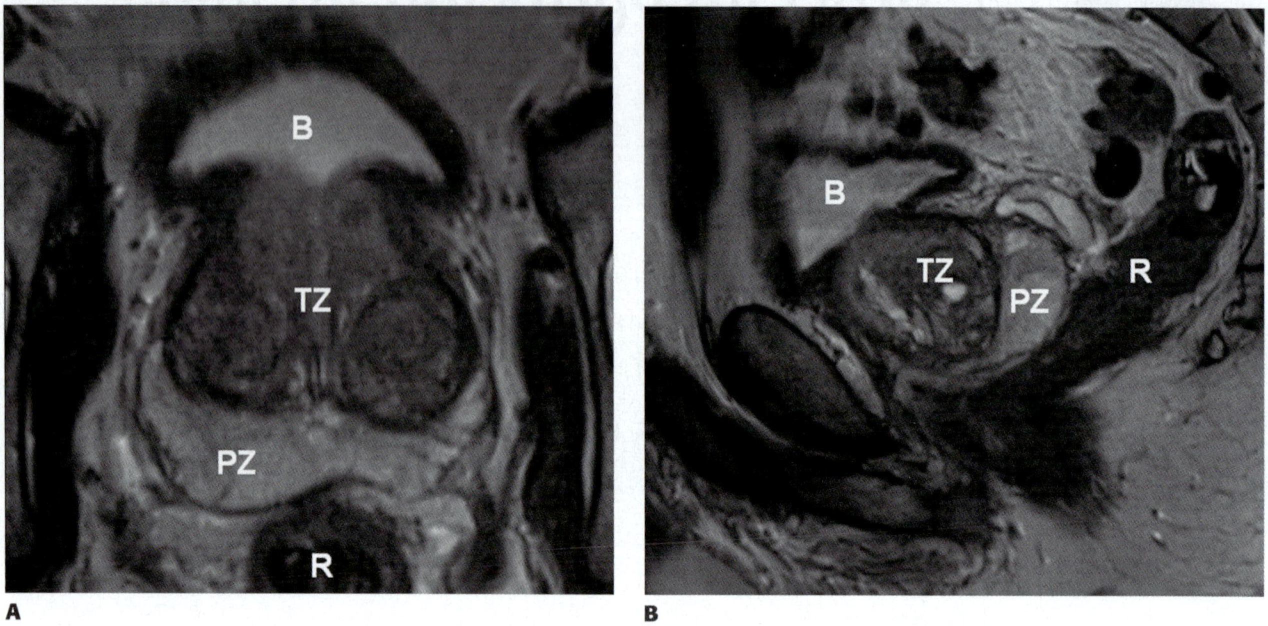

Figure 31-1. **Zonal anatomy of the prostate. A:** Axial T2-weighted MR image through the prostate. The healthy peripheral zone (PZ) has a higher signal intensity compared to the transition zone (TZ). The rectum (R) is posteriorly located from the prostate. The bladder (B) is anterior and cranially positioned from the prostate. **B:** Sagittal T2-weighted MR image through the prostate. The healthy peripheral zone (PZ) has a higher signal intensity compared to the transition zone (TZ). The rectum (R) is posteriorly located from the prostate. The bladder (B) is anterior and cranially positioned from the prostate.

a zonal distribution. Up to 70% to 80% of prostate cancer is located in the peripheral zone, whereas about 20% emerge in the transitional zone, and 10% in the central zone (Fig. 31-1).[20,21] Transition zone prostate cancers have a relatively lower Gleason score, local stage, and biochemical recurrence rate in comparison to cancers located in the peripheral zone.[22–24] Radiologically, in older patients, the transitional zone and central zone cannot be distinguished due to compression of the central zone by benign prostatic hyperplasia. Most transition zone tumors have additional tumor foci in the peripheral zone. Another aspect of the prostate anatomy that is relevant to radiologic imaging relates to the prostatic capsule. The prostate is surrounded by a thick layer of fibromuscular tissue corresponding to the capsule. The "true" prostatic capsule, however, is a thin (0.5 to 2 mm) layer of connective tissue located external to the peripheral zone. Around this layer there is the pelvic fascia, often called the "false" prostatic capsule.

Prostate MR Imaging

T1-Weighted MR Imaging

T1-weighted MR imaging has a very limited role for prostate cancer detection and localization. The T1-weighted contrast in the prostate is very low. Therefore, the zonal anatomy cannot be discerned using T1-weighted MR imaging (Fig. 31-2).

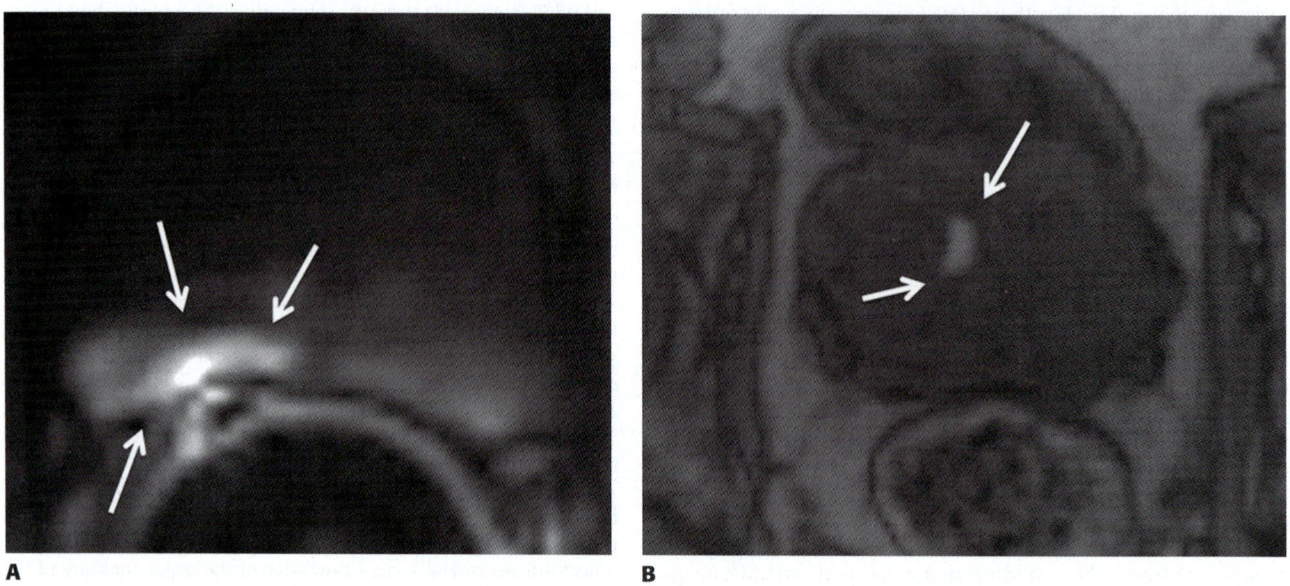

Figure 31-2. **A:** Area of high signal intensity (*arrows*) on a T1-weighted MR image in the right peripheral zone representing biopsy hematoma. **B:** Area of high signal intensity (*arrows*) on a T1-weighted MR image in the right transition zone representing biopsy hematoma.

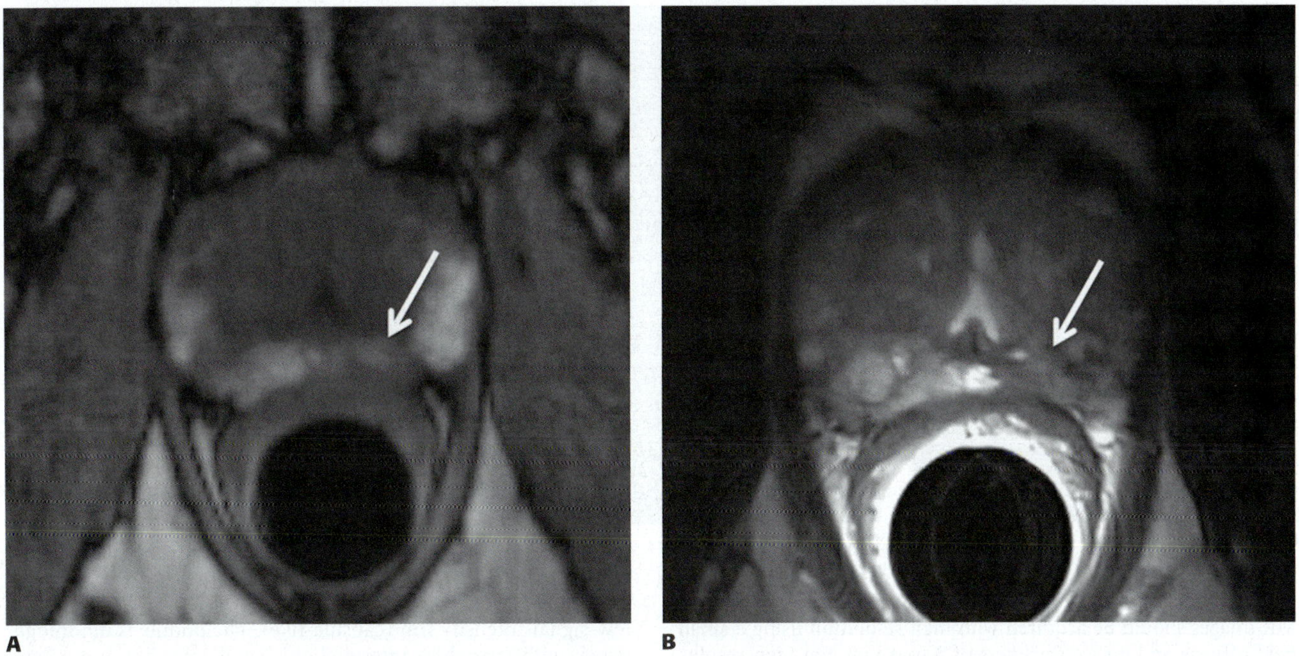

Figure 31-3. Hemorrhage exclusion sign in 61-year-old man with biopsy-proven prostate cancer in the left peripheral zone (apex). **A:** Axial T1-weighted MR image shows hemorrhage exclusion sign (*arrow*) in left peripheral zone. **B:** Axial T2-weighted image shows matching area of low signal intensity (*arrow*).

The T1-weighted sequence is applied for the detection of post-biopsy hemorrhage or artifacts. The latter can be a confounding factor on T2-weighted MR images.[25] However, the presence of excluded hemorrhage, which, in conjunction with a corresponding area of homogeneous low signal intensity at T2-weighted imaging, is highly accurate for cancer identification (Fig. 31-3).[26]

Anatomic T2-Weighted MR Imaging

Anatomical T2-weighted MR imaging is the cornerstone for interpretation of the prostate. The latter technique is helpful for zonal delineation and tumor detection and localization. High in plane resolution T2-weighted fast or turbo spin-echo sequences, performed with endorectal and/or external pelvic phased-array coils, are generally used to depict prostate anatomy (Fig. 31-4).[27]

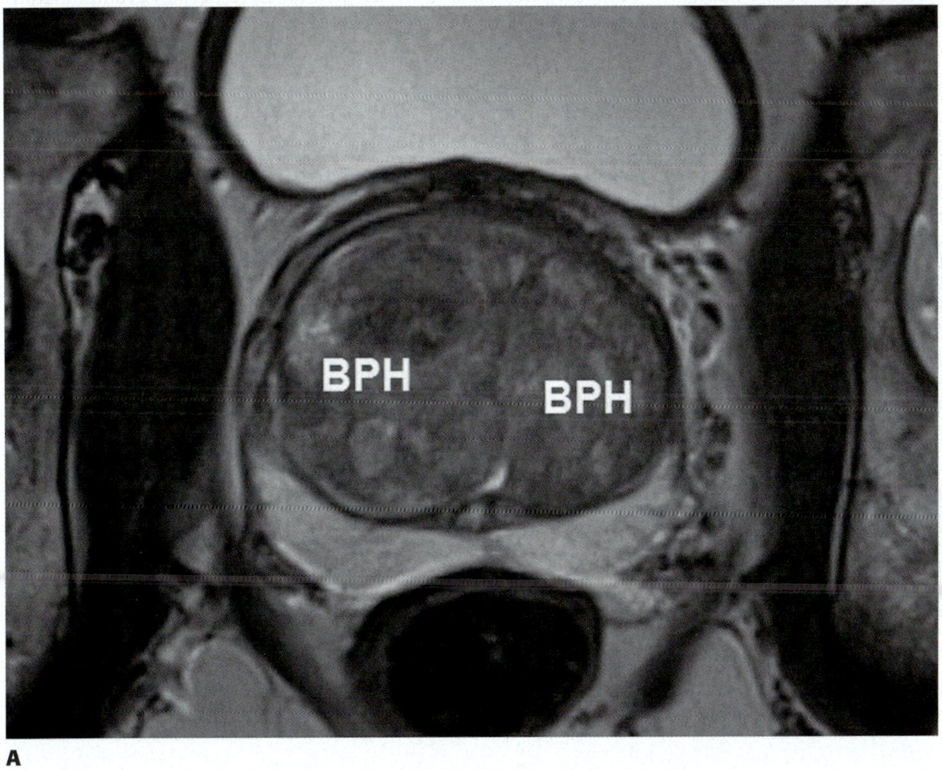

Figure 31-4. Healthy 56-year-old male with elevated PSA level of 20 ng/mL. Axial **(A)**, sagittal

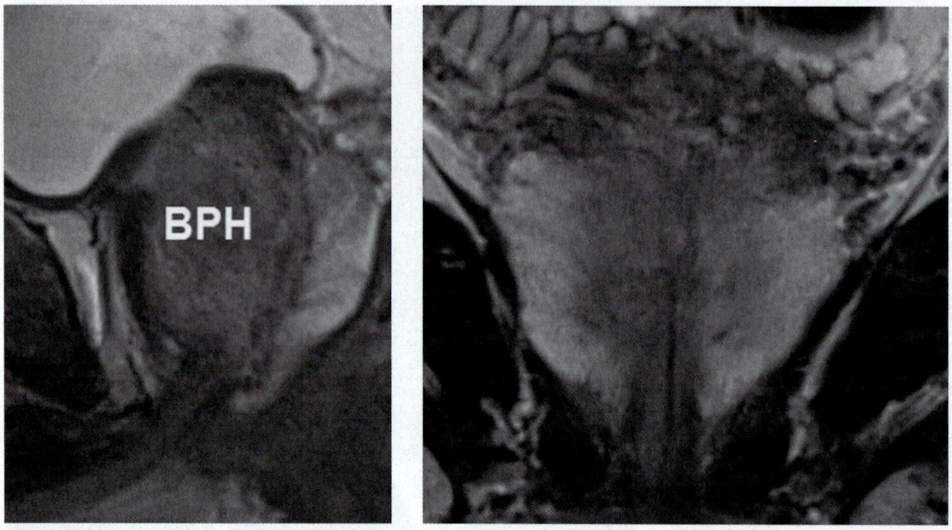

B C

Figure 31-4. (*Continued*) **(B)**, and coronal **(C)** T2-weighted MR image through the prostate. Extensive BPH is present in the transition zone. No signs of prostate cancer were present.

MR images should be acquired with high resolution using a small field of view and a slice thickness of 3 to 4 mm. On high-resolution T2-weighted MR images, the normal prostate can be divided into the peripheral zone that shows high signal intensity owing to its high water content, and the central gland (comprising central and transition zones) that has lower signal intensity.[28] The seminal vesicles demonstrated a high signal within the lumen. The seminal vesicle wall has a well-defined low-signal-intensity rim (Fig. 31-5).

In the elderly male, owing to variable extension of the transition zone due to benign prostatic hyperplasia, the size and signal intensity of the prostate transition zone may vary. Benign nodular hyperplasia of the prostate gives rise to nodular adenomas in the transition zone, and with time these will compress the central zone and forms a pseudocapsule; thus occupying the complete central gland. The peripheral zone is almost never affected by BPH and will retain its own histologic characteristics (Fig. 31-6). Benign prostatic hyperplasia is a round or oval nodule with a well-defined low-signal-intensity rim (capsule-like). The nodule is inhomogeneous with (variable) intermediate signal intensity and a low-signal-intensity rim that surrounds the expanded transition zone.[28] The typical nodular appearance of BPH on T2-weighted imaging will help in discriminating benign prostatic hyperplasia from prostate cancer. Because of transition zone expansion, the remainder of the compressed central zone is often indefinable on MR images.[27]

Prostate cancer can appear as an area of low signal intensity within the high signal intensity of a normal peripheral zone (Fig. 31-7). The degree of signal intensity on the T2-weighted MR image decrease may differ with the Gleason score.[29] Higher Gleason score components 4 or 5 have shown lower signal intensities on T2-weighted images than do lower Gleason score components 2 or 3. Unfortunately, not all prostate cancer foci appear as low signal intensity areas, and moreover prostatitis (especially granulomatous prostatitis), atrophy, or postbiopsy hemorrhage may mimic prostate

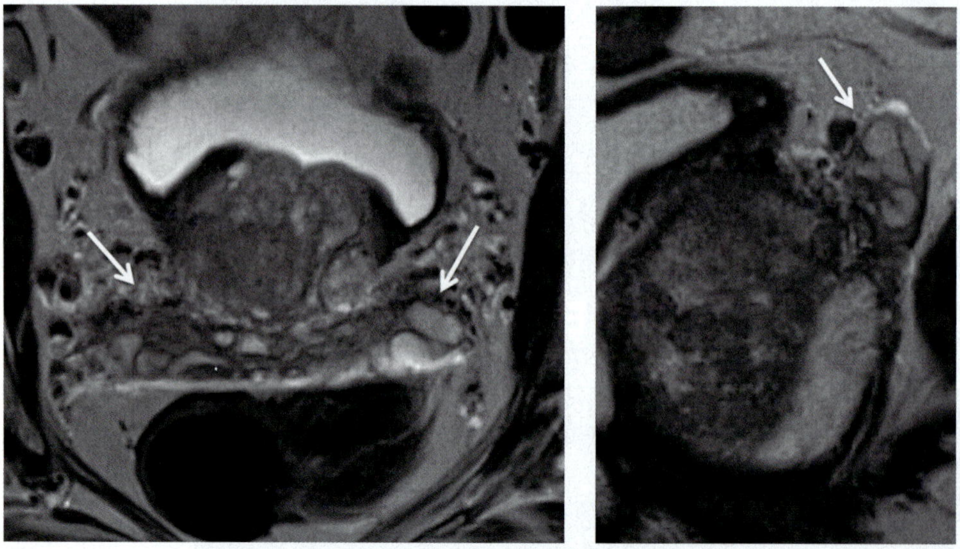

A B

Figure 31-5. Normal appearance of the seminal vesicles (*arrows*) in the axial **(A)** and sagittal **(B)** plane using T2-weighted MR imaging. The fluid filled lumen demonstrates high signal intensity.

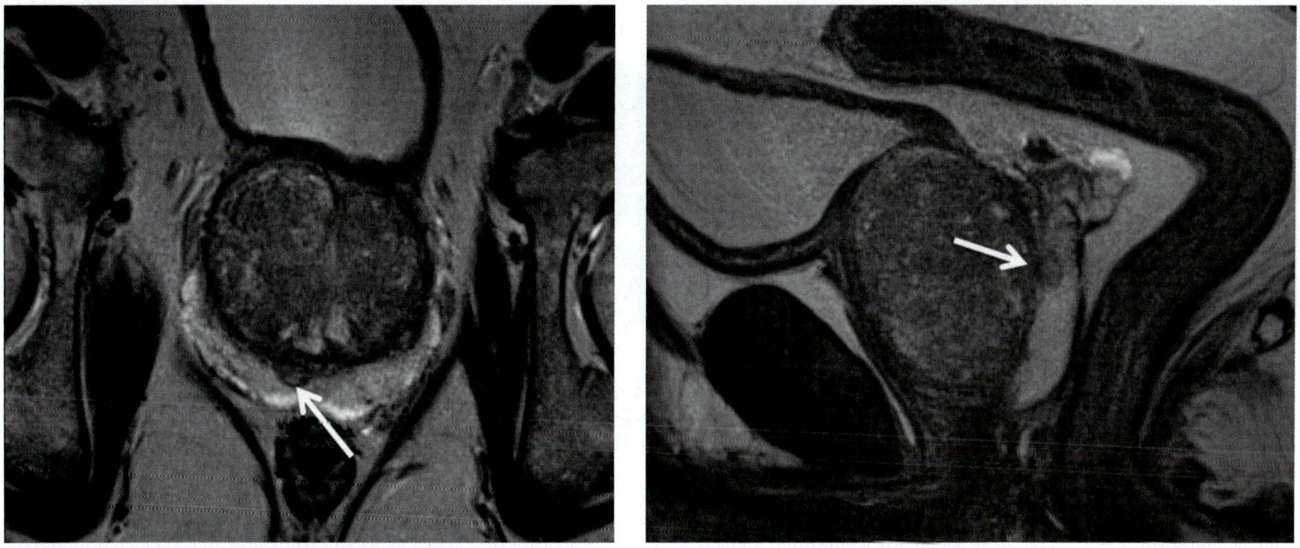

A B

Figure 31-6. (A, B) A well-circumscribed heterogeneous BPH nodule (*arrow*) in right midperipheral zone.

cancer (Fig. 31-8). To prevent false interpretation of T2-weighted images, MR imaging should be performed at least 4 weeks after prostatic biopsy. A rare subtype of prostate carcinoma, termed mucinous carcinoma, can appear as a hyperintense lesion on T2-weighted images because of its rich mucinous content. To increase the diagnostic accuracy, the addition of functional MR imaging techniques to anatomical T2-weighted MR imaging are needed.

Diffusion-Weighted Imaging

DWI explores the random motion of water molecules in the body. Water molecules exhibit random motion in tissue related to temperature (Brownian effect).[30] The movement of water molecules in biologic tissues is restricted because their motion is modified and limited by interactions with cell membranes and macromolecules.[31] Diffusion-weighted imaging can quantify this water motion in an indirect manner.[32] In biologic tissue, the DWI signal is derived from the motion of water molecules in the extracellular space, the intracellular space, and the intravascular space.[33,34]

DWI is obtained by measuring signal loss after a series of two motion-providing gradient pulses are added to both sides of a 180-degree refocusing RF pulse to enhance differences in molecular diffusion between tissues. The DWI pulse sequence labels hydrogen nuclei in space, of which most will be part of water molecules at any moment, and determines the length of the path that water molecules travel over a short period of time. However, DWI is not

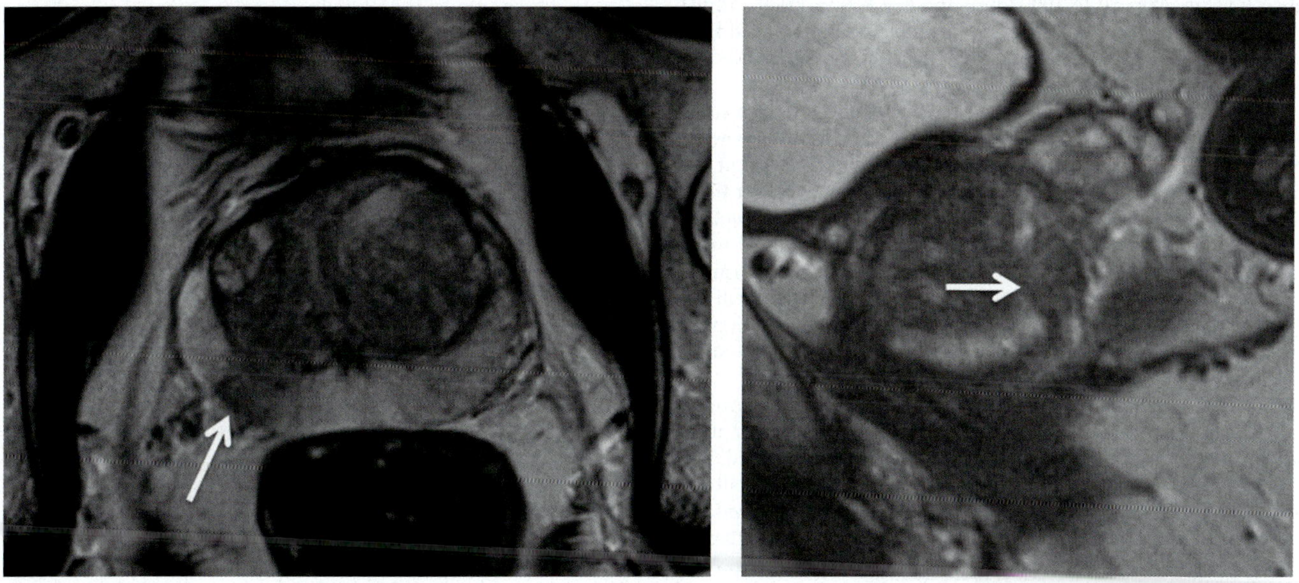

A B

Figure 31-7. A 63-year-old man with biopsy-proven prostate cancer with Gleason score of 7 in peripheral zone of right midprostate. **A:** Axial T2-weighted image illustrates focal low-signal-intensity nodule (*arrow*) in peripheral zone of right midprostate at site of biopsy-proven carcinoma. **B:** Sagittal T2-weighted image illustrates focal low-signal-intensity nodule (*arrow*) in peripheral zone of right midprostate at site of biopsy-proven carcinoma.

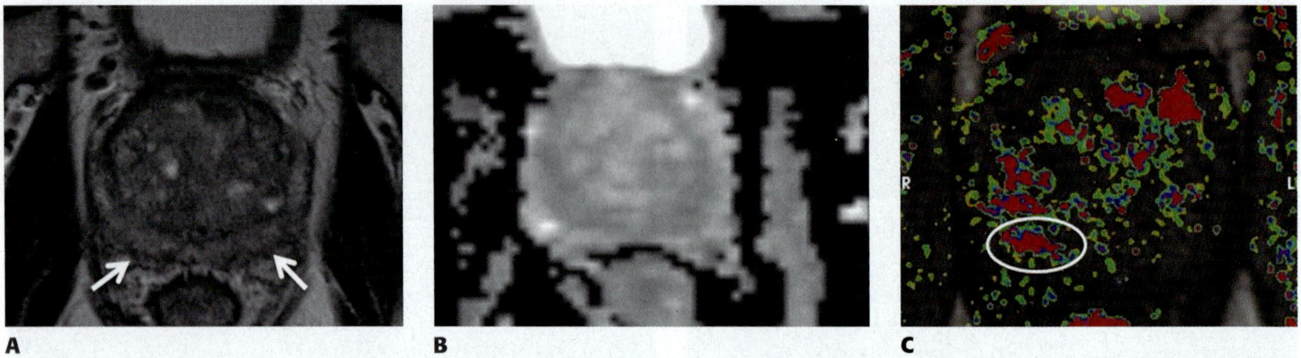

Figure 31-8. **A 54-year-old man with diffuse prostatitis (PSA level of 9.4 ng/mL). A:** Axial T2-weighted turbo spin-echo MR image shows diffuse low signal intensity within entire peripheral zone (*arrows*). **B:** ADC map calculated from a single-shot echo-planar DW image in three orthogonal diffusion gradients in the axial plane reveals intermediate-to-high ADC values. **C:** Fusion of axial T1-weighted image with color-encoded K_{trans} map delineates prostatitis area (*circle*).

able to determine the distance traveled by individual hydrogen nuclei, but is capable of estimating the mean distance traveled by all hydrogen nuclei in every voxel of imaged tissue. This quantification of proton diffusion properties in water is used to produce image contrast. Images that reflect proton diffusion are acquired by applying motion-encoding gradients, which cause phase shifts in moving protons, depending on the direction and quantity of their movement.[32]

The degree of restriction to water diffusion in biologic tissue is inversely correlated to the tissue cellularity and the integrity of cell membranes.[35,36] The motion of water molecules is more restricted in tissues with a high cellular density associated with numerous intact cell membranes (e.g., tumor tissue).[31] DWI has T2 and diffusion-weighted MR imaging characteristics. The signal intensity on the DWI represents a combination of signal on the $b = 0$ image and the dephasing due to water motion in the presence of the diffusion gradients. At low *b*-values, there is greater contribution from the $b = 0$ image and at higher *b*-values, contrast is determined more by relative diffusion.[37] DWI of the prostate is performed using at least two *b*-values ($b = 50$ to 100 s/mm^2 and $b = 800$ to 1,000 s/mm^2). A high *b*-value ($b \geq 1{,}000$ s/mm^2) is acquired or extrapolated from the former DWI sequence that may be helpful to pickup lesions within the transition zone.

Healthy prostate tissue in the peripheral zone is rich in tubular structures. This will allow for abundant self-diffusion of water molecules in their contents, and thus provides high apparent diffusion coefficient (ADC) values (Fig. 31-9). Prostate cancer tissue destroys the normal glandular structure of the prostate and replaces ducts. It also has a higher cellular density than does healthy prostate peripheral zone tissue. In most cases, the peripheral zone can be easily discriminated from the transition zone on DWI, as it will display relative higher ADC values.[38] On ADC maps, therefore, prostate cancer often shows lower ADCs in comparison to surrounding healthy peripheral zone prostate tissue (Fig. 31-10).[39–41]

Benign prostatic hyperplasia (BPH) is defined by hyperplasia of all cells that constitute the transition zone, with glandular, muscular, and fibrous compartments, more or less evenly involved. This nodular hyperplasia gives rise to inhomogeneous diffusion patterns and as tubular structures often remain in place, the increased cellular density of hyperplasia, which is far less predominant than in prostate carcinoma, might explain the observed reduction in ADC levels of the transition and central zone on DWI, due to decreased ratio of extracellular to intracellular volume (Fig. 31-11). However, as BPH has inhomogeneous diffusion characteristics, an increase in ADC has been observed as well.[42] DWI has to be read in conjunction with anatomical T2-weighted MR imaging.

Chronic prostatitis is histopathologic characterized by extracellular edema surrounding the involved prostatic cells with concomitant aggregation of lymphocytes, plasma cells, macrophages, and neutrophils in the prostatic stroma. This abundance in cells as compared to normal prostatic tissue may lead to a decreased ADC due to decreased extracellular to intracellular fluid volume ratio. Diffusion-weighted imaging is a noninvasive technique that shows differences between prostatitis and prostate cancer in both the peripheral zone and transition zone, although its usability in clinical practice is limited as a result of significant overlap in ADCs.[43]

Dynamic Contrast-Enhanced MR Imaging

The microvascular network formed by the capillaries supplies the tissues and permits their function. It provides a considerable surface area for exchanges between blood and tissues.[14] All pathologic conditions cause changes in the microcirculation.

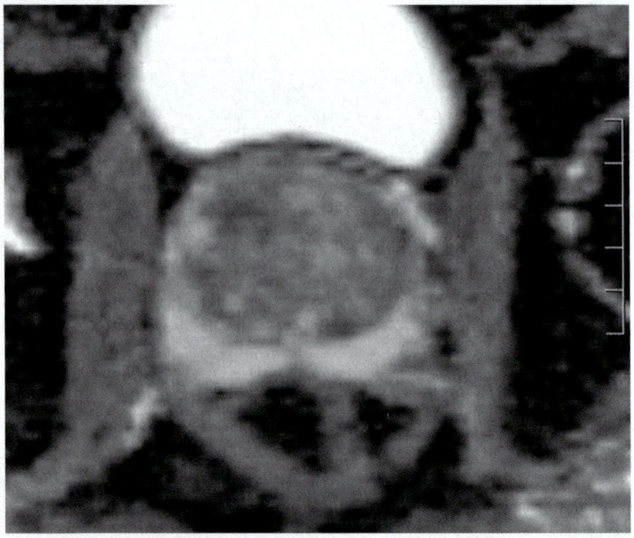

Figure 31-9. **A 64-year-old man with one negative TRUS biopsy session (PSA level of 6.4 ng/mL) underwent prostate MRI.** The ADC map calculated from a single-shot echo-planar DW image in three orthogonal diffusion gradients in the axial plane reveals high ADC values in the entire healthy peripheral zone.

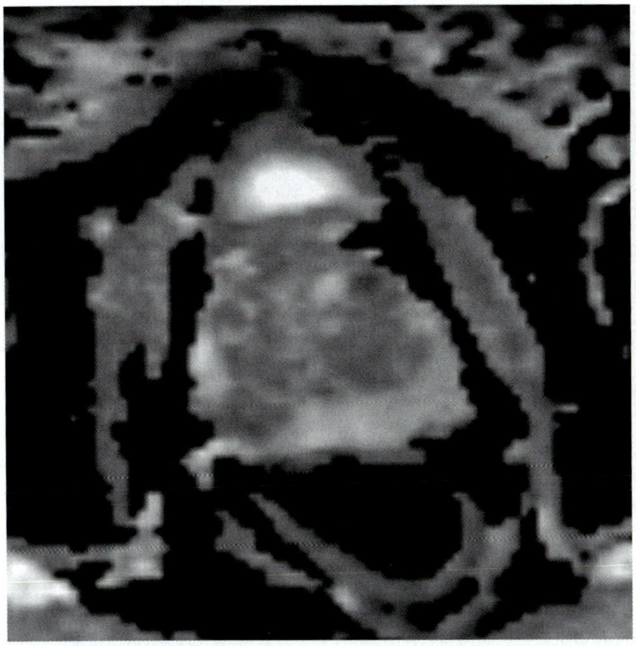

Figure 31-10. **A 68-year-old man with two negative TRUS biopsy sessions (PSA level of 10.2 ng/mL) underwent prostate MRI.** The ADC map calculated from a single-shot echo-planar DW image in three orthogonal diffusion gradients in the axial plane reveals low ADC values in the right midperipheral zone delineates prostate cancer lesion (*circle*).

For a tumor, one critical factor that affects development, growth, invasiveness, and progression into the metastatic form is the ability of the tumor to generate new blood vessels. Angiogenesis, the sprouting of new capillaries from existing blood vessels, and vasculogenesis, the de novo generation of new blood vessels, are the two primary methods of vascular expansion by which nutrient supply to tumor tissue is adjusted to match physiologic needs.[44] The importance of angiogenesis in prostate cancer is well established. A number of features are characteristic of malignant vasculature, many of which are amenable to study by DCE-MRI and DWI techniques. These include (a) spatial heterogeneity and chaotic structure; (b) poorly formed fragile vessels with high permeability to macromolecules because of the presence of large endothelial cell gaps, incomplete basement membrane, and relative lack of pericytes or smooth muscle association with endothelial cells; (c) arteriovenous shunting; (d) intermittent or unstable blood flow; and (e) extreme heterogeneity of vascular density with areas of low vascular density mixed with regions of high angiogenic activity.[45]

Dynamic susceptibility MR sequences (T2*-weighted) are sensitive to the vascular phase of contrast medium delivery, which reflect on tissue perfusion and blood volume. However, limited evidence is gathered for clinical application in the prostate. Sequences can also be designed to be sensitive to the presence of contrast medium in the extravascular extracellular space; thus reflecting on microvessel perfusion, permeability, and extracellular leakage space (so-called T1 or relaxivity-based methods).[46] The latter is the most common method applied in prostate MR imaging.

The three most important aspects of DCE-MRI include (a) intravenous contrast agent administration; (b) fast temporal resolution imaging of the entire prostate to visualize uptake and washout of the contrast agent; and (c) qualitative or quantitative estimation of signal intensity changes to determine the pharmacokinetic parameters of perfusion.[47] Dynamic contrast-enhanced MR imaging consists of a series of fast T1-weighted sequences covering the entire prostate before and after rapid injection of a bolus of a low molecular weight gadolinium chelate. DCE-MRI following the administration of low molecular weight contrast media (<1 kDa) is the most common imaging method for evaluating human tumor vascular function in situ.[48] Because the prostate as a whole is highly vascularized, a simple comparison of pre- and postgadolinium images is insufficient to discern prostate cancer.[46,49] A high first-pass extraction occurs in most normal prostate tissues, as well as in hyperplastic prostatic tissues and prostate cancer. In tumors, typically 12% to 45% of the contrast media leaks into the extravascular–extracellular space during the first pass.[50]

Assessment of signal intensity changes on T1-weighted dynamic contrast-enhanced MR images in order to estimate contrast agent uptake in vivo can be performed qualitatively, semiquantitatively, or quantitatively.

The *qualitative analysis* of signal intensity changes can be achieved by assessing the shape of the signal intensity–time curve.

The *semiquantitative* approach describing signal intensity changes by using a number of parameters such as: (a) the onset time of the signal intensity curve (t_0 = time from appearance in an artery to the arrival of contrast agent in the tissue of interest);

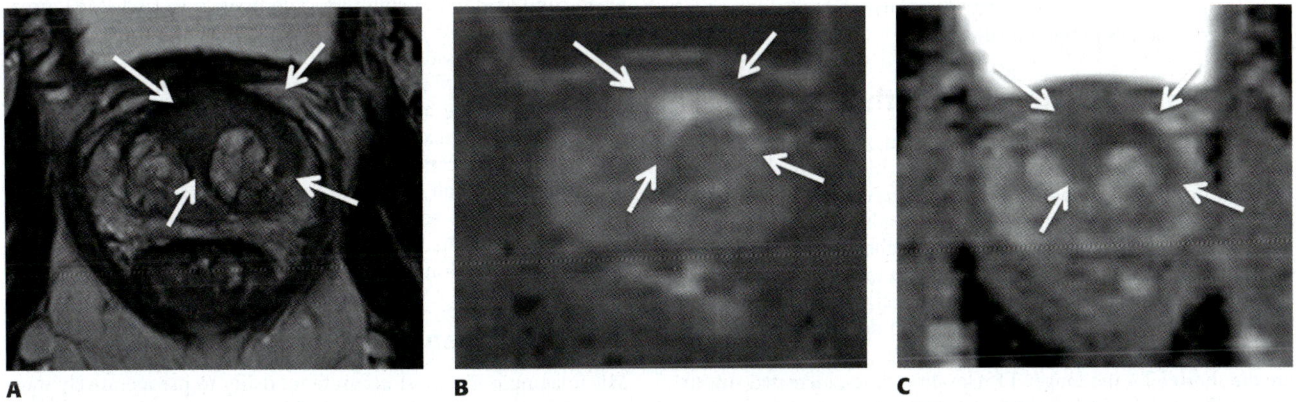

Figure 31-11. **Images in a 56-year-old male with a PSA level of 6.5 ng/mL and Gleason score 3 + 4 = 7 in the left transition zone of the prostate.** Transition zone cancer was clearly visible at MP-MRI. **A:** Axial T2-weighted turbo spin-echo image at base prostate level shows low homogeneous signal intensity extending from the anterior fibromuscular stroma into the left transition zone (*arrows*). **B:** Axial high *b*-value of 1,400 at the same level as **(A)** shows high homogeneous signal intensity extending from the anterior fibromuscular stroma into the left transition zone (*arrows*). **C:** Axial ADC map at the same level as **(A)**. Low ADC value is present in the left transition zone (*white arrows*).

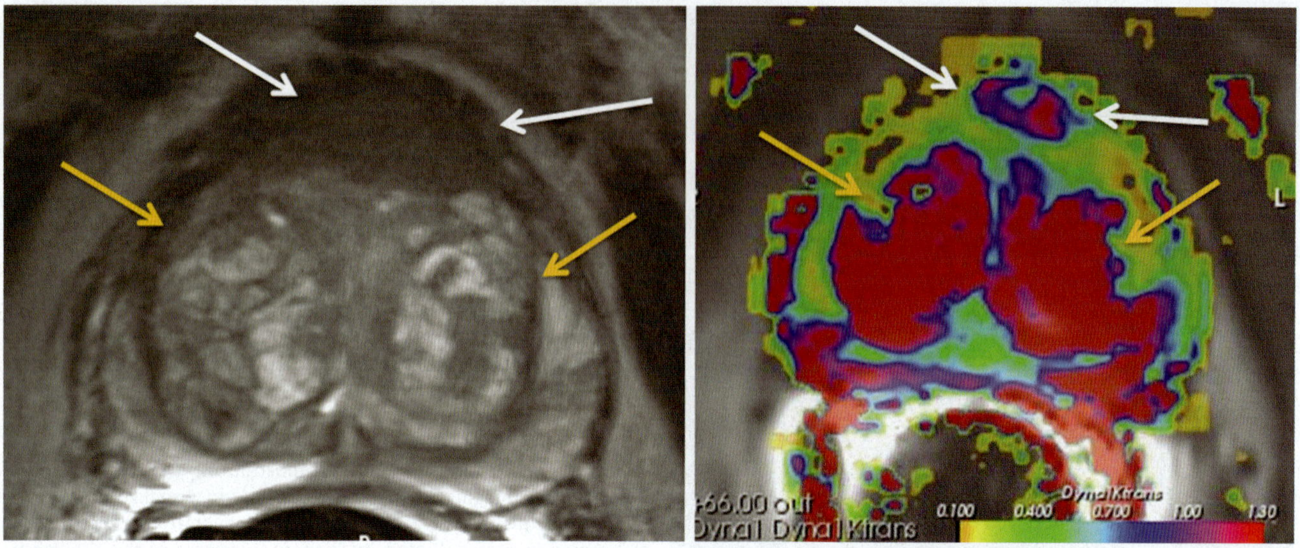

A B

Figure 31-12. A: Axial T2-weighted MR image with a clearly visible transition zone cancer (*white arrows*). **B:** Axial T1-weighted MR image at the same level as **(A)** with superimposed transfer constant parametric map. Enhancement of the prostate cancer lesion in the anterior transition zone (*white arrows*) and bilateral central gland (BPH nodules; *orange arrows*) is present.

(b) the slope and height of the enhancement curve (time-to-peak); (c) maximum signal intensity (peak enhancement); and (d) persistent delayed phase (type 1 curve), plateau delayed phase (type 2 curve), and washout delayed phase (type 3 curve).[46]

The *quantitative* approach using pharmacokinetic modeling, which is usually applied to changes in the contrast agent concentrations in tissue. Concentration–time curves are mathematically fitted by using one of many described pharmacokinetic models, and quantitative kinetic parameters are derived. These include: (a) transfer constant of the contrast agent (K_{trans}); (b) rate constant (K_{ep}); and (c) interstitial extravascular extracellular space (Ve) (Fig. 31-12).[46] The arterial input function used in the calculations also affects the reliability of the data obtained. In other words, robust methods for measuring the arterial input function are essential. Prostate cancer tends to enhance earlier, faster, and to a greater extent, and shows earlier contrast agent washout as compared with healthy prostate tissue.[49] Dynamic contrast-enhanced MR imaging is limited in the discrimination of cancer from prostatitis in the peripheral zone and from highly vascularized benign prostatic hyperplasia nodules in the transition zone.

1.5- and 3-T Field Strength

The increase signal-to-noise ratio obtained at 3 T compared to 1.5 T scanners resulted in improved image quality. Many of the differences between imaging at 1.5 and 3 T are the direct result of MR physical properties related to magnetic field strength changes. The signal-to-noise ratio is approximately two times higher at 3 T compared to 1.5 T. Probably, the most significant benefit is to decrease the acquisition time and/or increase the in-plane spatial resolution. The latter can be used to obtain enhanced anatomical details of the prostate. Potential drawbacks of clinical MR imaging at high field strengths are the shorter T2 and longer T1 relaxation times, increased susceptibility differences, dielectric effect, and the homogeneity of the magnetic field in the organ of interest. Increasing the spatial resolution at higher field could partially circumvent some of these issues.

A low molecular weight, extravascular and extracellular contrast agent (gadolinium chelate) shortens T1 relaxation of water and has high signal intensity on T1-weighted images. The T1 relaxation time of the tissues is prolonged at 3 T compared to 1.5 T. The relaxivity properties of gadolinium chelate are not significantly different at 1.5 than they are at 3 T. The longer T1-relaxation time of tissues and increased signal-to-noise ratio result in an increased contrast between tumor and normal tissue.[51]

In DCE-MRI, the signal-to-noise ratio increase can be used to improve the temporal resolution of dynamic measurements. Dynamic contrast-enhanced MR imaging is less accurate due to limitations of temporal and spatial resolution at 1.5 T. An increased temporal resolution may allow a more accurate estimation of the pharmacokinetic parameters.[52] Adjustments to dynamic contrast-enhanced MR imaging sequences for kinetic analysis are, however, necessary.[53]

Clinical Applications

Detection

There is an increased density of capillaries in prostatic carcinoma when compared with benign prostate tissue.[54] In DCE-MRI, prostate tumors present with strong enhancement compared to the healthy prostate tissue (Fig. 31-13). Prostate cancer enhancement appears earlier and washes out more quickly in comparison to normal tissue. The addition of dynamic contrast-enhanced MR imaging to anatomical imaging results in improved detection accuracies of prostate cancer. DCE-MRI can identify early-stage prostate cancer with high sensitivity and specificity and can predict the histologic grade to some extent.[55] DCE-MRI has high sensitivity, reported to be in the range of 74% to 96%, which is useful for the preliminary detection of tumors.[56]

Localization and Staging

MR imaging is the most accurate modality to preoperatively stage prostate cancer (stage T2 vs. stage T3, i.e., intra- and extraprostatic extension). MR imaging has a higher accuracy in the assessment of intraprostatic disease (stage T2), extracapsular extension, and seminal vesicle invasion (stage T3), as well as invasion of periprostatic structures (stage T4) compared to other imaging modalities. Apart from extracapsular extension, seminal vesicle invasion is an

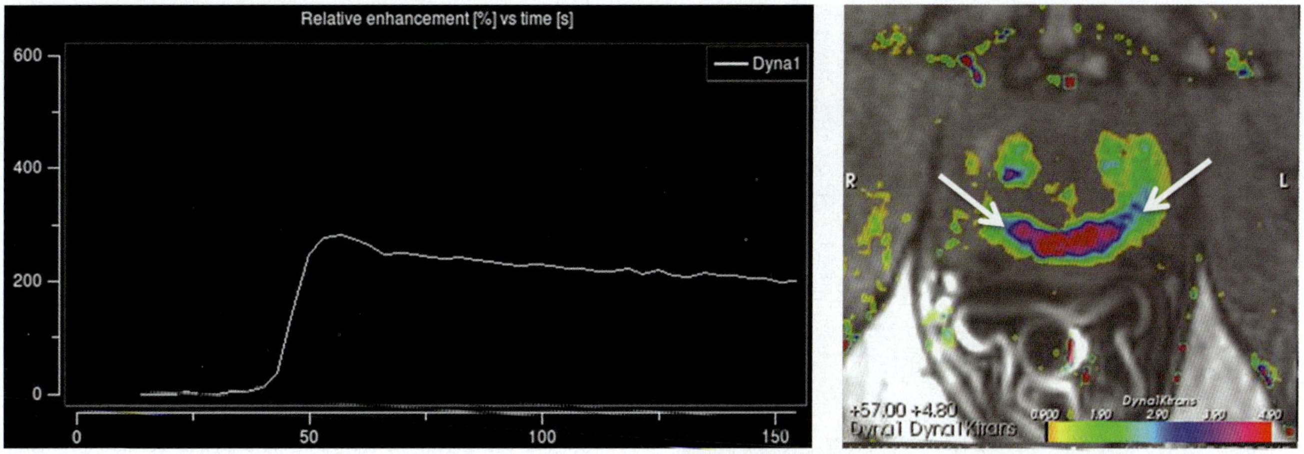

A B

Figure 31-13. Prostate cancers present with strong enhancement and fast washout compared to the healthy prostate tissue. **A:** A type 3 curve with washout is present in the left peripheral zone (**B**; *arrows*).

important prognostic factor, because it is associated with the highest rates of recurrence—second only to lymph node metastases.[57] MR imaging is also helpful to identify the invasion of adjacent organs (e.g., the bladder, pelvic floor muscles, and rectum). The addition of contrast results in more accurately detected tumors, capsular penetration, seminal vesicle invasion, and neurovascular bundle involvement compared to anatomical imaging.[58] The use of DCE-MRI in staging prostate cancer showed significant improvement in staging performance for the less experienced readers.[59] It may attract the readers eye to the area of interest, which may allow a more accurate evaluation of that area using high-resolution T2-weighted MR images.

Local Recurrence

Approximately 30% of patients who underwent radical prostatectomy will develop biochemical recurrent disease.[60,61] Biochemical failure, that is, a rising serum PSA in the absence of demonstrable metastases is widely accepted as an appropriate endpoint for defining treatment failure in men with localized prostate cancer. The serum PSA is routinely used to monitor disease recurrence after definitive therapy because biochemical recurrence antedates metastatic disease progression and prostate cancer–specific mortality by an average of 7 and 15 years, respectively.[62,63] Patients with biochemical recurrence after radical prostatectomy have an 88% 10-year overall survival rate compared to a 93% in males without signs of biochemical recurrence.

The workup of recurrent prostate cancer includes TRUS-guided prostate biopsy and a bone scintigraphy. TRUS-guided biopsy is invasive and has limited accuracy after radiation. The latter workup is performed, because there is no absolute PSA cutoff value to accurately predict on an individual basis, if one is dealing with local recurrence and/or systemic disease.

Following radical prostatectomy or radiation therapy, prostate evaluation with MR imaging is much more challenging. In a retrospective study, anatomical T2-weighted MR images were retrospectively examined in patients who were clinically validated of having postprostatectomy recurrence.[64] Clinical validation criteria for local recurrence were a positive biopsy result from the postprostatectomy fossa and a reduction in PSA level after salvage radiotherapy or serial MR images that showed at least a 20% increase in size of a suspicious pelvic soft tissue mass. Sensitivity and specificity for MR imaging detection of postprostatectomy recurrence were 95% and 100%, respectively.[64]

After external beam radiotherapy, prostatic tissue demonstrates diffuse low signal intensity on anatomical T2-weighted MR images with indistinct zonal anatomy and diffuse low T2 signal, which hinder tumor recurrence detection (Fig. 31-14). The contrast between benign irradiated tissues and recurrent cancer is therefore decreased, which makes detection of recurrence more difficult. For this reason, T2-weighted MR imaging is less helpful in localizing recurrence of prostate cancer. DCE-MRI is of added value in the detection of locally recurrent prostate cancer in either the postradiotherapy or prostatectomy patient. Initial results show promising value for DCE-MRI to depict postradiotherapy tumor recurrence, especially in the peripheral zone (Fig. 31-15).[65] Studies evaluating DCE-MRI after radiotherapy report sensitivities between 70% and

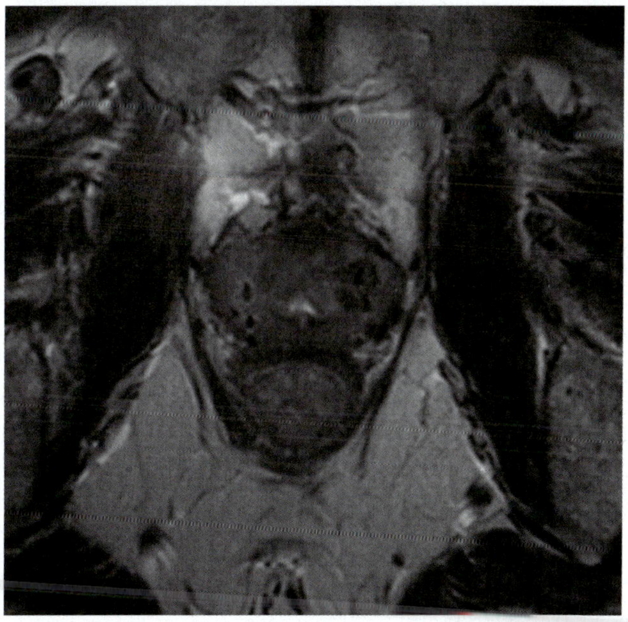

Figure 31-14. Axial T2-weighted MRI of a 75-year-old-male with a histopathologically proven prostate cancer (Gleason 9) 25 months after internal brachytherapy. The tumor is located in the left peripheral zone; however, it is not visible. Note that there is no zonal distinction visible.

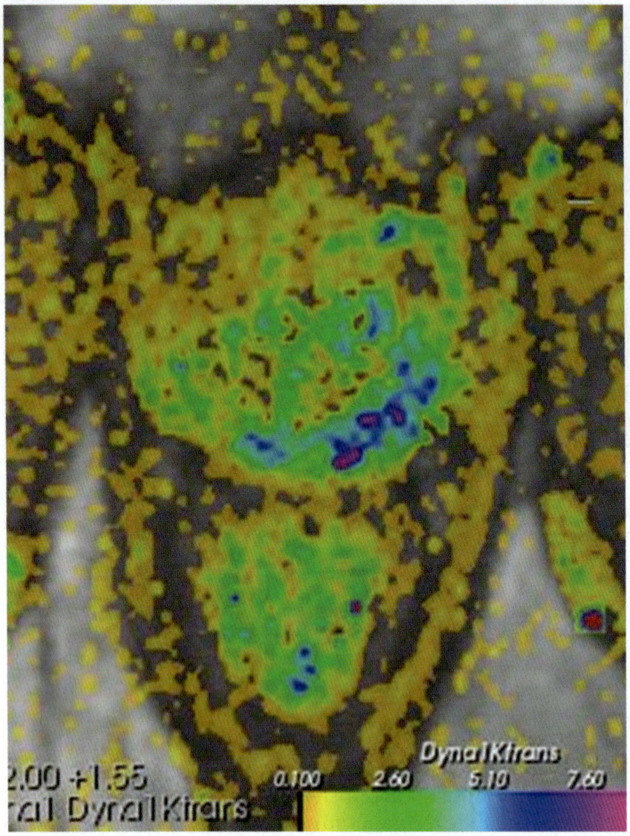

Figure 31-15. A 72-year-old patient with a local recurrent prostate cancer in the left peripheral zone. Postcontrast T1-weighted MRI demonstrates abnormal enhancement in the left peripheral zone, which is confirmed with MRI-guided biopsy. A Gleason 8 recurrent prostate cancer was diagnosed.

74% and a specificities between 73% and 85%.[66,67] Furthermore, the technique is valuable in detecting local recurrence occurring after radical prostatectomy with a sensitivity and specificity of 71% and 94%, respectively.[67]

REFERENCES

1. **Siegel R, Ma J, Zou Z, et al.** Cancer statistics, 2014. *CA Cancer J Clin* 2014;64(1):9–29.
2. **Loeb S, Bjurlin MA, Nicholson J, et al.** Overdiagnosis and overtreatment of prostate cancer. *Eur Urol* 2014;65(6):1046–1055.
3. **Krakowsky Y, Loblaw A, Klotz L.** Prostate cancer death of men treated with initial active surveillance: clinical and biochemical characteristics. *J Urol* 2010;184:131–135.
4. **Zlotta AR, Egawa S, Pushkar D, et al.** Prevalence of prostate cancer on autopsy: cross-sectional study on unscreened Caucasian and Asian men. *J Natl Cancer Inst* 2013;105(14):1050–1058.
5. **Pinto PA, Chung PH, Rastinehad AR, et al.** Magnetic resonance imaging/ultrasound fusion guided prostate biopsy improves cancer detection following transrectal ultrasound biopsy and correlates with multiparametric magnetic resonance imaging. *J Urol* 2011;186(4):1281–1285.
6. **Sciarra A, Panebianco V, Salciccia S, et al.** Modern role of magnetic resonance and spectroscopy in the imaging of prostate cancer. *Urol Oncol* 2011;29:12–20.
7. **Puech P, Sufana Iancu A, Renard B, et al.** Detecting prostate cancer with MRI: why and how. *Diagn Interv Imaging* 2012;93:268–278.
8. **Tamada T, Sone T, Higashi H, et al.** Prostate cancer detection in patients with total serum prostate-specific antigen levels of 4-10 ng/mL: diagnostic efficacy of diffusion-weighted imaging, dynamic contrast-enhanced MRI, and T2-weighted imaging. *AJR Am J Roentgenol* 2011;197:664–670.
9. **Hoeks CM, Barentsz JO, Hambrock T, et al.** Prostate cancer: multiparametric MR imaging for detection, localization, and staging. *Radiology* 2011;261(1):46–66.
10. **Turkbey B, Pinto PA, Mani H, et al.** Prostate cancer: value of multiparametric MR imaging at 3 T for detection—histopathologic correlation. *Radiology* 2010;255(1):89–99.
11. **Delongchamps NB, Rouanne M, Flam T, et al.** Multiparametric magnetic resonance imaging for the detection and localization of prostate cancer: combination of T2-weighted, dynamic contrast-enhanced and diffusion-weighted imaging. *BJU Int* 2011;107(9):1411–1418.
12. **Delongchamps NB, Beuvon F, Eiss D, et al.** Multiparametric MRI is helpful to predict tumor focality, stage, and size in patients diagnosed with unilateral low-risk prostate cancer. *Prostate Cancer Prostatic Dis* 2011;14(3):232–237.
13. **Scheenen TW, Futterer J, Weiland E, et al.** Discriminating cancer from noncancer tissue in the prostate by 3-dimensional proton magnetic resonance spectroscopic imaging: a prospective multicenter validation study. *Invest Radiol* 2011;46(1):25–33.
14. **Cuenod CA, Balvay D.** Perfusion and vascular permeability: basic concepts and measurement in DCE-CT and DCE-MRI. *Diagn Interv Imaging* 2013;94(12):1187–1204.
15. **Barry MJ.** Prostate-specific-antigen testing for early diagnosis of prostate cancer. *N Engl J Med* 2001;344:1373–1377.
16. **Costello LC, Franklin RB.** "Why do tumor cells glycolyze?": from glycolysis through citrate to lipogenesis. *Mol Cell Biochem* 2005;280:1–8.
17. **Franklin RB, Milon B, Feng P, et al.** Zinc and zinc transporter in normal prostate function and the pathogenesis of prostate cancer. *Front Biosci* 2005;10:2230–2239.
18. **Costello LC, Franklin RB.** The clinical relevance of the metabolism of prostate cancer; zinc and tumor suppression: connecting the dots. *Mol Cancer* 2006;5:17.
19. **Braun M, Perner S.** High-grade prostatic intraepithelial neoplasia: the only accepted prostate cancer precursor lesion. *Pathologe* 2011;32(suppl 2):237–241.
20. **McNeal JE.** Normal and pathologic anatomy of the prostate. *Urology* 1981;17:11–16.
21. **McNeal JE, Redwine EA, Freiha FS, et al.** Zonal distribution of prostatic adenocarcinoma. Correlation with histologic pattern and direction of spread. *Am J Surg Pathol* 1988;12:897–906.
22. **Augustin H, Erbersdobler A, Hammerer PG, et al.** Prostate cancers in the transition zone: Part 2; clinical aspects. *BJU Int* 2004;94:1226–1229.
23. **Greene DR, Wheeler TM, Egawa S, et al.** Relationship between clinical stage and histological zone of origin in early prostate-cancer—morphometric analysis. *Br J Urol* 1991;68:499–509.
24. **King CR, Ferrari M, Brooks JD.** Prognostic significance of prostate cancer originating from the transition zone. *Urol Oncol* 2009;27:592–597.
25. **White S, Hricak H, Forstner R, et al.** Prostate cancer: effect of postbiopsy hemorrhage on interpretation of MR images. *Radiology* 1995;195:385–390.
26. **Barrett T, Vargas HA, Akin O, et al.** Value of the hemorrhage exclusion sign on T1-weighted prostate MR images for the detection of prostate cancer. *Radiology* 2012;263(3):751–757.
27. **Hoeks CM, Barentsz JO, Hambrock T, et al.** Prostate cancer: multiparametric MR imaging for detection, localization, and staging. *Radiology* 2011;261(1):46–66.
28. **Hricak H, Williams RD, Spring DB, et al.** Anatomy and pathology of the male pelvis by magnetic resonance imaging. *AJR Am J Roentgenol* 1983;141(6):1101–1110.
29. **Wang L, Mazaheri Y, Zhang J, et al.** Assessment of biologic aggressiveness of prostate cancer: correlation of MR signal intensity with Gleason grade after radical prostatectomy. *Radiology* 2008;246(1):168–176.
30. **Lansberg MG, Norbash AM, Marks MP, et al.** Advantages of adding diffusion-weighted magnetic resonance imaging to conventional magnetic resonance imaging for evaluating acute stroke. *Arch Neurol* 2000;57:1311–1316.
31. **Koh DM, Collins DJ.** Diffusion-weighted MRI in the body: applications and challenges in oncology. *AJR Am J Roentgenol* 2007;188(6):1622–1635.
32. **Stejskal EO, Tanner JE.** Spin diffusion measurements: spin echoes in the presence of a time-dependent field gradient. *J Chem Phys* 1965; 42(1):288–292.
33. **Le Bihan D.** Molecular diffusion nuclear magnetic resonance imaging. *Magn Reson Q* 1991;7:1–30.
34. **Le Bihan D, Breton E, Lallemand D, et al.** Separation of diffusion and perfusion in intravoxel incoherent motion MR imaging. *Radiology* 1988;168:497–505.

35. **Guo Y, Cai YQ, Cai ZL, et al.** Differentiation of clinically benign and malignant breast lesions using diffusion- weighted imaging. *J Magn Reson Imaging* 2002;16:172–178.
36. **Gauvain KM, McKinstry RC, Mukherjee P, et al.** Evaluating pediatric brain tumor cellularity with diffusion-tensor imaging. *AJR Am J Roentgenol* 2001;177:449–454.
37. **Bammer R.** Basic principles of diffusion-weighted imaging. *Eur J Radiol* 2003;45:169–184.
38. **Somford DM, Fütterer JJ, Hambrock T, et al.** Diffusion and perfusion MR imaging of the prostate. *Magn Reson Imaging Clin N Am* 2008;16(4):685–695.
39. **Kumar V, Jagannathan NR, Kumar R, et al.** Apparent diffusion coefficient of the prostate in men prior to biopsy: determination of a cut-off value to predict malignancy of the peripheral zone. *NMR Biomed* 2007;20:505–511.
40. **Kim CK, Park BK, Lee HM, et al.** Value of diffusion-weighted imaging for the prediction of prostate cancer location at 3 T using a phased-array coil: preliminary results. *Invest Radiol* 2007;42:842–847.
41. **Tamada T, Sone T, Toshimutsu S, et al.** Age-related and zonal anatomical changes of apparent diffusion coefficient values in normal human prostatic tissues. *J Magn Reson Imaging* 2008;27:552–556.
42. **Ren J, Huan Y, Wang H, et al.** Diffusion-weighted imaging in normal prostate and differential diagnosis of prostate diseases. *Abdom Imaging* 2008;33(6):724–728.
43. **Nagel KN, Schouten MG, Hambrock T, et al.** Differentiation of prostatitis and prostate cancer by using diffusion-weighted MR imaging and MR-guided biopsy at 3 T. *Radiology* 2013;267(1):164–172.
44. **Padhani AR, Harvey CJ, Cosgrove DO.** Angiogenesis imaging in the management of prostate cancer. *Nat Clin Pract Urol* 2005;2:596–607.
45. **Hambrock T, Padhani AR, Tofts PS, et al.** Dynamic contrast-enhanced MR imaging in the diagnosis and management of prostate cancer. RSNA Categorical Course in Diagnostic Radiology. *Genitourinary Radiol* 2006;1:61–77.
46. **Huisman HJ, Engelbrecht MR, Barentsz JO.** Accurate estimation of pharmacokinetic contrast-enhanced dynamic MRI parameters of the prostate. *J Magn Reson Imaging* 2001;13(4):607–614.
47. **d'Arcy JA, Collins DJ, Padhani AR, et al.** Informatics in Radiology (infoRAD): Magnetic Resonance Imaging Workbench: analysis and visualization of dynamic contrast-enhanced MR imaging data. *Radiographics* 2006;26:621–632.
48. **Collins DJ, Padhani AR.** Dynamic magnetic resonance imaging of tumor perfusion. *IEEE Eng Med Biol Mag* 2004;23:65–83.
49. **Alonzi R, Padhani AR, Allen C.** Dynamic contrast enhanced MRI in prostate cancer. *Eur J Radiol* 2007;63(3):335–350.
50. **Daldrup HE, Shames DM, Husseini W, et al.** Quantification of the extraction fraction for gadopentetate across breast cancer capillaries. *Magn Reson Med* 1998;40(4):537–543.
51. **Nobauer-Huhmann IM, Ba-Ssalamah A, Mlynarik V, et al.** Magnetic resonance imaging contrast enhancement of brain tumors at 3 tesla versus 1.5 tesla. *Invest Radiol* 2002;37:114–119.
52. **Fütterer JJ, Scheenen TW, Huisman HJ, et al.** Initial experience of 3 Tesla endorectal coil magnetic resonance imaging and 1H-spectroscopic imaging of the prostate. *Invest Radiol* 2004;39:671–680.
53. **Wang J, Alsop DC, Li L, et al.** Comparison of quantitative perfusion imaging using arterial spin labeling at 1.5 and 4.0 Tesla. *Magn Reson Med* 2002;48:242–254.
54. **Bigler SA, Deering RE, Brawer MK.** Comparison of microscopic vascularity in benign and malignant prostate tissue. *Hum Pathol* 1993;24(2):220–226.
55. **Hara N, Okuizumi M, Koike H, et al.** Dynamic contrast-enhanced magnetic resonance imaging (DCE-MRI) is a useful modality for the precise detection and staging of early prostate cancer. *Prostate* 2005;62(2):140–147.
56. **Oto A, Yang C, Kayhan A, et al.** Diffusion-weighted and dynamic contrast-enhanced MRI of prostate cancer: correlation of quantitative MR parameters with Gleason score and tumor angiogenesis. *AJR Am J Roentgenol.* 2011;197(6):1382–1390.
57. **Blute ML, Bergstralh EJ, Iocca A, et al.** Use of Gleason score, prostate specific antigen, seminal vesicle and margin status to predict biochemical failure after radical prostatectomy. *J Urol* 2001;165(1): 119–125.
58. **Ogura K, Maekawa S, Okubo K, et al.** Dynamic endorectal magnetic resonance imaging for local staging and detection of neurovascular bundle involvement of prostate cancer: correlation with histopathologic results. *Urology* 2001;57(4):721–726.
59. **Fütterer JJ, Engelbrecht MR, Huisman HJ, et al.** Staging prostate cancer with dynamic contrast-enhanced endorectal MR imaging prior to radical prostatectomy: experienced versus less experienced readers. *Radiology* 2005;237(2):541–549.
60. **Djavan, B, Moul JW, Zlotta A, et al.** PSA progression following radical prostatectomy and radiation therapy: new standards in the new millennium. *Eur Urol* 2003;43:12–27.
61. **Khan MA, Han M, Partin AW, et al.** Long-term cancer control of radical prostatectomy in men younger than 50 years of age: update 2003. *Urology* 2003;62:86–91; discussion 91–92.
62. **Pound CR, Partin AW, Eisenberger MA, et al.** Natural history of progression after PSA elevation following radical prostatectomy. *JAMA* 1999;281:1591–1597.
63. **Freedland SJ, Humphreys EB, Mangold LA, et al.** Risk of prostate cancer-specific mortality following biochemical recurrence after radical prostatectomy. *JAMA* 2005;294:433–439.
64. **Sella T, Schwartz LH, Swindle PW, et al.** Suspected local recurrence after radical prostatectomy: endorectal coil MR imaging. *Radiology* 2004;231:379–385.
65. **Haider MA, Chung P, Sweet J, et al.** Dynamic contrast-enhanced magnetic resonance imaging for localization of recurrent prostate cancer after external beam radiotherapy. *Int J Radiat Oncol Biol Phys* 2008;70:425–430.
66. **Rouvière O, Valette O, Grivolat S, et al.** Recurrent prostate cancer after external beam radiotherapy: value of contrast-enhanced dynamic MRI in localizing intraprostatic tumor—correlation with biopsy findings. *Urology* 2004;63:922–927.
67. **Sciarra A, Panebianco V, Salciccia S, et al.** Role of dynamic contrast-enhanced magnetic resonance (MR) imaging and proton MR spectroscopic imaging in the detection of local recurrence after radical prostatectomy for prostate cancer. *Eur Urol* 2008;54:589–600.

CHAPTER

32 Perfusion CT Imaging in Oncology

Davide Prezzi, FRCR and Vicky Goh, MD, FRCR

Introduction

Dynamic contrast-enhanced CT imaging techniques (perfusion CT) enable clinicians to evaluate the functional blood supply to a tumor. From the subsequent changes in tumor and vascular enhancement following intravenous administration of an iodinated contrast agent, qualitative and quantitative parameters may be assessed that may quantify regional perfusion, blood volume, and microcirculatory changes. These tumor parameters provide prognostic or predictive information to the clinician and enable downstream treatment effects on the vasculature to be assessed. This technique was first described in the 1970s, but its clinical use has increased in recent years due to a combination of factors: technologic advances in acquisition and postprocessing methods facilitating its clinical implementation and a perceived clinical need, related to the use of therapeutic interventions in oncology. This chapter discusses the principles of perfusion CT techniques and their clinical application in oncology.

Principles of Perfusion CT

Contrast Agent Kinetics

Assessment of the functional vasculature of a tissue or organ of interest by dynamic contrast-enhanced computed tomography (CT), also known as perfusion CT, is based on the evaluation of intravenous contrast agent kinetics. In clinical practice low molecular weight (<1 kDa) iodinated contrast agents are used, which have negligible serum protein binding. Their distribution in the body is similar to that of extracellular fluid. Following a bolus intravenous injection, the contrast agent distributes rapidly within the vascular system (Fig. 32-1). As the contrast agent transits through a vascular bed, it passes from the intravascular to the extravascular extracellular compartment, with the exception of the brain, retina, and testis. The rate at which this occurs is determined by a number of factors including the rate of tissue delivery, vessel surface area, and the permeability of these vessels, which will differ between pathologic and normal tissue. There is subsequent return of contrast agent from the extravascular–extracellular compartment back into the intravascular compartment; its excretion is usually via the kidneys. Typically, there is insignificant passage of contrast agent into the intracellular compartment (<1%).

The differences in contrast agent kinetics between pathologic and normal tissues or organs can be exploited to provide specific information on the functional vasculature. By assessing the dynamic changes in vessel and tissue or organ enhancement over time following intravenous administration of an iodinated contrast agent, both qualitative and quantitative parameters that inform on the function of the vasculature may be assessed (Fig. 32-2). Qualitative parameters refer to descriptors of the enhancement-time curves. These include curve shape, time to peak enhancement, peak enhancement, or area under the enhancement-time curve (Fig. 32-3). These parameters will be influenced by technical and patient factors including contrast agent dose, contrast agent rate of administration, and cardiac output. Quantitative parameters are derived from kinetic modeling of the enhancement-time curves and are more physiology based. These include regional blood flow, blood volume, and extraction fraction or permeability surface area product (Table 32.1).

In tumors, these parameters may be obtained in a relatively robust manner (day-to-day reproducibility: coefficient of variation <25%) and may provide relevant clinical information to the clinician and enable treatment effects on the tumor vasculature to be assessed.[1] Regional blood flow, blood volume, and vascular leakage parameters within the tumor are interrelated and may vary with the underlying tumor environment. For example, (i) areas of high blood flow, blood volume, and leakage may reflect well-perfused areas with presence of shunting and areas of angiogenesis; (ii) areas of low blood flow, blood volume, and low leakage may represent areas of poor vascularization +/− necrosis; and (iii) areas of low blood flow, blood volume, and high leakage may represent poor perfusion regions with angiogenesis.

Biologic Correlates of Tumor Vascular Parameters

Tumor vascular parameters provide information regarding the delivery of oxygen and nutrients to the tumor, its functional "vascular density," and the rate of leakage from the capillaries or neovessels. These parameters may provide a surrogate measure of tumor angiogenesis and perfusion-related hypoxia.

Morphologic Characteristics of the Tumor Vasculature

The development of a viable tumor blood supply is essential to support tumor growth and proliferation.[2] This may occur through sprouting from preexisting vessels, de novo vascular formation through recruitment of circulating endothelial progenitor cells,

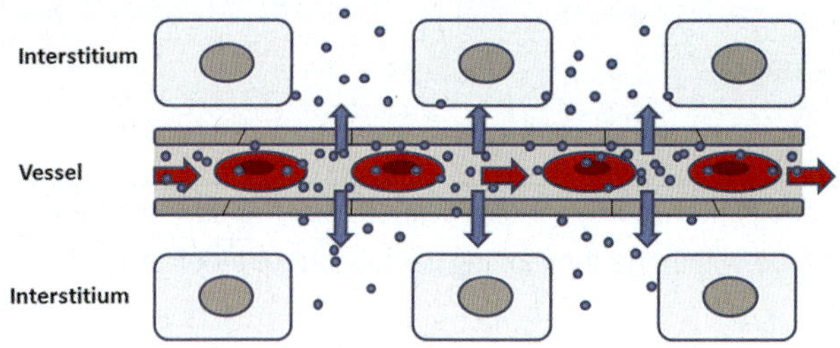

Figure 32-1. Distribution of contrast agent within the vascular bed of the organ of interest after intravenous administration.

and vessel cooption. The tumor microenvironment including hypoxia, glucose deprivation, and low pH plays an important role in the initiation of tumor angiogenesis via the activation of oncogenes and/or inactivation of tumor suppressor genes.[3]

In terms of morphology, the tumor vasculature appears functionally distinct and spatially heterogeneous. The vasculature lacks the usual hierarchical branching pattern and in general demonstrates greater vessel density at the tumor periphery. The vessels themselves are thin and tortuous, characterized by a relatively high endothelial cell proliferation rate, incomplete endothelium, relative absence of smooth muscle or pericyte investiture, and hyperpermeability resulting in high interstitial fluid pressure.

Immunohistochemistry Correlates of Perfusion CT Parameters

Microvessel density (MVD) and vascular endothelial growth factor (VEGF) are commonly used immunohistologic measures of angiogenesis. In a number of cancers including lung, renal, gastrointestinal, and pancreatic cancer, associations have been found between MVD and/or VEGF and various perfusion CT parameters. Most of the evidence relates to lung cancer. Typically, these correlations have been moderate: histologic analysis has been varied, based on different numbers of "hotspot" counts or from random areas of the whole tumor. There have also been negative studies, in part reflecting the heterogeneity of analyses and immunohistologic biomarkers used.[4]

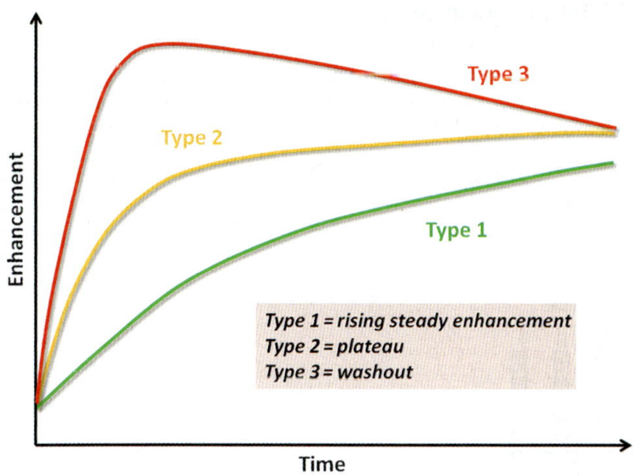

Figure 32-2. Qualitative assessment of enhancement-time curves. *Type 1*: Steady incremental enhancement; this pattern is usually seen in benign lesions. *Type 2*: Signal plateaus after a fast initial increase; this pattern may be seen in inflammatory lesions and some malignant tumors, for example, on treatment. *Type 3*: Fast initial enhancement followed by early washout; this pattern is typical of malignant tumors, due to increased microvessel density, hyperpermeability of the vasculature and arteriovenous shunting.

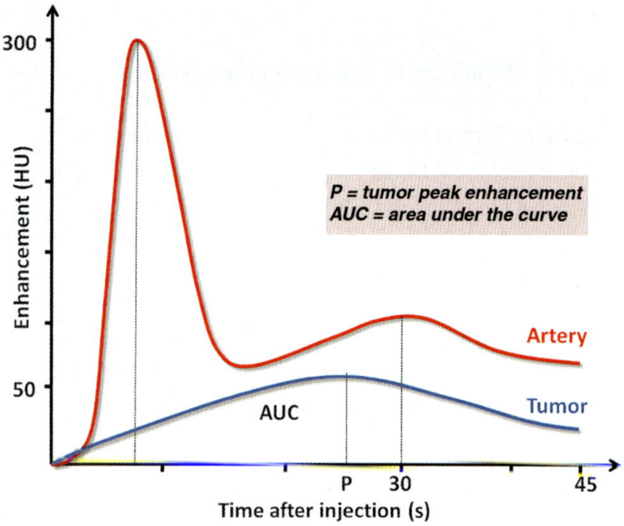

Figure 32-3. Enhancement-time curves for artery and tumor. The second arterial peak corresponds to the return of contrast agent from the extravascular–extracellular into the intravascular compartment.

With respect to the lung, peak CT enhancement in patients with solitary pulmonary nodules has been correlated significantly with both MVD and VEGF, irrespective of the benign or malignant nature of the nodules.[5] In patients with operable non–small cell lung cancer CT peak enhancement, blood flow, blood volume or permeability surface area product have been shown to have a moderate correlation with MVD: Li et al. found that the CT regional blood flow correlated with CD34 expression ($r = 0.715$; $p \leq 0.001$) assessed in six tumor regions: central (three regions) and peripheral (three regions).[6] Ma et al. have shown that CT peak enhancement and regional blood flow correlate with CD34 expression assessed in five hotspots in VEGF-positive but not VEGF-negative tumors.[7] Similarly, Sauter et al. have found a moderate correlation between extraction fraction and blood flow and CD34,[8] while Spira et al. have reported a positive association between MVD and blood flow and volume.[9] Peak enhancement, blood flow, and relative blood volume have also been shown to be significantly higher in VEGF-positive compared to VEGF-negative tumors.[7,10]

There have also been several pathologic correlative studies in abdominally sited cancers. In renal cell cancer an initial study in 24 patients showed a moderate correlation ($r = 0.60$) between peak enhancement and hotspot MVD (CD34).[11] More recently, a further small study ($n = 10$) where patients with renal cell cancer underwent volumetric perfusion CT prior to surgery has confirmed that regional blood flow and blood volume correlated significantly with MVD (CD34; $r = 0.600$ to 0.829); however, extraction fraction (measured as the transfer constant, K^{trans}) only demonstrated moderate correlations with MVD in nonnecrotic areas ($r = 0.550$).[12]

Moderate correlations ($r = 0.42$) between regional blood volume and hotspot MVD (CD34) have been found in gastric adenocarcinoma.[13] Similarly in colorectal cancer, moderate correlations between regional blood volume and permeability surface area product and nonhotspot MVD (CD34) have been shown.[14] In pancreatic adenocarcinoma, moderate correlations ($r = 0.49$) have also been found between MVD and peak enhancement in the arterial phase.[15]

Perfusion CT parameters may also inform on the presence of perfusion-related hypoxia. In lung cancer, blood volume measurements have been found to be negatively correlated to an exogenous marker of hypoxia (pimonidazole: $r = -0.48$).[16]

TABLE 32.1 Definition of Vascular Parameters

Vascular Parameter	Definition
Regional blood flow (BF)	Flow rate of whole blood through the vasculature of a defined tissue volume or mass
Regional blood volume (BV)	Volume of flowing whole blood within the functioning vasculature of a defined tissue volume or mass
Mean transit time (MTT)	Average time for blood to travel between the arterial inflow and the venous outflow, measured in seconds
Extraction fraction (EF)	Fraction of the whole blood contrast agent that is transferred to the extravascular extracellular space during a single passage of the contrast agent
Permeability surface area product (PS)	Product of permeability and total surface area of capillary endothelium in a unit volume or mass of tissue (mL/min/100 mL) and reflects the total diffusional flux across the capillaries into the extravascular extracellular space

However, one of the challenges of clinicopathologic correlative studies is the comparison of in vivo with ex vivo findings. Tacelli et al. have showed that the areas of low regional tumor blood volume but high permeability have higher CD34 expression (assessed in three hotspots in the nonnecrotic tumor portion) than areas of high regional tumor blood volume and high permeability: 72.1 versus 47.9, $p = 0.038$.[17] They postulated this difference could be related to the effect of the tumor microenvironment.[17]

Technical Aspects

Patient Preparation

Prior to the examination, patients should be well hydrated and have a normal renal function. For studies involving abdominal organs such as the liver, pancreas, and bowel, recent food intake may affect organ perfusion, and fasting prior to CT may be appropriate. If an oral contrast agent is required, water or a negative oral contrast agent is preferred to positive contrast agents. An antiperistaltic drug (e.g., glucagon or hyoscine-*N*-butylbromide) is advisable for studies of the bowel.

Keeping the patient well informed concerning the CT acquisition will improve the quality of the study. Clear instructions should be given, for example, regarding the need to stay still, breathing instructions for any breath-held studies, cessation of swallowing during the acquisition for head and neck studies, and warnings of the potential effects induced by the intravenously administered contrast agent including a hot flush.

Contrast Agent Administration

The dose and manner in which contrast agents are administered may influence parameter quantification. Kinetic modeling benefits from a bolus injection of contrast agent, at an injection rate of at least 4 mL/s via a large bore intravenous cannula, usually sited in the antecubital fossa. Injection rates beyond 10 mL/s appear to confer no additional benefit for quantification. The total injected iodine dose should be within the range of 12 to 18 g. It is important that the iodine concentration administered is not less than 300 mg/mL. Conversely, if iodine concentrations are greater than 350 mg/mL the contrast agent must be warmed to body temperature prior to injection, as the higher viscosity will slow the actual injection rate. The volume of contrast agent will depend on the iodine concentration used.[1]

CT Data Acquisition

With current state-of-the-art technology, an entire organ may be encompassed with a high spatial resolution and a high temporal acquisition sampling rate. To ensure accurate quantification, a sampling rate of 2 seconds or less should be used (Fig. 32-4).

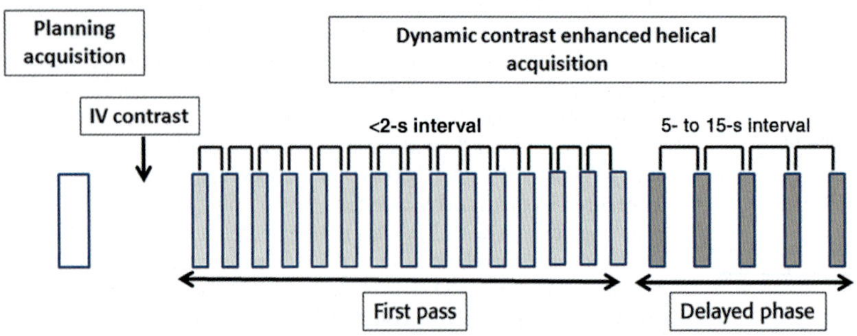

Typical acquisition parameters	Kilovoltage	mA	Contrast agent concentration & volume
Head & neck	80–100	<150	Intravenous administration: >4 mL/s Concentration: >300 mL/mg iodine Typical volumes: 30–60 mL
Thorax	80–100	<150	
Abdomen & pelvis	100–120	<150	

Figure 32-4. Schema showing typical perfusion CT acquisition for tumor evaluation and suggested contrast agent injection rate.

For the initial perfusion phase, an acquisition duration of 45 seconds is adequate; for the interstitial phase at least five additional time points are recommended, the sampling rate ranging from 5 to 15 seconds depending on the kinetic model applied.[1] As the concentration of iodine within blood vessels and tissues is proportional to the resultant increase in attenuation, temporal changes in attenuation can be analyzed using standard kinetic models without prior conversion to iodine concentration.

Motion Correction and Image Registration

For target areas located in motion susceptible sites, breath-holding during the first pass study will reduce motion artifact and voxel displacement. For longer-duration studies, motion correction/image registration may compensate for motion artifact, and this is incorporated into commercial software platforms, for example, based on a nonrigid deformable registration technique.[18]

Quantification of Vascular Parameters

The vascular parameters that can be quantified include regional blood flow, blood volume, and extraction fraction or permeability surface area product (Table 32.1). Different mathematical models may be applied to derive these. Commonly used tracer kinetic modeling includes "Maximum initial slope", "Patlak" and "Distributed parameter analysis" (Table 32.2). In practice, quantification using commercial platforms requires a region of interest to be placed within an input artery (to generate an arterial input function [AIF]) and for the lesion(s) of interest. From the arterial and tissue enhancement-time curves that are displayed by the software, quantitative parametric maps are generated for each pixel (or voxel) representing a parameter value (Fig. 32-5). While volume-of-interest analysis, encompassing the whole tumor, may be the least susceptible to observer error and experience, and provide a global evaluation of perfusion and angiogenesis, this may not best reflect the heterogeneity within a tumor, particularly if this demonstrates areas of necrosis, calcification or hemorrhage, as these are "averaged" in the process.[19]

What Is an Appropriate Target Lesion?

In practice, it is important to choose an appropriate target lesion(s). Ideally, this should be greater than 2 cm and not in close proximity to large vessels (e.g., superior vena cava or aorta), heart or diaphragm in order to reduce artifacts. For lesions located in motion susceptible sites, breath-holding techniques (+/− initial hyperventilation), and/or the use of motion correction/image registration will reduce motion artifacts. For target lesions located within the bowel, the use of a standard antiperistaltic (Buscopan or Glucagon) will reduce the motion related to peristalsis. It is also important to select an appropriate artery to derive the AIF. The vessel chosen must be of sufficient size to prevent partial volume averaging occurring secondarily due to pulsation or movement artifact (including peristalsis) or laminar flow within the vessel. If this is the case this will influence and change the arterial time-attenuation curve. It is assumed that the arterial time-attenuation curve of the artery in the field of view is identical to the vessel supplying the tumor. This is only valid if there is no significant stenosis of the artery or other major feeding vessels.

Clinical Implementation

Quality Assurance and Quality Control

The ready availability of perfusion CT software on commercial reporting workstations has facilitated clinical implementation. However, in addition to standard quality assurance that tests the performance of the CT scanner, quality control procedures should be in place for perfusion CT, particularly where longitudinal studies are planned and robust quantification is required, for example, in the clinical trial setting.[1] Quality control refers to the processes needed to maintain quality. Standardization of acquisition, analysis and reporting protocols should be implemented, where possible. These acquisition, radiation dose, data processing, and reporting protocols should be recorded for each patient allowing audit to be undertaken. The use of phantom calibration, assessment of image quality (contrast to noise ratio), and, in clinical trials, central data review should be undertaken of at least 10% of the dataset.

Radiation Dose

The cancer risk associated with perfusion CT has to be balanced against the potential benefits derived from quantification of tumor vascularity. Imaging should comply with the ALARA (As Low As Reasonably Achievable) principle. The radiation dose of a perfusion CT acquisition is dependent on the temporal frequency of the acquisition, volume of coverage, kilovoltage, and milliampere selected.[20] The risk significance of a radiation exposure from perfusion CT will depend to some extent on the clinical circumstance. For example, the risk significance will be relatively inconsequential in the context of radiation therapy where the therapy dose is much higher than the diagnostic perfusion CT.

The CT acquisition should be tailored to the research or clinical question or clinical context. A maximal acceptable dose should be assigned for the acquisition ensuring that satisfactory signal to noise characteristics can be obtained. In general, it is good practice to ensure that a maximum effective dose of 20 mSv for a volume of tissue measuring 4 cm in the craniocaudal direction is not exceeded.[1] The effective dose is obtained by multiplying the dose length product (DLP, mGy/cm),provided by the CT scanner, and the appropriate conversion factor (mSv/mGy/cm). The DLP and CT Dose Index by volume ($CTDI_{vol}$) of perfusion CT studies should be recorded in the patient record.

TABLE 32.2 Summary of the Commonly Applied Kinetic Models

Kinetic Model	Compartments	Assumptions	Quantitative Parameter
Johnson-Wilson distributed parameter	Dual	Constrained input function	Regional blood flow, blood volume, permeability surface area product
Patlak	Dual	One-way transfer Well-mixed compartments	Extraction fraction, blood volume
Maximum slope	Single	No venous outflow	Regional blood flow

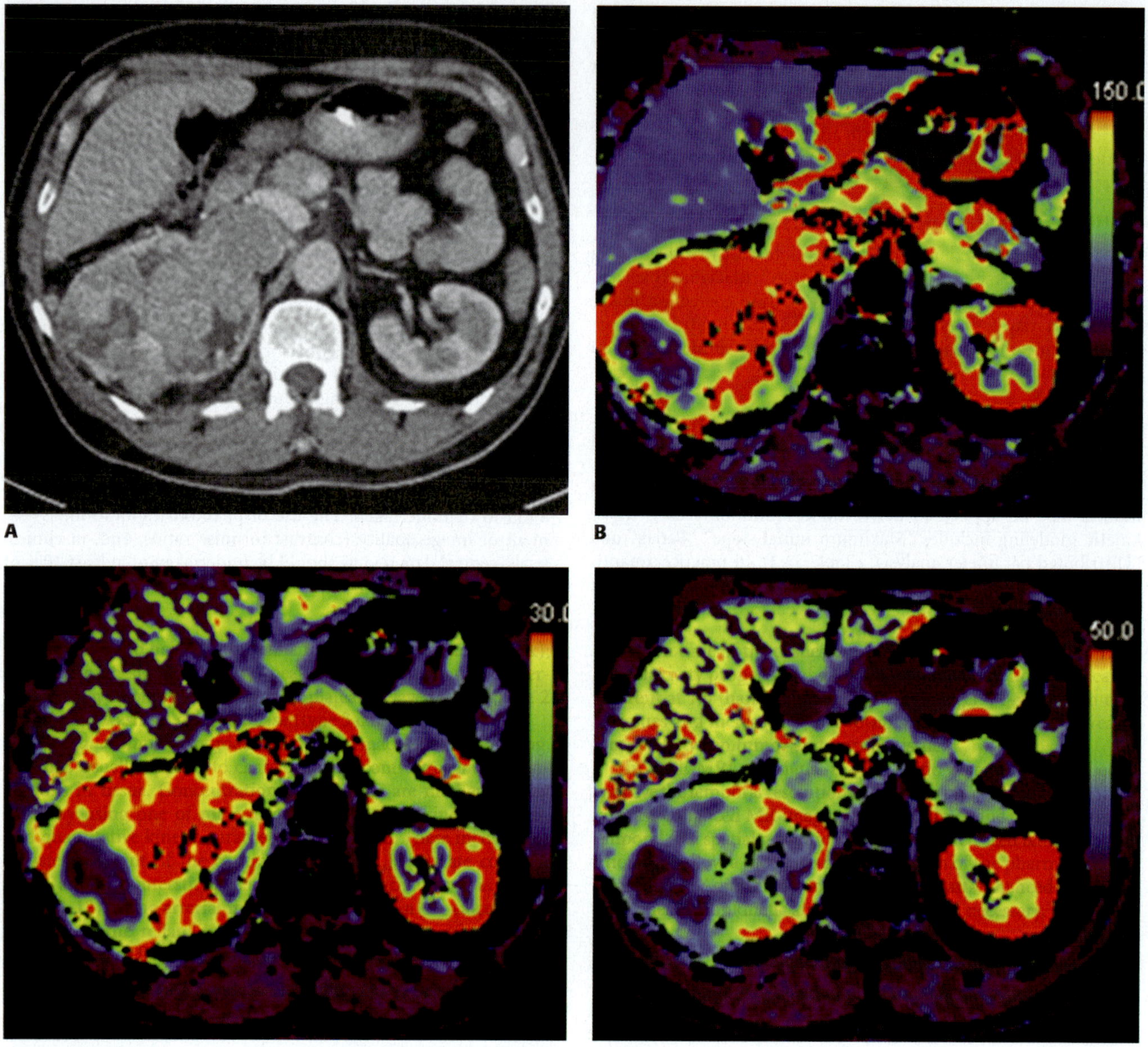

A B C D

Figure 32-5. **CT image of a renal tumor (A) and corresponding parametric maps of regional blood flow (B), blood volume (C), and extraction fraction (D) are shown.** The tumor demonstrates heterogeneous blood flow and blood volume.

It is also important in the context of repeated measurements that intra- and interobserver variability is limited. In general intraobserver is better than interobserver agreement,[21] in concordance with other studies of observer agreement using traditional morphologic measures of response;[22] where appropriate a single observer should analyze serial examinations in the same patient.

Clinical Applications

In oncologic practice, its main role remains the evaluation of the effectiveness of drugs that target the tumor vasculature, particularly in the context of clinical trials.[23] However, by exploiting the differences in perfusion parameters between tumor and normal tissues, and reflecting perfusion and angiogenesis, perfusion CT may also assist lesion characterization, delineation of tumor extent, tumor phenotyping, and prognostication.

Response Assessment

Quantitative parameters derived from perfusion CT may be used to monitor the effects of a variety of treatments. These include chemotherapy with standard and novel agents (antiangiogenic drugs, vascular disrupting agents, and immunotherapy), radiotherapy, and interventional oncologic procedures such as embolization of the tumor vascular supply or radiofrequency ablation. Early evidence has shown that a common long-term effect of treatment is a reduction in perfusion CT parameters following treatment completion, although in the short-term there may be a variable vascular effect related to the therapeutic mechanism of action (Table 32.3).

With standard chemotherapy, which affects actively replicating cells via DNA damage or interruption of DNA repair, this effect is thought to reflect the loss of angiogenic cytokine support following cell death.[52] With antiangiogenic therapies, differing vascular effects

TABLE 32.3 **Summary of Clinical Trials Using Perfusion CT as a Tumor Response Biomarker**

Author	Cancer	Therapy	Parameters/Change with Therapy	Year
Targeted agents				
Thomas et al.[19]	Solid tumors	Endostatin	BF, BV/decrease	2003
Willett et al.[24]	Rectal	Bevacizumab	BF, BV/decrease	2004
Xiong et al.[25]	Solid tumors	SU6668	BF, BV/decrease	2004
McNeel et al.[26]	Solid tumors	MEDI-522	MTT/increase	2005
Faria et al.[27]	Renal	Thalidomide	BF, BV/decrease	2007
Meijerink et al.[28]	Solid tumors	AZD2171/Gefitinib	BF/decrease	2007
Ng et al.[29]	NSCLC	Combretastatin/RT	BV/decrease	2007
Ng et al.[30]	Solid tumors	*N*-nitro-L-arginine	BV/decrease	2007
Koukorakis et al.[31]	Colorectal	Bevacizumab	BF, BV/decrease	2007
Fournier et al.[32]	Renal	Tyrosine kinase inhibitors	BF, BV/decrease	2010
Lind et al.[33]	NSCLC	Sorafenib/Erlotinib	BF/decrease	2010
Schlemmer et al.[34]	GIST	Imatinib/sunitinib	HPI/decrease	2011
Ng et al.[35]	Carcinoid	Bevacizumab/Interferon	BF, BV/decrease	2011
Fraioli et al.[36]	NSCLC	CC + bevacizumab	BF, PS/decrease	2011
Jiang et al.[37]	HCC	Bevacizumab	BF, BV, PS/decrease; MTT/increase	2012
Anzidei et al.[38]	Colorectal	CC + bevacizumab	PS/increase	2012
Frampas et al.[39]	HCC	Sorafenib/sunitinib	BV, BF/no significant change	2013
Tacelli et al.[40]	NSCLC	CC +/– bevacizumab	TVV, TEF/decrease	2013
Sacco et al.[41]	HCC	Sorafenib	MTT/increase	2013
Standard therapy				
Gandhi et al.[42]	Oropharynx	Cisplatin/5FU	BF, BV/decrease	2006
Sahani et al.[43]	Colorectal	Chemoradiation	BF, BV, PS/decrease	2005
Bellomi et al.[44]	Colorectal	Chemoradiation	BF, BV, PS/decrease	2007
Petralia et al.[45]	Head and neck	Cisplatin/5FU	BF, BV/decrease	2009
Wang et al.[46]	NSCLC	Chemoradiation	BF, BV, PS/decrease	2009
Squillaci et al.[47]	Renal	Cryoablation	BF, BV, PS/decrease	2009
Ng et al.[48]	Renal	Interferon	BF/increase	2010
Jahnsen et al.[49]	Colorectal	Chemoradiation	BV, PS/decrease	2010
Curvo-Semedo et al.[50]	Rectal	Chemoradiation	BF/decrease; MTT/increase	2012
Yang et al.[51]	HCC	Chemoembolization	HAP, TLP, HPI/decrease	2012

CC, conventional chemotherapy; BF, blood flow; BV, blood volume; PS, permeability surface area product; MTT, mean transit time; NSCLC, non–small cell lung cancer; HCC, hepatocellular carcinoma; HAP, hepatic arterial perfusion; HPI, hepatic perfusion index; m, metastatic; RT, radiation treatment; TVV, tumor vascular volume; TEF, total tumor extravascular flow; TLP, total liver perfusion.

may be seen depending on the mechanism of action of the drug under investigation and timing of the scan. An initial effect may be a decrease in vascular permeability and reduction in interstitial fluid pressure, with normalization of function of the vasculature resulting in a transient increase in tumor blood flow.[53] In the longer term, with subsequent pruning of the vasculature, a reduction in regional blood flow, blood volume, and vascular permeability may be elicited (Fig. 32-6). With vascular disrupting agents, which target the proliferating immature vasculature +/– the mature vasculature a rapid shutdown in tumor vascularization may occur that is usually transient and reversible within 24 to 48 hours. This may be followed by a rebound revascularization.[54] With radiotherapy, the acute effects are related to an initial inflammatory effect; the permeability is related to microvascular damage, which can lead to tumor shrinkage.[55] With interventional procedures perfusion CT parameters may provide evidence of effective treatment or the need for further procedural attempts for optimal therapeutic effect.[56]

In early-phase clinical trials, these quantitative parameters may provide insight into drug pharmacodynamics.[57] Tumor angiogenesis is an attractive target for anticancer therapy. For drug

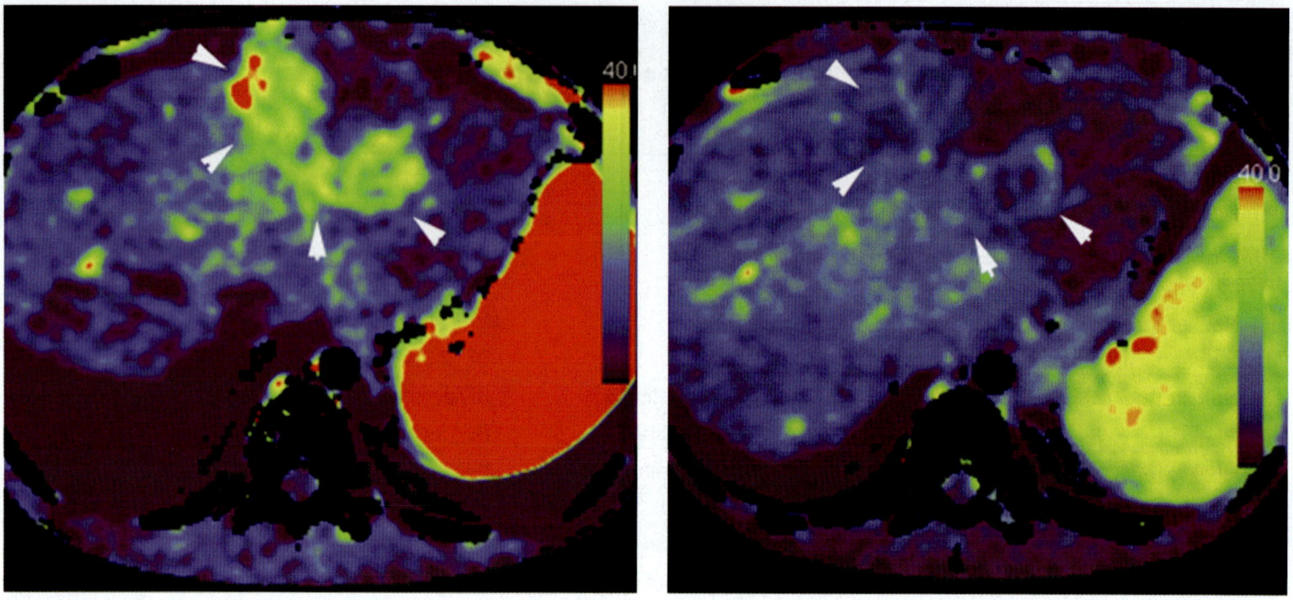

Figure 32-6. Axial image showing a decrease in vascularization measured by arterial liver perfusion before **(A)** and after **(B)** sorafenib, a tyrosine kinase inhibitor, in a hepatocellular carcinoma.

development, results from such trials may inform on "go-no-go" pharma decisions, as well as appropriate dosages to be taken into further stages. In recent years, different therapeutic agents have been developed and licensed including antibodies targeting VEGF (e.g., bevacizumab) and small molecule tyrosine kinase inhibitors (e.g., sunitinib, sorafenib, pazopanib). These agents have been shown to be effective in clinical trials in several cancers including metastatic colorectal cancer,[58] metastatic renal cell cancer,[59,60] and hepatocellular cancer[61] with a modest improvement in objective benefit (progression-free survival or overall survival).

Perfusion CT for Lesion Characterization and Phenotyping

Apart from its role in response assessment, perfusion CT techniques may aid lesion characterization and augment assessment of tumor biology, providing an imaging "phenotype" either as a single modality[9] or when combined with 18F-FDG-PET/-CT,[62–64] where perfusion parameters are combined with metabolic parameters. As mentioned previously, the differences in tumor and normal tissue vascularization are related to the structural and functional differences in tumor and normal vessels, although there may be an overlap in the vascular characteristics of inflammation and cancer. There are exceptions: for example, pancreatic tumors, where lower perfusion is typically observed in first pass studies compared to the normal pancreatic parenchyma.[65–68] A similar reduction in vascularization is also seen in inflammatory pancreatitis[66,69] and chronic pancreatitis,[66,70] but this may be to a lesser extent than tumors.[71]

In the lung both semiquantitative and quantitative measures may improve the characterization of solitary pulmonary nodules. Malignant lesions typically have a higher rate of enhancement and faster washout on the enhancement-time curves compared with benign lesions. Absence of enhancement is a strong predictor of benignity[72]; using a threshold of 15 HU or greater, sensitivity, specificity, and accuracy for malignancy can be 98%, 58%, and 77%, respectively.[72] In terms of quantitative parameters, Zhang et al. found in 65 patients with solitary pulmonary nodules that the mean perfusion value of malignant nodules was significantly higher than in benign nodules (70 vs. 10 mL/min/100 mL, respectively).[73] Similarly, Sitartchouk et al. found that perfusion and blood volume were significantly higher in malignant than benign solitary pulmonary nodules.[74] However, inflammatory nodules also demonstrate elevated perfusion values, reducing specificity.[75] The addition of vascular permeability measurements has the potential to improve differentiation of malignant and inflammatory nodules: Ma et al. found that permeability was significantly higher in cancer compared with inflammatory nodules.[7]

In the context of cirrhosis, perfusion CT has the potential to improve detection and characterization of hepatocellular carcinoma. In a rat model of hepatocellular carcinoma, Fournier et al. demonstrated that perfusion CT allowed for early tumor detection: arterial blood flow was high with a sensitivity and specificity of detection of 86% and 65% within 11 weeks of tumor induction, even though only 7% was visible by eye.[76] Hepatocellular carcinoma typically shows an increase in arterial liver perfusion.[77–79]

In the colon, assessment of regional vascular parameters may help in distinguishing cancer from diverticular disease. Their features may overlap in terms of clinical symptoms and morphologic imaging, and distinction between colon cancers and diverticular disease based on these characteristics can be challenging, particularly as up to 30% of colon cancers are coincident with diverticular disease. Vascular parameters such as regional blood flow, blood volume, and permeability surface area product are highest in cancer: regional blood flow and blood volume had a sensitivity of 80% and specificity of 75% and 70%, respectively, for differentiating cancer from acute diverticulitis, which is better than that achieved using established CT morphologic criteria.[80]

Perfusion CT techniques have also been applied to characterize lymph nodes, where it may potentially provide additional information to size, and aid differentiation between malignant and benign lymph nodes either as a single modality[81] or combined with 18F-FDG-PET/CT.[63,82,83] These have included the assessment of mediastinal lymph nodes in lung cancer,[63] squamous cell cancer of the head and neck,[81] and breast cancer.[84] Metastatic nodes typically demonstrate higher perfusion than benign nodes.

Perfusion CT as a Prognostic and Predictive Biomarker

This remains an exploratory area for perfusion CT but clinically promising, as tumor angiogenesis and tumor hypoxia may be adverse prognostic factors. A few studies have addressed the question whether perfusion CT can provide additional information to current tumor staging strategies. Some correlative studies have assessed whether perfusion CT parameters may reflect tumor type, grade, or stage in a number of cancers including hepatocellular carcinoma,[85] NSCLC,[6,7,86] and colorectal cancer.[87,88] Higher-grade hepatocellular carcinomas have been shown to have higher perfusion measurements than lower grade.[85] In primary colorectal tumors, permeability surface area product is increased in patients with metastatic disease compared with tumors without evidence of metastases at staging.[88] With a correlation between permeability surface area product and MVD,[14] this finding supports the theory that greater angiogenesis in colorectal cancer may be associated with a higher likelihood of metastatic disease.

Perfusion CT parameters have also shown promise in terms of predicting outcome at staging. Regional blood flow, as a marker of overall tumor perfusion and an indirect marker of hypoxia, may be an important prognostic biomarker. A study in primary esophageal cancer treated with chemoradiation found that overall survival was lower in patients with lower baseline blood flow.[89] A rectal cancer study has also produced similar results.[87] This is consistent with our current understanding of tumor evolution, which proposes that tumor hypoxia may be associated with a more aggressive tumor type, with supportive evidence found in other cancers including extracranial head and neck[90] and cervical cancer.[91] In a small study of colorectal cancer patients treated with surgery and followed up until presentation with metastatic disease, baseline regional blood flow was found to be substantially lower in patients who developed subsequent metastases in comparison to patients who remain disease free.[88]

It is hypothesized that a higher regional blood flow ensures better tumor oxygenation and potentially increases radiosensitivity and enables better delivery of the chemotherapeutic agents. Several studies have shown that tumors which have a lower regional blood flow are more likely to be poor responders to chemotherapy and radiotherapy treatment. This was shown to be the case in renal cell carcinoma, where the baseline enhancement blood flow and blood volume were significantly lower in patients who did not respond to treatment.[32,92] This is also the case for head and neck squamous cell carcinoma, where lower regional blood flow values are associated with a higher radiotherapy failure rate.[90,93] Similar results have been shown for antiangiogenic therapy, where higher baseline quantitative parameters are associated with a higher response rate.[37,94] With locoregional procedures, such as laser-induced thermotherapy for lung tumors[95] and radiofrequency ablation or transarterial chemoembolization for liver tumors,[57,96] perfusion CT may predict for technical success immediately after treatment. Hegenscheid et al. have suggested that lung tumors with perfusion measurements which do not change after therapy are likely to have progressive disease.[95]

Summary

In summary, perfusion CT is a robust technique for imaging the functional tumor vasculature. With current state-of-the-art technology, whole-organ regional blood flow, blood volume, and vascular leakage can be investigated: this can encompass more than a single target lesion. In early-phase clinical trials, perfusion CT may provide evidence of an early vascular response prior to size change. In wider clinical practice, perfusion CT may have a role in the assessment of response to locoregional therapy, conventional chemo- and radiotherapy, as well as antiangiogenic agents licensed for clinical use. Perfusion CT may also aid lesion characterization and has shown potential as a prognostic and predictive biomarker. As technologic improvements in CT continue to evolve, clinical applications are likely to further expand.

REFERENCES

1. **Miles KA, Lee TY, Goh V, et al. Experimental Cancer Medicine Centre Imaging Network Group.** Current status and guidelines for the assessment of tumour vascular support with dynamic contrast-enhanced computed tomography. *Eur Radiol* 2012;22:1430–1441.
2. **Folkman J.** The role of angiogenesis in tumour growth. *Semin Cancer Biol* 1992;3:65–71.
3. **Hanahan D, Folkman J.** Patterns and emerging mechanisms of the angiogenic switch during tumourigenesis. *Cell* 1996;86:353–364.
4. **Goh V, Rodriguez-Justo M, Engledow A, et al.** Assessment of the metabolic flow phenotype of primary colorectal cancer: correlations with microvessel density are influenced by the histological scoring method. *Eur Radiol* 2012;22:1687–1692.
5. **Yi CA, Lee KS, Kim EA, et al.** Solitary pulmonary nodules: dynamic enhanced multidetector row CT study and comparison with vascular endothelial growth factor and microvessel density. *Radiology* 2004;233: 191–199.
6. **Li Y, Yang ZG, Chen TW, et al.** Peripheral lung carcinoma: correlation of angiogenesis and first-pass perfusion parameters of 64-detector row CT. *Lung Cancer* 2008;61:44–53.
7. **Ma SH, Le HB, Jia BH, et al.** Peripheral pulmonary nodules: relationship between multi-slice spiral CT perfusion imaging and tumor angiogenesis and VEGF expression. *BMC Cancer* 2008;8:186.
8. **Sauter AW, Winterstein S, Spira D, et al.** Multifunctional profiling of non-small cell lung cancer using 18F-FDG PET/CT and volume perfusion CT. *J Nucl Med* 2012;53:521–529.
9. **Spira D, Neumeister H, Spira SM, et al.** Assessment of tumor vascularity in lung cancer using volume perfusion CT (VPCT) with histopathologic comparison: a further step toward an individualized tumor characterization. *J Comput Assist Tomogr* 2013;37:15–21.
10. **Tateishi U, Kusumoto M, Nishihara H, et al.** Contrast-enhanced dynamic computed tomography for the evaluation of tumor angiogenesis in patients with lung carcinoma. *Cancer* 2002;95:835–842.
11. **Wang JH, Min PQ, Wang PJ, et al.** Dynamic CT evaluation of tumor vascularity in renal cell carcinoma. *AJR Am J Roentgenol* 2006;186:1423–1430.
12. **Reiner CS, Roessle M, Thiesler T, et al.** Computed tomography perfusion imaging of renal cell carcinoma: systematic comparison with histopathological angiogenic and prognostic markers. *Invest Radiol* 2013;48(4):183–191.
13. **Yao J, Yang ZG, Chen HJ, et al.** Gastric adenocarcinoma: can perfusion CT help to noninvasively evaluate tumor angiogenesis? *Abdom Imaging* 2011;36:15–21.
14. **Goh V, Halligan S, Daley F, et al.** Colorectal tumor vascularity: quantitative assessment with multidetector CT—do tumor perfusion measurements reflect angiogenesis? *Radiology* 2008;249:510–517.
15. **Hattori Y, Gabata T, Matsui O, et al.** Enhancement patterns of pancreatic adenocarcinoma on conventional dynamic multi-detector row CT: correlation with angiogenesis and fibrosis. *World J Gastroenterol* 2009;15:3114–3121.
16. **Mandeville HC, Ng QS, Daley FM, et al.** Operable non-small cell lung cancer: correlation of volumetric helical dynamic contrast-enhanced CT parameters with immunohistochemical markers of tumor hypoxia. *Radiology* 2012;264:581–589.
17. **Tacelli N, Remy-Jardin M, Copin MC, et al.** Assessment of non-small cell lung cancer perfusion: pathologic-CT correlation in 15 patients. *Radiology* 2010;257:863–871.
18. **Saddi KA, Chefd'hotel C, Cheriet F.** Large deformation registration of contrast-enhanced images with volume preserving constraint. In: Pluim JPW, Reinhardt JM, eds. *Proceedings of SPIE: Medical Imaging 2007—Image Processing*. Vol. 6512. Bellingham, WA: International Society for Optical Engineering; 2007: 651203.
19. **Thomas JP, Arzoomanian RZ, Alberti D, et al.** Phase I pharmacokinetic and pharmacodynamics study of recombinant human endostatin in patients with advanced solid tumors. *J Clin Oncol* 2003;21:223–231.
20. **Goh V, Dattani M, Farwell J, et al.** Radiation dose from volumetric helical perfusion CT of the thorax, abdomen or pelvis. *Eur Radiol* 2011;21:974–981.
21. **Ng QS, Goh V, Fichte H, et al.** Lung cancer perfusion at multi-detector row CT: reproducibility of whole tumor quantitative measurements. *Radiology* 2006;239:547–553.
22. **Erasmus JJ, Gladish GW, Broemeling L, et al.** Inter- and intraobserver variability in measurement of non-small cell carcinoma lung lesions: implications for assessment of tumor response. *J Clin Oncol* 2003;21:2574–2582.

23. **Goh V, Ng QS, Miles KA.** Computed tomography perfusion imaging for therapeutic assessment: has it come of age as a biomarker in oncology? *Invest Radiol* 2012;47:2–4.
24. **Willett CG, Boucher Y, di Tomaso E, et al.** Direct evidence that the VEGF-specific antibody bevacizumab has antivascular effects in human rectal cancer. *Nat Med* 2004;10:145–147.
25. **Xiong HQ, Herbst R, Faria SC, et al.** A phase I surrogate endpoint study of SU6668 in patients with solid tumours. *Invest New Drugs* 2004;22:459–466.
26. **McNeel DG, Eickhoff J, Lee FT, et al.** Phase I trial of a monoclonal antibody specific for integrin (MEDI-522) in patients with advanced malignancies, including an assessment of tumour perfusion. *Clin Cancer Res* 2005;11:7851–7860.
27. **Faria SC, Ng CS, Hess KR, et al.** CT quantification of effects of thalidomide in patients with metastatic renal cell carcinoma. *Am J Roentgenol* 2007;189:378–385.
28. **Meijerink MR, van Cruijsen H, Hoekman K, et al.** The use of perfusion CT for the evaluation of therapy combining AZD2171 with gefitinib in cancer patients. *Eur Radiol* 2007;17:1700–1713.
29. **Ng QS, Goh V, Carnell D, et al.** Tumor antivascular effects of radiotherapy combined with combretastatin a4 phosphate in human non-small-cell lung cancer. *Int J Radiat Oncol Biol Phys* 2007;67:1375–1380.
30. **Ng QS, Goh V, Carnell D, et al.** Effect of nitric-oxide synthesis on tumour blood volume and vascular activity: a phase I study. *Lancet Oncol* 2007;8:111–118.
31. **Koukourakis MI, Mavanis I, Kouklakis G, et al.** Early antivascular effects of bevacizumab anti-VEGF monoclonal antibody on colorectal carcinomas assessed with functional CT imaging. *Am J Clin Oncol* 2007;30:315–318.
32. **Fournier LS, Oudard S, Thiam R, et al.** Metastatic renal carcinoma: evaluation of anti-angiogenic therapy with dynamic contrast enhanced CT. *Radiology* 2010;256:511–518.
33. **Lind JS, Meijerink MR, Dingemans AM, et al.** Dynamic contrast enhanced CT in patients treated with sorafenib and erlotinib for non-small-cell lung cancer: a new method for monitoring treatment? *Eur Radiol* 2010;20:2890–2898.
34. **Schlemmer M, Sourbron SP, Schinwald N, et al.** Perfusion patterns of metastatic gastrointestinal stromal tumor lesions under specific molecular therapy. *Eur J Radiol* 2011;77:312–318.
35. **Ng CS, Charnsangavej C, Wei W, et al.** Perfusion CT findings in patients with metastatic carcinoid tumors undergoing bevacizumab and interferon therapy. *Am J Roentgenol* 2011;196:569–576.
36. **Fraioli F, Anzidei M, Zaccagna F, et al.** Whole-tumor perfusion CT in patients with advanced lung adenocarcinoma treated with conventional and antiangiogenetic chemotherapy: initial experience. *Radiology* 2011; 259:574–582.
37. **Jiang T, Kambadakone A, Kulkarni NM, et al.** Monitoring response to antiangiogenic treatment and predicting outcomes in advanced hepatocellular carcinoma using image biomarkers, CT perfusion, tumor density, and tumor size (RECIST). *Invest Radiol* 2012;47:11–17.
38. **Anzidei M, Napoli A, Zaccagna F, et al.** Liver metastases from colorectal cancer treated with conventional and antiangiogenetic chemotherapy: evaluation with liver computed tomography perfusion and magnetic resonance diffusion-weighted imaging. *J Comput Assist Tomogr* 2012;35:690–696.
39. **Frampas E, Lassau N, Zappa M, et al.** Advanced hepatocellular carcinoma: early evaluation of response to targeted therapy and prognostic value of perfusion CT and dynamic contrast enhanced-ultrasound. Preliminary results. *Eur J Radiol* 2013;82:e205–e211.
40. **Tacelli N, Santangelo T, Scherpereel A.** Perfusion CT allows prediction of therapy response in non-small cell lung cancer treated with conventional and anti-angiogenic chemotherapy. *Eur Radiol* 2013;23:2127–2136.
41. **Sacco R, Faggioni L, Bargellini I, et al.** Assessment of response to sorafenib in advanced hepatocellular carcinoma using perfusion computed tomography: results of a pilot study. *Dig Liver Dis* 2013;45:776–781.
42. **Gandhi D, Chepeha DB, Miller T, et al.** Correlation between initial and early follow-up CT perfusion parameters with endoscopic tumor response in patients with advanced squamous cell carcinomas of the oropharynx treated with organ-preservation therapy. *Am J Neuroradiol* 2006;27:101–106.
43. **Sahani DV, Kalva SP, Hamberg LM, et al.** Assessing tumor perfusion and treatment response in rectal cancer with multisection CT: initial observations. *Radiology* 2005;234:785–792.
44. **Bellomi M, Petralia G, Sonzogni A, et al.** CT perfusion for the monitoring of neo-adjuvant chemoradiation therapy in rectal carcinoma. *Radiology* 2007;244:486–493.
45. **Petralia G, Preda L, Giugliano G, et al.** Perfusion computed tomography for monitoring induction chemotherapy in patients with squamous cell carcinoma of the upper aerodigestive tract: correlation between changes in tumor perfusion and tumor volume. *J Comput Assist Tomogr* 2009;33:552–559.
46. **Wang J, Wu N Cham MD, et al.** Tumor response in patients with advanced non-small-cell lung cancer: perfusion CT evaluation of chemotherapy and radiation therapy. *Am J Roentgenol* 2009;193:1090–1096.
47. **Squillaci E, Manenti G, Ciccio C, et al.** Perfusion CT monitoring of cryoablated renal cell tumors. *J Exp Clin Cancer Res* 2009;28:138.
48. **Ng CS, Wang X, Faria SC, et al.** Perfusion CT in patients with metastatic renal cell carcinoma treated with interferon. *Am J Roentgenol* 2009;194:166–171.
49. **Jahnsen MH, Aerts HJ, Kierkels RG, et al.** Tumor perfusion increases during hypofractionated short course radiotherapy in rectal cancer: sequential perfusion CT findings. *Radiother Oncol* 2010;94:156–160.
50. **Curvo-Semedo L, Portilha MA, Ruivo C, et al.** Usefulness of perfusion CT to assess response to neoadjuvant combined chemoradiotherapy in patients with locally advanced rectal cancer. *Acad Radiol* 2012;19:203–213.
51. **Yang L, Zhang XM, Tan BX, et al.** Computed tomographic perfusion imaging for the therapeutic response of chemoembolization for hepatocellular carcinoma. *J Comput Assist Tomogr* 2012;36:226–230.
52. **Lissoni P, Fugamalli E, Malugani F, et al.** Chemotherapy and angiogenesis in advanced cancer: vascular endothelial growth factor (VEGF) decline as predictor of disease control during taxol therapy in metastatic breast cancer. *Int J Biol Markers* 2000;15:308–311.
53. **Jain RK.** Normalization of tumor vasculature: an emerging concept in antiangiogenic therapy. *Science* 2005;307:58–62.
54. **Hinnen P, Eskens FA.** Vascular disrupting agents in clinical development. *Br J Cancer* 2007;96:1159–1165.
55. **Garcia-Barros M, Paris F, Cordon-Cardo C, et al.** Tumour response to radiotherapy regulated by endothelial cell apoptosis. *Science* 2003;300: 1155–1159.
56. **Chen G, Ma DQ, He W, et al.** Computed tomography perfusion in the evaluating the therapeutic effect of transarterial chemoembolization for hepatocellular carcinoma. *World J Gastroenterol* 2008;14:5738–5743.
57. **Parulekar WR, Eisenhauer EA.** Phase I trial design for solid tumour studies of targeted non-cytotoxic agents: theory and practice. *J Natl Cancer Inst* 2004;96:990–997.
58. **Hurwitz H, Fehrenbacher L, Novotny W, et al.** Bevacizumab plus irinotecan, fluorouracil, and leucovorin for metastatic colorectal cancer. *N Engl J Med* 2004;350:2335–2342.
59. **Escudier B, Eisen T, Stadler WM, et al.** Sorafenib in advanced clear-cell renal-cell carcinoma. *N Engl J Med* 2007;356:125–134.
60. **Motzer RJ, Hutson TE, Tomczak P, et al.** Sunitinib versus interferon alfa in metastatic renal-cell carcinoma. *N Engl J Med* 2007;356:115–124.
61. **Llovet JM, Ricci S, Mazzaferro V, et al.** Sorafenib in advanced hepatocellular carcinoma. *N Engl J Med* 2008;359:378–390.
62. **Goh V, Engledow A, Rodriguez-Justo M, et al.** The flow-metabolic phenotype of primary colorectal cancer: assessment by integrated 18F-FDG PET/perfusion CT with histopathologic correlation. *J Nucl Med* 2012;53:687–692.
63. **Sauter AW, Spira D, Schulze M, et al.** Correlation between [(18)F]FDG PET/CT and volume perfusion CT in primary tumours and mediastinal lymph nodes of non-small-cell lung cancer. *Eur J Nucl Med Mol Imaging* 2013;40(5):677–684.
64. **Ippolito D, Capraro C, Guerra L, et al.** Feasibility of perfusion CT technique integrated into conventional (18)FDG/PET-CT studies in lung cancer patients: clinical staging and functional information in a single study. *Eur J Nucl Med Mol Imaging* 2013;40:156–165.
65. **Kandel S, Kloeters C, Meyer H, et al.** Whole-organ perfusion of the pancreas using dynamic volume CT in patients with primary pancreas carcinoma: acquisition technique, post-processing and initial results. *Eur Radiol* 2009;19:2641–2646.
66. **Delrue L, Blanckaert P, Mertens D, et al.** Tissue perfusion in pathologies of the pancreas: assessment using 128-slice computed tomography. *Abdom Imaging* 2011;37:595–601.
67. **Delrue L, Blanckaert P, Mertens D, et al.** Assessment of tumor vascularization in pancreatic adenocarcinoma using 128-slice perfusion computed tomography imaging. *J Comput Assist Tomogr* 2011;35:434–438.

68. **Klauss M, Stiller W, Fritz F, et al.** Computed tomography perfusion analysis of pancreatic carcinoma. *J Comput Assist Tomogr* 2012; 36:237–242.
69. **Tsuji Y, Hamaguchi K, Watanabe Y, et al.** Perfusion CT is superior to angiography in predicting pancreatic necrosis in patients with severe acute pancreatitis. *J Gastroenterol* 2010;45:1155–1162.
70. **Arikawa S, Uchida M, Kunou Y, et al.** Assessment of chronic pancreatitis: use of whole pancreas perfusion with 256-slice computed tomography. *Pancreas* 2012;41(4):535–540.
71. **Lu N, Feng XY, Hao SJ, et al.** 64-slice CT perfusion imaging of pancreatic adenocarcinoma and mass-forming chronic pancreatitis. *Acad Radiol* 2011;18:81–88.
72. **Swensen SJ, Viggiano RW, Midthun DE, et al.** Lung nodule enhancement at CT: multicenter study. *Radiology* 2000;214:73–80.
73. **Zhang M, Kono M.** Solitary pulmonary nodules: evaluation of blood flow patterns with dynamic CT. *Radiology* 1997;205:471–478.
74. **Sitartchouk I, Roberts HC, Pereira AM, et al.** Computed tomography perfusion using first pass methods for lung nodule characterization. *Invest Radiol* 2008;43:349–358.
75. **Ohno Y, Koyama H, Matsumoto K, et al.** Differentiation of malignant and benign pulmonary nodules with quantitative first-pass 320-detector row perfusion CT versus FDG PET/CT. *Radiology* 2011;258: 599–609.
76. **Fournier LS, Cuenod CA, de Bazelaire C, et al.** Early modifications of hepatic perfusion measured by functional CT in a rat model of hepatocellular carcinoma using a blood pool contrast agent. *Eur Radiol* 2004;14:2125–2133.
77. **Ippolito D, Sironi S, Pozzi M, et al.** Perfusion computed tomographic assessment of early hepatocellular carcinoma in cirrhotic liver disease: initial observations. *J Comput Assist Tomogr* 2008;32:855–858.
78. **Ippolito D, Sironi S, Pozzi M, et al.** Perfusion CT in cirrhotic patients with early stage hepatocellular carcinoma: assessment of tumor-related vascularization. *Eur J Radiol* 2010;73:148–152.
79. **Ippolito D, Capraro C, Casiraghi A, et al.** Quantitative assessment of tumour associated neovascularisation in patients with liver cirrhosis and hepatocellular carcinoma: role of dynamic-CT perfusion imaging. *Eur Radiol* 2012;22:803–811.
80. **Goh V, Halligan S, Taylor SA, et al.** Differentiation between diverticulitis and colorectal cancer: quantitative CT perfusion measurements versus morphologic criteria—initial experience. *Radiology* 2007;242: 456–462.
81. **Trojanowska A, Trojanowski P, Bisdas S, et al.** Squamous cell cancer of hypopharynx and larynx—evaluation of metastatic nodal disease based on computed tomography perfusion studies. *Eur J Radiol* 2012;81:1034–1039.
82. **Veit-Haibach P, Schmid D, Strobel K, et al.** Combined PET/CT-perfusion in patients with head and neck cancers. *Eur Radiol* 2013; 23:163–173
83. **Bisdas S, Spicer K, Rumboldt Z.** Whole-tumor perfusion CT parameters and glucose metabolism measurements in head and neck squamous cell carcinomas: a pilot study using combined positron-emission tomography/CT imaging. *AJNR Am J Neuroradiol* 2008;29:1376–1381.
84. **Liu Y, Bellomi M, Gatti G, et al.** Accuracy of computed tomography perfusion in assessing metastatic involvement of enlarged axillary lymph nodes in patients with breast cancer. *Breast Cancer Res* 2007;9:R40.
85. **Sahani DV, Holalkere NS, Mueller PR, et al.** Advanced hepatocellular carcinoma: CT perfusion of liver and tumor tissue—initial experience. *Radiology* 2007;243:736–743.
86. **Tateishi U, Nishihara H, Tsukamoto E, et al.** Lung tumors evaluated with FDG-PET and dynamic CT: the relationship between vascular density and glucose metabolism. *J Comput Assist Tomogr* 2002;26:185–190.
87. **Hayano K, Shuto K, Koda K, et al.** Quantitative measurement of blood flow using perfusion CT for assessing clinicopathological features and prognosis in patients with rectal cancer. *Dis Colon Rectum* 2009;52:1624–1629.
88. **Goh V, Halligan S, Wellsted DM, et al.** Can perfusion CT assessment of primary colorectal adenocarcinoma blood flow at staging predict for subsequent metastatic disease? A pilot study. *Eur Radiol* 2009;19:79–89.
89. **Hayano K, Okazumi S, Shuto K, et al.** Perfusion CT can predict response to chemoradiation therapy and survival in oesophageal squamous cell carcinoma: initial results. *Oncol Rep* 2007;18:901–908.
90. **Hermans R, Meijerink M, Van den Bogaert W, et al.** Tumor perfusion rate determined non-invasively by dynamic computed tomography predicts outcome in head-and-neck cancer after radiotherapy. *Int J Radiat Oncol Biol Phys* 2003;57:1351–1356.
91. **Haider MA, Milosevic M, Fyles A, et al.** Assessment of the tumor microenvironment in cervix cancer using dynamic contrast enhanced CT, interstitial fluid pressure and oxygen measurements. *Int J Radiat Oncol Biol Phys* 2005;62:1100–1107.
92. **Han KS, Jung DC, Choi HJ, et al.** Pretreatment assessment of tumor enhancement on contrast-enhanced computed tomography as a potential predictor of treatment outcome in metastatic renal cell carcinoma patients receiving antiangiogenic therapy. *Cancer* 2010;116:2332–2342.
93. **Bisdas S, Rumboldt Z, Wagenblast J, et al.** Response and progression-free survival in oropharynx squamous cell carcinoma assessed by pretreatment perfusion CT: comparison with tumor volume measurements. *AJNR Am J Neuroradiol* 2009;30:793–799.
94. **Wang J, Wu N, Cham MD, et al.** Tumor response in patients with advanced non-small cell lung cancer: perfusion CT evaluation of chemotherapy and radiation therapy. *AJR Am J Roentgenol* 2009;193:1090–1096.
95. **Hegenscheid K, Behrendt N, Rosenberg C, et al.** Assessing early vascular changes and treatment response after laser-induced thermotherapy of pulmonary metastases with perfusion CT: initial experience. *AJR Am J Roentgenol* 2010;194:1116–1123.
96. **Ippolito D, Bonaffini PA, Ratti L, et al.** Hepatocellular carcinoma treated with transarterial chemoembolization: dynamic perfusion-CT in the assessment of residual tumor. *World J Gastroenterol* 2010;16:5993–6000.

CHAPTER

33 Musculoskeletal Perfusion Imaging

George R. Matcuk Jr, MD

Introduction

Musculoskeletal disorders contribute greatly to health care system costs because of their high prevalence and impact on disability, with arthritis and back pain alone affecting over 100 million individuals and costing more than $200 billion per year.[1] New advances in minimally invasive surgical techniques, image-guided interventions, and other therapeutic options have spurred interest in new methods of noninvasive imaging methods capable of diagnosing disease at its earliest stages. Although they have yet to be implemented in routine clinical practice, perfusion imaging techniques have been investigated and show promise for musculoskeletal applications, including for the evaluation of normal versus abnormal bone marrow and muscle; assessment of avascular necrosis, synovitis, and chondrosis; and evaluation of musculoskeletal tumors, including recurrence and therapy response.

Techniques

Dynamic contrast-enhanced (DCE) techniques can be applied to the musculoskeletal system using magnetic resonance (MR), computed tomography (CT), or ultrasound (US) in a similar manner to other areas of the body, allowing assessment of perfusion and vascularity, which will only be briefly reviewed here.

MR perfusion imaging after the intravenous administration of gadolinium-based contrast agents is the most commonly used technique and is made possible by the development of ultrafast T1-weighted gradient echo–based pulse sequences with fat saturation, such as the fast low angle shot (FLASH) sequence.[2–5] MR has the advantage of high contrast resolution and can be done at the time of routine clinical imaging, where MR is the gold standard for imaging of most musculoskeletal disorders. An MR angiography sequence with sparse k-space sampling has been successfully implemented as a DCE-MRI technique, which eases adding this technique as part of a routine clinical MRI tumor protocol.[6]

Dynamic CT following the intravenous administration of iodinated contrast agents can likewise be used for musculoskeletal perfusion imaging, with the potential for higher resolution imaging and easier assessment of greater three-dimensional volumes of tissue, but at the cost of radiation dose to the patient.[7] Dynamic CT may be the modality of choice for musculoskeletal perfusion imaging when the lesion is small and involves cortical bone, susceptibility artifacts limit MR, or contraindications to MR, such as a pacemaker exists.

Contrast-enhanced ultrasound (CEUS) utilizing microbubble contrast agents can also be used to assess perfusion, offering real-time dynamic imaging, which can be useful for visualizing very early or late enhancement patterns that may be missed with CT or MR and the additional ability to perform multiple repeat injections and observations as part of a single examination without radiation and contrast-related nephrotoxicity. However, the microbubble fragility and Doppler-related artifacts have limited their clinical usage. Additionally, the inability of ultrasound to penetrate bone limits the musculoskeletal applications.[8]

For superficial structures such as the hand and wrist, optical perfusion imaging techniques are also possible following intravenous administration of fluorescent compounds such as indocyanine green (ICG).[9]

Data obtained from these DCE techniques regardless of modality used can be analyzed using both qualitative and quantitative methods. Regions of interest (ROI) chosen within a lesion can be compared to ROIs of normal structures such as uninvolved muscle or bone marrow. Visual analysis of shapes or patterns of time–intensity curves (TIC) can be used to qualitatively characterize perfusion as one of seven described types (Fig. 33-1).[10] Further assessment of the TIC can include measurements of the maximum enhancement (ME), rate of early enhancement (REE), area under the curve (AUC), time to peak (TTP) enhancement, and initial slope of increase, although these values are sensitive to variations between acquisition protocols and sequence parameters. Quantitative parameters of vascular permeability (k_{trans}) can also be extracted from these data.

Bone Marrow

Characterization of bone marrow using perfusion imaging techniques is one of the most common musculoskeletal applications and is an area of active investigation and the subject of numerous recent publications.[11]

Normal Marrow and Osteoporosis

Hematopoietic (red) marrow is more vascular than fatty (yellow) marrow, and therefore, younger patients (with a high percentage of red marrow within their vertebra) demonstrate greater perfusion than older patients.[12–14] Women demonstrate a higher marrow perfusion rate than men younger than 50 years, but then show

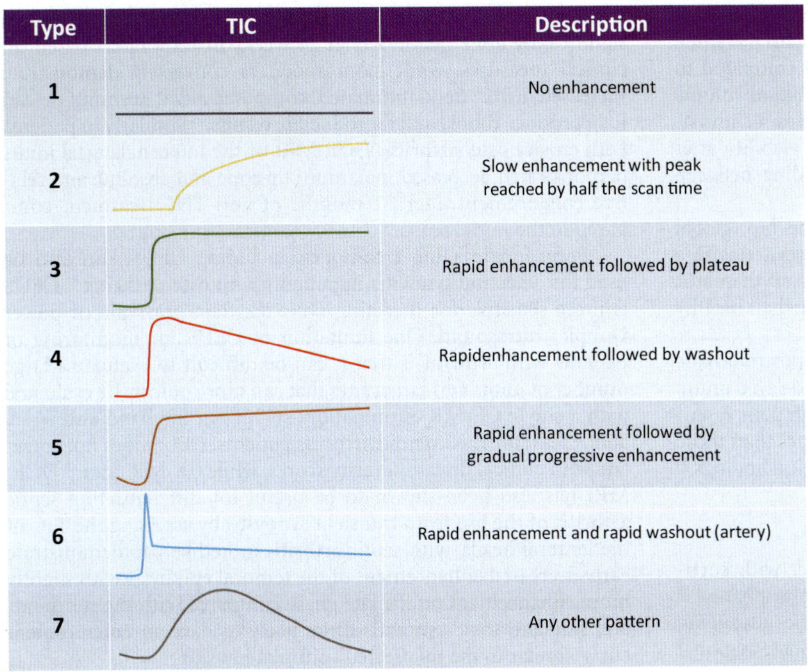

Figure 33-1. DCE perfusion imaging time–intensity curve patterns.

a more marked decrease than men older than 50 years.[12] These differences related to age and gender are likely related to associated decreases in bone mineral density and increased fat fraction, with osteopenic bone demonstrating decreased marrow perfusion relative to bone with normal density and further reduction in mean enhancement slope of osteoporotic bone on DCE-MR.[15–18] There are also small but significant differences in marrow perfusion between vertebral levels, with decreased perfusion from upper to lower lumbar levels, possibly related to increased stresses on lower levels.[19] Hypertension may also influence marrow perfusion, with decreased femoral head and proximal shaft perfusion demonstrated in hypertensive compared to normotensive rats.[20] However, differences in perfusion parameters in bone marrow based on age and fat fraction are small, there is wide variation between individuals, and they are unlikely to confound changes related to malignancy or treatment.[21]

Vertebral Compression Fractures

For acute osteoporotic vertebral compression fractures, perfusion parameters including plasma flow (PF), plasma volume (PV), extraction flow (EF), and mean transit time (MTT) are increased relative to healthy vertebral bone marrow.[17,22] The increased perfusion in fractures is thought to be related to reparative neovascularization.[17] Perfusion levels of normal vertebra are not significantly changed in patients with compression fractures at other levels.[12]

Extensive research efforts have centered on using imaging to differentiate benign (osteoporotic) versus malignant vertebral compression fractures.[23–34] Signal intensities and morphologic features on routine MR pulse sequences alone do not offer a high degree of specificity in differentiating between these entities. Contrast-enhancement and diffusion-weighted imaging (DWI) increase sensitivity and specificity, with positive and negative predictive values (NPVs) of 90%.[28] MR perfusion imaging techniques have also shown promise as an additional tool, with spots of high plasma flow demonstrating higher interstitial volume, extracellular volume, and extraction flow in osteoporotic fractures compared to malignant fractures, with a specificity of 92%; however there were no significant differences in perfusion parameters in regions of increased MTT.[35]

Myeloproliferative Disorders and Malignancy

Perfusion imaging techniques can also be used to help differentiate normal marrow from marrow involvement by diffuse bone marrow disease, which can sometimes be difficult on anatomic imaging in young patients or adults with red marrow reconversion or in cases of early dissemination. Analysis of time–intensity curves in patients with aplastic anemia showed a lower peak value with slower washout compared to normal marrow.[36] Myeloproliferative disorders including essential thrombocytopenia and polycythemia vera may demonstrate no significant differences in perfusion parameters compared to normal patients, although patients with myelofibrosis do demonstrate increased marrow perfusion.[36,37]

In hematologic malignancies, multiple myeloma, lymphoma, and metastatic disease, TIC analysis demonstrated earlier and steeper enhancement with faster wash-out of abnormal compared to normal marrow, even in areas where differences were not apparent on conventional MR images, probably related to neoangiogenesis.[38–40] For patients with treated hematologic malignancies, the peak enhancement ratio has been shown to be significantly lower in patients in remission compared to those with recurrence.[39] In patients with acute myelogenous leukemia (AML) in remission, perfusion parameters may help predict relapse-free and overall survival.[41] Likewise, decreased perfusion parameters can indicate a treatment response for multiple myeloma and bone marrow metastases.[42–47]

Osteonecrosis

Interest in early detection of acute avascular necrosis (AVN) was one of the first musculoskeletal applications of MR perfusion imaging, with lack of enhancement of avascular marrow demonstrated in a dog model before morphologic changes could be identified on routine MR sequences.[48] Steroids have been implicated as one of the causative agents of osteonecrosis, and decreased femoral perfusion parameters after intravenous administration of a single dose of methylprednisolone in a rabbit model were demonstrated in 56% at 5 days and 83% at 14 days.[49]

In a study of patients with avascular necrosis of the femoral head, there was an increase in peak enhancement of the femoral head with progressive osteonecrosis on DCE-MRI, although there was a delayed time-to-peak enhancement in patients with increased intramedullary pressure but normal MRI (grade 0) compared to controls.[50] These findings are likely due to increased blood volume and reactive bone marrow edema with resultant stasis. Contrast-enhanced MRI may also help predict femoral head viability after femoral neck fracture, aiding the clinician in deciding between joint-preserving therapy versus arthroplasty.[51]

In patients with developmental dysplasia of the hip, global decreased enhancement after closed reduction is associated with a higher risk of AVN.[52] In patients with systemic lupus erythematosus without AVN, femoral head perfusion was higher than healthy controls.[53]

Perfusion imaging can also be useful for assessing posttraumatic avascular necrosis. In a study of patients with scaphoid delayed union or nonunion, DCE-MRI of the proximal fragments with poor vascularity demonstrated lower peak enhancement and slopes than those with good vascularity, with strong correlation with surgical findings.[54]

Paget Disease

Paget disease of bone is a disorder of bone turnover with cortical and trabecular thickening and elevated alkaline phosphatase.[55] Pagetoid bone is hypervascular, especially along the advancing peripheral zone, and DCE-MRI can be used to evaluate regional microcirculation.[56] MR perfusion imaging has also shown significant reduction in regional bone perfusion in Paget disease following bisphosphonate therapy.[57]

Stress Reaction and Bone Marrow Edema

DCE-MRI has been used to assess stress reactions of the pelvis and lower extremities. Higher slope and maximum enhancement values of the time–intensity curves were demonstrated when MRI revealed a fracture line, callus, or adjacent muscle edema, although there was no significant correlation for periosteal or marrow changes alone.[58] Perfusion abnormalities have also been demonstrated in subchondral bone associated with bone marrow edema, with a decreased eliminate rate constant (k_{el}) reflecting a longer residence time of the contrast medium within the interstitial compartment.[59] These subchondral perfusion changes have been shown to temporally precede eventual bone and cartilage lesions of osteoarthritis in an experimental guinea pig model. In another study, significant increases in the relative rate of enhancement (RER) in areas of bone marrow edema on DCE-MRI in rheumatoid arthritis patients relative to uninvolved bone and reductions in RER after antitumor necrosis factor (TNF) alpha therapy preceded changes in conventional Rheumatoid Arthritis MRI Scoring (RAMRIS).[60]

Synovitis

With the development of new disease-modifying antirheumatic drugs (DMARDs), there has been increased interest in being able to diagnosis and follow active synovitis associated with inflammatory arthritides prior to the development of radiographic changes, such as joint space narrowing and erosive changes. Although ultrasound and routine contrast-enhanced MRI can demonstrate synovitis and early erosive changes, perfusion imaging techniques offer additional quantitative information and may better assess early treatment response.[61–63] MR synovial perfusion parameters have been shown to be able to accurately differentiate clinically active from inactive disease in juvenile idiopathic arthritis (JIA) patients, with clinically active patients more often demonstrating a type 4 (fast enhancement followed by a wash-out phase) TIC pattern.[64] Quantitative analysis of optical or MR perfusion imaging of synovitis in patient with inflammatory arthritis has shown that the REE decreases significantly after treatments at 24 weeks in responders based on clinical measures, while nonresponders conversely demonstrate increased REE.[9] Semiautomated computer-aided techniques can help produce robust and reproducible results.[65] Similarly in patients with erosive osteoarthritis, DCE-MRI of the interphalangeal joints demonstrated decreased maximum upslope and absolute and relative enhancement after 12 months of anti-TNF treatment compared to the initial scans.[66]

Perfusion imaging techniques, including CEUS, can also be used for detecting synovitis in patients with osteoarthritis.[67] CEUS is more sensitive for detecting synovitis than grayscale or power Doppler ultrasound. One limitation of CEUS for monitoring of patients with arthritis is that it can be difficult to evaluate a large number of joints and target sites that can more quickly be evaluated with a single CE-MR examination, such as in the hand and wrist, and at least for rheumatoid arthritis patients, CEUS does not correlate with clinical disease severity scores, while CE-MR does.[68] DCE-MRI has also been shown to be useful for differentiating septic arthritis of the hip from transient synovitis by assessing the TIC of the femoral heads, with septic arthritis more likely to demonstrate early decreased enhancement of the femoral epiphysis with slightly more enhancement on the late phase compared with the contralateral side and toxic synovitis more likely to have an enhancement curve similar to the unaffected contralateral side.[69]

Muscle and Tendon

Perfusion imaging techniques can be applied to assess skeletal muscle pathology. DCE-MRI has shown that there are decreased enhancement values in sarcopenic rats related to aging, despite the fact that there is no significant difference in T2 relaxation.[70] Assessment of skeletal muscle microcirculation has also been performed using dynamic CEUS, with evaluation before, during, and after tourniquet arterial occlusion of the thigh demonstrating decreased arterial perfusion reserve in patient with peripheral artery disease and type 2 diabetes mellitus.[71,72] The same technique can be used to demonstrate improved muscular perfusion after peripheral arterial disease treatment (angioplasty and/or thromboendarterectomy).[73] CEUS has also been used to demonstrate increased first-pass blood flow in denervated muscle in a rabbit model.[74] DCE-MRI has been used in a rat model to evaluate muscle ischemia–reperfusion injury, demonstrating a heterogeneous postischemic profile with areas of both increased enhancement (14% to 76%) and other areas with no reflow (5% to 77%), indicating that muscle reperfusion after prolonged ischemia (4 hours) may be incomplete.[75]

Although any tendon can potentially be evaluated using dynamic perfusion techniques, most research has focused on the rotator cuff, particularly with CEUS. Evaluation of the supraspinatus tendon in asymptomatic volunteers demonstrated significantly lower peak enhancement within the articular medial margin compared to the bursal or lateral margins.[76] There is also a significant decrease in regional supraspinatus blood flow in patients younger than 40 compared to those older than 40 and significant increase in blood flow with exercise in all patients.[77] CEUS may be useful for the evaluation of vascularity following rotator cuff repair. Although the repaired tendon is relatively avascular at short- to intermediate-term follow-up, there is relative increased blood flow in the peribursal region and bone anchor site.[78,79]

Tumors

One of the first and primary uses of perfusion imaging has been for the evaluation of tumors and treatment response. DCE imaging techniques have also been applied extensively to the evaluation of musculoskeletal lesions.

Benign Versus Malignant

DCE-MRI has been used to attempt to differentiate benign from malignant bone and soft tissue masses. For osseous lesions, perfusion parameters cannot accurately differentiate benign from malignant lesions; however, there is better promise for differentiating benign from malignant soft tissue tumors.[80] A start of enhancement within 6 seconds, peripheral pattern of enhancement, and arterial type of enhancement pattern (early onset with rapidly progressive enhancement) are all features more often associated with malignancy, with the start of enhancement demonstrating the highest sensitivity (91%) and the pattern of enhancement demonstrating the highest specificity (97%). However, malignant tumors do not always demonstrate all three of these features, and benign tumors may occasionally demonstrate one or more of these features. For example, synovial sarcoma will often only consistently demonstrate an early start of enhancement but can often have other TIC patterns and diffuse enhancement.[81] Conversely, benign schwannomas and aggressive fibromatosis may demonstrate early enhancement.[80] In another study evaluating DCE-MRI of soft tissue tumors, combining enhancement within the first minute, E(max/1), within the second minute, E(max/2), and the steepest slope of enhancement, overall accuracy for differentiating benign from malignant lesions was 95.5%.[82]

Certain histologic subtypes of bone tumors do demonstrate characteristic TIC patterns. Malignant bone tumors typically demonstrate very early and high wash-in with fast wash-out; giant cell tumor has fast and high wash-in with fast wash-out but then a plateau trend; inflammatory-like lesions (osteoid osteoma, Brodie abscess, eosinophilic granuloma) have moderate wash-in, plateau, then moderate wash-out; benign cartilaginous lesions show slow (venous) wash-in and a plateau trend.[83] Placing multiple separate ROI within the same bone tumor can allow determination of variance of the mean slope values, demonstrating the heterogeneity of vascularity, with malignant tumors demonstrating more variability than benign tumors.[84] This technique could also potentially be used for biopsy planning purposes to target the most vascular/viable portion of the lesion and is even feasible under MR guidance.[85]

CEUS has also been used to characterize soft tissue masses. Four perfusion patterns have been described: P1 = nonenhancing or only rim enhancement of a pseudocapsule; P2 = peripherally enhancing with central nonenhancement; P3 = diffusely enhancing with scattered nonenhancing areas; and P4 = completely, homogeneously enhancing mass.[86] Malignant lesions demonstrate a P2 or P3 enhancement pattern with a 100% sensitivity, but only a 70% specificity. Combining lesion localization (deep to the superficial fascia), size (>3.3 cm), and perfusion pattern (P2 or P3) yielded a sensitivity of 89%, specificity of 85%, PPV of 86%, and NPV of 88% for malignancy. However, quantitative CEUS data did not prove reliable for differentiating benign from malignant soft tissue masses due to substantial overlap. CEUS also may be useful for targeting and increasing yields on ultrasound-guided biopsy of musculoskeletal tumors.[87]

CT perfusion has been used for the evaluation of suspected osteoid osteoma. All osteoid osteomas have early enhancement with a delay between nidus and arterial peak below 30 seconds.[88] Most (80%) of the other benign and malignant osteoid osteoma mimickers demonstrated slow and progressive enhancement (Fig. 33-2), but nearly half of the remainder demonstrated perfusion patterns similar to osteoid osteomas.

Treatment Response

One of the advantages of perfusion imaging is that it provides additional qualitative and quantitative parameters to assess response to neoadjuvant radiation or chemotherapy that may be inapparent on conventional anatomic imaging. In particular, most sarcomas often do not demonstrate significant decreases in tumor size in response to treatment, making evaluation of treatment response by World Health Organization (WHO) or Response Evaluation Criteria in Solid Tumors (RECIST) criteria less effective.[89] The Choi response criteria, which were developed for evaluating treatment response in gastrointestinal stromal tumors, take into account decrease in attenuation on CT and have less dependence on decrease in tumor size and have also been applied to evaluation of sarcomas, applying decreased enhancement on MRI as a surrogate for decreased attenuation on CT.[90] However, early after treatment, sarcomas may sometimes show no decrease in size or may even have a mild increase in size due to intratumoral hemorrhage or necrosis, even when there is a clinical and histopathologic response to treatment. Perfusion imaging techniques are likely to become more important for evaluating tumor response, as many new target cancer therapies are cytostatic rather than cytotoxic, meaning a good tumor response may be associated with predominantly a decrease in perfusion or metabolism without a major reduction in tumor size.[89]

DCE-MRI has been used to demonstrate chemotherapy response in soft tissue sarcomas. In one early study, volume measurements correctly predicted tumor response in 6 of 10 patients, but DCE-MRI correctly predicted response in 8 of 10 patients, with early and rapid progressive enhancement correlated histologically with viable tumor and late and gradual or no enhancement associated with necrosis or granulation tissue.[91] Tumor blood flow (TBF) estimation by deconvolution analysis of DCE-MRI data has been shown to be decreased in both bone and soft tissue sarcomas with a good response (>90% necrosis) to chemotherapy.[92]

Investigation of sarcoma neoadjuvant chemotherapy treatment response with CEUS is currently being conducted at our institution. In our preliminary studies, CEUS demonstrated the amount of viable vascularized tumor tissue better than grayscale or Doppler imaging techniques alone. In one case, qualitative and quantitative analysis of an undifferentiated pleomorphic sarcoma demonstrated marked

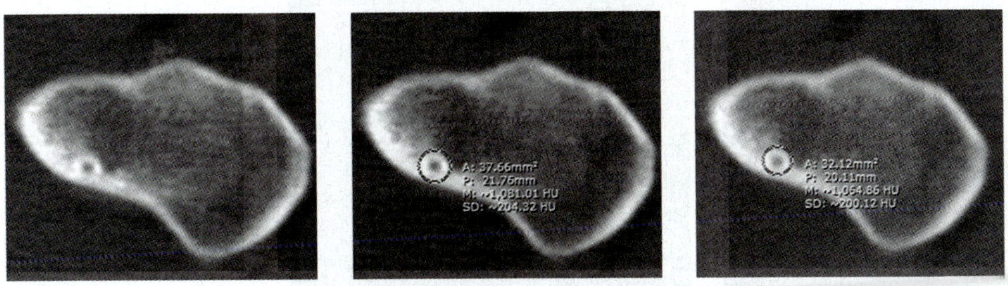

A B C

Figure 33-2. A 22-year-old woman with left hip pain and a cortically based lytic lesion of the posterior femoral neck, concerning for an osteoid osteoma. Axial CT images of the lesion **(A)** and with region of interests drawn showing the mean attenuations on pre- **(B)** and postcontrast images **(C)** demonstrate no enhancement, indicating that this lesion is simply a benign bone cyst and not an osteoid osteoma.

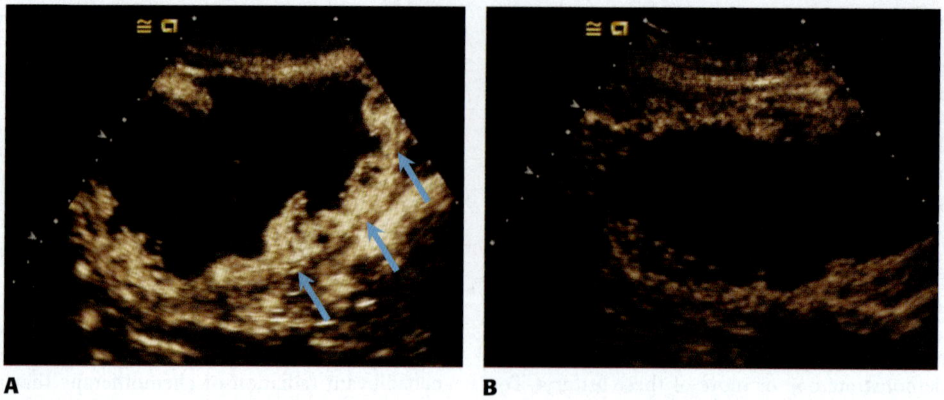

Figure 33-3. **A 58-year-old man with biopsy-proven right thigh undifferentiated pleomorphic sarcoma (UPS).** A contrast-enhanced ultrasound (CEUS) after two cycles of neoadjuvant chemotherapy (NAC) demonstrates significant residual enhancing tumor (*blue arrows*, **A**). A repeat CEUS after five cycles of NAC **(B)** demonstrates marked decreased size and enhancement of this residual tumor volume, indicating a treatment response. (Case courtesy of Mittul Gulati, MD. University of Southern California.)

decreased enhancing residual tumor after five cycles of neoadjuvant chemotherapy, compared to after only two cycles (Fig. 33-3).

Tumor Recurrence

DCE-MRI may have value in evaluating postoperative patient for tumor recurrence. In one study with DCE-MRI, subtraction images better demonstrated recurrences than routine sequence in 10 of 98 patients, although four cases were less well seen and only one case was seen only on the subtraction images.[93] DCE-MRI in a case of Ewing sarcoma of the right distal femur with a pathologic fracture predicted the early tumor response, absence of recurrence, presence of necrosis, and lack of fracture healing.[94] Although conventional MRI imaging is usually sensitive for sarcoma recurrence, in one study, the specificity was only 52%, as it can be difficult to distinguish tumor recurrence from postsurgical inflammation and fibrosis.[95] However, the specificity increased to 97% with the addition of DCE-MRI, with recurrences demonstrating an arterial type enhancement pattern. However, in this study, all patients had negative margins at surgery and were at least 6 months postoperative. In our experience, care must be taken when evaluating for recurrence in the early postoperative period, as granulation tissue may sometimes demonstrate an arterial type enhancement pattern that can be mistaken for residual or recurrent tumor (Fig. 33-4).

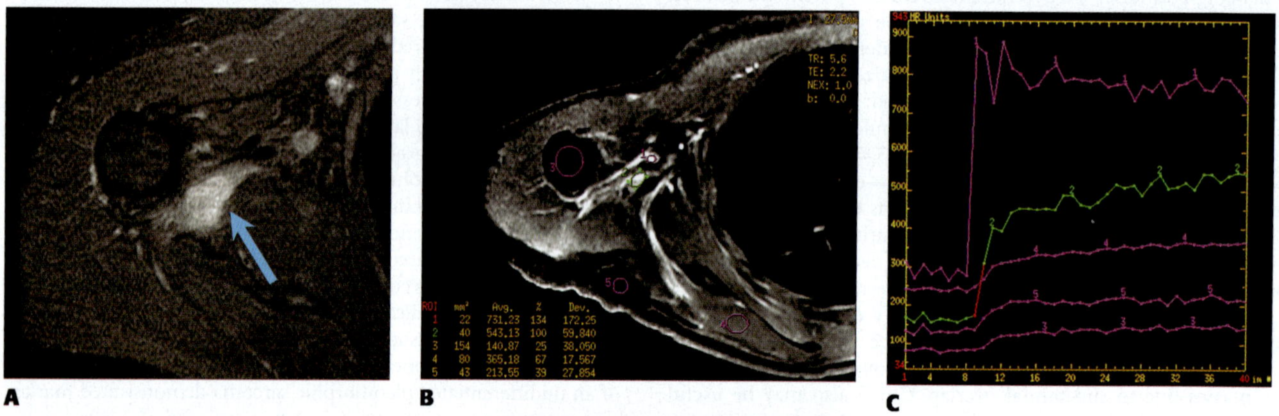

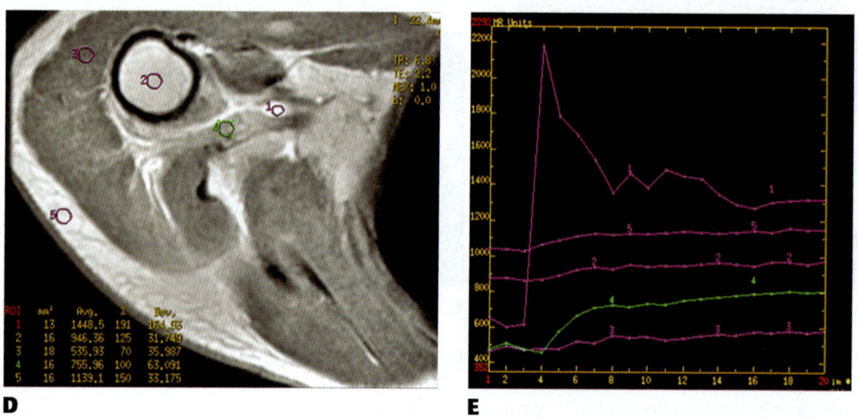

Figure 33-4. **A 33-year-old woman with right axillary neurofibroma.** Preoperative postcontrast T1 fat-saturated MR image **(A)** demonstrates the enhancing mass (*arrow*) arising from the axillary nerve. DCE-MRI within 3 months of surgery **(B)** demonstrates a TIC pattern with an early and rapid rise **(C,** *green line 2***)** similar to the arterial pattern **(C,** *top line 1***)**, concerning for residual or recurrent tumor. However, a follow-up DCE-MRI 4 months after the first **(D)** demonstrates that the TIC pattern **(E,** *green line 4***)** now has a slower and less rapid rise and plateau, consistent with evolving postoperative granulation tissue.

REFERENCES

1. **Ma VY, Chan L, Carruthers KJ.** Incidence, prevalence, costs, and impact on disability of common conditions requiring rehabilitation in the United States: stroke, spinal cord injury, traumatic brain injury, multiple sclerosis, osteoarthritis, rheumatoid arthritis, limb loss, and back pain. *Arch Phys Med Rehabil* 2014;95:986–995.e981.
2. **Konez O, Bis KG, Shirkhoda A, et al.** Gradient-echo perfusion imaging of musculoskeletal abnormalities with contrast-enhanced two-dimensional fat-saturation FLASH. *J Magn Reson Imaging* 1997;7:895–902.
3. **Verstraete KL, Dierick A, De Deene Y, et al.** First-pass images of musculoskeletal lesions: a new and useful diagnostic application of dynamic contrast-enhanced MRI. *Magn Reson Imaging* 1994;12:687–702.
4. **Erlemann R, Vassallo P, Bongartz G, et al.** Musculoskeletal neoplasms: fast low-angle shot MR imaging with and without Gd-DTPA. *Radiology* 1990;176:489–495.
5. **Erlemann R, Reiser MF, Peters PE, et al.** Musculoskeletal neoplasms: static and dynamic Gd-DTPA—enhanced MR imaging. *Radiology* 1989; 171:767–773.
6. **Fayad LM, Mugera C, Soldatos T, et al.** Technical innovation in dynamic contrast-enhanced magnetic resonance imaging of musculoskeletal tumors: an MR angiographic sequence using a sparse k-space sampling strategy. *Skeletal Radiol* 2013;42:993–1000.
7. **Barfett J, Velauthapillai N, Jaskolka JD.** Perfusion in peripheral musculoskeletal structures from dynamic volumetric computed tomography using an en bloc approach. *J Comput Assist Tomogr* 2010;34:626–632.
8. **Chang KV, Lew HL, Wang TG, et al.** Use of contrast-enhanced ultrasonography in musculoskeletal medicine. *Am J Phys Med Rehabil* 2012; 91:449–457.
9. **Meier R, Thuermel K, Noel PB, et al.** Synovitis in patients with early inflammatory arthritis monitored with quantitative analysis of dynamic contrast-enhanced optical imaging and MR imaging. *Radiology* 2014;270:176–185.
10. **Lavini C, de Jonge MC, van de Sande MG, et al.** Pixel-by-pixel analysis of DCE MRI curve patterns and an illustration of its application to the imaging of the musculoskeletal system. *Magn Reson Imaging* 2007;25:604–612.
11. **Biffar A, Dietrich O, Sourbron S, et al.** Diffusion and perfusion imaging of bone marrow. *Eur J Radiol* 2010;76:323–328.
12. **Chen WT, Shih TT, Chen RC, et al.** Vertebral bone marrow perfusion evaluated with dynamic contrast-enhanced MR imaging: significance of aging and sex. *Radiology* 2001;220:213–218.
13. **Vande Berg BC, Malghem J, Lecouvet FE, et al.** Magnetic resonance imaging of the normal bone marrow. *Skeletal Radiol* 1998;27:471–483.
14. **Vande Berg BC, Malghem J, Lecouvet FE, et al.** Magnetic resonance imaging of normal bone marrow. *Eur Radiol* 1998;8:1327–1334.
15. **Griffith JF, Yeung DK, Antonio GE, et al.** Vertebral bone mineral density, marrow perfusion, and fat content in healthy men and men with osteoporosis: dynamic contrast-enhanced MR imaging and MR spectroscopy. *Radiology* 2005;236:945–951.
16. **Griffith JF, Yeung DK, Tsang PH, et al.** Compromised bone marrow perfusion in osteoporosis. *J Bone Miner Res* 2008;23:1068–1075.
17. **Biffar A, Schmidt GP, Sourbron S, et al.** Quantitative analysis of vertebral bone marrow perfusion using dynamic contrast-enhanced MRI: initial results in osteoporotic patients with acute vertebral fracture. *J Magn Reson Imaging* 2011;33:676–683.
18. **Wang YX, Zhang YF, Griffith JF, et al.** Vertebral blood perfusion reduction associated with vertebral bone mineral density reduction: a dynamic contrast-enhanced MRI study in a rat orchiectomy model. *J Magn Reson Imaging* 2008;28:1515–1518.
19. **Hillengass J, Stieltjes B, Bauerle T, et al.** Dynamic contrast-enhanced magnetic resonance imaging (DCE-MRI) and diffusion-weighted imaging of bone marrow in healthy individuals. *Acta Radiol* 2011;52:324–330.
20. **Zhang YF, Wang YX, Griffith JF, et al.** Proximal femur bone marrow blood perfusion indices are reduced in hypertensive rats: a dynamic contrast-enhanced MRI study. *J Magn Reson Imaging* 2009;30:1139–1144.
21. **Breault SR, Heye T, Bashir MR, et al.** Quantitative dynamic contrast enhanced MRI of pelvic and lumbar bone marrow: effect of age and marrow fat content on pharmacokinetic parameter values. *AJR Am J Roentgenol* 2013;200:W297–W303.
22. **Biffar A, Sourbron S, Schmidt G, et al.** Measurement of perfusion and permeability from dynamic contrast-enhanced MRI in normal and pathological vertebral bone marrow. *Magn Reson Med* 2010;64:115–124.
23. **Thawait SK, Kim J, Klufas RA, et al.** Comparison of four prediction models to discriminate benign from malignant vertebral compression fractures according to MRI feature analysis. *AJR Am J Roentgenol* 2013;200:493–502.
24. **Cho WI, Chang UK.** Comparison of MR imaging and FDG-PET/CT in the differential diagnosis of benign and malignant vertebral compression fractures. *J Neurosurg Spine* 2011;14:177–183.
25. **Tokuda O, Harada Y, Ueda T, et al.** Malignant versus benign vertebral compression fractures: can we use bone SPECT as a substitute for MR imaging? *Nucl Med Commun* 2011;32:192–198.
26. **Wang KC, Jeanmenne A, Weber GM, et al.** An online evidence-based decision support system for distinguishing benign from malignant vertebral compression fractures by magnetic resonance imaging feature analysis. *J Digit Imaging* 2011;24:507–515.
27. **Tang G, Liu Y, Li W, et al.** Optimization of b value in diffusion-weighted MRI for the differential diagnosis of benign and malignant vertebral fractures. *Skeletal Radiol* 2007;36:1035–1041.
28. **Bhugaloo A, Abdullah B, Siow Y, et al.** Diffusion weighted MR imaging in acute vertebral compression fractures: differentiation between malignant and benign causes. *Biomed Imaging Interv J* 2006;2:e12.
29. **Fu TS, Chen LH, Liao JC, et al.** Magnetic resonance imaging characteristics of benign and malignant vertebral fractures. *Chang Gung Med J* 2004;27:808–815.
30. **Maeda M, Sakuma H, Maier SE, et al.** Quantitative assessment of diffusion abnormalities in benign and malignant vertebral compression fractures by line scan diffusion-weighted imaging. *AJR Am J Roentgenol* 2003;181:1203–1209.
31. **Chan JH, Peh WC, Tsui EY, et al.** Acute vertebral body compression fractures: discrimination between benign and malignant causes using apparent diffusion coefficients. *Br J Radiol* 2002;75:207–214.
32. **Finelli DA.** Diffusion-weighted imaging of acute vertebral compressions: specific diagnosis of benign versus malignant pathologic fractures. *AJNR Am J Neuroradiol* 2001;22:241–242.
33. **Moulopoulos LA, Yoshimitsu K, Johnston DA, et al.** MR prediction of benign and malignant vertebral compression fractures. *J Magn Reson Imaging* 1996;6:667–674.
34. **Yuh WT, Zachar CK, Barloon TJ, et al.** Vertebral compression fractures: distinction between benign and malignant causes with MR imaging. *Radiology* 1989;172:215–218.
35. **Geith T, Biffar A, Schmidt G, et al.** Quantitative analysis of acute benign and malignant vertebral body fractures using dynamic contrast-enhanced MRI. *AJR Am J Roentgenol* 2013;200:W635–W643.
36. **Katsuya T, Inoue T, Ishizaka H, et al.** Dynamic contrast-enhanced MR imaging of the water fraction of normal bone marrow and diffuse bone marrow disease. *Radiat Med* 2000;18:291–297.
37. **Courcoutsakis N, Spanoudaki A, Maris TG, et al.** Perfusion parameters analysis of the vertebral bone marrow in patients with Ph(1) (−) chronic myeloproliferative neoplasms (Ph(neg) MPN): a dynamic contrast-enhanced MRI (DCE-MRI) study. *J Magn Reson Imaging* 2012;35:696–702.
38. **Moulopoulos LA, Maris TG, Papanikolaou N, et al.** Detection of malignant bone marrow involvement with dynamic contrast-enhanced magnetic resonance imaging. *Ann Oncol* 2003;14:152–158.
39. **Zhang L, Mandel C, Yang ZY, et al.** Tumor infiltration of bone marrow in patients with hematologic malignancies: dynamic contrast-enhanced magnetic resonance imaging. *Chin Med J (Engl)* 2006;119:1256–1262.
40. **Zha Y, Li M, Yang J.** Dynamic contrast enhanced magnetic resonance imaging of diffuse spinal bone marrow infiltration in patients with hematological malignancies. *Korean J Radiol* 2010;11:187–194.
41. **Chen BB, Hsu CY, Yu CW, et al.** Dynamic contrast-enhanced MR imaging measurement of vertebral bone marrow perfusion may be indicator of outcome of acute myeloid leukemia patients in remission. *Radiology* 2011;258:821–831.
42. **Kayhan A, Yang C, Soylu FN, et al.** Dynamic contrast-enhanced MR imaging findings of bone metastasis in patients with prostate cancer. *World J Radiol* 2011;3:241–245.
43. **Bauerle T, Merz M, Komljenovic D, et al.** Drug induced vessel remodeling in bone metastases as assessed by dynamic contrast enhanced magnetic resonance imaging and vessel size imaging: a longitudinal in vivo study. *Clin Cancer Res* 2010;16:3215–3225.
44. **Dafni H, Kim SJ, Bankson JA, et al.** Macromolecular dynamic contrast-enhanced (DCE)-MRI detects reduced vascular permeability in a prostate cancer bone metastasis model following anti-platelet-derived growth factor receptor (PDGFR) therapy, indicating a drop in vascular endothelial growth factor receptor (VEGFR) activation. *Magn Reson Med* 2008;60:822–833.

45. **Hillengass J, Wasser K, Delorme S, et al.** Lumbar bone marrow microcirculation measurements from dynamic contrast-enhanced magnetic resonance imaging is a predictor of event-free survival in progressive multiple myeloma. *Clin Cancer Res* 2007;13:475–481.
46. **Montemurro F, Russo F, Martincich L, et al.** Dynamic contrast enhanced magnetic resonance imaging in monitoring bone metastases in breast cancer patients receiving bisphosphonates and endocrine therapy. *Acta Radiol* 2004;45:71–74.
47. **Moehler TM, Hawighorst H, Neben K, et al.** Bone marrow microcirculation analysis in multiple myeloma by contrast-enhanced dynamic magnetic resonance imaging. *Int J Cancer* 2001;93:862–868.
48. **Nadel SN, Debatin JF, Richardson WJ, et al.** Detection of acute avascular necrosis of the femoral head in dogs: dynamic contrast-enhanced MR imaging vs spin-echo and STIR sequences. *AJR Am J Roentgenol* 1992;159:1255–1261.
49. **Hayashi S, Fujioka M, Ikoma K, et al.** Evaluation of femoral perfusion in a rabbit model of steroid-induced osteonecrosis by dynamic contrast-enhanced MRI with a high magnetic field MRI system. *J Magn Reson Imaging* 2014. [Epub ahead of print].
50. **Chan WP, Liu YJ, Huang GS, et al.** Relationship of idiopathic osteonecrosis of the femoral head to perfusion changes in the proximal femur by dynamic contrast-enhanced MRI. *AJR Am J Roentgenol* 2011;196:637–643.
51. **Lang P, Mauz M, Schorner W, et al.** Acute fracture of the femoral neck: assessment of femoral head perfusion with gadopentetate dimeglumine-enhanced MR imaging. *AJR Am J Roentgenol* 1993;160:335–341.
52. **Tiderius C, Jaramillo D, Connolly S, et al.** Post-closed reduction perfusion magnetic resonance imaging as a predictor of avascular necrosis in developmental hip dysplasia: a preliminary report. *J Pediatr Orthop* 2009;29:14–20.
53. **Bluemke DA, Petri M, Zerhouni EA.** Femoral head perfusion and composition: MR imaging and spectroscopic evaluation of patients with systemic lupus erythematosus and at risk for avascular necrosis. *Radiology* 1995;197:433–438.
54. **Ng AW, Griffith JF, Taljanovic MS, et al.** Is dynamic contrast-enhanced MRI useful for assessing proximal fragment vascularity in scaphoid fracture delayed and non-union? *Skeletal Radiol* 2013;42:983–992.
55. **Seton M.** Paget disease of bone: diagnosis and drug therapy. *Cleve Clin J Med* 2013;80:452–462.
56. **Libicher M, Kasperk C, Daniels M, et al.** Dynamic contrast-enhanced MRI in Paget's disease of bone—correlation of regional microcirculation and bone turnover. *Eur Radiol* 2008;18:1005–1011.
57. **Libicher M, Kasperk C, Daniels-Wredenhagen M, et al.** Dynamic contrast-enhanced MRI for monitoring bisphosphonate therapy in Paget's disease of bone. *Skeletal Radiol* 2013;42:225–230.
58. **Kiuru MJ, Pihlajamaki HK, Perkio JP, et al.** Dynamic contrast-enhanced MR imaging in symptomatic bone stress of the pelvis and the lower extremity. *Acta Radiol* 2001;42:277–285.
59. **Aaron RK, Dyke JP, Ciombor DM, et al.** Perfusion abnormalities in subchondral bone associated with marrow edema, osteoarthritis, and avascular necrosis. *Ann N Y Acad Sci* 2007;1117:124–137.
60. **Hodgson R, Grainger A, O'Connor P, et al.** Dynamic contrast enhanced MRI of bone marrow oedema in rheumatoid arthritis. *Ann Rheum Dis* 2008;67:270–272.
61. **Jeromel M, Jevtic V, Sersa I, et al.** Quantification of synovitis in the cranio-cervical region: dynamic contrast enhanced and diffusion weighted magnetic resonance imaging in early rheumatoid arthritis—a feasibility follow up study. *Eur J Radiol* 2012;81:3412–3419.
62. **Boss A, Martirosian P, Fritz J, et al.** Magnetic resonance spin-labeling perfusion imaging of synovitis in inflammatory arthritis at 3.0 T. *MAGMA* 2009;22:175–180.
63. **Watrin-Pinzano A, Loeuille D, Goebel JC, et al.** Quantitative dynamic contrast enhanced MRI of experimental synovitis in the rabbit knee: comparison of macromolecular blood pool agents vs Gadolinium-DOTA. *Biomed Mater Eng* 2008;18:261–272.
64. **Hemke R, Lavini C, Nusman CM, et al.** Pixel-by-pixel analysis of DCE-MRI curve shape patterns in knees of active and inactive juvenile idiopathic arthritis patients. *Eur Radiol* 2014;24:1686–1693.
65. **Boesen M, Kubassova O, Parodi M, et al.** Comparison of the manual and computer-aided techniques for evaluation of wrist synovitis using dynamic contrast-enhanced MRI on a dedicated scanner. *Eur J Radiol* 2011;77:202–206.
66. **Jans L, De Coninck T, Wittoek R, et al.** 3 T DCE-MRI assessment of synovitis of the interphalangeal joints in patients with erosive osteoarthritis for treatment response monitoring. *Skeletal Radiol* 2013;42:255–260.
67. **Song IH, Althoff CE, Hermann KG, et al.** Knee osteoarthritis. Efficacy of a new method of contrast-enhanced musculoskeletal ultrasonography in detection of synovitis in patients with knee osteoarthritis in comparison with magnetic resonance imaging. *Ann Rheum Dis* 2008;67:19–25.
68. **Stramare R, Coran A, Faccinetto A, et al.** MR and CEUS monitoring of patients with severe rheumatoid arthritis treated with biological agents: a preliminary study. *Radiol Med* 2014;119:422–431.
69. **Kim EY, Kwack KS, Cho JH, et al.** Usefulness of dynamic contrast-enhanced MRI in differentiating between septic arthritis and transient synovitis in the hip joint. *AJR Am J Roentgenol* 2012;198:428–433.
70. **Nicolato E, Farace P, Asperio RM, et al.** Dynamic contrast-enhanced magnetic resonance imaging of the sarcopenic muscle. *BMC Med Imaging* 2002;2:2.
71. **Amarteifio E, Wormsbecher S, Demirel S, et al.** Assessment of skeletal muscle microcirculation in type 2 diabetes mellitus using dynamic contrast-enhanced ultrasound: a pilot study. *Diab Vasc Dis Res* 2013; 10:468–470.
72. **Amarteifio E, Weber MA, Wormsbecher S, et al.** Dynamic contrast-enhanced ultrasound for assessment of skeletal muscle microcirculation in peripheral arterial disease. *Invest Radiol* 2011;46:504–508.
73. **Amarteifio E, Krix M, Wormsbecher S, et al.** Dynamic contrast-enhanced ultrasound for assessment of therapy effects on skeletal muscle microcirculation in peripheral arterial disease: pilot study. *Eur J Radiol* 2013;82:640–646.
74. **Goyault G, Bierry G, Holl N, et al.** Diffusion-weighted MRI, dynamic susceptibility contrast MRI and ultrasound perfusion quantification of denervated muscle in rabbits. *Skeletal Radiol* 2012;41:33–40.
75. **Loerakker S, Oomens CW, Manders E, et al.** Ischemia-reperfusion injury in rat skeletal muscle assessed with T2-weighted and dynamic contrast-enhanced MRI. *Magn Reson Med* 2011;66:528–537.
76. **Adler RS, Fealy S, Rudzki JR, et al.** Rotator cuff in asymptomatic volunteers: contrast-enhanced US depiction of intratendinous and peritendinous vascularity. *Radiology* 2008;248:954–961.
77. **Rudzki JR, Adler RS, Warren RF, et al.** Contrast-enhanced ultrasound characterization of the vascularity of the rotator cuff tendon: age- and activity-related changes in the intact asymptomatic rotator cuff. *J Shoulder Elbow Surg* 2008;17:96S–100S.
78. **Cadet ER, Adler RS, Gallo RA, et al.** Contrast-enhanced ultrasound characterization of the vascularity of the repaired rotator cuff tendon: short-term and intermediate-term follow-up. *J Shoulder Elbow Surg* 2012;21:597–603.
79. **Adler RS, Johnson KM, Fealy S, et al.** Contrast-enhanced sonographic characterization of the vascularity of the repaired rotator cuff: utility of maximum intensity projection imaging. *J Ultrasound Med* 2011; 30:1103–1109.
80. **van der Woude HJ, Verstraete KL, Hogendoorn PC, et al.** Musculoskeletal tumors: does fast dynamic contrast-enhanced subtraction MR imaging contribute to the characterization? *Radiology* 1998;208:821–828.
81. **van Rijswijk CS, Hogendoorn PC, Taminiau AH, et al.** Synovial sarcoma: dynamic contrast-enhanced MR imaging features. *Skeletal Radiol* 2001;30:25–30.
82. **Tuncbilek N, Karakas HM, Okten OO.** Dynamic contrast enhanced MRI in the differential diagnosis of soft tissue tumors. *Eur J Radiol* 2005;53:500–505.
83. **Barile A, Regis G, Masi R, et al.** Musculoskeletal tumours: preliminary experience with perfusion MRI. *Radiol Med* 2007;112:550–561.
84. **Kawakami Y, Kunisada T, Sugihara S, et al.** New approach for assessing vascular distribution within bone tumors using dynamic contrast-enhanced MRI. *J Cancer Res Clin Oncol* 2007;133:697–703.
85. **Parkkola RK, Mattila KT, Heikkila JT, et al.** Dynamic contrast-enhanced MR imaging and MR-guided bone biopsy on a 0.23 T open imager. *Skeletal Radiol* 2001;30:620–624.
86. **Loizides A, Peer S, Plaikner M, et al.** Perfusion pattern of musculoskeletal masses using contrast-enhanced ultrasound: a helpful tool for characterisation? *Eur Radiol* 2012;22:1803–1811.
87. **Loizides A, Widmann G, Freuis T, et al.** Optimizing ultrasound-guided biopsy of musculoskeletal masses by application of an ultrasound contrast agent. *Ultraschall Med* 2011;32:307–310.
88. **Gondim Teixeira PA, Lecocq S, Louis M, et al.** Wide area detector CT perfusion: can it differentiate osteoid osteomas from other lytic bone lesions? *Diagn Interv Imaging* 2014;95:587–594.

89. **Tirkes T, Hollar MA, Tann M, et al.** Response criteria in oncologic imaging: review of traditional and new criteria. *Radiographics* 2013;33:1323–1341.
90. **Stacchiotti S, Collini P, Messina A, et al.** High-grade soft-tissue sarcomas: tumor response assessment—pilot study to assess the correlation between radiologic and pathologic response by using RECIST and Choi criteria. *Radiology* 2009;251:447–456.
91. **van Rijswijk CS, Geirnaerdt MJ, Hogendoorn PC, et al.** Dynamic contrast-enhanced MR imaging in monitoring response to isolated limb perfusion in high-grade soft tissue sarcoma: initial results. *Eur Radiol* 2003;13:1849–1858.
92. **Kajihara M, Sugawara Y, Sakayama K, et al.** Evaluation of tumor blood flow in musculoskeletal lesions: dynamic contrast-enhanced MR imaging and its possibility when monitoring the response to preoperative chemotherapy-work in progress. *Radiat Med* 2007;25: 94–105.
93. **Vanel D, Shapeero LG, Tardivon A, et al.** Dynamic contrast-enhanced MRI with subtraction of aggressive soft tissue tumors after resection. *Skeletal Radiol* 1998;27:505–510.
94. **El Khadrawy AM, Hoffer FA, Reddick WE.** Ewing's sarcoma recurrence vs radiation necrosis in dynamic contrast-enhanced MR imaging: a case report. *Pediatr Radiol* 1999;29:272–274.
95. **Del Grande F, Subhawong T, Weber K, et al.** Detection of soft-tissue sarcoma recurrence: added value of functional MR imaging techniques at 3.0 T. *Radiology* 2014;271:499–511.

CHAPTER

34 Contrast-Enhanced Ultrasound: Clinical Applications

Harshawn Malhi, MD, Raymond Azab, MD,
Vinay Duddalwar, MD, FRCR, and Edward G. Grant, MD, FACR

Introduction

The clinical application of non cardiac contrast-enhanced ultrasound (CEUS) has been steadily gaining traction over the past decade. Traditionally, ultrasound (US) without the use of perfusion agents sufficed given the intrinsically high contrast between blood and solid tissue and the effective ability of color Doppler to quantify hemodynamic parameters such as direction and velocity of blood flow. With the advent of newer and more sophisticated contrast agents, these fundamental capabilities have allowed for superior visualization of the microcirculation, once a domain restricted to angiography, contrast-enhanced computed tomography (CECT) and contrast-enhanced magnetic resonance (CEMR) imaging. Contrast use in US can provide a detailed analysis of vascular structures and allow for imaging of lesions and organs in real time. The advantages of CEUS include a real-time dynamic imaging modality with a good safety profile and a contrast agent that is not nephrotoxic. In addition, it is indispensable in patients with critical renal function that may have contraindications to receiving CECT or CEMR imaging. This chapter will provide a survey of the current clinical applications and potential future uses of CEUS on selected organs.

Contrast Agents

The most common indication for performing a CEUS examination is the characterization of a focal visceral mass. Malignancy induced angiogenesis allows for tumor growth, which in turn can be exploited to aid in diagnosing tumors. The detection of tumoral neovascularization is one of the fundamental aspects of oncologic imaging. It is from this basic principle that several contrast US agents arose.

The US contrast agents in use today consist of second-generation agents composed of tiny bubbles of a perfluorocarbon gas contained within a stabilizing shell made from a lipid or protein, commonly referred to as microbubble contrast agents. These microbubbles are smaller than red blood cells, and thus they avoid filtration in the lungs and the heart. They are true "blood pool" agents in the sense that they do not diffuse through the vascular endothelium (as compared to the contrast agents of CT and MRI).

Microbubble contrast agents are useful in that the perfluorocarbon gas is highly echogenic and provides contrast from the background tissue. These agents also interact with image processing. The major determinant of this interaction is the peak negative pressure of the transmitted US pulse, reflected by the mechanical index (MI). When exposed to a low MI, the agents display stable nonlinear oscillations in the presence of the US beam pulse, which generate harmonics of the transmitted frequency, including a frequency double that of sound emitted by the transducer, the second harmonic. The bubbles can undergo irreversible destruction, if the MI is raised to a sufficient level. This produces a brief but bright US echo.

Breast

The primary utility of CEUS in the breast is oncologic. Angiogenesis plays a key role in the breast cancer growth and metastasis. Vascular morphology varies between benign and malignant lesions. Malignant lesions contain irregular and tortuous vessels that are peripherally based, whereas benign lesions have a smooth contour[1,2] (Fig. 34-1). Color and power Doppler US is limited in that it cannot evaluate the microvasculature architecture of breast lesions.[3] Compared with Doppler US, CEUS offers better sensitivity in the visualization of pathologic microvessels in neoplastic tissue.[4]

Several studies have been published demonstrating the effectiveness of CEUS in differentiating malignant from benign breast lesions by capitalizing on tumor angiogenesis. A study by Wan et al.[5] using second-generation contrast agents compared both the contrast enhancement pattern (qualitative analysis) and contrast enhancement kinetic analysis (quantitative analysis) of 91 breast lesions with histopathologic correlation. Malignant lesions more often showed heterogeneous and centripetal enhancement, whereas benign lesions mainly showed homogeneous and centrifugal enhancement. For quantitative analysis, malignant lesions showed significantly higher and more rapid enhancement than benign lesions. The time to peak (TTP) was also significantly shorter for malignant lesions. Studies have also shown that, following contrast administration, invasive breast carcinomas exhibit earlier TTP and more rapid washout. These aggressive lesions were associated with established predictors of poor prognosis. Importantly, studies have also demonstrated that CEUS kinetics can discriminate benign from malignant breast lesions similar to CEMRI, which is currently the gold standard imaging modality for evaluating tumor angiogenesis.[6–9]

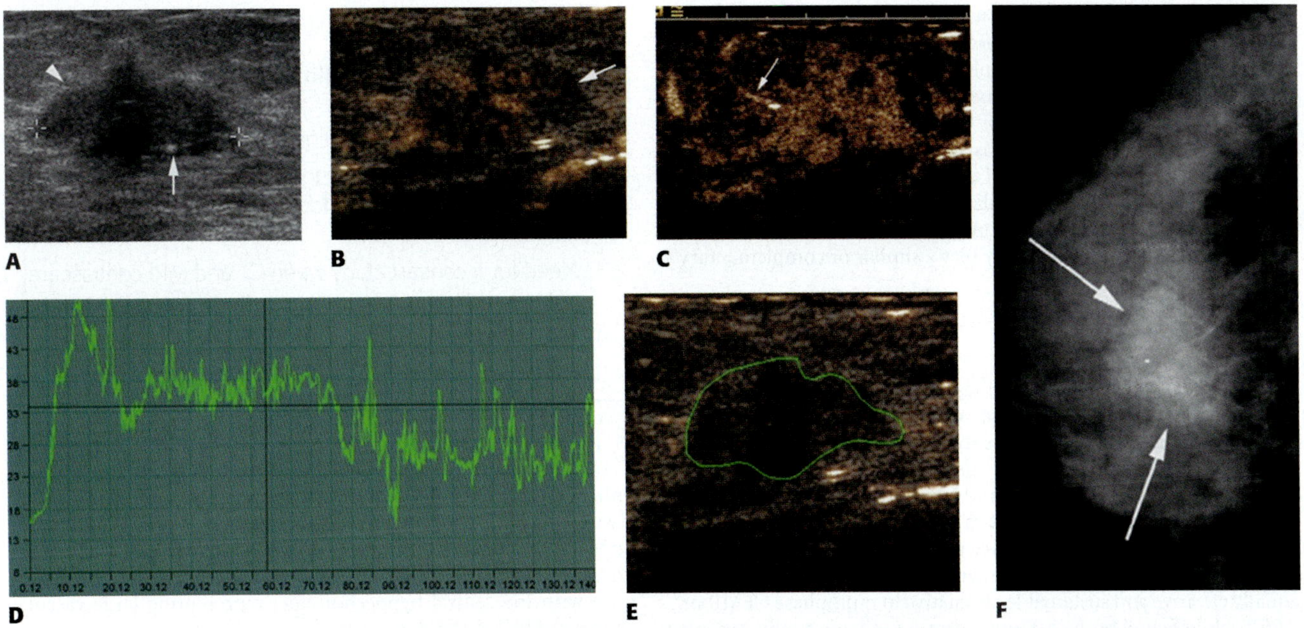

Figure 34-1. A 66-year-old woman with a 23-mm ductal infiltrative carcinoma of the right breast (note: Figures A–F are of the same mass). **A:** Conventional US. Spiculated mass, classified as BIRADS 5. Infiltrative feature is suspected because of the echogenicity of the surrounding fat (*arrowhead*). Microcalcifications are also visible within the tumor (*arrow*). **B:** Conventional US with superimposed CEUS. The tumor is strongly enhances after injection with peripherally located vessels. A poorly enhancing portion of the lesion corresponds to necrosis (*arrow*). **C:** CEUS of the lesion without superimposed conventional US. Details of enhancement are well depicted. Tumoral feeding artery is visible outside of the lesion (*arrows*). **D:** Dynamic curve of enhancement after injection. Enhancement is rapid (time to peak = 10 seconds) with a washout phase (total time: 2 minutes). These characteristics are commonly seen in cases of ductal infiltrative carcinoma. **E:** Drawn region of interest (ROI) to obtain enhancing curves. **F:** Mammogram. Craniocaudal view of the right breast. The hypervascular nodule corresponds to a spiculated dense mass visible in the center of the breast (*arrow*). Analysis of the contours is more difficult on mammogram due to the high density of the breast. Reprinted with permission from Balleyguiera C, Opolonb P, Mathieuc MC, et al. New potential and applications of contrast-enhanced ultrasound of the breast: own investigations and review of the literature. *Eur Radiol* 2009;69:14–23.

Several studies have reported that the potential of CEUS in the evaluation of tumor perfusion before and after neoadjuvant chemotherapy. Traditionally, decrease in tumor volume has been used to evaluate response, but changes in tumor vascularity can also be utilized for assessment.[10–12] Specifically, CEUS can demonstrate decreases in overall tumor perfusion, peak intensity, and size following neoadjuvant therapy (Fig. 34-2). Despite these promising results, CEMRI remains the gold standard for evaluating tumor response following neoadjuvant therapy.[13]

CEUS may also be of value in depicting tumor recurrence after initial treatment, specifically differentiating tumor recurrence versus postsurgical scar. Scars may appear as suspicious lesions

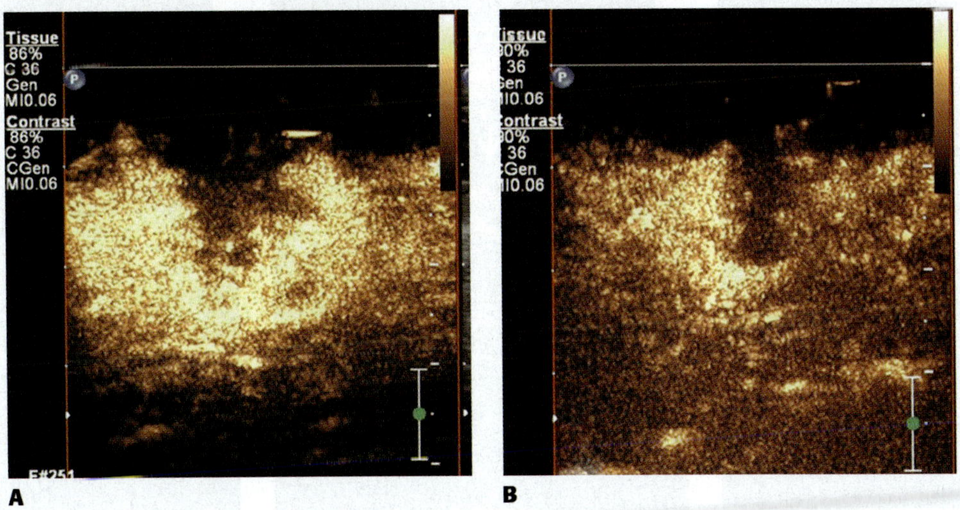

Figure 34-2. CEUS of a 28-mm malignant breast lesion before and after neoadjuvant chemotherapy (NAC). **A:** CEUS showing heterogeneous enhancement with a local blood perfusion defect in the center thought to represent tumor necrosis. **B:** After three cycles of NAC, CEUS shows a reduction in overall tumor size and a decrease in enhancement intensity. (Reprinted with permission from Cao X, Xue J, Zhao B. Potential application value of contrast-enhanced ultrasound in neoadjuvant chemotherapy of breast cancer. *Ultrasound Med Biol* 2012;38:2065–2071.)

on conventional US, often hypoechoic with posterior shadowing, similar to many malignant tumors.[10] In essence, recurrent tumors will demonstrate angiogenesis (enhancement), whereas scars demonstrate minimal to no enhancement.

In summary, the exact role of CEUS in the spectrum of oncologic imaging for breast tumors is still evolving and has yet to be standardized. Currently, CEMRI is the gold standard modality utilized to evaluate tumor vascularity and angiogenesis, response to neoadjuvant therapy, and recurrence after resection. CEUS of breast lesions thus may eventually play a similar or complementary role to CEMRI.[10]

Liver

The characterization of focal liver lesions has long been a challenging and essential part of medical imaging. CT attenuation, MRI signal, and echogenicity on conventional US taken alone are often nonspecific characteristics. The distinguishing feature of many lesions remains their vascularity and hemodynamic qualities. These unique enhancement characteristics are afforded by the dual blood supply of the liver by the hepatic artery (25% to 30%) and the portal vein (70% to 75%). CEUS has become increasingly accepted as an equally effective and sustainable alternative to multiphase CEMR or CECT while saving both cost and harmful radiation to the patient. Currently, several established indications exist for the clinical use of CEUS in the liver (Table 34.1).

TABLE 34.1 **Uses of Contrast Ultrasound in the Liver**

1. Incidental findings on routine ultrasound.
2. Lesion(s) or suspected lesion(s) detected with US in patients with a known history of a malignancy, as an alternative to CT or MRI.
3. Need for a contrast study when CT and MRI contrast are contraindicated.
4. Inconclusive MRI/CT.
5. Inconclusive cytology/histology results.

Hemangioma: Cavernous and Flash

Histologically, hemangiomas consist of multiple vascular channels lined by a single layer of endothelium and separated by fibrous septa. Cavernous hemangiomas are the most common benign tumors of the liver, occurring in approximately 4% of the population. The vast majority of hemangiomas are small and asymptomatic, usually discovered incidentally. Potentially malignant lesions such as hypervascular metastases or hepatocellular carcinoma (HCC) can have a similar sonographic appearance to hemangiomas. Sonographically, the typical appearance of a hemangioma is homogeneously hyperechoic, possibly with posterior acoustic enhancement. Of note, echogenicity is relative to the background tissue; thus, in the setting of hepatic steatosis, a hemangioma may appear hypo- or isoechoic relative to the echogenic fatty liver parenchyma.[14] Larger hemangiomas may be heterogeneous in appearance with the central hypoechoic foci representing large vascular spaces or fibrous collagen scars.

On CEUS, hemangiomas will initially demonstrate the typical peripheral globular nodular enhancement. This is followed by the centripetal progression of the enhancement until the entire lesion is enhancing and hyperechoic compared to the background liver parenchyma (Fig. 34-3). This enhancement usually persists into the portal venous phase and may last for several minutes.[15] Smaller "flash" hemangiomas will demonstrate diffuse immediate arterial enhancement that will often persist on the later phases.[16]

Focal Nodular Hyperplasia

Focal nodular hyperplasia (FNH) is the second most common benign liver mass and does not carry malignant potential. They are most common in women of childbearing age. Histologically, these lesions represent developmental hyperplastic lesions thought to be

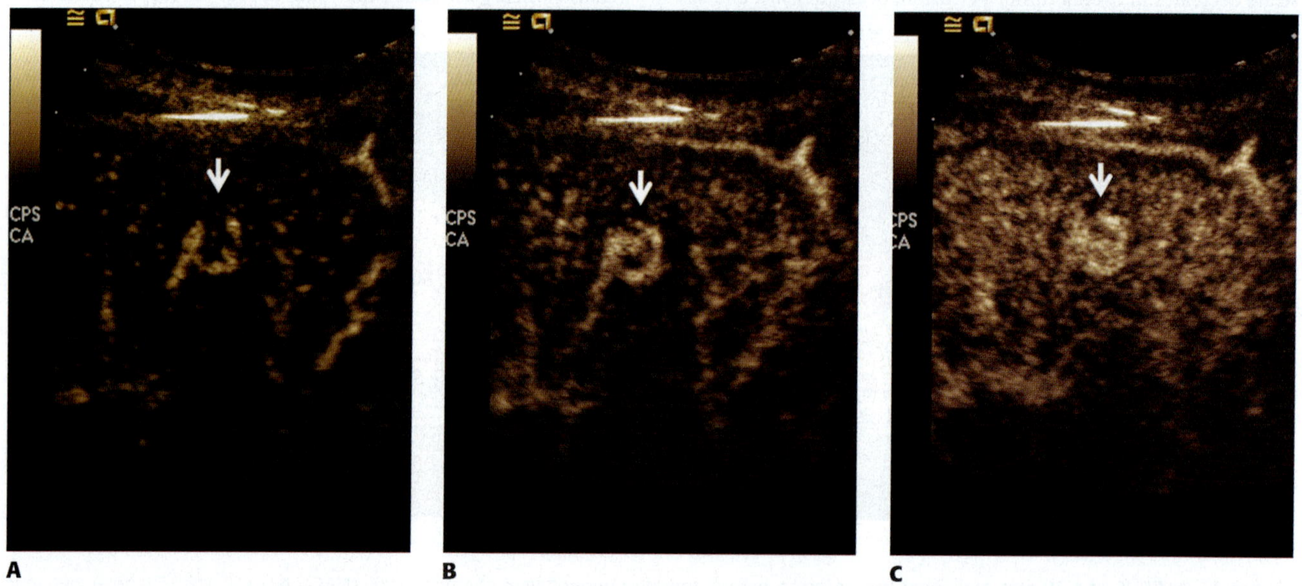

Figure 34-3. Hepatic hemangioma demonstrating progressive centripetal filling on three consecutive CEUS images (*arrows*). **A:** Early peripheral nodular filling. **B:** Progressive centripetal contrast enhancement of the hemangioma. **C:** Near complete enhancement of the hemangioma.

related to a focal congenital vascular malformation.[17] This results in a histologic mix of abnormally arranged non neoplastic hepatocytes, Kupffer cells, biliary ducts, and components of portal triads. Similarly to hemangiomas, FNH is usually asymptomatic and discovered incidentally.

Sonographically, FNH can be very subtle, often referred to as the "stealth lesion." This is in large part because histologically, FNH is essentially hyperplastic normal liver tissue; and therefore, shares similar echogenicity to the normal hepatic parenchyma. If seen, a FNH will be typically made apparent by the displacement of normal surrounding vasculature and subtle contour abnormalities rather than an inherent difference in the echogenicity of the lesion. The typical linear or stellar central scar seen in FNH is usually hypoechoic, though occasionally hyperechoic.[18] On Doppler US, well-developed peripheral and central blood vessels may be seen coursing through a well-circumscribed central scar.

On CEUS, FNH is hypervascular in the arterial phase (predominately within the central scar) and enhances more than the background liver parenchyma. Additionally, a large feeding vessel can often be seen on the arterial phase. This is followed by the centrifugal filling direction in the portal venous phase (in contrast to the centripedal filling seen in hemangiomas). Enhancement is sustained in the portal venous phase with equal or greater enhancement than the background liver tissue (Fig. 34-4). Occasionally, an unenhanced scar may be seen in both the arterial and portal venous phases. Usually, the conventional US and CEUS findings of FNH are fairly specific, and no further imaging is needed. If further clarification is required, a sulfur colloid scan or biopsy may be performed to confirm the diagnosis.

Adenoma

Adenomas are tumors consisting of normal to slightly atypical hepatocytes, which occasionally contain bile ducts, Kupffer cells, calcification, and fat, thus making their appearance highly variable on imaging. They can range in size from 8 to 15 cm and are associated with females using oral contraceptives. Although typically asymptomatic, adenomas are known to present with severe pain in the setting of hemorrhage or infarction. This complication can ultimately result in rupture, hemoperitoneum, and shock, making the management of incidentally detected adenomas slightly more complicated. Small adenomas are often managed conservatively, whereas large or growing adenomas may be resected to avoid the potential complications of rupture.

As mentioned above, the histologic variability of adenomas makes their imaging characteristics equally varied and their sonographic appearance nonspecific. They may be hyperechoic, hypoechoic, isoechoic, or heterogeneous. In regards to their vascularity, adenomas can demonstrate well-defined intralesional blood vessels (usually venous), and can therefore be indistinguishable from FNH based on their conventional US and Doppler appearance.[19] Sulfur colloid studies are often used to differentiate between the two given the characteristic cold appearance of adenomas (due to the relative lack of Kupffer cells) in opposition to FNH that appears hot.

CEUS is a useful tool in helping discriminate between these two hypervascular lesions that are managed differently. Adenomas will typically be hypervascular on the arterial phase just as FNH, though usually to a lesser extent[20] (Fig. 34-5). The distinguishing factor, however, is the centripetal filling pattern seen on the subsequent phases with adenomas. This is in contrast to the centrifugal filling pattern of FNH.

Regenerative/Dysplastic Nodules

Regenerative and dysplastic nodules both occur in the setting of cirrhosis. Regenerative nodules represent benign localized proliferation of liver parenchyma (with normal hepatocellular function and Kupffer cells) within a cirrhotic liver in response to liver injury. These nodules may progress to become dysplastic nodules, which are premalignant and classified further as low or high grade based on degree of dysplasia.

Regenerative and dysplastic nodules are often sonographically occult. When seen, they can have any degree of echogenicity. On CEUS, regenerative nodules will usually show similar arterial phase and portal venous phase vascularity and enhancement to the remainder of the cirrhotic liver. Dysplastic nodules may demonstrate transient arterial phase hypovascularity followed by isovascularity.[21] Both regenerative and dysplastic nodules are usually supplied by the portal venous system.

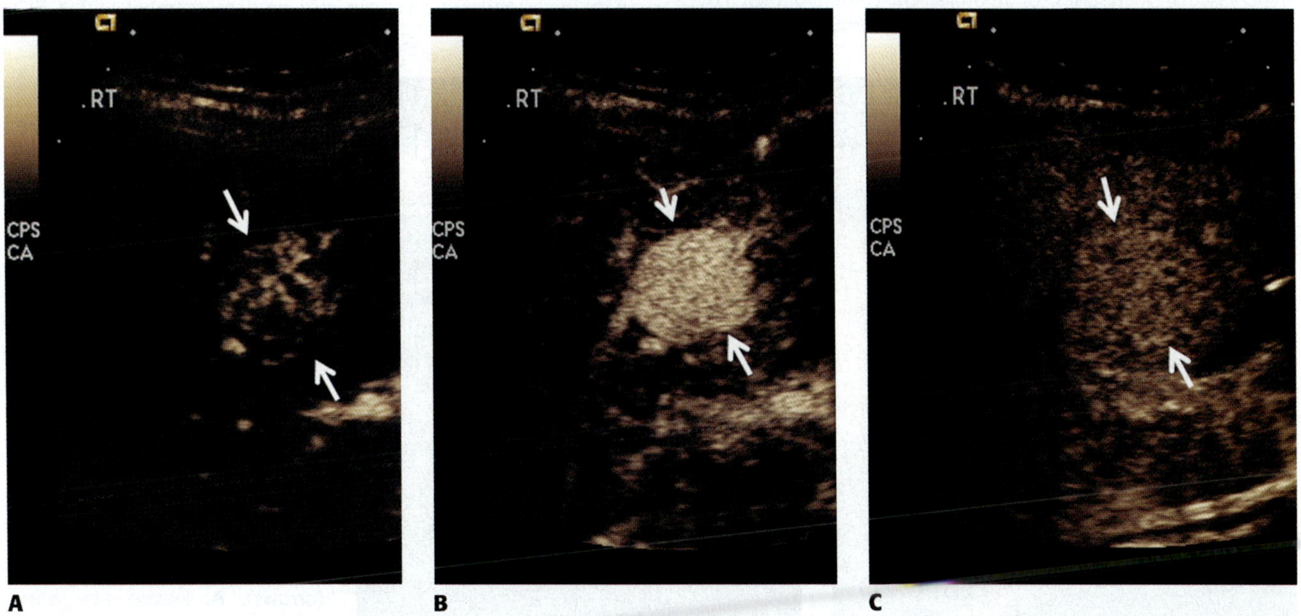

Figure 34-4. Focal nodular hyperplasia (FNH) on three consecutive CEUS images (*arrows*). **A:** Early hypervascular enhancement within the central scar. **B:** Subsequent centrifugal direction of contrast enhancement. **C:** Sustained mild enhancement on the portal venous phase.

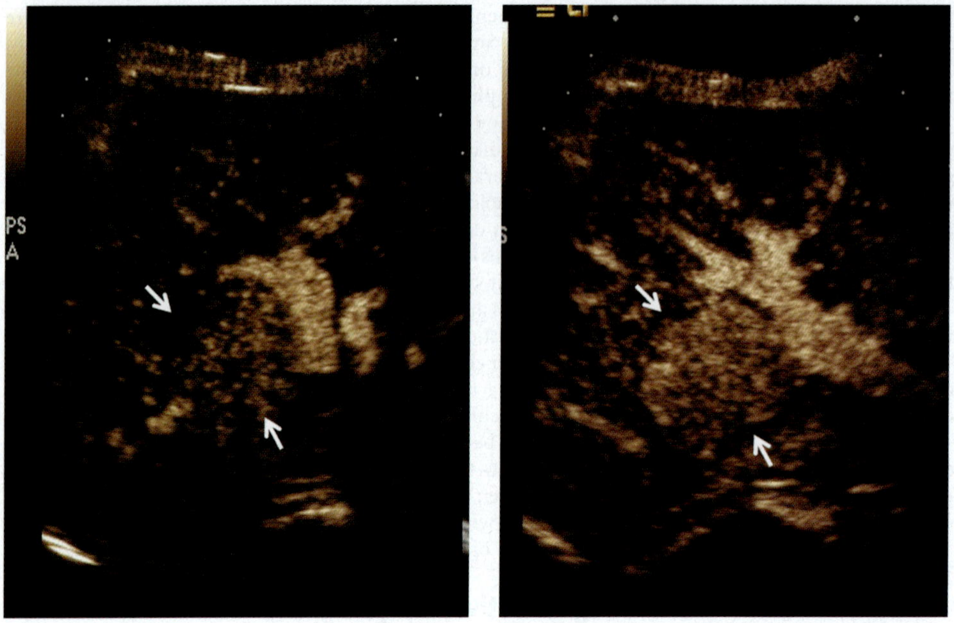

A B

Figure 34-5. Hepatic adenoma (*arrows*). **A:** Hypervascular early central enhancement on the arterial phase, typically less intense than focal nodular hyperplasia. **B:** Centripetal filling pattern seen on more delayed phase.

Hepatocellular Carcinoma

HCC is the most common primary visceral malignancy in the world, accounting for 80% to 90% of all primary liver malignancies. It is predominantly seen in males (5:1) and in the setting of cirrhosis (alcoholic and viral).[18] Although usually solitary tumors, HCCs may also be multifocal or infiltrative in nature. Particular evaluation of the portal venous system is necessary as tumor thrombus is a common complication. Sonographically, HCC is variable in appearance. When larger in size, they often have mixed echogenicity due to tumor necrosis and hypervascularity. Conversely, smaller lesions are usually solid and appear hypoechoic. HCCs can also be hyperechoic, if there is fatty metamorphosis or sinusoidal dilation. Small hyperechoic HCCs can therefore simulate hemangiomas, hypervascular metastases, or lipomas. On color Doppler, HCCs usually show hypervascularity and tumor shunting.

On CEUS, HCCs demonstrate the classic and characteristic arterial enhancement owing to arterial neovascularity (Fig. 34-6). This is followed by decreased portal venous flow ("washout") as also seen on four-phase CEMRIs and CECTs. The arterial phase may exhibit dysmorphic vessels with intervening regions of necrosis or scarring. The portal venous phase demonstrates washout with the lesion appearing hypoechoic compared to the background liver parenchyma. Given the unique and easily identifiable enhancement pattern of HCC, CEUS may contribute to the surveillance of suspicious lesions detected in patients with known predisposing factors. Of note, several atypical variations of enhancement patterns of HCCs have been described, including arterial phase hypovascularity with delayed or no enhancement and arterial enhancement without washout.[21]

Tumor thrombus in the portal or hepatic veins contains malignant neovascularity that can also be demonstrated with CEUS.

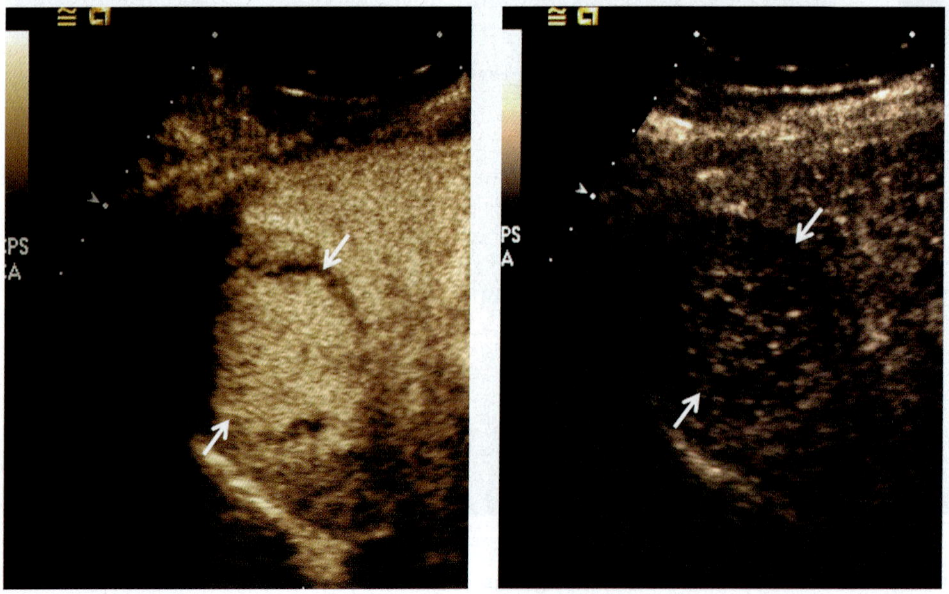

A B

Figure 34-6. Hepatocellular carcinoma (HCC) demonstrating arterial enhancement and washout (*arrows*). **A:** Intense early arterial enhancement. **B:** Contrast washout of HCC on later phase (4-minute delay).

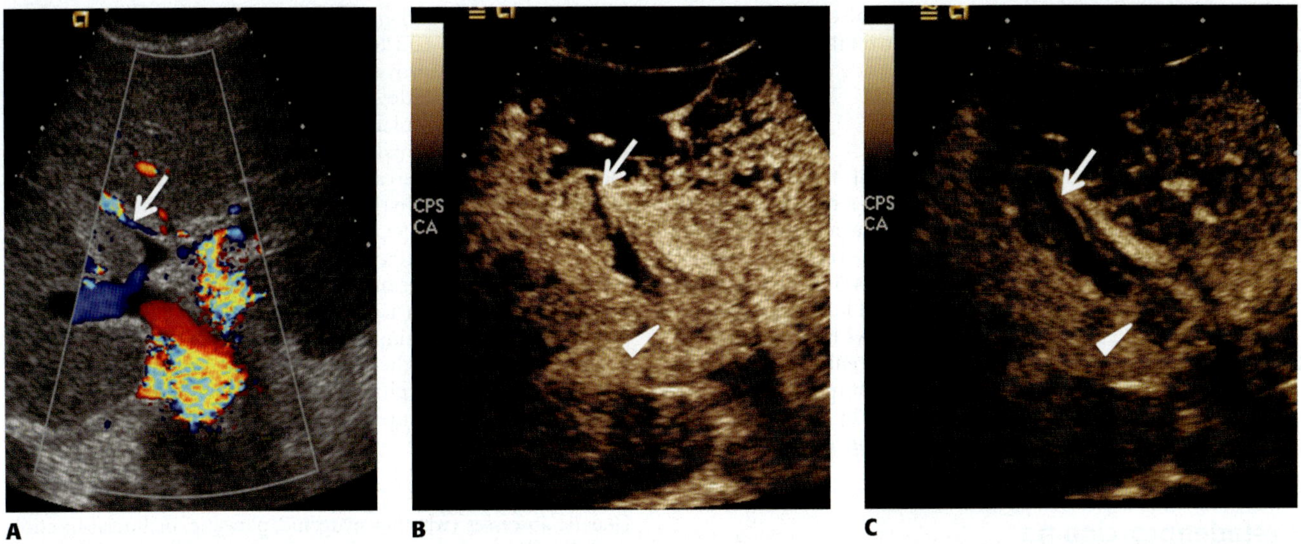

Figure 34-7. **Malignant portal vein thrombus from hepatocellular carcinoma. A:** Thrombus within the left portal vein (*arrow*), unclear if bland or malignant on unenhanced color Doppler image. **B:** CEUS images demonstrating enhancement of the malignant thrombus (*arrow*). Thrombus is identified extending into the main portal vein (*arrowhead*). **C:** Thrombus washout.

The enhancement patterns should be similar to the tumor from which it originated and will have a different appearance than a normally enhancing vessel (an arterial tumor blush rather than discrete vessels)[22] (Fig. 34-7). A marked washout in the portal and late phases may occur in metastatic portal vein thrombosis, up to an anechoic appearance, resembling bland thrombus in this vascular phase (Fig. 34-8).

Fibrolamellar HCC is a histologic subtype of HCC, which is often seen in younger patients and is not associated with chronic liver disease. These tumors are usually solitary and well encapsulated. Similar to HCC, fibrolamellar HCCs can have variable sonographic appearances. Common findings include punctate calcifications and a hyperechoic central scar. On CEUS, fibrolamellar HCCs will typically demonstrate heterogeneous arterial enhancement secondary to necrosis with washout on the portal venous phase.

Cholangiocarcinoma

Cholangiocarcinomas are the second most common primary hepatic tumor after HCC. They are highly malignant and occur primarily in the sixth and seventh decades of life. Histologically, cholangiocarcinomas are usually adenocarcinomas arising from the bile duct epithelium. They can arise peripherally or centrally in the liver with the hilar variant known as a Klatskin tumor. Given their biliary origin, both variants may cause proximal biliary ductal dilation secondary to luminal obstruction.

Sonographically, cholangiocarcinomas usually appear as a mixed echogenicity mass with associated biliary ductal dilatation. On CEUS, most cholangiocarcinomas show peripheral irregular rim-like enhancement with heterogeneous central hypoenhancement during the arterial phase, followed by characteristic

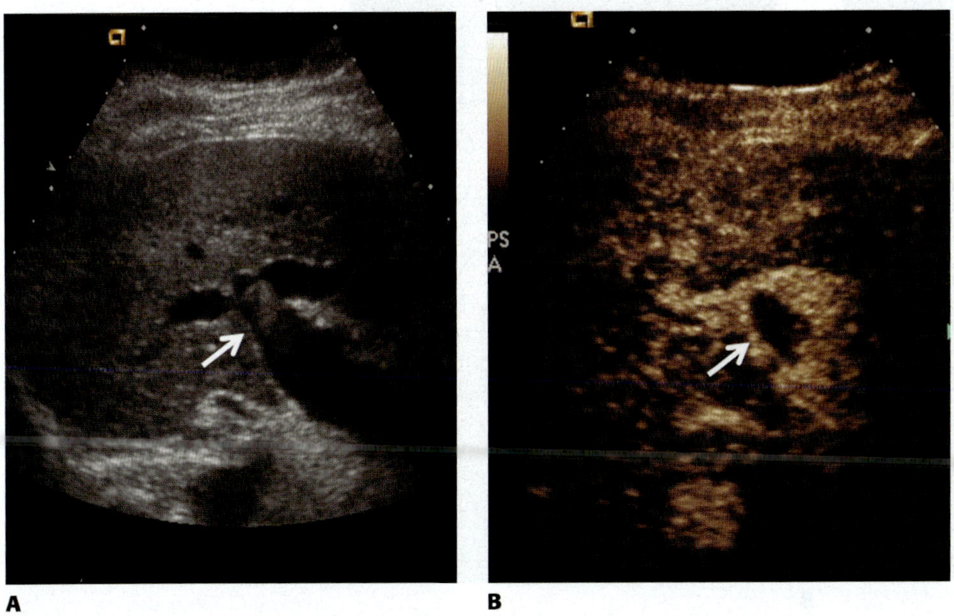

Figure 34-8. Bland thrombus CEUS (*arrows*). **A:** Grayscale image demonstrating echogenicity within the bifurcation of the main portal vein, representing a nonocclusive thrombus. **B:** Corresponding contrast-enhanced image during the portal venous phase demonstrates nonenhancement of a bland thrombus.

washout on portal and late phases. Minimal enhancement of irregularly thickened bile ducts may be seen on the portal venous phase.

Angiosarcoma

Angiosarcomas are extremely rare malignant tumors typically occurring in the 6th and 7th decades. There is a reported association with certain carcinogens (thoratrast, arsenic, and polyvinyl chloride).[23] There are several morphologic types including a single mass, multifocal hypervascular masses, or diffuse infiltration of the liver. Early metastatic spread to the spleen and lung are common. Sonographically, these tumors are almost always heterogeneous in appearance and demonstrate diffuse arterial enhancement with CEUS, given their moderately hypervascular nature, which persists into the venous phase. They are typically fed by large peripheral vessels with centripetal flow, similar to the enhancement pattern of hemangiomas on CEUS.

Cystadenocarcinoma

Cystadenocarcinomas are rare malignant or premalignant cystic tumors that likely arise from the ectopic nests of primitive biliary tissue. They are typically complex, multilocular cystic masses with septations and mural calcifications. Sonographically, cystadenocarcinomas appear as large, well-defined multiloculated anechoic masses with highly echogenic septa. Nodular components may or may not be present, because they are largely avascular, minimal enhancement is seen with CEUS; however, abnormal enhancing vessels may be seen peripherally or within the septa.

Metastases

Metastases are the most common liver tumor in the United States, up to 20 times more common than HCC.[18] Metastatic lesions to the liver most commonly originate from primary tumors of the gallbladder, colon, stomach, pancreas, breast, and lung. Sonographically, they may be hypo-, iso-, or hyperechoic depending on their vascularity. They may or may not have a hypoechoic halo representing surrounding edema, as can also be seen with HCC. Many metastatic lesions are of similar echogenicity to the background liver, making their detection difficult or impossible. CEUS is an effective method to help combat this problem and improve lesion visibility on US. On CEUS, the appearance of metastatic disease on the arterial phase is variable depending on the vascularity of the lesion. Hypovascular metastases (i.e., gastrointestinal tumors, lung) are hypoenhancing on the arterial phase, whereas hypervascular metastases (i.e., neuroendocrine tumors, thyroid, renal) are hyperenhancing on the arterial phase (Fig. 34-9). The portal venous and late phases are often more useful in detecting and characterizing metastases. On these phases, metastases often become more apparent as hypoenhancing defects. Taken together, this means that hypervascular metastases may have a similar enhancement pattern to HCC, with hyperenhancement on the arterial phase and washout on the portal venous and delayed phases. When detected initially on US, the diagnosis can be confirmed with tissue sampling.

Abscess

Hepatic abscesses (whether pyogenic, parasitic, or fungal in etiology) may demonstrate a rim-like enhancement pattern, which may persist or fade to background on the delayed phases. If the abscess center is liquefied, it will not enhance and will appear as a persistent hypoechoic defect on delayed phases. Occasionally, enhancing septae may be seen within the central defect[16] (Fig. 34-10).

Post Procedure Monitoring (Local Ablative Treatment)

Percutaneous ablation therapy has become a mainstay for the management of selected patients with liver malignancies. The follow up of these treated lesions is essential to determine residual disease with the goal being complete necrosis of the mass. Follow up can be done with CEUS and requires careful comparison to pretreatment imaging. Live scanning through the entire treated lesion is necessary to look for persistent enhancing portions of tissue within or surrounding the treated lesion. For hypovascular malignancies, the completeness of treatment can be assessed by comparing the pretreatment lesion and location of volume with that of the post treatment necrotic region (Fig. 34-11). For this reason, obtaining a pretreatment CEUS of the lesion to be ablated is of high utility.

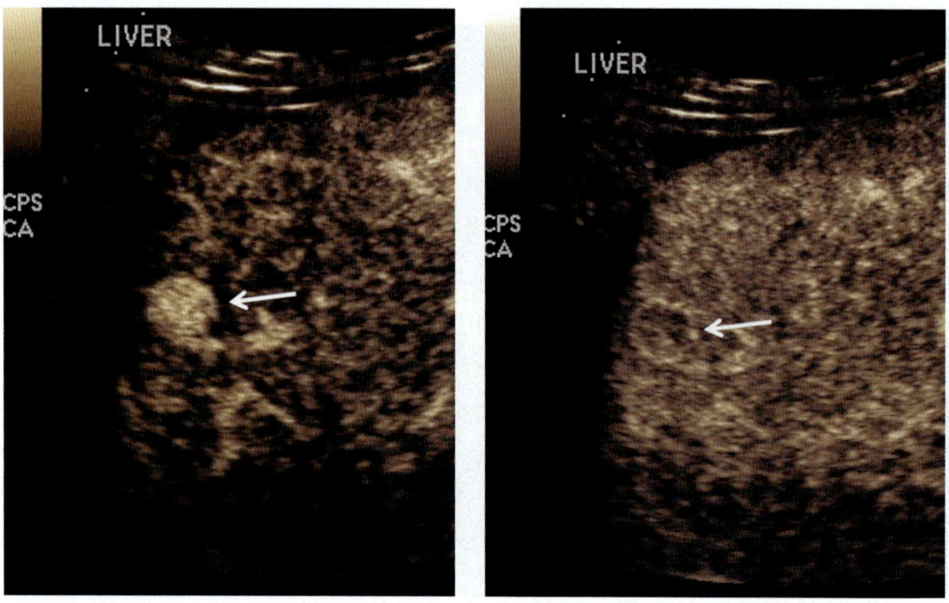

A B

Figure 34-9. Renal cell carcinoma metastasis to the liver (*arrows*). **A:** Arterial phase contrast-enhanced image demonstrates rapid enhancement (10 seconds). **B:** Rapid early washout is also present (20 seconds).

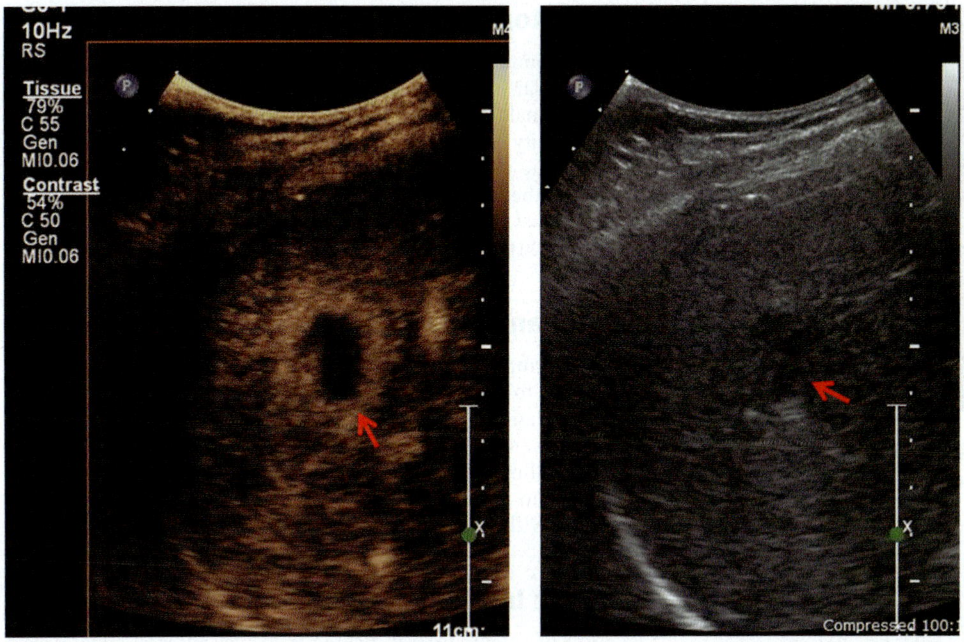

A B

Figure 34-10. Hepatic abscess (*arrows*). **A:** Rim-like enhancement pattern of a hepatic abscess with central nonenhancing defect. **B:** Hazy, ill-defined appearance of hepatic abscess on grayscale image with posterior acoustic enhancement.

Of note, normal peripheral uniform enhancement can be seen in the postablative setting for up to 30 days.[16] Careful considerations should be made before misinterpreting this normal peripheral lesion hyperemic halo as residual disease. Comparison to pretreatment imaging is often helpful as well in the characterization of the enhancement itself with nodular or irregular enhancement raising suspicion for residual disease (Fig. 34-12). If residual tumor is suspected, the patient may be referred for retreatment of the residual disease.

Spleen

Splenic pathology is uncommon, and thus, CEUS of this organ has been less utilized and studied than say, for example, the liver. A majority of the previously published work with CEUS and the spleen has been to characterize focal lesions. Overall, studies have shown that on a majority of splenic lesions found on conventional US, CEUS evaluation of these lesions can be used as a first-line test in differentiating between benign and malignant lesions. A small proportion of the remaining indeterminate lesions can be further evaluated with MRI, CT, and nuclear medicine scintigraphy.

Hemangiomas

Hemangiomas are the most common splenic primary tumor with a prevalence of 0.3% to 14% at autopsy. Although usually small (<2 cm) and incidentally detected on imaging, hemangiomas may occasionally be large (i.e., cavernous hemangiomas) and present as a palpable mass or after they have ruptured and bleed, similar to their hepatic counterparts. On conventional US, hemangiomas are usually round avascular echogenic lesions. In large cavernous hemangiomas, atypical features may be present such as cystic change and calcifications.

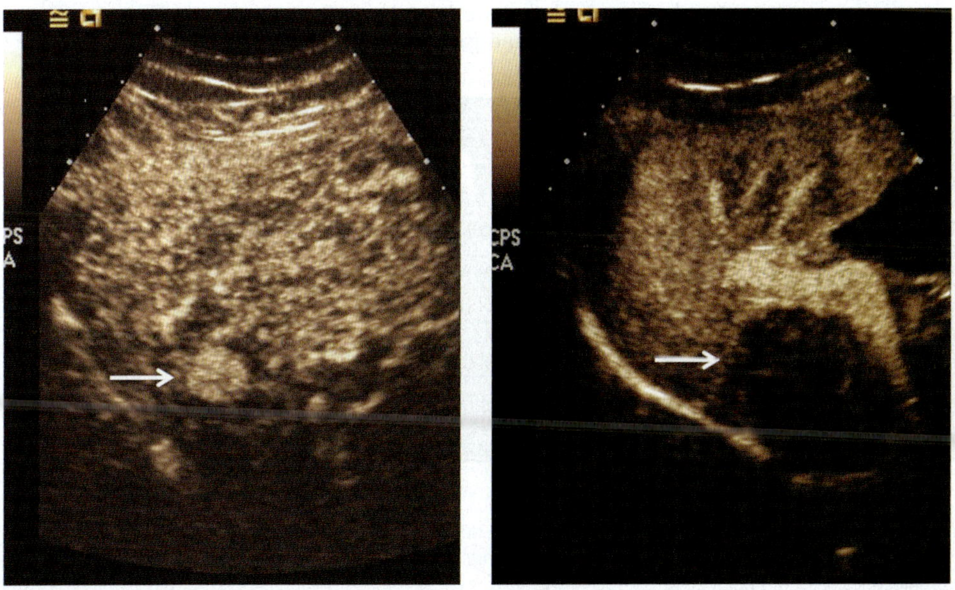

A B

Figure 34-11. Hepatocellular carcinoma (HCC) before and after radiofrequency ablation (RFA) (*arrows*). **A:** Arterially enhancing HCC within the right hepatic lobe. **B:** CEUS image demonstrating no residual arterial enhancement and a large devascularized defect after RFA.

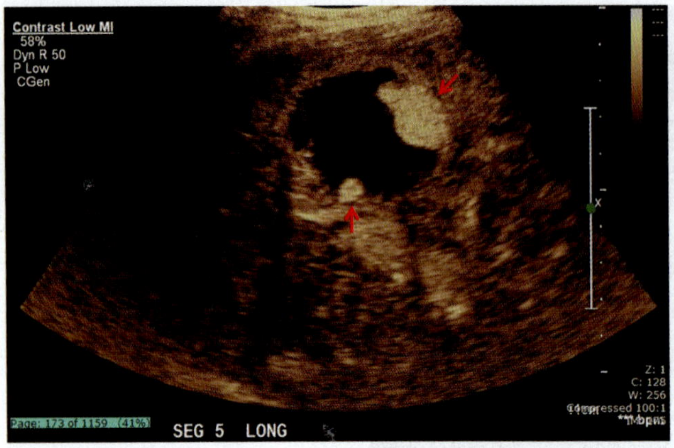

Figure 34-12. Partially treated hepatocellular carcinoma with two regions of peripheral mural nodular enhancement (*red arrows*).

Following administration of US contrast agents, hemangiomas typically enhance diffusely in the arterial phase. Unlike hepatic hemangiomas, splenic hemangiomas rarely demonstrate an early peripheral nodular enhancement (Fig. 34-13). Enhancement can be either homogenous or heterogeneous with retention of contrast into the delayed phase, eventually becoming isoechoic to the background normal splenic parenchyma. Hemangiomas can rarely show washout in the delayed phase; however, this generally occurs late, unlike the early rapid washout seen with malignant lesions.[24–27]

Cystic Lesions

Primary cysts of the spleen can be divided into two general categories, either parasitic (i.e., echinococcosis infection) or nonparasitic (epithelial). Secondary cysts result from trauma and contain blood, debris, and possibly mural calcification. The diagnosis of a simple primary epithelial simple cyst is straightforward on conventional US. CEUS of simple cysts demonstrates nonenhancement and lack the peripheral enhancement that can be seen in infectious or neoplastic cystic lesions. Echinococcus or hydatid cysts are seen in the spleen in only 5% of individuals infected with this parasite. They may be anechoic or have heterogeneous echogenicity on conventional US. Following CEUS, hydatid cysts demonstrate peripheral but not internal enhancement.[24]

Hamartomas

Splenic hamartomas (also known as splenomas, splenadenomas, and nodular hyperplasia of the spleen) are rare benign lesions. On conventional US, they are usually homogeneous solid masses. Their echogenicity is hyperechoic compared to the background normal splenic parenchyma. Despite their hypervascularity on color Doppler, these lesions demonstrate variable enhancement following contrast enhancement, thus limiting the diagnostic utility of this modality.[24]

Lymphangioma

Splenic lymphangiomas may occur in isolation or secondary to multisystem organ involvement. On conventional US, this benign and rare lesion appears as a cystic structure with septations, calcifications, and internal echogenic debris. Ranging in size from a few millimeters to several centimeters, lymphangiomas demonstrate no intrinsic vascularity with color Doppler and do not enhance with CEUS.[24]

Splenic Infarction

Causes of splenic infarct include sickle cell disease, hyperviscosity syndromes, emboli, myeloproliferative disorders, trauma, and iatrogenic (i.e., embolization or postsurgical). On conventional US, an acute infarct appears ill-defined, usually peripheral, hypoechoic, and wedge-shaped. CEUS may aid in confirming the diagnosis of a splenic infarct. Following contrast administration, infarcts do not enhance, are well defined with often better appreciation of the wedge-shaped nature when compared to conventional US scanning alone.[24,27,28]

Splenic Abscess

Common organisms infecting the spleen include *Mycobacterium tuberculosis*, and *Candida*, virtually confined to immunosuppressed patients. On conventional US, candidiasis has been described as demonstrating a "bull's eye" appearance with several lesions ranging from 0.5 to 2 cm in size. The conspicuity of these lesions against the normal splenic parenchyma improves following the administration of contrast. On conventional US, Gram-negative and Gram-positive bacterial abscesses may be hypoechoic have irregular walls, septations, and contain internal debris and gas. Bacterial abscesses have a variable appearing

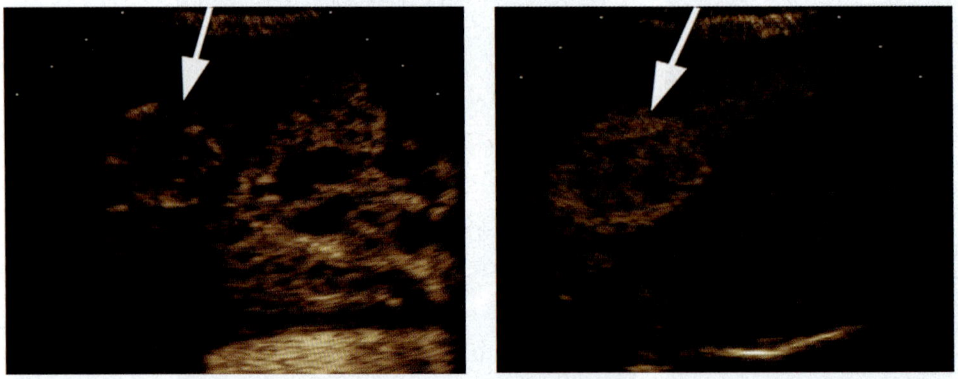

A B

Figure 34-13. Splenic hemangioma (*arrows*). **A:** CEUS examination showed peripheral nodular enhancement in early arterial phase (**A**, 9 s). **B:** Persistent hyperenhancement in late parenchymal phase (**B**, 184 s). (Reprinted with permission from Yu X, Yu J, Liang P, et al. Real-time contrast-enhanced ultrasound in diagnosing of focal spleen lesions. *Eur Radiol* 2012;81:430–436.)

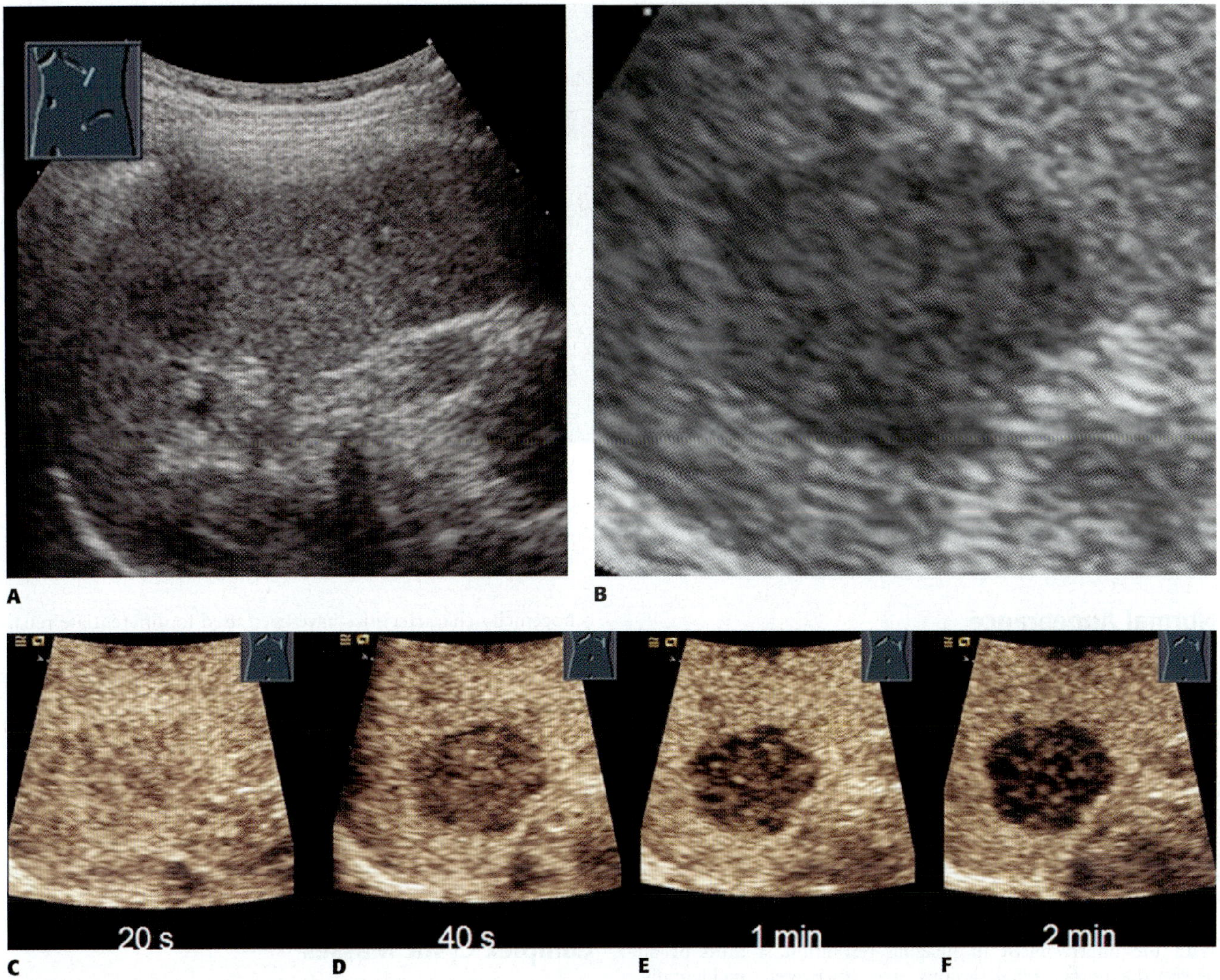

Figure 34-14. Patient with low-grade non-Hodgkin's lymphoma. **A:** A well-delineated focal hypoechoic lesion was seen on conventional US. **B:** Detailed view of the lesion. **C:** CEUS image reveals homogeneous isoechoic enhancement during the arterial phase. **D–F:** CEUS image reveals homogeneous hypoechoic enhancement during the subsequent parenchymal (delayed) phase. (Reprinted with permission from Gorg C, Weide R, Schwerk WB. Malignant splenic lymphoma: sonographic patterns, diagnosis and follow-up. *Clin Radiol* 1997;52:535–540.)

following contrast administration with some authors reporting no enhancement and others describing rim enhancement. Clinical correlation is important in this situation as tumor with central necrosis, but a viable and enhancing peripheral rind can have a similar appearance.[24,25,27–29]

Lymphoma

The spleen is involved in 30% to 40% of cases of systemic lymphoma. Typical conventional US appearances of lymphoma include hypoechoic nodules of various sizes or infiltrating disease. Following contrast administration, lymphoma typically demonstrates homogenous isoenhancing or hypoenhancing lesions relative to background splenic parenchyma in the arterial phase. On more delayed images, the lesions become more hypoenhancing and conspicuous when compared to the background spleen (Fig. 34-14). Late phase imaging may demonstrate fine enhancing regions relative to the normal splenic parenchyma thought to represent microcirculation within the tumor.[24–31]

Metastasis

Malignant neoplasms of the pancreatic tail, colon, and stomach may directly invade the spleen. Malignancies that may metastasize to the spleen hematogenously include melanoma, breast, and lung cancer. The most common appearance of a metastasis on conventional US is a hypoechoic lesion. Following administration of contrast, splenic metastasis typically show enhancement slightly less than or similar to that of background splenic parenchyma followed by rapid washout (Fig. 34-15). Delayed phase imaging may demonstrate enhancing regions thought to represent microcirculation of viable tumor, similar to lymphoma. Given the similar appearances, metastasis cannot be differentiated from the lymphoma on CEUS imaging alone.[24,27,32]

Renal

The use of CEUS in the kidney is evolving and maturing. Current uses include evaluating the general vascular perfusion of the kidney and to its most publicized use—the evaluation of focal renal masses[15,33] (Table 34.2).

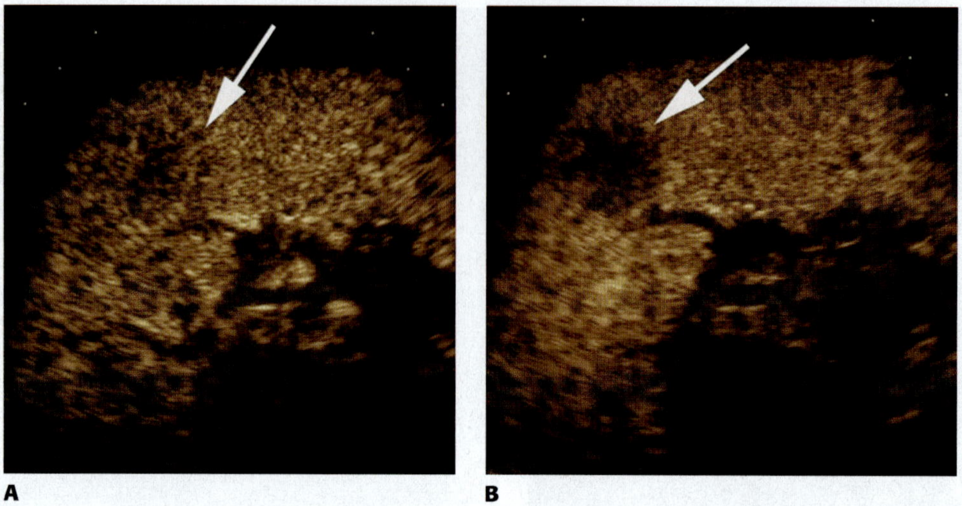

Figure 34-15. Splenic metastasis on CEUS examination (*arrows*). **A:** The lesion demonstrates heterogeneous hypoenhancement in arterial phase. **B:** Distinct hypoenhancement is noted in the parenchymal (delayed) phase. (Reprinted with permission from Yu X, Yu J, Liang P, et al. Real-time contrast-enhanced ultrasound in diagnosing of focal spleen lesions. *Eur Radiol* 2012;81:430–436.)

Normal Appearance

The renal cortex normally enhances rapidly in the arterial phase, followed by successive perfusion of the medulla, and then subsequently, a more homogenous appearance corresponding to the nephrographic phase as seen on CECT or CEMRI. The enhancement gradually fades, secondary to reduced contrast within the circulation. While there is a fair amount of potential in evaluation of the renal perfusion and the blood flow quantification, this has not yet translated into routine clinical use[34,35] (Fig. 34-16).

Evaluation of Focal Renal Masses

With the improvement in imaging resolution, a third of all newly diagnosed renal lesions are discovered incidentally. Characterization of these lesions are important for management and CEUS is a good option to help resolve diagnostic dilemmas, especially in patients with abnormal renal function. While a difference in echogenicity is well demonstrated by conventional US imaging, CEUS adds the factor of differential vascularity and enhancement, and helps in evaluating masses and mass-like lesions in the kidneys. Enhancement patterns in combination with echogenicity characteristics have been used to differentiate renal masses into benign, indeterminate, and malignant categories.[36]

TABLE

34.2 Uses of Contrast Ultrasound in the Kidney

1. Characterization of renal masses.
   a. Evaluation and characterization of renal pseudotumors versus true mass lesions.
   b. Characterization of complex mass lesions.
   c. Characterization of renal cysts.
2. Renal ischemia and perfusion.
3. Abdominal/renal trauma.
4. Guidance of renal biopsy and ablative procedures.

Renal Cell Carcinoma

Renal cell carcinomas (RCCs) are the most common malignant renal neoplasm and the eighth most common malignancy affecting adults. On conventional US, these masses are heterogeneously hypoechoic or isoechoic. On CEUS, RCCs have been reported to be heterogeneously hypervascular. Other recited features include early enhancement washout on the delayed phase and the presence of a pseudocapsule[36] (Fig. 34-17).

Complex Cystic Masses

Complex cystic masses have variable malignant potential depending upon the presence of certain characteristics such as septal enhancement, number and thickness of septations, wall thickness, and the presence or absence of mural nodules. The role of CEUS in delineating these features has been studied with good results. CEUS can also be used to classify cysts through Bosniak grading.[37,38] The presence and nature of contrast-enhanced septations, and nodular protuberances can help differentiate a benign cyst from an indeterminate or neoplastic cyst (Fig. 34-18).

Angiomyolipomas

Angiomyolipomas (AMLs) are benign mesenchymal tumors of the kidney. They are predominately isolated but can be large, multiple, and bilateral in patients with a history of tuberous sclerosis. AMLs are usually asymptomatic, but larger (>4 cm) lesions can hemorrhage. On conventional US, AMLs are commonly hyperechoic. On CEUS, AMLs tends to enhance peripherally and centrally enhance less than the normal cortex.[36]

Oncocytomas

Oncocytoma is the most common benign solid renal tumor, but unfortunately, it shares many of the imaging features also seen in RCC. Conventional US may demonstrate a well-defined, homogeneous, and hypoechoic to isoechoic solid mass, with or without an echogenic central scar. CEUS features of oncocytoma include early

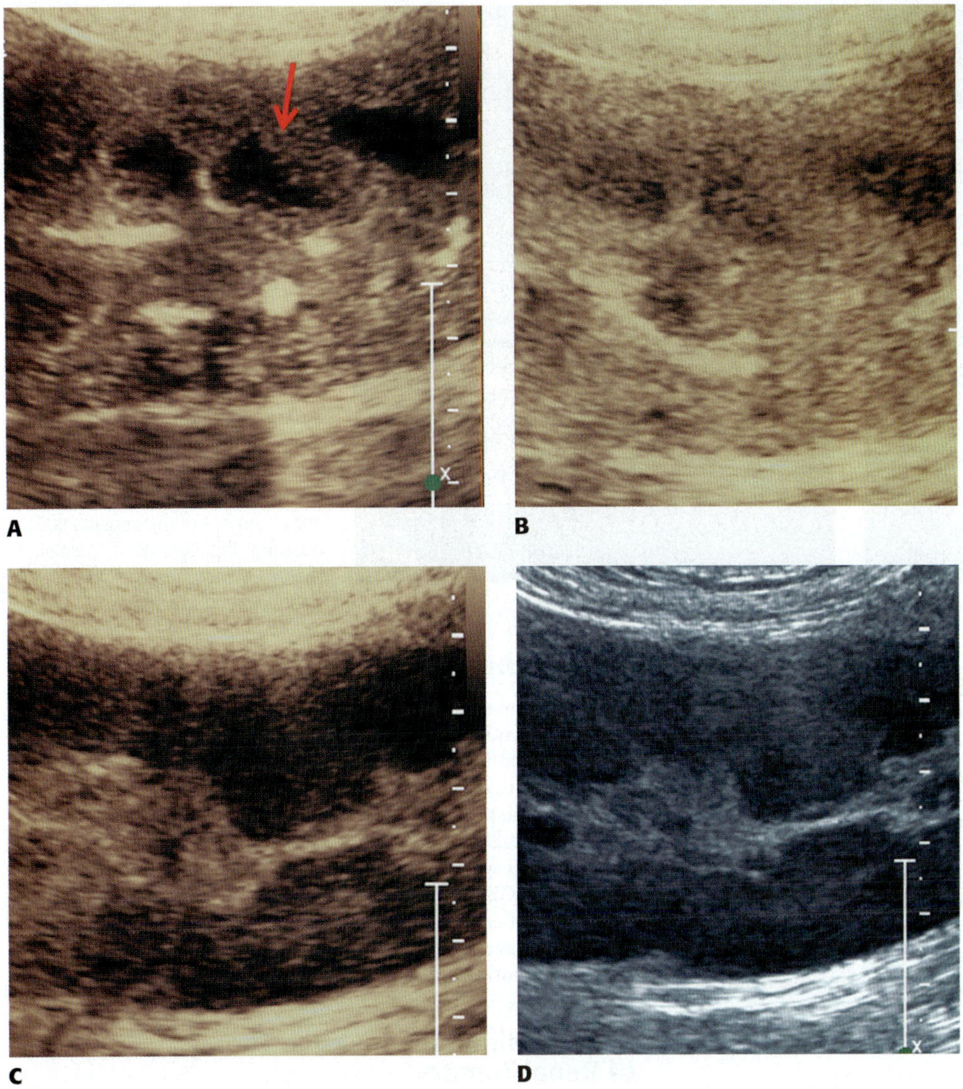

Figure 34-16. **Appearance of renal cortex and medulla after contrast injection. A:** Early arterial phase following contrast injection: normal renal cortex enhances early with renal pyramids well seen as relative areas hypoperfusion at this stage (*red arrow*). **B:** Nephrographic phase equivalent: there is a more homogenous appearance to the entire kidney. **C:** Late phase: appearance of the kidney is similar to normal grayscale US images. **D:** Grayscale image of normal kidney.

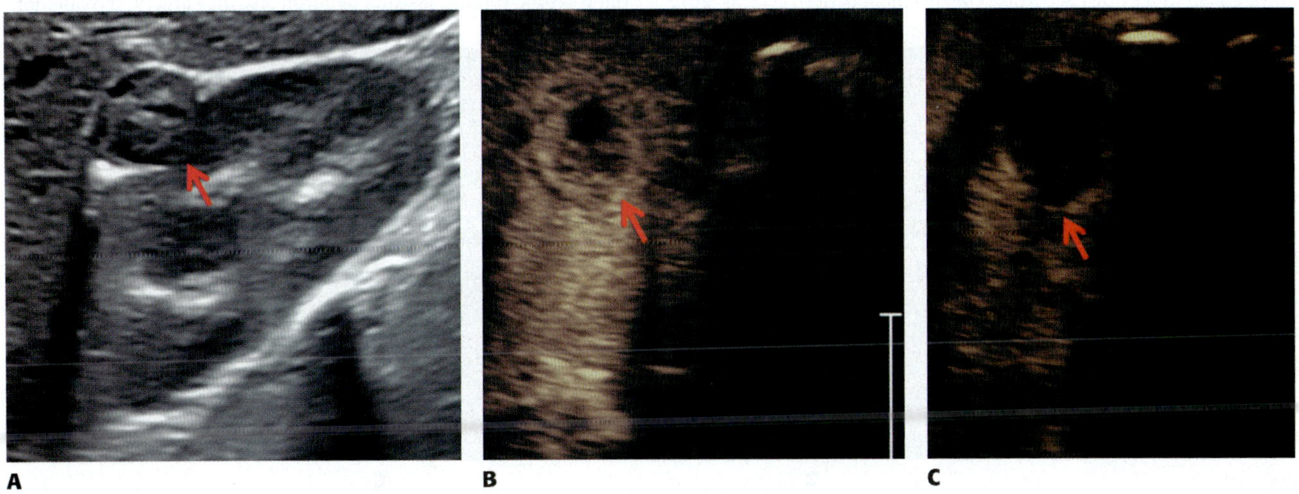

Figure 34-17. A 29-year-old female with a right-sided renal mass (*red arrows*). **A:** Grayscale image reveals an exophytic mass arising from the right interpole. **B:** Early phase CEUS image demonstrates very early enhancement with a nonenhancing center. **C:** Late-phase image reveals significant washout compared to cortex. On biopsy this was a renal cell (clear cell type) carcinoma.

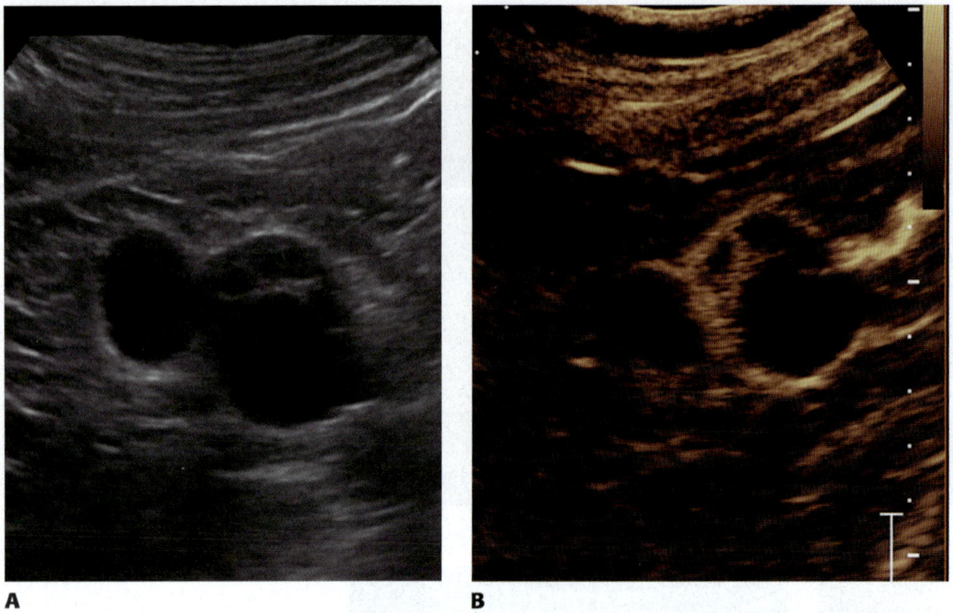

Figure 34-18. A 56-year-old male with a complex renal cyst. **A:** Gray-scale imaging reveals a nodular thickened complex septation along the margin of the larger cyst. **B:** Following contrast injection, there is marked enhancement of the septations. This classifies the cyst as a Bosniak III lesion. On resection, this was a cystic clear cell renal carcinoma.

enhancement, enhancement greater than adjacent cortex, and rapid washout (Fig. 34-19). The well-described avascular scar depicted on CT and MR has also been reported.[39]

Evaluation of Pseudotumors

A renal pseudotumor is a mass that simulates a tumor on imaging but is composed of non neoplastic tissue. CEUS can help differentiate a pseudotumor from a true renal mass. The ability to evaluate dynamic contrast enhancement and kinetics is crucial for demonstrating the presence of a renal pseudotumor such as a hypertrophied column of Bertin. The concordance of the enhancement pattern within the cortex and the characteristic location helps in diagnosing this lesion.[40]

Metastases

Metastasis to the kidney is uncommon. The main diagnostic dilemma is to distinguish it from a primary renal tumor. Metastasis does not have a characteristic pattern on CEUS but tends to be hypovascular in comparison to the normal cortical enhancement pattern (Fig. 34-20).

Renal Ischemia/Infarction

Renal ischemia/infarction results from reduced or a complete lack of perfusion to the kidney. The underlying etiologies include thromboembolism (most common), aortic or renal artery dissection, vasculitis, iatrogenic, and renal vein thrombosis. CEUS aids in evaluating the presence and extent of renal parenchymal ischemia, and therefore, can be used in the evaluation of suspected infarction. Renal infarcts will appear as wedge-shaped areas of nonperfusion. In addition, CEUS can help in the differentiation of nonperfused and hypoperfused organs. This is critical in the evaluation of a failing transplanted kidney.[41] There is, however, no current role in the routine evaluation and screening for renal artery stenosis.[42]

Role in Minimally Invasive Therapy of Renal Tumors

While the standard therapy of suspected RCC is nephrectomy or nephron-sparing open surgery, minimally invasive treatments (laproscopic/robotic-assisted nephron sparing surgery, cryoablation,

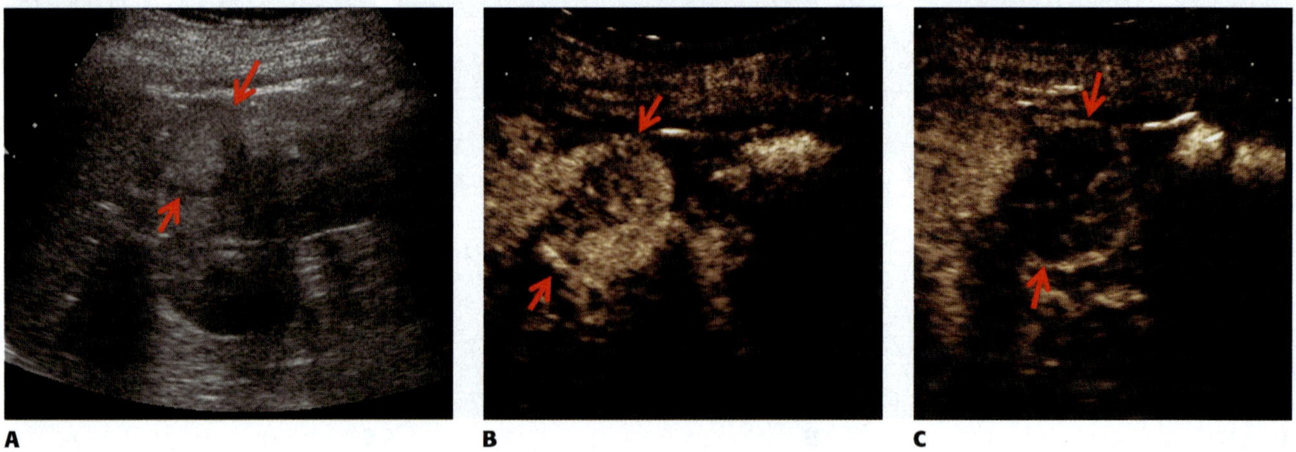

Figure 34-19. A 64-year-old female with a mass in the right kidney (*red arrows*). **A:** Hyperechoic mass in the right kidney which is well marginated. **B:** Following contrast inject, there is early enhancement of the majority of the mass with a nonenhancing area in the center. **C:** Delayed images reveal an early washout from the majority of the mass. Surgical pathology revealed oncocytoma.

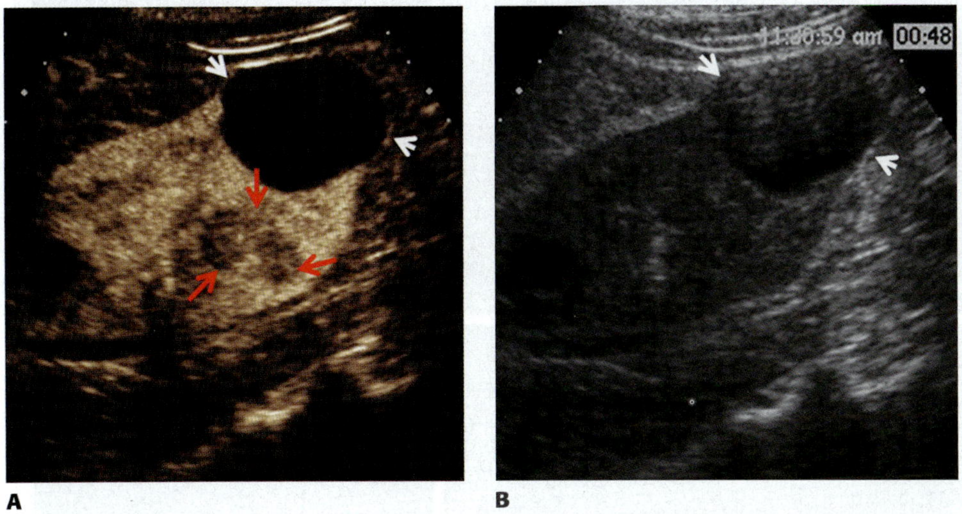

Figure 34-20. A 78-year-old male with metastatic melanoma. **A:** Image following CEUS reveals poorly defined relatively hypovascular focal lesion (*red arrows*). Incidental note is made of a Bosniak I simple cyst (*arrowheads*). **B:** Grayscale images unable to identify the focal lesion.

and radiofrequency ablation) have emerged as viable treatment alternatives in selected cases. There is an established role of CEUS in the evaluation of renal masses during and following minimally invasive treatments to monitor completeness of therapy and for the detection of disease recurrence.[43,44]

Role in Trauma

CEUS has been used in the emergency room setting to help evaluate cases of abdominal trauma. It may assist in diagnosing lesions such as hematomas, and also assess the perfusion of the kidney in suspected cases of more proximal arterial injury.[42,45]

Role in Infection

An abnormal finding on conventional US will be seen in only around 20% of patients with bacterial pyelonephritis. When positive findings of pyelonephritis are discovered on sonography, they can include renal enlargement, hydronephrosis, loss of the corticomedullary differentiation (i.e., increased renal cortical echogenicity), and abscess formation. Gas identified in the renal parenchyma aids in diagnosing emphysematous pyelonephritis. CEUS can assist in differentiating focal pyelonephritis from mass lesions and aids in delineating abscesses[42] (Fig. 34-21).

Contrast Quantification in the Kidney

While absolute measurements of volumetric blood flow on CEUS are not feasible in a practical sense, measurement of contrast kinetics such as TTP and time to washout can be used to obtain pathophysiologic quantifiable information. Potentially, this could increase the specificity of CEUS and also supplement diagnostic information available from qualitative CEUS.[46,47] Its role is yet to be evaluated clinically. Early work has shown promise in renal perfusion evaluation, renal transplant evaluation, revascularization procedures, and for evaluation of masses, as described above (Fig. 34-22).

Bowel

The primary utility of CEUS in bowel imaging lies in the evaluation of inflammatory bowel disease, specifically Crohn disease (CD). CD is a chronic inflammatory disease with alternating periods of acute inflammation and remission. Given these characteristics, adequate treatment requires periodic assessment of inflammatory activity as well as possible transmural complications.[48] An important complication is development of fibrotic scarring of the intestinal wall that can result in symptomatic (bowel obstructive) strictures and stenosis[49] (Fig. 34-23).

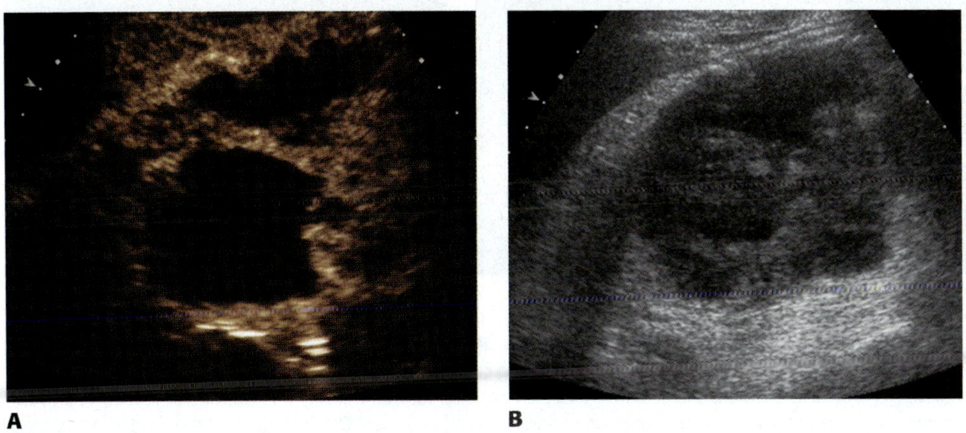

Figure 34-21. A 59-year-old male patient status postrenal transplant and complex peritransplant fluid collection found to represent an abscess. **A:** CEUS image demonstrates enhancing septations and loculations. **B:** Grayscale image alone does not demonstrate septations as readily.

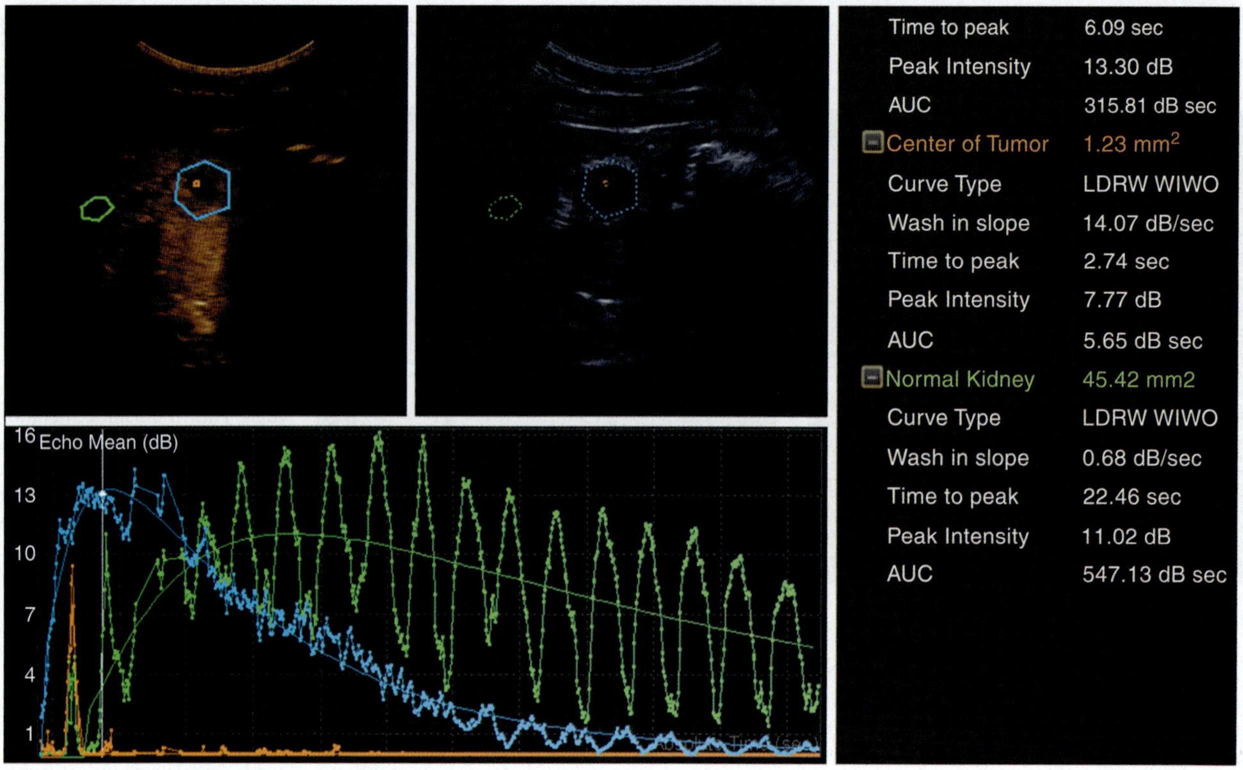

Figure 34-22. Contrast kinetics on a renal cell carcinoma same case as Figure 34-17. This shows region of interest 1 (ROI 1) (**blue**), which is in the tumor enhances earlier and more than normal renal cortex (ROI 3, **green**). The center of the tumor is necrotic (ROI 2, **orange**).

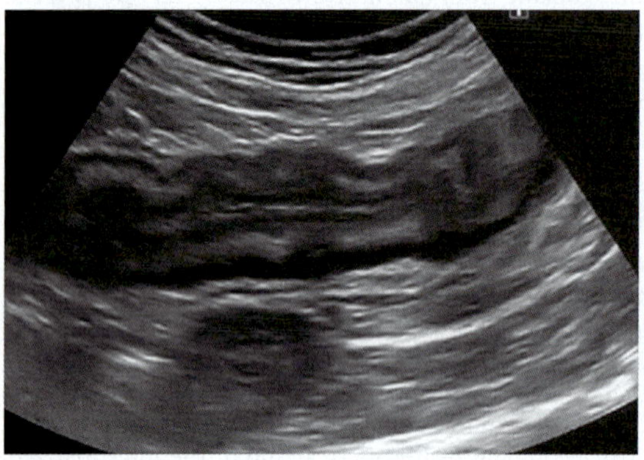

A

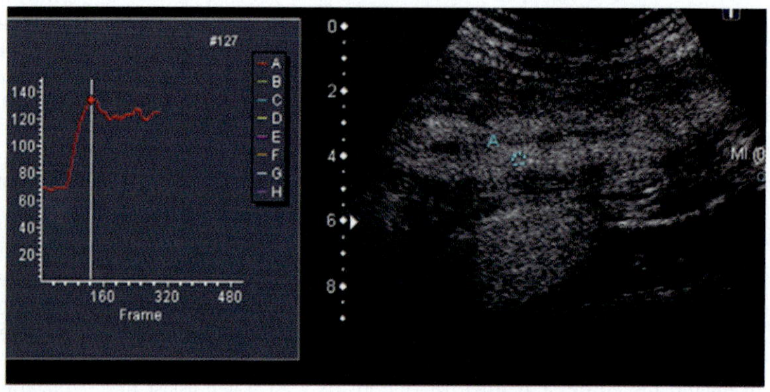

B

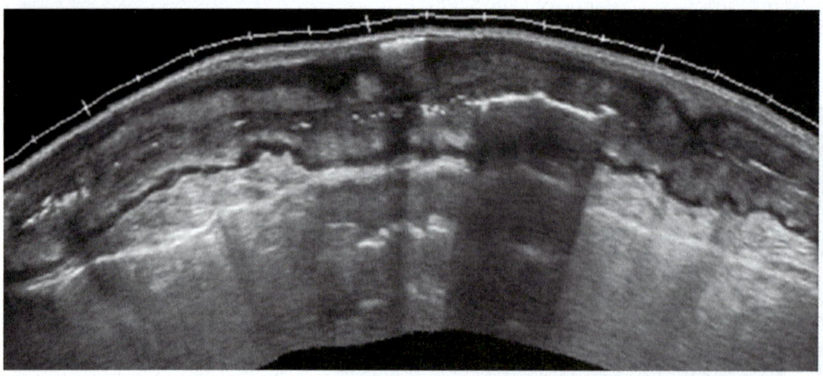

C

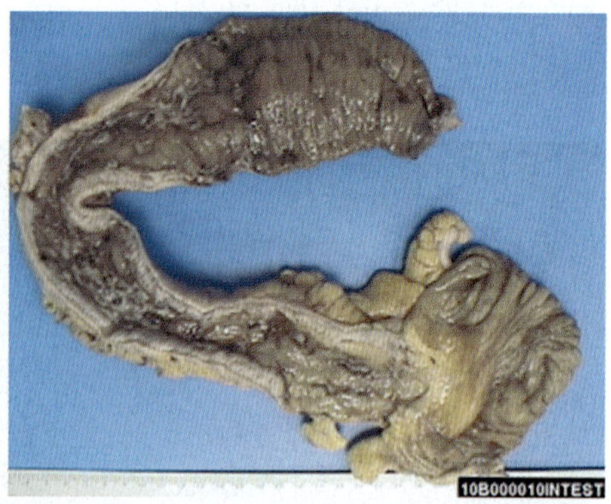

D

Figure 34-23. A 43-year-old woman with Crohn disease and severe ileal stenosis/stricture. **A:** Longitudinal conventional US scan of the intestinal thickened segment before contrast administration. **B:** Measurement of bowel wall vascularity following contrast administration in a manually defined ROI, obtaining the brightness–time curves over a period of 40 s. In this case, absolute and percentage of increase of enhancement was 64% and 93%, respectively (baseline value 69, maximum value 133). **C:** Longitudinal conventional US compound scan of the surgical specimen. **D:** Photograph of the divided gross specimen confirms the presence of mural thickening of a long ileal segment with congested mucosa, eroded appearance, and abundant linear ulcers that tend to converge over the entire surface. (Reprinted with permission from Ripollés T, Rausell N, Paredes JM, et al. Effectiveness of contrast-enhanced ultrasound for characterization of intestinal inflammation in Crohn's disease: a comparison with surgical histopathology analysis. *J Crohns Colitis* 2013;7:120–128.)

Ultrasonography, CT enterography, and MRI enterography can be used to determine the anatomic location and length of diseased bowel.[50–53] Conventional US imaging in the acute inflammatory phase of CD may demonstrate diffuse edema involving the bowel wall with loss of bowel wall layer visualization. In the chronic phase, the bowel wall layers are visible and the bowel wall is usually thickened. Chronic strictures manifest as thickened and rigid bowel segments with dilation of the bowel more proximally.[54]

The introduction of CEUS has enabled assessment of bowel wall microcirculation, which is intrinsically associated with the inflammatory process in CD.[55] Several studies have demonstrated significant relationships between measurements obtained from CEUS and clinical or endoscopic indices of disease activity, whereas others have failed to reproduce similar results.[49,55,56] Possibilities of these incongruent results may be related to interobserver variability of enhancement patterns and overlapping appearances of active/acute and fibrotic/chronic CD.[54,55] In general however, following administration of contrast, patients with active disease may demonstrate early transmural enhancement initiating in the mucosa and eventually involving the entire bowel wall.[55] Differentiating chronic fibrotic strictures from acute inflammatory strictures is difficult with CEUS as there are overlapping features and the rapid inflow of contrast does not allow for confident evaluation of specific enhancement patterns.[54]

An additional emerging application of CEUS in CD is to differentiate responders from nonresponders during specific pharmacologic treatment. Studies have demonstrated that quantitative (i.e., TTP and time–intensity curves) parameters applied to the areas of interest rather than qualitative assessment (visual interpretation) is useful to discover treatment responders. In general, patients responding to medical treatment demonstrate reducing bowel wall vascularity. Given the relapsing course of this disease and need for frequent monitoring, this application of bowel CEUS has potential to be used in conjunction with clinical indices to evaluate the efficacy of medical therapy.[54]

REFERENCES

1. **Less JR, Skalak TC, Sevick EM, et al.** Microvascular architecture in a mammary carcinoma: branching patterns and vessel dimensions. *Cancer Res* 1991;51:265–273.
2. **Kedar RP, Cosgrove D, McCread VR, et al.** Microbubble contrast agent for color Doppler US: effect on breast masses—work in progress. *Radiology* 1996;198:679–686.
3. **Schroeder RJ, Bostanjoglo M, Rademaker J, et al.** Role of power Doppler techniques and ultrasound contrast enhancement in the differential diagnosis of focal breast lesions. *Eur Radiol* 2003;13:68–79.
4. **Delorme S, Krix M.** Contrast-enhanced ultrasound for examining tumor biology. *Cancer Imaging* 2006;6:148–152.
5. **Wan C, Du J,Fang H, et al.** Evaluation of breast lesions by contrast enhanced ultrasound: qualitative and quantitative analysis. *Eur Radiol* 2012;81:444–450.
6. **Botond KS, Saracco A, Tánczos E, et al.** Correlation of contrast-enhanced ultrasound kinetics prognostic factors in invasive breast cancer. *Eur Radiol* 2013;23:3228–3236.
7. **Caproni N, Marchisio F, Pecchi A, et al.** Contrast-enhanced ultrasound in the characterization of breast masses: utility of quantitative analysis in comparison with MRI. *Eur Radiol* 2010;20:1384–1395.
8. **Hata T, Takahashi H, Watanabe K, et al.** Magnetic resonance imaging for preoperative evaluation of breast cancer: a comparative study with mammography and ultrasonography. *J Am Coll Surg* 2004;198:190–197.
9. **Ricci P, Cantisani V, Ballesio L, et al.** Benign and malignant breast lesions: efficacy of real time contrast-enhanced ultrasound vs. magnetic resonance imaging. *Ultraschall Med* 2007;28:57–62.
10. **Balleyguiera C, Opolonb P, Mathieuc MC, et al.** New potential and applications of contrast-enhanced ultrasound of the breast: own investigations and review of the literature. *Eur Radiol* 2009;69:14–23.
11. **Vallone P, D'Angelo R, Filice S, et al.** Color-Doppler using contrast medium in evaluating the response to neoadjuvant treatment in patients with locally advanced breast carcinoma. *Anticancer Res* 2005;25:595–600.
12. **Cao X, Xue J, Zhao B.** Potential application value of contrast-enhanced ultrasound in neoadjuvant chemotherapy of breast cancer. *Ultrasound Med Biol* 2012;38:2065–2071.
13. **Stuhrmann M, Aronius R, Schietzel M.** Tumor vascularity of breast lesions: potentials and limits of contrast-enhanced Doppler sonography. *Am J Roentgenol* 2000;175:1585–1589.
14. **Marsh JI, Gibney RG, Li DK.** Hepatic hemangioma in the presence of fatty infiltration: an atypical sonographic appearance. *Gastrointest Radiol* 1989;14:262–264.
15. **Wilson SR, Burns PN.** Microbubble enhanced ultrasound imaging: what role? *Radiology* 2010;257:24–39.
16. **Claudon M, Cosgrove D, Albrecht T, et al.** Guidelines and good clinical practice recommendations for contrast enhanced ultrasound (CEUS)—update 2008. *Ultraschall Med* 2008;29:28–44.
17. **Wanless IR, Mawdsley C, Adams R.** On the pathogenesis of focal nodular hyperplasia of the liver. *Hepatology* 1985;5:1194–1200.
18. **Rumack C, Wilson S, Charboneau J, et al.** *The liver, diagnostic ultrasound.* 4th ed. Philadelphia, PA: Elsevier Mosby; 2011:78–145.
19. **Golli M, Van Nhieu JT, Mathieu D, et al.** Hepatocellular adenoma: color Doppler and pathologic correlations. *Radiology* 1994;190:741–744.
20. **Kim TK, Jank HJ, Burns PN, et al.** Focal nodular hyperplasia and hepatic adenoma: differentiation with low mechanical index contrast-enhanced sonography. *AJR Am J Roentgenol* 2008;190:58–66.
21. **Jang HG, Kim TK, Burns PN, et al.** Enhancement patterns of hepatocellular carcinoma at contrast-enhanced US: comparison with histologic differentiation. *Radiology* 2007;244:898–906.
22. **Claudon M, Dietrich C, Choi B, et al.** Guidelines and Good Clinical Practice Recommendations for Contrast Enhanced Ultrasound (CEUS)—update 2012. A WFUSMB-EFSUMB initiative in cooperation with representatives of AFSUMB, AIUM, ASUM, FLAUS and ICUS. *Ultrasound Med Biol* 2013;39:187–210.
23. **Kew MC.** Tumors of the liver. In: Zakim D, Boyer TD, eds. *Hepatology: a textbook of liver disease.* Philadelphia, PA: Saunders; 1982:1048–1084.
24. **Harvey C.** Contrast media, ultrasound, application in focal splenic lesions. In: Baert A, ed. *Encyclopedia of imaging, volume 1.* Berlin, Germany: Springer; 2008:528–531.
25. **Stang A, Keles H, Hentschke S, et al.** Differentiation of benign from malignant focal splenic lesions using sulphur hexafluoride-filled microbubble contrast-enhanced pulse-inversion sonography. *AJR Am J Roentgenol* 2009;193:709–721.
26. **Herbay A, Barreiros AP, Ignee A, et al.** Contrast-enhanced ultrasonography with sonovue: differentiation between benign and malignant lesions of the spleen. *J Ultrasound Med* 2009;28:421–434.
27. **Sutherland T, Temple F, Galvin A, et al.** Contrast-enhanced ultrasound of the spleen: an introduction and pictorial essay. *Insights Imaging* 2011;2:515–524.
28. **Yu X, Yu J, Liang P, et al.** Real-time contrast-enhanced ultrasound in diagnosing of focal spleen lesions. *Eur Radiol* 2012;81:430–436.
29. **Catalano O, Sandomenico F, Matarazzo I, et al.** Contrast-enhanced sonography of the spleen. *AJR Am J Roentgenol* 2005;184:1150–1156.
30. **Gorg C, Weide R, Schwerk WB.** Malignant splenic lymphoma: sonographic patterns, diagnosis and follow-up. *Clin Radiol* 1997;52:535–540.
31. **Picardi M, Soricelli A, Pane F, et al.** Contrast-enhanced harmonic compound US of the spleen to increase staging accuracy in patients with Hodgkin lymphoma: a prospective study. *Radiology* 2009;251:574–582.
32. **Schön CA, Görg C, Ramaswamy A, et al.** Splenic metastases in a large unselected autopsy series. *Pathol Res Pract* 2006;202:351–356.
33. **Cokkinos DD, Antypa EG, Skilakaki M, et al.** Contrast enhanced ultrasound of the kidneys: what is it capable of? *Biomed Res Int* 2013;2013:13.
34. **Wei K, Le E, Bin JP, et al.** Quantification of renal blood flow with contrast-enhanced ultrasound. *J Am Coll Cardiol* 2001;37:1135–1140.
35. **Kishimoto N, Mori Y, Nishiue T, et al.** Renal blood flow measurement with contrast-enhanced harmonic ultrasonography: evaluation of dopamine-induced changes in renal cortical perfusion in humans. *Clin Nephrol* 2003;59:423–428.
36. **Barr RG, Peterson C, Hindi A.** Evaluation of indeterminate renal masses with contrast-enhanced US: a diagnostic performance study. *Radiology* 2013,271.133–142.
37. **Nicolau C, Bunesch L, Sebastia C.** Renal complex cysts in adults: contrast-enhanced ultrasound. *Abdom Imaging* 2011;36:742–752.
38. **Quaia E, Bertolotto M, Cioffi V, et al.** Comparison of contrast-enhanced sonography with unenhanced sonography and contrast-enhanced CT in the diagnosis of malignancy in complex cystic renal masses. *AJR Am J Roentgenol* 2008;191:1239–1249.

39. **Wu Y, Du L, Li F, et al.** Renal oncocytoma: contrast-enhanced sonographic features. *J Ultrasound Med* 2013;32:441–448.
40. **Correas JM, Claudon M, Tranquart F, et al.** The kidney: imaging with microbubble contrast agents. *Ultrasound Q* 2006;22:53–66.
41. **Bertolotto M, Martegani A, Aiani L, et al.** Value of contrast-enhanced ultrasonography for detecting renal infarcts proven by contrast enhanced CT. A feasibility study. *Eur Radiol* 2008;18:376–383.
42. **Piscaglia F, Nolsøe C, Dietrich CF, et al.** The EFSUMB guidelines and recommendations on the clinical practice of contrast enhanced ultrasound (CEUS): update 2011 on nonhepatic applications. *Ultraschall Med* 2012;33:33–59.
43. **Chen Y, Huang J, Xia L, et al.** Monitoring laparoscopic radiofrequency renal lesions in real time using contrast-enhanced ultrasonography: an open-label, randomized, comparative pilot trial. *J Endourol* 2013;27:697–704.
44. **Meloni MF, Bertolotto M, Alberzoni C, et al.** Follow-up after percutaneous radiofrequency ablation of renal cell carcinoma: contrast-enhanced sonography versus contrast-enhanced CT or MRI. *Am J Roentgenol* 2008; 191:1233–1238.
45. **Valentino M, Serra C, Zironi G, et al.** Blunt abdominal trauma: emergency contrast enhanced sonography for detection of solid organ injuries. *Am J Roentgenol* 2006;186:1361–1367.
46. **Greis C.** Quantitative evaluation of microvascular blood flow by contrast-enhanced ultrasound (CEUS). *Clin Hemorheol Microcirc* 2011; 49:137–149.
47. **Dietrich CF, Averkiou MA, Correas JM, et al.** An EFSUMB introduction into dynamic contrast-enhanced ultrasound (DCE-US) for quantification of tumour perfusion. *Ultraschall Med* 2012;33:344–351.
48. **Stange EF, Travis SP, Vermeire S, et al.** European evidence based consensus on the diagnosis and management of Crohn's disease: definitions and diagnosis. *Gut* 2006;55:1–15.
49. **Ripollés T, Rausell N, Paredes JM et al.** Effectiveness of contrast-enhanced ultrasound for characterization of intestinal inflammation in Crohn's disease: a comparison with surgical histopathology analysis. *J Crohns Colitis* 2013;7:120–128.
50. **Parente F, Greco S, Molteni M, et al.** Modern imaging of Crohn's disease using bowel US. *Inflamm Bowel Dis* 2004;10:452–461.
51. **Panés J, Bouzas R, Chaparro M, et al.** Systematic review: the use of ultrasonography, computed tomography and magnetic resonance imaging for the diagnosis, assessment of activity and abdominal complications of Crohn's disease. *Aliment Pharmacol Ther* 2011;34:125–145.
52. **Bodily KD, Fletcher JG, Solem CA, et al.** Crohn's disease: mural attenuation and thickness at contrast-enhanced CT enterography—correlation with endoscopic and histologic findings of inflammation. *Radiology* 2006;238:505–516.
53. **Siddiki HA, Fidler JL, Fletcher JG, et al.** Prospective comparison of state-of-the-art MR enterography and CT enterography in small-bowel Crohn's disease. *AJR Am J Roentgenol* 2009;193:113–121.
54. **Quaia E.** Contrast-enhanced ultrasound of the small bowel in Crohn's disease. *Abdom Imaging* 2013;38:1005–1013.
55. **Wong DD, Forbes GM, Zelesco M, et al.** Crohn's disease activity: quantitative contrast-enhanced ultrasound assessment. *Abdom Imaging* 2012; 37:369–376.
56. **Girlich C, Jung EM, Iesalnieks I, et al.** Quantitative assessment of bowel wall vascularisation in Crohn's disease with contrast-enhanced ultrasound and perfusion analysis. *Clin Hemorheol Microcirc* 2009;43:141–148.

CHAPTER

35 Pediatric Applications of Perfusion Ultrasound

Karl Muchantef, MD, Thomas Scholbach, Dr. med. habil, and Ricardo Faingold, MD

Introduction

Knowledge of blood flow and tissue perfusion can influence clinical decisions and patient management in a gamut of disease processes. Many diseases are associated with perfusion changes, such as inflammatory processes, organ failure, transplant rejection, arterial stenosis, tumor growth and necrosis, hypoperfusion, and ischemia. The Doppler shift of ultrasound (US) frequency can be used to depict blood flow velocity and to quantify it. US and Doppler techniques are currently very popular and have many advantages over other modalities with potential in perfusion mapping: computed tomography (radiation exposure), magnetic resonance imaging (cost, availability, length of exam, sedation in young children), and nuclear medicine (limited morphologic information, radiation).

Several publications using color Doppler sonography (CDS) assessed quantification of tissue perfusion by counting color Doppler signals in still images.[1–3] There are also reports on the use of quantitative Doppler signal analysis with and without contrast-enhancing agents.[4–9] Despite such developments, it is not a simple task to obtain blood flow and tissue perfusion data in a reliable, noninvasive, inexpensive, and radiation-free manner. This chapter discusses the most currently used Doppler techniques (color Doppler, power Doppler, pulsed Doppler, and contrast-enhanced US) and also the potential of perfusion quantification with dynamic CDS or dynamic tissue perfusion measurement (DTPM) in children. Spectral Doppler velocity measurements and resistive index (RI) are still the basis of many scientific medical investigations of perfusion, despite offering a limited representation of actual tissue perfusion, as detailed below.

Color and Power Doppler

Color Doppler uses red and blue shades to depict blood flow toward or away from the transducer (according to equipment settings), with differing shades representing differing velocities of motion. The color hue assigned to a pixel results from the angle-dependent Doppler frequency shift returning from that pixel. By convention, higher velocities of blood flow are assigned a brighter color hue. The measured US frequency shift is displayed as an array of colors within a gray-scale image, depicting the local velocity of blood flow. Color Doppler hence provides an image with tissue morphology depicted in gray scale and blood flow depicted by color.[10,11] Power Doppler imaging depicts the strength of the Doppler-shifted signal rather than the frequency shift of that signal. That is to say, the color hue depicted relates mainly to the volume of moving blood, rather than the velocity and direction of the flow. Directional information is lost in power Doppler imaging; its advantage is increased sensitivity to low flow as compared to color Doppler.[11]

Spectral Doppler

In the case of spectral Doppler imaging, a time velocity tracing depicts variations in blood flow velocity at a point within a vessel during the cardiac cycle. Spectral Doppler analysis has gained tremendous popularity and found many clinical applications. Using the spectral tracing, the RI may be calculated from the equation:

$$\mathrm{RI} = (\mathrm{PSV} - \mathrm{EDV}) / \mathrm{PSV},$$

where PSV is the peak systolic velocity, and EDV is the end-diastolic velocity. This ratio describes the relative degree of velocity drop during a complete heart cycle. The RI calculation is independent of the angle of insonation; the RI expresses the ratio of two velocities, both identically affected by the Doppler angle.

The RI is sometimes interpreted as a parameter of blood flow itself. It is often assumed that a high RI signifies a low perfusion state and an increasing RI indicates decreasing perfusion; however, this is not necessarily the case.[12] RI relies upon only two velocity measurements (PSV and EDV) obtained at a single point in a single vessel. As a surrogate measure of tissue perfusion, RI measurements disregard a crucial point: tissue viability depends not only on the pulsatility of blood flow or the resistance against it but also on blood flow volumes (Table 35.1).

Contrast-Enhanced Ultrasound

Microbubble-based intravenous contrast agents are not routinely used in pediatric imaging in North America. Intravenously injected microbubbles enhance US backscatter by producing harmonic frequencies that are multiples of the transmitted frequency and therefore increase the US signal from flowing blood, particularly in the arterial system and microvasculature.[10] Level of saturation and velocity to reach the level of saturation are obtained with dedicated software. Contrast-enhanced ultrasound (CEUS) has many clinical applications,[13–15] some of which are discussed later (Table 35.2).

TABLE 35.1 Resistive Index

Measures one point in one vessel
Velocity information usually available
Cardiac cycle dynamics preserved
Noninvasive
Unlimited observation time
Inexpensive
Fast acquisition

Dynamic Tissue Perfusion Measurement

A software-based DTPM technique is capable of extracting dynamic (changing with heart cycle) flow data of perfusion signals from color Doppler sonographic videos. Perfused area and actual local perfusion velocity within an arbitrarily chosen region of interest (ROI) are extracted automatically by software from a sonographic video (PixelFlux, Chameleon-Software, Leipzig, Germany).[16] No ECG gating is required, and the software recognizes the variation of flow and is able to stablish the cardiac cycle based on a pattern.

The guiding idea behind DTPM is to quantify tissue perfusion by referring to all relevant parameters that influence the total amount of blood passing through a tissue section during a complete heart cycle. These are the mean perfusion velocity of all vessels and the mean perfused area of the tissue section under investigation. Both are directly proportional to the amount of transported blood. Both do also change significantly during one complete cardiac cycle. It is therefore necessary to start with the measurement of these two basic parameters at the beginning of a heartbeat and to continue in as short time intervals as possible to the end of the heartbeat. This is important because significant differences between momentary systolic and diastolic perfusion may exist even in tiny vessels.

From these data, a mean perfusion velocity, as well as a mean perfused area, are calculated thus referring all measurement to the very basic rhythm of perfusion—one complete heart cycle. By multiplication of these mean values—mean perfused area and mean perfusion velocity—mean perfusion intensity is calculated. Mean perfusion intensity thus also refers to the area of the tissue section that is captured by the ROI of the current investigation: mean velocity (v) of all pixels is multiplied by the area (A) of all colored pixels contained with the ROI and divided by the total area of the ROI (colored pixels plus gray-scale area of nonperfused tissue). Thereby, the mean flow intensity value of the ROI (I) is calculated.

$$I[\text{cm/s}] = A\left[\text{cm}^2\right] \times v[\text{cm/s}] / A_{\text{ROI}}\left[\text{cm}^2\right]$$

Following this algorithm, a dynamic (with respect to the ever-changing values during a full heart cycle) mean perfusion intensity can be calculated of a tissue section in a freehand or geometrically standardized ROI (Fig. 35-1).

As with any measurement, a crucial point is standardization—in DTPM, it is the presetting of the US equipment. Color Doppler frequency as well as gain have to be kept constant for comparable investigations. Color flow velocity settings may be changed to avoid aliasing if necessary. The software recognizes the change of color scale values automatically (Table 35.3).

TABLE 35.2 Contrast-Enhanced Ultrasound

Measures enhancement in an ROI
Velocity information not available
Cardiac cycle dynamics not preserved
Invasive
Limited observation time
Expensive
Slow acquisition, requires postprocessing

Practical Issues Regarding DTPM

Spectral Doppler, color Doppler, and power Doppler sonography are often used to assess blood flow and provide an estimate of organ perfusion. Quantitative evaluation of blood flow with CDS using pixel count per square centimeter has been described in assessment of bowel perfusion.[1,2] There are also reports on the use of quantitative Doppler signal analysis with and without contrast-enhancing agents.[5–9] However, it may be time-consuming and difficult to reproduce in the clinical and research settings. Evaluation of Doppler spectral waveform is helpful in determining the characteristics of blood flow patterns, which are affected by the metabolic status of the organ supplied by that vessel, hemodynamic status, and age of the patient.[17] DTPM offers a standardized, quantitative assessment of tissue perfusion within a definable ROI. Data are extracted over the cardiac cycle and flow parameters obtained.

Applications of Doppler US and DTPM

To demonstrate the broad applicability of Doppler US and DTPM, some examples of clinical applications are given below in infants, children, and adolescents.

Infants

Assessment of blood flow and organ perfusion in infants has been traditionally done by spectral Doppler and sometimes by CDS.[2,17,18] Recent use of CDS with tissue perfusion quantification has shown that this technique is promising and with great potential as a noninvasive tool in the research setting and clinical practice.[19,20]

Kidneys

The use of RI is well established in the evaluation of the kidneys. It is well known that RI of renal arteries varies in the first 12 months of life. They are usually measured in the arcuate or interlobar arteries. In term infants, the RI ranges from 0.6 to 0.8, although in premature babies, RI may reach 0.9 in the renal arteries. The hemodynamic status and the structural and functional immaturity of the kidneys in neonates are responsible for these changes.[17]

Acute kidney injury (AKI) has been associated with perinatal asphyxia, hypotension, or cardiac failure. It may develop with or without changes in creatinine levels or urine output. Decreased blood flow velocity in the renal arteries with pulsed Doppler imaging has been described in severe hypoxic–ischemic injury (HII).[3] CDS evaluation of renal parenchyma[20] appears to be a useful tool for quantification of renal perfusion in AKI (Fig. 35-2).

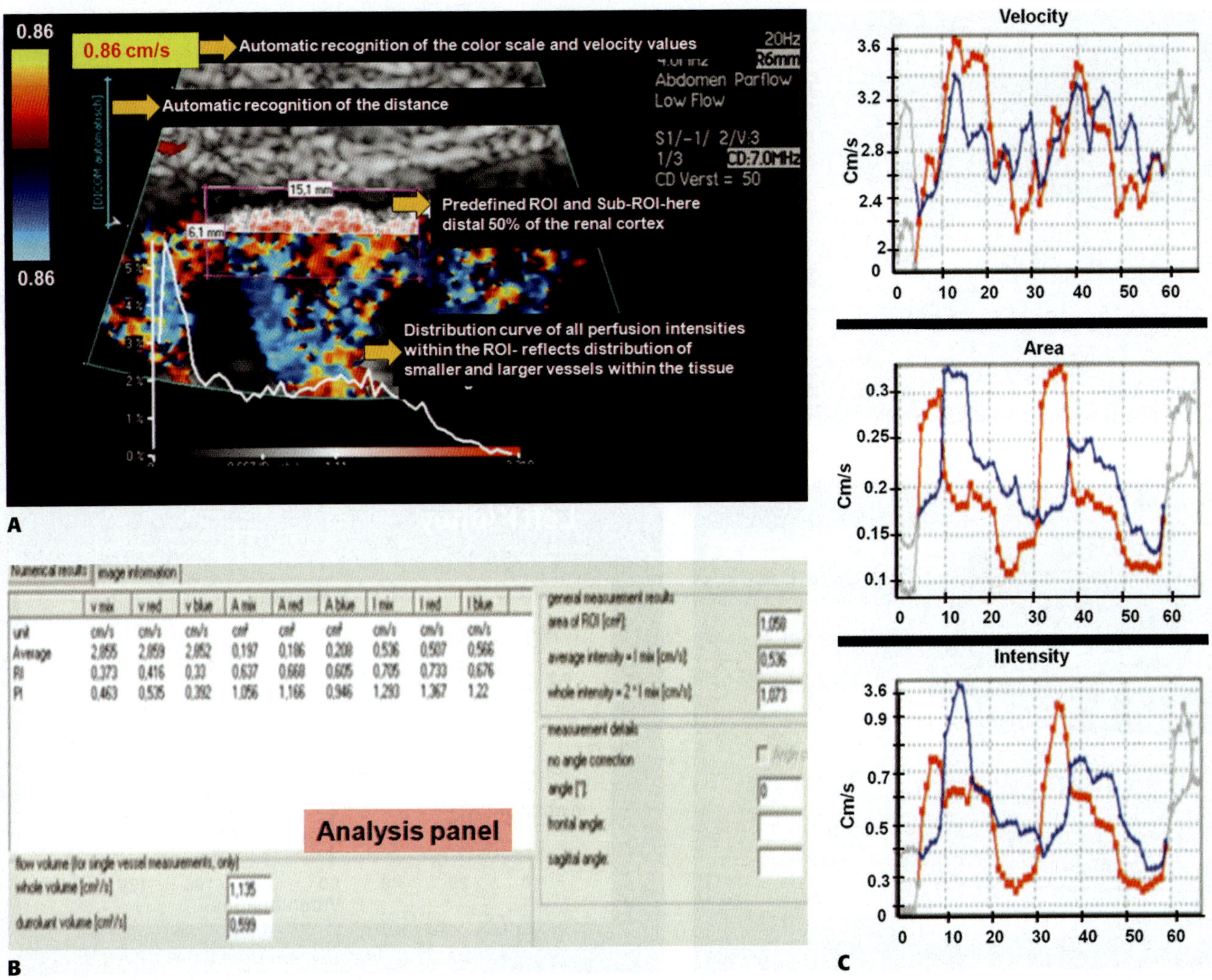

Figure 35-1. Tissue perfusion of the renal cortex. **A:** A standardized region of interest (ROI) is defined with a sub-ROI defining the distal 50% of the cortex. Each ROI contains colored pixels and nonperfused tissue. Numerical description of vessel distribution according to their perfusion intensities with associated distribution curve is included (*white curve*). **B:** Tables of dynamic tissue perfusion measurement (DTPM) results are shown in analysis panel and in **(C)**. Time course diagrams of relevant perfusion parameters (*graphs*).

Bowel

US Doppler interrogation of the gastrointestinal tract is useful for assessment of superior mesenteric artery (SMA) Doppler waveform and intestinal perfusion. The flow pattern in the SMA is of high resistance in the fasting state and becomes of low resistance with loss of reversal of diastolic flow in the postprandial state.[17] In normal fasting neonates, bowel wall perfusion usually ranges from one to nine color Doppler signals per centimeter square (mean = 3.78, standard error of mean = 0.20).[2]

TABLE 35.3 Tissue Perfusion Measurement
Measures perfusion of all vessels in an ROI
Velocity information available
Cardiac cycle dynamics preserved
Noninvasive
Unlimited observation time
Inexpensive
Fast acquisition, requires postprocessing

Necrotizing Enterocolitis

Intestinal mural perfusion can be assessed directly, in real time at the bedside, with CDS. In 2005, the use of color Doppler was described to assess bowel wall perfusion in necrotizing enterocolitis (NEC).[2] In neonates with NEC, color Doppler US revealed three types of flow in the bowel wall: normal, increased, and absent. Normal CDS flow corresponded to the values obtained in control infants. CDS flow was considered increased when certain types of hyperemic flow pattern were different from the normal neonates. They were described as follows: "circular" flow pattern around the bowel; a "Y" pattern of distal mesenteric and subserosal vessel; and parallel CDS lines or a "zebra" pattern due to increased flow in mucosal folds. CDS perfusion was considered absent when no mural CDS signals were demonstrated (Fig. 35-3). These nonperfused bowel loops were correlated with abdominal x-rays (AXR) and with laparotomy and

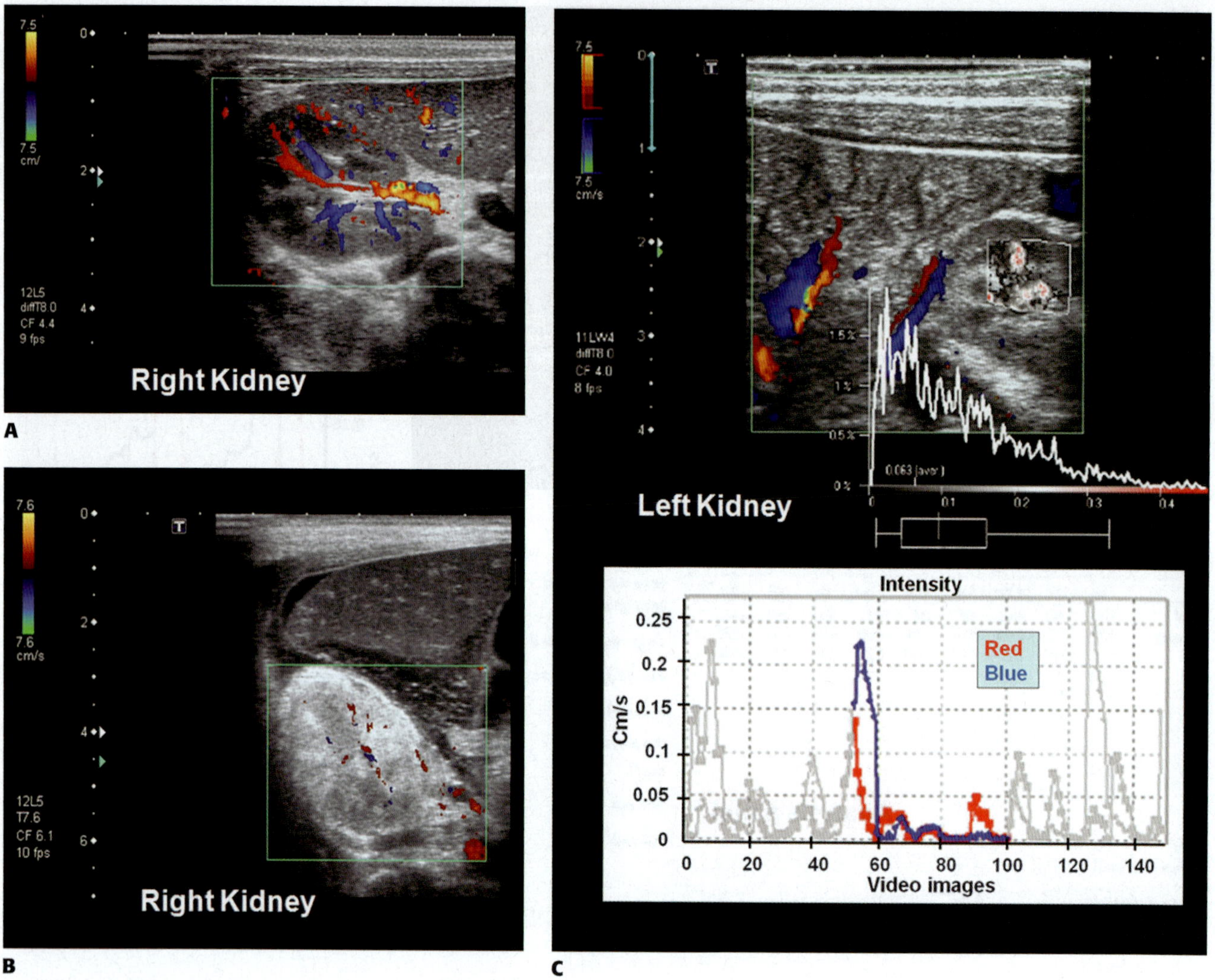

Figure 35-2. Renal perfusion with color Doppler sonography (CDS). **A:** A 2-day-old boy. Perfusion with CDS shows normal parenchymal flow. **B:** A 1-day-old boy. CDS shows decreased perfusion within hyperechogenic parenchyma. **C:** A 2-day-old girl. DTPM with quantification of ROI using dedicated software and renal perfusion intensity curve shows values of 0.15 cm/s, indicating preserved flow. *Red* and *blue curves* represent blood flow toward and away from transducer during dynamic CDS measurements.

pathologic specimens. The sensitivity of CDS to detect gangrenous bowel was 100% compared to 40% for AXR.[2]

Intestinal Hypoxic–Ischemic Injury

Asphyxia may result in perinatal hypoxia, hypercarbia, and acidosis. It may cause redistribution of blood flow with an increase in the flow to the brain, heart, and adrenal glands and a decrease to the kidneys, bowel, and skin. Multiple organ failure has been reported in more than 50% of infants with severe perinatal asphyxia.[18]

It has been reported that pulsed Doppler interrogation in the SMA is altered in neonates with perinatal asphyxia. They showed a significant decrease in the mean blood flow velocities and increase in RI in severe HII.[18]

Evaluation of intestinal mural blood flow with CDS and dynamic CDS or DTPM has been described as preserved intramural perfusion and increased or decreased bowel perfusion. In a retrospective pilot study, we evaluated 28 neonates using DTPM. We were able to assess intramural perfusion of a specified ROI and observed a trend toward a decreased bowel wall perfusion (Fig. 35-4) during the first 24 hours of life in 7 nonsurvivors compared to 21 survivors (0.040 ± 0.015 cm/s $\times$ 0.052 ± 0.029 cm/s).[21]

Therefore, assessment of the mesenteric circulation and bowel perfusion in perinatal asphyxia may have a role in predicting outcomes and understanding the pathophysiology of bowel injury in HII.

Brain

Normal cerebral blood flow (CBF) changes over time particularly in neonates. Cerebral perfusion corresponds to up to 25% of cardiac output in healthy infants. CBF is affected by cardiac output and also with variations of pO_2 and pCO_2, for example, patients with patent ductus arteriosus may have CBF changes according to the severity of the disease. There is a physiologic increase in CBF during the first days of life, with corresponding increase in PSV and EDV. In premature neonates, resistive indices are known to be higher than in term neonates. The normal RI of intracranial arteries in term infants in the first day of life has been described to be 0.726 with a standard deviation of 0.057.[22]

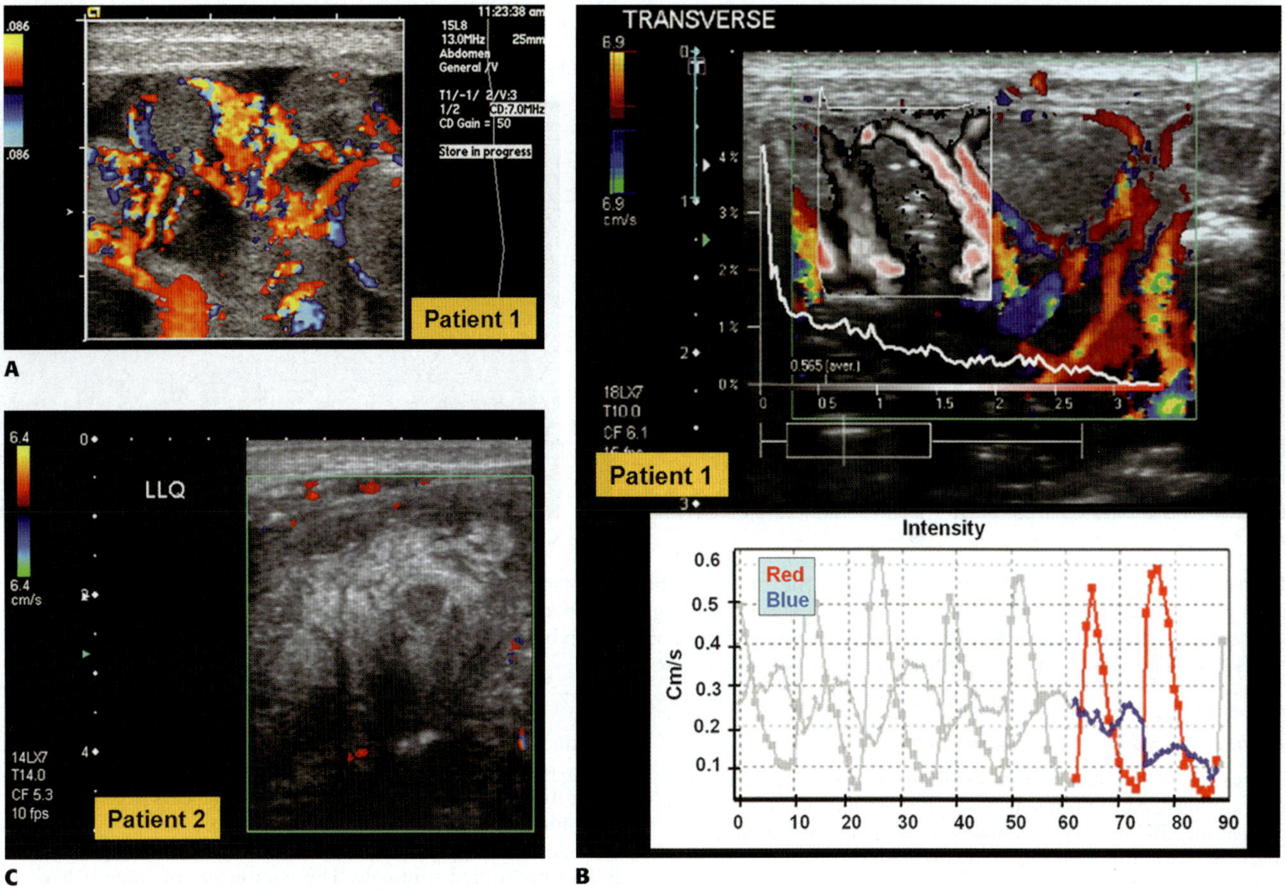

Figure 35-3. Ultrasound images of the intestine in neonates with necrotizing enterocolitis (NEC). **A:** High-resolution CDS transverse mage shows mixed pattern with "circular" and "zebra" patterns due to viable hyperemic perfusion pattern in bowel loops. **B:** DTPM with quantification of ROI using dedicated software and intestinal perfusion intensity curve shows values of 0.6 cm/s, indicating hyperemic flow in NEC. The patient did well clinically. **C:** Different patient: CDS transverse image shows featureless loops of bowel with absent perfusion in a premature baby with severe NEC confirmed by laparotomy to be gangrenous bowel.

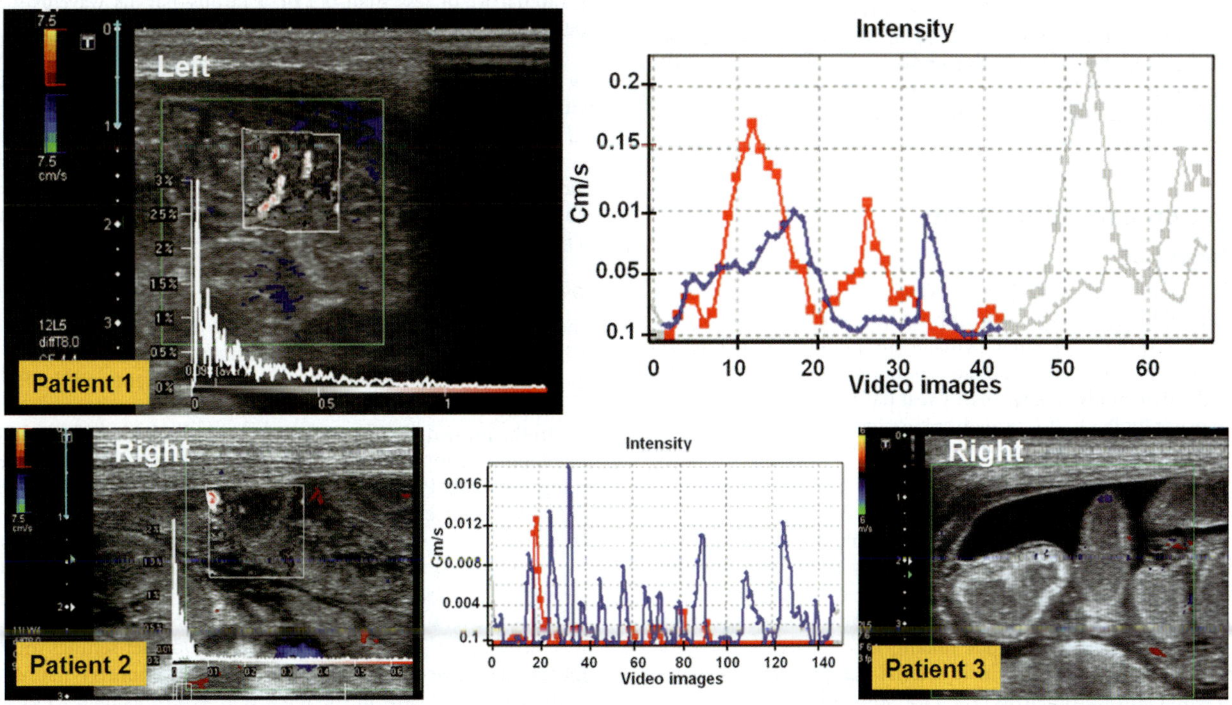

Figure 35-4. Intestinal color Doppler sonography and hypoxic–ischemic injury (HII). Patient 1 (*upper row*), a 1-day-old girl; DTPM demonstrates preserved bowel wall flow with quantification of ROI using dedicated software. Intestinal perfusion intensity curve with values of up to 0.17 cm/s. Patient 2 (*lower row*), a 2-day-old boy; DTPM shows decreased perfusion and corresponding intestinal perfusion intensity curve with values of up to 0.013 cm/s. Patient 3 (*lower row*); CDS shows some decrease in bowel perfusion and edematous bowel wall with associated ascites in a different infant.

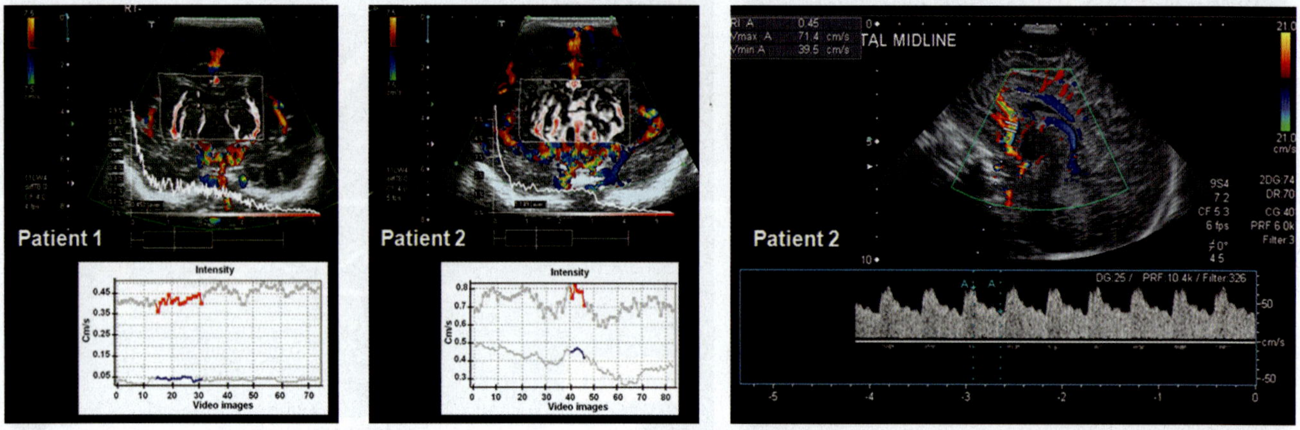

A B C

Figure 35-5. Hypoxic–ischemic encephalopathy (HIE) in two patients. **A:** Patient 1: A 1-day-old boy with mild HIE. DTPM shows ROI in basal ganglia to calculate cerebral perfusion intensity, and corresponding perfusion intensity curve with perfusion up to 0.45 cm/s. **B,C:** Patient 2: A 1-day-old girl with severe HIE. **B:** DTPM demonstrates very increased perfusion in basal ganglia (0.9 cm/s). **C:** Demonstrates pulsed Doppler interrogation with decreased intracranial resistive index (RI) in neonate with severe HIE.

Perinatal Asphyxia and Hypoxic–Ischemic Injury

The causes of hypoxic–ischemic encephalopathy (HIE) are complex and related to multiple factors. They are thought to be due to changes in CBF by a combination of systemic hypotension, abnormal cerebral autoregulation leading to cerebral hypoperfusion, and subsequent HII.[18,20] During the postasphyxiated period, an increase in CBF within the first few hours of life may last for hours or days. This period is known as reperfusion phase and may be responsible for reperfusion brain injury.

In neonates with HIE, increased CBF velocities up to three times more than controls with decrease in RI of the intracranial arteries to 0.5 or less, measured at 12 to 72 hours of life, have been described in severe HII.[18,23] In a retrospective pilot study,[19] cerebral perfusion intensity with DTPM of basal ganglia values were significantly higher in the 7 nonsurvivors (Fig. 35-5) compared to 23 survivors (0.226 ± 0.221 vs. 0.111 ± 0.082 cm/s; $p = 0.02$). In neonates, at risk for stroke, CDS may also be used for assessment of luxury perfusion.

Children and Adolescents

Kidneys

Normally, the peak systolic flow velocity in the main renal arteries should be up to 180 cm/s, with diastolic forward flow of 25 to 50 cm/s.[17] At the renal parenchyma, there should be a brisk systolic upstroke with an acceleration index of greater than 300 cm/s^2. Most consider that children older than 1 year have an RI similar to that of normal adults, 0.5 to 0.7, though some suggest that adult values are realized later in childhood.[24,25]

Renal Artery Hypertension

Hypertension in children is usually secondary to parenchymal renal disease or lesions of the renal artery itself, with fibromuscular dysplasia as the most common cause of renal artery disease in children.[26–28] Additional causes of pediatric renin–angiotensin-mediated hypertension include inflammatory arteritis, congenital aortic coarctation, and extrinsic arterial compression (as may be seen with neurofibromatosis type 1), among others.

Imaging of the main renal artery for hypertension has focused on two parameters: PSV and renal-to-aortic velocity ratio. As mentioned, 180 cm/s is considered the upper limit for normal PSV. A ratio of 3.5 is considered the upper limit for the normal renal artery-to-aorta ratio.[17] These criteria are well established in adult populations, though their diagnostic performance is largely unknown in children.

Spectral Doppler imaging at the level of the renal parenchyma is also performed routinely. The parameters of interest here are acceleration time and RI, as detailed above. These parameters may be limited by their normal variability in health kidneys.[29,30] While the role of US in the evaluation of pediatric renal artery stenosis remains controversial,[31] a recent study of 35 pediatric patients found a sensitivity of 90% and specificity of 68% for detecting a vascular cause for hypertension in high-risk individuals when an intrarenal RI of less than 0.5 or a tardus–parvus waveform was identified[32] (Fig. 35-6).

Contrast-enhanced US has been studied in adult populations for the diagnosis of renal artery stenosis.[33,34] Studies suggest that with the addition of contrast agent, the positive and negative predictive values of US in these patients are increased. DTPM may also contribute to the diagnosis of renal artery stenosis as diminished perfusion may be demonstrated at the level of the renal cortex, where the renin-secreting juxtaglomerular apparatus is located (Fig. 35-6).

Renal Transplantation

The normal RI of a transplanted kidney in a pediatric recipient is 0.5 to 0.8.[35] When grafting adult kidneys into pediatric patients, an inverse correlation between size of the recipient and the RI was found.[35]

In the immediate posttransplant period, certain expected findings should be appreciated; transient anastomotic edema may cause mildly elevated PSV, turbulent flow, and diminished RI.[36] Graft edema may conversely result in increased RI with diminished diastolic flow.[36]

In children, graft thrombosis is the leading cause of transplant loss in the 1st year, accounting for 35% of 1st year losses and 18% of all losses.[37] Arterial thrombosis may be diagnosed by US, noting that hyperacute rejection may be a mimic, and Doppler settings must be optimized for detection of low flow. Venous thrombosis is manifested by the absence of flow in the renal vein as well as high RI or even reversal of flow in the artery; associated graft edema is expected.

Renal artery stenosis is a late vascular complication seen in transplantation. With the exception of two studies that we know of,[38,39]

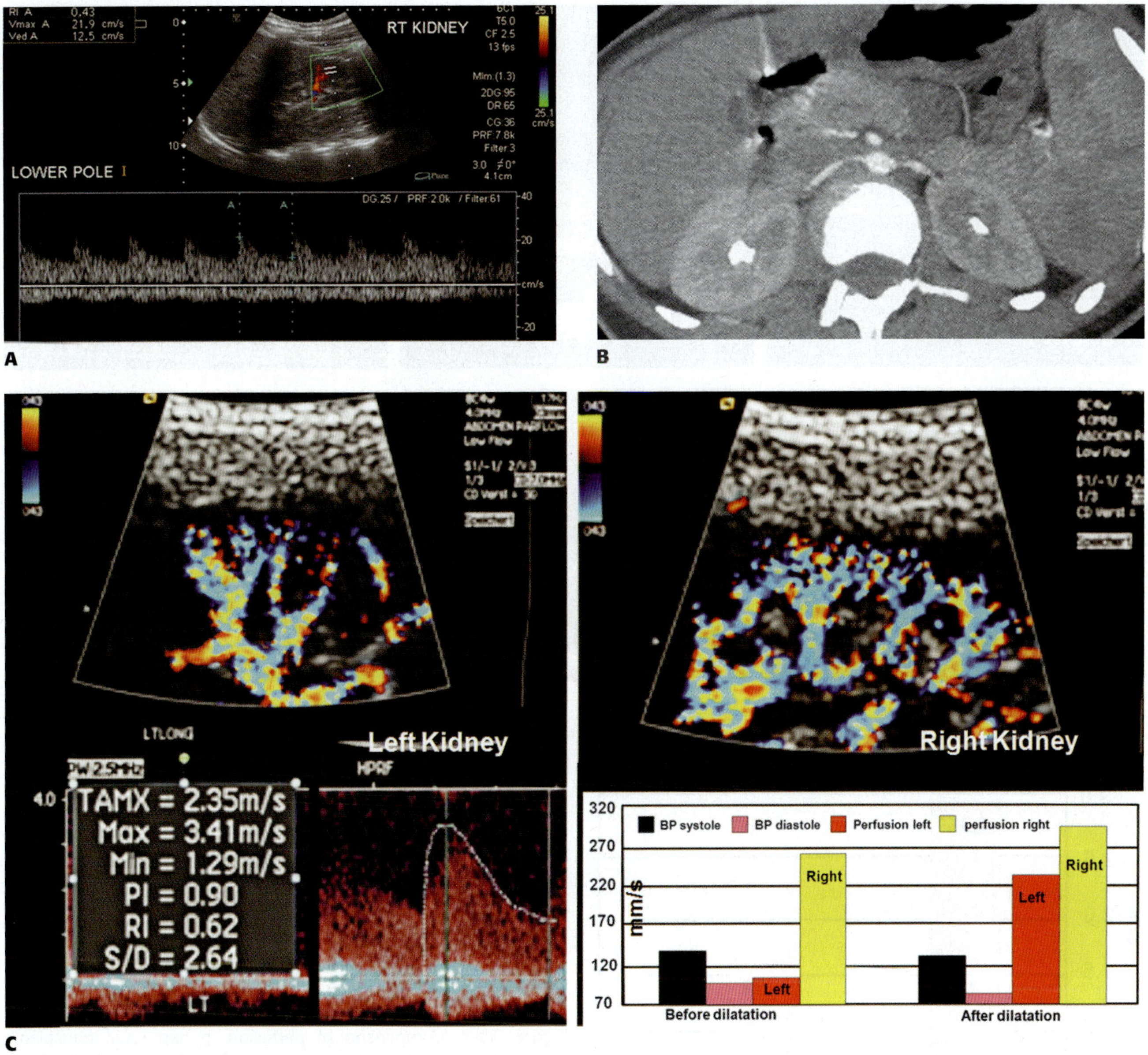

Figure 35-6. Renal artery stenosis. Screening US from a 12-year-old female with hypertension **(A)** shows a RI of 0.43. Oblique axial maximum intensity projection image from CT angiography **(B)** shows bilateral proximal renal artery stenosis. Findings were confirmed at angiography (not shown); angioplasty was performed with resulting resolution of hypertension. DTPM from a different patient **(C)** shows the left and right kidneys, respectively. Flow spectrum of the stenotic left renal artery shows a maximum flow velocity of 341 cm/s. DTPM perfusion intensity measurements and diastolic/systolic blood pressure before and after angioplasty are shown on the lower panel.

the work relating to posttransplant arterial stenosis has been performed in adults and extrapolated to children. It is our practice to use the same cutoff values for PSV and renal artery-to-iliac artery ratio as is used in native kidneys: 180 cm/s and 3.5, respectively.

Unfortunately, the common causes of delayed intrinsic graft dysfunction—cyclosporine toxicity, allograft rejection, and acute tubular necrosis—all result in a nonspecific elevation in resistive indices.[36,40]

The role of DTPM in the setting of renal transplant follow-up has been evaluated. A study of 78 adult renal transplant recipients showed a correlation of tissue perfusion measurements with histologic features of peritubular inflammation and interstitial fibrosis.[41] A DTPM study of 38 renal transplants in children and young adults showed a marked decline in cortical perfusion as early as 1 year after transplant.[42] This decline was more marked in the peripheral 50% of the cortex (Fig. 35-7). In parallel, the perfusion pulsatility was rising in these transplants with decreasing cortical perfusion. Moreover, in a recent publication, DTPM was shown to have predictive value in anticipating the survival of transplant function.[43]

Diabetic Nephropathy

DTPM has been studied in assessing renal microvascular damage in pediatric patients with type 1 diabetes mellitus and apparently normal renal function without microalbuminuria.[44] In a study of 92 pediatric patients as compared to 71 healthy control subjects, it was found that perfusion in the peripheral aspect of the cortex was 31% decreased in the diabetes group relative to controls.

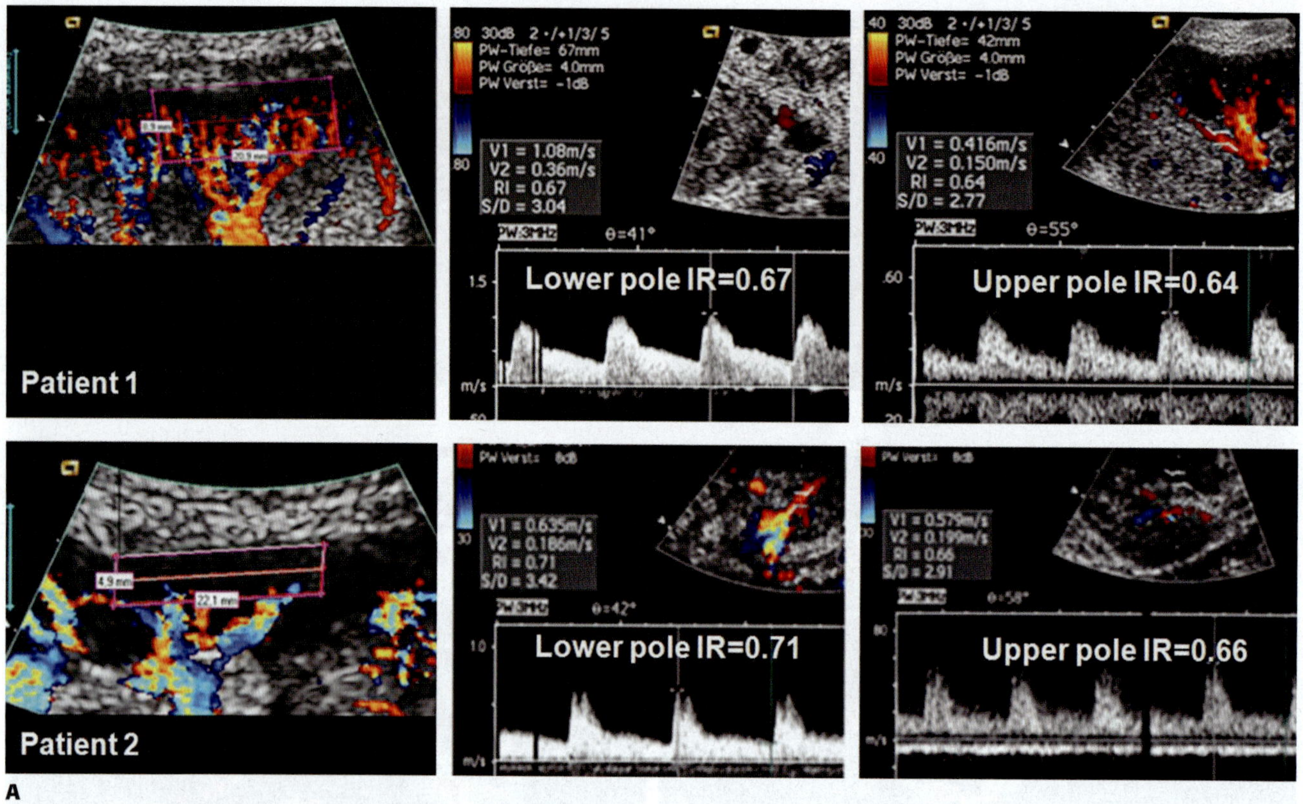

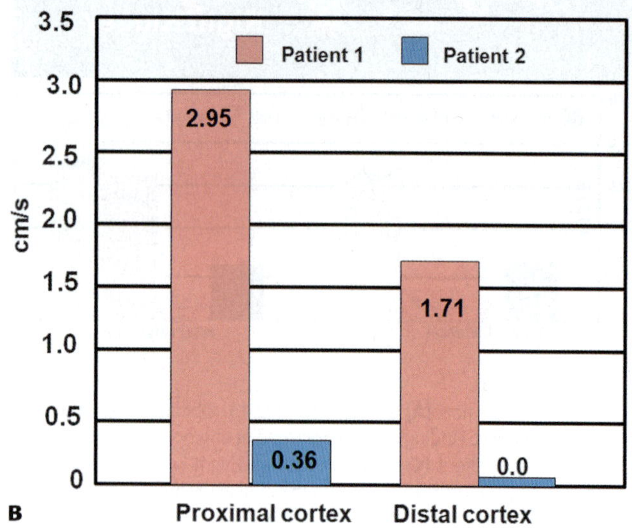

Figure 35-7. **Comparison of perfusion in two renal transplants with differing function. A:** Patient 1: Well-functioning transplant with good cortical vascularization and normal serum creatinine. Patient 2: Insufficient transplant with total loss of peripheral cortical microvasculature and elevated creatinine. Resistive indices are similar in both transplants. **B:** Perfusion intensity graph shows the values for the proximal and distal renal cortices of the two patients.

Bowel

In clinical practice, evaluation of patients with inflammatory bowel disease relies upon clinical, laboratory, endoscopic, and imaging parameters, as appropriate. Doppler US can play a role in decision making and management. A recent meta-analysis demonstrated no significant difference in the diagnostic accuracy among US, MRI, and CT in the evaluation of patient's with inflammatory bowel disease[45] (Fig. 35-8).

Blood flow in normal pediatric splanchnic arteries has been described. Bowel inflammation results in increased volume of splanchnic blood flow with a concomitant decrease in RI.[46–49] Maconi et al.[49] found no relation between splanchnic hemodynamics and disease activity, though they do report decreased RI in all patients with Crohn's relative to control subjects. As expected, there is also correlation between the presence of Crohn disease and elevated levels of portal venous blood flow.[49] In their study of 92 pediatric patients, Spalinger et al.[1] found a correlation between vessel density measured in the bowel wall by CDS, bowel wall thickness, and disease activity in Crohn patients.

Contrast-enhanced US in the setting of Crohn's has been well studied, with several potential clinical applications identified. Contrast-enhanced US has proven effective in differentiating hypervascular inflammatory stenoses from hypovascular fibrotic

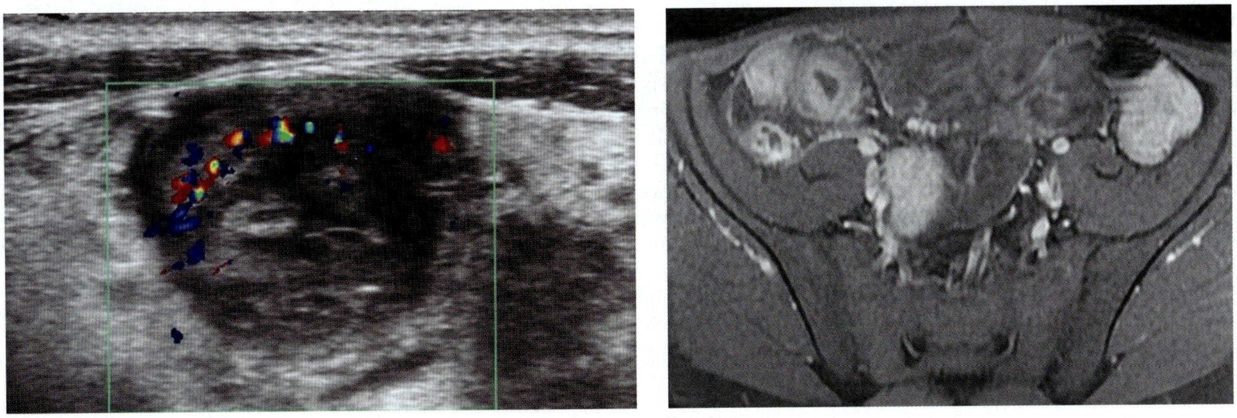

A B

Figure 35-8. Crohn disease in a 16-year-old male. **A:** CDS shows hyperemia and mural thickening involving the cecum. **B:** Contrast-enhanced T1 with fat saturation MR sequence shows thickening and hyperenhancement of the terminal ileum, cecum, and appendix.

stenoses.[50] Monitoring treatment effect is also possible by CEUS. Quantitative changes in the pattern of enhancement in successfully treated bowel have been shown after pharmacologic treatment.[51] Further, residual hyperemia of a thickened bowel wall after treatment may portend relapse.[52]

DTPM has been studied in the setting of Crohn disease. In a report of 14 children with Crohn disease as compared to 34 healthy children, it was found that mean flow velocity in regions of diseased small and large bowel were significantly elevated in Crohn patients.[53] Mean small bowel flow velocity in Crohn disease was 0.095 cm/s versus 0.025 cm/s in control subjects, whereas large bowel mean flow velocity was 0.082 cm/s compared to 0.012 cm/s in healthy controls.

In a study of 12 pediatric patients with ulcerative colitis, colonic wall perfusion as measured by DTPM was significantly correlated with histopathologic changes as diagnosed from biopsy specimens.[54]

Altered mesenteric flow is also present in celiac disease. A study of 23 children found that PSVs in the SMA were higher in untreated celiac patients relative to healthy controls and to treated celiac patients.[55] The PSV in the treated group was found to be similar to that of normal patients.

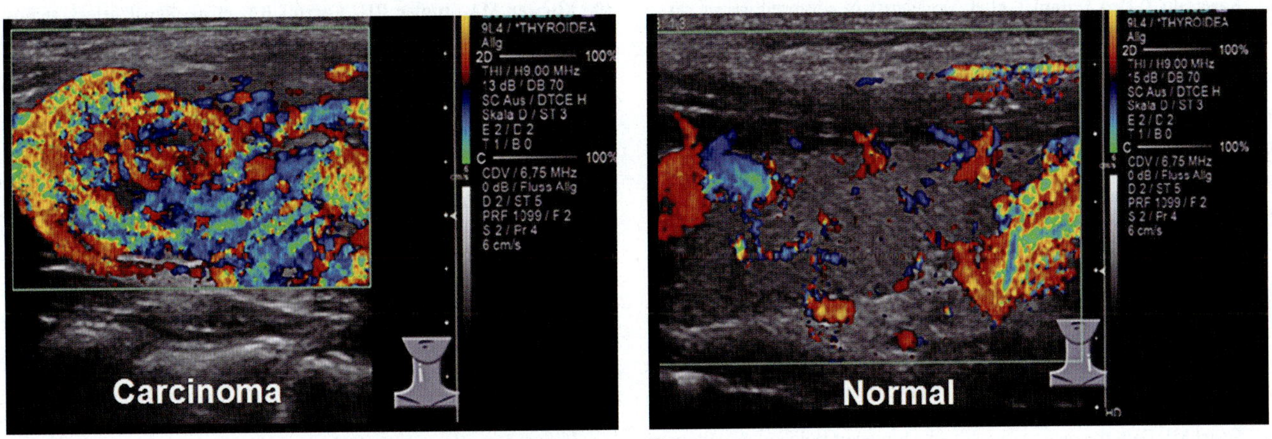

A B

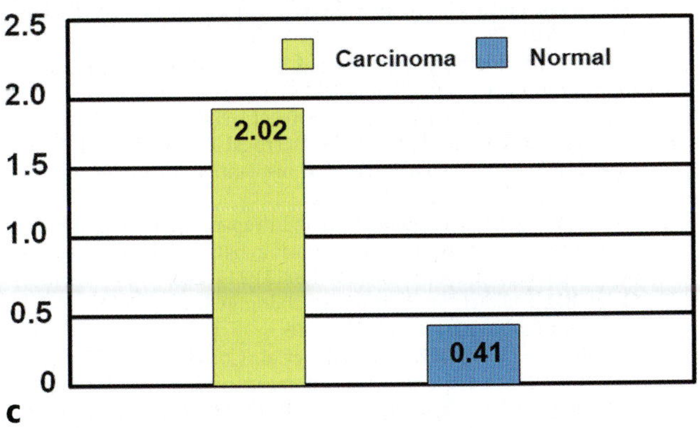

C

Figure 35-9. Perfusion ultrasound in a child with thyroid carcinoma. DTPM demonstrates increased perfusion intensity in thyroid carcinoma **(A)** compared to normal **(B)**. **C:** Perfusion intensity in the lesion is measured at 2.02 cm/s, whereas the background thyroid shows a perfusion intensity of 0.41 cm/s.

Tumors

Tumor perfusion can be evaluated by DTPM; tumoral ischemia, hypoperfusion, or hyperemia may be revealed (Fig. 35-9). This is potentially important information as tumor hypoxia has been correlated with chemo- and radioresistance of certain tumors.[56–58] In a series of metastatic squamous cell tumors of the head and neck, it was found that tumor perfusion as measured by DTPM was correlated with a direct measure of tumor oxygenation; hypoxic tumors had significantly lower perfusion than normally oxygenated ones.[59]

The clinical application of DTPM in the oncology setting is in the early phases of investigation, with considerable research required before a defined clinical role for DTPM in the routine management of these patients is established.

Disclosures

Drs. Karl Muchantef and Ricardo Faingold have no disclosures.

Dr. Thomas Scholbach and his son Dr. Jakob Scholbach developed the PixelFlux technique and software and both own the Chameleon Software company.

REFERENCES

1. **Spalinger J, Patriquin H, Miron MC, et al.** Doppler US in patients with crohn disease: vessel density in the diseased bowel reflects disease activity. *Radiology* 2000;217(3):787–791.
2. **Faingold R, Daneman A, Tomlinson G, et al.** Necrotizing enterocolitis: assessment of bowel viability with color doppler US. *Radiology* 2005;235(2):587–594.
3. **Schroder RJ, Bostanjoglo M, Hidajat N, et al.** Analysis of vascularity in breast tumors—comparison of high frequency ultrasound and contrast-enhanced color harmonic imaging. *Rofo* 2002;174(9):1132–1141.
4. **Kawasaki T, Ueo T, Itani T, et al.** Vascularity of advanced gastric carcinoma: evaluation by using power doppler imaging. *J Gastroenterol Hepatol* 2001;16(2):149–153.
5. **Kuwa T, Cancio LC, Sondeen JL, et al.** Evaluation of renal cortical perfusion by noninvasive power doppler ultrasound during vascular occlusion and reperfusion. *J Trauma* 2004;56(3):618–624.
6. **Lassau N, Koscielny S, Opolon P, et al.** Evaluation of contrast-enhanced color doppler ultrasound for the quantification of angiogenesis in vivo. *Invest Radiol* 2001;36(1):50–55.
7. **Ogura O, Takebayashi Y, Sameshima T, et al.** Preoperative assessment of vascularity by color Doppler ultrasonography in human rectal carcinoma. *Dis Colon Rectum* 2001;44(4):538–546; discussion 546–538.
8. **Stoeckelhuber BM, Wiesmann M, Kreft B, et al.** Perfusion imaging of the kidney using contrast-enhanced phase-inversion ultrasound. *Rontgenpraxis* 2004;55(5):167–174.
9. **Krix M, Weber MA, Krakowski-Roosen H, et al.** Assessment of skeletal muscle perfusion using contrast-enhanced ultrasonography. *J Ultrasound Med* 2005;24(4):431–441.
10. **Siegel MJ.** *Pediatric sonography*. 4th ed. Lippincott Williams & Wilkins; 2011.
11. **Boote EJ.** AAPM/RSNA physics tutorial for residents: topics in US: doppler US techniques: concepts of blood flow detection and flow dynamics. *Radiographics* 2003;23(5):1315–1327.
12. **Perrella RR, Duerinckx AJ, Tessler FN, et al.** Evaluation of renal transplant dysfunction by duplex doppler sonography: a prospective study and review of the literature. *Am J Kidney Dis* 1990;15(6):544–550.
13. **Taylor GA.** Potential pediatric applications for US contrast agents: lessons from the laboratory. *Pediatr Radiol* 2000;30(2):101–109.
14. **Fleischer AC, Niermann KJ, Donnelly EF, et al.** Sonographic depiction of microvessel perfusion: principles and potential. *J Ultrasound Med* 2004;23(11):1499–1506.
15. **Darge K.** Contrast-enhanced US (CEUS) in children: ready for prime time in the United States. *Pediatr Radiol* 2011;41(11):1486–1488.
16. Chameleon-Software. PixelFlux. http://www.chameleon-software.de
17. **Chavhan GB, Parra DA, Mann A, et al.** Normal Doppler spectral waveforms of major pediatric vessels: specific patterns. *Radiographics* 2008;28(3):691–706.
18. **Ilves P, Lintrop M, Talvik I, et al.** Changes in cerebral and visceral blood flow velocities in asphyxiated term neonates with hypoxic-ischemic encephalopathy. *J Ultrasound Med* 2009;28:1471–1480.
19. **Faingold R, Cassia GS, Saint-Martin C.** Cerebral perfusion measurements using dynamic color doppler sonography in neonates with Hypoxic Ischemic Encephalopathy (HIE) treated with therapeutic hypothermia. *Pediatric Radiol* 2011;(I):S250–S310. NE252–NE253.
20. **Cassia GS, Faingold R, Bernard C, et al.** Neonatal hypoxic-ischemic injury: sonography and dynamic color Doppler sonography perfusion of the brain and abdomen with pathologic correlation. *AJR Am J Roentgenol* 2012;199(6):W743–W752.
21. **Cassia GS, Faingold R.** Hypoxic ischemic injury: intestinal appearances and perfusion measurements using ultrasound and dynamic color doppler sonography in neonates submitted to therapeutic hypothermia. *Pediatric Radiol* 2011;41(1):S250–S310. FN259.
22. **Allison JW, Faddis LA, Kinder DL, et al.** Intracranial resistive index (RI) values in normal term infants during the first day of life. *Pediatr Radiol* 2000;30(9):618–620.
23. **Liu J, Cao HY, Huang XH, et al.** The pattern and early diagnostic value of Doppler ultrasound for neonatal hypoxic-ischemic encephalopathy. *J Trop Pediatr* 2007;53(5):351–354.
24. **Kuzmic AC, Brkljacic B, Ivankovic D, et al.** Doppler sonographic renal resistance index in healthy children. *Eur Radiol* 2000;10(10):1644–1648.
25. **Vade A, Subbaiah P, Kalbhen CL, et al.** Renal resistive indices in children. *J Ultrasound Med* 1993;12(11):655–658.
26. **Robitaille P, Lord H, Dubois J, et al.** A large unilateral renal artery aneurysm in a young child. *Pediatr Radiol* 2004;34(3):253–255.
27. **Park SH, Chi JG, Choi Y.** Primary intimal fibroplasia with multiple aneurysms of renal artery in childhood. *Child Nephrol Urol* 1990;10(1):51–55.
28. **Bartosh SM, Aronson AJ.** Childhood hypertension. An update on etiology, diagnosis and treatment. *Pediatr Clin North Am* 1999;46(2):235–252.
29. **Kliewer MA, Hertzberg BS, Keogan MT, et al.** Early systole in the healthy kidney: variability of Doppler US waveform parameters. *Radiology* 1997;205(1):109–113.
30. **Kliewer MA, Tupler RH, Carroll BA, et al.** Renal artery stenosis: analysis of Doppler waveform parameters and tardus-parvus pattern. *Radiology* 1993;189(3):779–787.
31. **Kurian J, Epelman M, Darge K, et al.** The role of CT angiography in the evaluation of pediatric renovascular hypertension. *Pediatr Radiol* 2013;43(4):490–501; quiz 487–499.
32. **Castelli PK, Dillman JR, Kershaw DB, et al.** Renal sonography with Doppler for detecting suspected pediatric renin-mediated hypertension—is it adequate? *Pediatr Radiol* 2014;44(1):42–49.
33. **Ciccone MM, Cortese F, Fiorella A, et al.** The clinical role of contrast-enhanced ultrasound in the evaluation of renal artery stenosis and diagnostic superiority as compared to traditional echo-color-Doppler flow imaging. *Int Angiol* 2011;30(2):135–139.
34. **Melany ML, Grant EG, Duerinckx AJ, et al.** Ability of a phase shift US contrast agent to improve imaging of the main renal arteries. *Radiology* 1997;205(1):147–152.
35. **Gholami S, Sarwal MM, Naesens M, et al.** Standardizing resistive indices in healthy pediatric transplant recipients of adult-sized kidneys. *Pediatr Transplant* 2010;14(1):126–131.
36. **Nixon JN, Biyyam DR, Stanescu L, et al.** Imaging of pediatric renal transplants and their complications: a pictorial review. *Radiographics* 2013;33(5):1227–1251.
37. **Smith JM, Stablein D, Singh A, et al.** Decreased risk of renal allograft thrombosis associated with interleukin-2 receptor antagonists: a report of the NAPRTCS. *Am J Transplant* 2006;6(3):585–588.
38. **del Valle SY, Lorente Ramos RM, Berrocal Frutos T, et al.** Vascular complications in pediatric renal transplant: echographic diagnosis. *An Esp Pediatr* 1999;50(3):263–268.
39. **Toma P, Lucigrai G, Magnano G, et al.** Intraparenchymal renal Doppler: the indirect signs of renal artery stenosis in native and transplanted kidneys in childhood. *Radiol Med* 1994;88(3):244–248.
40. **Coley BD.** Pediatric applications of abdominal vascular Doppler: Part II. *Pediatr Radiol* 2004;34(10):772–786.
41. **Scholbach T, Wang HK, Yang AH, et al.** Correlation of histopathology and dynamic tissue perfusion measurement (DTPM) in renal transplants. *BMC Nephrology* 2013;14:143. http://www.biomedcentral.com/1471-2369/14/143.

42. **Scholbach T, Girelli E, Scholbach J.** Tissue pulsatility index: a new parameter to evaluate renal transplant perfusion. *Transplantation* 2006;81(5):751–755.
43. **Scholbach T, Wang HK, Yang AH, et al.** Prognostic value of dynamic tissue perfusion measurements in transplanted kidneys. *Open J Organ Transplant Surg* 2014;4:1–5.
44. **Scholbach T, Vogel C, Bergner N.** Color doppler sonographic dynamic tissue perfusion measurement demonstrates significantly reduced cortical perfusion in children with diabetes mellitus type 1 without microalbuminuria and apparently healthy kidneys. *Ultraschall Med* 2014;35(5):445–450.
45. **Horsthuis K, Bipat S, Bennink RJ, et al.** Inflammatory bowel disease diagnosed with US, MR, scintigraphy, and CT: meta-analysis of prospective studies. *Radiology* 2008;247(1):64–79.
46. **Sjekavica I, Barbaric-Babic V, Krznaric Z, et al.** Assessment of Crohn's disease activity by doppler ultrasound of superior mesenteric artery and mural arteries in thickened bowel wall: cross-sectional study. *Croat Med J* 2007;48(6):822–830.
47. **Di Sabatino A, Armellini E, Corazza GR.** Doppler sonography in the diagnosis of inflammatory bowel disease. *Dig Dis* 2004;22(1):63–66.
48. **Sigirci A, Baysal T, Kutlu R, et al.** Doppler sonography of the inferior and superior mesenteric arteries in ulcerative colitis. *J Clin Ultrasound* 2001;29(3):130–139.
49. **Maconi G, Parente F, Bollani S, et al.** Factors affecting splanchnic haemodynamics in Crohn's disease: a prospective controlled study using Doppler ultrasound. *Gut* 1998;43(5):645–650.
50. **Kratzer W, von Tirpitz C, Mason R, et al.** Contrast-enhanced power Doppler sonography of the intestinal wall in the differentiation of hypervascularized and hypovascularized intestinal obstructions in patients with Crohn's disease. *J Ultrasound Med* 2002;21(2):149–157; quiz 158–149.
51. **Quaia E, Migaleddu V, Baratella E, et al.** The diagnostic value of small bowel wall vascularity after sulfur hexafluoride-filled microbubble injection in patients with Crohn's disease. Correlation with the therapeutic effectiveness of specific anti-inflammatory treatment. *Eur J Radiol* 2009;69(3):438–444.
52. **Ripolles T, Martinez MJ, Barrachina MM.** Crohn's disease and color Doppler sonography: response to treatment and its relationship with long-term prognosis. *J Clin Ultrasound* 2008;36(5):267–272.
53. **Scholbach T, Herrero I, Scholbach J.** Dynamic color Doppler sonography of intestinal wall in patients with Crohn disease compared with healthy subjects. *J Pediatr Gastroenterol Nutr* 2004;39(5):524–528.
54. **Scholbach T, Hormann J, Scholbach J.** Dynamic tissue perfusion measurement in the intestinal wall—correlation with ulcerative colitis. *J Med Ultrasound* 2010;18(2):62–70.
55. **Ertem D, Tuney D, Baloglu H, et al.** Superior mesenteric artery blood flow in children with celiac disease. *J Pediatr Gastroenterol Nutr* 1998;26(2):140–145.
56. **Lin SC, Chien CW, Lee JC, et al.** Suppression of dual-specificity phosphatase-2 by hypoxia increases chemoresistance and malignancy in human cancer cells. *J Clin Invest* 2011;121(5):1905–1916.
57. **Wen YA, Stevens PD, Gasser ML, et al.** Downregulation of PHLPP expression contributes to hypoxia-induced resistance to chemotherapy in colon cancer cells. *Mol Cell Biol* 2013;33(22):4594–4605.
58. **Wu YC, Ling TY, Lu SH, et al.** Chemotherapeutic sensitivity of testicular germ cell tumors under hypoxic conditions is negatively regulated by SENP1-controlled sumoylation of OCT4. *Cancer Res* 2012;72(19):4963–4973.
59. **Scholbach T, Scholbach J, Krombach GA, et al.** New method of dynamic color doppler signal quantification in metastatic lymph nodes compared to direct polarographic measurements of tissue oxygenation. *Int J Cancer* 2005;114(6):957–962.

INDEX

Note: Page numbers in *italics* denote figures; page numbers followed by a "t" denote tables